Brief Table of Contents

SPECIAL FEATURES

- Neurobiology Figures
- Developmental and Life Span Tables and Figures
- DSM-IV Criteria Boxes and Tables
- Research Studies and Abstracts
- Controversy Boxes
- Differential Diagnosis Tables

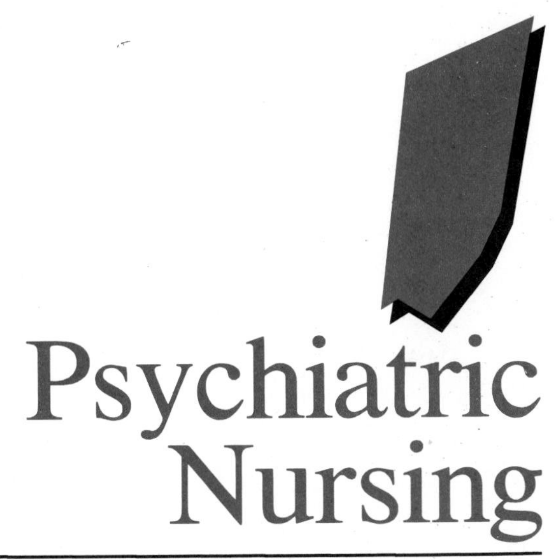

Psychiatric Nursing

Biological and Behavioral Concepts

Psychiatric Nursing

Biological and Behavioral Concepts

EDITED BY
DEBORAH ANTAI-OTONG, M.S., R.N.,C.S.
Psychiatric Clinical Specialist and Educational Consultant
Director, Employee Assistance Program
Department of Veterans Affairs Medical Center

Faculty Associate
Texas Woman's University

Formerly Instructor
El Centro Community College
Dallas, Texas

NEUROBIOLOGY EDITOR
GAIL KONGABLE, M.S.N., C.N.R.N., C.C.R.N.
Assistant Professor in Research
Department of Neurosurgery
University of Virginia Health Sciences Center
Charlottesville, Virginia

Neurobiological Illustrations by Marie T. Dauenheimer, M.A.

W.B. SAUNDERS COMPANY
A Division of Harcourt Brace & Company

Philadelphia London Toronto
Montreal Sydney Tokyo

W.B. Saunders Company
A Division of
Harcourt Brace & Company

The Curtis Center
Independence Square West
Philadelphia, Pennsylvania 19106

Library of Congress Cataloging-in-Publication Data

Psychiatric nursing: biological and behavioral concepts / edited by Deborah Antai-Otong.
p. cm.
ISBN 0–7216–3778–7
1. Psychiatric nursing. 2. Behavior therapy. I. Antai-Otong, Deborah.
[DNLM: 1. Psychiatric Nursing—methods. 2. Behavior Therapy—nurses' instruction. WY 160 P97238 1995]
RC440.P7537 1995
610.73′68—dc20
DNLM/DLC 94-25346

Cover art by Robert Hochgertel

A Note on the Cover
Mental illness is a shattering experience. It affects all aspects of a person's life, from one's day-to-day sense of well-being to one's effectiveness at work, from relationships with family members to interactions with strangers. Therapy for even the mildest of mental illnesses is often prolonged, certainly more time consuming and tentative than treatments for purely physical problems like tonsillitis or even appendicitis, which can be addressed with a brief and definitive surgical procedure. It is both this ''shattering'' concept and the complex ramifications for care that the author and editors have sought to represent in the cover design.

PSYCHIATRIC NURSING:
Biological and Behavioral Concepts
ISBN 0–7216–3778–7

Printed in the United States of America

Last digit is the print number: 9 8 7 6 5 4 3 2 1

To my best friend and incredible husband, Okon,
who has supported me throughout this magnificent endeavor.

About the Author

Deborah Antai-Otong's contribution to psychiatric nursing encompasses both the clinical and educational realms. She has been a clinical psychotherapist for the past 15 years, specializing in women's issues such as depression, early childhood trauma, addictive disorders, and couples and marital therapy. Her experience ranges from being a crisis therapist at a local mental health center to serving as a psychiatric clinical specialist overseeing a psychiatric triage unit at a major metropolitan medical center.

A prolific author and program speaker, Deborah has contributed articles and chapters to numerous nursing journals and textbooks, and has delivered more than 200 presentations to a wide variety of audiences on topics as diverse as posttraumatic stress disorder, empowerment, and managing change and transition. She has participated in various psychiatric nursing committees, and has taught at both the undergraduate and graduate levels. A member of Sigma Theta Tau, she currently serves as President of the Texas Nurses Association, District Four, and recently served as Chairperson of the ANCC Test Development Committee for Clinical Specialist in Adult Psychiatric–Mental Health Nursing.

List of Contributors

Deborah Antai-Otong, M.S., R.N.,C.S.
Psychiatric Clinical Specialist and Educational Consultant; Director, Employee Assistance Program, Department of Veterans Affairs Medical Center; Faculty Associate, Texas Woman's University, Dallas, Texas

Linda Funk Barloon, M.S., R.N.,C.
Clinical Nurse Specialist, Children's Mercy Hospital, Kansas City, Missouri

Holly Berchin, M.S.N., R.N.,C.S.
Adjunct Faculty, Kent State University School of Nursing, Kent, and University of Akron, College of Nursing, Akron; Coordinator of the Eating Disorders Program and Psychiatric Consultation Liaison Nurse—Clinical Nurse Specialist, Children's Hospital Medical Center, Akron, Ohio

Johnnie Bonner, M.S., R.N.
Clinical Nurse Specialist, Department of Veterans Affairs Medical Center, Dallas, Texas

Margaret Brackley, Ph.D., R.N.,C.S.
Associate Professor, University of Texas Health Science Center at San Antonio; Clinical Associate, Department of Psychiatry, University Hospital; and Family Nurse Practitioner, University Health System Downtown Nurses' Prenatal Clinic, San Antonio, Texas

Kathleen C. Buckwalter, Ph.D., R.N.
Professor, University of Iowa College of Nursing; Associate Director of Research Development and Utilization, University of Iowa Hospitals and Clinics, Iowa City, Iowa

Martha Buffum, D.N.Sc., R.N.,C.S.
Assistant Clinical Professor, Department of Mental Health, Community, Administrative Nursing, School of Nursing, University of California, San Francisco; Associate Chief of Nursing Service for Research, Department of Veterans Affairs Medical Center, San Francisco, California

Linda Garand, M.S., R.N.,C.S.
Doctoral Student and Research Associate, University of Iowa College of Nursing, Iowa City, Iowa

Janie Rehschuh Gilkison, M.S.N., R.N.
Guest Faculty, Psychiatric Mental Health Nursing, Collin County Community College, McKinney; Staff Nurse, Health Services Department, Dallas Public Schools, Dallas, Texas

Christine Grant, Ph.D., R.N.
Assistant Professor of Psychiatric Mental Health Nursing, University of Pennsylvania, Philadelphia, Pennsylvania

Geri Richards Hall, M.A., A.R.N.P., C.S.
Gerontology Clinical Nurse Specialist, University of Iowa Hospitals and Clinics, Iowa City, Iowa

Ada Lynne Hendricks, M.S., R.N.
Clinical Nursing Instructor, University of Kansas School of Nursing, Kansas City, Kansas; Evening Supervisor, Two Rivers Psychiatric Hospital, Kansas City, Missouri

Gail Kongable, M.S.N., C.N.R.N., C.C.R.N.
Assistant Professor in Research, Department of Neurosurgery, University of Virginia Health Sciences Center, Charlottesville, Virginia

Susan L. W. Krupnick, M.S.N., C.A.R.N., C.S.
Adjunct Lecturer, University of Pennsylvania School of Nursing; Psychiatric Consultation Liaison Nurse, Hospital of the University of Pennsylvania Health Care System, Philadelphia, Pennsylvania

Erika Madrid, D.N.Sc., R.N.,C.S.
Assistant Professor, Nursing Department, Holy Names College, Oakland, California

Melissa Barker Neathery, M.S.N., R.N.
Instructor, Baylor University School of Nursing; Clinical Coordinator, Green Oaks at Medical City Day Hospital, Dallas, Texas

Rose M. Nieswiadomy, Ph.D., R.N.
Professor, Texas Woman's University, Dallas Center, Dallas, Texas

Catherine Pawlicki, M.S.N., R.N.,C.S.
Adjunct Faculty, University of Kansas Graduate Program in Nursing, Kansas City, and Wichita State University Graduate Program in Nursing, Wichita; Associate Director of Nursing, The Menninger Clinic, and Director of the Psychodynamic Nursing Program, The Karl Menninger School of Psychiatry and Mental Health Science, Topeka, Kansas.

Duane F. Pennebaker Ph.D., A.R.N.P., F.N.A.P., F.R.C.N.A.
Associate Professor and Director, Nursing Program, University of Washington—Bothell, Bothell, Washington

Kay Perry, M.S.N., R.N.,C.S., A.R.N.P.
Menninger Partial Hospital Services, Kansas City, Missouri

Ardyce A. Plumlee, M.N., R.N., C.A.R.N.
Assistant Professor (Retired), University of Kansas School of Nursing, Kansas City, Kansas

Christine McCormick Pries, M.A., A.R.N.P., C.S.
Associate Director, Research, Evaluation, and Community Relations, Vera French Community Mental Health Center, Davenport, Iowa

Hope Quallo, M.S., R.N.,C.S.
Clinical Associate, University of Rochester; Advanced Practice Nurse and Therapist, Department of Psychiatry, Adult Ambulatory Clinic, University of Rochester Medical Center, Rochester, New York

Joy A. Riley, D.N.Sc., R.N.,C.S.
Lecturer, Indiana University School of Nursing; Executive Director, Schizophrenia Treatment and Rehabilitation (STAR), Inc., Indianapolis, Indiana

Martha Bledsoe Sanford, Ph.D., R.N.
Associate Professor, Baylor University School of Nursing, Dallas, Texas

Bess Stewart, Ph.D., R.N., F.A.A.N.
Associate Professor and Assistant Dean for Doctoral Studies, University of Texas Health Science Center at San Antonio School of Nursing, San Antonio, Texas

Jacqueline M. Stolley, M.A., R.N.,C.
Research Associate and Doctoral Student, University of Iowa College of Nursing, Iowa City, Iowa

Nancy R. Tommasini, M.S.N., R.N.,C.S.
Assistant Professor, Psychiatric–Mental Health Nursing Program, Yale University School of Nursing; Psychiatric Consultation-Liaison Nurse Specialist, Yale–New Haven Hospital, New Haven, Connecticut

Sylvia Anderson Whiting, Ph.D., R.N.,C.S.
Associate Professor, South Carolina State University College of Nursing, South Carolina State University, Orangeburg, South Carolina

List of Reviewers

Susan Elizabeth Alden, Ph.D., R.N.
College of Nursing
Teikyo Marycrest University
Davenport, Iowa

Mary Elaine Allen, Ph.D., R.N.,C.S.
College of Nursing
University of Oklahoma
Oklahoma City, Oklahoma

Jill S. Anderson, Ph.D., R.N.,C.S.
College of Nursing
University of Illinois at Chicago
Chicago, Illinois

Gretchen E. Bagley, M.S.N., M.A., R.N., F.N.P.
Department of Nursing
Pikes Peak Community College
Colorado Springs, Colorado

Lorna Mill Barrell, Ph.D., R.N.
College of Nursing
Virginia Commonwealth University
Richmond, Virginia

Jesse E. Bateau, M.S.N., R.N.,C.S.
College of Nursing
Wayne State University
Detroit, Michigan

Pamela J. Bender, M.S.N., R.N.
Clinical Research Department
Southern New Jersey Medical Institute
Stratford, New Jersey

Andrea C. Bostrum, Ph.D., R.N.
Kirkhof School of Nursing
Grand Valley State University
Allendale, Michigan

Geraldine T. Caron, Ed.D., R.N.
Private Practice
Consulting Staff
Psychedelic and Chemical Dependency Units
Lower Keys Hospital and DePoo Hospital
Key West, Florida

Catherine Caston, M.A.N., M.R.E.
Ph.D. Candidate
Lecturer and Clinical Teacher
B.S.N. Program
School of Nursing
Louisiana State University Medical Center
New Orleans, Louisiana

Sharon Lee Evers, M.S.N., R.N.,C.S.
School of Nursing
Columbus College
Columbus, Georgia

Marian Farrell, Ph.D., R.N.C.
College of Nursing
University of Scranton
Scranton, Pennsylvania

Deborah L. Finfgeld, Ph.D., R.N.
Associate Professor
College of Nursing
Illinois Wesleyan University
Bloomington, Illinois

Helen T. Geyer, B.S.Pharm., C.S.
SUNY Health Science Center at Brooklyn
Brooklyn, New York

Carolyn Anne Green, Ed.D., R.N.
School of Nursing
Solano College
Suisun City, California

Claire Griffin-Francell, M.S., R.N.
President
Southeast Nurse Consultants, Inc.
Atlanta, Georgia

Janice Harvey, M.S.N., R.N.,C.S.
Psychiatric Nursing Department
University of Utah Hospital
Salt Lake City, Utah

Cheryl Hilgenberg, M.S., R.N.
Assistant Professor
College of Nursing
Milliken University
Decatur, Illinois

Sharon K. Holmberg, Ph.D., R.N.
University of Rochester
School of Nursing
Rochester, New York

Dorothy J. Irvin, M.S.N., R.N.,C.S.
School of Nursing
St. John's College
Springfield, Illinois

Alice R. Kempe, M.Ed., M.S.N., Ph.D.
School of Nursing
Ursuline College
Pepper Pike, Ohio

Linda Nance Marks, Ed.D., R.N., A.N.P.
College of Nursing
University of Texas at Arlington
Arlington, Texas

Marjorie Fay Rash Miller, M.S.H.Ed., M.S.N., R.N.
Dean of Health Occupations Division
Professor of Nursing
College of Nursing
Vincennes University
Vincennes, Indiana

Carolyn W. Mosley, M.N., R.N.
B.S.N. Program
School of Nursing
Louisiana State University Medical Center
New Orleans, Louisiana

Carol J. Nelson, M.S.N., R.N.
Nursing Department
Spokane Community College
Spokane, Washington

Maryann Nihart, M.A., R.N.,C.S.
Turning Point Center for Depression
San Francisco, California
Partner, Professional Growth Facilitators
San Clemente, California

Alice Parkinson, M.S., R.N.
Assistant Professor
College of Nursing
University of Utah
Salt Lake City, Utah

Mariamma J. Pyngolil, M.S.N., A.R.N.P., C.S.
Broward General Medical Center
Fort Lauderdale, Florida

Linda E. Reese, M.A., R.N.
School of Nursing
The College of Staten Island
Staten Island, New York

Louise Suit, Ed.D., R.N.
College of Nursing
Harding University
Searcy, Arkansas

Patricia R. Teasley, M.S.N., R.N.,C.S.
School of Nursing
Columbus College
Columbus, Georgia

William R. Whetstone, Ph.D., R.N.
Statewide Nursing Program
Division of Nursing
California State
University–Dominguez Hills
Carson, California

Sylvia Anderson Whiting, Ph.D., R.N.,C.S.
College of Nursing
South Carolina State University
Orangeburg, South Carolina

Judy G. Winterhalter, D.N.Sc., R.N.,C.S.
Associate Professor, Graduate Nursing
School of Nursing
Gwynedd-Mercy College
Gwynedd Valley, Pennsylvania

Preface

Psychiatric nursing is at a crossroads. The biological and medical research of recent years has developed a large and increasing body of information concerning the neurobiological sciences that nursing in this Decade of the Brain must recognize and assimilate. The alternative is the reduction of the nurse's place in this most caring of all disciplines and its usurpation by others in the mental health arena such as psychologists and social workers.

NEUROBIOLOGICAL CONCEPTS

Psychiatric Nursing: Biological and Behavioral Concepts fully recognizes the advances in neurobiology and attempts to place this new knowledge in a learning context for students and clinicians. The text includes extensive discussion of neurobiological concepts relating to both physiology and pathophysiology, with a specially designed art program whose development was overseen by a research neuroscience nurse.

LIFE SPAN CONSIDERATIONS

It is important to view mental health, mental illness, and neuropathology in the context of growth and development. Rather than relegating this topic to one or two isolated chapters, *Psychiatric Nursing* includes life span considerations as a theme throughout. ''Across the Life Span'' text discussions and special life span tables address the causes and manifestations of specific disorders and their therapies in relation to the developmental stage of the client.

ROLE OF THE NURSE

Given the increased research activity in mental health and mental illness and its impact on client care, the participation of the nurse as a member of the mental health care team is undergoing increasing scrutiny and adaptation. For this reason, the role of the nurse in both general and advanced practice is explored in discussions that incorporate both the problem-solving tools available in the nursing process and the newly published *Diagnostic and Statistical Manual of Mental Disorders* (4th Edition) classification. Throughout the text, collaboration with other health care providers and with clients for self-care is stressed.

ORGANIZATION

Unit I, Perspectives and Principles, provides a general overview of psychiatric nursing, from the history and delineation of the discipline to cultural attitudes concerning mental health and psychiatric care. Ethical and legal issues are also addressed in this section. The last three chapters discuss the nurse–client relationship, the classification of mental disorders, and general principles of crisis intervention.

The psychopathologies are presented in depth in *Unit II, Response to Stressors Across the Life Span.* Each discussion includes the role of the nurse in working with the client, developmental considerations involving the condition, and neurobiological as well as psychosocial bases of the problem. Each chapter also provides at least one case study and nursing care plan demonstrating the place of different forms of therapy in the treatment of the disorder.

The therapies themselves become the focus for *Unit III, Therapeutic Interventions*. Individual, family, group, milieu, and community approaches to psychiatric illness are discussed, along with psychopharmacological and other somatic therapies.

Finally, *Unit IV, Advanced Psychiatric Nursing Practice*, explores in greater depth the specific roles of psychiatric nursing in general nursing practice as well as in specialized practice such as psychiatric liaison nursing. The place of research in psychiatric nursing is addressed, and the text concludes with a general framework for developing psychiatric nursing skills in light of the changing expectations of the profession.

PEDAGOGIC FEATURES

Each chapter in the book begins with a Chapter Outline and Chapter Objectives, which give the reader an overview of the chapter. A list of Key Terms is also provided; these terms are defined within the chapter as well as in a Glossary at the back of the book. Suggestions for Clinical Conferences at the end of each chapter provide ideas for projects and discussion groups related to the subject matter in the chapter. The Chapter Summary at the conclusion of each chapter as well as the Study Questions at the end of each unit aid review and self-testing. Answers to the Unit Study Questions are supplied in an appendix at the end of the book. (Rationales for the answers are included in the accompanying Instructor's Manual.)

INSTRUCTOR ANCILLARIES

An Instructor's Manual accompanies this text. It includes the following features: Chapter orientation, key terms, lecture topic suggestions, a chapter/lecture outline, chapter objectives, prerequisite knowledge required for the chapter, extra background information, teaching strategies, audiovisual support materials related to the chapter topic, answers with rationales for the Unit Study Questions in the textbook, transparency masters, and a test bank of approximately 500 items. The test bank is also available on the ExamMaster computer program.

SUMMARY

Psychiatric nursing continues to expand in the wake of technological advances and socioeconomic and legislative changes. Understanding the complexity of mental illness is critical to recognizing not only the behaviors characterizing psychiatric disorders but also the biological and psychosocial factors underlying adaptive and maladaptive responses. It is hoped that this text will enable all nurses and nursing students to collaborate with clients and other health care providers to formulate continuous and comprehensive care in a variety of clinical settings.

DEBORAH ANTAI-OTONG, M.S., R.N.,C.S.

Acknowledgments

Completing this book feels great! My inspiration to embark on this endeavor arose from the support and encouragement I received from my family, colleagues, and editors.

My appreciation for their support is immense. I want to acknowledge some remarkable people. First, I want to express a special thanks to my terrific children, Derek and Leslie, who probably felt neglected at times. Their patience and endurance are greatly valued and appreciated. They are indeed "a mother's pride."

Second, a special thanks goes to my friends and colleagues who made writing this book exciting. Their contributions underscore their commitment and expertise in psychiatric–mental health nursing.

Third, I want to thank Rosanne Hallowell and Denise Black Gold, Developmental Editors at W.B. Saunders, who have been extremely supportive. Their expertise and patience have been a vital part of this book's completion. I also want to extend my appreciation and thanks to my copy editor, Sue Reilly. Her continuous supportive attitude, guidance, knowledge, and creativity enhanced the completion of this text.

Finally, a very special thanks to my editor and dear friend, Dan Ruth. His enthusiasm, vision, and encouragement have played a tremendous role in the evolution of this book. I thank him for giving me a chance to make a difference in psychiatric nursing. His friendship is truly valued and revered.

DEBORAH ANTAI-OTONG, M.S., R.N.,C.S.

Contents

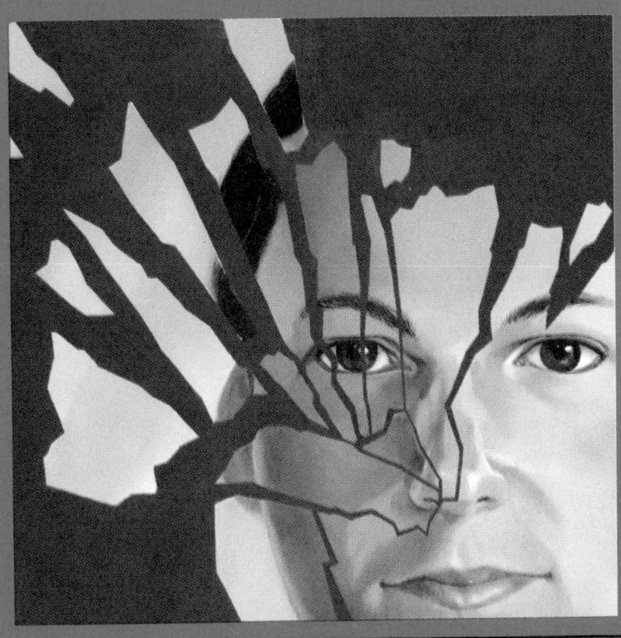

U N I T

1

Perspectives and Principles

CHAPTER 1

History of Psychiatric–Mental Health Nursing

DEBORAH ANTAI-OTONG, M.S., R.N.,C.S.

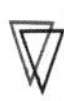

OUTLINE

CHAPTER OBJECTIVES

Upon completion of this chapter, you will be able to:

1. Discuss the impact of society, economics, and religion on attitudes toward mental illness.
2. Describe the evolution of psychiatry.
3. Discuss the evolution of psychiatric–mental health nursing.
4. Analyze the role and purpose of professional organizations such as the American Nurses Association and the National League for Nursing in relation to psychiatric–mental health nursing.
5. Discuss the future of psychiatric–mental health nursing.
6. Evaluate the influence of technological and neurobiological advances on psychiatric–mental health nursing.
7. Recognize the significance of biological and behavioral interface on psychiatric–mental health nursing.

KEY TERMS

Decade of the Brain
Deinstitutionalization
Mental health movement
Moral treatment
National Institute of Mental Health
Neurobiology
Psychotropics

THE EVOLUTION OF PSYCHIATRIC–MENTAL HEALTH CARE

Methods of treating clients who are mentally ill have been evolving over the past century: from driving out evil spirits and confinement to the milieu therapy of today and primary mental health care of tomorrow. This evolution is partly a reflection of changes in the philosophical and theoretical foundations of treatment as well as economic concerns. Scientific and technological advances of the past few decades have also influenced the treatment of psychiatric clients by enhancing our knowledge of the brain's structure and function and our understanding of the biochemical and genetic bases of many psychiatric disorders. These discoveries are providing hope for clients, their families, and advocates for the mentally ill.

As we embark on the twenty-first century, people are experiencing enormous stresses associated with changes in economic conditions and societal structures as well as rapid advances in scientific technology. Consequently, there has been a concurrent increase in demand for psychiatric–mental health services. Approximately 10 to 15 percent of the general population have some form of mental illness, for which about one third seek treatment (Iscoe & Harris, 1984; Reiger et al., 1988). The resulting strain on the health care system is compounded by the current health care crisis, with gaps in services to the poor and uninsured, who are most in need of mental health services. The lack of preventive care associated with limited access to the health care system further compromises people's abilities to cope effectively with crises.

In addition, there is a growing population of older adults and those with chronic illness, both mental and physical. The global epidemic of acquired immunodeficiency syndrome (AIDS), with women and children increasingly at risk, is yet another factor that is increasing the demand for services. Changes in the structure of hospitals, shorter hospital stays, and an imbalance in the supply of health care providers (with an overabundance of physicians and a persistent shortage of nurses) place other burdens on an already overwhelmed health care system (American Nurses Association [ANA], 1991).

All these factors add new dimensions to the scope of psychiatric nursing practice. Psychiatric–mental health nurses will continue to have pivotal roles in identifying clients at risk, in assessing client responses to stress across the life span, and in developing therapeutic interventions. In addition, as the health care delivery system evolves in response to the current crisis, nurses must continue to be at the forefront of client advocacy, encouraging clients and families to be active partners in their health care. Neurobiological research will continue to challenge nurses to rethink the causes and treatment of mental illness, to develop strategies for integrating the neurobiological and psychosocial aspects of psychiatric–mental health nursing, to develop innovative measures to meet the needs of clients, and to redefine the nurse's role through research and education.

Mental illness has always been an integral part of human existence. Throughout history, the plight of the mentally ill has often depended on the cultural and religious beliefs of the civilization in which they lived.

EARLY HISTORY

During ancient times, insanity was associated with sin and demonic possession. Healers were summoned to extract these unseen spirits through rituals and by the use of herbs, ointments, and precious stones. Mental illness was often perceived as incurable, and treatment of the insane was sometimes inhumane and brutal.

THE MIDDLE AGES

Throughout the Middle Ages, mentally ill people who were not cared for within their families were often imprisoned or forced to live on the streets and beg for food. For more humane treatment, they depended on the charity of religious groups, who dispensed alms and ran almshouses and general hospitals where the insane were admitted.

The first mental asylum was the Hospital of St. Mary of Bethlehem, from which the term *bedlam* was coined. Built in London, England, during the fourteenth century, Bethlehem was conceived as a sanctuary or refuge for the destitute and afflicted and became the model for similar institutions elsewhere.

THE FIFTEENTH THROUGH SEVENTEENTH CENTURY PERIOD

Skepticism about the curability of mental illness, rampant during the Middle Ages, continued during this period. Asylums became repositories for prolonged enclosure of the chronic mentally ill. Conditions were deplorable. Because the insane were thought to have no feelings and were believed to lack understanding, they were treated more like animals than human beings. Men and women were not given separate quarters, and violent inmates were placed with those who were convalescing or tranquil. The inhabitants were poorly clothed and fed, often chained and caged, and deprived of heat and sunlight (Conolly, 1968; Ellenberger, 1974).

Care in these institutions was custodial and administered by attendants who were poorly treated. Their wages were meager, less than the amount paid to domestic workers and laundresses. They had to sleep on wards and rarely received respite from continual care responsibilities. These working conditions made it difficult to attract and keep attendants (Scull, 1982).

During the latter part of the seventeenth century, American colonists of European origin carried their perceptions and superstitions about the mentally ill from their home countries. Deep-rooted ideas about the mentally ill and witchcraft culminated in witch hunts and executions, such as those that occurred in Salem, Massachusetts. The Salem hysteria persisted for many years and interfered with the transition to humane treatment of those who were mentally ill.

THE EIGHTEENTH CENTURY

The French and American revolutions, inspired by the desire to broaden the rights of humankind and bring freedom and fair treatment to all, provided the catalyst for transforming society's attitudes toward the mentally ill and poor. A myriad of today's social concerns originated during this century, including campaigns for the abolition of slavery and the championing of equal rights for women and care for the impoverished.

Benjamin Rush (1745–1813). The American physician Benjamin Rush was a forerunner in bringing attention to the plight of those with mental disorders. He emphasized the need for pleasant surroundings and diversional and **moral treatment** for the mentally ill. (*Moral treatment* refers to humane care of persons with mental illness. This approach surmises that mental illness is "curable" under benevolent conditions.)

Some of Rush's treatments, such as bloodletting and the administration of cold and hot baths, harsh purgatives and emetics, were considered controversial. He believed that the inducement of fright or shock would cause the mentally ill to regain their sanity. He was credited with inventing the tranquilizer chair and the gyrator. The principle of the tranquilizer chair, on which the mentally ill person's extremities were strapped down, was that a reduction in motor activity and pulse rates produced calming effects. The gyrator was a form of shock therapy, consisting of a rotating, swinging platform onto which the person was strapped and moved at a high speed. The idea was to increase cerebral circulation, the major focus of Rush's theories and therapies.

Rush's advocacy for humane treatment and his concerns for the mentally ill became the basis for his 1812 publication of *Medical Inquiries and Observations upon the Disease of the Mind,* the first American treatise on psychiatry. This document was considered to be the authoritative work on the topic for several decades. Rush later came to be known as the father of American psychiatry.

Philippe Pinel (1745–1826). Another concerned physician and advocate for humane treatment of the mentally ill during this era was the Frenchman Philippe Pinel, who advocated kindness and moral treatment. His perceptions and concerns about the dire living conditions and brutal treatment of these people influenced the new social consciousness of his era.

Pinel's greatest impact came after he was placed in charge of a large hospital for the insane, Bicerte. He proved that releasing the insane from chains and providing moral treatment improved their prospect. His compassionate endeavors brought about sweeping changes in French institutions for the mentally ill and reformation of societal attitudes toward those with mental illness, creating optimism about its curability.

William Tuke (1732–1822). Another pioneer during this century was William Tuke, an English merchant and devout member of the Society of Friends. He began a 4-generation dynasty that advocated humane treatment of the mentally ill. He abhorred the deplorable conditions of several asylums, including Bethlehem, and his services were often sought in developing humane conditions in mental institutions. Tuke's descendants played major roles in increasing public awareness of the vile living conditions and treatment of those with mental illness. His efforts were instrumental in raising money to establish homes, including the York Retreat, that provided comfort, security, and safety for the mentally ill.

Franz Anton Mesmer (1734–1815). Another approach to treatment of the mentally ill was mesmerism, named after the Austrian physician Franz Anton Mesmer. He renewed the art of suggestive healing that stemmed from the ancient use of trances that later became the basis of hypnosis. Mesmer and his followers used a form of hypnotism, a dreamlike trance, to explore the basis of neurosis. His techniques, which he attributed to "animal magnetism," were used to effect cures.

THE NINETEENTH CENTURY: THE EMERGING ROLE OF THE PSYCHIATRIC NURSE

In the nineteenth century, a movement began in Europe and the United States that championed a reformation of ideas in establishing state hospitals. The evolution of psychiatric–mental health nursing (Table 1–1) marks its beginning with the building of the first psychiatric hospital in America at Williamsburg, Virginia, in 1773. In

TABLE 1–1
The Evolution of Psychiatric Nursing

DATES AND EVENTS	TYPE OF MENTAL HEALTH TREATMENT	ROLE OF PSYCHIATRIC NURSE	HISTORICAL FIGURES	SIGNIFICANT CONTRIBUTIONS
1773: First psychiatric hospital in America at Williamsburg, Virginia	Custodial care provided by nonnursing attendants	Essentially nonexistent	Florence Nightingale stressed the significance of emotional support	Nightingale's *Notes on nursing* was published in 1859
1882: First training school for nursing of the mentally ill established at McLean Asylum, Waverly, Massachusetts (first humane treatment established)	Primarily consisted of custodial care	Nurses attempted to create a safe, kind, clean environment	Linda Richards was the first graduate psychiatric nurse in the United States	Richards was instrumental in establishing nursing education in psychiatric and general hospitals
1920s–1940s, including World War II (1943): Postwar casualties (including increased mental illness) increased funding for advanced training in psychiatry. National Mental Health Act of 1946 increased funding and stimulated advanced training and research preparation of psychiatric nurses. NIMH began offering "integration grants" to promote integration of mental health and behavioral concepts into clinical practice	Care focused on a disease model rather than the client. Primarily "curative care"	Nursing care paralleled the medical or disease model. Primarily "maternal" and companion role with custodial care. Some nurses were involved in advanced practice and worked in community mental health centers, inpatient settings, academic institutions, and private practice	Harriet Bailey published the first psychiatric nursing textbook, *Nursing mental disease* (1920), which focused on the disease rather than the client	
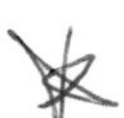 1950s–1960s: NLN-ANA coalition recommended sanctioned integration of psychiatric nursing into clinical experience in generic curricula. Advent of psychotropic drugs (1950s). Comprehensive Mental Health Act of 1960 increased federal funding to build community mental health centers, which led to the development of community psychiatry. Deinstitutionalization began in 1963; chronically ill clients were released to community mental health centers	Psychotropics replaced restraints and seclusion. Decentralization began, with a focus on improved client care. Deinstitutionalization began with a move of clients from state and long-term facilities to community-based services. Focus was on primary prevention. Major treatment involved inpatient, partial hospitalization, and day hospitals	Emphasis on therapeutic relationship, nursing process, and research. In the 1960s, psychiatric nurses continued to have an undifferentiated role and were involved in creating a therapeutic environment (milieu therapy). Major focus was on primary prevention and community-based treatment: ► interdisciplinary collaboration ► use of various treatment modalities, such as crisis intervention, supportive therapy, and psychotherapies The role of psychiatric nursing in community-based settings continued to be unclear	Major nursing contributions were made by Hildegard Peplau, Gwen Tudor, June Mellow, and Ida Orlando, who stressed the importance of the interpersonal or therapeutic relationship. Additionally, Theresa Muller focused on the significance of coping with everyday stresses. Madeline Leininger (1969) stressed the importance of community-based care within various cultures and societies. Aguilera & Messick (1970) integrated Caplan's crisis intervention concepts into nursing practice	Peplau's (1952) book, *Interpersonal relations in nursing*, delineated the role of psychiatric nursing. Mellow (1967) and Tudor (1952) published clinical studies of nursing and interpersonal relationships. ANA Division on Psychiatric and Mental Health Nursing Practice published the *Statement on psychiatric nursing practice* (1967). Aguilera & Messick published the first edition of *Crisis intervention: Theory and methodology* (1970). Shirley Smoyak's book, *The psychiatric nurse as a family therapist* (1970), stressed the significance of treating clients within their social contexts.

TABLE 1–1
The Evolution of Psychiatric Nursing *Continued*

DATES AND EVENTS	TYPE OF MENTAL HEALTH TREATMENT	ROLE OF PSYCHIATRIC NURSE	HISTORICAL FIGURES	SIGNIFICANT CONTRIBUTIONS
1970s and 1980s: A decrease in federal funding for advanced psychiatric–mental health nursing training, education, and research led to decreased psychiatric clinical experiences. 1989: U.S. Congress proclaimed 1990s as the "Decade of the Brain"	Focus continued on community-based services and increased on technological advances and neurobiology in the study of mental illness. Late 1980s experienced increased inpatient psychiatric treatment with evidence of abuse within private psychiatric settings, which led to increases in health care costs	Psychiatric nurses in advanced practice began using an array of psychotherapeutic approaches, including various psychotherapies, behavior modification, cognitive therapy, and prescriptive authority and performing research. Treatment focused on psychogeriatric and pediatric nursing; trauma throughout the life span; and severe personality disorders	Major nursing leaders continued to define nursing practice within a changing health care system. Major focus included various age groups, prevention and health promotion, and outcome identification. Other areas of concern included researching outcomes and the effectiveness of nursing interventions	The 1976 ANA *Statement on psychiatric and mental health nursing practice* defined the standards of psychiatric nursing practice. The 1982 ANA *Standards of psychiatric and mental health nursing practice* delineated specific outcome criteria for clinical practice in the specialty.
1990s–2000: Continued advances in technology and understanding of mental illness within domains of neurobiology (genetics, brain mapping, neurotransmitters, and psychopharmacology). Health care reform focuses on primary health care, prevention, and community-based treatment and services	Present focus on prevention, community-based services, and primary prevention using various approaches such as mental health centers, partial hospitalization, day care centers, home health, and hospice care	Advanced nurse practitioners continue to provide various psychotherapeutic interventions. Increased emphasis on researching client outcomes and improving the quality of cost-effective client care	Various nursing organizations are uniting to present a strong and cohesive posture to maximize benefits from proposed health care reforms in the 1990s and beyond	ANA recently revised its *Statement on psychiatric–mental health clinical practice and standards of psychiatric–mental health clinical nursing practice* (1994).

Data from Chamberlain, 1983; Peplau, 1989; Sills, 1973.

1817, the McLean Asylum in Massachusetts became the first U.S. institution that provided humane treatment for the mentally ill.

Before this period, care was administered primarily by attendants because the psychiatric nursing role had not yet been established. Increased concern and sensitivity to the needs of the mentally ill generated a demand for better educated attendants to care for severely disturbed clients.

Shattuck (1948), a noted physician, wrote in his report on the 1850 Sanitary Commission of Massachusetts that nurses play a greater role in caring, preventing disease, and promoting health than do physicians.

This progressive attitude waned with the decline in public resources and the influx of poor European immigrants, which compounded social stress and poor living conditions. These factors placed people at risk for mental illness. The increased incidence of mental illness was met with little public concern for humanitarian care, apathy coupled with poor public funding, and increased brutality and malevolence toward the mentally ill. Conditions in jails and mental institutions became deplorable, and the need for reform was urgent.

Dorothea Lynde Dix (1802–1887). Dorothea Lynde Dix, at the time a retired Massachusetts schoolteacher, led the crusade that brought these conditions to the attention of the public and the legislative bodies. She discovered deplorable, inhumane treatment of the jailed mentally ill while substituting for a theology student who was scheduled to visit them. She was appalled by the miserable conditions of prisoners who were chained, caged, and deprived of heat. The frigid Massachusetts weather made the lack of heat and sunlight deadly and heartless. Her undertakings revitalized humane treatment of the mentally ill.

Renewed public and legislative concern improved standards of care for the mentally ill, which led to a proliferation in state hospitals. Unfortunately, the number of state hospitals was insufficient to meet the tremendous needs of the mentally ill, and care remained primarily custodial at the end of the nineteenth century.

THE TWENTIETH CENTURY: THE ERA OF PSYCHIATRY

The dawning of the twentieth century in the United States found that improved societal attitudes promoted sensitivity toward the mentally ill. These changes endured and reflected society's increasing concern for others. Likewise, legislators ultimately responded to these changes by developing widespread measures for welfare reform and enacting child labor laws. These transformations encouraged medicine to take the lead and explore the basis of mental illness through scientific and clinical studies.

Several major breakthroughs in the evolution of psychiatric care emerged during the twentieth century. Exploration of the reasons for mental disease accelerated with contributions from numerous theoreticians and researchers, who laid the foundation for understanding and demystifying mental illness.

Adolph Meyer (1866–1950). In 1902, Adolph Meyer, a psychiatrist from Sweden, initiated the psychobiological theory and dynamic concept of psychiatric care. He focused on physical and emotional maturational changes. He emphasized the need to study the person's whole environment to determine the effects on the total personality. His psychobiological theory centered on treatment rather than disease, and it integrated biochemical, genetic, psychosocial, and environmental stresses with mental illness. He accepted the concept that mental disease resulted from the client's maladaptation to his or her environment. Meyer introduced the concept of common-sense psychiatry, which was based on ways that clients could realistically improve their life situations (Lewis, 1974).

Clifford Beers (1876–1943). Clifford Beers, a former mental client, contributed to preventive care through his classic work, *A Mind that Found Itself*, which was published in 1908. His writings provided a descriptive account of his tormenting experiences in mental institutions. He played a major role in establishing the mental hygiene movement in New Haven, Connecticut, in 1908 and in promoting the early detection of mental illness. National recognition and adoption of this movement began the following year.

Emil Kraepelin (1856–1926). Emil Kraepelin, a noted psychiatrist from Munich, devised a classification of mental disorders that gave momentum to the advancement of psychiatry. His work shifted from an emphasis on research in the pathobiological laboratory to the observation and study of conditions known as *dementia praecox* and *mania*.

Eugen Bleuler (1857–1939). At the end of the nineteenth century, Swiss psychiatrist Eugen Bleuler, one of Kraepelin's students, coined the term *schizophrenia* and included among its characteristics the four A's: *a*pathy, *a*ssociative looseness, *a*utism, and *a*mbivalence. His noted treatise, "Dementia Praecox or the Group of Schizophrenias," delineated the complexity of schizophrenia.

Sigmund Freud (1856–1939). During this period, a Viennese neurologist named Sigmund Freud was credited with the development of theories of psychoanalysis, psychosexuality, and neurosis. He revolutionized psychiatry through his use of psychoanalysis, a method that serves as the basis for treatment and a theory for personality development and greater understanding of human behavior. He popularized the use of the term *catharsis*, dream interpretations, and explanations for hysteria. His contribution stimulated the development and rationale for research and established the basis of modern psychoanalytical therapy. This technique focused on increasing awareness of the unconscious aspects of the client's personality.

Carl Gustav Jung (1875–1961). Carl Gustav Jung, a Swiss psychiatrist, broke with Freud and developed his own theory of the origins of neurosis. He was one of the earliest neo-Freudians who later founded the field of analytical psychology. Jung proposed and developed the concepts of extroverted and introverted personality. He integrated spiritual concepts, reasoning, and mysticism with the creative notion of human beings. He felt more optimistic about human character than did Freud and minimized the relevance of early life experiences.

Karen Horney (1885–1952). Karen Horney, a prominent psychoanalyst who was another neo-Freudian, objected to Freud's notion that neurosis and personality development were based on biological drives. Her theory suggested that neurosis stems from cultural factors and impaired interpersonal relationships. Overall, neo-Freudian theorists broadened the psychodynamic concepts and stressed the impact of disturbed interpersonal relationships in maladaptive responses. Furthermore, they minimized the biological factors of mental illness.

Numerous studies examining the relationship among biochemical, genetic, and psychosocial reactions were initiated in the early twentieth century. These included clinical studies in psychiatry and neurology, such as Hans Selye's (1956) stress and general adaptation syndromes. Psychosomatic medicine also emerged and gained prominence during the mid-twentieth century (Alexander, 1950).

Harry Stack Sullivan (1892–1949). Harry Stack Sullivan (1953) postulated the hypothesis of interpersonal theory and stimulated the development of multidisciplinary approaches to psychiatric and milieu therapy. He believed that anxiety interfered with the ability to cope and communicate effectively, resulting in mental illness. He surmised that anxiety could be reduced through a meaningful interpersonal relationship that stressed the process of effective communication. His interpersonal theory influenced psychiatric–mental health nursing practice and has become an integral part of nursing education.

Other Contributions. In 1952, the American Psychiatric Association published the *Diagnostic and Statistical Manual of Mental Disorders*. This manual provided a new and comprehensive classification of mental disorders. (The evolution of this manual is discussed in Chapter 7.)

The importance of the nurse's "therapeutic use of self" was advanced in 1952 by publication of Hildegard Peplau's text, *Interpersonal Relations in Nursing: A Conceptual Framework for Psychodynamic Nursing*. Peplau's theory stemmed primarily from the interpersonal theory of Harry Stack Sullivan, but she expanded it with her own concepts and applied them to nursing. Her work provided the first theoretical framework for psychiatric–mental health nurses and defined nursing as an interactive, exploratory, caring, and health-promotion process. Peplau delineated four overlapping phases of the nurse–client relationship: orientation, identification, exploration, and resolution. Peplau asserted that all nurse–client interactions are opportunities to build a mutual understanding and to identify goals that have an impact on client outcomes and responses.

Other theoretical approaches to psychiatric–mental health nursing have emerged from Peplau's early work. June Mellow, Gwen Tudor, and Ida Jean Orlando are examples of nurses who have made major contributions to psychiatric–mental health nursing. Their theoretical strategies also paralleled the development of concepts such as therapeutic relationships and positive client outcomes.

The Advent of Somatic Therapies

Somatic therapy is synonymous with *biological* therapy. These therapies were introduced in the late 1930s and included hypoglycemic shock to treat schizophrenia. Other treatment modalities included metrazol shock, electroshock, and psychosurgery (primarily frontal lobotomy). Psychosurgery was a radical treatment approach that was used to manage anxiety in clients with agitation and psychotic disorders. Somatic therapies brought optimism to psychiatry and revolutionized psychiatric nursing, because the clients required physical and custodial nursing care.

Psychotropics emerged in the 1950s with the advent of chlorpromazine (Thorazine) and imipramine (Tofranil). These agents revolutionized the treatment of mental illness and generated tremendous change in the role of psychiatric–mental health nursing; they calmed clients and reduced the need for other somatic therapies, such as insulin and electroconvulsive shock therapies. The optimism generated by new psychodynamic approaches and these major tranquilizers led to the community mental health movement of the 1960s.

The Mental Health Movement

During the mid-twentieth century, numerous strides were made to improve services for the mentally ill (Table 1–2). The **mental health movement** gained support and progressed in the form of federal provisions that gave authority to the U.S. Public Health Service to address mental health. These impelling changes gained momentum from experiences in treating soldiers following World War (WW) II. The result was the passage of the National Mental Health Act of 1946.

The mental health movement gained momentum during the WW II period; psychiatry finally progressed from its primitive stage of confinement and brutality to one that emphasized the need for interpersonal relations. The role of nursing evolved at the same time and was transformed from that of custodial care to more active participation on the mental health team. This new role broadened the scope of nursing practice. Increased public acceptance, awareness, and understanding after WW II provided a climate that fostered restoration of the psychological wartime casualties. WW II served as a pivotal point in the transition of nursing practice. Nurses, because of their increased visibility associated with caring for the wounded, attained respect for their innovative contributions to patient care (Stevens & Henrie, 1966).

The nation pulled together; there was increased sensitivity and optimism in support of mental health professions, such as psychiatry, nursing, social work, and psychology. The basis of legislative efforts, such as the 1961 President's Commission on Mental Illness and Health, established by President Eisenhower, and later the Federal Community Mental Health Centers legislation during the Kennedy and Johnson administrations, emphasized prevention, primary care, and rehabilitation. Proponents of this legislation hoped to reduce long-term hospitalization or institutionalization and to develop comprehensive community-based services.

Deinstitutionalization and Community-Based Care. **Deinstitutionalization** of the mentally ill followed these legislative initiatives, and it was fueled by the notion that institutions were unhealthy for the mentally ill. The Community Mental Health Centers Act of 1963 was an attempt to release chronically ill clients from institutions and place them back into community rehabilitation settings (Bassuk & Gerson, 1978).

Gerald Caplan's (1961) contributions in identifying primary, secondary, and tertiary prevention had an impact on psychiatric nursing as it emerged from the back wards of institutions to community-based settings. He believed that the incidence and severity of mental illness could be minimized by using preventive measures such as early case finding, diagnosis, and crisis intervention. Caplan's work was consistent with the intent of the mental health movement, which sought to provide comprehensive psychiatric services for clients, families, communities, and various cultures.

Historically, psychiatric nursing interventions centered on illness rather than prevention and health promotion. Leininger (1969, 1973) described the shift from hospital-based to community-based care as one of the "most significant trends" (p. 2) in the care and treatment of the mentally ill. Leininger noted that primary prevention is critical to minimizing and reducing the prevalence of mental illness. She added that this process involves understanding and researching unique in-

TABLE 1–2
The Mental Health Movement: 1940s–1990s

DATES AND EVENTS	CHANGES
1946: Passage of the Mental Health Act	Authorized formation of National Institute of Mental Health, which supported research of ► crisis intervention ► psychiatric diagnoses ► prevention and treatment of mental illness
1961: President's Commission on Mental Illness and Health	Legislative support for educating mental health professionals, including nurses, social workers, psychiatrists, and psychologists
1963: Passage of the Community Mental Health Centers Act	Deinstitutionalization (chronically mentally ill released from institutions to community rehabilitation centers)
1970–1980: Explosion of interest in biological markers and the neurobiological basis of mental illness and treatment	Advent of third-generation psychotropics. Increased popularity of biological therapies
1990s: Decade of the Brain	Advances in technology and neurobiology. Identification of Innovative diagnostic studies, especially for schizophrenia and mood disorders
1990s–Twenty-First Century: Impelling social and economical changes. Health care reforms	Soaring rate of homelessness. Lack of legislative funding for primary, secondary, tertiary prevention. Global AIDS epidemic. Recognition of the need for systematized health care delivery. Growing high risk for mental illness among pregnant women, children, elderly, substance abusers, victims of violence

dividual needs and responses to stress within various cultures and societies.

How would psychiatric nursing be integrated into the community mental health movement? Three key issues had an impact on this process: (1) nursing education and experience, (2) nursing role and function, and (3) the relationship of nursing with other mental health disciplines (DeYoung et al., 1983; Leininger, 1969).

Several research groups attempted to identify these dilemmas along with possible solutions. The first was a national survey of the psychiatric nurse's role in outpatient clinics, which discovered that fewer than 10 percent of nurses were included as part of the mental health team (Glittenberg, 1963). Inconsistent educational preparation, which varied from associate to doctoral preparation, complicated the perception of the nurse in community-based facilities. Additionally, other disciplines did not respect the advanced training of master's- and doctoral-prepared nurses, further compromising their attraction to the specialty. Furthermore, the study found that more than half of nurses participated in the initial assessment, co-therapy, and home visits (Glittenberg, 1963). Another study, conducted at Maimonides Medical Center from 1963 to 1968, concluded that most psychiatric nurses functioned as generalists, and many believed that their role on the mental health team was underrated or ancillary (Stokes et al., 1969). Additionally, these findings suggested that the psychiatric nurse was an invaluable resource and member of the mental health team, regardless of educational preparation. Both studies suggested the need to increase dialogue and collaboration with other disciplines to promote understanding and comprehensive mental health services.

New Psychotherapies. Sweeping changes in the 1960s also created opportunities for innovative psychotherapies that centered on self-actualization (Abraham Maslow), transactional analysis (Eric Berne), and gestalt therapy (Fritz Perls). These therapies overshadowed strategies associated with pure psychoanalysis. They broke with traditional long-term psychotherapy and evolved in a decade when people wanted variety and quick solutions to old problems. These therapies provided seemingly quick solutions that put people "in touch with themselves" and focused on the "here and now" rather than early life experiences as proposed by pure psychoanalytical theory. Theorists asserted that these strategies produced self-actualization and responsibility for life choices.

Biological Aspects of Mental Illness. The 1970s and 1980s produced an explosion of interest in the biological aspects of mental illness. Researchers focused on **neurobiology,** biological markers, and genetic bases for mental illness and on changing treatment modalities. The new generation of antidepressants and anxiolytics emerged during the latter decade. The early 1980s also ushered in a decade of reduced federal allocations for community mental health services and decreased the mandated services from 12 to 5 (see Chapter 25). By 1984, mental health centers were no longer funded. Reduction in funding has had far-reaching effects on the mental health movement. It has contributed to the widening gap between those who can afford health care and those who cannot. Lack of adequate funding has led to fragmentation of community mental health services, a lack of coordination in aftercare or rehabilitation, and duplication of services owing to a lack of coordinated services.

The 1990s: The Decade of the Brain. In 1989, the U.S. Congress declared the 1990s "the Decade of the Brain." This declaration was based on the fact that 50 million Americans are affected by disorders that involve the brain, ranging from familial illnesses to prenatal trauma to affective and addictive disorders. The need for knowledge and expertise in biological and psychological sciences will continue to be essential, because this knowledge provides the basis of development and use of psychopharmacological agents and psychotherapeutic interventions. Since the late 1980s, the expansion of technological advances, such as brain imaging, has provided the capability of direct examination of the living brain. These techniques, which assess brain structure and some aspects of brain function, include computed tomography, positron emission tomography, magnetic resonance imaging, and single-photon emission computed tomography.

The Future. As psychiatry enters the twenty-first century, nurses and other mental health professionals will be challenged to deal with a new world. Such changes will include a need for expanded knowledge and skills in genetic engineering; continued growth of the elderly population; advances in telecommunications; and advances in space exploration (Naisbitt, 1982; Naisbitt & Aburdene, 1990). Technological and psychological adaptations to these developments are transitions into the future.

Numerous social changes have already begun, such as those in Europe, the Middle East, and East European countries. Major changes include decision making by the people rather than by the government. Increased violence in certain regions has contributed to increased injury and death among ethnic populations. Poverty and illnesses are rampant among many of the war-torn countries of Eastern Europe. These social changes affect human relations and human coping patterns. Lifestyle changes and changing attitudes toward the mentally ill continue to parallel society's participation in economic, social, and legislative issues. The enormous cost of and poor access to health care continue to coincide with the increased risk for chronic debilitating illnesses and a decline in primary prevention. Nurses must continue to be actively involved in promoting health (Parse, 1992).

PSYCHIATRIC NURSING EDUCATION: EVOLUTION OF A SPECIALTY

Looking to the future of psychiatric–mental health nursing involves reviewing the evolution of societal issues that affect individual responses to stress. Psychiatric nursing has evolved from a role in which the primary concern was providing a clean, humane environment to one in which assessing stress responses and establishing, promoting, and evaluating interventions that deal with these responses are paramount. Nurses play pivotal roles in determining and promoting the developmental progression of clients toward the establishment of mental health.

The unique contribution of the nurse in caring for the mentally ill has been well documented throughout the ages. Before the eighteenth century, the attitude and nature of servants or attendants were recognized as important in creating relaxed, calm surroundings for those with mental illness. The advent of moral treatment involved recognizing and treating the mentally ill as human beings.

Nursing care of the mentally ill was extremely limited during the early part of the nineteenth century because nurses lacked formal training and education. Custodial care remained the primary mode of treatment within institutions. Much was accomplished because of the work of Linda Richards, the first graduate nurse in America (1873), who collaborated with Dr. Edward Cowles of McLean Asylum and persevered in the establishment of several schools in general and mental hospitals. Their efforts were instrumental in organizing the first formal training for nursing of the mentally ill in the United States in 1882. This was a 2-year training program that focused mainly on custodial care and placed little emphasis on developing psychosocial skills—custodial care centered on providing for safety and physical needs. The use of male attendants to control clients and protect nurses continued. Richards (1911) stressed the need for students to take courses in state hospitals and develop prudence and compassion, which, she emphasized, were essential nursing qualities.

These early accomplishments laid the foundation of psychiatric nursing, and it provided men with their first opportunity to become trained nurses. Until then, men were not allowed to enter nursing because there was concern that they were not as nurturing as women (Mericle, 1983).

Training for mental health nurses was significant because it provided care other than incarceration for treatment of mental illness. The role of nursing until 1937 remained custodial and under the auspices of medicine rather than nursing. Nurses were not held in high esteem by their peers.

Before the National Mental Health Act of 1946, there was no systematic effort to address the needs of the mentally ill. This legislation supported increased funding for training of mental health professionals to reduce the prevalence of mental disorders through understanding and prevention. Increased funding and societal efforts to support humane treatment for the mentally ill allowed university nursing schools to strengthen their curricula. These endeavors increased the number of trained psychiatric–mental health nurses available to promote the quality of psychiatric nursing education in undergraduate schools (baccalaureate level) and integrate concepts throughout the nursing curricula. Nursing schools began to transform their modified "maternal" or custodial role to therapeutic and preventive perspectives.

Another milestone in the evolution of psychiatric nursing was the formation of the National League for Nursing (NLN) in 1952. This organization was also concerned with the education and training of nurses in the mental health area, and as a result, the Mental Health and Psychiatric Advisory Service was formed. Kathleen Black, a registered nurse, was its first director. Representatives from this service acted as educational consultants for nursing schools nationwide.

NURSING THEORISTS

Hildegard Peplau

In 1952, Peplau's publication of *Interpersonal Relations in Nursing: A Conceptual Framework for Psychodynamic Nursing* influenced nursing practice (see earlier discussion of Peplau's contribution to psychiatric nursing). The foundation of her theory came from Harry Stack Sullivan's postulates. Her concepts and perspectives were developed into nursing theory that became the basis of interpersonal processes in nursing. These were related to the promotion of healthy adaptation to life stressors.

June Mellow and Gwen Tudor

Other theorists during the 1950s included June Mellow, who developed concepts in nursing theory based on work with clients with schizophrenia. She stressed the influence of the nurse–client relationship and the nursing process on client outcomes. Furthermore, Gwen Tudor (1952) defined psychiatric nursing as an interpersonal process of observation, intervention, and evaluation. Tudor described three major functions of the nurse as a facilitator of communication, social interaction, and client needs. She believed that mental illness resulted from impaired communication, social interaction, and self-care. Additionally, she stressed the significance of social context and its impact on the nurse's attitude and response to the client's needs and subsequent mental health. Contributions from these nurses were instrumental in legitimizing the role of psychiatric nursing and establishing the foundation for current therapeutic interventions (see Table 1–1).

NATIONAL INSTITUTE OF MENTAL HEALTH

In 1954, the **National Institute of Mental Health** (NIMH) supported a pilot program to integrate behavioral concepts and psychiatric content into undergraduate curricula. It also identified the shortage of psychiatric–mental health nurses trained to care for emotionally disturbed children and the need for primary prevention of mental illness. Opportunities for trained psychiatric–mental health nurses flourished during the 1950s and 1960s, evolving within nursing and becoming an integral part of the profession. The role of the psychiatric clinical specialist during this era focused on the need for advanced preparation built on the foundation of behavioral and nursing concepts. Additionally, nursing leaders expressed the need for doctoral training and research. The federal government's role has been critical in identifying the need for and supporting the preparation of nurses in psychiatric–mental health nursing (Chamberlain, 1983).

AMERICAN NURSES ASSOCIATION

The American Nurses Association (ANA) was established in 1893. This organization later stressed the importance of including clinical preparation in psychiatric nursing as part of training for nursing students. McLean and several other Boston hospitals provided clinical settings for this training.

The ANA has also had a major impact on the evolution of psychiatric–mental health nursing. It has been instrumental in providing the foundation of psychiatric–mental health nursing practice as we know it today. In 1967, the ANA's Division on Psychiatric–Mental Health Nursing published the *Statement on Psychiatric Nursing Practice*. It validated the significance and impact of psychiatric nursing education and the diversity of this discipline in meeting the needs of the mentally ill. These 1967 standards advocated that nurses define and develop nursing practice based on theory, experience, research, and prevention, using the nursing process. Additionally, the statement played a vital role in the historical development of psychiatric–mental health nursing education and practice.

In the fall of 1974, the Executive Committee of the Division on Psychiatric–Mental Health Nursing appointed an ad hoc committee to revise the *Statement* to meet ANA's commitment to maintain high standards of nursing practice and improve the quality of nursing care. Furthermore, the ad hoc committee decided to increase the consumer's understanding of the psychiatric–mental health nurse by clarifying the relationship between education, experience, and specialties. The following major themes evolved from this committee's efforts (ANA, 1976):

- The strong trend toward community-based, short-term treatment models, with a concomitant emphasis on deinstitutionalization
- Emphasis on the assurance of quality care

TABLE 1–3
Milestones in Child and Adolescent Psychiatry: 1890s–1990s

1890: PSYCHOLOGY
- Interest in the nervous child
- School phobias
- Residential care for poor (asylum, workhouse, reformatory)

1895: ADOLPH MEYER
- Stressed preventive care and the need for formal training in child psychiatry
- Initiated Kanner's research of childhood psychiatry
- Stressed the appraisal of psychobiological and social factors to increase understanding of mental illness in children and families (Kanner, 1935)

1906: PSYCHOANALYSIS AND PSYCHODYNAMICS
Focus on assessment and treatment
- Impact of family on child
- Play therapy (Isaacs, 1961)
- Child psychotherapy
- White House Conference on Children (1909) announced goals of developing strong, innovative program to care for emotionally disturbed children

1920s–1930s: CHILD GUIDANCE MOVEMENT
Social reforms: development of community services for children
- Focus on prevention of juvenile delinquency
- First child guidance clinic
- Development of teaching department on child psychiatry in hospitals
- White House Conference on Child Health and Protection proclaimed that emotionally ill child has the right to live in a world that does not separate him or her from others (Kanner, 1955)

1940s–1960s: POST–WORLD WAR II REFORMS
- Identification of large numbers of severely disturbed children
- Increased institutionalization in punitive establishments, homes, and special schools (interdisciplinary approach)

1970s: FAMILY THERAPY
Educational opportunities flourished

1980s
Child and adolescent psychiatric–mental health nursing came of age
- Certification became available
- Advocates for children and adolescents

1990s: DECADE OF THE BRAIN
- Surge in family studies of mood disorders, schizophrenia, and other mental disorders

LATE 1970s TO PRESENT
- Decreased federal funding for children
- Reduced support of childhood nutritional programs, education, and day care

- Significant development in the arena of litigation and mental services

The ANA established a certification program in 1973 to provide an objective and credible means of recognizing professional expertise in the specialty for both functional and clinical domains of nursing. More than 80,000 registered nurses since 1975 have been certified through the American Nurses Credentialing Center (ANCC). Certification has allowed nurses to compete within the health care delivery system as distinguished health care providers (ANCC, 1993).

In 1976, the ANA established two levels of professional nurses: baccalaureate and advanced practice. In psychiatry, the advanced level was initially established as the clinical specialist in adult psychiatric–mental health nursing. This was later followed by the clinical specialist in child and adolescent psychiatric–mental health nursing. (See Table 1–3 for a review of the milestone events in the development of child and adolescent psychiatry from the 1890s to the present.)

In 1989, the ANA Commission on Organizational Assessment and Renewal recommended that ANCC be considered a distinct agency used by the ANA for credentialing purposes. Credentialing programs are based on the ANA's Congress for Nursing Practice. The goals of the ANCC entail "promoting and enhancing public health by certifying nurses and accrediting organizations using ANA standards of nursing practice, nursing services, and continuing education" (ANCC, 1993, p. 3). By 1998, a minimum of a bachelor of science or higher degree in nursing will be a prerequisite for the initial certification process for the generalist.

The 1994 publication, *A statement of psychiatric–mental health clinical nursing practice and standards of psychiatric–mental health clinical practice*, represents a collaboration of various psychiatric nursing organizations that delineates the role of the generalist and the advanced-practice psychiatric nurse (ANA, 1994).

PSYCHIATRIC NURSING JOURNALS

Other landmarks from the 1960s to the 1980s included the advent of psychiatric nursing journals: *Perspectives in Psychiatric Care* (1963), *Journal of Psychosocial Nursing and Mental Health Services* (1963), *Issues in Mental Health Nursing* (1979), and *Archives of Psychiatric Nursing* (1987).

FEDERAL FUNDING OF PSYCHIATRIC NURSING EDUCATION

Chamberlain (1983) identified the impact of 1960s federal spending on the evolution of psychiatric–mental health nursing as having achieved the following results:

- More master's-level psychiatric nursing programs
- More practicing master's-prepared nurses
- Greater interest in the integration of mental health concepts in baccalaureate nursing program curricula
- Development of continuing education programs that focused on psychiatric nursing concepts
- Diversity of NIMH master's and doctoral program graduates in service delivery settings (i.e., administrators, faculty, practitioners, and research)

Legislative allocation of funds for psychiatric–mental health education peaked in 1969, when there was a major setback in appropriating financial support for both undergraduate and graduate psychiatric nursing programs. This trend has continued through the 1970s and into the 1990s, despite increased community demands to treat the mentally ill.

AMENDMENTS TO THE COMMUNITY MENTAL HEALTH ACT

The 1975 amendments to the Community Mental Health Centers Act of 1963 addressed the need for the least restrictive care, changes in the commitment process, and deinstitutionalization of the mentally ill. The amendments were adopted by passage of the Mental Health Act of 1980 and the National Plan for the Chronically Ill in 1981. This legislation centered on increasing remission and decreasing exacerbation of symptoms by providing continuity of care in U.S. communities and health care organizations. The result of this legislation was that nurses were often replaced with other health care professionals and attendants to run units and direct client care. The trend toward replacing registered nurses with paraprofessionals reflects increasing health care costs and lack of access to care.

TRENDS IN PSYCHIATRIC NURSING

Psychiatric health care systems are influenced by the social and economic climate of the times. Before and during the nineteenth century, these systems were predominantly paternalistic and closed (Peplau, 1989). During the 1960s and 1970s, changes within health care facilities paralleled the deinstitutionalization of mental health care. Social concerns for the mentally ill and legislative support for preventive interventions were the basis of funding and training for advanced-practice psychiatric–mental health nurses. Before the 1980s, mental health facilities comprised primarily clients with chronic mental illness.

The 1980s drastically changed psychiatric nursing in several ways. Initially, there was a noticeable decrease in funding of traineeships from the NIMH. A lack of funding led to a decrease in advanced-level psychiatric–mental health nurses. Second, there was an enormous growth in freestanding psychiatric facilities that resulted in client abuse and misuse of health care to fill empty beds. Finally, an outcry from clients, their families, and client advocacy groups led to numerous investigations and a subsequent decrease in the number of psychiatric admissions and eventual closure of psychiatric units and hospitals. These changes affected job security and increased job loss of nurses working in the private sector. Psychiatric nurses can have an impact on these transitions by becoming proactive in societal, economic, and legislative activities that affect their practice.

Future trends of psychiatric nursing will be determined by a number of factors. As psychiatric–mental health nursing moves into the next century, it is challenged to meet the complex demands of advanced technology, telecommunications, and societal and economic changes. Research will continue to direct and provide the basis for understanding mental illness in areas such as neurobiology, psychodynamics, and exploration of life span issues. New lifestyle patterns will continue to affect societal, economic, and legislative norms.

CONCEPTS OF PRACTICE

Other solutions include integrating complex concepts into nursing practice. Expanding neurobiological and technological advances and psychosocial factors are major issues that presently confront psychiatric nurses. Angela McBride (1990) supported this notion and urged psychiatric–mental health nurses to reexamine their future roles in meeting societal needs. She advocated integrating research-based practice with the revaluing of biological knowledge and becoming fundamentally reassociated with care and caring.

McBride (1990) also suggested that the research agenda for psychiatric nurses is an important component of integrating biological concepts into practice. Areas that need change include the following:

- Closing the gap of nursing knowledge regarding the relevance of the neurobiology of mental illness
- Implementing the NIMH agenda
- Revamping nursing curricula to interface biological and behavioral sciences

McBride further stressed the importance of nurses' reassociating themselves with caring, described as the following:

- Being responsive to clients rather than being judgmental
- Using the concept of nurturing as one that encompasses the protection of client rights
- Having a health care system that fosters effective communication at all levels
- Exploring the ethical issues and values associated with the professional commitment of working with mentally ill clients

Other nursing leaders support these concepts and advocate increased collaboration within psychiatric nursing practice, academia, specialties, and organizations to confront complex issues and factors affecting psychiatric–mental health nursing in the next decade (Pothier et al., 1990).

DIRECTIONS FOR NURSING EDUCATION

Nurse educators and psychiatric–mental health nurses must be active participants in the transformation of the health care agenda for the twenty-first century. Their concerted efforts are critical to the success of integrating and expanding neurobiological advances into practice and understanding social changes that affect the mental health of their clients. The future of psychiatric–mental health nursing depends on these endeavors.

Changes in nursing curricula can be made by integrating topics such as circadian rhythms, neurological assessment, factors that affect client compliance, early signs and symptoms of violence, and the neurobiological basis of mental illness (McBride, 1990).

SOCIETAL CHANGES

As the health care system strives to improve access to care for populations at risk, such as women, children, low-income groups, the homeless, and the elderly, psychiatric nurses will be confronted with the need to redefine their role. The incidence of mental illness is increasing, especially among the chronically ill and those misusing substances. Society is faced with severe challenges because of deteriorating social structures, a global epidemic of AIDS, and increased violence and poverty levels (ANA, 1991). Unemployment continues to increase, and family breakdown affects all levels of society. These situations increase the incidence of crisis and mental illness among people across the life span.

Nurses are on the front line of health care, and they are the chief advocates for health promotion from the time clients enter until they leave treatment. Complex client needs require psychiatric–mental health nurses to integrate neurobiological, psychosocial, developmental, and holistic concepts into their practice so that they can effectively and efficiently assess, direct, and evaluate health care. The ability to measure the effectiveness of these interventions is critical to health promotion.

HEALTH CARE REFORM

Current health care reform proposals suggest a return to community and primary health care. This provides a window of opportunity for psychiatric–mental health nurses to redefine their roles as major providers in a changing health care system (ANA, 1994; Billings, 1993b). Nursing interventions that promote health and prevention are critical to expanded hospital- and community-based care. Many clients will be treated in community facilities such as day hospitals, private practices, hospices, home health programs, partial hospitals, and mental health centers. The range of interventions includes case management, psychoeducation, prescriptive authority, psychotherapy, medication clinics, and dual diagnoses (clients diagnosed with distinct dual disorders, such as a mental illness and chemical addiction). A continued lack of funding impels nurses and other health care professionals to maximize resources and develop innovative treatments to meet the present and future needs of a society under tremendous stress.

COLLABORATION OF NURSING ORGANIZATIONS

As psychiatric–mental health nursing moves into the twenty-first century, other significant changes are occurring. A new partnership within a number of major psychiatric nursing organizations reflects the bid of those organizations to collaborate and revolutionize the scope and standards of psychiatric–mental health nursing practice with the ANA. Major nursing organizations engaging in this endeavor include the Coalition for Psychiatric Nursing, the ANA Council on Psychiatric–Mental Health Nursing, the American Psychiatric Nurses Association, the Association of Child and Adolescent Psychiatric Nurses and the Society for Education and Research in Psychiatric–Mental Health Nursing. This effort at unity will enable psychiatric–mental health nurses to form a powerful and collaborative partnership among organizations. This tone is crucial to making successful changes within a transforming society and health care system and responding effectively to the needs of the psychiatric–mental health nurse and the consumer (Billings, 1993a; Krauss, 1993).

► CHAPTER SUMMARY

Historically, the treatment and the perception of the mentally ill have been influenced by religious and social norms. Treatment has varied from brutal, inhumane torture in asylums to community-based psychotherapy. Psychiatric nurses did not exist before 1882, at which time McLean Asylum in Massachusetts began the first formal training of psychiatric nurses.

The practice of psychiatric–mental health nursing has continued to evolve, and it has become far removed from that of custodian and controller. It has emerged as a specialty that requires the integration of neurobiological and behavioral concepts. McBride (1990) stressed that the future of psychiatric–mental health nurses hinges on their willingness to appreciate these concepts, develop research-based practice, and integrate caring into their practice.

The challenges of the twenty-first century will continue to mirror the impact of societal, economic, and legislative factors on people throughout the life span. Psychiatric–mental health nurses can rise to the occasion by identifying clients at risk, participating in research endeavors to enhance practice, and developing effective treatment approaches. Overall, this process involves redefining the role of psychiatric–mental health nursing within a health care system in crisis and seeing nurses place themselves in key positions to direct client care.

Suggestions for Clinical Conferences

1. Identify several recent and past psychiatric nursing leaders, and compare their contributions to psychiatric–mental health nursing.
2. Compare the impact of the mental health movement to present changes in health care.
3. Trace the evolution of psychiatric–mental health care from the Middle Ages to the 1990s.

4. Invite a clinical specialist to discuss the role of the National Institute of Mental Health and psychiatric–mental health research.

References

Aguilera, D., & Messick, J. (1970). *Crisis intervention: Theory and methodology*. St. Louis: C. V. Mosby.

Alexander, F. (1950). *Psychosomatic medicine: Its principles and applications*. New York: Norton.

American Nurses Association. (1967). *Statement on psychiatric nursing practice*. Kansas City, MO: Author.

American Nurses Association. (1976). *Statement on psychiatric and mental health nursing practice*. Kansas City, MO: Author.

American Nurses Association. (1982). *Standards of psychiatric and mental health nursing practice*. Kansas City, MO: Author.

American Nurses Association. (1991). *Nursing agenda for health care reform*. Kansas City, MO: Author.

American Nurses Association. (1994). *Statement on psychiatric–mental health clinical nursing practice and standards of psychiatric–mental health clinical nursing practice*. Washington, DC: American Nurses Publication.

American Nurses Credentialing Center. (1993). *American Nurses Credentialing Center catalog* (p. 3). Washington, DC: Author.

American Psychiatric Association. (1952). *Diagnostic and statistical manual of mental disorders*. Washington, DC: Author.

Bailey, H. (1920). *Nursing mental diseases*. New York: Macmillan.

Bassuk, E. L., & Gerson, S. (1978). Deinstitutionalization and mental health services. *Scientific American, 238*(2), 46–53.

Beers, C. (1908). *A mind that found itself*. New York: Doubleday.

Billings, C. V. (1993a). Forging professional partnerships. *American Nurses Association Council Perspectives, 2*(3), 8.

Billings, C. V. (1993b). The "possible" dream of mental health reform. *The American Nurse, 25*(2), 5–9.

Caplan, G. (1961). *An approach to community mental health*. New York: Basic Books.

Chamberlain, J. G. (1983). The role of the federal government in the development of psychiatric nursing. *Journal of Psychosocial Nursing and Mental Health Services, 21*(4), 11–18.

Conolly, J. (1968). *The construction and government of lunatic asylums*. London: Dawsons of Pall Mall.

DeYoung, C. D., Tower, M., & Glittenberg, J. (1983). Out of uniform and into trouble . . . again. Thorofare, NJ: Slack.

Ellenberger, H. F. (1974). Psychiatry from ancient to modern times. In S. Areti (Ed.), *American handbook of psychiatry* (2nd ed., pp. 3–27). New York: Basic Books.

Glittenberg, J. A. (1963). The role of the nurse in outpatient psychiatric clinics. *The American Journal of Orthopsychiatry, 39,* 1.

Isaacs, S. (1961). Obituary: Melanie Klein 1882–1960. *Journal of Child Psychology and Psychiatry, 2,* 1–4.

Iscoe, I., & Harris, L. C. (1984). Social and community interventions. *Annual Review of Psychology, 35,* 333–360.

Kanner, L. (1935). *Child psychiatry*. Springfield, IL: Charles C Thomas.

Krauss, J. (1993). *Health care reform: Essential mental health services*. Washington, DC: American Nurses Association.

Leininger, M. (1969). Community psychiatric nursing: Trends, issues, and problems. *Perspectives in Psychiatric Care, 7*(1), 10–20.

Leininger, M. (1973). *Contemporary issues in mental health nursing*. Boston: Little, Brown.

Lewis, N. C. D. (1974). American psychiatry from its beginnings to World War II. In S. Areti (Ed.), *American handbook of psychiatry* (2nd ed., pp. 28–42). New York: Basic Books.

Mellow, J. (1967). Evolution of nursing therapy through research. *Psychiatric Opinion, 4*(1), 15–21.

McBride, A. B. (1990). Psychiatric nursing in the 1990s. *Archives of Psychiatric Nursing, 4*(1), 21–28.

Mericle, B. P. (1983). The male as psychiatric nurse. *Journal of Psychosocial Nursing and Mental Health Services, 21*(11), 28–34.

Naisbitt, J. (1982). *Megatrends*. New York: Warner Books.

Naisbitt, J., & Aburdene, P. (1990). *Megatrends 2000: Ten directions for the 1990s*. New York: Morrow.

Nightingale, F. (1859). *Notes on nursing*. London: Harrison & Sons.

Parse, R. R. (1992). Nursing knowledge for the 21st century: An international commitment. *Nursing Science Quarterly, 5*(9), 8–12.

Peplau, H. E. (1952). *Interpersonal relations in nursing*. New York: Putnam.

Peplau, H. E. (1989). Future directions in psychiatric nursing from the perspective of history. *Journal of Psychosocial Nursing and Mental Health Services, 27*(2), 18–27, 25–28, 39–40.

Pothier, P. C., Stuart, G. W., Puskar, K., & Babich, K. (1990). Dilemmas and direction for psychiatric nursing in the 1990s. *Archives of Psychiatric Nursing, 5*(5), 284–291.

Reiger, D. A., et al. (1988). One-month prevalence of mental disorders in the United States. *Archives of General Psychiatry, 45*(11), 977–986.

Richards, L. A. (1911). *Remininiscences of Linda Richards*. Boston: Barrows.

Scull, A. T. (1982). *Museums of madness*. London: Penguin Education.

Selye, H. (1956). *The stress of life*. New York: McGraw-Hill.

Shattuck, L. (1948). *Report of the sanitary commission of mental health—1850*. Cambridge: Harvard University Press.

Sills, G. M. (1973). Historical developments and issues in psychiatric–mental health nursing. In M. L. Leininger (Ed.), *Contemporary issues in mental health nursing* (pp. 125–136). Boston: Little, Brown.

Smoyak, S. (1975). *The psychiatric nurse as a family therapist*. New York: John Wiley.

Stevens, L. F., & Henrie, D. D. (1966). A history of psychiatric nursing. *Bulletin of the Menninger Clinic, 30*, 32–38.

Stokes, G. A., Williams, F. S., Davidites, R. M., Bulbulyen, A., & Ullman, M. (1969). *The roles of psychiatric nurses in community mental health practice: A giant step*. New York: Faculty Press.

Sullivan, H. S. (1953). *The interpersonal theory of psychiatry*. New York: Norton.

Tudor, G. E. (1952). A sociopsychiatric nursing approach to intervention in a problem of mutual withdrawal on a mental hospital ward. *Psychiatry: Journal for the Study of Interpersonal Processes, 15*(2), 193–217.

U. S. Congress. (1989). Decade of the brain proclamation. Public Law 101–158 (HJ Res. 174). July 25, 1989, 130 STAT. 152–154.

CHAPTER 2

Concepts of Psychiatric Care: Therapeutic Models

MARTHA SANFORD, Ph.D., R.N.

OUTLINE

CHAPTER OBJECTIVES

Upon completion of this chapter, you will be able to:

1. Identify the basic concepts of each theory discussed in the chapter.
2. Discuss the assumptions concerning the contributing factors that lead to mental disorders.
3. Understand the importance of using theories in practice.
4. Discuss how each theory suggests a person can be helped.
5. Identify the stages of growth and development as identified in various theories.
6. Compare and contrast the developmental stages according to various theorists.
7. Describe the implications of theories for nurses.
8. Discuss the assumptions about people derived from each theory.
9. Use concepts from the theories to design interventions.
10. Assess cognitive distortions used by yourself and clients.
11. Describe the client outcomes suggested by each theory.

KEY TERMS

Anima
Animus
Archetypes
Chronobiology
Circadian rhythms
Classic conditioning
Cognitive processes
Defense mechanisms
Drive
Ego
Entropy
Equifinality
Eros
Id
Inferiority complex
Infradian rhythms
Libido
Modeling
Negentropy
Operant conditioning
Persona
Personification
Reinforcement
Repression
Schemata
Shadow
Superego
Thanatos
Theory
Ultradian rhythms
Zeitgeber

What are therapeutic models, and why do we need to study them? Models give us structures that we can use to visualize phenomena. Therapeutic models guide our thinking about phenomena. When we care for clients with complex mental and physical disorders, we need some framework for organizing our thinking about the manifestations, the development, and the treatment of the disorders. Once we have a structure for observing disorders, we can begin to develop theories about how the disorders develop and how they can be treated.

Theory develops from observations by individuals and groups of individuals as they study humans and their environments. We see relationships between cause and effect. As patterns of relationships begin to emerge repeatedly, scholars then acknowledge support of theories.

Nurses use theories to direct assessment and to suggest interventions and causes. Theories from a variety of professional fields have implications for nursing care. Nurses may not find any single theory adequate for practice, but they will find useful concepts and principles from several theories. Each theory is an attempt to establish a scientific method for studying the individual as a living, social being. Each theory contributes to a language with which to examine and communicate human action. This chapter briefly examines major concepts of the most commonly used theories.

PSYCHOANALYTICAL THEORY

Freud's psychoanalytical theory addresses the relationships among inner experiences, behavior, social roles, and functioning (Arlow, 1989). This theory proposes that conflicts among unconscious motivating forces affect behavior. People usually do not like conflict and therefore develop certain structures of the mind, or ways of responding, to maintain equilibrium and keep conflicts from causing too much discomfort. The defensive process of **repression** keeps conflicts out of the realm of awareness, thus avoiding discomfort and pain. Repression is an unconscious process that requires energy to keep thoughts out of awareness.

DRIVES

Sigmund Freud (1952), often called the father of psychoanalysis, viewed humans as stimulus driven, responding to both internal and external stimuli. The perceived stimulus produces a drive, or instinct. **Drive** is a state of excitation in response to stimuli. These drives are instinctual urges and impulses arising from biological and psychological needs. The drive produces mental activity that seeks gratification, or discharge, resulting in a decrease in tension.

The psychoanalytical theory assumes that humans have two primary drives or forces: the drive toward life (eros) and the drive toward death (thanatos). **Eros** includes instincts concerned with self-preservation and survival of the species. **Thanatos** is expressed as aggression or hate, which can be directed inwardly (as in suicide) or outwardly (as in murder).

STRUCTURE OF PERSONALITY

Freud proposed hypothetical structures—the id, the ego, and the superego—to explain his observation that behaviors result from conflicts among the needs of the individual, the restrictions of the environment, and internalized moral values (Fig. 2–1).

The **id** represents psychological energy, or **libido**. Freud says this energy is primarily a sexual and aggressive drive. The id is the first structure to develop in the personality, and it operates on the pleasure principle to reduce tension. For example, a hungry infant reflexively sucks to receive nourishment, thus reducing its hunger. Id is also characterized by primary process thinking, a mode of thought that is primarily imagery. It is irrational and not based on reality. Hallucinations of psychotic clients are examples of primary process thinking.

The **ego** is the chief executive officer of the mind. It mediates between the drives, forces, or conflicts of the id and the superego. It maintains a reality orientation for the person. It keeps the strong forces of the superego from being extremely inhibitive and the id from causing the person to become overly exhibitionistic. The ego operates on the reality principle and is charac-

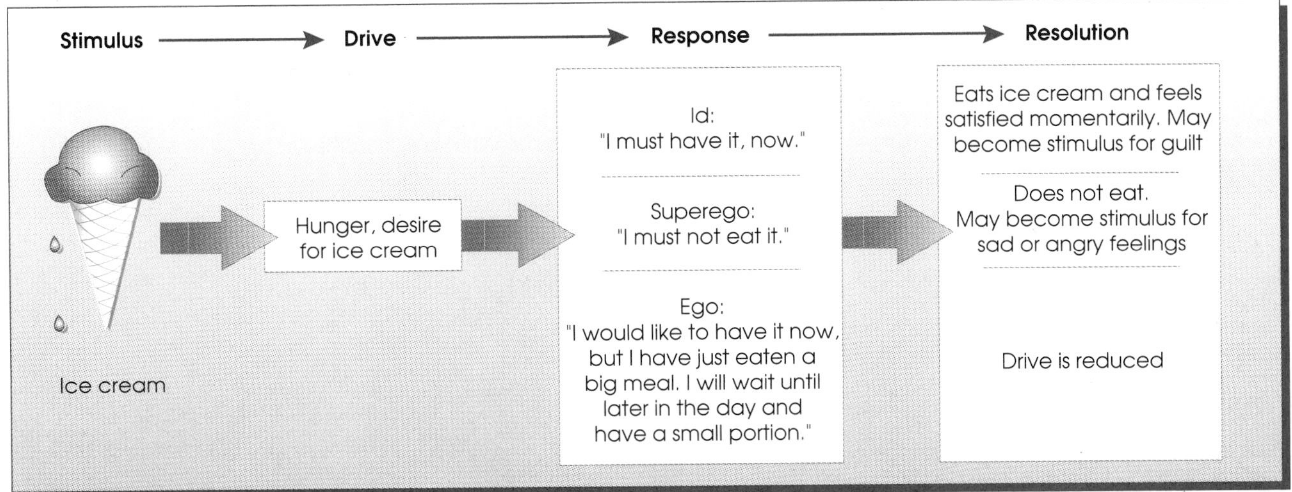

FIGURE 2–1
Example of operation of the id, ego, and superego in resolving conflicts. The resolution depends on which force predominates.

terized by secondary process thinking, which is logically oriented in time and distinguishes between reality and unreality. As such, it provides a means of delaying gratification of needs. The ego is partially under conscious control, whereas the id is unconscious.

The **superego** has two main functions, based on reward and punishment. It is the superego that rewards moral behavior and punishes actions that are not acceptable by creating guilt. The superego is our conscience, a residue of internalized values and moral training of early childhood. An overly strict superego may lead to extremes of guilt and anxiety.

The ego manages the sexual and aggressive drives of the id, keeping them from being destructive. Anxiety results when the ego cannot mediate against the unconscious drives. Anxiety is a warning to the ego of an emerging danger. **Repression** is the first line of defense against unacceptable, painful, and unwanted memories. Repression is an unconscious process that keeps unacceptable impulses out of awareness and prevents these impulses from becoming conscious. The energy associated with these impulses, or drives, is not changed or sublimated into something else but requires extra energy to keep the drive out of awareness. Some repressed conflicts break through awareness and are defended against in other ways.

DEFENSE MECHANISMS

Anna Freud (1937), Sigmund Freud's daughter, further explicated the **defense mechanisms**. Vaillant (1977), in his analysis of data from a 30-year study of a cohort of healthy male college students, classified the defense mechanisms in a hierarchy from psychotic to healthy (Table 2–1). The defense mechanisms have two aspects. First, they keep unwanted thoughts out of awareness and use energy to do this. Second, energy cannot be contained indefinitely; therefore, some defense mechanisms allow the energy to be discharged, as in reaction formation, projection, and sublimation. Defense mechanisms are the methods used by the ego to fight instinctual outbursts of the id and superego.

PSYCHOSEXUAL THEORY OF DEVELOPMENT

The psychoanalytical theory proposes that adult character traits, behaviors, and thinking processes are a result of crucial events in the developmental years. The personality is almost completely formed by 5 years of age. During the various stages, the child is motivated by the need for pleasure and derives that pleasure by stimulating the various erogenous zones of the body or by being stimulated by the parents in their handling. Each stage is localized in specific bodily zones (Table 2–2).

The *oral stage* of development begins at birth, extending about 18 months. During this stage, stimulation of the mouth, such as in sucking, biting, and swallowing, is the primary source of satisfaction. Not getting needs met at this stage may produce problems with eating and habits such as smoking and biting nails. A wide range of adult behaviors, from excessive optimism to sarcasm, cynicism, and pessimism, have been attributed to problems during this stage. Fixation at this stage is characterized by narcissism and incorporation of loved objects (the instinctual behavior that motivates the person to receive gratification by symbolically swallowing the important other) (Fenichel, 1945).

During the *anal phase* (18 months to 3 years of age), sexual gratification shifts to the anus. This occurs during the period of toilet training. The child is concerned with retaining and letting go of feces. Problems occurring in the resolution of this phase may result in rebelliousness and a exaggerated need to be in control. If the fixation is with retention or holding in, the adult may be excessively neat, clean, and compulsive. If expulsion is

TABLE 2–1
Vaillant's Four Levels of Defense Mechanisms

LEVEL	DEFENSE	EXAMPLE
Level I Psychotic mechanisms: these mechanisms are common in healthy individuals before age 5	Delusional projection: frank delusions about external reality, usually of a persecutory type	Example: "The Devil is devouring my heart"
	Denial: denial of external reality, including the use of fantasy as a substitute for other people	Example: "I will make a new him in my own mind"
	Distortion: grossly reshaping external reality to suit inner needs	Example: hallucinations, wish-fulfilling delusions, and megalomaniacal beliefs
Level II Immature mechanisms: common in healthy individuals ages 3 to 15, in character disorder, and in adults in psychotherapy. They may change with improved interpersonal relationships or with repeated and forceful interpretation during long therapy	Projection: attributing one's own unacknowledged feeling to others	Example: prejudice, rejections of intimacy, suspicion, and injustic collecting
	Schizoid fantasy: tendency to use fantasy and to indulge in autistic retreat for the purpose of conflict resolution and gratification	Example: avoidance of intimacy and use of eccentricity to repel others
	Hypochondriasis: the transformation of reproach toward others arising from bereavement, loneliness, or unacceptable aggressive impulses into, first, self-reproach and then complaints of pain, somatic illness, and neurasthenia	Example: chronic pain syndromes
	Passive-aggressive behavior: aggression toward others expressed indirectly and ineffectively through passivity or directed against the self	Example: procrastinations, failures, illnesses that affect others more than self
	Acting out: direct expression of an unconscious wish or impulse in order to avoid being conscious of the effect that accompanies it. Acting out involves chronically giving in to impulses in order to avoid the tension that would result were there any postponement of instinctual expressions	Example: using behavior or delinquent or impulsive acts to avoid being aware of one's feelings. Chronic use of drugs, perversion, self-inflicted injury to relieve tension
Level III Neurotic defenses: These mechanisms are common in healthy individuals aged 3 to 90, in neurotic disorder, and in mastering acute adult stress. These defenses can be changed by brief therapy	Intellectualization: thinking about instinctual wishes in formal, affectively bland terms and not acting on them. The idea is in consciousness, but the feeling is missing. Vaillant believes intellectualization includes mechanisms of isolation, rationalization, ritual, undoing, restitution, and magical thinking	Example: paying attention to the inanimate to avoid intimacy with people, or paying attention to external reality to avoid expression of inner feelings
	Repression: seemingly inexplicable naivete, memory lapse, or failure to acknowledge input from a selected sense organ. The feeling is in consciousness, but the idea is missing. It blocks conscious perception of instinct feelings	Example: a man who weeps, but does not know for whom he weeps
	Displacement: the redirection of feelings toward an object relatively less cared for than the person or situation arousing the feelings	Example: practical jokes, with hidden hostile intent, phobias, hysterical conversion reactions, and some prejudice
	Reaction formation: behavior in a fashion diametrically opposed to an unacceptable instinctual impulse	Example: overtly caring for someone else when one wishes to be cared for oneself
	Dissociation: temporary but drastic modification of one's character or of one's sense of personal identity to avoid emotional distress	Example: fugues, hysterical conversion reactions, a sudden unwarranted sense of superiority, counterphobic behavior in order to block out anxiety

►TABLE 2–1
Vaillant's Four Levels of Defense Mechanisms *Continued*

LEVEL	DEFENSE	EXAMPLE
Mature mechanisms: These mechanisms are common in healthy individuals ages 12 to 90	Altruism: vicarious but constructive and instinctually gratifying service to others	Example: philanthropy and well-repaid service to others
	Humor: overt expression of ideas and feelings without individual discomfort or immobilization and without unpleasant effect on others	Example: jokes and games
	Sublimation: indirect or attenuated expression of instincts without either adverse consequences or marked loss of pleasure	Example: expressing aggression through pleasurable games, sports, and hobbies

From Vaillant, G. E. (1977). *Adaptation to life.* Boston: Little, Brown.

the problem, the adult may be dirty, wasteful, and extravagant.

During the *phallic stage*, which occurs at the end of the third or fourth year, erotic gratification shifts to the genital region. The child becomes sexually attracted to the parent of the opposite sex and fears the parent of the same sex, who is now perceived as a rival. The child overcomes this conflict by identifying with the parent of the same sex. Object love at this stage is ambivalent and may affect object relations in adult life.

The early school-age years (6 to 12 years) constitute a period of quiescence Freud called *latency*. The child begins to submit to the demands of the superego and sublimate instincts. The way the person handles the internal and external demands becomes, for better or for worse, consolidated during this time.

At the start of adolescence, the final stage, called the *genital stage,* begins. Heterosexual behavior is evident, and the person undertakes various activities in preparation for marriage and family.

APPLICATION TO NURSING

It is important for nurses to understand that the role of unconscious conflict is the motivation of behavior. When we are tempted to ask "Why did you . . . ?" we are reminded that often the person cannot identify the motivation because it is unconscious.

Psychoanalytical theory has demonstrated the central role of anxiety in dysfunctional behavior. Nurses must be aware of clients' mechanisms that defend against instinctual demands and anxiety. When we recognize that a client is using a defense mechanism, we know that the anxiety must be reduced before the defenses can be disengaged.

SOCIAL THEORIES

ERIK ERIKSON

Erik Erikson was a student of Anna Freud. Unlike Freud, Erikson (1963) believed that a person's social view of self is more important than libidinal urges. Erikson's optimistic outlook on human growth and development speaks to new opportunities for particular strengths to develop at each stage. These strengths emerge when each crisis is met and must be continuously upheld throughout life to be useful. The task of identity is seen as the major task of life. All previous tasks are fundamental to self-discovery, and all adult tasks are predicated on comfortable resolution of identity.

Erikson believed that human institutions evolved along with the human species and that a particular institutional form can be related to each developmental stage (Table 2–3). Erikson did not identify an institution for the last stage. Perhaps he believed that no society had progressed far enough to produce such an institution.

CARL JUNG

Carl Jung (1967) differed with Freud on the nature of the unconscious. He postulated a collective unconscious containing the universal memories and history of all humans. The collective unconscious is that part of unconscious material that is universal in humans, in contrast with the personal unconscious that is determined by individual personal experience. From his study of international myths, folklore, and art, Jung discovered common, repeated images that he called ***archetypes***. The collective unconscious contains symbolic access to archetypes, which serve as its building blocks. An archetype can be a mythical figure, such as the Hero, the Nurturing Mother, the Powerful Father, or the Wicked Witch. Other powerful archetypes are the persona and the shadow. The **persona** is the public personality, the aspects of self that one reveals to others, the role that society expects one to play. The persona is frequently at variance with true identity. The **shadow** archetype reflects the prehistoric fear of wild animals and represents the animal side of human nature. The shadow contains the opposite of what we feel ourselves to be.

Two of the most important archetypes are those of men and women themselves. Jung recognized that hu-

TABLE 2–2
Freud's Stages of Psychosexual Growth and Development

STAGE OF DEVELOPMENT	CRITICAL EXPERIENCES	DEVELOPMENTAL TASK	MAJOR CHARACTERISTICS	OTHER POSSIBLE PERSONALITY TRAITS
Oral (birth–18 months)	Weaning	Establishing trust	Autoeroticism, narcissism, omnipotence, pleasure principle, frustration, dependence	Fixation at the oral stage is associated with passivity, gullibility, and dependence, the use of sarcasm, and the development of orally focused habits (e.g., smoking, nail biting)
Anal (18 months–3 years)	Toilet training	Developing sphincter control, self-control, feeling of autonomy	Reality principle, fear of loss of object love, approval and disapproval, beginning superego development	Fixation associated with anal retentiveness (stinginess, rigid thought patterns, obsessive-compulsive disorder) or anal expulsive character (messiness, destructiveness, cruelty)
Phallic (3–5 years)	Oedipal conflict, castration anxiety	Establishing sexual identity, beginning socialization	Differentiation between the sexes, superego more internalized	Unresolved outcomes may result in difficulties with sexual identity and with authority figures
Latency* (6–12 years)	Peer group experience, intellectual growth	Group identification	Superego influence in erotic interests, immense intellectual development	Fixations can result in difficulty in identifying with others and in developing social skills, resulting in a sense of inadequacy and inferiority
Prepuberty and adolescence* (12–15 years)	Established heterosexual relationships	Developing social control over instincts	Identity, turmoil, consideration of needs of others	
Genital (15 years–adult)	Sexual maturity	Resolving dependence–independence conflict	Heterosexual relations	Inability to negotiate this stage could result in difficulties in becoming emotionally and financially independent, lack of strong personal identity and future goals, and inability to form satisfying intimate relationships

*The latency and prepuberty and adolescence stages of psychosexual development were not included in Freud's original description of development. Anna Freud (1946) extended Freud's works when she described developments in these periods of life.

TABLE 2–3
Erikson's Eight Stages of Ego Development

STAGES	NUCLEAR CONFLICT	STRENGTHS	INSTITUTION
1. Oral–sensory (birth to one year)	1. Trust–mistrust	1. Drive and hope	1. Religion
2. Muscular–anal (1–3 years)	2. Autonomy–doubt, shame	2. Self-control and willpower	2. Law and order
3. Locomotor–genital (3–5 years)	3. Initiative–guilt	3. Direction and purpose	3. Education and economic
4. Latency (6–11 years)	4. Industry–inferiority	4. Method and competence	4. Technology
5. Adolescence (12–18 years)	5. Identity–role confusion	5. Devotion and fidelity	5. Ideology
6. Young adulthood (19–35 years)	6. Intimacy–isolation	6. Affiliation and love	6. Ethics
7. Adulthood (35–50 years)	7. Generativity–stagnation	7. Production and care	7. Generative succession
8. Maturity (50+ years)	8. Ego integrity–despair		8. Unnamed

mans are psychologically bisexual, that is, that "masculine" and "feminine" qualities are to be found in both sexes. The **anima** represents the feminine archetype in men, and the **animus** represents the masculine archetype in women. A man understands the nature of woman by virtue of his anima, and a woman understands a man by virtue of her animus. Problems can arise, though, if a member of either gender projects an idealized archetype onto the other and does not accept the real personality of the individual.

In Jung's view, motivation comes not only from past conflicts but also from future goals and the need for self-fulfillment. There are two basic personality orientations: *introversion*, which describes the person who is focused inward, cautious, shy, timid, and reflective; and *extroversion*, which describes the person who is outgoing, sociable, assertive, and energetic. Jung believed that the healthy personality maintains a balance in all spheres—male and female, introversion and extroversion, conscious and unconscious—and has the ability to accept the past and strive for the future.

APPLICATION TO NURSING

Most nursing theories have a developmental perspective derived from Erikson and other such theorists. Assessing the developmental stage of clients gives us direction in designing interventions (Table 2–4). If the client is distant and suspicious, we know that we are going to work on developing a sense of trust in the nurse–client relationship. We know that interventions for a 16-year-old girl with a newborn will be different from interventions for a 30-year-old woman with a newborn. The 16-year-old girl is faced with having to construct an identity as a mother before she has consolidated her identity as a woman.

Jung emphasized the importance of symbolism, rituals, and spirituality. When we enter a client's environment, we see symbols of importance to the person. We become aware of the client's rituals of self-care. When clients' rituals interfere with growth and health, we look for the conflicts and anxiety behind the behaviors.

INTERPERSONAL SOCIAL THEORY

ALFRED ADLER

Alfred Adler (Ansbacher & Ansbacher, 1956), another psychoanalyst, departed from Freudian theory by emphasizing the conscious as the core of personality. He believed that personality is shaped by one's social environments and interactions and that people actively guide their own growth and development.

Adler proposed that inferiority feelings are the stimulus for growth, but an **inferiority complex** prevents people from solving life's problems. An inferiority complex is an exaggeration of feelings of inadequacy and insecurity resulting in defensiveness and neurotic behavior. Feelings of inferiority arise from being organically inferior, by being spoiled and then having to meet rejection, or by being neglected. When people strive for improvement, superiority, or perfection, tension increases, and more energy must be expended. Each person creates a unique pattern of striving for superiority that is learned from early parent–child interaction.

According to Adler, all people must solve three categories of problems during their lifetime: problems involving behavior toward others, problems of occupation, and problems of love. He described four basic styles that people use in working through these problems: avoiding, expecting to get everything from others, dominating others, and cooperating with others. Healthy people are characterized by self-reliance and cooperatively working with others within the culture.

▶TABLE 2–4
Stages of Development: Comparison of Freud's, Erikson's and Piaget's Theories

	FREUD	ERIKSON	PIAGET
Old age		Integrity vs. despair	
Middle age		Generativity vs. self-absorption	
Early adulthood		Intimacy vs. isolation	
17 yrs	Genital		Formal operations
16 yrs ↑		Identity vs. role confusion	
9 yrs			Concrete operations
8 yrs ↑	Latency	Industry vs. inferiority	
4 yrs ↑	Phallic	Initiative vs. guilt	
2 yrs	Anal	Autonomy vs. shame & doubt	Preoperational thought
1 yr	Oral	Trust vs. mistrust	Sensorimotor

Courtesy of Chris McCormick Pries, A.R.N.P.

HARRY STACK SULLIVAN

Harry Stack Sullivan (1940) studied traditional psychoanalysis but focused on interpersonal relationships instead of the unconscious. He believed that the cultural environment greatly shapes the personality and that personality development does not end at 5 years of age but continues until young adulthood. Sullivan extended the description of personality development through stages. He emphasized the importance of the development of the self-concept and discussed how this progresses through adolescence. He called this development of the self-system *personification*. Personification includes all related attitudes, feelings, and concepts about oneself or another acquired from extensive experience. The persona is what one is talking about when one refers to "I" or "me." The development of the persona begins in infancy with perceiving the mother as good or bad. As the self begins to differentiate, the infant comes to perceive the mother as both good and bad.

The persona, or self-concept, begins with the idea of a "good me," "bad me," and "not me." The good me is perceived when the mother is rewarding the infant. The bad me arises in response to the negative experiences with the mother. The not me arises out of extreme anxiety that the child rejects as a part of the self. As development proceeds, the child integrates these personas into a realistic view of self.

Sullivan emphasized the importance of peers and reciprocal relationships to the developing child and adolescent. When a child learns patterns of responding that hinder interpersonal relationships and cause others to respond negatively, the child experiences intense anxiety that further interferes with social relationships (Table 2–5). These ways of responding are primarily communication patterns. Sullivan (1971) believed that if communication patterns between individuals, groups, and nations could be changed, then each of those entities could be changed.

KAREN HORNEY

Karen Horney's (1937) key concept was that of basic anxiety, the feeling of isolation and helplessness in a potentially hostile world. Because people are dependent on each other, she believed, they often find themselves in a state of anxious conflict when others do not treat them well. Insecure, anxious children develop personality patterns to help them cope with their feelings of isolation and helplessness. They may become aggressive as a way of protecting what little security they do have. They may become too submissive, or they may become selfish and self-pitying as a way of gaining attention or sympathy.

In general, people relate to each other in one of three ways: (1) they can move toward others, seeking love,

TABLE 2–5
Sullivan's Stages of Healthy Interpersonal Development from Birth to Maturity

PHASE	LEVEL OF INTERACTING, COMMUNICATING, AND COMPREHENDING
Infancy	Experiences maternal tenderness and intuits material anxieties. Struggles to achieve feelings of security and to avoid anxiety
Childhood	Modifies actions to suit social demands in sex-role training, peer play, family events. Uses movement and language to avoid anxiety
Juvenile	Learns to accept subordinate to authority figures outside the family. More concept of self-status and role
Preadolescence	Capable of participating in genuine love relationships with others. Develops consideration and concerns outside the self
Early adolescence	Heterosexual contacts enter into personal relationships. Attempts to integrate sex with other personal relationships
Late adolescence	Masters expression of sexual impulses. Forms satisfying and responsible associations. Uses communication skills to protect self from conflicts with others

Data from Sullivan, H. S. (1953). In H. S. Perry & M. L. Gawal (Eds.), *Interpersonal theory of psychiatry.* New York: W. W. Norton.

support, and cooperation; (2) they can move away from others, trying to be independent and self-sufficient; or (3) they can move against others, being competitive, critical, and domineering. Ideally, the healthy personality balances all three orientations. Problems arise when people become locked into only one mode: too weak-willed and self-denying, afraid to offend anyone; too independent, afraid to admit dependency; or too hostile, afraid to express affection.

APPLICATION TO NURSING

The interpersonal theories suggest that we assess and develop interventions for social systems as well as the self-system. These theories suggest that nurses strengthen support systems; foster interpersonal relationships; strengthen the client's belief system; and facilitate faith, hope, and love.

BEHAVIORAL THEORIES

Behavioral theories do not address the unconscious or the self-concept as do the psychosocial theories of personality. In behavioral theories the emphasis is on the behaviors of the person. These theories assume a learning model of human behavior that differs from the intrapsychic or disease model of mental disorders. Behaviors, both normal and abnormal, are assumed to be learned.

Differences in human behavior are accounted for by the experiences in the person's life that initiate a response. The human being is like a machine that operates according to fixed laws. Behavior can be controlled by the kind and extent of **reinforcement** that follows a particular behavior. A behavior that is reinforced will likely be repeated. A person is best understood by observing what he or she does in a particular situation.

B. F. SKINNER

B. F. Skinner (1953), a prominent behavioral theorist in America, identified two kinds of behavior: respondent and operant. Respondent behavior occurs when a known and specific stimulus elicits a response. Respondent behaviors can be simple, as in a reflex action, or learned, such as those behaviors involved in conditioning. Operant behaviors are those that obtain a response or reinforcement from the environment or from another person.

All aspects of behavior are controlled through reinforcement; therefore, a person is a product of past reinforcements. Past experiences are important only to the degree that they are still active in directly contributing to the client's present distress. For example, a toddler who falls down steps may have a lifelong fear of going up a flight of steps or may develop a fear of heights.

Some psychologists trained in the behavioral school began to believe that behavior was not merely the product of environmental stimuli. In the social learning approach, **cognitive processes** mediate the influence of environmental events on behavior by determining what stimuli are attended to, perceived, and interpreted. Rotter (1954) added the belief that the likelihood that a particular behavior will occur is influenced by the person's expectancy that the behavior will lead to goal attainment and the values attached to those goals. In other words, people generally choose actions that they expect will lead to valued goals. In the instance of the toddler, when confronted by a flight of stairs, she may choose not to go up because she does not want to feel anxious.

BANDURA AND WALTERS

Bandura and Walters (1963) placed emphasis on the role of **modeling** in learning behaviors. Many social responses and personality characteristics are acquired simply by imitating or copying the behavior of the models one observes. Modeling typically involves a social situation and a social relationship (the model and the imitator). The model can be an actual person, a film, or a cartoon representation. Modeling, or imitation, can produce rapid acquisition of social behaviors. Learning does not require direct, or external, reinforcement of imitated behavior. The person merely "tries on" the behavior.

Bandura (1977) also emphasized the importance of internal reinforcement. A person who is able to reinforce his or her own behavior has a sense of self-efficacy. *Self-efficacy* refers to the expectation that one can effectively cope with and master situations, achieving desired outcomes through one's own personal efforts.

CONDITIONING

Basic concepts of behavioral theories derive from stimulus, response, and reinforcement. In **classic conditioning,** the reinforcement is the presenting stimulus that causes the response. If a neutral stimulus is paired with the reinforcing stimulus repeatedly, the neutral stimulus will become a reinforcing stimulus producing the same response. The original stimulus is called the *unconditioned stimulus* and the original response is called the *unconditioned response*. The neutral stimulus becomes the conditioned response, and the response then becomes the conditioned response. An example of classic conditioning is Pavlov's experiments with dogs, which learned to salivate at the sound of a tone that had been previously presented at the same time as meat powder on the tongue.

Operant conditioning occurs when behavior is produced without any observable external stimulus. The person's response is seemingly spontaneous in that it is not related to any known observable stimulus. Operant behavior operates on the person's environment resulting in a reward. An example is the bell that rings when a person fails to buckle the seat belt. The person puts on the seat belt, and the bell stops ringing. The operant behavior is the act of putting on the seat belt in expectation of a reward. The reinforcement occurs when the bell stops ringing. This example is also an example of negative reinforcement. The response in classic conditioning does not operate on the environment, and the reinforcement comes before instead of after the response.

When a person's behavior is rewarded, the behavior will likely be repeated. Behavior is strengthened by positive and negative reinforcement; it is weakened by punishment. *Positive reinforcement* refers to an increase in the frequency of a response followed by a favorable event. Reinforcement involves a contingency between behavior and the reinforcing event. *Negative reinforcement* refers to an increase in behavior as a result of avoiding, or escaping from, an aversive event that one would have expected to occur had the escape behavior not been emitted. *Punishment* is an aversive event contingent on a response. The result is a decrease in the frequency of that response. *Extinction* refers to the cessation or removal of a response.

To learn new behaviors, reinforcement in animal studies may be presented in several ways. The behavior can be rewarded each time the behavior occurs, at fixed intervals, or at a fixed ratio. None of these is what actually happens. Realistically, rewards are random and are the most potent form of reinforcement. The shorter the interval between reinforcements, the more rapidly the animals will respond. Conversely, as the interval between reinforcements gets longer, the rate of animal response decreases.

The frequency of reinforcement also affects the extinguishing of a response. Behaviors are extinguished more quickly when reinforced continuously and the reinforcement is then stopped than when reinforced intermittently. Animals on a fixed-ratio schedule respond much faster than those on a fixed-interval schedule. Responding faster on fixed-interval reinforcement does not make any difference; the animal may press the bar for food 5 times or 50 times and it will still be reinforced only when the predetermined interval has passed.

A fixed-ratio schedule of payment is used in industry in situations when a worker's pay depends on the number of units produced or a salesperson's commission on the number of items sold. This reinforcement schedule is effective as long as the ratio is not set too high and the reinforcement is worth the effort.

Other reinforcement schedules include variable ratios, variable intervals, and mixed schedules (Skinner, 1963).

APPLICATION TO NURSING

Nurses can use classic conditioning to initiate a behavior and operant conditioning to ensure that the behavior is repeated. In classic conditioning, the reward comes before the behavior, and in operant conditioning, the reward comes after the behavior. The difficulty with applying behavior modification to humans is finding the appropriate reinforcement. In nursing, we seldom know our clients well enough to discern reinforcers or how to initiate a response that can be reinforced. This theory sounds simple and straightforward, but it requires ingenuity, imagination, and perceptual skill to implement.

One of the best reinforcements nurses can use is the "placebo effect"—an attitude of optimistic concern and belief in the efficacy of the intervention.

COGNITIVE THEORIES

AARON BECK

Aaron Beck (1991) is one of the foremost proponents of cognitive psychology. Cognitive theories emphasize the mental processes involved in knowing. The field looks at how we direct our attention, perceive, think, remember, solve problems, form mental images, and arrive at beliefs. Cognitive researchers study how people explain their own behavior, understand a sentence, do arithmetic, solve intellectual problems, reason, form opinions, and remember events. These mental processes de-

TABLE 2–6
Beck's Common Cognitive Distortions

- Arbitrary inference: the process of drawing a specific conclusion in the absence of evidence to support the conclusion. The evidence may be contrary to the conclusion
- Selective abstraction: focusing on a detail taken out of context, ignoring more salient features of the situation, and conceptualizing the whole experience on the one detail
- Overgeneralization: the pattern of drawing a general rule or conclusion from one or more isolated incidents and applying the concept across the board to related and unrelated situations
- Magnification and minimization: errors in evaluating the significance or magnitude of an event that are so gross as to constitute a distortion
- Personalization: the proclivity to relate external events to oneself when there is no basis for making such a connection
- Absolutist (dichotomous) thinking: places all experiences in one of two opposite categories; for example, flawless or defective, immaculate or filthy, saint or sinner. In describing himself, the patient selects the extreme negative categorization

From Beck, A. T., Rush, A. J., Shaw, B. F., & Emery, G. (1979). *Cognitive therapy of depression* (p. 14). New York: Guilford Press.

termine, to a great extent, emotional and behavioral responses.

A basic assumption of cognitive theories is that personality is shaped by **schemata.** Schemata are cognitive structures, or patterns, that consist of the person's beliefs and assumptions. Schemata develop early in life from personal experiences and become active in response to stressful situations. Schemata influence people to interpret certain life situations in a biased way. Starting with preferential selection of data to which the person attends, through the evaluation, interpretation, and recall from short-term memory, activated schemata, or biases, determine the content of cognitive processing. These schemata even influence retrieval from long-term memory. According to this theory, these biases produce the symptoms of various psychological disturbances. Clients with cognition of themes of loss or defeat are likely to be depressed. A client with an anxiety disorder interprets situations as dangerous. In paranoid conditions the person selectively interprets themes of abuse or interference. Exaggerated interpretations of personal gain characterize clients with mania (Beck, 1991). Beck identifies six common cognitive distortions that result in dysfunctional behavior (Table 2–6).

ALBERT ELLIS

Albert Ellis (1973) called his cognitive theory *rational emotive therapy* (RET). He believed that irrational thoughts cause maladaptive behavior. An activating event or situation (A) arises that is threatening to the person. Because the person has a certain belief (B), an emotional response or consequence (C) occurs (Fig. 2–2). RET modifies the underlying irrational beliefs (D) to change the emotional consequence.

Beck and Ellis disagree on certain issues. Beck views the cognition as dysfunctional rather than irrational. Ellis believes the irrational belief causes the dysfunctional behavior, whereas Beck believes the cognitions are symptoms rather than the cause of the disorder. The activation of the schemata is the mechanism by which the depression or anxiety or aggression develops but is not the cause. Biological, genetic, stress, and personality factors combine to predispose people to various disorders.

Therapy helps the person recognize the connections among cognition, affect, and behavior. Reality-oriented interpretations for the biased cognition are substituted for the distorted thoughts. This requires identifying and altering the dysfunctional beliefs that predispose one to distort experiences. Excessive dysfunctional behavior and distressing emotions found in various psychiatric disorders are exaggerations of normal adaptive processes (Beck, 1976, 1991).

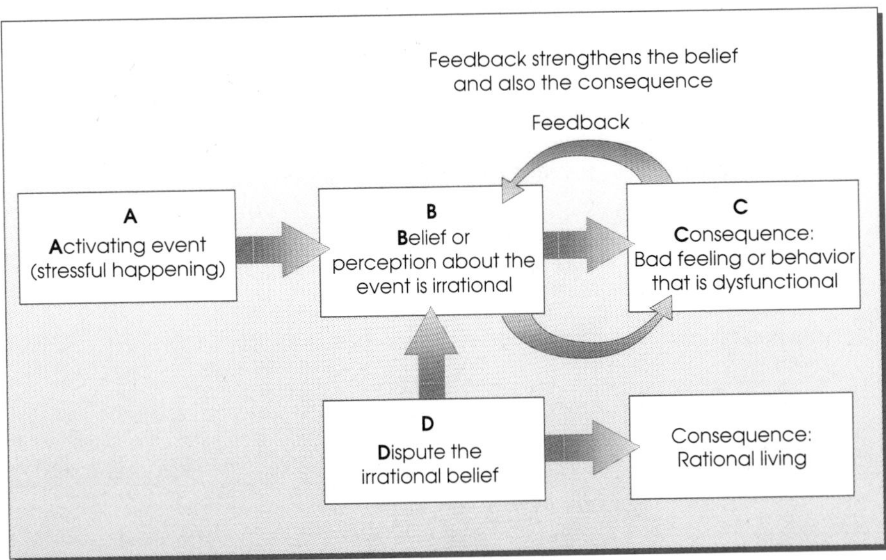

FIGURE 2–2
Ellis's ABCs of rational emotive therapy.

COGNITIVE THERAPY

Cognitive therapy addresses the person's cognitive organization and structure, which are biologically and socially influenced. Therapy helps modify assumptions that maintain maladaptive behaviors, distortion in logic, and systematic biases in thinking. The therapist and the client together construct "counters" to the cognitive distortions. A counter is a statement that counteracts or negates the thought. This theory does not yet identify the factors that produce a shift in the information processing to the negative and what factors maintain the shift.

Research over the last 30 years supports certain aspects of the theory (Beck, 1991). Outcome studies support the effectiveness of the therapy in the outpatient treatment of unipolar depression, anxiety disorders, and panic disorder. A meta-analysis of 27 studies (Dobson, 1989) showed the efficacy of cognitive therapy in unipolar depression and its superiority to other treatments, including antidepressant drugs. The National Institute of Mental Health collaborative study of the treatment of depression has shown the superiority of cognitive therapy in comparison with antidepressant drug and interpersonal therapy (Shea et al., 1990). Other studies showed the efficacy of the therapy in treating anxiety disorders (Beck, 1976; Butler et al., 1991; Sokol et al., 1989).

JEAN PIAGET

Cognitive theories also address human development. Whereas the psychoanalytical theorists addressed psychosexual development and Erikson described social development, Jean Piaget (Inhelder & Piaget, 1958) proposed a sequence of cognitive development that emphasized the relationship between action and thought (see Table 2–4). Piaget began his research on children in the early 1920s. He studied the responses of children and young people to various tasks concerning physical phenomena. On the basis of the responses, Piaget and his coworkers developed a theory for interpreting the development of universal patterns of reasoning. They identified stages that are characterized by distinctive features in the patterns of a person's reasoning (Table 2–7). Piaget proposed that each stage serves as a precursor to all succeeding stages, so that reasoning develops sequentially, always from the less effective to the more effective stage. This progression is not necessarily at the same rate for every person, and people do not progress through the stages exhibiting all the reasoning characteristics of a particular stage. Reasoning develops gradually, at a particular time showing the features of stage 1 on some problems while exhibiting certain features of stage 2 on others. The stage concept is more useful for classifying reasoning patterns than for describing the overall intellectual behavior of a particular person at a given time.

TABLE 2–7
Piaget's Stages of Cognitive Development

PERIOD	CHARACTERISTICS OF THE PERIOD	MAJOR CHANGE OF THE PERIOD
Sensorimotor (0–2 years)	—	
Stage 1 (0–1 month)	Reflex activity only; no differentiation	Development proceeds from reflex activity to representation and sensorimotor solutions to problems
Stage 2 (1–4 months)	Hand–mouth coordination: differentiation via sucking reflex	
Stage 3 (4–8 months)	Hand–eye coordination: repeats unusual events	
Stage 4 (8–12 months)	Coordination of two schemata; object permanence attained	
Stage 5 (12–18 months)	New means through experimentation—follows sequential displacements	
Stage 6 (18–24 months)	Internal representation: new means through mental combinations	
Preoperational (2–7 years)	Problems solved through representation: language development (2–4 years); thought and language both egocentric: cannot solve conservation problems	Development proceeds from sensorimotor representation to prelogical thought and solutions to problems
Concrete operational (7–11 years)	Reversibility attained; can solve conservation problems—logical operations developed and applied to concrete problems; cannot solve complex verbal problems	Development proceeds from prelogical thought to logical solutions to concrete problems
Formal operational (11 years–adulthood)	Logically solves all types of problems—thinks scientifically; solves complex verbal problems; cognitive structures mature	Development proceeds from logical solutions to concrete problems to logical solutions to all classes of problems.

The first stage is called *sensorimotor.* This stage is characteristic of children's thinking from birth to about 2 years of age. The young infant appears to think that the only objects that exist are the objects that can be seen. As the child grows in experience, he or she develops an awareness of the permanence of material objects. Information is obtained through the senses and motor action.

The preoperational stage moves through three periods between the ages of 2 and 7 years. In the first period, children can differentiate an image or a word from what it stands for (e.g., a chair) and can name an object not in sight. As children begin to speak, they develop representational thought and can grasp several events as a whole, whereas at the level of sensorimotor intelligence, successive actions and perceptual states are linked one by one. On the one hand, children can differentiate image and language from action and reality; on the other, they lack causal reasoning. Interaction with the physical world is essential to intellectual development in the first two periods.

Between the ages of 4 and 5½ years, children are more able to examine and set about a specific task, adapt their intelligence to it, and reason about more difficult everyday problems. However, a distinct characteristic of thought at this stage is their tendency to center on some striking feature of the object about which they are reasoning to the exclusion of other relevant aspects. Distorted reasoning is the result. Each situation is viewed egotistically, from a personal point of view. Between the ages of 5 and 6 years, the rigid and irreversible intellectual structures begin to become more flexible, and children begin the transition to the third stage of thought.

Concrete operational thought extends from about 7 years of age to pubescence (see Table 2–7). Operations are mental actions that have a definite and strong structure. At this stage, children's logical thoughts extend only to objects and events of first-hand reality. Children are able to consider two contrasting features, for example, height and width, that may balance and compensate for any distortion brought about by concentrating on one aspect of the situation. As children approach 7 or 8 years of age, they can begin to look at their own thinking and monitor it. They can look at alternative actions that will achieve the same outcome.

The fourth stage, formal operational, is characterized by formal reasoning (see Table 2–7). Children become better at organizing and structuring data with the methods of concrete operational thought. They become aware that such methods do not lead to a logically exhaustive solution to their problems. These children can use hypotheses and deduction, can accept an unproven hypothesis, are able to deduce its consequences in the light of other known information, and then verify empirically whether, in fact, those consequences occur. They can reflect on their own reasoning to look for inconsistencies. They can check their results in numerical calculations against order-of-magnitude estimates. Piaget called these abilities *combinatorial reasoning, control of variables, functional relationships,* and *probabilistic correlations.*

Developmental theories suggest that all facets of development follow a predictable pattern (Maier, 1969) that is orderly and can readily be described by criteria marking distinct developmental phases. Childhood is distinctly different from adulthood in all areas of human functioning. Cognitive, behavioral, psychosocial, cultural, and spiritual development are interrelated and interdependent, leading toward integration and maturity. When the needs of children are compromised, development may not progress. The person grows physically, but other development is impaired.

APPLICATION TO NURSING

Cognitive theories are a rich source for nursing intervention. Strategies detailed in the writings of the practitioners are practical and useful. Basic cognitive distortions are easy to recognize and learn. The difficult part is helping the client develop effective counters, or statements that counteract the destructive self-talk.

Piaget's theory of cognitive development helps nurses recognize impaired development and provide a relationship that facilitates the person's accomplishment of developmental tasks. It is not uncommon that medical treatment cannot proceed because psychosociocultural and spiritual needs are not being met. Developmental stage based on an assessment of behavior, cognition, and belief patterns must be identified if the nurse is to plan interventions likely to achieve a healthful outcome. Cognitive development is not emphasized as much as social development, but it is equally important. Assessing knowledge level and client teaching needs is a part of nursing care, and cognitive theory can give direction in planning care.

NEUROBIOLOGICAL THEORIES

An important theory of modern psychiatric therapy is that all behavior is a reflection of brain function and all thought processes represent a range of functions orchestrated by nerve cells (neurons) in the brain. Just as the brain controls complex behaviors such as normal feeling, learning, thinking, and speaking, it is the origin of disorders of affect (emotion), perception, and cognition (thought) that characterize neurotic and psychotic illnesses.

Neurons and glial cells are the two most abundant cell types in the brain. Neurons consist of a cell body, specialized appendages called *dendrites,* and an *axon* (Fig. 2–3). Neurons respond to an internal or external stimulus by generating chemical or electrical signals (impulses) that collectively create thought and action. Dendrites are the receptor filaments of impulse transmission from other neurons. The axon extends to the neighboring neurons to carry on the information in a manner

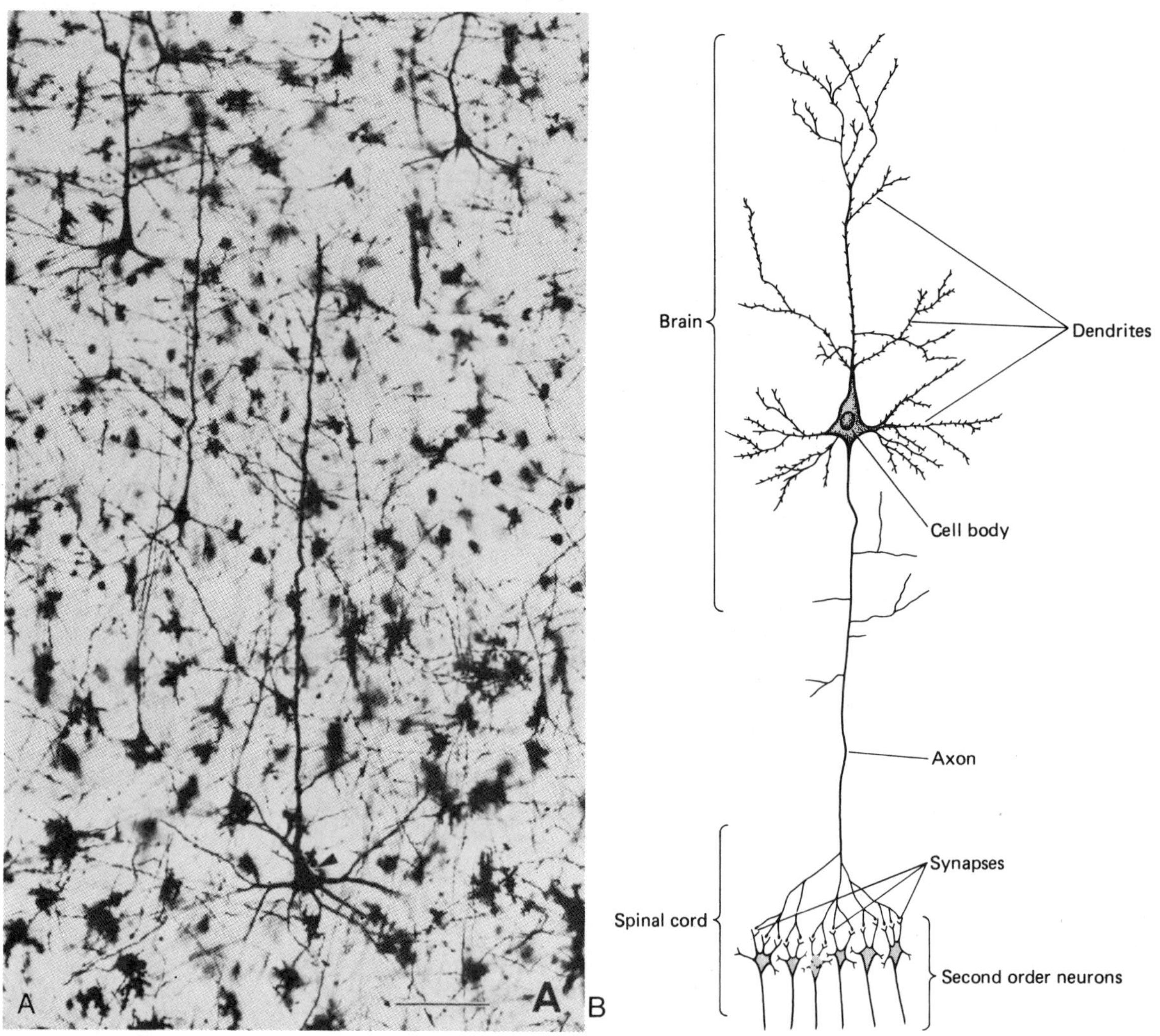

FIGURE 2–3
A, Medium-sized pyramidal neuron from the human cerebral cortex. The bar represents 100 μm. *B,* Structure of a large neuron of the brain, showing its important functional parts. (*A* from Burt A. M. [1993]. *Textbook of neuroanatomy* [p. 34]. Philadelphia: W. B. Saunders; *B* from Guyton A. C. [1991]. *Basic neuroscience* [2nd ed., p. 86]. Philadelphia: W. B. Saunders.)

similar to electrical conduction. At the end of the axon, the impulse jumps across the gap to the next dendrite. This region between the axon and the dendrite of two neurons is the *synapse* (Fig. 2–4) (see Chapter 26 for detailed discussion of the neuron anatomy and physiology).

Brain regions are specialized for different functions (see Fig. 2–4). Multiple layers of neurons make the cortex, or brain surface, and their axons reach into the subcortical brain to form a connection between related but separate parts of the cortex. These dense numbers of neurons in the cortex contribute to its gray appearance and are called *gray matter,* whereas the axons travel in bundles, or "tracts," in the subcortical white matter.

Clusters of specialized neurons are organized spatially within the brain. Cognitive function is primarily located in the frontal lobe cortex, motor and sensory function in the parietal lobes, and affective processes in the temporal lobes and limbic system. Receiving and responding to stimuli requires integration of the activity of many of these specialized areas, some of which are isolated from each other but connected by an elaborate system of tracts that carry impulses between the functional areas. The specific nature of the information and response is a function of the cells recruited to carry the impulse and the type of chemical signal (neurotransmitter) produced at the synapse. Imbalances in these chemical signals (neurotransmitters) are believed to be the primary origin of mental disorders.

Neurobiological theory of mental disorders suggests that cognitive and emotional dysfunctions result from multiple causes, such as genetic influences, nutrition, infectious processes, and other pathological conditions that contribute to neurotransmitter imbalances in the brain. These neurochemical disruptions may contribute to the abnormal cognitive and emotive responses that characterize mental illness.

NEUROENDOCRINE RESEARCH

Studies of brain function in persons with mental disorders indicate that there are abnormalities in the amount of neurotransmitters produced or available to receptor sites. Normally, neurons communicate through neurotransmitters synthesized at the end of the axon. As the electrical impulse moves to the terminal plate of the axon, the transmitter substance is released into the synaptic cleft (see Figs. 2–3 and 2–4). Receptor sites on the receiving neuron (postsynaptic neuron) pick up the neurotransmitter substance that, in turn, causes the receiving neuron to activate. Once the neurotransmitter is released, it is either taken up in the receptor site and deactivated by enzymes or taken back up into the presynaptic axon. This process and the transmitter chemicals involved are key elements in understanding the medications used to treat mental illnesses and their effect on the transmitters at the receptor sites to alleviate symptoms.

Four important neurotransmitters are dopamine, norepinephrine (NE), serotonin, and gama-aminobutyric acid (GABA) (Table 2–8). These neurochemicals are synthesized in the axon terminals, where they are released.

Dopamine. Dopamine is primarily responsible for fine motor movement, sensory integration, and emotional behavior. Dopamine is metabolized by monoamine oxidase (MAO). Several types of dopamine receptors exist (D_1, D_2, and D_3) and carry out different degrees of stimulation or inhibition of the postsynaptic response. Hyperactivity of the dopaminergic system is implicated in schizophrenia and mania, whereas hypoactive dopamine systems are believed to contribute to depression (Sacher et al., 1978). Dopamine action is discussed in more detail in Chapter 12.

Norepinephrine. NE is also known as *noradrenaline*. It is closely related to its precursor dopamine and is secreted primarily by noradrenergic neurons in the locus ceruleus in the pons, but also in scattered neuron bundles in the cerebral cortex, limbic system, amygdala, thalamus, and hypothalamus (see Chapter 10 and Fig. 10–1). NE is the precursor to adrenaline, the main ingredient in the sympathetic "fight or flight" response to a real or perceived threat. Two classes of noradrenergic receptors (alpha and beta) exist to mediate different postsynaptic responses to NE release. NE transmission and uptake are impaired in a variety of neuropsychiatric disorders, but primarily the anxiety and addiction types (see Chapters 10 and 17).

Serotonin. Serotonergic neuron cell bodies are located in the upper pons raphe nuclei. These neurons project to the basal ganglia, the limbic system, and the cerebral cortex (see Chapter 9 and Fig. 9–1). They modulate awakeness and alertness and are known to influence the transmission of sensory pain. Serotonin dysregulation has been implicated in mood disorders, anxiety, violence, and schizoaffective disorders.

Gamma-aminobutyric Acid. GABA is an inhibitory neurotransmitter that serves as the brain's modulator. GABA receptors throughout the brain counteract the effects of the excitatory neurotransmitters norepinephrine and dopamine, preventing disorganized and frenzied responses to stimuli and dampening emotional arousal. A person with low levels of GABA or fewer GABA receptors is theoretically more susceptible to anxiety disorders (see Chapter 10 and Fig. 10–1).

Psychopharmacologic Agents and Neurotransmitters. Psychotherapeutic drugs are prescribed to manipulate the processes of neurotransmitter production and absorption to reestablish "normal" neurochemical balance. For example, antidepressants increase the amount of NE and serotonin in the synaptic cleft. The tricyclic antidepressants block the reuptake of NE and serotonin, thus leaving more transmitter substance in the synaptic cleft to activate other neurons. MAO inhibitors block the metabolism of NE and serotonin in the synaptic cleft. A side effect of antidepressants is sedation and postural hypotension due to blockade of $alpha_1$ receptors.

Manipulation of one aspect of neurotransmitter action may create physical symptoms related to the altered transmitter levels. For example, side effects of antidepressents are sedation and postural hypotension due to blockade of $alpha_1$-receptors. Antipsychotic medication blocks dopamine receptors but also contributes to the motor system problems such as pseudoparkinsonism and other dyskinesias (see Chapter 12 and Fig. 12-1).

Summary. Neuropsychiatric disorders are not simply a result of too little or too much neurotransmitter substance. Levels and combinations fluctuate with important brain function, individual responses, and processes of growth and aging. Many questions remain regarding transmitter dysregulation in psychiatric disorders. Increased knowledge of the therapeutic action of psychodynamic drugs has contributed to much of the current understanding of neurotransmitter involvement.

DATA FROM DIAGNOSTIC TECHNOLOGIES

Recent advancement in brain imaging technology has provided information to improve our understanding of the actual electrical and chemical processes of brain function and metabolism. Discoveries of the molecular and cellular activities of the neuron clarify the role of the brain and the neurotransmitters in translating neurophysiological events into behavior, thought, and emotion. Radiological and metabolic measurements have demonstrated structural abnormalities in persons with abnormal behaivor, thought, and expressed emotion patterns of mental illness. For example, data from positron emission tomography have revealed reduced blood flow in the frontal lobe during cognitive testing in some

CEREBRAL CORTEX (Lateral View)

The cerebral cortex consists of several layers of billions of nerve cells called *neurons (see Figure 2-3)*. These neurons are specialized for functions such as movement and sensation (parietal cortex), vision (occipital cortex), speech and hearing (temporal cortex), and mentation (frontal cortex). Axons extend from the neurons and merge into bundles (nerve fibers) to make up the white matter. These fibers connect the neurons of specialized cortical areas to related and complementary areas of the brain, facilitating integrated processing of information and complex responses.

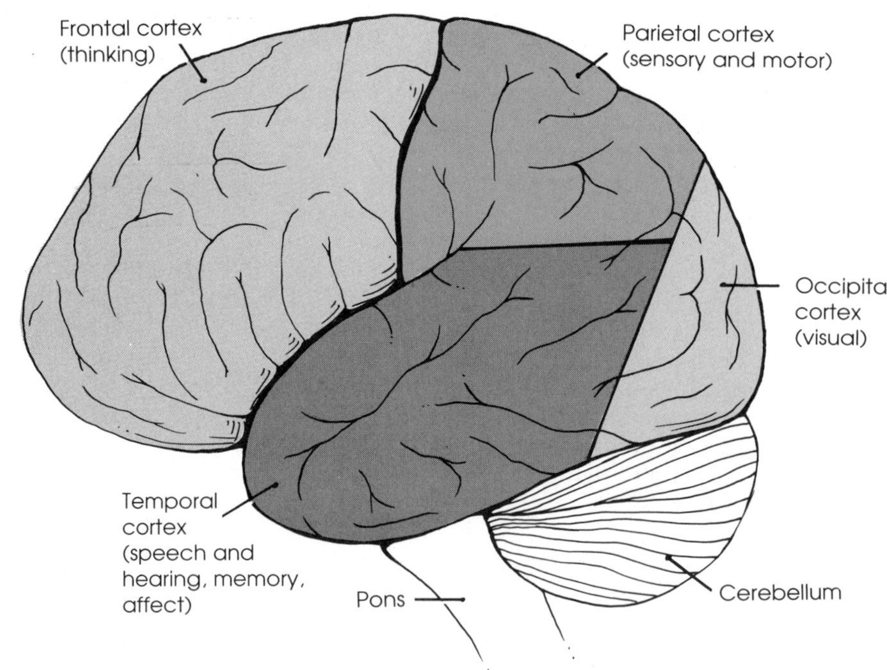

LIMBIC SYSTEM AND BRAIN STEM

Posterolateral View of Brain Stem

DIENCEPHALON
MIDBRAIN
PONS
MEDULLA
Thalamus
Hypothalamus
Ventral tegmental dopaminergic area
Mesolimbic dopaminergic system
Locus ceruleus
Rostral raphe nuclei
Lateral tegmental norepinephrine cell system
Caudal (lower) raphe nuclei

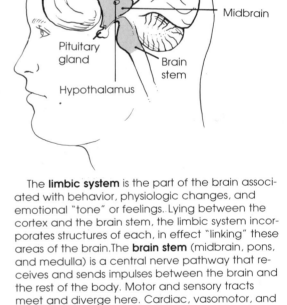

Limbic system
Midbrain
Pituitary gland
Brain stem
Hypothalamus

The **limbic system** is the part of the brain associated with behavior, physiologic changes, and emotional "tone" or feelings. Lying between the cortex and the brain stem, the limbic system incorporates structures of each, in effect "linking" these areas of the brain.The **brain stem** (midbrain, pons, and medulla) is a central nerve pathway that receives and sends impulses between the brain and the rest of the body. Motor and sensory tracts meet and diverge here. Cardiac, vasomotor, and respiratory centers are also nearby. The *hypothalamus* influences these vital tracts and centers for normal physiologic maintenance, and also plays a role, along with the *pituitary gland*, in producing stress and anxiety responses. The *locus ceruleus*, the *dopaminergic and norepinephrine systems*, and the *raphe nuclei* are groupings of neurons that produce neurotransmitters important in brain function.

FIGURE 2–4
Neurobiological concepts basic to the understanding of psychiatric disorders. (Illustration concept: Gail Kongable, M.S.N., C.N.R.N., C.C.R.N., Department of Neurosurgery, University of Virginia Health Sciences Center. Illustration by Marie T. Dauenheimer.)

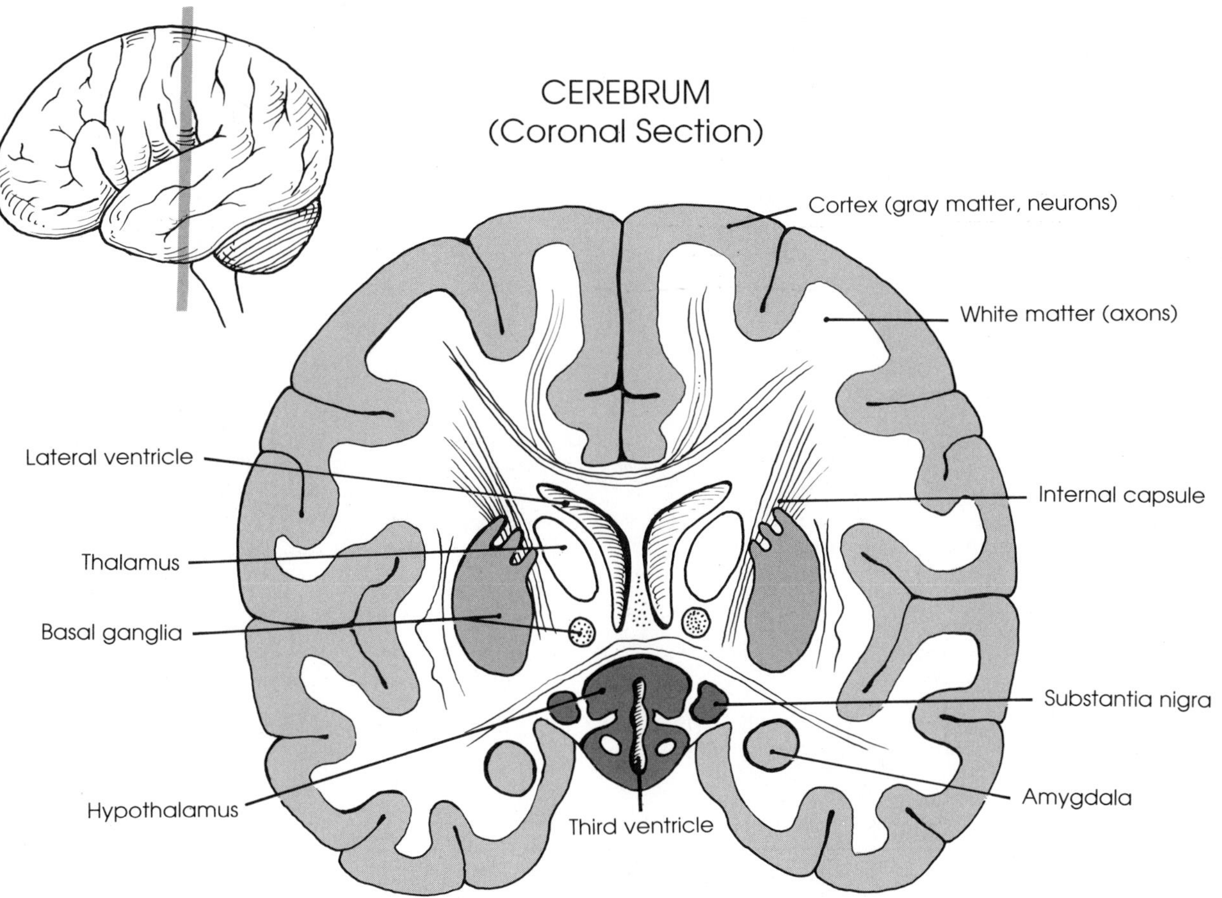

The basal ganglia are nests of neurons located deep in the subcortical white matter. They control fine motor activity, particularly of the arms and legs. Bundles of nerve fibers from the motor cortex pass through tracts in the internal capsule and deliver impulses to the midbrain, thalamus, hypothalamus, pituitary gland (hypophysis), and limbic system located nearby. Abnormal information processing in these areas results in the characteristic behaviors of anxiety disorders, mood disorders, abnormal stress responses, endocrine disorders, and symptoms associated with schizophrenia.

SYNAPSES AND NEUROTRANSMITTERS

The **synapse** is the junction between one neuron and the next. Impulses (electrical or chemical) begin in the cell body of one neuron in response to stimuli and travel along the axon to an adjacent neuron.

Neurotransmitters are the chemical substances that transfer an impulse from one neuron to another. Each neuron can secrete several different transmitter substances at its synapse. The synaptic vesicles, which store the neurotransmitters, migrate to the presynaptic membrane of the transmitting neuron, where they release the neurotransmitter into the synaptic space (synaptic cleft). The neurotransmitter diffuses across the synaptic space to the postsynaptic membrane of the target neuron. Receptor sites on the postsynaptic membrane take up the neurotransmitters, and in this way the impulse is transferred to the next neuron.

Neurotransmitter dysfunction plays a role in a number of psychiatric disorders, including mood disorders, anxiety states, and schizophrenia.

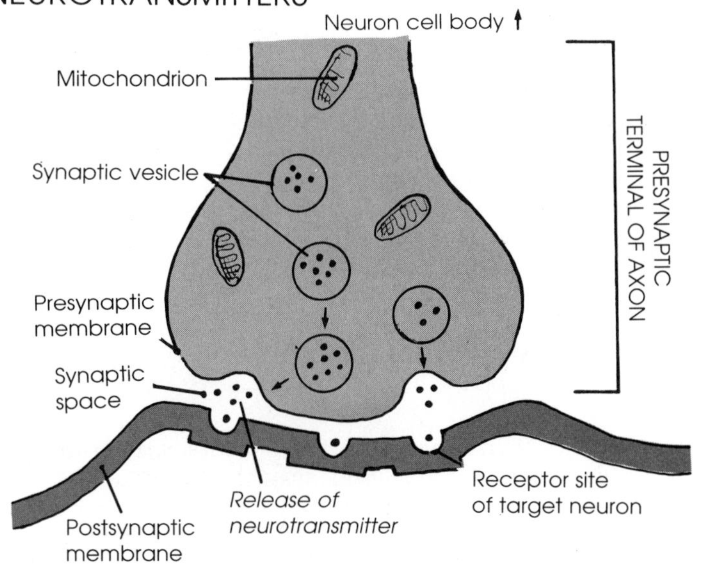

TABLE 2–8
Important Neurotransmitters in Mental Illness

	CONTROL, EFFECT, OR RESPONSE	SITES OF SECRETION	IMPORTANT IN THESE DISORDERS
Biogenic Amines			
Dopamine	Fine movement, sensory integration, emotional behavior	► Nigrostriatum (substantia nigra) ► Mesolimbic and limbic systems ► Posterior pituitary	► Bipolar disorder ► Schizophrenia
Noradrenaline	"Fight or flight" response (sympathetic system)	► Locus ceruleus ► Adrenal medulla ► Amygdaloid body	► Certain mood disorders ► Addictions
Serotonin	Temperature, sleep, hunger, consciousness, behavior	► Raphe nuclei ► Hypothalamus	► Certain mood disorders ► Anxiety ► Personality disorders ► Schizoaffective disorders
Amino Acids			
Gamma-aminobutyric acid	Inhibitory	► Throughout cerebral cortex	► Anxiety states
Neuropeptides			
Hypothalamic hormones: ephinephrine, histamine	Alertness; inflammatory response	► Hypothalamus ► Adrenal medulla	► Stress response ► Anxiety states
Pituitary hormones: vasopressin, growth hormone, thyroid-stimulating hormone, corticotropin	Blood pressure regulation, cellular renewal, healing, stimulation of thyroxine secretion to control metabolism; corticosteroid release	► Pituitary gland	► Endocrine disorder with associated depressed mood

persons with schizophrenia (Paulman et al, 1990). Computed tomography and magnetic resonance imaging have shown enlarged ventricles, cortical thinning, and temporal lobe atrophy in some persons with schizophrenia (Brown et al., 1986; Shelton & Weinberger, 1986; Suddath et al., 1989).

Other case reports have shown that people with anxiety disorders and multiple personality disorders have different patterns of brain functioning. In multiple personality disorder, the different personalities appear to use different areas of the brain. Obsessive-compulsive disorder appears to be influenced by abnormal functioning of the basal ganglia–limbic-cortical circuits (Baxter, 1990). Temporal lobe atrophy and dysfunction of the limbic system are implicated in panic disorder. Although these findings suggest a possible cause and are used as diagnostic evidence for the diagnosis, they are not established diagnostic criteria and serve as hypotheses for further research.

PRENATAL AND OBSTETRICAL RESEARCH

Structural specialization in the brain occurs early in fetal development of the neural system. At about 4½ months' gestation, large numbers of specialized neurons migrate toward their specific destinations. Organized cell arrays of cell bodies are achieved before birth in the cortex and islands (nuclei) within the deeper regions of the brain. It is possible that these neurons migrate errantly or become disorganized in persons with mental illness, specifically schizophrenia (Conrad et al., 1991). Irregularities in the size of the nuclei and the neurons and myelin sheath have been discovered (Benes, 1989). Torrey and Kaufman (1986) suggested that this damage may be due to an in utero infectious process. Studies in Finland (Mednick et al., 1988) and another in England (O'Callaghan et al., 1991) showed that after the 1957 pandemic of Asian flu, there was a significant increase in the number of births of people who later developed schizophrenia. Another study in the United States demonstrated that persons with schizophrenia were more likely to have been born in the late winter or early spring months, suggesting an infectious process (DeLisi et al., 1986).

Obstetrical complications may contribute to the risk of developing schizophrenia (McNeil & Kay, 1978). The clients with schizophrenia who have a history of obstetrical complications develop the disorder an average of 5 years earlier than those without such a history (Lewis & Murray, 1987).

GENETICS

Mental illness may be transferred genetically, just as other familial traits. Twin studies and family histories reveal a genetic vulnerability toward the development of mood disorders, anxiety disorders, schizophrenia, and other major mental disorders (Tienari, 1975; Torrey, 1992).

Twin studies have shown that certain personality traits are genetically transmitted, such as temperament, introversion, and extroversion (Pogue-Geile & Rose, 1985). Researchers are producing evidence that brain pathways determining behavior patterns in men and women differ because of the different hormones produced by each sex (Bouchard, 1984; Ehrhardt & Meyer-Bahlberg, 1981; MacLusky & Naftolin, 1981; McEwen, 1981; Rubin et al., 1981).

Recent physiological studies have suggested that persons experiencing recurrent panic attacks may have a genetically determined carbon dioxide hypersensitivity in brain stem–mediated autonomic nervous system control. This is based on the discovery that hyperventilation occurs first followed by an increase in heart rate (Papp et al., 1989). Temporal lobe abnormality has also been implicated in panic disorders, causing people to experience psychosensory symptoms similar to those seen in temporal lobe epilepsy (Boulenger et al., 1986). These findings have supported the efforts to determine genetic or structural origins for many of the other mental disorders.

Twin studies in schizophrenia suggest that not everyone who inherits a tendency for schizophrenia will become ill. Only those subjected to physical stress—such as a virus, head injury, and birth complications—are at risk of developing schizophrenia. Gottesman and Bertelsen (1989) traced 150 children of Danish twins. In some sets of twins studied, only one had schizophrenia. These researchers found that the risk of schizophrenia was about the same—1 in 6—in the children of people with the disease and in children of their unaffected genetically identical twins. In children of unaffected fraternal twins of schizophrenic clients, only 1 in 50 had the disease. Similar findings occur in bipolar disorders.

The incidence of schizophrenia and the age of onset of the disorder are similar throughout the world and across a variety of cultures and geographic areas that have wide differences in perinatal mortality rates and prevalence of serious infectious illness, lending credence to the genetic theory. Gender differences exist in incidence and severity of mental illness as well. Men with schizophrenia have a far worse outcome than do women and more frequently exhibit classic and negative symptoms of the disorder (Salokangas & Stengard, 1990). Researchers are investigating a group of genes, rather than just one, that may predispose people to major mental disorders (Tienari, 1975; Torrey, 1992).

IMMUNE SYSTEM STUDIES

Increasing physiological evidence proves that the brain and the immune system communicate directly and indirectly through a complex array of hormones and neurotransmitters. Pituitary hormones affect the cells of the immune system, and the sympathetic nerves penetrate into the lymph nodes and spleen (Agius et al., 1991). Many studies show that stress may predispose some persons to illness via an immune system effect (Irwin & Strausbaugh, 1991). Stress-related disorders are associated with either a decrease in immunologic competence or an alteration in the regulation of the immune system (Melnechuk, 1988) (see Chapter 11).

Many of the immune system disorders such as systemic lupus erythematosus and multiple sclerosis include depression, emotional lability, nervousness, and confusion in the symptomatology, giving rise to the hypothesis that certain psychiatric symptoms arise from abnormal immune processes. Studies of immune system functioning in schizophrenia have shown increases in certain immune cells and products (Rapaport & McAllister, 1991). This was especially true in research done before the administration of antipsychotic medication. Antipsychotic agents inhibit the binding of the anti–human leukocyte antigen (HLA) antibodies to lymphocytes. HLAs are part of the system used by lymphocytes to recognize and process foreign material. HLAs are associated with autoimmune disorders such as ankylosing spondylitis, rheumatoid arthritis, narcolepsy, multiple sclerosis, diabetes, and systemic lupus erythematosus.

ENDOCRINE STUDIES

Endocrine studies of depressed persons have shown functional differences in the hypothalamic-pituitary-thyroid axis compared with healthy subjects and dysthymic clients. Changes occur in thyroid-stimulating hormone (TSH) and thyroid hormones subsequent to dexamethasone administration (Kjellman et al., 1993).

This is demonstrated in the fact that persons with endocrine disorders often also have symptoms of mental disorders. Depression is common in persons with hyperadrenalism (Cushing's syndrome) and hypoadrenalism (Addison's disease). Hyperthyroidism causes anxiety, and hypothyroidism may result in depression. Both hypoparathyroidism and hyperparathyroidism are associated with anxiety and depression. Hypomania and depression often follow administration of corticotropin. See Chapter 9 for further discussion.

Alternative therapies such as phototherapy have an antidepressant effect in the treatment of seasonal affective disorder, suggesting that depression may be due to a neuroendocrine imbalance related to changes in light and temperature in the external environment (Bielski et al., 1992).

CHRONOBIOLOGY

Often what affects one body system can affect other systems directly or indirectly. This is especially true of the interaction of the nervous, endocrine, and immune systems.

Many mental disorders, especially the mood disorders, are accompanied by problems in biological rhythms. **Chronobiology** is the field of science that studies the rhythms of life. Biological phenomena fluctuate over time in response to internal and external factors. Internal rhythms in humans are believed to be controlled by the suprachiasmatic nucleus within the hypothalamus (Moore, 1988). Individual factors such as genetics, arrangement of neural pathways, and age and gender of the person affect the rhythmic patterns.

Rhythms external to humans influence the internal rhythms as well. The external rhythm that sets, or synchronizes, the internal rhythm is called ***a zeitgeber.*** The process by which these zeitgebers synchronize the internal clock to the period of the zeitgeber is called *entrainment.* An example of entrainment is the sleep–wake cycle. People have regular times for sleeping and waking based on external factors such as school and work. Processes that alter some aspect of a biological rhythm, with the exception of the rhythm's period, are called *maskers.* Drinking coffee to stay awake to study for an examination is an example of masking. The coffee can mask the rhythm of mental alertness by creating a brief period of alertness at a time when the person is normally ready for sleep.

The interrelationships among the many rhythms of life are quite complex. Many biological activities rise and fall in rhythmic patterns. Biological rhythms that repeat approximately every 24 hours are called ***circadian rhythms.*** Body temperature, hormone secretion, the immune system, sleep and wakefulness, and the cardiovascular and other body systems all exhibit circadian rhythms.

Disturbances in these rhythms of life are exhibited in mood disorders. Depression is often characterized by marked disturbances in the daily sleep–wake cycle and disturbances in rapid-eye-movement (REM) and non-REM sleep.

Recent research indicates that light, especially bright light, is effective in shifting human circadian rhythms and can alleviate some depression in seasonal affective disorder (Terman et al., 1989). Changes in amplitudes of temperature and TSH circadian rhythms also occur in depression. The most consistent abnormal finding is an advance in the timing of the nadir of the cortisol secretion in depression. All these events are influenced by the pituitary-thyroid-adrenal axis.

Some scientists are investigating the implications circadian rhythms have for the timing of surgery and the administration of drugs in an effort to optimize their therapeutic effects.

SUMMARY

Mental disorders are most likely caused by a variety of factors. A genetic factor seems indicated, but children who have an illness or injury or who grow up in families with few resources and poor coping skills are at greater risk than children who have better support systems. The difficulty in forming conclusions about the causes of mental disorders relates to the nature of the research itself. Brain studies are done on animals or on humans post mortem. There is no way to tell what the brain was like before the disorder developed. With the newer imaging techniques, researchers can see what is taking place in the brain at the time of the scan. The scans are done on people who have a particular disorder as well as normal control subjects, but the number of persons that can be studied is limited due to time and cost. At some point, research studies must include people before and after the disorder becomes apparent. The question remains about which comes first, the structural problems or the learned ways of behaving, thinking, feeling, and believing. Do the neuroendocrine problems in depression come before the depression, or does the sense of helplessness and hopelessness cause the neuroendocrine problems? Is the propensity for anxiety inherited, or is it learned? Each theory is convincing when studied in depth, and a piece of the truth emerges. However, to understand the etiology of mental disorders, one must take into account the valid points from all the theories.

Nursing is diagnosing and treating responses to health problems. These responses are mediated by perception. The most effective nursing care addresses the perceptual system of the client and discovers ways to change unhealthy patterns.

SYSTEMS THEORY

Systems theory is a way of viewing a person, families, groups, and society. Several theories of nursing are based on systems theory, warranting a brief overview of its concepts.

BASIC CONCEPTS

General systems theory was introduced in 1928 by Ludwig von Bertalanffy (1968). Although it began as a theory for explaining biological systems, other scientific disciplines found it useful as well.

In general systems theory, a system is a set of components or units interacting with each other within a boundary that filters the kind and the rate of flow of inputs and outputs to and from the system. Systems have both structure and function. For example, the body is the structure, but also the body has a multitude of functions. Systems can be open or closed. Open systems are open to the exchange of matter, energy, and information with their environment. Biological and social systems are open systems. Open systems move in the direction of greater differentiation, elaboration, and a higher level of organization. The system can be explained only as a totality or whole. Holism, or synergism, is the concept that the whole is not just the sum of the parts but is something different from the parts.

Systems have boundaries that separate them from their environments. The open system has permeable boundaries between itself and a broader suprasystem. The closed system has rigid, impenetrable boundaries. Boundaries are easily defined in physical and biological systems but are difficult to delineate in social systems such as organizations. Boundaries keep out what is not necessary or desirable to the system and bring in the necessary and desirable resources.

In a dynamic relationship with the environment, the open system receives various inputs. Inputs are the resources needed by the system. Inputs are transformed in a process called *throughput* and are exported as output.

Closed systems engender **entropy**. As entropy increases, the system fails. Entropy is a movement toward disorder, lack of resource transformation, and death. An example is when the body fails to function, the person can no longer use inputs and dies.

Negentropy, or negative entropy, is a process of more complete organization and ability to transform resources, of increasing complexity and higher organization. It is the process of building up, whereas entropy is the process of running down. An example of negentropy is the learning process. Information is an input, learning is the throughput, or the higher organizational complexity. The result can be referred to as negentropy. In terms of the nursing process, entropy can be equated with health problems and negentropy with healthful outcomes or state of greater organization.

Open systems seek equilibrium and homeostasis through the continuous inflow of materials, energy, and information. The concept of feedback is important in understanding how a system maintains a steady state. Information concerning the outputs or the process of the system is fed back as an input into the system, perhaps leading to changes in the transformation process and future outputs. Feedback can be both positive and negative. Negative input is information that suggests the system is deviating from a steady state. An example of this is pain.

Systems are arranged in hierarchies. A system is composed of subsystems of a lower order and is also part of a suprasystem. Open systems are further characterized by **equifinality,** which suggests that goals or purposes may be achieved with different initial conditions and in different ways. Individuals and social systems can accomplish objectives with diverse inputs and with varying internal activities. Closed systems are mechanistic with a direct cause-and-effect relationship between the initial condition and the final state.

APPLICATION TO NURSING

Each client is viewed holistically as a system functioning within a system. The client cannot be treated in isolation. If the client is to achieve a steady state, then boundaries, input, output, and throughput must be addressed. Throughput is what happens to the input before it is exported. In humans, throughput is what happens to food between ingestion and elimination. It is what happens between sensation and observable behavior. The goal of treatment is to achieve equilibrium, to manage resources positively, and to change the throughput processes such as changing perception.

A general systems theory perspective offers a philosophy that recognizes change, growth, learning, and the interrelatedness of all living systems. Humans are viewed as holistic, goal-directed, self-maintaining, self-creating persons of intrinsic worth, capable of self-reflection on their own uniqueness. This perspective also provides an ecological view of persons as interrelated, interdependent, interacting, complex organisms constantly influencing and being influenced by the environment. In systems theory, mental illness is viewed as a result of disordered social systems as well as a psychoneuroimmunoendocrine system gone awry.

HUMAN NEED THEORY

BASIC CONCEPTS

All theories about human development and behavior address human needs, but Abraham Maslow's (1943, 1970) explication of human needs fits well into nursing's focus.

Needs motivate the behavior of a person. According to Maslow, a basic need is inactive or functionally absent in the healthy person. If basic needs are not met, illness is likely to occur. When needs are met, health occurs.

According to Maslow, needs are hierarchical, with the lower level needs being critical to survival. The needs at the lower levels must be met before the needs at the higher levels can be met (Fig. 2–5).

Maslow also specified cognitive and aesthetic needs. Cognitive needs include the need to know and understand, to be curious, to explain, to organize, to analyze, and to look for relations and meanings. The aesthetic needs include the needs for order, symmetry, closure, and beauty.

APPLICATION TO NURSING

Recognition of human needs is crucial to nursing care. The behavior of the client will give clues to needs. The nurse then must orchestrate interventions to facilitate need fulfillment.

Human need theory has been useful to nursing in organizing curricula and in assessing and giving care, but it may have contributed to the emphasis on the physiological needs. The need to maintain life and physical integrity is the first priority when life and physical integrity are threatened. However, the nurse's role does not stop with meeting only physiological needs. Meeting physiological needs is not enough now that the role of

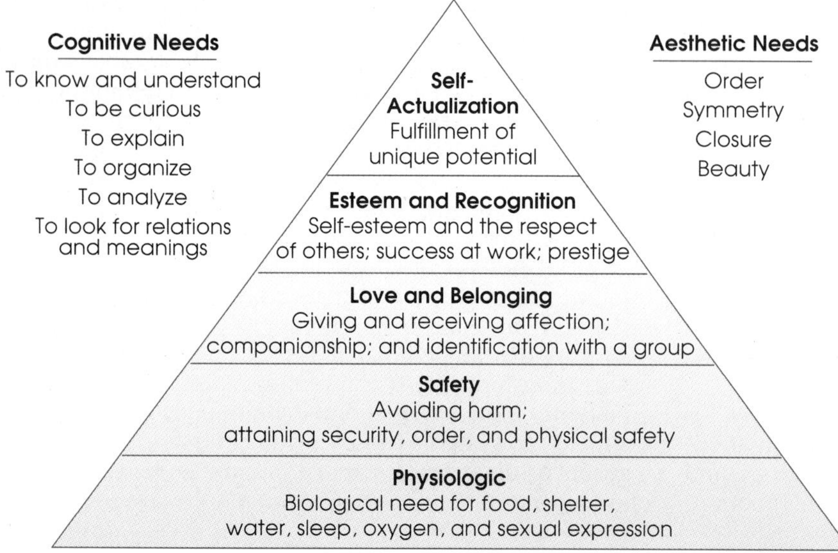

FIGURE 2–5
Maslow's hierarchy of needs. Maslow postulated that if basic needs are not met, illness is likely to occur. Maslow also specified cognitive and aesthetic needs.

perception in altering physiological processes is being explicated.

THE WELLNESS–ILLNESS CONTINUUM

BASIC CONCEPTS

Before the 1960s, nursing used the definition of health provided by the World Health Organization (1947) stating that health is a state of complete physical, mental, and social well-being and not merely the absence of disease or infirmity. In 1961, Halbert Dunn first published his classic text, *High Level Wellness*, and changed the focus to levels of wellness instead of disease. He viewed health and illness as dynamic and moving along a continuum rather than circumscribed states.

High-level wellness is an integrated method of functioning oriented toward maximizing the potential of which the person is capable, within the environment where he or she is functioning. High-level wellness occurs when the physical and psychosocial needs are met in ways that support maximum functioning and leave the person with an energy reserve from which to draw. Low-level wellness or severe illness is the inability of people to meet their needs in a way that allows them to function and that depletes their energy reserve.

The concepts basic to Dunn's model are totality, uniqueness, energy, inner and outer worlds, and self-integration and energy use (Table 2–9).

For a person to use energy in maintaining high-level wellness, the person must function in an integrated way. When the person faces change, he or she must make changes using energy efficiently. For example, when a person has a flulike illness and temperature of 103°F, he or she will take measures to conserve physical energy so that the physical resources needed to combat the illness are available. The person may seek psychosocial support to conserve energy but will not, if functioning in an integrated manner, run a marathon.

APPLICATION TO NURSING

The wellness–illness model emphasizes a holistic view of health. Mental health and illness also exist on a con-

TABLE 2–9
Basic Concepts of Dunn's Model of Wellness–Illness

- Totality: integration of the physical and psychosocial components into a unified whole. The person must be viewed as a whole. Each aspect of a person is interdependent on all other aspects
- Uniqueness: each person's life experiences, genetic make-up, and developmental processes come together to make an individual unlike any other
- Energy: the environment must provide people with a constant source of energy to meet their physical and psychosocial needs
- Self-integration: all parts of the personality must be balanced and linked
- Energy use: How a person uses energy affects the level of wellness and illness
- Inner and outer worlds: a person's experiences, both inner and outer and past and present, influence that person's behavior

Adapted from Dunn, H. L. (1972). *High level wellness* (7th ed.). Arlington, VA: Beatty.

tinuum and are not separate from physical health and illness.

Nurses work with people experiencing all levels of wellness and illness, with the goal of helping others achieve an optimal level of wellness. The nurse identifies positive and negative aspects of wellness, builds on positive attributes, and reduces negative factors. The nurse helps the person conserve energy and make the most efficient use of available energy. Working together, the nurse and the client resolve conflicts between the person and the environment and within the self to maintain integrity. This theory emphasizes the need for nurses to be vigilant in treating the whole person and not merely addressing the physiological needs.

NURSING THEORIES AND MODELS

A theory is an organized set of statements related to significant questions in a discipline communicated into a meaningful whole. It is a picture of reality that describes, explains, predicts, or prescribes responses, events, situations, conditions, or relationships. Theories have concepts relating to the discipline's phenomena. These concepts relate to each other to form theoretical statements. Theoretical statements are based on repeated observations over time.

Theories are made up of assumptions, concepts, propositions, and exemplars that form the foundation for a discipline or profession. Theory provides goals for practice, defines the boundaries of practice, and describes the behaviors for members of the profession (Riehl-Sisca, 1989). Nursing theory provides the nurse with goals for assessment, diagnosis, and intervention and, as a result, makes practice more efficient and effective. The language of nursing theory provides a common ground for communication. It describes scientific principles to accurately predict the consequences of care and the range of client responses.

The major concepts in nursing theory have been identified as human beings, nursing, health, and the environment. Generally, *human beings* are described as holistic and interactive, a developing system in interaction with the environment. The description of *nursing* includes the nursing process, the recipient of care, and the role of the nurse. The goal of nursing takes some form of assisting, restoring, maintaining, enhancing, or promoting optimal health. The *environment* includes various aspects of society: events, conditions, and elements that make up the client's surroundings. The health care system is part of the environment. Most theories address the internal environment as well. *Health* is depicted as a state of wellness or optimal functioning. Internal and external environments are determinants of the health state.

In the following theories, you will notice how each describes the four concepts. This is merely a brief overview of the conceptual framework of nursing.

NEUMAN'S SYSTEMS MODEL

Person. People are a unique composite of characteristics within a normal given range of response. Each person in a state of wellness or illness is a dynamic composite of the interrelationship of physiological, psychological, sociocultural, and developmental variables. People maintain harmony and balance with their environment by a process of interaction and adjustment.

Each person has a basic structure or central core of survival factors unique to the individual but in a range common to other humans, such as temperature, genetic response pattern, ego structure, and strengths and weaknesses of body organs. The central core is protected from stressors by concentric rings. The outside ring is the normal line of defense—a normal range of responses that evolves over time. An inner ring consists of a flexible line of defense—a dynamic, rapidly changing protective buffer that prevents stressors from breaking through the normal line of defense.

Nursing. Nursing is a unique profession concerned with all the variables affecting a person's response to stressors. The nurse seeks the highest potential level of stability for each client and assesses the client's response to stressors and the relationship of the environment to the client's reactions. The nurse assists individuals, families, and groups to attain or maintain a maximum level of wellness by interventions directed toward reducing stress, strengthening the line of defense, and maintaining a reasonable degree of adaptation.

Health. Wellness is the ability of a person's flexible line of defense to maintain equilibrium against any stressor. Any variances in wellness occur when stressors are able to penetrate the flexible line of defense. Health is seen on a continuum, depending on the degree of need fulfillment. Not getting needs met results in a reduced state of wellness. A stressor is anything that attempts to penetrate a person's normal line of defense to cause disequilibrium.

Environment. The environment includes all internal and external factors. *The internal* environment is the flexible line of defense against stressors, such as the body's immune response pattern. The *external* environment is the normal line of defense and consists of coping ability, lifestyle, and developmental stage (Neuman, 1980).

OREM'S SELF-CARE MODEL

Person. The person is a total being with universal developmental needs and is capable of continuous self-care. The person is a unity that can function biologically, symbolically, and socially. Persons have the ability to perform self-care—activities that people initi-

TABLE 2–10
Peplau's Model of Interpersonal Theory: Basic Concepts and Their Interrelationships

	NURSING is related to:	**PERSON is related to:**	**HEALTH is related to:**	**ENVIRONMENT is related to:**	**INTERPERSONAL RELATIONSHIPS (I.P.R.'s) are related to:**
PERSON	Nursing is a process between persons (nurse and patient).				
HEALTH	Health is the goal of nursing.	Health is within the person.			
ENVIRONMENT	Environment provides the context of nursing.	The person is within the environment.	The environment can be health promoting or illness maintaining.		
INTERPERSONAL RELATIONSHIPS (I.P.R.'s) (Nurse–Patient + Other)	I.P.R.'s are the crux or essential processes of nursing.	Persons develop through I.P.R.'s.	I.P.R.'s contribute to a person's health and a person's health will in turn influence ongoing I.P.R.'s.	The environment forms the context of I.P.R.'s.	
COMMUNICATION (Verbal & Nonverbal)	Communication is an essential component of nursing.	Communication is a transaction between persons.	Communication facilitates health by contributing to I.P.R.'s.	Communication occurs within the context of the environment and is part of the environment.	Communication occurs within interpersonal relationships.
PATTERN INTEGRATION	Pattern Integration occurs in nursing to create change.	Pattern Integration occurs between persons as an interaction of individual patterns.	Pattern Integration can facilitate health by contributing to ongoing I.P.R.'s.	Pattern Integration is a part of the environment.	Pattern Integration occurs within interpersonal relationships.
ROLES	Roles are the means for conducting nursing.	Roles are used by the nurse to promote health within the patient.	Roles are used by the nurse to promote health.	Roles are used in the context of the environment.	Roles are used within interpersonal relationships.
THINKING (includes self-understanding & preconceptions)	Thinking occurs in nursing as a prerequisite.	Thinking is used by persons to process experience.	Self-understanding can promote health. Preconceptions can impede or promote health depending on their impact on interpersonal relationships.	Thinking occurs in the person within the environment.	Self-understanding can promote I.P.R.'s. Preconceptions can promote or hinder I.P.R.'s & vice versa.
LEARNING	Learning occurs in nursing as a consequent.	Learning is an interpersonal process used for growth.	Learning promotes health.	Learning occurs in the person within the environment.	Learning occurs within the context of I.P.R.'s. The interactions between learning and I.P.R.'s can enhance or hinder each other.
COMPETENCIES	Competencies develop as a consequence of nursing.	Competencies are skills developed within persons.	The development of competencies promotes health.	Competencies occur in the person within the environment.	Competencies can assist in the development of I.P.R.'s.
ANXIETY	Anxiety occurs in nursing.	Anxiety occurs as a result of perceived personal threat.	Anxiety impedes health at severe or panic levels.	Anxiety occurs in the person within the environment.	Anxiety impedes the development of relationships at severe or panic levels.

From Forchuk, C. (1990). Peplau's theory: Concepts and their relations. *Nursing Science Quarterly, 4*(2), 58–59.

COMMUNICATION is related to:	PATTERN INTEGRATION is related to:	ROLES are related to:	THINKING is related to:	LEARNING is related to:	COMPETENCIES are related to:
Pattern Integration and communication occur together in interpersonal relationships					
Roles require communication	Roles are used by the nurse as part of the pattern integration.				
Thinking is mediated through symbols (language). Changes in verbal communication reflect changes in thinking and vice versa.	Thinking occurs within the person and therefore indirectly interacts with pattern integration.	Thinking is required to implement appropriate roles.			
Communication promotes learning and learning can then promote future communication.	Learning occurs within the person and therefore indirectly interacts with pattern recognition.	Learning occurs with successful implementation of nurse roles, particularly the counsellor and teacher roles.	Thinking is a prerequisite for learning and learning, in turn, assists thinking.		
Communication promotes the development of competencies.	Competencies occur within the person and therefore indirectly interact with pattern integration.	Competencies are developed through successful implementation of nurse roles, particularly the counsellor and teacher roles.	Competencies are both a prerequisite for thinking and further develop through thinking.	Competencies are learned by developing skills and capacities.	
Anxiety impedes communication at severe or panic levels.	Anxiety occurs in the person and therefore indirectly interacts with pattern integration.	Anxiety at severe or panic levels will limit the appropriate roles to be used.	Anxiety impedes thinking when at severe or panic levels.	Anxiety impedes thinking when at severe or panic levels.	Anxiety at severe or panic levels impedes the development of competencies.

ate and perform on their own behalf to maintain life, health, and well-being. The ability to care for oneself is self-care agency; the ability to care for others is dependent-care agency. Agency means action. Self-care is undertaken to meet three types of self-care requisites: universal, developmental, and health deviation.

Nursing. Nursing consists of deliberate and purposeful actions to provide assistance to those who are unable to meet health-related self-care needs. The nurse is required to design, create, provide, and manage systems of therapeutic care to a person with self-care deficits until the person can care for himself or herself. In chronic poor health or disability, the nurse seeks to stabilize or minimize the effects.

Health. Health is a state of being whole, sound, and fully integrated. It includes physiological and psychophysiological mechanisms in relation to and in interaction with other humans.

Environment. Orem presented a limited view of the environment that includes the factors and conditions that can be manipulated in caring for clients. The individual and the environment form an integrated functional whole or system (Orem, 1980).

ORLANDO'S NEEDS-ORIENTED THEORY

Person. People are developmental beings with needs and are unique in their responses, thoughts, and feelings.

Nursing. Nursing consists of finding out and meeting the client's immediate need for help to avoid, relieve, diminish, or cure the person's sense of helplessness, to the end that the patient experiences an increased sense of well-being and an improvement in behavior. The nurse assesses behavior and its meaning, shares these perceptions, and explores the meanings with the client.

Health. Health is a sense of adequacy or well-being, comfort, and fulfilled needs (Orlando, 1961).

Environment. Orlando did not define the environment.

ROY'S ADAPTATION MODEL

Person. Roy describes a person as a biopsychosocial being in constant interaction with a changing environment. To cope with a changing world, the person uses both innate and acquired mechanisms that are biopsychosocial in origin. Health and illness are one inevitable dimension of the person's life. To respond positively to environmental changes, the person must adapt. Adaptation is a result of the stimulus one is exposed to and the adaptation level. The person has four modes of adaptation: physiological needs, self-concept, role function, and interdependence.

Nursing. The goal of nursing is to contribute to the person's health, quality of life, and dying with dignity by promoting adaptation in each of the four modes. Nurses assess behavior and the stimuli that influence adaptation. Interventions manage these stimuli and enhance the interaction of the person with the environment.

Health. Health is a state and a process of being and becoming an integrated, whole person. It is a reflection of the level of adaptation. Lack of integration represents lack of health.

Environment. The environment includes conditions, circumstances, and influences that surround and affect the development and behavior of the person. These influencing factors are categorized as focal, contextual, and residual stimuli. The changing environment stimulates the person to make adaptive responses (Roy, 1984).

PEPLAU'S INTERPERSONAL THEORY

In nursing, and especially psychiatric nursing, perhaps the most influential theorist has been Hildegard Peplau (1952). A survey of psychiatric nurses (Hirschmann, 1989) showed that one half used this theory as a foundation for practice. Peplau's work has influenced every aspect of nursing so that her work is now considered "public domain." She introduced nursing to the importance of the interpersonal relationship and communication strategies, the nursing process, the concept of nursing diagnosis, and more. The concepts that are important in her theory are also important concepts in other psychosocial theories; therefore, they may serve as a summary of how nurses can help clients. Table 2–10 identifies the concepts and shows how these concepts are interrelated.

Person. Persons are described as unique in experiences, beliefs, expectations, and patterns of relating to others. The client is viewed "as a person responding in the situation and in relation to whatever or whoever is in it with him or her—illusory or real" (Peplau, 1952, p. 270). The client includes individuals, groups, families, and communities.

Nursing. "Nursing is a significant, therapeutic, interpersonal process. It functions co-operatively with other human processes that make health possible for individuals in communities. . . . Nursing is an educative instrument, a maturing force, that aims to promote forward movement of personality in the direction of creative, constructive, productive, personal and community living" (Peplau, 1952, p. 16). The focus of nursing is the "reactions of the client to the circumstances of illness or health problems, thus overlapping medicine only when dealing with disease process directly" (Peplau, 1969, p. 37).

Health. Health "is a word symbol that implies forward movement of personality and other ongoing human processes in the direction of creative, constructive, productive, personal, and community living" (Peplau, 1952, p. 12).

Environment. The environment includes the physiological, psychological, and social fluidity that is the context of the nurse–client relationship (Peplau, 1952). Peplau recognized the positive contribution that a therapeutic milieu and a supportive environment make to health.

►CHAPTER SUMMARY

Nurses provide care to individual clients and to groups. This is an expansive mandate that requires broad skills. Nurses develop an expertise in caring for unique persons in unique circumstances.

Centuries of observations of human functioning provide a data base on which nurses can establish their practice. This chapter provides an introduction to major concepts important to nursing care. Each theory discussed is a unique field of study unto itself, but nurses can feel confident that the concepts are based on repeated observations over time.

Nursing is an applied science that uses concepts from the study of humans in a variety of disciplines, including medicine, psychology, sociology, anthropology, ecology, political science, mathematics, and philosophy. We use the concept of wholeness from Dunn's (1961) concept of high-level wellness. We use the structure of systems theory to organize data to show relationships, to suggest ways to manage interventions, and to manage the environment. We use theories of personality development to understand behavior and thinking and to give us strategies for interventions.

Ideas about how people think and behave and what we can do to foster homeostasis, integrity, or adaptation are addressed differently by the various theories discussed in this chapter. Psychoanalytical theory gives us a language and a structure for thinking about thought and behavior. Interpersonal theories emphasize the importance of social and environmental relationships. Behavioral theories give us potent methods for changing behavior. Cognitive theories provide ways to change thinking. All theories propose to foster a higher level of wellness, integrity, adaptation, or negentropy. When nurses are faced with a client problem, they go to the theories for ideas for causes and interventions. For example, a nurse is in contact with an angry client, one who is refusing care. The nurse knows the person is anxious about something. What clues can he or she discover that will point to the cause? Using systems theory, the nurse will look for inputs and outputs. He or she will examine boundaries and what the client is doing with inputs. Knowing the principle of equifinality (more than one way to skin a cat), the nurse may try a variety of maneuvers to reduce strain on the system. Drawing from behavioral theory, he or she will reinforce appropriate behaviors and ignore or set limits on inappropriate ones. Using cognitive theories, the nurse will look for distorted thoughts and help the client see the fallacy and discover realistic cognition.

Nursing theories provide a structure more suited to the care we give. Several nursing theories are based on systems theory. Other theories are incorporated into nursing theories to explain relationships that point to interventions. All nursing theories take into account growth and development, human needs, and interpersonal relationships.

Nurses are becoming comfortable in selecting a nursing theory for practice. Standards of care require it. Which particular theory a nurse uses is influenced by her educational experience or her place of employment. New and developing knowledge can be structured within the chosen theory that, in turn, provides the basis for lifelong learning. We know from learning theories that new data are incorporated into an existing structure. In this sense, each nurse's practice is based on a particular theory, whether it is implicit (developed from the nurse's own practice) or explicit (one consciously adopted from the profession).

Suggestions for Clinical Conferences

1. Choose one theory, and use it to assess, diagnose, and develop interventions to reach desired outcomes.
2. Observe nursing interventions used by nurses, and relate those interventions to one of the theories discussed.
3. Compare client outcomes with outcomes suggested by various theories.
4. Discuss each student's view of the concepts of person, health, nursing, and environment.
5. Discuss the feelings engendered by the nurse–client relationship.
6. Discuss the difficulties in using theories in practice.

References

Agius, M. A., Glasg, F. R., & Arnason, B. G. (1991). Autoimmune neurological diseases and their potential relevance to psychiatric diseases. In J. Gorman & R. Kertzner (Eds.), *Psychoimmunology update* (pp. 9–29). Washington, DC: American Psychiatric Press.

Ansbacher, H. L., & Ansbacher, R. R. (1956). *The individual psychology of Alfred Adler: A systematic presentation in selections from his writings*. New York: Basic Books.

Arlow, J. A. (1989). Psychoanalysis. In R. J. Corsini & D. Wedding (Eds.), *Current psychotherapies* (4th ed.). Itasca, IL: F. E. Peacock.

Bandura, A. (1977). *Social learning theory*. Englewood Cliffs, NJ: Prentice-Hall.

Bandura, A., & Walters, R. H. (1963). *Social learning and personality development*. New York: Holt.

Baxter, L. R. (1990). Brain imaging as a tool in establishing a theory of brain pathology in obsessive-compulsive disorder. *Journal of Clinical Psychiatry, 51*(Suppl. 2), 22–25.

Beck, A. T. (1976). *Cognitive therapy and the emotional disorders*. New York: International Universities Press.

Beck, A. T. (1991). Cognitive therapy: A 30-year retrospective. *American Psychologist, 46*(4), 368–375.

Beck, A. T., Rush, A. J., Shaw, B. F., & Emery, G. (1979). Cognitive therapy of depression. New York: Guilford.

Benes, F. M. (1989). Myelination of cortical-hippocampal relay during late adolescence. *Schizophrenia Bulletin, 15,* 213–226.

Bielski, R. J., Mayor, J., & Rice, J. (1992). Phototherapy with broad-spectrum white fluorescent light: A comparative study. *Psychiatry Research, 43,* 167–175.

Bouchard, T. J. (1984). Twins reared together and apart: What they tell us about human diversity. In S. W. Fox (Ed.), *Individuality and determinism*. New York: Plenum.

Boulenger, J. P., Bierer, L. M., Uhde, T. W., Silberman, E. K., & Post, R. M. (1986). Psychosensory phenomena in panic and affective disorder. In C. Shagass, R. C. Josiassen, W. H. Bridger, W. J. Weiss, D. Stoff, & G. H. Simpson (Eds.), *Biological psychiatry* (pp. 462–465). New York: Elsevier.

Brown, R., Colter, N., Corsellis, J. A., Crow, T. J., Frith, C. D., Jagoe, R., Johnstone, E. C., & Marsh, L. (1986). Postmortem evidence of structural brain changes in schizophrenia. *Archives of General Psychiatry, 43,* 36–42.

Butler, G., Fennell, M., Robson, P., & Gelder, M. (1991). Comparison of behavior therapy and cognitive behavior therapy in the treatment of generalized anxiety disorder. *Journal of Consulting Clinical Psychology, 59*(1), 167–175.

Conrad, A. J., Abebe, T., Austin, R., Forsythe, S., & Schechel, A. B. (1991). Hippocampal pyramidal cell disarray in schizophrenia as a bilateral phenomenon. *Archives of General Psychiatry, 40,* 413–417.

Davis, J. M. (1978). Dopamine theory of schizophrenia: A two-factor theory. In L. C. Wynne, R. L. Cromwell, & S. Matthysse (Eds.), *The nature of schizophrenia: New approaches to research and treatment* (pp. 105–115). New York: Wiley.

DeLisi , L. E., Crow, T. J., & Hirsch, S. R. (1986). The third biannual winter workshops on schizophrenia. *Archives of General Psychiatry, 43,* 706–711.

Dobson, K. S. (1989). A meta-analysis of the efficacy of cognitive therapy for depression. *Journal of Clinical Psychology, 57*(3), 414–419.

Dunn, H. L. (1961). *High level wellness*. Arlington, VA: Beatty.

Ehrhardt, A. A., & Meyer-Bahlberg, H. F. (1981). Effects of prenatal sex hormones on gender-related behavior. *Science, 211,* 1312–1318.

Ellis, A. (1973). *Rational-emotive therapy*. In R. J. Corsini (Ed.), *Current psychotherapies*. Itasca, IL: Peacock.

Erikson, E. H. (1963). *Childhood and society* (2nd ed.). New York: W. W. Norton.

Fenichel, O. (1945). *The psychoanalytic theory of neurosis*. New York: W. W. Norton.

Forchuk, C. (1990). Peplau's theory: Concepts and their relations. *Nursing Science Quarterly, 4*(2), 54–60.

Freiberg, K. L. (1983). *Human development: A life-span approach* (2nd ed.). Monterey, CA: Wadsworth.

Freud, A. (1937). *The ego and the mechanisms of defense*. London: Hogarth Press.

Freud, A. (1946). *The ego and mechanisms of defense* (C. Baines, Trans.). New York: International Universities Press.

Freud, S. (1952). New introductory lectures on psychoanalysis. In M. J. Adler (Ed.), *Great books of the western world: Vol. 54. Freud* (W. J. H. Sprott, Trans.). Chicago: William Benton, Encyclopaedia Britannica. (Original work published 1932)

Gottesman, I. I., & Bertelsen, A. (1989). Confirming unexpressed genotypes for schizophrenia: Risks in the offspring of Fischer's Danish identical and fraternal discordant twins. *Archives of General Psychiatry, 46*(5), 478–480.

Hirschmann, M. (1989). Psychiatric and mental health nurses' beliefs about therapeutic paradox. *Journal of Child and Adolescent Psychiatric–Mental Health Nursing, 2*(1), 7–13.

Horney, K. (1937). *The neurotic personality of our time*. New York: W. W. Norton.

Inhelder, B., & Piaget, J. (1958). *The growth of logical thinking from childhood to adolescence*. New York: Basic Books.

Irwin, M. R., & Strausbaugh, H. (1991). Stress and immune changes in humans: A biopsychosocial model. In J. Gorman & R. Kertzner (Eds.), *Psychoimmunology update*. (pp. 55–79). Washington, DC: American Psychiatric Press.

Jung, C. (1967). *Collected works*. Princeton, NJ: Princeton University Press.

Kjellman, B. F., Thorell, L., Orhagen, T., d'Elia, G., & Kagedal, B. (1993). The hypothalamic-pituitary-thyroid axis in depressive patients and healthy subjects in relation to the hypothalamic-pituitary-adrenal axis. *Psychiatry Research, 47*(1), 7–21.

Lewis, S. W, & Murray, R. M. (1987). Obstetric complications, neurodevelopmental deviance, and risk of schizophrenia. *Journal of Psychiatric Research, 21,* 413–421.

MacLusky, N. J., & Naftolin, F. (1981). Sexual differentiation of the central nervous system. *Science, 211,* 1294–1303.

Maier, H. W. (1969). *Three theories of child development*. New York: Harper & Row.

Maslow, A. H. (1943). A theory of human motivation. *Psychological Review, 50,* 370.

Maslow, A. H. (1970). *Motivation and personality* (2nd ed.). New York: Harper & Row.

McEwen, B. S. (1981). Neural gonadal steroid actions. *Science, 211,* 1303–1311.

McNeil, T. F., & Kay, L. (1978). Obstetric factors in the development of schizophrenia. In L. C. Wynne, R. L. Cromwell, & S. Matthysse (Eds.), *The nature of schizophrenia* (pp. 401–429). New York: Wiley.

Mednick, S., Machon, R. A., & Huttunen, M. O. (1988). Adult schizophrenia following prenatal exposure to an influenza epidemic. *Archives of General Psychiatry, 45,* 189–192.

Melnechuk, T. (1988). Emotions, brain, immunity and health: A review. In M. Clynes & J. Panksepp (Eds.), *Emotions and psychopathology* (pp. 181–247). New York: Plenum.

Moore, R. Y. (1988). The suprachiasmatic nucleus and the mammalian circadian system. In W. T. Hekkens, G. A. Kerkhos, & W. J. Rietveld (Eds.), *Advances in the biosciences: Trends in chronobiology* (Vol. 73). Oxford: Pergamon Press.

Neuman, B. (1980). The Betty Neuman health care systems model: A total person approach to patient problems. In J. P. Riehl and C. Roy (Eds.), *Conceptual models for nursing practice* (2nd ed.). East Norwalk, CT: Appleton-Century-Crofts.

Neuman, B. (1980). *The Neuman systems model*. East Norwalk, CT: Appleton-Century-Crofts.

O'Callaghan, E., Sham, P., Takei, N., Glover, G., & Murray, R. M. (1991). Schizophrenia after prenatal exposure to 1957 A2 influenza epidemic. *Lancet, 1,* 1248–1250.

Orem, D. E. (1980). *Nursing: Concepts of practice* (2nd ed.). New York: McGraw-Hill.

Orlando, I. J. (1961). *The dynamic nurse–patient relationship*. New York: G. P. Putnam.

Papp, L. A., Goetz, R. R., Cole, R., Klein, D. F., Jordon, F., Liebowitz, M. R., Fyer, A. J., Hollander, E., & Gorman, J. M. (1989). Hypersensitivity to carbon dioxide in panic disorder. *American Journal of Psychiatry, 146,* 779–781.

Parry, B. L., Berga, L. L., Kripke, D. F., & Gillin, J. C. (1980). Melatonin and phototherapy in premenstrual depression. In D. K. Hayes, J. E. Pauly, & R. J. Reiter (Eds.), *Chonobiology: Its role in clinical medicine, general biology and agriculture* (Part B, pp. 35–43). New York: Wiley-Liss.

Paulman, R. G., Devous, M. D., Sr., Gregory, R. R., Herman, J. H., Jennings, L., Bonte, F. J., Nasrallah, H. A., & Raese, J. D. (1990). Hypofrontality and cognitive impairment in schizophrenia: Dynamic single-photon tomography and neuropsychological assessment of schizophrenic brain function. *Biological Psychiatry, 27*(4), 377–99.

Peplau, H. (1952). *Interpersonal relations in nursing*. New York: Putnam.

Peplau, H. (1969). Theory: The professional dimension. In C. M. Norris (Ed.), *Proceedings of the first nursing theory conference* (pp. 33–46). Kansas City, KS: University of Kansas Medical Center.

Pogue-Geile, M. F., & Rose, R. J. (1985). Developmental genetic studies of adult personality. *Developmental Psychology, 21*(3), 547–557.

Rapaport, M. H., & McAllister, C. G. (1991). Neuroimmunologic factors in schizophrenia. In J. Gorman & R. Kertzner (Eds.), *Psychoimmunology update* (pp. 31–55). Washington, DC: American Psychiatric Press.

Riehl-Sisca, J. (1989). *Conceptual models for nursing practice* (3rd ed.). Norwalk, CT: Appleton & Lange.

Rotter, J. B. (1954). *Social learning and clinical psychology*. Englewood Cliffs, NJ: Prentice-Hall.

Roy, C. (1984). *An introduction to nursing: An adaptation model* (2nd ed.). Englewood Cliffs, NJ: Prentice-Hall.

Rubin, R. T., Reinisch, J. M., & Hasket, R. F. (1981). Postnatal gonadal steroid effects on human behavior. *Science, 211*, 1318–1324.

Sachar, E. J., Gruen, P. H., Altman, N., Langer, G., & Halpern, F. S. (1978). Neuroendocrine studies of brain dopamine blockade in humans. In L. C. Wynne, R. L. Cromwell, & S. Matthysse (Eds.), *The nature of schizophrenia: New approaches to research and treatment* (pp. 95–104). New York: Wiley.

Salokangas, R. K., & Stengard, E. (1990). Gender and short-term outcome in schizophrenia. *Schizophrenia Research, 3*, 333–345.

Shea, M. T., Pilkonis, P. A., Beckham, E., Collins, J. F., Elkin, I., Sotsky, S. M., & Docherty, J. P. (1990). Personality disorders and treatment outcome in the NIMH Treatment of Depression Collaborative Research Program. *American Journal of Psychiatry, 147*(6), 711–718.

Shelton, R. C., & Weinberger, D. R. (1986). Computerized tomography in schizophrenia: A review and synthesis. In H. A. Nasarallah & D. R. Weinberger (Eds.), *Handbook of schizophrenia: Vol. 1. The neurology of schizophrenia* (pp. 207–250). Amsterdam: Elsevier.

Skinner, B. F. (1963). Operant behavior. *American Psychologist, 18*, 503–515.

Skinner, B. F. (1953). *Science and human behavior*. New York: Macmillan.

Sokol, L., Beck, A. T., Greenberg, R. L., Wright, F. D., & Berchick, R. J. (1989). Cognitive therapy of panic disorder: A nonpharmacological alternative. *Journal of Nervous and Mental Disorders, 177*(12), 711–716.

Suddath, R. L., Casanova, M. F., Goldberg, T. E., Daniel, D. G., Kelsoe, J. R., Jr., & Weinberger, D. R. (1989). Temporal lobe pathology in schizophrenia: A quantitative magnetic resonance imaging study. *American Journal of Psychiatry, 146*(4), 464–472.

Sullivan, H. S. (1940). *Conceptions of modern psychiatry*. New York: W. W. Norton.

Sullivan, H. S. (1971). *The fusion of psychiatry and social science*. New York: W. W. Norton.

Terman, M., Terman, J. S., Quitkin, F. M., McGrath, P. J., Stewart, J. W., & Rafferty, B. (1989). Light therapy for seasonal affective disorder: A review of efficacy. *Neuropsychopharmacology, 2*, 1–22.

Tienari, P. (1975). Schizophrenia in Finnish male twins. In M. H. Lader (Ed.), *Studies of schizophrenia*. Ashford, Kent: Headley Brothers.

Torrey, E. F. (1992). Are we overestimating the genetic contribution to schizophrenia? *Schizophrenia Bulletin, 18(2)*, 159–170.

Torrey, E. F., & Kaufman, C. A., (1986). Schizophrenia and neuroviruses. In H. A. Nasarallah & D. R. Weinberger (Eds.), *Handbook of schizophrenia: Vol. 1. The neurology of schizophrenia* (pp. 361–376). Amsterdam: Elsevier.

Vaillant, G. E. (1977). *Adaptation to life*. Boston: Little, Brown.

von Bertalanffy, L. (1968). *General systems theory*. New York: Braziller.

Wehr, T. A. (1988). Chronobiology of affective illness. In W. T. Hekkens, G. A. Kerhos, & W. J. Rietveld (Eds.), *Advances in biosciences: Trends in chronobiology* (Vol. 73). Oxford: Pergamon Press.

World Health Organization. (1947). *Constitution*. Geneva: WHO.

Yates, M., Leake, A., Candy, J., Fairbairn, A. F., McKeith, I. G., & Ferrier, I. N. (1990). 5-HT_2 receptor changes in major depression. *Biological Psychiatry, 27*, 489–496.

C H A P T E R

Cultural Considerations

BESS STEWART, Ph.D., R.N.,C.S., F.A.A.N.

OUTLINE

CHAPTER OBJECTIVES

Upon completion of this chapter, you will be able to:

1. Define the following terms: culture, subculture, race, ethnicity, cultural relativism, and acculturation.
2. Discuss the influence of culture on the health beliefs and practices of individuals.
3. Describe the cause of mental illness as defined in a cultural context.
4. Discuss cultural life span issues from infancy to older adulthood.
5. Discuss the psychiatric–mental health nurse's role in providing culture-specific care.

KEY TERMS

Acculturation
Cultural relativism
Culture
Enculturation
Ethnicity
Race
Subculture

The past three decades have witnessed the emergence of interest in and the study of cultural issues related to health care. Two events converged in the 1960s to focus attention on the need for culturally sensitive mental health services for economically disadvantaged minority populations (Rogler & Malgady, 1987). The first was the rise of the civil rights movement, and the second was the increased immigration of various cultural groups to the United States. The beliefs, values, and health practices of these groups differ significantly from those of a nurse educated in the biomedical model. However, for much of the past two decades, the cultural aspects of psychiatric–mental health care have been ignored. The cultural literature clearly documents that **culture** shapes the perception of reality and strongly influences behavior and psychological disorders (Kiev, 1972). Different cultures reinforce different behaviors and provide acceptable ways for their expression. Thus, the cultural context delineates the types of adjustment to stress that are used. Culture also influences which behaviors are considered deviant and then, in turn, partially determines the types of adjustments. To work effectively with clients from various cultures, it is imperative that nurses become familiar with the beliefs, values, and dysfunctional and help-seeking behaviors of different cultural groups. Such knowledge is crucial in implementing culture-specific psychiatric nursing care. By acknowledging cultural differences and similarities, psychiatric nurses increasingly heighten their clinical sensitivity in dealing with clients from different cultures. This commonly leads to adopting a style of practice that reflects an appreciation of how cultural elements affect the process and outcome of mental health interventions.

OVERVIEW OF CULTURE AND BEHAVIOR

The link between culture and mental health dates back to the early twentieth century. In 1893, Emil Kraepelin (1856–1926) described the syndrome he named *dementia praecox,* based on his observations of clients he identified as suffering from "madness." Kraepelin (1906) was a visionary who sought to demonstrate that this syndrome could be recognized in non-Western cultures. Consequently, he traveled to the Far East and reported that he could identify cases of dementia praecox in Java, a culture vastly different from his own. Since Kraepelin's pioneering transcultural investigations, psychiatrists from the West who have worked in non-Western cultures have also been able to identify schizophrenia in a variety of countries.

Sigmund Freud also had a strong influence on the relationship between culture and mental illness. Freud's concepts of personality development were outgrowths of his development of psychoanalysis as a method for dealing with mental illness. He emphasized that infant and early childhood experiences were the most influential factors in personality development. Margaret Mead (1928) and Ruth Benedict (1934) used Freud's basic premises about early childhood development to demonstrate the way in which cultures differ from one another in moral systems, child rearing, sex role behavior, and types of mental disorder. Mead (1928) was able to demonstrate that in American culture, adolescent girls experience a period of crisis and search for identity but that Samoan girls experience no such crisis.

Benedict (1934) was also concerned with the way in which child-rearing practices relate to adult personality and later-life behavior. She noted that in some societies there is a sharp demarcation between what is expected of a child and what is expected of an adult. For example, in American culture, at some point a child is said to become an adult and is treated differently. In other societies, there is no break at all; the life cycle is perceived as a continuous process in which children are given increasing responsibility and independence as they move toward adulthood.

In the 1960s Leininger began her efforts to promote the need to consider nursing within a cultural context (Leininger, 1979), which are only now beginning to yield significant results (Giger & Davidhizer, 1991). The introduction of cultural concepts to psychiatric nursing will have a profound impact on nursing as health care moves into the twenty-first century.

BASIC CONCEPTS OF CULTURE

Culture is a term used to refer to the way of life of a people. It emphasizes the holistic, integrated way of life, including behavior. Culture shapes the perception of reality and strongly influences societal norms or conflicts, behaviors, and psychological disorders (Kiev, 1972). Culture is accumulated and diverse, and it has the following basic characteristics:

- Culture is learned—it is passed down from generation to generation through the process of enculturation.
- Culture is shared—almost everything one does is patterned after the actions of the larger groups of which one shares membership.
- Culture is a whole or a system—the parts are interrelated in complex ways.
- Culture is cumulative—knowledge is stored and passed from one generation to the next.
- Culture is diverse—basic problems of life are solved by cultural means, but there is never only one solution.

Many solutions are found among various races and ethnic groups. People are born into a family, where they learn to internalize rules of behavior and depend on others for approval. Although these cultural rules exist, it is individuals who interpret them and either act according to those rules or choose to break them (Schusky & Culbert, 1978).

A ***subculture*** is a group of people that share values and beliefs that are not common to all members of their larger cultural group (Boyle & Andrews, 1989).

A ***race*** is a subgroup of people possessing a definite combination of physical characteristics of a genetic origin, the combination of which distinguishes the subgroup as different from other subgroups. Race and ethnicity are often used interchangeably, but they do not consistently have the same meaning (Giordano, 1973).

Ethnicity is a group classification in which members share a unique social and cultural heritage passed from one generation to the next. It involves customs, language, religion, and other cultural factors. Racial differences may or may not be germane to ethnic differences.

Cultural relativism is the concept that recognizes that characteristics of another culture should be approached with respect. It refers to the differences in beliefs, feelings, behaviors, traditions, and social practices that are found among diverse peoples of the world (Schusky & Culbert, 1978).

Acculturation refers to changes that result from contact between two or more autonomous cultures. Acculturation has traditionally been considered a process that involves the absorption of new cultural customs (Schusky & Culbert, 1978).

Enculturation is the process by which culture is learned and acquired by particular individuals (Schusky & Culbert, 1978).

Beliefs. Beliefs are basic assumptions, ideas, feelings, or convictions that are accepted as truth by people within a culture. Beliefs are conceived to have three types of components: (1) cognitive, which represents knowledge held with some certainty about what is good or bad, right or wrong, or desirable or undesirable; (2) affective, which arouses intense feelings; and (3) behavioral, which leads to action or activity. Beliefs are conditioned by culture, but all beliefs are not equally important; therefore, the more central a belief, the more a change in that belief will be resisted.

Attitudes. Attitudes are feelings toward a person, an object, or an idea that include cognitive, affective, and behavioral elements. Attitudes are relatively enduring sets of beliefs formed by past experiences and learned through the process of enculturation, predisposing one to respond in a certain manner.

Value Orientation. Values are common beliefs shared by members of a group or society. Values may be learned through formal teaching or informal role modeling. Cultural values shape decisions made by people concerning matters of health and illness. Rather than reflecting the values of any one member of a cultural group, a cultural value system "represents what is expected, required or forbidden within a given culture; [it is this] system criteria by which conduct is judged and sanctions applied" (Albert, 1968, p. 16).

Kluckhohn and Strodtbeck (1961) defined value orientation as a complex entity that gives order and direction to human activity as it relates to the solution of "common human problems." They further suggested that although in all cultures some members will hold different value orientations from the group, dominant value orientations can be identified for specific cultural groups. Kluckhohn and Strodtbeck (1961) identified four major value orientations and their possible solutions, as follows:

1. Man–nature orientation: This problem involves the relationship of people with nature and supernature. The three types of solutions are mastery over nature, subjugation to nature, and harmony with nature.
2. Time orientation: This problem is concerned with the temporal focus of human life. The three types of solutions are the future, the present, and the past.
3. Activity orientation: This problem is concerned with the various modes of human activity. The three types of solutions toward human activity are being, being-in-becoming, and doing.
4. Relational orientation: This problem is concerned with a person's relationship to other people. The three types of solutions are collateral, lineal, and individualistic (Tripp-Reimer, 1984).

CULTURE AND PSYCHOPATHOLOGY: THEORIES AND ISSUES

The definition of mental illness takes the normal, expected, and acceptable behavior in a culture as a baseline; any unconscious or uncontrollable deviance from the baseline is viewed as abnormal behavior or mental illness. Anthropologists who study forms of mental illness cross-culturally use two major categories to distinguish disorders: (1) behavioral disorders that are caused by brain damage, and (2) behavioral disorders in which there is no apparent brain damage. The latter category is subdivided into (a) psychoses, such as schizophrenia, depression, and paranoia, and (b) neuroses of a variety of types. Although symptoms of mental illness vary from culture to culture, there are no universal theories that explain these deviations.

Causes of Mental Illness. Relatively little is known about major mental disorders among different cultural groups, and it is appropriate to assume that the same biological factors are involved. However, certain risk factors that predispose to mental illness in the general population may be questionable when applied to certain cultural groups. Family structure and dynamics, socioeconomic levels, educational opportunities, and cognitive–linguistic frameworks all are different (McEnany, 1991). Other vulnerable groups, such as infants and children, adolescents, and the elderly, may have pressing mental health needs as well.

BIOCHEMICAL INFLUENCES

There is a paucity of research in the area of cultural and biological causes of mental illness. Two theories of causality predominate in the literature, but the linkage between causation and culture has yet to be explored.

Depression. It has been postulated that depressive illness may be associated with a deficiency of the neurotransmitters norepinephrine, serotonin, and dopamine at certain receptor sites in the brain. The medical approach to discussing depression from a cultural perspective has focused on the universality of the human central nervous system and the association between affect and structural chemical changes in the central nervous system (Gold et al., 1988a, 1988b).

Western depression is defined by *somatic* symptoms, such as tearfulness, weight gain or loss, sleep disturbance, and *psychological* symptoms, such as dysphoric mood, guilt, and suicidal thoughts. In other cultures, somatic complaints are characterized by the expression of personal and social distress in an idiom of bodily complaints and medical help-seeking (Lin et al., 1985). This does not mean that people from other cultures do not experience depressive illness, but it does indicate that they have different ways of expressing it (see Chapter 9 for an in-depth discussion of depression.)

Schizophrenia. Most researchers agree that biological factors play a significant role in the cause of schizophrenia; however, no single neurochemical has been found to underlie the diverse behaviors and progressive loss of affective responses. One hypothesis suggests that there is a malfunction in the system that regulates dopaminergic function. A second hypothesis implies an association among low-platelet monoamine oxidase levels and paranoid symptoms and chronic schizophrenia (Reynolds, 1989).

There has been an increased interest in the role of biological determinants, particularly those considered to be genetic. The strongest evidence of the role of genetics in schizophrenia comes from the research of Cancro (1982) and Liberman et al. (1984). They concluded that stressful life events can precipitate schizophrenia in genetically predisposed persons.

The cause of schizophrenia remains unclear. Most researchers support the concept of multiple causation. Liberman et al. (1984) stated that "schizophrenic symptoms" occur when noxious social events combine with pre-existing vulnerability to produce sensory overload, hyperarousal, and impaired processing of social stimuli. Cultural influences on the development of schizophrenia have yet to be confirmed (see Chapter 12 for further discussion of schizophrenia).

INCIDENCE AND PREVALENCE OF SPECIFIC DISORDERS ACROSS CULTURES

Cultural differences are the focus of many mental health researchers concerned with the incidence and prevalence of specific disorders across cultures. However, most psychiatric literature dealing with the prevalence of mental illness in non-Western cultures has relied on anecdotal reports by authors who have spent brief periods in non-Western cultures observing certain behaviors, then commenting on the differences from Western culture.

To study the frequency of a particular mental illness in a variety of cultures, it is important to identify the illness wherever it appears, and unless mental health professionals agree on their definitions of symptoms, it is impossible to know whether or not the same condition is being discussed. Agreement on the definition of symptoms is an essential prerequisite to studying variations in the prevalence of psychiatric illness in different cultures. Psychotic and neurotic behaviors may be socially acceptable in one culture and not in another. If a psychiatric disorder has the same incidence and prevalence in two different cultures, it can be either the product of biological manifestations that are common to humans or the consequence of environmental factors shared by the two cultures. The more diverse the cultures in which similar or identical illness manifests, the more likely that biological factors are the cause. On the other hand, differences in the manifestation of an illness in a number of cultures may be caused by environmental factors exerting an influence on the form of illness.

Features of illness that do not vary from culture to culture have been designated *culture free*, whereas those that do vary with culture have been termed *culture bound*. Culture-bound features of mental illness that are confined to a particular culture and are not evident in others imply the impact of cultural factors rather than a common heritage among human beings (Flaskerud, 1989) (Table 3–1).

Increased need to meet the needs of diverse populations has prompted the inclusion of a section on culture-bound syndromes in the *Diagnostic and Statistical*

TABLE 3–1
Culture-Bound Syndromes in Mental Illness

	CULTURE-BOUND SYNDROME	WESTERN SYMPTOMS
African American	"Nervous breakdown"	Anxiety, sadness, tension, irrational anger, hearing voices, inability to carry out activities of daily living
Hispanic American	*Nervios* (nerves)	Palpitations, weakness, dizziness, headaches
	Ataque (fits)	Hyperventilation, fits of violence, catatonia, salivation
	Susto (fright)	Weakness, anxiety, fear
Asian American	*Sia chit* (lose mind, nervous breakdown)	Sadness, crying, difficulty sleeping, fright, panic, various physical symptoms
	Ba (crazy or insane)	Hearing voices, dangerous behavior; impaired thought, memory, logic, or intelligence
	Neurasthenia	Headache, various aches and pains, pressure and heaviness in the head, morbid fears, tremors, hopelessness, irritability
	Posttraumatic stress disorder	Depression and traumalike symptoms from being refugees

TABLE 3–2
Outline for Cultural Formulation

MAJOR COMPONENTS OF CULTURAL CONSIDERATIONS	NURSING IMPLICATIONS
▸ Cultural identity of the client	▸ Appreciation of diversity is a major component of holistic nursing care. Understanding the client's uniqueness (e.g., language, family rituals, and health practices) enables the nurse to plan an individualized plan of care
▸ Cultural explanation for the client's illness	▸ Understanding a cultural explanation of symptoms decreases inappropriate labeling (e.g., description of physical or psychosocial symptoms, family reaction, coping patterns, and response to mental illness) and helps the nurse intervene appropriately
▸ Cultural factors associated with the psychosocial environment and level of functioning	▸ These data are also relevant to assessing the impact of psychosocial stressors, family and individual coping, and interactional patterns (e.g., several generations living in one home or neighborhood, financial and psychosocial resources)
▸ Cultural components of the nurse–client relationship	▸ The nurse needs to appreciate his or her uniqueness (culture, ethnic background, and socioeconomic status) to appreciate that quality in the client
▸ Cultural assessment (basis of diagnosis and plan of care)	▸ Nurses need to develop an assessment tool that integrates cultural, psychosocial, and biological components. This would be the best approach to using the nursing process to identify cultural needs through the nurse–client relationship and initiating culture-bound interventions and a comprehensive plan of care

Data from American Psychiatric Association. (1994). *Diagnostic and statistical manual of mental disorders* (4th ed., pp. 843–844). Washington, DC: Author.

Manual of Mental Disorders, Fourth Edition (DSM-IV) (APA, 1994). A number of clinicians were unfamiliar with these culture-bound practices, beliefs, and behaviors. Historically, these clinical presentations were identified with psychopathology rather than culture-bound syndromes. The DSM-IV depicts three areas of information germane to various cultural presentations: (1) specific clinical presentations that are included in the DSM-IV classifiction; (2) a delineation of culture-bound syndromes and a glossary in Appendix I; and (3) a template of cultural formulation designed to increase sensitivity in the application of various diagnostic criteria (Table 3–2).

Culture-bound disorders are generally thought of as folk or traditional illnesses. However, neurasthenia, a mental disorder, was originally thought to be of neurological or biological origin by American psychiatrists but is now seen in China and frequently diagnosed by Chinese psychiatrists. Symptoms of the disorder include headache, pressure and heaviness in the head, aches and pain, hopelessness, morbid fears, insomnia, and poor appetite (Kleinman, 1982).

Another diagnosis commonly used, especially among African Americans, is "nervous breakdown," referring to mental illness in general. The diagnosis seems to imply that the nerves have worn out (Flaskerud, 1989).

A final example of culture-bound symptoms is *susto*, or magical fright. *Susto* can be caused by any disturbing experience that causes part of the self to separate from the body. It is believed that the spirit leaves the body and cold air rushes in to take over. If not cured in the early stages, the client may experience continuous periods of malaise, loss of appetite, and listlessness (Holland, 1978). In addition to a psychic upset, somatic complaints such as anxiety, depressed mood, and agitation are experienced.

CULTURAL IMPACT ON DEVELOPMENT ACROSS THE LIFE SPAN

Erik Erikson (1963) was a pioneer in including the social and cultural aspects in the context of developmental theory. He described the psychosocial development of the human being on a continuum from birth to death, and he identified four major phases in life: childhood, adolescence, adulthood, and old age. Erickson emphasized that culture is the interplay of customs and that children's play helps resolve conflicts or developmental crises.

Each developmental task has a challenge that must be solved and attitudes and abilities to be developed. Erikson believed that if the crisis is not worked through, the opportunity to resolve it may occur later. The outcomes of each stage can be positive or negative and will affect the identity or the self throughout life. Erikson's life span theory is important to psychiatric nurses' understanding of ethnic cultural groups' responses to illness. The forces that operated in a person during childhood will continue to operate into that person's adulthood. In addition, developmental crises that have not been resolved may affect the coping and adaptive responses to stress.

Life span theories are based on the assumption that attitudes and behavioral responses found in behavioral pathology are related to and stem from normal biosocial behavior. Some theorists stress that it is difficult to extinguish behaviors learned in early childhood because of parental influences and reinforcement, stating that anxieties generated during infancy and childhood do not change with age and they cannot be altered. It is even suggested that self-image developed in childhood becomes a self-fulfilling prophecy. The following sections describe the cultural impact on developmental processes.

INFANCY

The developing infant is subject to influences of culture from the moment of conception. The parent's perception of illness, religious values, language, perception of others' religious values, childbearing patterns, and health practices all are modeled for the infant. This perception, in turn, helps shape the child's view of the world. The child takes cues for behavior from observing and imitating family members. The perceptions then are incorporated into the self-concept (Martinez, 1978). The overall self-concept of a person is often determined by the mother–child attachment called *bonding*. The emotional bond is considered crucial for optimal physical and emotional development of the child. Studies have shown that if there is interference in the process of attachment, later problems in behavior, failure to thrive, and child abuse are likely to occur (Biehler, 1981; Drotar, 1985).

CHILDHOOD AND ADOLESCENCE

Like the infant, the young child is shaped by the cultural values and beliefs of the family. It is at this stage of development that family rituals are introduced and the child is socialized in those rituals. Separation anxiety is a major developmental crisis, and the parental response to this crisis is of major significance to future responses to anxiety.

Hispanic American families tend to adopt a more relaxed attitude toward the achievement of developmental tasks; there is a basic acceptance of the child's individuality. They seem less pressured than Caucasian parents to achieve developmental goals. The family is usually close knit and demands loyalty. Some studies (Martinez, 1988) have suggested that this close-knit family structure protects the Hispanic American child from maladaptive emotional disturbances, yet some Hispanic Americans experience depression or may manifest behavioral problems, or both. Hispanic American children with depression usually present with somatic complaints such as nausea and vomiting, stomachaches, and headaches. Children with these symptoms may be taken to a *curandera,* who will probably diagnose the problem as *empacho* rather than a mental illness. The *curandera* is a folk healer who is used by family members across the age continuum and who is customarily consulted for the treatment of five traditional folk illnesses: *mal de ajo* (evil eye), *empacho, caida de mollera* (fallen fontanelle), *susto*, and *mal puesto* or *mono clavado* (hex). Folk healers treat physical illnesses as well as mental illnesses such as anxiety, depression, and even neurotic and psychotic symptoms (Gomez & Gomez, 1985).

The Chinese American family has also been described as a close-knit social unit that provides its members with support, security, and a means for meeting emotional needs (Fong, 1985). Family loyalty, unquestioning allegiance, and total subordination to one's elders and superiors are expected. Children are taught that strong and negative feelings are not to be openly expressed. Individuality is not supported; achievement is for the family. Shame and all misfortune affect not only the individual but the family as well (Kleinman, 1980).

According to Louie (1985), the departure of younger generations from traditional family belief systems is the greatest stressor in the Chinese American family. Chang (1991) found that traditional Chinese American values are eroding rapidly owing to the acculturation process. Many children do not show elders the traditional respect, and many elders can no longer count on their children for support.

Cultural differences in rates and manifestations of mental illness are found in young children from other cultures as well. Weisz et al. (1987) compared psychosocial differences between children in Thailand and the Unites States and found striking differences. Thai children are socialized to be nonaggressive, peaceful, polite, and deferent, whereas in the United States, independence and competitiveness are encouraged. Children in Thailand are referred for psychological treatment of "overcontrolled syndrome" (fearfulness, sleep problems, and somatic complaints), whereas in the United States children are referred for treatment of "undercontrolled syndrome" (fighting, aggressive behavior, and disobedience).

Children from non-Western cultures and African Americans frequently describe minority status as a stressor (Gibson & Ogbu, 1991). Southeast Asian refugees with catastrophic life changes have experienced severe stress since coming to this country. A series of losses, which include for some the loss of country, home, family members, and friends, has severely impaired their ability to cope (Fox, 1991).

ADULTHOOD

Adulthood presents unique challenges for people and encompasses maturation, socialization, and culturally sanctioned obligations. This is the time in their life span when men and women are expected to make significant decisions with lifelong implications: separating from the family of origin, getting married, rearing children, and making career decisions. These decisions are played out in a cultural context and can place tremendous stress on the person. For an example, see the accompanying Research Study display on stress-related family change among Vietnamese refugees. The timing of the tasks, the ritual of transition, the themes, the coping mechanisms, and the meaning attached to these different stages vary from culture to culture. These tasks become internalized and translated into psychological expectations for self and others (Falicov & Karrer, 1980). Fail-

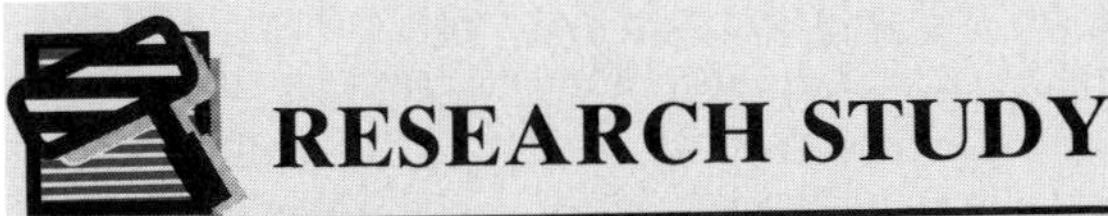

RESEARCH STUDY

Stress-Related Family Change Among Vietnamese Refugees

Fox, P.G. (1991). *Journal of Community Health Nursing, 8*(1), 45–56.

Study Problem or Purpose

The purpose of the study was to identify changes in the structural and functional dimensions of family life of Vietnamese refugees and to determine the amount of stress experienced because of these changes.

Methods

Thirty Vietnamese refugee women aged 25 to 57 years, all of whom were married to their present spouses in Vietnam, were interviewed using an open-ended interview technique. A Vietnamese research assistant was used to translate from English to Vietnamese. To evaluate the interview guide, trial interviews were conducted with these Vietnamese women in the sample. The guide proved satisfactory and was used in an intensive, semistructured interview. Socioeconomic data were collected on each woman and her spouse. Data were also collected on the affective dimensions of the spousal relationship, the amount and quality of time spent together, shared activities, the frequency and types of disagreements, and the amount of stress felt due to life circumstance.

Findings

A significant finding was that because of structural changes in shifting from an open family system to a closed family system, there followed functional changes in family relations. For example, decision making was now confined to the spousal couple, because they no longer had the duty to seek advice and consent from the parental families. In addition, women tended to continue to hold the attitude that their husbands had the legitimate right to make final family decisions. Most indicated that if they held differing opinions, they would withdraw from conflict to maintain harmony within the family. Working wives expressed more satisfaction with their relationships, whereas nonworking wives expressed feelings of social isolation, loneliness, and often fear. These feelings decreased the women's capacity to deal with daily life events and frequently led to feelings of despair and depression.

Implications

Changes in the functional and structural dimensions of the Vietnamese refugee's spousal relationship holds implications for psychiatric nurses, as the person's general health as well as mental health are at risk. Women who experienced a decrease in spousal affection and support acknowledged stress in all areas of their lives. The psychiatric nursing assessment of the client must include family functioning, so that empirical, culturally based interventions can be developed.

---

ure to adequately fulfill these tasks frequently leads to feelings of frustration, failure, and, subsequently, depression. In some cultural groups, such as Asian, Italian, Greek, and Puerto Rican Americans, the father is the authoritarian head of the family, and everyone is expected to respect him. Young adults experience extreme anxiety and stress when they attempt to challenge old traditions, especially the father's authority (Rotunno & McGoldrick, 1982). In Hispanic American society, the nuclear family is imbedded in the extended family network. Immigration patterns frequently mean separation from this extended family network. When this occurs, the Hispanic American wife experiences stress owing to relocation and loss of family and friends; this is often expressed as somatic complaints, usually masking depression (Falicov & Karrer, 1980).

The onset of many psychiatric disorders in African American adults tends to occur in late adolescence and the early 20s. The behaviors frequently exhibited by this group that may require psychiatric interventions include suicidal gestures, violence directed toward self, or violence directed toward others, such as sexual assult and homicide. The major mental disorders diagnosed in this group are affective illness, adjustment disorder, and schizophrenia (Baker, 1988). Substance abuse, particularly alcohol, remains a concern throughout the life cycle. African Americans frequently experience feelings of sadness, anxiety, and anger. This anger is frequently acted out in destructive ways within the community and has been referred to as "black-on-black" crime (Baker, 1988).

OLDER ADULTHOOD

The striking increase in the number of people 65 years of age and older has emerged as one of the greatest health care issues of the 1990s. A more significant factor is that more elderly are from culturally diverse groups, especially African American. This size of this group will increase substantially over the next decade. Not only basic health services but also mental health services will be required (Kermis, 1986).

Mental health for the older person is complex, because mental disorders can be the result of physical, social, or emotional distress or dysfunction (Hogstel, 1990). Poor health is identified by the elderly as the problem that most concerns them (Burnside, 1988), and poor health is likely to result in anxiety and depression.

Depression is the most common mental health problem in older adults. Although the symptoms are similar to those in younger adults, many older adults tend to deny depressed mood and instead have multiple somatic complaints, especially the minority elderly and the elderly from non-Western cultures (Lefley, 1990; Rosenbaum, 1989).

Although there are few sources of information available on mental health, aging, and culture, it is appropriate to assume that the degree of acculturation, the socioeconomic status, and the perceptions of mental illness and its impact on the family will need to be considered when planning care for the minority elderly, because this group makes the most extensive use of family and informal support networks as their physical and mental health needs change. The elderly in most minority cultural groups tend to be community dwelling, usually living with a family member. Only about 1 percent are hospitalized for psychiatric treatment. They tend to underutilize the mental health delivery system and are therefore only intermittently assisted in the mental health arena. Various factors have combined to produce this state of affairs, including inadequate reimbursement for mental health services, fragmented federal policies, and lack of access in many poor communities (Kermis, 1986).

PSYCHOPHARMACOLOGY AND CULTURE

To provide optimal care to clients, it is important that psychiatric nurses be cognizant of differences in responses to medications among various cultural and ethnic groups. Although cultural differences in response to psychotropic medications have been under review for the past decade, few objective data can be found in the literature. These objective comparisons of psychotropic medications in clients from different cultures have been hindered significantly by problems in designing culturally equivalent diagnostic and evaluation tools. Therefore, it has been difficult to ensure comparable data on diagnoses, severity of illness, and degree of improvement among clients from different cultural groups. However, according to Lin et al. (1986), there is large-scale usage of psychotropics in many different countries. This testifies to the clinical usefulness of psychotropic drugs in controlling psychiatric symptoms in various cultures.

Studies on the relationship between culture and psychopharmacology indicate that differences in dosages do exist, especially between Western and non-Western cultures. It has been suggested that these variations may be accounted for by differences in body size, body weight, and fat distribution (Lin & Finder, 1983).

Side effects of psychotropic medications appear to be quite problematic for non-Western cultures. For example, Asian clients tend to experience severe extrapyramidal side effects, especially with neuroleptics. African American clients taking tricyclic antidepressants have been reported to develop delirium and experience severe extrapyramidal side effects from higher dosages of haloperidol, as compared with their Caucasian counterparts.

Because consideration of the effect of culture on psychotropic medication dosage and side effects is in its infancy, it is important for psychiatric nurses to perform a thorough assessment of the client and remain alert to potential problems. There is a serious need for research in this area.

NEUROLEPTICS

Early studies on cultural differences in psychotropic drug response suggested that Europeans received lower dosages of several neuroleptics than did Americans. More recent studies indicated that clients from non-Western cultures such as India, Pakistan, China, Japan, and Indonesia also receive lower dosages of neuroleptics and show clinical improvement at these lower dosages, as compared with Americans and Europeans (Allen et al., 1977, 1980). Consistent with these international reports, it has been observed that Asian Americans also respond to lower dosages of neuroleptics (Lawson, 1986; Lin & Finder, 1983; Lin et al., 1986). Young African American males respond well to lower dosages of neuroleptics and generally report more extrapyramidal symptoms when placed on high dosages of haloperidol decanoate (haloperidol injection) (Campinha-Bacote, 1991). These findings place the young African American male at high risk for developing neuroleptic malignant syndrome or tardive dyskinesia unless dosages are monitored.

ANTIDEPRESSANTS

Data on cultural differences in the use of antidepressants are inconsistent. Rudorfer et al. (1984) found that Asians used much lower dosage ranges than their American counterparts. Other studies have also indicated that compared with Caucasians, the therapeutic dosages for antidepressants may be lower for Hispanic Americans, African Americans, and Puerto Rican Americans (Marcos & Cancro, 1982; Rudorfer & Robbins, 1982).

LITHIUM

In comparing cultural variations in the management of manic behavior, Yang (1985) found that Chinese clients responded well to lower dosages of lithium (mean lithium blood levels of 0.4 to 0.8 mEq/L) as compared with Caucasian clients (who required a mean lithium blood level of 0.5 to 1.2 mEq/L) to maintain a therapeutic response. This finding indicates that there are significant differences in the level of brain receptor response to lithium between the two groups (Lin et al., 1986).

CULTURAL CONSIDERATIONS FOR SELECTED POPULATIONS

Five cultural groups are presented here because they may offer the greatest challenges to psychiatric nurses in planning culture-specific care. The five groups include (1) African Americans, (2) Hispanic Americans, (3) Puerto Rican Americans, (4) Asian Americans, and (5) Native Americans.

AFRICAN AMERICANS

African Americans consult with extended family, their kin, or their minister when faced with stress and problems. They are reluctant to seek mental health care because reliance on the extended family is easier and less humiliating; however, when family resources are depleted, they will seek other services, including mental health. They may initially mistrust the nurse as an outsider and consider the nurse as an intruder into their intimate affairs (Baker, 1987, 1988; Bell & Mehta, 1979; McGoldrick et al., 1982). These concerns are usually demonstrated by missed appointments or by being reluctant to speak freely about themselves.

In view of increased stress and deprivation as part of the African American life experience, there is a high percentage of debilitating mental disorders in this cultural group. Baker (1988) noted that schizophrenia is the leading diagnosis for African Americans admitted to inpatient services, whereas depressive illness ranked second. This diagnosis tends to range across the age continuum (Bell & Mehta, 1981; Jones & Gray, 1986).

A broad range of psychological disorders noted in African American children is considered to be related to racial differences (Baker, 1988), but the prevalence of these disorders tends to be high among children from lower socioeconomic groups, making it apparent that poverty is an overriding factor. Hyperkinesis, pica, learning disabilities, and aggressive behavior are commonly seen in African American children (Bullough & Bullough, 1972, 1982). Often, these children are given the diagnosis of hyperactive or attention deficit disorder and, in some instances, diagnosed as being mentally retarded. In recent years, however, more African American children and adolescents are being given the diagnosis of bipolar disorder. There is also the possibility that some of the children diagnosed as hyperactive and destructive may indeed have been misdiagnosed and may also belong in the diagnostic category of bipolar disorder (Tharp, 1991).

HISPANIC AMERICANS

It is generally presumed that Hispanic Americans have a greater need for mental health services than the general population because of additional stress from acculturation pressure, poverty, language barriers, limited education, and discrimination. However, there is substantial documentation that Hispanic Americans are underrepresented in mental health facilities and generally have low rates of psychosis. Moreover, differences have been found in the types and severity of psychopathology in Hispanic Americans as compared with Caucasians. Hispanics tend to display more affective and fewer paranoid symptoms. This discrepancy between high-risk factors and a low prevalence of psychoses and low utilization of mental health resources has mental health practitioners perplexed. One explanation suggests that Hispanics have different cooperative criteria than Caucasians for perceiving and evaluating psychological difficulties. A second explanation for the low prevalence of psychoses in Hispanics is that the social and familial structure of the Hispanic family life buffers people from conflicts with the larger society and is generally protective of their mental health. It is believed that Hispanics rarely face crises alone, and their close-knit extended family serves as anxiety-sharing and anxiety-reducing mechanisms in stressful situations (Falicov, 1982; Jenkins, 1988; Masden, 1969).

A third factor cited as contributing to the low rates of reported psychopathology among Hispanic Americans is the psychological and behavioral attributes of folk illness. These illnesses are regarded as "diseases of adaptation," which affords people the opportunity to satisfy repressed drives or to avoid stress from role conflict or failure (Falicov, 1982; Martinez, 1988). The stress-alleviating and preventive functions of these disorders coincide with the dynamics of Hispanic American folk psychiatry or *curanderismo* (Kiev, 1968). There are differences of opinion among investigators about how widespread the beliefs in *curanderismo* and the associated folk illness, particularly *susto* and *mal puesto*; however, they occur frequently enough to merit attention by mental health workers. *Susto* is believed to occur when a person is frightened by a traumatic event and the soul leaves the body, leaving the person weak, scared, and anxious. Belief in *mal puesto* may be used defensively to deny the existence of a mental disorder (Martinez, 1988). Hispanic Americans vary in the degree of acculturation—some have moved away from their ethnic minority groups, whereas some steadfastly cling to values and beliefs of their country of origin. A significant number of Hispanic Americans maintain elements of both cultures. In times of stress, these cultural elements may co-mingle and give rise to unusual and idiosyncratic manifestations in the face of psychopathology and stress. A significant number maintain elements of both cultures (American and Hispanic).

PUERTO RICAN AMERICANS

Puerto Rican clients express psychological distress through somatic symptoms and complaints. In times of stress, they may return to their old neighborhood to be with their family and chat with friends. This is an adaptive response to stress that is often helpful (Ramos-McKay et al., 1988).

Because Puerto Rican women are traditionally responsible for the preservation of the family, they often experience the stress of role conflict, acculturation, and changes in family structure. Puerto Rican women seek help more often than Puerto Rican men and do so with a variety of physical complaints combined with anxiety and symptoms of depression (Garcia-Preto, 1982). They often complain of marital conflicts and problems with the rejection of parental cultural values by adolescent children (Garcia-Preto, 1982). In the traditional Puerto Rican family, the father is recognized as the authority, whereas the wife and children are submissive. The nuclear family is closely aligned with the supportive extended family system. Individualism and independence from the family are not traditional Puerto Rican values, and mental health problems are viewed as family problems. Families on the mainland as well as families on the island use the extended family systems in times of crises. According to Canino and Canino (1982), the extended family is used as a buffer against the stress of adaptation to immigration.

A significant number of Puerto Ricans believe in spiritism (*espiritismo,* i.e., a belief system consisting of an invisible world populated by spirits). These spirits can penetrate the visible world and attach themselves to human beings (Ramos-McKay et al., 1988). *Espiritismo* is provided as a form of mental health therapy consistent with the Puerto Rican concept of mental health. *Espiritismas* (healers) who work with the client communicate in the same language, describing the problems in psychosomatic fashion and accepting the client's symptoms as described (Comas-Diaz & Duncan, 1985). Furthermore, the *espiritismas* also include the extended family in the healing process. Most Puerto Ricans do not separate physical well-being from psychological well-being. For example, anxiety can be expressed as headaches or "pain in the brain."

Marcos and Cancro (1982) stated that most mentally ill Hispanic American clients present emotional symptoms in language that emphasizes physical complaints, such as shortness of breath, palpitations, dizziness, and headaches. Puerto Ricans from the lower socioeconomic group experience environmental stress that frequently leads to a diagnosis of affective disorder and substance abuse rather than psychotic disorder. The concept of the Puerto Rican syndrome, or *ataque,* as a phenomenon involving symptoms of mutism, catatonic posturing, hyperventilation, and bizarre behavior has been suggested as being the equivalent to a conversion disorder that is used as a coping strategy or defense mechanism against psychotic disorder. Suicidal gestures and attempts are prevalent among Puerto Ricans. These are believed to be responses to the Puerto Ricans' tendency to repress anger and aggression. Generally, the people who attempt suicide have no previous psychiatric symptoms, nor do they exhibit clinical depression.

Psychiatric nurses working with Puerto Ricans who adhere to traditional cultural values should include the client's extended family as well as the immediate family and significant others in planning care. Psychiatric nurses need to be aware of possible suicide attempts, especially by women, and explore with them more effective ways of dealing with their anger. Assertiveness training should be incorporated, because this has been found to be useful with some Puerto Ricans (Comas-Diaz & Duncan, 1985).

ASIAN AMERICANS

Asian Americans constitute a highly diverse and complex group and have been viewed as an upwardly mobile population with few psychological problems and therefore not in need of mental health services. However, recent research (Lin, 1983; Sue & McKinney, 1975) has suggested that the lack of utilization of mental health service does not necessarily reflect a lack of need. According to Sue and Morishima (1982), many Asian Americans who experience psychological distress tend to seek help from medical rather than mental health professionals. Physiological explanations of distress are usually sought for symptoms such as headaches, loss of appetite, difficulty in sleeping, allergies, digestive problems that are also associated with depression, and anxiety. Several explanations have been offered for the lack of Asian Americans seeking mental health care. According to Tsai et al. (1980), the person's view of the cause of mental distress may encourage him or her to attempt to solve problems without letting family members know the true extent of the distress. Asian Americans generally believe that mental health can be maintained by the avoidance of bad thoughts and the exercise of willpower. Such explanations logically guide people to attribute psychological distress to personal weakness. Behaviorally and cognitively, the person may try to shut down any distressing thoughts and feelings, which may further exacerbate distress. Stigma and shame may also arise over the experience of mental distress. Experiencing mental distress and changes in the ability to function may lead Asian Americans to feel that they have failed to achieve what their family expects of them. Further disgrace may be experienced if the person were to seek help outside the family. Help-seeking outside the family is still kept close to the cultural community. This is usually done in three phases: priests are approached first, then public sources, and professional psychiatric help last. Similarly, a family may not seek help for psychiatric problems within the family, because of the anticipated disgrace or the impression that their parenting skills are lacking (Root, 1985; Sue, 1988). Because of the pervasive influence of China on the development of Asia, Chinese health practices influence the belief systems of most people in Southeast Asia, and Chinese folk remedies, including acupuncture, massages, and herbal medicines, are widely sought among most Asian Americans. Folk remedies are related to Chinese theories of health as a state of balance among the components of the body and the body with the environment. Illness prevention and treatment involve the balance of *yin* and *yang* to ensure health. Many Asian Americans use folk medicines for a wide variety of illnesses, including mental illness, and may take them simultaneously with medications prescribed by mental health professionals.

NATIVE AMERICANS

Native Americans constitute one of the most impoverished ethnic groups in the United States. Native Americans also experience the effects of social discrimination and the past relocation of communities from traditional lands to distant and often barren reservation sites (Nelson et al., 1992). These difficult life circumstances appear to be closely associated with a higher incidence and greater severity of mental disorders among Native Americans. Depression is the most common mental disorder among Native Americans, including young children. Depression is frequently complicated by severe anxiety and the use of alcohol and other drugs (Nelson et al., 1992). Low self-esteem, substance abuse, and life frustrations often lead to violent behavior among some tribes. These behaviors include child physical and sexual abuse, spouse abuse, elder abuse, and suicide (May, 1988a, 1988b).

Although the issue of Native American alcohol abuse is complicated, according to Brod (1975), alcohol remains a major mental health problem for many Native Americans. It has been reported that the suicide, homicide, and accidental death rates among some Native American adolescents are higher than the national average (Nelson et al., 1992). It has been suggested that many accidental deaths associated with known depression and alcohol use and single-vehicle accidents are actually suicidal deaths.

Other common mental health problems of Native Americans are major anxiety, including panic disorder, psychosomatic disorders, and emotional problems resulting from disturbed interpersonal and family relationships (Neligh, 1990).

The Native American belief system plays an important part in the treatment of physical and mental illness. This belief system is based on maintaining harmony and thus preserving health. When disruptions or imbalances occur, illness results. The illness may manifest itself in mental, physical, or spiritual realms (Avery, 1991). The restoration of a healthy state is achieved through correction of imbalances. These corrective measures usually involve a ceremony. For healing specific ailments, there are several ceremonies, ranging from the 9-day-long Yeibeichei dance to elaborate healing ceremonies or "sings." There are also chemical and physical cures consisting of botanical medicines. In addition, there are many Native American healers with specialty areas such as sand painters, chanters, ceremonial specialists, and diagnosticians (Avery, 1991). Although not all Native Americans practice traditional medicine, a considerable percentage of the population does. Information on specific Native American medical practices is scarce because most Native Americans hold their medical practices sacred and they fear being ridiculed. Nursing interventions should focus on tribe-specific knowledge of beliefs and values rather than generalizing about all Native Americans.

BARRIERS TO EFFECTIVE CULTURE-SPECIFIC CARE

It is well documented that many minority and cultural groups underutilize mental health services. Many factors have been identified as contributing to this phenomena, such as racism, economic disadvantages, language, and client fears and beliefs about the causes of distress and expectations about recovery. Asian Americans have dropout rates that far exceed that of other ethnic groups.

Sue and McKinney (1975) suggested that premature termination may be related to communication problems, confusion over how therapy works, and conflict with the values of the therapist. Baker (1988) cited similar factors in dealing with the African American client. According to Baker, the client brings a well-honed ability to "read" verbal and nonverbal behavior and thus is able to sense if the therapist is anxious, uncomfortable, or rejecting. Once the client has identified a hostile or nonsupportive environment, he or she will probably leave and not return. If the client perceives this problem during an inpatient admission, he or she will generally become noncommunicative.

Language barriers and insufficient income provide a double barrier to accessibility to services and the availability of problem-solving strategies. It has been suggested that for the Hispanic American client, it is important to have an adequate number of Spanish-speaking personnel to provide care. This will be even more necessary in the future because the Hispanic population is the fastest increasing cultural group in the United States.

THE NURSE'S ROLE

PROVIDING CULTURE-SPECIFIC NURSING CARE

Although health beliefs and practices may be shared among people from the same cultural group, each client also remains an individual who may subscribe to cultural norms in varying degrees (Leininger, 1979). Several factors may contribute to the variation in health beliefs and practices of persons within the cultural group; these include education, level of acculturation, socioeconomic status, and previous experience with biomedical services. Therefore, it is imperative that the psychiatric nurse evaluate these factors in each individual client to determine the needs of each client and the relevance of cultural aspects of his or her psychiatric care. Because standard goals for therapy may be incongruent with cultural values, the following guidelines may facilitate the initial therapeutic contact with the client:

1. Find out what the client's beliefs are about mental and emotional problems. Determine how other similar problems in the family have been addressed. This provides information on the implicit rules of the family as well as their level of acculturation.
2. Explain the therapeutic plan, and identify the types of changes that need to occur and who will be involved. Some clients, because of their cultural context, expect the health care provider to be an authority and to tell them what to do to feel better. This enhances the client's trust in the nurse.
3. If possible, use concrete methods when approaching problem solving. Many clients come to therapy hoping to be able to leave with answers to their problems. Concrete examples help the client become unstuck.
4. Place appropriate time limits on the helping relationship to decrease the possibility of overdependence (Root, 1985).

Culture-specific nursing care involves the nurse's effective integration of the client's ethnic and cultural background into the nursing process–based client care. According to Orque et al. (1983), the idea of culture-specific care uses the same steps as the nursing process. Providing culture-specific care requires from the nurse the same rigor, discipline, and the use of nursing sciences as would be used to deliver care to any client. However, despite technical competence, nursing interventions may prove ineffective if the nurse is unwilling to understand culturally different clients.

According to Foster (1990) and Stewart (1991), culture-specific care means taking into account factors in the client's history that may influence diagnosis. Because deviant behavior may or may not signal mental illness, it would be prudent for the nurse to have an understanding of the client's explanation for his or her symptoms. Eliciting the client's explanation of his problem in a nonjudgmental fashion can serve to improve health care and to satisfy the expectations with which the clients sought medical attention (Kleinman et al., 1978). Because culture intensively influences a person's behavior, the nurse needs to understand the client's cultural orientation and to incorporate this into the delivery of psychiatric nursing care. Additionally, it is important to have knowledge of the level of acculturation to be able to make an assessment of what is normal or abnormal. Because cultures are so diverse, it is difficult for the nurse to know all aspects of each client's culture.

Tripp-Reimer and Afifi (1989) identified two processes nurses can use to improve communication in most instances: cultural assessment and cultural negotiation. A cultural assessment is a systematic appraisal of the beliefs, values, and practices needed to determine the context of client needs and to tailor appropriate psychiatric nursing interventions. During the first stage of the assessment, the nurse determines the client's ethnicity, the degree of affiliation with the ethnic group, the pattern of decision making, and the preferred communication style. Subsequently, the nurse elicits cultural information that is problem specific (e.g., mental health issues). The nurse can also determine the client's reasons for seeking care, notions about the problem, and previous and anticipated treatment. The last stage of the assessment is directed at gaining detailed cultural factors that may influence intervention strategies (Tripp-Reimer & Afifi, 1989).

The second process is cultural negotiation. This can be thought of as acts of translation in which messages, instructions, and belief systems are linked and processed between the professional and lay models of health problems and preferred treatment. The client's views are elicited regarding the illness experience. Attention is given to providing scientific information while acknowledging that the client may hold different views. Psychiatric nurses who are competent in cultural assessment and negotiation will likely be successful in gaining the client's trust and cooperation (Fong, 1985).

Although understanding the cultural implications is necessary for appropriate psychiatric care, caution must be used not to overgeneralize or stereotype clients on the basis of their ethnic heritage. Knowledge of cultural variations can serve as background cues for obtaining additional information. It must not be assumed that client needs are in all ways based on ethnicity.

Townsend (1991) has developed guidelines that are appropriate and can be adapted to the needs of clients from diverse cultural groups. The plans are intended to be used as guidelines for the construction of care plans that must be individualized to meet the needs of each client based on assessment. According to Townsend (1991), information presented with each diagnosis should include the following:

- Definition
- Possible cause
- Defining characteristics
- Goals and objectives
- Interventions, with rationale
- Desired client outcomes or evaluations

THE NURSING PROCESS

The nursing process is the framework for nursing practice and is the appropriate vehicle to help nurses provide culturally relevant care to a culturally diverse population. The nursing process is composed of assess-

Nursing Care Plan 3-1 The Client with Depression (Mrs. Liu)

▶ **Nursing Diagnosis:** Ineffective Individual Coping

▶ Mrs. Liu, a 35-year-old married Chinese American woman who recently immigrated to the United States, was admitted to an inpatient psychiatric unit with a diagnosis of depression. She had been very erratic at home, either being sullen or crying and yelling. She expressed a desire to kill herself and stated, "They think I am crazy because I am crying. I am crying because I have a headache, toothache, and stomachache." She was given a diagnosis of depression.

OUTCOME IDENTIFICATION	NURSING ACTIONS	RATIONALES	EVALUATION
1. By [date], client makes plans that reflect desire to live.	1. Demonstrate a therapeutic nurse–client relationship through brief, frequent contact and an accepting attitude.	1. An accepting attitude conveys to the client that the client is worthwhile. Trust is enhanced.	*Goal met:* Client decreases the number of and frequency of somatic complaints.
2. By [date], client identifies alternative coping behaviors.	2. Assist client to identify ways of coping, and assist in problem solving.	2. Low self-worth may interfere with client's perception of own problem-solving ability. Assistance may be required.	Client discusses beliefs in folk healing practices. Client begins to talk about alternative coping strategies.
3. By [date], client verbalizes feeling of shame and understanding of her diagnosed mental illness.	3. Demonstrate acceptance and understanding of cultural norms regarding the shame of mental illness.	3. Acceptance of client's beliefs and values enhances feelings of self-worth and decreases feelings of shame.	Client verbalizes awareness of own coping abilities. Client participates in all activities.
4. By [date], client identifies functional support systems.	4. Explore, with client and family, cultural folk practices for healing—those known about and/or those tried by the client.	4. Knowledge of client's cultural beliefs allows the nurse to deliver culture-specific care.	
5. By [date], client voluntarily spends time with other clients on unit.	5. Reinforce appropriate behaviors.	5. Positive reinforcement enhances self-esteem and encourages repetition of desirable behaviors.	

ment, nursing diagnosis, planning, implementation, and evaluation. Through the use of the nursing process, clients are helped to communicate their needs and to cope. Boyle and Andrews (1989) identified five purposes for focusing on cultural concepts in nursing practice, as follows:

1. To identify cultural needs
2. To understand the cultural context of the client and family
3. To use culture-sensitive nursing strategies to meet mutual goals
4. To have the skills to use the resources of a variety of cultural subsystems within the community
5. To have the ability to learn from and respond to culturally diverse situations

The major purpose of the collection of cultural data is to gain greater insight into the nature and behavior of clients and the problems they encounter in health promotion. Strategies for coping with illness are also more relevant and focus on cultural aspects (Boyle & Andrews, 1989). The nursing diagnosis should be a statement that accurately reflects the client's health state. Plans are made and implemented, mutually derived goals are determined, and significant others included when appropriate. Precise behavioral objectives provide a basis for subsequent evaluation of what was done or what will be done, who will do it, and when the goal will be accomplished.

Although cultural information should be included during the assessment phase so that a culturally relevant and accurate diagnosis can be made, cultural data are

Nursing Care Plan 3-2 The Client with Schizophrenia (Mr. Enrique)

► **Nursing Diagnosis:** Sensory-Perceptual Alterations related to visual and auditory distortions

► Mr. Enrique, a 39-year-old married man living with his wife and three children, is an unskilled laborer who has not worked for 9 years because he could not perform his duties. He was diagnosed as emotionally disturbed and is on disability insurance. He has deteriorated over the past 6 months and is now hospitalized with a diagnosis of schizophrenia. During the psychiatric interview, he admitted to "seeing and hearing things," reported having severe insomnia, and requested medication to sleep. During the interview he admitted seeing *calojes*, which are animals (souls), and he expressed fear that they are after him.

OUTCOME IDENTIFICATION	NURSING ACTIONS	RATIONALES	EVALUATION
1. By [date], client will demonstrate accurate perception of the environment by responding appropriately to stimuli.	1. Frequently orient client to reality and surroundings.	1. Client safety is jeopardized during periods of disorientation.	*Goal met:* Client demonstrates accurate perception of the environment.
2. Client will discuss content of hallucinations within [date].	2. Use simple explanations and face-to-face interactions when communicating with patient.	2. Face-to-face communication is most effective in dealing with client experiencing perceptual distortions. Simple explanations allow the client to focus on one idea at a time.	Client is able to verbalize ways in which to correct inaccurate perceptions and restore reality to the situation. Client is able to refrain from responding to false sensory perceptions.
3. Client will be able to define and test reality, eliminating sensory misperceptions by [date].	3. Give positive feedback when thinking and behavior are clear; do not negate cultural belief.	3. Positive reinforcement enhances self-esteem and encourages repetition of desirable behaviors.	

Nursing Care Plan 3-3 The Client with Anxiety (Maria)

▶ **Nursing Diagnosis:** Self-Esteem Disturbance

▶ Maria, a 21-year-old Hispanic American, has recently become withdrawn and quieter than usual. She has been crying frequently and has begun talking to herself. She states, "I want to die." A year ago her boyfriend rejected her. Her parents are older and more traditional. When they first noticed her change in behavior, particularly washing her hands excessively, they thought she might have a hex (*mal puesto*) and took her to a *curandera* to have it removed. As her symptoms progressed, she was admitted to an inpatient psychiatric unit.

OUTCOME IDENTIFICATION	NURSING ACTIONS	RATIONALES	EVALUATION
1. By [date], client will verbalize feelings of self-worth.	1. Spend time with client to establish trusting relationship.	1. Trust enhances therapeutic interaction.	*Goal met:* Client expresses feeling of self-worth.
2. By [date], client will identify alternative coping strategies.	2. Develop an understanding of clients cultural beliefs about folk medicine and folk practices.	2. Patient may be unaware of the relationship between physical symptoms and emotional problems.	Client has decreased number of somatic complaints. Client discusses cultural beliefs about folk medicine.
3. By [date], client will identify functional support systems.	3. Refer client and family to community support group from same culture.	3. An accepting attitude conveys to client that you respect his or her cultural beliefs.	Client begins to talk about coping strategies that have worked in the past.
4. By [date], client will verbalize a desire to live.	4. Assess for plan to self-harm. Provide a safe environment.	4. Patient safety is a nursing priority.	Client able to demonstrate adaptive coping techniques that enhance self-worth. Client verbalizes will not harm self.

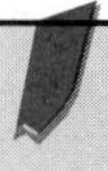

Nursing Care Plan 3-4 The Client with Schizoaffective Disorder (Mr. Williams)

► **Nursing Diagnosis:** Self-Esteem Disturbance

► Mr. Williams, a 32-year-old married African American man, was admitted to an inpatient psychiatric unit. He was tearful and distraught and reported suicidal ideation. He also reported accusatory auditory hallucinations, and he had used alcohol before admission. A substance abuse history was obtained. Client began drinking at age 13 to be "just like dad." He has a prior history of disorderly conduct, and his family has given up on him. His wife has just given birth to a son, and he fears that he can't be a good father. He was given a diagnosis of schizoaffective disorder.

OUTCOME IDENTIFICATION	NURSING ACTIONS	RATIONALES	EVALUATION
1. By [date], client will discuss fear of failure.	1. Encourage client to verbalize fears. Provide a safe environment.	1. Verbalization of fears in a nonthreatening environment may help client come to terms with long unresolved issues. Patient safety is a nursing priority.	*Goal met:* Client shows positive expressions and reactions to culture-specific nursing interventions. Client able to verbalize adaptive coping strategies to use in place of substances. Client able to verbalize support people from whom to seek help when strong urge for substance abuse occurs.
2. By [date], client will exhibit increased feelings of self-worth by setting realistic goals.	2. Assist client to focus on positive aspects of self.	2. Low self-worth may interfere with client's perception of self. Assistance may be required.	
3. By [date], client will exhibit increased feelings of self-worth by making positive statements about himself.	3. Assign client to work with a therapist from same culture, preferably an African American man.	3. The therapist from the same culture and gender may enhance the client's feelings of acceptance and self-worth.	
4. By [date], client verbalizes need for help regarding substance abuse.	4. Explore with client community resources to learn parenting skills.	4. Community resources and support groups may be necessary to maintain self-esteem.	

► TABLE 3–3
Guidelines for Psychiatric Nursing Interventions in a Cultural Context

1. Understand your own cultural values and biases.
2. Acquire a basic knowledge of cultural values, health beliefs, and practices of cultural groups you routinely serve.
3. Be respectful of, interested in, and understanding of other cultures without being judgmental.
4. Establish rapport, and show a genuine concern for the client.
5. Ask questions in several ways to cross-check on the information obtained.
6. Adjust the style of the interaction to complement the differences in age between yourself and the client.
   a. Adopt a serious, respectful attitude toward elderly clients.
   b. Make a special effort to be informal when working with young clients.
7. Use open-ended questions rather than those that elicit yes or no responses.
8. Ask the client how he or she prefers to be addressed.
9. Avoid slang, technical jargon, and complex sentences.
10. Build on cultural practices, reinforcing those that are positive and promoting change only in those that are harmful.

important at all phases of the nursing process. As nurses become more experienced in dealing with clients from various cultures, they become cognitively aware of cultural influences on mental illness and develop acceptable ways to approach problems in a particular cultural group. Table 3–3 outlines some guidelines for psychiatric nursing interventions in a cultural context.

The accompanying Nursing Care Plans provide examples of how to provide nursing care in a cultural context among diverse cultural groups.

► CHAPTER SUMMARY

Cultural patterns associated with ethnic heritage often guide the client in determining how to express distress, when to seek help, and from whom to seek help. In many cultural groups, the family is an important point of reference as a microcosm of cultural heritage and identity.

Presenting problems need to be understood, diagnosed, and treated with knowledge of the cultural context of the person seeking help. Nursing's role includes collecting cultural data, making culture-specific nursing diagnoses, planning appropriate care, and evaluating interventions based on knowledge of the client's culture.

Cultural knowledge needs to be used to augment, clarify, explain, and assist the nurse in attaining client goals. Collecting information about the client's cultural background allows the psychiatric nurse to modify planned interventions to meet the client's needs.

Suggestions for Clinical Conferences

1. Discuss the way that culture influences the definition, form, and incidence of socially deviant behavior. Give examples to illustrate.
2. Discuss the meaning of the term *culture-bound syndrome,* and give examples of this condition. Support answers with appropriate citation of sources in the literature.
3. In the study of culture, it is important to differentiate among the concepts of culture, race, and ethnicity. Discuss these concepts and their implications for nursing practice.
4. Discuss the relationship between culture and mental illness.
5. Discuss how acculturation impacts the nurse–client relationship. Cite relevant literature.

References

Albert, E. M. (1968). Values: II. Value systems. In D. L. Sills (Ed.), *International encyclopedia for the social sciences.* New York: Macmillan/Free Press.

Allen, J. J., Rack, P. H., & Vaddadi, K. S. (1977). Differences in effects of clomipramine on English and Asian volunteers. *Postgraduate Medical Journal, 4,* 79–86.

Allen, P., Rack, P. H., & Vaddadi, K. S. (1980). Ethnic differences in drug response. *Postgraduate Medicine Journal, 1,* 46–49.

American Psychiatric Association. (1994). *Diagnostic and statistical manual of mental disorders* (4th ed.): Washington, DC: Author.

Avery, C. (1991). Native-American medicine: Traditional healing. *Journal of the American Medical Association, 265*(17), 2271–2273.

Baker, F. M. (1988). Afro-Americans. In L. Comas-Diaz & E. H. Griffith (Eds.), *Clinical guidelines in cross cultural mental health.* New York: John Wiley & Sons.

Baker, F. M. (1987). The Afro-American life cycle: Success, failure, and mental illness. *Journal of the National Medical Association, 79*(6), 625–633.

Bell, C. C., & Mehta, H. (1979). Misdiagnosis of black patients with manic-depressive illness: I. *Journal of the National Medical Association, 72,* 141–145.

Bell, C. C., & Mehta, H. (1981). Misdiagnosis of black patients with manic-depressive illness: II. *Journal of the National Medical Association, 73,* 101–107.

Benedict, R. (1934). *Patterns of culture.* New York: Mentor Books.

Biehler, R. (1981). *Child development: An introduction.* Boston: Houghton Mifflin.

Boyle, J. S., & Andrews, M. M. (1989). *Transcultural concepts in nursing.* Glenview, IL: Little, Brown.

Brod, T. (1975). Alcoholism as a mental health problem of Native-Americans. *Archives of General Psychiatry, 32,* 1385–1391.

Bullough, V. L., & Bullough, B. (1982). *Health care for other Americans.* New York: Appleton-Century-Crofts.

Bullough, B., & Bullough, V. L. (1972). *Poverty, ethnic identity, and health care.* New York: Appleton-Century-Crofts.

Burnside, I. (1988). *Nursing the aged* (3rd ed.). New York: McGraw-Hill.

Campinha-Bacote, J. (1991). Community mental health services for the underserved: A culturally specific model. *Archives of Psychiatric Nursing, 5*(4), 229–235.

Cancro, R. (1982). The role of genetic factors in the etiology of schizophrenia disorders. In L. Grinspoon (Ed.), *Psychiatry 1982: Annual review.* Washington, DC: American Psychiatric Press.

Canino, G., & Canino, A. I. (1982). Culturally syntonic family therapy for migrant Puerto Ricans. *Hospital and Community Psychiatry, 33*(4), 299–303.

Chang, K. (1991). Chinese Americans. In J. N. Giger & R. E. Davidhizar (Eds.), *Transcultural nursing: Assessment and intervention* (pp. 359–377). St. Louis: C. V. Mosby.

Comas-Diaz, L., & Duncan, J. W. (1985). The cultural context: A factor in assertiveness training with mainland Puerto Rican women. *Psychology of Women Quarterly, 9*(4), 463–475.

Drotar, D. (Ed.). (1985). *New directions in failure to thrive implications for research and practice.* New York: Plenum Press.

Erikson, E. (1963). *Childhood and society* (2nd ed.). New York: W. W. Norton.

Falicov, C. J. (1982). Mexican families. In M. McGoldrick, J. Pearce, & J. Giordano (Eds.), *Ethnicity and family therapy* (pp. 134–163). New York: Guilford Press.

Falicov, C. J., & Karrer, A. (1980). Cultural variations in the family life cycle: The Mexican-American family. In Carter & M. McGoldrick (Eds.), *The family life cycle: A Framework for family therapy.* New York: Gardner Press.

Flaskerud, J. (1989). Transcultural concepts in mental health nursing. In J. S. Boyle & M. M. Andrews (Eds.), *Transcultural concepts in nursing care.* Glenview, IL: Scott, Foresman.

Fong, C. (1985). Ethnicity and nursing practice. *Topics in Clinical Nursing, 7*(3), 1–10.

Foster, S. W. (1990). The pragmatics of culture: The rhetoric of difference in psychiatric nursing. *Archives of Psychiatric Nursing, 4*(5), 292–297.

Fox, P. G. (1991). Stress related to family change among Vietnamese refugees. *Journal of Community Health Nursing, 8*(1), 45–56.

Garcia-Preto, N. (1982). Puerto Rican families. In M. McGoldrick, J. Pearce, & J. Giordano (Eds.), *Ethnicity and family therapy* (pp. 164–186). New York: Guilford Press.

Gibson, M., & Ogbu, J. (Eds.) (1991). *Minority status and schooling: A comparative study of immigrants and involuntary minorities.* New York: Garland Press.

Giger, J. N., & Davidhizer, R. E. (1991). *Transcultural nursing.* St. Louis: C. V. Mosby.

Giordano, J. (1973). *Ethnicity and mental health.* New York: Institute of Pluralism and Group Identity.

Giordano, J., & Giordano, J. P. (1977). *The ethno-cultural factor in mental health: A literature review and bibliography.* New York: Institute on Pluralism and Group Identity.

Gold, P. W., Goodwin, F. K., & Chrousos, G. P. (1988a). Clinical and biochemical manifestations of depression: I. Relation to the biology of stress. *New England Journal of Medicine, 319*(6), 348–353.

Gold, P. W., Goodwin, F. K., & Chrousos, G. P. (1988b). Clinical and biochemical manifestations of depression: II. Relation to the biology of stress. *New England Journal of Medicine, 319*(7), 413–420.

Gomez, G. E., & Gomez, E. A. (1985). Folk healing among Hispanic Americans. *Public Health Nursing, 2*(4), 245–249.

Hogstel, M. O. (1990). *Geropsychiatric nursing.* St. Louis: C. V. Mosby.

Holland, W. (1978). Mexican-American medical beliefs. In R. Martinez (Ed.), *Hispanic culture and health care: Fact, fiction, folklore.* St. Louis: C. V. Mosby.

Jenkins, J. H. (1988). Ethnopsychiatric interpretations of schizophrenic illness: The problem of nervios within Mexican-American families. *Culture, Medicine and Psychiatry, 12,* 301–329.

Jones, B. E., & Gray, M. A. (1986). Problems in diagnosing schizophrenia and affective disorders among Blacks. *Hospital and Community Psychiatry, 37*(1), 61–65.

Kermis, M. D. (1986). *Mental health in late life: An adoptive process.* Boston: Jones & Bartlett.

Kiev, A. (1968). *Curanderismo: Mexican-American folk psychiatry.* New York: Free Press.

Kiev, A. (1972). *Transcultural psychiatry.* New York: Free Press.

Kleinman, A. (1980). *Patients and healers in the context of culture.* Berkeley: University of California Press.

Kleinman, A. (1982). Neurasthenia and depression: A study in somatization and culture in China. *Culture and Medicine Psychiatry, 6,* 117–190.

Kleinman, A. M., Eisenberg, L., & Good, B. (1978). Culture, illness, and care: Clinical lessons from anthropologic and cross-cultural research. *Annals of Internal Medicine, 88,* 251–258.

Kluckhohn, F. R., & Strodtbeck, F. (1961). *Variation in value orientations.* New York: Row and Patterson.

Kraepelin, E. (1906). *Lectures on clinical psychiatry.* London: Baillierie, Tindall & Cox. (Thomas Johnson translation).

Lawson, W. B. (1986). Racial and ethnic factors in psychiatric research. *Hospital and Community Psychiatry, 37,* 50–54.

Lefley, H. (1990). Culture and chronic mental illness. *Hospital and Community Psychiatry, 41*(3), 277–286.

Leininger, M. (Ed.). (1979). *Transcultural nursing.* New York: Masson International Nursing Publications.

Liberman, Marshall, B. D., Marder, S. R., Dawson, M. E., Nuechterlein, K. H., & Doane, J. A. (1984). The nature and problem of schizophrenia. In A. S. Bellack (Ed.), *Schizophrenia: Treatment, management and rehabilitation.* Orlando: Grune and Stratton.

Lin, K., Poland, R. E., & Lesser, I. M. (1986). Ethnicity and pharmacology. *Culture, Medicine and Psychiatry, 10,* 151–165.

Lin, K. M., & Finder, E. (1983). Neuroleptic dosages for Asians. *American Journal of Psychiatry, 140,* 490–491.

Lin, L. E., Carter, U. B., & Klienman, A. M. (1985). An exploration of somatization among Asian refugees and immigrants in primary care. *American Journal of Public Health, 75,* 1080–1084.

Lin, T. Y. (1983). Psychiatry and Chinese culture. *Western Journal of Medicine, 139*(6), 58–63.

Louie, K. B. (1985). Providing health care to Chinese clients. *Topics in Clinical Nursing, 7*(3), 18–25.

Marcos, L. R., & Cancro, R. (1982). Pharmacotherapy of Hispanic depressed patients: Clinical observations. *American Journal of Psychotherapy, 36*(4), 505–512.

Martinez, C. (1988). Mexican-Americans. In L. C. Comos-Diaz & E. H. Griffith (Eds.), *Cross-cultural mental health.* New York: John Wiley.

Martinez, R. A. (1978). *Hispanic culture and health care: Fact, fiction, folklore.* St. Louis: C. V. Mosby.

Masden, W. (1969). Mexican Americans and Anglo Americans: A comparative study of mental health in Texas. In S. C. Ploa & R. B. Edgerton (Eds.), *Changing perspectives in mental illness.* New York: Rinehart & Winston.

May, P. (1988a). *An annotated bibliography of American Indian suicide.* Rockville, MD: Indian Health Service.

May, P. (1988b). Mental health and alcohol abuse indications of Indian Health in the Albuquerque area. *American-Indian Alaska-Native Mental Health Service Review, 2,* 33–46.

McEnany, G. W. (1991). Psychobiology and psychiatric nursing: A philosophic matrix. *Archives of Psychiatric Nursing, 5*(5), 255–261.

McGoldrick, M., Pearce, J., & Giordano, J. (1982). Ethnicity and family therapy: An overview. In *Ethnicity and family therapy* (pp. 3–30). New York: Guilford Press.

Mead, M. (1928). *Coming of age in Samoa.* New York: William Morrow.

Mead, M. (1934). *Sex and temperament in three primitive societies.* New York: Mentor Books (Reprint).

Neligh, G. (1990, Summer). *Mental health programs for American Indians: Their logic, structure, and function.* National Center for American Indian/Alaska Native Mental Health Research.

Nelson, S., McCoy, G., Stetter, M., & Vondenwager, W. (1992). An overview of mental health services for American Indians and Alaska natives in the 1990's. *Hospital and Community Psychiatry, 43*(3), 257–261.

Orque, M., Block, D., & Monrroy, L. S. (1983). *Ethnic nursing care.* St. Louis: C. V. Mosby.

Ramos-McKay, J., Comas-Diaz, L. C., & Rivera, L. A. (1988). Puerto Ricans. In L. C. Comos-Diaz, & E. H. Griffith (Eds.), *Cross-cultural mental health.* New York: John Wiley.

Reynolds, G. P. (1989). Beyond the dopamine hypothesis. *British Journal of Psychiatry, 155,* 305–316.

Rogler, L. H., & Malgady, R. G. (1987). What do culturally sensitive mental health services mean? *American Psychologist, 42*(6), 565–570.

Root, M. P. (1985). Guideline for facilitating therapy with Asian-American clients. *Psychotherapy, 22*(21), 349–355.

Rosenbaum, J. N. (1989). Depression: Viewed from a transcultural nursing theoretical perspective. *Journal of Advanced Nursing, 14*(7), 7–12.

Rotunno, M., & McGoldrick, M. (1982). Italian families. In M. McGoldrick, J. Pearce, & J. Giordano (Eds.), *Ethnicity and family therapy* (pp. 340–363). New York: Guilford Press.

Rudorfer, M. V., Lane, E. A., Chang, W. H., Zhang, M., & Potter, W. Z. (1984). Desipramine pharmacokinetics in Chinese and Caucasian volunteers. *British Journal of Clinical Pharmacology, 17,* 433–440.

Rudorfer, M. V., & Robbins, E. (1982). Amitriptyline overdose: Clinical effects on tricyclic antidepressant plasma levels. *Journal of Clinical Psychiatry, 43,* 457–460.

Schusky, E. L., & Culbert, T. P. (1978). *Introducing culture* (3rd ed.). Englewood Cliffs, NJ: Prentice Hall.

Stewart, B. (1991). A staff development workshop on cultural diversity. *Journal of Nursing Staff Development, 7*(4), 6–9.

Sue, S. (1988). Psychotherapeutic services for ethnic minorities. *American Psychologist, 43*(4), 301–308.

Sue, S., & McKinney, H. (1975). Asian Americans in the community health care system. *American Journal of Orthopsychiatry, 41,* 111–118.

Sue, S., & Morishima, J. K. (1982). *The mental health of Asian Americans.* San Francisco: Jossey-Bass.

Tharp, R. G. (1991). Cultural diversity and treatment of children. *Journal of Consulting and Clinical Psychology, 59*(6), 799–812.

Townsend, M. C. (1991). *Nursing diagnosis for psychiatric nursing: A pocket guide for care plan construction* (2nd ed.). Philadelphia: F. A. Davis.

Tripp-Reimer, T. (1984). Cultural assessment. In J. P. Bellock & P. A. Bamford (Eds.), *Nursing assessment: A multidimensional approach.* Monterey, CA: Wadsworth.

Tripp-Reimer, T., & Afifi, L. A. (1989). Cross-cultural perspective on patient teaching. *Nursing Clinics of North America, 24*(3), 613–618.

Tsai, M., Teng, L. N., & Sue, S. (1980). Mental status of Chinese in the United States. In A. Kleinman & T. Y. Lin (Eds.), *Normal and deviant behavior in Chinese culture.* Hingham, MA: Reidel Press.

Weisz, J. R., Suwanlert, S., Chaiyasit, W., Weiss, B., Achenbach, T. M., & Walter, B. R. (1987). Epidemiology of behavioral and emotional problems among Thai and American Children. *Journal of the American Academy of Child and Adolescent Psychiatry, 26,* 890–897.

Yang, Y. Y. (1985). Prophylactic efficacy of lithium and its effective plasma levels in Chinese bipolar patients. *Acta Psychiatrica Scandinavia, 71,* 171–175.

CHAPTER

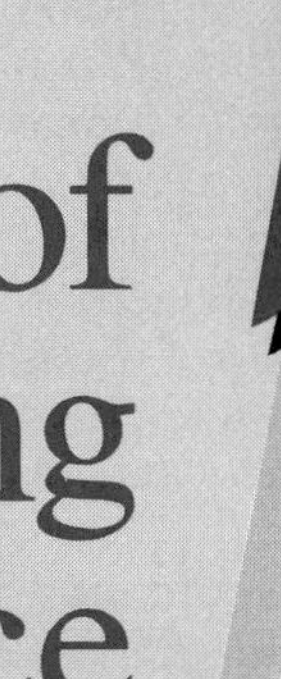

Foundations of Psychiatric Nursing Practice

DEBORAH ANTAI-OTONG, M.S., R.N.,C.S.

OUTLINE

Mental Health Promotion: An Integral Aspect of Psychiatric Nursing
- Primary Prevention
- Secondary Prevention
- Tertiary Prevention

The Impact of Stress on Client Response
- Stress and Mental Illness
- Neurobiological and Behavioral Responses to Stress
- Determinants of Response to Stress

Life Span Issues: Stress and the Developmental Process

Essential Qualities of the Psychiatric Nurse
- Therapeutic Use of Self
- Genuineness and Warmth
- Empathy
- Acceptance
- Maturity and Self-Awareness
- Leadership

The Psychiatric Nurse as a Member of the Mental Health Team
- Generalist and Advanced-Practice Roles
- The Role of the Psychiatric Nurse Today
- Future Trends
- The Mental Health Team

Using the Nursing Process in Psychiatric Settings
- Factors Determining the Effectiveness of the Nursing Process
- The Nursing Process and Standards of Care

Chapter Summary

CHAPTER OBJECTIVES

Upon completion of this chapter, you will be able to:

1. Analyze the role of nurses in primary, secondary, and tertiary prevention.
2. Define the collaborative process between nurses and clients.
3. Identify essential qualities of psychiatric–mental health nurses.
4. Discuss the significance of empathy.
5. Describe the roles of mental health team members.

KEY TERMS

Collaboration
Empathy
Empowerment
Mental health team
Primary prevention
Secondary prevention
Self-awareness
Stress
Tertiary prevention

Psychiatric nursing has evolved over the past decade in tandem with socioeconomic changes and neurobiological discoveries. Nurses are actively involved in integrating these changes into their practice and research endeavors. Linking mental illness with brain function and psychosocial factors is complex and requires an appreciation of genetic, endocrine, and immunological factors that affect client responses. The complexity of mental illness challenges psychiatric nurses to understand and integrate neurobiological processes into interventions that restore and maintain health.

Health promotion is a major domain of psychiatric nursing and includes assessment of client strengths and reinforcement of adaptive responses. Activities that facilitate this process include health teaching, stress management, and crisis intervention.

This chapter discusses the major concepts of psychiatric nursing that include mental health promotion, stress and adaptation, life span factors, therapeutic use of self, **collaboration**, and the nursing process.

MENTAL HEALTH PROMOTION: AN INTEGRAL ASPECT OF PSYCHIATRIC NURSING

Promoting mental health is a major goal of psychiatric nurses. *Mental health* refers to an adaptation to distress by mobilizing internal and external resources to minimize tension. The mentally healthy client is independent, has high self-esteem, and is able to form meaningful interpersonal relationships.

In contrast, *mental illness* refers to maladaptive responses to distress and an inability to mobilize resources. Maladaptation increases tension, and the client becomes overwhelmed. The mentally ill client is often dependent, has low self-esteem, and forms meaningful interpersonal relationships only with difficulty. Recognizing adaptive and maladaptive coping patterns is crucial to health promotion, because nurses can intervene appropriately to minimize the deleterious effects of mental illness.

Health promotion and prevention must begin as early as the prenatal period and continue through older adulthood. Preventive measures need to foster a sense of well-being and self-actualization throughout the life span. Specific interventions may include education, stress management in children and adolescents, parenting classes, and assisting older adults in adjusting to retirement (WHO, 1986).

As psychiatric nurses move into the twenty-first century, they will be faced with enormous opportunities to identify and care for clients at risk for mental illness. High-risk groups include the elderly poor, those with acquired immune deficiency syndrome (AIDS)-related illnesses, substance abusers, and victims of violence. Unemployment, homelessness, and disintegration of families also increase vulnerability to mental illness. Societal stressors, coupled with a lack of adequate access to health care, further compromise and increase the risk of mental illness (ANA, 1991a). Psychiatric nurses are challenged to respond to tremendous societal demands, identify vulnerable populations, and collaborate with clients, families, and mental health professionals to mobilize resources that promote health.

TABLE 4–1
Populations at Risk for Mental Illness

- Those with familial or genetic predisposition to mental illness, such as clients with a family history of affective or mood disorders and schizophrenia
- Those with poor access to health care
- Those disadvantaged, i.e., homeless and poor
- Those undergoing significant lifestyle changes, i.e., pregnant adolescent
- Those misusing substances
- Victims of violence
- Elderly poor

The role of psychiatric nursing continues to parallel compelling changes in client populations, socioeconomic trends, neurobiological advances, and health care reform. Identifying clients at risk (Table 4–1) and providing early interventions are major nursing goals.

Sweeping societal changes and health care reforms demand a new way of caring for the mentally ill. An increasing number of mentally ill clients are being discharged after shorter inpatient stays into communities with inadequate services. A number of these clients become homeless, substance abusers, and victims of crime. Treatment often consists of "Band Aid" approaches provided in emergency departments and community shelters. Psychiatric nurses can adjust to these changes by collaborating with clients, mental health professionals, and community service workers to create innovative treatment modalities and outcomes. Preventive measures must be a major aspect of outcomes and interventions. Three areas of prevention are advocated in caring for mentally ill clients: primary, secondary, and tertiary.

PRIMARY PREVENTION

Primary prevention is the first stage of care, and it involves using measures that prevent mental illness and provide cost-effective interventions. These interventions are used to counteract circumstances or conditions that are potentially harmful. They generate coping skills and other measures that reduce vulnerability to illness and promote health (Caplan, 1964).

During the past decade, there has been a resurgence of interest in prevention by the World Health Organization (WHO, 1988). This organization identified an agenda of "Health for All—2000" that calls for measures to prevent mental, neurological, and psychosocial disorders. Areas of interest include protecting the developing brain, minimizing predisposition to illness, and increasing resistance to disease (Cooper, 1990, Dupont, 1989; WHO, 1987).

Psychiatric nurses can incorporate primary prevention measures into practice initially by identifying persons at risk and, later, by reinforcing existing adaptive coping responses. Interventions that protect the developing brain include genetic counseling, maternal immunization against rubella, and prenatal and parenting classes. Parenting classes need to focus on child rearing, the importance of early immunization, and proper nutrition for nursing mothers and children.

Education is a key component of primary prevention, and it can be used to minimize predisposition to illness and increase resistance to disease. Teaching prospective parents to avoid prolonged separation, child abuse, and battering is an example of primary prevention. Other teaching measures include educating families about the acute and long-term effects of substance abuse, the risks of sexually transmitted diseases, problem solving and conflict resolution skills, and the importance of wearing protective head gear (when riding bicycles) and seat belts (in cars) to minimize head trauma.

Overall, nurses can use primary preventive measures to collaborate with clients and families and to promote adaptive coping measures that minimize the risk of mental illness Furthermore, these measures must be culturally sensitive and congruent with the client's belief system. When clients do not respond to primary preventive interventions, symptoms of mental illness are likely to evolve and require aggressive treatment.

SECONDARY PREVENTION

Secondary prevention is the second stage in which measures are used to curtail disease processes. They focus on early detection, case finding, and priority interventions (WHO, 1980). Psychiatric nurses participate in this process by assessing the nature and degree of client response, identifying available resources, and implementing measures that reduce symptoms and mobilize adaptive coping responses. Collaboration with clients, families, and other mental health professionals is also a crucial part of secondary prevention.

Case management is a good example of secondary prevention. Psychiatric–mental health nurses can use this comprehensive approach to support client strengths, facilitate the highest level of functioning, and facilitate growth toward optimal health. Additionally, it can be used to provide supportive therapy and to monitor client responses to medication and other interventions. Case management can be used in both inpatient and outpatient settings to provide continuity of care (ANA, 1994).

The following interventions are also examples of how case management can be used to establish secondary prevention:

- Medication maintenance
- Education
- Crisis intervention
- Screening for early detection of developmental and emotional disturbances in childhood and adolescent populations
- Screening for cognitive and affective disorders in older adult populations

Once client symptoms are identified and interventions are initiated, treatment focuses on minimizing long-term disability.

TERTIARY PREVENTION

Tertiary prevention is the third stage of prevention, and measures are used to minimize relapse and chronic disability and to restore clients to their optimal level of function. Adaptation, restoration, reintegration, and aftercare are major components of tertiary prevention. Nursing interventions involve promoting an understanding of the impact of stress, medication compliance, and maladaptive responses on mental illness. These measures include stress management, education, relapse prevention, crisis intervention, fostering of adaptive coping behaviors, and reinforcement of client strengths.

In summary, primary, secondary, and tertiary prevention are the foundation of health promotion. The processes involve identifying high-risk groups, intervening when maladaptive responses are identified, and minimizing the deleterious effects of mental illness.

THE IMPACT OF STRESS ON CLIENT RESPONSE

STRESS AND MENTAL ILLNESS

The link between stress and mental illness remains a mystery despite enormous technological discoveries concerning the brain. Early theorists sought to define stress as the basis of adaptive responses and a part of human existence. Stress remains a vital part of adaptation, and its relationship to mental illness continues to bewilder clients and clinicians.

Stress refers to a stimulus or demand that generates disruption in homeostasis or produces a reaction. A stressor is a source of stress. Stress can produce adaptive and maladaptive responses. Studying for a test, contesting a divorce, winning a lottery, and having a baby are examples of stressful situations. Psychosocial stress is usually created by unexpected or unusual occurrences, whereas neurobiological stress may be caused by disturbances in biochemical processes (see Chapter 7 for a more detailed discussion of stress).

Hospitalization and other forms of treatment place enormous stress on clients. They are often forced to comply with unfamiliar daily routines, such as when to eat, sleep, and bathe. Treatments such as electroconvulsive therapy and medications pose the risk of adverse reactions and increase feelings of helplessness, loss of control, fear, and frustration. Nurses must be sensitive to these reactions and assist the client in coping with them. Exploring the meaning of various responses helps clients and nurses develop effective interventions that reduce stress.

NEUROBIOLOGICAL AND BEHAVIORAL RESPONSES TO STRESS

Stress is manifested by neurobiological and behavioral responses. Neurobiological responses to stress include activation of the hypothalamus-pituitary-adrenal (HPA) axis, which arouses the autonomic nervous system (see Fig. 11–1 in Chapter 11). Stimulation of the autonomic nervous system prepares the person for "fight or flight." Physical manifestations of stress include increased heart and respiratory rates, increased visual acuity, and diaphoresis. Behavioral responses are determined by the client's repertoire of coping skills and may include anger, uncooperativeness, or perceptual and sensory disturbances. What determines how one responds to stress?

DETERMINANTS OF RESPONSE TO STRESS

Response to stress is influenced by internal and external resources. Internal resources include personality traits, coping patterns, and biological processes. External resources include the number and severity of stressors and social support.

Internal Resources. Personality traits determine a person's appraisal of events, self-esteem, tolerance to stress, and ability to form meaningful relationships.

Coping patterns may be short-term or long-term. Short-term patterns reduce stress to a tolerable level. Examples include the person who takes alprazolam (Xanax) prior to a presentation or drinks after a heated argument. Long-term patterns refer to behaviors that relieve stress for an extended period. An example is the husband who seeks treatment for substance abuse and participates in an aftercare program to maintain abstinence.

Biological responses to stress are determined by the person's cognitive processes, genetic predisposition, developmental stage, and biochemical processes that influence the appraisal of an event. One person's stress may be uneventful to another. Primary appraisal is based on cognitive processes that determine how one is able to manage it (Lazarus, 1966). When a situation is appraised as threatening, the usual responses are anxiety, fear, anger, agitation, or denial. Threatening situations generally stimulate the HPA axis, which is equivalent to autonomic nervous system arousal. Neuroendocrine processes are mobilized to maintain biological stability or homeostasis. Secondary appraisal involves exploring available resources and options for coping with the event (Lazarus, 1966).

External Resources. Support systems are essential components in the successful resolution of stress. They are defined as close relationships with others that foster support, protection, and self-reliance during stressful periods. The quality of these relationships influences susceptibility to maladaptive responses and buffers people against distress.

Managing stress is a complex process that involves mobilizing internal and external resources. Overall, the impact of stressors on human behavior is determined by a person's ability to use a repertoire of adaptive coping skills to maintain homeostasis or equilibrium. The following clinical examples demonstrate cognitive appraisal and biological responses.

Clinical Example: The Client with Agoraphobia

John is afraid of open spaces and crowds. His psychological appraisal of these situations is that they are frightening and threatening. His biological responses include increased heart rate, shortness of breath, diaphoresis, dry mouth, lightheadedness, and bouts of confusion. Behavioral responses are avoidance of crowds, social isolation, and possibly suicidal gestures. John seeks psychiatric therapy for agoraphobia. Treatment strategies include biological intervention with a benzodiazepine, such as lorazepam, and psychotherapeutic interventions, including cognitive therapy and desensitization.

Clinical Example: The Client with an Adjustment Disorder with Depressed Mood

Marsha's cognitive appraisal of the event of divorce is failure and uncertainty about the future and her family's reaction to it. Her biological responses include depressed mood, loss of appetite, and decreased energy and motivation, and her behavioral responses include social isolation, irritability, and agitation. She seeks crisis intervention at a local woman's center. She mobilizes her support systems by her professional contacts and by talking to friends and family who validate, support, and accept her feelings and decisions. She focuses on her strengths, and her self-esteem increases. This case shows the importance of support systems during stressful events.

LIFE SPAN ISSUES: STRESS AND THE DEVELOPMENTAL PROCESS

Human beings are constantly interacting with their internal and external environments to maintain homeostasis. Development is a major part of this process because of its potential for modifying and changing behavior. As the person develops, certain patterns of organization occur, namely, developmental stages. These stages are predetermined by genetic, neurobiological, and psychosocial factors. They determine how one's needs are met, and they lay the foundation for adaptive processes.

Stress plays a crucial role in the developmental process, because each stage requires adequate coping skills to master age-specific tasks that prepare for subsequent stages. A repertoire of adaptive coping behaviors is vital to mastering developmental tasks, and failure to achieve it usually triggers or precipitates illness or maladaptive responses. For example, the infant who fails to master trust is at risk of developing poor self-esteem and may have problems forming meaningful relationships throughout the life span. In contrast, the infant who has loving parents and masters trust is likely to have high self-esteem and develop meaningful relationships in adult life.

In summary, development is a dynamic process that places enormous stress on people. The potential for growth and maturity is determined by the available resources and adaptive coping skills that foster mastery of age-specific tasks (see Chapter 7 for a more detailed discussion of stress across the life span).

ESSENTIAL QUALITIES OF THE PSYCHIATRIC NURSE

Psychiatric nurses have the unique role of helping clients in distress. Continuous care and monitoring of client responses enable nurses to provide distinct psychiatric interventions. This unique role allows the nurse to assess client response to stressful situations. Distressed clients may use adaptive or maladaptive behaviors to reduce tension. Assessing their needs compels nurses to understand the role of neurobiological, psychosocial, and behavioral variables on human response. This knowledge helps psychiatric nurses develop effective interventions, outcomes, and evaluations that facilitate adaptive behaviors in the mentally ill.

The foundation of client interventions, outcomes, and evaluations stems from the therapeutic relationship between the nurse and the client. The unique nature of the therapeutic relationship requires certain qualities in the nurse. The seven essential qualities include therapeutic use of self, genuineness, warmth, **empathy**, acceptance, maturity, and **self-awareness** (Table 4–2). These qualities enable nurses to assess the complex needs of the mentally ill through therapeutic relationships.

THERAPEUTIC USE OF SELF

The heart of psychiatric nursing is the therapeutic use of self. *Therapeutic use of self* refers to forming a trusting relationship that provides for the comfort, safety, and acceptance of the client. Active listening, self-awareness, mutuality, and effective communication are elements of this concept. This relationship begins when the nurse approaches the client with genuine interest and concern and continues throughout treatment. As the relationship evolves, the client feels less threatened and frequently seeks out the nurse for reassurance and support. Therapeutic relationships help clients recognize their strengths and maladaptive responses.

TABLE 4–2
Essential Qualities of Psychiatric Nurses

► Therapeutic use of self	► Acceptance
► Genuineness	► Maturity
► Warmth	► Self-awareness
► Empathy	

GENUINENESS AND WARMTH

The second and third essential qualities of psychiatric nurses are genuineness and warmth. Genuineness implies a sense of openness, realness, and a lack of defensiveness (Truax & Carkhuff, 1967), and it conveys a congruency between verbal and nonverbal behaviors in nurses and clients.

Freud (1912) stressed the curative properties of warmth, and he associated it with respect, acceptance, and positive regard for clients in distress. Warmth imparts consistency, kindness, patience, and caring for clients (Menninger, 1947). It can be conveyed only if it is genuine. Psychiatric nurses must convey genuineness and warmth as major aspects of the therapeutic use of self. These qualities are tools that foster the expression of feelings and thoughts in distressed clients. Sharing of feelings allows nurses to accurately interpret client responses.

EMPATHY

The fourth nursing quality is empathy. A number of theorists have defined empathy as a crucial aspect of therapeutic relationships. The first ones were Truax and Carkhuff (1967), who asserted that empathy occurs when the nurse successfully assumes "the internal frame of reference of the client" (p. 285) and "experiences client feelings as if they were his own" (p. 313). In other words, the nurse "walks a mile in the client's shoes" and experiences the world from his or her emotional perspective without being emerged or overwhelmed by the experience. Empathy allows nurses to perceive and communicate more accurately with clients.

The second theorist was Ehmann (1971), who defined empathy "as a means to share and experience the feelings of the patient" (pp. 75–76). Empathy is a powerful communication tool that conveys "I am with you, and I have a sense of what you are experiencing." During the empathic process, the nurse never totally loses his or her identity. The therapeutic use of empathy facilitates a deeper understanding of the client's situation while it helps the client move toward self-awareness, feelings, and their meaning (Table 4–3).

An example of empathy is noted in the following situation:

Nurse–Client Dialogue

CLIENT: I cannot talk about the rape (client begins to cry).

TABLE 4–3
Ehmann's Empathy Process: The Client Who Has Experienced Trauma (Rape)

PHASES	CHARACTERISTICS	NURSE'S BEHAVIOR
Identification	Absorption in client's situation (temporary) Allows nurse to establish a sense of similarity	Attentive to client's expression of shame and guilt after rape
Incorporation	The act of merging the client's experience with the nurse's	Imagines what the client must be going through
Reverberation	Interaction of the nurse and client experiences	Feels sadness for client; reaches out and touches client when she cries
Detachment	Separation or withdrawal of subjective involvement and resumption of one's own identity	Hands client a tissue, stating "This must be very difficult for you to talk about"

NURSE: I know this must be very difficult for you to talk about.
CLIENT: I shouldn't have gone out with Jimmy because I've never trusted him.
NURSE: It sounds like you are blaming yourself.
CLIENT: Well, who else can I blame?
NURSE: You are not responsible for what happened.

The nurse's response conveys caring and genuine concern for the client's distress. The nurse understands what she must be going through without allowing the client's overwhelming sadness to affect her.

Empathy is often confused with sympathy. Sympathy differs from empathy because it interferes with formation of therapeutic relationships. Sympathy blurs boundaries between the nurse and the client, making it difficult for each of them to distinguish his or her feelings from those of the other (Katz, 1963). Sympathy is feeling or sharing the identical concerns of another. Empathy fosters autonomy and self-care, whereas sympathy encourages dependency.

ACCEPTANCE

The fifth nursing quality is acceptance. Acceptance suggests neither approval nor disapproval but tolerance and appreciation of the client as a human being regardless of gender, culture, religion, or socioeconomic status. Client attributes are received without judgment. Therapeutic relationships use acceptance to create environments that encourage expression of feelings, thoughts, and behaviors. Acceptance and tolerance of differences in others require maturity and self-awareness, which are the sixth and seventh essential qualities of psychiatric nurses.

MATURITY AND SELF-AWARENESS

Maturity plays a major role in the nurse's ability to tolerate differences and be responsive to client needs. It also suggests that the nurse is aware of certain responses to given situations or clients that interfere with objectivity. Self-awareness of certain feelings or reactions, such as anger, protectiveness, dependency, and anxiety, helps the nurse assist clients with similar issues. Maturity and self-awareness are crucial to the promotion of client safety, comfort, and appreciation for individual attributes, capacities, and limitations.

Psychiatric–mental health nurses are confronted with the daily responsibility of assessing, intervening, and evaluating client responses to stress. Client interactions, especially those exhibiting maladaptive responses, such as demanding behavior, verbal abuse, and uncooperativeness, generate various reactions in nurses. Client responses to stress vary and include treatment modalities and hospitalization.

Psychiatric nurses need to identify the meaning of their own stress and develop strategies that increase personal and professional growth. Increased client demands, coupled with the persistent nursing shortage and uncertainty about health care reforms, increase the stress in psychiatric nurses. Increased stress often generates feelings of powerlessness and apathy. Suggested strategies include nurse support or supervision groups that create climates of empathy, caring, and opportunities to explore the meaning of specific reactions to clients and various clinical situations.

Support groups can assist nurses in the following tasks:

- Exploring the meaning of negative or overly protective reactions to specific client behaviors
- Learning how to take care of themselves by attending to their biological and psychosocial needs, both personal and professional
- Using stress reduction and progressive relaxation techniques
- Enhancing altruism among colleagues
- Developing effective problem-solving, conflict-resolution, and communication skills.

Self-awareness is the foundation of exploring nurses' reactions to specific clients and clinical situations. Nurses need to be aware of themselves in relation to others. Support or supervision groups are crucial to personal and professional growth. The complexity of mental illness and the human response to others compels psychiatric nurses to create workplace environments that help them manage stress effectively.

LEADERSHIP

On inpatient units, psychiatric nurses provide 24-hour care for clients, but their power is often minimized by themselves and others. In community-based settings, psychiatric nurses also provide direct and indirect care of clients. Leadership skills are essential in these settings because astute problem solving and decision making have immediate impact on the well-being of clients. Nurses must be supported by management and administration in developing and maintaining leadership skills that create a sense of power and pride in their contributions to the health care system. All nurses are potential leaders, regardless of their responsibilities. Leadership behaviors include empowerment, directing client care, monitoring client outcomes, and collaborating with clients and other mental health professionals.

Empowerment refers to a sense of inner strength, confidence, and self-worth. Strategies that enhance effective communication, problem solving, and conflict resolution are major areas of empowerment. Developing leadership skills must be an integral aspect of professional development, beginning with the student experience and continuing with the practice experience. Students working with clients in the psychiatric areas must be able to learn leadership behaviors from experienced nurses to develop their own sense of leadership and promote professional growth.

The role of psychiatric nurses is greatly influenced by their ability to integrate leadership skills into their practice. Building leadership skills begins in nursing school, and these skills are enhanced by clinical experiences and role models. Developing leadership skills at various levels is a mechanism for attracting the novice and retaining the experienced psychiatric nurse. As nurses move from inpatient setting to primary caregiver roles, collaboration with other mental health professional becomes more crucial to developing effective treatment. Sound leadership skills are equally important in communicating and resolving conflicts effectively.

Psychiatric nurses need to explore issues that affect them in the workplace. The ability to manage stressful situations is determined by self-esteem, confidence, and a sense of power. Survival in the workplace rests on self-awareness and the ability to use leadership skills effectively to collaborate with clients and colleagues.

THE PSYCHIATRIC NURSE AS A MEMBER OF THE MENTAL HEALTH TEAM

The concept of nursing has always existed in association with the role of caretaker, surrogate, and nurturer. Psychiatric nursing has come of age and emerged from the role of custodian or attendant from the back wards of asylums and state institutions to a role that is theory based and includes evaluating, orchestrating, and collaborating in the care of the mentally ill.

GENERALIST AND ADVANCED-PRACTICE ROLES

Changes in the role of the psychiatric nurse parallel the changes in psychiatry, and as the twenty-first century approaches, the neurobiological aspects of mental illness will receive increasing attention. The American Nurses Association (ANA, 1994) has delineated two levels of psychiatric–mental health nursing practice: basic (or generalist) and advanced practice. Roles concur with specific educational preparation, clinical experiences, specialty, and certification. The basic-level nurse is a baccalaureate-prepared registered nurse who is clinically prepared to care for clients with mental illness. Certification as a mental health nurse validates clinical competence.

In comparison, the advanced-practice registered nurse is master's or doctorally prepared in psychiatric–mental health nursing, commands the advanced knowledge and theory of mental illness needed to resolve complex mental health problems, and academically supervises graduate students (ANA, 1994).

Traditionally, psychiatric nurses have incorporated holistic concepts in the nursing process. An increased emphasis on brain function and its impact on client behavior suggests that psychiatric nurses need to redefine their roles to understand and meet the complex needs of the mentally ill. Integrating biological concepts into nursing practice does not negate the significance of psychosocial concepts, but it provides a comprehensive appreciation of clients as whole systems with complex needs.

THE ROLE OF THE PSYCHIATRIC NURSE TODAY

Psychiatric nurses are vital members of the **mental health team**. They actively direct and evaluate client responses to stress across the life span. Their continuous monitoring of clients experiencing crises further employs the nurse's input to intervene and create environments that minimize maladaptive responses and promote mental health. The impact of these interventions on client outcomes is often minimized by psychiatric nurses and other mental health professionals.

Psychiatric nurses need to appreciate their role in various mental health settings. This process can initially be accomplished by recognizing the importance of daily interventions and client responses. The agitated client who calms down after the nurse establishes trust and explains that the oral lorazepam (Ativan) will reduce irritability is an example of a frequently used psychiatric nursing intervention. Understanding the effects of benzodiazepines on the nervous system helps nurses recognize the impact of medication on client behavior. As the student nurse observes this nurse–client interaction, the student can learn about therapeutic interactions.

Student supervision is another mechanism that establishes the significance of psychiatric nurses. It helps students appreciate the specialty of psychiatric nursing while integrating certain skills into their educational process. As students recognize the importance of the nurse's place on the mental health team, they can emulate basic therapeutic interventions, such as active listening, therapeutic interactions, and effective communication and understand the complexity of mental illness.

The role of psychiatric nursing stems from its responsibility in promoting and restoring mental health. Primary prevention can be used to identify high-risk groups and provide health education. The nurse can intervene at this stage by using secondary prevention to restore health and to halt the disease process or deterioration.

Secondary prevention can be initiated during an acute phase on inpatient, emergency departments, or homeless shelters. As clients respond to interventions and health is restored, the psychiatric nurse is concerned with preventing deleterious effects of mental illness. This stage is referred to as *tertiary prevention*.

The role of the nurse in tertiary prevention is to prevent disability and promote rehabilitation and health maintenance. Aftercare programs such as Alcoholics Anonymous, Narcotics Anonymous, and Cocaine Anonymous are examples of tertiary programs. Nurses may also be involved in education programs for the mentally ill and focus on medication compliance, dual diagnoses, stress management, and coping skills. Prescription authority enables advanced-practice registered nurses to collaborate with the physician and support clients on maintenance medications and to evaluate their response over time through direct observation and drug levels (see Chapter 26 for a detailed description of prescriptive authority).

FUTURE TRENDS

Understanding the complex nature of mental illness compels nurses to integrate major nursing concepts with newer biological components. Appreciation of the expansion of advances in studies of brain function is crucial to recognizing the complexity of mental illness. Numerous studies show the genetic predisposition, anatomical or structural alterations, and biochemical processes in the brain as major components of mental illness.

As psychiatric–mental health nursing moves into a decade in which correlates of mental illness with brain function are being established, nurses need to review and expand their knowledge of physical processes of the nervous system. This knowledge will enhance their ability to develop effective client outcomes and interventions that restore health and prevent illness. Integrating biological concepts into nursing practice also means that nurses can use a repertoire of knowledge based on caring, psychosocial, and cultural factors to help clients in distress. Case management is a role component that enables nurses in various clinical settings to support and facilitate the client's highest level of function. Crisis intervention, problem solving, education, and collaboration with various mental health professionals and community resources are major aspects of case management (ANA, 1994).

As psychiatric nurses define and redirect their roles within a changing health care system, they must be able to adapt to the movement from acute inpatient settings to community-based care. In the near future, inpatient psychiatric care will consist of shorter hospital stays that are limited to acute care, medication stabilization, and research. Health care is evolving into community-based treatment in which nurses are primary caregivers. How will a changing health care system affect the role of psychiatric nurses?

Socioeconomic changes and proposed health care reform are prompting health care systems to re-examine how they provide service to clients. Care for the mentally ill has changed drastically since deinstitutionalization in the 1960s. Community services for the mentally ill have failed to meet the need, and the mentally ill represent a large portion of the homeless population.

THE MENTAL HEALTH TEAM

As previously discussed, the role of the psychiatric nurse has varied over the years, evolving from a custodian role to one that directs, manages, and collaborates with others to promote health. However, in spite of this evolution, the role of psychiatric nursing is still unclear to many consumers and mental health professionals. Nurses must continue to educate through active dialogue, emphasizing their strength and diversity as health care providers.

Educating mental health professionals and consumers begins when psychiatric nurses actively participate in client care as members of the mental health team. Mental health teams are interdisciplinary groups usually led by a psychiatrist or other professional, such as a psychiatric nurse.

The mental health team provides a collaborative approach to client care. Collaboration maximizes resources and provides enormous opportunities to assess clients as the members reduce fragmentation and dehumanization. The team generates treatment planning that incorporates input from various disciplines such as nursing, psychiatry, psychology, social services, and occupational therapy, and from mental health aides to meet the complex needs of the mentally ill and their families.

Psychiatrist. Psychiatrists are physicians who have specialized in psychiatry. These health care practitioners may be certified by the American Board of Psychiatry and Neurology and are responsible for making psychiatric diagnoses and prescribing treatment. Other responsibilities include prescribing psychotropics or other medication and providing medical treatment, such as electroconvulsive therapy. Psychiatrists are also responsible for directing research such as drug trials and for providing psychotherapy and supervision for medical students.

Clinical Psychologist. Clinical psychologists have a doctorate in psychology and are generally involved in administering and interpreting psychological or neuropsychological testing that assists the mental health team in diagnosing psychiatric conditions. Psychologists also participate in psychotherapy, biofeedback, and behavioral modification.

Psychiatric Social Worker. Psychiatric social workers are graduates of a master's program and are involved in identifying and dealing with social issues that affect clients and their families and mobilizing community resources. They also gather psychosocial data on admission and provide crisis intervention and psychotherapy.

Occupational Therapist. Occupational therapists are graduates of a master's or doctoral program in occupational therapy. They are primarily involved in providing an assortment of arts and craft activities that help clients express intrapsychic and interpersonal responses. They also assist clients in gaining skills needed to perform activities of daily living such as hand–eye coordination and vocational skills. Activities focus on altering the course of illness. Often, the client's relationship with the occupational therapist is more therapeutic than the activity itself.

Mental Health Worker or Psychiatric Aide. Mental health workers or psychiatric aides provide direct care to clients. There are no formal mental health educational requirements for this position. These practitioners are important members of the mental health team, and they play a vital role in maintaining a therapeutic milieu under the supervision of the professional registered nurse.

The Collaborative Process. Overall, the mental health team identifies complex client needs based on input from all members of the team. The collaborative process involves an active participation by members of the team and the consumer or client. These endeavors foster health care environments that promote holistic approaches to client care through communication; sharing of innovative ideas; impacting on total quality management; and fostering creativity, autonomy, and accountability. The mental health team establishes the tone, foundations, and milieus that promote a sense of trust and respect for similarities and differences among professionals to assess client needs, develop outcomes, and evaluate consumers' response to treatment (ANA, 1982).

Rising health care costs and shifts in health care delivery systems from impatient to community-based services require innovative and collaborative approaches to maximize resources and provide quality care. Case management is an example of this approach, and it is rapidly becoming a popular concept among various mental health professionals. Case management enables the mental health team to identify potential and anticipated discharge needs and referrals; work with clients and families in their homes and communities to promote self-care; and convey a long-term commitment to clients. Overall, the collaborative process provides quality, comprehensive, outcome-oriented care.

USING THE NURSING PROCESS IN PSYCHIATRIC SETTINGS

During the 1960s, interpersonal and scientific perspectives of psychiatric nursing were developed. Leaders in this endeavor included Orlando, Neuman, Roy, and others who emphasized the integration of cognitive, interpersonal, and technical skills of nursing practice (see Chapter 2 for more information on leading nursing theorists). Dramatic changes have occurred over the past 30 years. Changes have evolved through the application of scientific methods to several conceptual models or theoretical frameworks, such as Maslow's hierarchy of needs, Erikson's developmental stages, and Roy's adaptation model. These models have improved psychiatric nurses' understanding of client responses to internal and external environments by directing the nursing process. Additionally, nursing continues to progress toward application of scientific methods through the nursing process.

As nurses approach the twenty-first century, they must appreciate the neurobiological link with mental illness. Enormous technological discoveries concerning the brain and other biochemical processes provide unique opportunities for psychiatric nurses to integrate biological and behavioral concepts into practice. Current biological trends suggest the need to assess and identify specific client outcomes and to determine the effectiveness of interventions.

American Nurses Association. The ANA has played a major role in developing standards of practice since the 1960s. In 1967, the association attempted to define psychiatric nursing when it published the *Statement on Psychiatric Mental Health Nursing Practice*. This publication traced the historical milestones of psychiatric nursing practice and education. Later, the ANA (1973) gave credence to the nursing process by publishing the first *Standards of Nursing Practice*. The 1970s highlighted the professional autonomy and accountability of nursing, and the development of nursing standards exemplified the association's commitment to the scientific approach to the nursing process. The evolution of the nursing process has reflected trends that have defined nursing (Griffith & Christensen, 1982).

Another ANA milestone came in 1982 when it published the *Standards of Psychiatric and Mental Health Nursing Practice*. This document symbolized the ANA's continued commitment to develop the nursing process and improve the quality of care. These standards modified previous ones defined by the Division of Psychiatric and Mental Health Nursing Practice in 1973.

The emergence of the 1990s, the Decade of the Brain, finds that the ANA has again maintained its commitment to psychiatric nursing by publishing *A Statement on Psychiatric–Mental Health Clinical Nursing Practice and Standards of Psychiatric–Mental Health Clinical Nursing Practice* (1994). These standards incorporate and acknowledge the expansion of advances in neurobiology as a major component of mental illness. They also delineate the role of psychiatric nurses as either generalist or advanced practice. Other issues discussed include the move toward a changing health care system that focuses on nurses as primary care providers in outpatient settings.

FACTORS DETERMINING THE EFFECTIVENESS OF THE NURSING PROCESS

The importance of the nursing process has been exemplified by the ANA's commitment to improve it over time. The nursing process is an interactive problem-solving approach to systematically effecting change in clients. Nurses can use this process to organize and assess clients' needs and outcomes. The effectiveness of the nursing process is influenced by the following factors:

- Mutuality
- Therapeutic nurse–client relationship
- The nurse's communication style
- The nurse's educational level (knowledge of behavioral and neurobiological sciences)
- The nurse's clinical experience
- The client's developmental stage

Mutuality refers to the nurse–client interactive participation in decision making. Mutual respect between the nurse and the client is crucial to therapeutic interactions. This relationship fosters individuality, autonomy, and partnership in developing effective treatment outcomes. It is the basis of the nursing process. Nurses can maximize client resources and promote self-actualization and the restoration of health through mutuality. Effective interactions stem from effective communication between the nurse and the client.

Effective communication enables the nurse to gather data and assess client problems or diagnoses. Communication styles and patterns vary and are shaped by cultural, socioeconomic, neurobiological, and developmental stage factors. Effective communication enhances collaboration with clients and other mental health professions in defining effective treatment strategies and evaluating client responses.

Other factors determine how clients are assessed, including educational level and clinical experience. These factors influence theoretical frameworks or models used to diagnose or assess data and establish client outcomes. A comparison between a generalist and an advanced-practice psychiatric nurse can be seen in the following example of the depressed client. The generalist nurse may elicit questions that center on the client's reasons for seeking treatment, whereas the advanced practitioner may seek answers to early childhood factors that play a role in client's present symptoms.

Life span, or developmental, issues is the final factor that determines the effectiveness of the nursing process. These variables determine age-specific tools, questions, or approaches used to assess symptoms and develop client outcomes. Assessing children requires data about playmates, social interactions, and school performance. Parents are key participants in the child's treatment planning. In contrast, older adults are assessed for cognitive performances, suicidal risk, prescription overuse, and support systems.

THE NURSING PROCESS AND STANDARDS OF CARE

The nursing process is a critical part of psychiatric nursing. It has evolved over the past three decades to provide a viable nursing tool used to assess the client's needs, develop client outcomes, and evaluate the effectiveness of interventions. As we move into the next decade, assessing and anticipating the complex client needs will continue to rise. Recently, critical thinking concepts have been defined and integrated into the nursing process. Application of knowledge, use of astute judgment, and evaluation of complex client responses are part of this process. Furthermore, autonomous and creative thinking help nurses use the nursing process to provide quality and continuous care (Wilkinson, 1992).

The ANA delineates standards of care as those professional activities in which psychiatric nurses use the nursing process to assess, diagnose, plan, implement, and evaluate various forms of care. (Table 4–4 lists the ANA standards and the nursing behaviors that define them as applied to psychiatric–mental health nurses. Table 4–5 lists the ANA Standards of Professional Performance as applied to psychiatric–mental health nurses as well as clinical nurses in general.)

Theory-Based Practice

The clinical example of Mr. Jones demonstrates how the nursing process and standards of care can be used to identify client responses and develop a plan of care.

Clinical Example: Mr. Jones

Mr. Jones, a 55-year-old man, presents with symptoms of decreased appetite and sleep, increased irritability and agitation, and social isolation. He is seeking evaluation in an outpatient psychiatric triage unit and is accompanied by his wife of 30 years.

Assessment

Standard I: Assessment. *The psychiatric–mental health nurse collects client health data.*

During the initial step of the nursing process, the psychiatric–mental health nurse collects data. This process encompasses engaging the client in an interview that allows nurses to observe verbal and nonverbal communication. Factors that affect data collection include the quality of the nurse–client relationship, developmental stage, culture, educational level, communications skills and language, mental status, and cognitive

TABLE 4–4
ANA Standards of Psychiatric–Mental Health Nursing Practice

STANDARD I. ASSESSMENT
The psychiatric–mental health nurse collects client health data.

STANDARD II. DIAGNOSIS
The psychiatric–mental health nurse analyzes the assessment data in determining diagnoses.

STANDARD III. OUTCOME IDENTIFICATION
The psychiatric–mental health nurse identifies expected outcomes individualized to the client.

STANDARD IV. PLANNING
The psychiatric–mental health nurse develops a plan of care that prescribes interventions to attain expected outcomes.

STANDARD V. IMPLEMENTATION
The psychiatric–mental health nurse implements the interventions identified in the plan of care.

STANDARD V-A. COUNSELING
The psychiatric–mental health nurse uses counseling interventions to assist clients in improving or regaining their previous coping abilities, fostering mental health, and preventing mental illness and disability.

STANDARD V-B. MILIEU THERAPY
The psychiatric–mental health nurse provides, structures, and maintains a therapeutic environment in collaboration with the client and other health care providers.

STANDARD V-C. SELF-CARE ACTIVITIES
The psychiatric–mental health nurse structures interventions around the client's activities of daily living to foster self-care and mental and physical well-being.

STANDARD V-D. PSYCHOBIOLOGICAL INTERVENTIONS
The psychiatric–mental health nurse uses knowledge of psychobiological interventions and applies clinical skills to restore the client's health and prevent further disability.

STANDARD V-E. HEALTH TEACHING
The psychiatric–mental health nurse, through health teaching, assists clients in achieving satisfying, productive, and healthy patterns of living.

STANDARD V-F. CASE MANAGEMENT
The psychiatric–mental health nurse provides case management to coordinate comprehensive health services and ensure continuity of care.

STANDARD V-G. HEALTH PROMOTION AND HEALTH MAINTENANCE
The psychiatric–mental health nurse employs strategies and interventions to promote and maintain mental health and prevent mental illness.

STANDARD V-H. PSYCHOTHERAPY
The certified specialist in psychiatric–mental health nursing uses individual, group, and family psychotherapy, child psychotherapy, and other therapeutic treatments to assist clients in fostering mental health, preventing mental illness and disability, and improving or regaining previous health status and functional abilities.

STANDARD V-I. PRESCRIPTION OF PHARMACOLOGIC AGENTS
The certified specialist uses prescription of pharmacologic agents in accordance with the state nursing practice act, to treat symptoms of psychiatric illness and improve functional health status.

STANDARD V-J. CONSULTATION
The certified specialist provides consultation to health care providers and others to influence the plans of care for clients, and to enhance the abilities of others to provide psychiatric and mental health care and effect change in systems.

STANDARD VI. EVALUATION
The psychiatric–mental health nurse evaluates the client's progress in attaining expected outcomes.

TABLE 4–5
Standards of Professional Performance

Standard I: Quality of Care
Standard II: Performance Appraisal
Standard III: Education
Standard IV: Collegiality
Standard V: Ethics
Standard VI: Collaboration
Standard VII: Research
Standard VIII: Resource Utilization

function. The young child is likely to have more difficulty expressing feelings than is the young adult. Additionally, clients with cognitive impairment, such as those with schizophrenia and dementia, also have difficulty organizing their thoughts and responding effectively during assessments.

Data collection is based on various theoretical frameworks that enable the nurse to interpret, validate, and organize findings and set up a plan of care. Various data collection tools may be used (see Fig. 6–2 in Chapter 6). Data are collected from various sources, such as clients, significant others, and other mental health professionals.

Data collected from Mr. Jones include changes in sleeping, eating, and concentration patterns over the past 6 weeks. He also reports losing his job several months ago after being employed 20 years. He fears he will not be able to find employment because of his age. His wife corroborates his story and expresses concerns about his present behavioral changes.

Nursing Diagnosis

Standard II: Diagnosis. *The psychiatric–mental health nurse analyzes the assessment data in determining diagnoses.*

Diagnoses are synonymous with client problems. The criteria for psychiatric nursing diagnoses include recognizing and identifying patterns of response or actual or potential mental illness and mental health defined within the scope of psychiatric–mental health nursing practice. Furthermore, diagnosing involves making inferences and using sound judgment regarding client problems.

Diagnoses comply with accepted classification systems developed by the North American Nursing Diagnosis Association that are used in clinical settings to identify client actual and potential adaptive and maladaptive responses. They are validated by clients, significant others, and other mental health professionals. These findings are documented to promote identification of client outcomes, care plans, and research (ANA, 1994).

Data from the case history suggest that Mr Jones is depressed. The findings include

- Ineffective Individual Coping
- Sleep Pattern Disturbance
- Impaired Social Interaction
- High Risk for Violence: Self-Directed
- Self-Esteem Disturbance

See the accompanying Nursing Care Plan.

Outcome Identification and Planning

Standard III: Outcome Identification. *The psychiatric–mental health nurse identifies expected outcomes individualized to the client.*

Standard IV: Planning. *The psychiatric–mental health nurse develops a plan of care that prescribes interventions to attain expected outcomes.*

The major treatment intent of identification of client outcomes is health promotion and restoration, that is, what the client can expect from nursing interventions or treatment. Client outcomes must be realistic, attainable, therapeutic, individualized, measurable, and cost effective.

An individualized plan of care directs therapeutic interventions that facilitate the successful resolution of client problems by restoring physical and mental health, preventing illness, and effecting rehabilitation. It is a blueprint that guides nurses and mental health professionals in identifying client outcomes, effective treatment options, and client activities and delegates specific function of the mental health team. The nurse's role is determined by educational level, clinical experience, and certification.

For instance, all nurses are trained to use the nursing process, but specific interventions require specialized training, certification, and educational preparation. The generalist nurse is a baccalaureate-prepared registered nurse who is primarily involved in promoting health restoration, assessing maladaptive responses, improving coping behaviors, and preventing further maladaptation. This is generally accomplished by managing the client's basic needs such as activities of daily living, maintaining a therapeutic milieu, practicing case management, administering psychotropics, and assessing client response and milieu therapy. Community functions may include home visits, case management, and joining the crisis team of a mental health center or homeless shelter.

In contrast, the advanced-practice nurse is a master's or doctorally prepared nurse who has acquired in-depth knowledge of human behaviors and complex causal factors. This nurse is able to apply this knowledge and solve complex problems involved in mental health and mental illness. Specific interventions often consist of an assortment of psychotherapy, unit management, private practice, consultation and liaison functions, and prescriptive authority. Regardless of the nurse's role, collaboration with clients, families, and other mental health professionals broadens the scope of practice, the effectiveness of treatment, and the evaluation of client responses.

Implementation

Standard V: Implementation. *The psychiatric–mental nurse implements the interventions identified in the plan of care.*

After the nurse assesses the client, identifies the problems or nursing diagnoses, establishes client outcomes, and develops a plan of care, how will he or she implement the plan? Application of knowledge and testing hypotheses are critical components of implementation and intervention. An array of interventions can be used to promote health and minimize the deleterious effects of mental illness. Specific interventions are determined by the identified client needs and may include milieu therapy, stress management, education, behavior modification, and various psychotherapies.

Implementation is an open, dynamic process, and interventions are continuously being monitored by client responses. This process enhances nurse–client collaboration, maximizes resources, and minimizes the fragmentation of health care services.

Evaluation

Standard VI: Evaluation. *The psychiatric–mental health nurse evaluates the client's progress in attaining expected outcomes.*

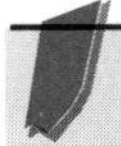

Nursing Care Plan 4-1 The Depressed Client (Mr. Jones)

Nursing Diagnosis: High Risk for Violence: Self-Directed

OUTCOME IDENTIFICATION	NURSING ACTIONS	RATIONALES	EVALUATION
1. By [date], client verbalizes feelings rather than acting on them.	1a. Establish rapport. Encourage expression of feelings. 1b. Maintain safe environment. Assess level of dangerousness. 1c. Observe for mood changes. Notify physician of changes in behavior.	1a. Establishes therapeutic interaction. Conveys empathy, caring, and interest. 1b. Provides safety and control and decreases acting out behaviors. 1c. Change in mood increase risk of dangerousness.	*Goal met:* Nurse forms therapeutic relationship. Client expresses feelings. Client does not express suicidal ideations or act on thoughts.

Nursing Diagnosis: Ineffective Individual Coping

OUTCOME IDENTIFICATION	NURSING ACTIONS	RATIONALES	EVALUATION
1. By [date], client develops realistic perception of present stressor(s).	1a. Explore meaning of recent job loss and other stressors. 1b. Understand meaning of present stressors.	1a. Helps client understand self and present responses. 1b. Validates understanding of meaning of presenting symptoms.	*Goal met:* Client returns to pre-crisis level of functioning. Client develops adaptive coping skills. Client's self-esteem increases.
2. By [date], client develops enduring adaptive coping skills.	2. Assist in identifying strengths and coping skills.	2. Places focus on positive attributes and increases self-esteem.	

Nursing Diagnosis: Sleep Pattern Disturbance

OUTCOME IDENTIFICATION	NURSING ACTIONS	RATIONALES	EVALUATION
1. By [date], client's normal sleeping patterns return to optimal level.	1a. Assess normal sleeping patterns. 1b. Maintain quiet environment. 1c. Provide comfort measures.	1a. Helps nurse identify normal sleeping patterns. 1b and c. Promotes rest, sleep.	*Goal met:* Client's normal sleeping patterns are maintained.

Nursing Diagnosis: Self-Esteem Disturbance

OUTCOME IDENTIFICATION	NURSING ACTIONS	RATIONALES	EVALUATION
1. By [date], client verbalizes three positive attributes and increased self-esteem.	1a. Provide successful experiences. 1b. Convey acceptance and empathy. 1c. Encourage active participation in treatment.	1a–c. Positive, successful experiences increase confidence and self-esteem.	*Goal met:* Client's self-esteem increases. Client is able to explore options to deal with present stressors.

Criterion-focused evaluations are standards by which nursing interventions are measured. The decision to continue interventions and continuously monitor client responses is a major nursing role in caring for persons with mental illness.

As the client's health status changes, so does the nursing care. The complexity of mental illness and client responses challenges nurses to use sophisticated evaluation measures to assess client needs. The acutely ill client experiencing hallucinations, delusions, and agitation requires immediate relief of these symptoms. Major nursing interventions include establishing trust, administering medication to reduce anxiety and agitation, maintaining nutrition, and promoting self-care. Acutely ill clients have numerous needs and require ample nursing care. In contrast, when acute symptoms are alleviated, nursing care decreases and often involves decreased monitoring. Specific interventions may include individual or marital therapies, discharge planning, stress management, and education. Overall, nursing care is a dynamic process that varies with client needs, cost effectiveness, available resources, and the preparedness of the nurse.

Summary of the Nursing Process

The nursing process is the foundation of nursing because it provides a systematic and scientific approach to identifying client needs and potential outcomes. Opportunities to promote health reduce the deleterious effects of mental illness. Psychiatric–mental health nurses can maximize the effects of this process by collaborating with members of the mental health team to identify and respond to clients in distress.

►CHAPTER SUMMARY

Psychiatric nursing is an integral aspect of nursing practice, and psychiatric nurses use therapeutic interactions to establish rapport and to foster a sense of safety and security of clients in distress. Integrating clinical thinking principles into the nursing process enables nurses to use a systematic means of identifying adaptive and maladaptive responses in clients experiencing stress.

As psychiatric nursing moves into the next decade, it faces enormous challenges. Major changes include health care reforms, staggering increases in the incidence of violence, family disintegration, and increases in the number of people vulnerable to mental illness, such as substance abusers, the aging poor, the homeless, and those with AIDS. Additional changes include an expansion in technological studies of the brain and its impact on mental illness. Psychiatric nurses are confronted with these changes and with caring for sicker clients who lack adequate access to health care.

What does the future hold for psychiatric nurses? The ANA has taken a major step and exemplified its commitment to psychiatric nursing and the complex needs of the mentally ill by proposing new standards that integrate biological components into traditional holistic approaches to psychiatric nursing practice. Psychiatric nurses need to continue redefining their role within traditional psychiatric and community settings that incorporate the primary caregiver role. The success of these endeavors depends on the ability of nurse leaders, educators, researchers, and practitioners to redefine their roles and integrate biological and traditional nursing concepts into practice.

Suggestions for Clinical Conferences

1. Present case histories, and discuss how the the case relates to primary, secondary, and tertiary prevention.
2. Role-play clinical situations; assess self-awareness and explore feelings.
3. Arrange for a presentation by a psychiatric clinical specialist to discuss the diversity of the role in clinical and community settings.
4. Discuss the essential qualities of the psychiatric–mental health nurse.

References

American Nurses Association (1967). *Statement on psychiatric and mental health nursing practice*. Kansas, MO: Author.

American Nurses Association. (1973). *Standards of nursing practice*. Kansas City, MO: Author.

American Nurses Association. (1982). *Standards of psychiatric and mental health nursing practice*. Kansas City, MO: Author.

American Nurses Association. (1991a). *Nursing agenda for health care reform*. *Kansas* City, MO: Author.

American Nurses Association. (1991b). *Standards of clinical nursing practice*. Washington, DC: Author.

American Nurses Association. (1994). *Statement on psychiatric–mental health nursing clinical practice and standards of psychiatric–mental health clinical nursing practice*. Washington, DC: American Nurses Publishing.

Caplan, G. (1964). *Principles of preventive psychiatry*. New York: Basic Books.

Cooper, B. (1990). Epidemiology and prevention in the mental health field. *Social Psychiatry and Psychiatric Epidemiology*, *25*, 9–15.

Dupont, A. (1989). Factors influencing the incidence of mental retardation and their implications. In B. Cooper & T. Helgasom (Eds.), *Epidemiology and the prevention of mental disorders* (pp. 327–337). London: Rutledge.

Ehmann, V. E. (1971). Empathy: Its origins, characteristics, and process. *Perspectives in Psychiatric Care*, *9*(2), 72–80.

Freud, S. (1912). *The dynamics of transference* (standard ed., 12; pp. 97–108). London: Hogarth Press.

Griffith, J. W., & Christensen, P. J. (1982). *Nursing process: Application of theories, frameworks, and models*. St Louis: C. V. Mosby.

Katz, R. L. (1963). *Empathy: Its nature and uses*. London: Free Press of Glencoe.

Lazarus, R. S. (1966). *Psychological stress and the coping process*. New York: McGraw-Hill.

Menninger, K. A. (1947). *The human mind* (3rd ed.). New York: Alfred A. Knopf.

Truax, C. B., & Carkhuff, R. R. (1967). *Towards effective counseling and psychotherapy*. Chicago: Aldine.

Wilkinson, J. M. (1992). *Nursing process: A critical thinking approach*. Redwood City, CA: Addison-Wesley.

World Health Organization. (1980). *Changing patterns in mental health care: Copenhagen reports on a working group*. EURO Reports and Studies, 25, WHO, Regional Office for Europe, Copenhagen, Denmark.

World Health Organization. (1985). *Targets for health for all*. WHO, Regional Office for Europe, Copenhagen, Denmark.

World Health Organization. (1988). *Prevention of mental, neurological, and psychosocial disorders*. WHO Regional Office for Europe, Copenhagen, Denmark.

CHAPTER

Legal and Ethical Issues

ADA LYNNE HENDRICKS, M.S., R.N.
LINDA FUNK BARLOON, M.S., R.N.,C.

OUTLINE

CHAPTER OBJECTIVES

Upon completion of this chapter, you will be able to:

1. Discuss the history of legal and ethical changes in mental health treatment.
2. Understand and use ethical principles in decision making.
3. Have a working knowledge of U.S. mental health laws and their application to the psychiatric population.
4. Discuss client rights and the application of rights in the clinical setting.
5. Identify legal and ethical issues impacting the psychiatric nurse today and in the future.

KEY TERMS

Advocacy
Against medical advice
Autonomy
Beneficence
Bioethics
Civil commitment
Competency
Deinstitutionalization
Elopement
Ethics
Justice
Mental illness
Negligence
Philosophy
Standards
Tort law
Values

Psychiatric nurses are routinely involved in the complex life events of clients that are often complicated by legal and ethical issues. Not only must they make legal and ethical decisions for themselves, they also must guide and support clients as they struggle with these same issues (Wilkinson, 1987). It is critical, therefore, that nurses have the necessary tools to accomplish these objectives. In adapting to the frequent changes in the health care system and the world around them, clients depend on nurses to assist them in finding access to the most effective care possible (Nixon, 1992). An understanding of the legal and ethical issues and the ability to address them influence the care provided by psychiatric nurses.

LEGAL ISSUES IN PSYCHIATRY: HISTORICAL PERSPECTIVES

Both clients and health care providers are aware of their legal rights now more than ever before (Nixon, 1992). Nurses have a responsibility to be aware of the legal and ethical rights of their clients, because consumers depend on nurses to understand the system and aid in their care. Many changes in psychiatric care have occurred throughout history, and this care continues to alter as dispersing of available knowledge, refashioning of the psychosocial environment, and shifting of the political climate impact the mental health care system (see Table 5–1 for a historical overview.)

In colonial times, Americans used English common law to decide how to handle the mentally ill. Methods of treatment included arrests, beating, placement in prisons, poor houses, or cages. In 1751, the Pennsylvania Colonial Assembly passed a law establishing a hospital for the poor who were sick and for the mentally ill. It was the first hospital known to have a philosophy of curing the mentally ill rather than simply housing them. Even so, clients were restrained and beatings were frequent. The insane were believed not to feel heat or cold and therefore were unprotected from the weather (Dice, 1987). There were no laws protecting the liberty of the mentally ill. To initiate hospitalization, a relative or friend could obtain an order for admission from a hospital manager or physician, resulting in the client being forcibly detained in the hospital. The hospital could earn extra revenue by displaying clients and charging a fee for the public's entertainment (Dice, 1987).

At that time, mental health caregivers thought it necessary to attempt to domesticate the spirits of the mentally ill. Dr. Benjamin Rush, known as the Father of Psychiatry, invented two mechanical restraint devices. He believed in physical punishment; however he was humane by the standards of the time. Rush required attendants to pay attention to personal hygiene and show respect for clients. He succeeded in separating the men and women into different buildings (Dice, 1987).

During the early decades of the nineteenth century, a few states passed laws requiring that the mentally ill could be kept in prison only a short time or during emergencies (Dice, 1987). During the 1840s, Dorothea Dix traveled around Massachusetts and Rhode Island visiting the mentally ill who were living in jails and almshouses due to inadequate space in asylums. She found conditions in which the insane were tied, chained, or placed in iron collars in dirty, dark, unheated cells. Some victims froze to death, and others were maimed by caretakers. Dix brought her findings to lawmakers and the public, who were horrified at the inadequate living conditions. As a result an asylum was enlarged to provide more space in a more appropriate facility. She was responsible for starting 32 public and private facilities to care for the mentally ill. Dix worked toward social reform in caring for the emotionally ill and became convinced that the cause of mental illness could be reversed (Sanders & DuPlessis, 1985).

In the 1860s, Mrs. E. P. W. Packard was committed to psychiatric hospitalization owing to accusations by her husband, Rev. Theophilus Packard. After being discharged, Mrs. Packard traveled nationally, accusing her husband of conspiring to have her locked up unnecessarily. She believed that the allegedly insane should be incarcerated not based solely on the opinions of others but on the behavior of the individual (Weiner & Wettstein, 1993). This resulted in new laws that were the foundation of the commitment laws in place until the reforms of the 1960s and 1970s.

In the 1870s, legislation that protected the community from the mentally ill was passed; these laws permitted people to be committed indefinitely. The revised criteria resulted in an increase in the percentage growth of hospitalized mentally ill at a rate of twice the percentage growth of the American population as a whole between

TABLE 5–1
Historical Overview of Legal Events in Psychiatric Care

1751	The first mental hospital was established in the American colonies with a philosophy for curing the mentally ill.
Early 1800s	A few states made laws that the mentally ill could be kept in prison only for a short time or in an emergency.
1840s	Dorothea Dix traveled and conducted public hearings about conditions for the insane.
1860s	Efforts of Mrs. E. P. W. Packard, a victim of involuntary commitment, resulted in new commitment laws.
1870s	Stricter laws were passed to commit clients indefinitely or release them.
1903–1950	The number of hospitalized mentally ill clients increased at twice the rate of growth of the American population.
1946	The National Mental Health Act of 1946 was passed, and National Institute of Mental Health was created.
1960s	Client rights movement evolved from the Civil Rights movement.
1963	The Community Mental Health Centers Act of 1963 resulted in a 75% decrease in the number of clients in state hospitals. Many clients had difficulty adjusting because of poor continuity of care.
1970s	The U.S. Supreme Court ruled that the right to legal counsel applies to mentally ill.
1980s	Medication administration policies in most states and territorial jurisdictions established a client's right to refuse medication.

1903 and 1950. Despite the difficulties described, state-operated facilities and other hospitals provided care that was unavailable outside these institutions (Dice, 1987).

Increasing interest in mental health occurred at the time of both World Wars because of the large number of returning veterans with emotional problems. The National Mental Health Act of 1946 was passed, the National Institute of Mental Health was created, and the goals for the future of mental health were set as the nation became more aware of its citizens with psychiatric problems (Betrus & Hoffman, 1992).

The terms *psychiatric* and *mental health* first came into use during the 1950s (Betrus & Hoffman, 1992). With new techniques that were developed, new psychotropic medication, as well as the changing political climate, mental health reformers were able to visualize hope for a community-based mental health system rather than state-operated mental hospitals (Dice, 1987).

The Community Mental Health Centers Act of 1963 provided an opportunity for people to receive outpatient treatment or short-term hospitalization in community mental health centers close to their city or town (Dice, 1987). This act resulted in a change in the education of nurses to focus on community mental health (Betrus & Hoffman, 1992). Between 1955 and 1980, the number of clients in state mental hospitals decreased by more than 75%, partly because states were no longer required to provide the funding to care for the mentally ill outside the hospital setting. This was to encourage the use of community mental health resources. If clients were discharged from the hospital, federal Medicaid funds would provide financial support for their care. Clients who were discharged into the community had difficulty adjusting outside the hospital because of poor continuity of care. Often, these clients ended up in other institutionalized settings, in poor living conditions, or even on the streets (Dice, 1987).

During the 1960s, increasing concern with the rights of psychiatric clients resulted from the Civil Rights movement, the availability of legal services, public disgust with the conditions in mental institutions, and an assertion by the mentally ill of their legal rights. The 1960s' liberal philosophy of equality, self-determinism, and liberty provided the framework that influenced developments such as client rights, confidentiality, informed consent, and **deinstitutionalization**. These changes in the delivery of treatment created challenges that affect mental health therapy even today (Freitas & Pieranunzi, 1990; Garritson, 1988).

Other changes in the 1970s and 1980s affected the rights of the mentally ill. After the U.S. Supreme Court ruled that a person accused of a capital offense has a right to legal counsel and acknowledged that the Constitution emphasizes the right to liberty, the right to legal counsel was successfully applied to the mentally ill (McFadyen, 1989). The psychiatric client has constitutional rights explicitly protected by the Constitution that are not relinquished because of psychiatric status. These rights include freedom of speech, the right to due process, freedom from cruel and unusual punishment, and the right to equal protection under the law. The psychiatric client also has rights that are considered fundamental rights, for example, the right to marry, the right to choose one's own fate, and entitlements that are provided by state and federal statutes, such as civil commitment procedures (Bloom & Asher, 1982). These legal rights set the foundation from which decisions are made. The rights of psychiatric clients are explored further in this chapter.

ETHICAL DECISION MAKING IN PSYCHIATRIC NURSING

Along with legal parameters, psychiatric nurses have ethical obligations that impact their practice. Nurses use professional judgment in determining what is right and best for clients, and they often face ethical dilemmas. An understanding of basic ethical principles and guidelines for analyzing issues is a valuable resource in ethical decision making.

ETHICAL CONCEPTS

The branch of **philosophy** called **ethics** is concerned with the examination of moral judgments and decisions about conduct. The term *ethics* is derived from the Greek word *ethos,* which means conduct or character. The terms *ethics* and *morals* are often used interchangeably. **Bioethics** is ethics applied to health care (Davis & Aroskar, 1991).

There are two traditional ethical positions: (1) deontology and (2) utilitarianism, or teleology. In the deontological approach, an act has an inherent moral significance, and decisions are based on adherence to certain principles without regard to consequences. An example of using this method is never telling a lie, regardless of the consequences. The utilitarian approach focuses on the consequences of actions and is concerned with maximizing the greatest good and least harm for the most people. With this reasoning, telling a lie is justified if the outcome results in the most good (Davis & Aroskar, 1991).

Principles are general rules that guide conduct and decision making. Ethical principles include **beneficence**, autonomy, **justice**, and fidelity (Table 5–2).

PROFESSIONAL ETHICS IN NURSING

In applying ethical reasoning, nurses may use moral principles in decision making. Nursing, like other health professions, has codes of ethics to guide its practice. Originally, nurses followed ethical standards associated with the religious orders with which nurses were allied. In the late 1800s, the Florence Nightingale Pledge was created to reflect the ethical principles of the nurses trained by Nightingale. Its tenets included treating the client rather than the disease and loyalty to the profes-

Table 5–2
Examples of Ethical Principles

Beneficence (Nonmaleficence): People should promote good, do no harm, and prevent harm.
Autonomy: People have the right to make their own decisions based on their values; each person is unique yet interdependent with others.
Justice: People should be treated fairly, and the disadvantaged must be protected. Benefits should be equitably distributed.
Fidelity: People should be faithful to their duties and obligations.

Data from Eriksen, J. (1989). Steps to ethical reasoning. *Canadian Nurse 85*(7), 23–24; and Davis, A. J., & Aroskar, M.A. (1991). *Ethical dilemmas and nursing practice* (3rd ed.). Norwalk, CT: Appleton & Lange.

sion (Davis & Aroskar, 1991). Since that time, nurses have continued to develop statements of **standards** to guide professional practice and to symbolize the **values** of the profession. In 1985, the American Nurses Association (ANA) revised its Code for Nurses, which was originally adopted in 1950 (Table 5–3). The ANA code establishes standards of practice to which nurses are held accountable.

ETHICAL DILEMMAS AND A DECISION-MAKING MODEL

Despite principles and standards of conduct, nurses still face ethical dilemmas. An ethical dilemma is a situation that involves deciding between equally unsatisfactory alternatives, often with conflicting principles. For example, a nurse may support the autonomy of a mentally ill client to make decisions, but the client's refusal of treatment may be harmful. Many hospitals have ethics committees (of which nurses are vital members) that may be used in situations involving ethical dilemmas. Eriksen (1989) outlined areas of knowledge to be used as an aid in ethical decision making (Table 5–4). Nurses need to discuss dilemmas with coworkers and acquire knowledge and skill to make good professional choices. Standards of conduct and principles are useful tools for nurses to help justify moral actions taken.

Psychiatric nurses become involved in ethical decision making with clients because of the intimate nature of the nurse–client relationship. For example, a nurse may struggle with the need to obtain parental consent for an adolescent to be treated for substance abuse while realizing that the client may refuse to participate if it means telling her parents. Similarly, a nurse may wonder if a client who consents to the use of antipsychotic agents truly understands the risks and is in fact clinically competent to make that decision. Table 5–5 outlines some topics of ethical concern in psychiatric nursing practice.

The use of a decision-making model may be helpful in analyzing a situation; however, nurses should be cautioned not to expect simplistic solutions to ethical dilemmas. The following model is a guide to ethical decision making (Kentsmith et al., 1986):

TABLE 5–3
American Nurses Association Code for Nurses with Interpretive Statements

1. The nurse provides services with respect for human dignity and the uniqueness of the client unrestricted by considerations of social or economic status, personal attributes, or the nature of health problems.
2. The nurse safeguards the client's right to privacy by judiciously protecting information of a confidential nature.
3. The nurse acts to safeguard the client and the public when health care and safety are affected by the incompetent, unethical, or illegal practice of any person.
4. The nurse assumes responsibility and accountability for individual nursing judgments and actions.
5. The nurse maintains competence in nursing.
6. The nurse exercises judgment and uses individual competence and qualifications as criteria in seeking consultation, accepting responsibilities, and delegating nursing activities to others.
7. The nurse participates in activities that contribute to the ongoing development of the profession's body of knowledge.
8. The nurse participates in the profession's efforts to implement and improve standards of nursing.
9. The nurse participates in the profession's efforts to establish and maintain conditions of employment conducive to high-quality nursing care.
10. The nurse participates in the profession's efforts to protect the public from misinformation and misrepresentation and to maintain the integrity of nursing.
11. The nurse collaborates with members of the health professions and other citizens in promoting the community and national efforts to meet the health care needs of the public.

Reprinted with permission from *Code for Nurses with Interpretive Statements*, © 1985, American Nurses Association, Washington, DC.

Table 5–4
Areas of Knowledge Required for Ethical Decision Making in Nursing

Knowledge of oneself and one's values: Recognize own beliefs and values so that decisions are personally acceptable.
Knowledge of the facts: Obtain and understand relevant facts and options of each situation.
Knowledge of standards: Seek familiarity with Code for Nurses, which outlines expectations of profession.
Knowledge of the law: Know legal aspects and societal values that apply to nursing care.
Knowledge of philosophy: Seek an understanding of principles of ethical reasoning.

Data from Eriksen, J. (1989). Steps to ethical reasoning. *Canadian Nurse, 85*(7), 23–24.

Table 5–5
Topics of Ethical Concern in Psychiatric Nursing Practice

- Impact of labeling clients with psychiatric diagnoses
- Prohibitive cost of some psychotropic medication
- Restricted access to care
- Clients who may be considered least desirable (i.e., violent, chemically dependent, and indigent)
- Faddish versus effective treatment
- Subjective nature of making determinations such as defining mental illness, competency, and insanity
- Genetic counseling for clients with mental illnesses with possible genetic components
- Balancing protection of the client with fostering of autonomy
- Balancing individual rights with the protection of others
- Balancing the benefits of drug treatment with the risks

1. *Review the facts*. What are the facts of the situation? What information is fact, and what is an assumption or emotional reaction? What additional information is needed, and what is the best source of information?

2. *Review the ethical issues*. What, if any, ethical issues are involved? What ethical aspects are in conflict?

3. *Look at options*. What are the options? What are the consequences of each option? What are the moral justifications for each option? What other factors such as professional codes and laws affect the options?

4. *Choose an option and act*. Have the options and their consequences been carefully considered? What is the nature of the ends and the means of the decision? How does the action reflect the ethical principles reviewed?

5. *Evaluate*. How well was the case analyzed? Were the consequences of the action accurately predicted? Was the action justified?

The following case study illustrates the application of this model.

Case Study: Applying an Ethical Decision-Making Model

An adult client with a history of alcohol and cocaine dependence requested admission to a chemical-dependence treatment unit of a private facility. The client had been treated at this facility four times in the past year and had been discharged against medical advice on all four occasions. The treatment team met to discuss whether or not to readmit this client. Although this is not an exhaustive list, the team raised the following issues.

Reviewing the Facts

Why does the client want to be readmitted? What was the course of previous treatments? What were the circumstances of previous discharges against medical advice? What is different at this time? What are the client's supports? What is the client's motivation for treatment? How have we differentiated between fact and assumption? What other information can the client provide? What information can others (such as family members and Alcoholics Anonymous sponsors) provide?

Reviewing the Ethical Issues

How do ethical principles such as beneficence, autonomy, and fidelity relate to this case? What is our responsibility to this client? What personal values of team members come into play? How do the relationships of team members with the client relate to this case? Are there other issues that might influence the decision, such as the client's position in the community and his financial status? What are the conflicting ethical principles?

Looking at Options

What are the possible choices of action? What treatment alternatives are available in the community? What changes in the treatment plan can be made if the client is admitted (such as having the client work with the team to develop a daily contract and anticipatory planning for substance withdrawal)? What immediate and long-term consequences can we predict for each option? What legal and institutional constraints affect the decision? Should the hospital ethics committee be consulted?

Choosing an Option

After carefully analyzing the case, the team will choose a course of action that seems most "right."

The nurse may examine an ethical dilemma and use a systematic approach to come to a moral decision, but it is not always in the nurse's power to carry out that decision. Wilkinson (1987) defined this inner turmoil of not being able to act on an ethical decision as moral distress:

> *Because of their conflicting loyalties and responsibilities—to licensing bodies, employing institutions, physicians, other nurses, patients, and patients' families—nurses are especially prone to suffer moral distress.* (p. 16)

Carpenter (1991) suggested, based on research findings, that problems with ethical decision making may be an important factor in the stress associated with nursing. It may also affect the nurse's self-concept and attitude toward the nursing profession and whether the nurse changes to a different career.

THE NURSE AS CLIENT ADVOCATE

Advocacy means defending a cause or pleading a case in another's behalf (Bloom & Asher, 1982). Client advocacy involves recognizing and enforcing client rights, both legal and human. Legal rights are "claims that would be currently backed by law if the case went to court," and human rights are claims that are "critical to maintaining human dignity but have not yet attained legal recognition" (Annas, 1992, p. 7).

Advocacy takes many forms. Informally, a nurse may become an advocate by ensuring that the client's voice is heard and by educating clients about the health care system and their rights within the system. Some institutions have client advocates who address grievances and help resolve them. Client advocates may also function in case management roles in an attempt to provide adequate mental health services for the client (Annas, 1992). Advocates not only work to correct mistreatment but are proactive to prevent rights violations (Smoyak, 1986).

As an advocate, the nurse holds the interests of the client above the interests of others, and at times the nurse may have divided loyalties. Fully protecting the client's rights requires a high degree of professional autonomy in practice to empower the nurse to put the client first (Bernal, 1992).

Legal advocacy is concerned with changing the way society responds to the mentally ill through the legal system. The field of mental health disability law developed in the 1960s, and since that time there has been a proliferation of litigation aimed at defining and protecting the rights of the mentally disabled (Carty, 1992). Nurses can influence the development of this type of law by contacting legislative officials about health care issues and lobbying through professional nursing organizations and public service groups (Wakefield, 1993).

Many health care organizations have adopted statements regarding client rights. The Joint Commission on Accreditation of Healthcare Organizations (JCAHO), a private accrediting agency, outlines standards for client rights that include respect and dignity, privacy, and the right of the client to know the identity of caregivers. The American Hospital Association and many individual health institutions have adopted policies concerned with client rights (Annas, 1992) (see the section on client rights later in this chapter).

Health care continues to move away from a paternalistic model, in which the health team knows what is best for the client, to a model that views clients as consumers and emphasizes client rights (Valentine et al., 1990). An understanding of the law and an ability to communicate with clients, physicians, lawyers, and administrators are basic qualifications for the nurse who is an effective client advocate (Annas, 1992).

DEFINING MENTAL ILLNESS

In the general population the term ***mental illness*** is used indiscriminately, but legally the term has more specific, yet difficult-to-define criteria. Although most states have statutes that attempt to define mental illness, there is some variation from state to state (Weiner & Wettstein, 1993). A mental illness may be defined as "a disability severe enough to warrant hospitalization, continued treatment, or monitoring" (Weiner, 1990, p. 153). Mental illnesses may involve a loss of contact with reality and nonpsychotic disorders that cause significant impairment in functioning and emotional distress (Bennett, 1986). Some states specifically exclude diagnoses such as mental retardation, other developmental disabilities, alcoholism, and substance abuse from the legal definition of mental illness (Weiner & Wettstein, 1993).

U.S. MENTAL HEALTH LAWS

There are a number of sources of law with which the psychiatric nurse must be familiar that mandate the treatment of the mentally ill. Among them are constitutional and statutory laws that are enacted by federal or state legislative bodies. Also, federal and state agencies such as the U.S. Department of Health and Human Services and state mental health agencies mandate rules and regulations that have the same authority as law. It is important for the nurse to be aware that many laws affecting the mentally ill vary from state to state (Weiner & Wettstein, 1993). Other accrediting agencies such as the JCAHO also influence the care of mentally ill clients. This section outlines the various admission criteria for psychiatric hospitalization and reviews the laws that pertain to the rights of the mentally ill client.

ADMISSION CATEGORIES

Voluntary Hospitalization

Voluntary commitment to a psychiatric hospital occurs when a person meeting admission criteria freely chooses to be hospitalized. Approximately half of the admissions to state mental health facilities are voluntary (Weiner & Wettstein, 1993). A client may feel pressured into treatment by family members or health care professionals because of the threat of involuntary commitment. For an admission to be considered voluntary, the client must be informed of the physical conditions and the expectations of the institution, the admission process, and alternatives to hospitalization (Bloom & Asher, 1982). Persons who are incapable of giving informed consent may not be admitted on a voluntary basis (*Zinermon v. Burch*, 1990). A voluntary client may leave the hospital at will; however, many states have laws that allow the client to be detained if the client meets the criteria for involuntary commitment, namely danger to self or others (Cushing, 1988) (see the section on discharge later in this chapter).

Involuntary Hospitalization (Commitment)

The state has the authority to require the hospitalization of an unwilling person when that person meets the requirements of the **civil commitment** standards. The ability of the state to hospitalize a person without consent is at the center of legal and ethical debates regarding the rights of the mentally ill. The goal of the civil commitment process is to balance the individual right to freedom with the protection of mentally ill people who are unable to care for themselves and the protection of society (Weiner & Wettstein, 1993) (Fig. 5–1). For a client to be involuntarily committed for psychiatric treatment, there must be "clear and convincing" evidence of imminent danger to the client or others (*Addington v. Texas*, 1979). The "clear and convincing" standard is a lower standard of evidence than in criminal cases, which require evidence "beyond a reasonable doubt" (Bloom & Asher, 1982). Table 5–6 lists criteria that states use for involuntary commitment.

Often, it is a family member or mental health professional who identifies when a person is in need of hospitalization. If the person is unwilling to be hospitalized, a petition must be filed with the state's attorney in the county in which the person resides explaining why the person should be involuntarily committed. A civil commitment hearing must take place to determine if the

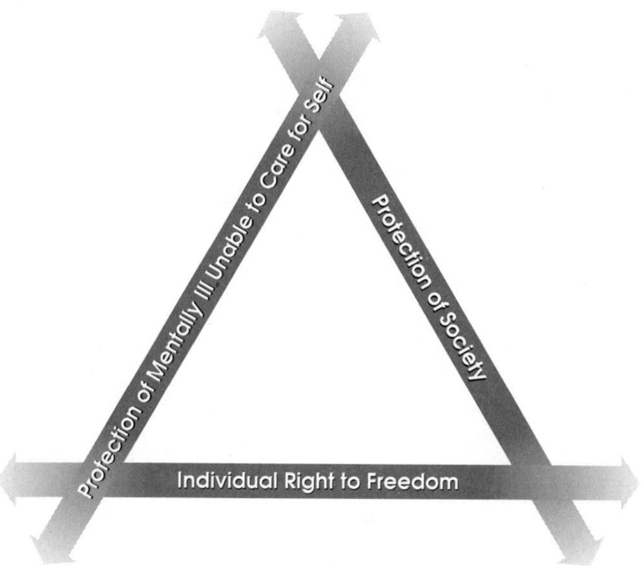

FIGURE 5–1
The civil commitment process attempts to balance three civil rights: the individual right to freedom, the protection of society, and the protection of the mentally ill from inflicting harm on themselves.

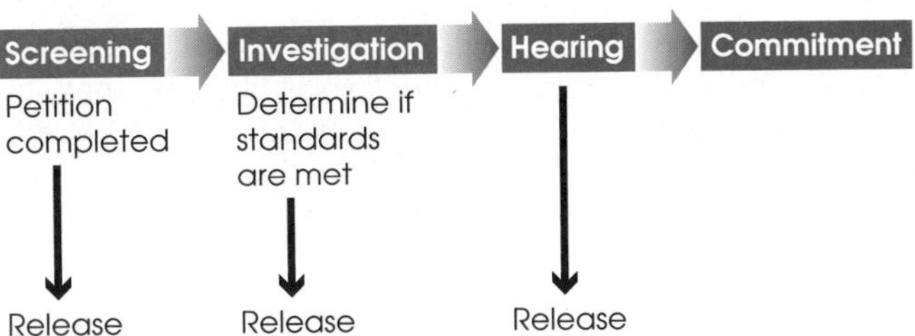

FIGURE 5–2
The civil commitment process. (Adapted from *American Journal of Psychiatry, 144*[2], 193–196, 1987. Copyright 1987, the American Psychiatric Association. Reprinted by permission.)

person meets civil commitment standards (Fig. 5–2; also see the section on due process later in this chapter). The conditions of senility, epilepsy, alcoholism, or drug dependence in themselves are not sufficient grounds for commitment—the person must also meet civil commitment requirements (Bennett, 1986).

As involuntary clients are hospitalized and then are stabilized by medication or other therapies, they no longer meet the standards for commitment and may be released or given the option of voluntary hospitalization. These persons are often part of the "revolving door" of mental health care, where they move in and out of hospitals. Some states now have outpatient commitment in an effort to stabilize persons with acute symptoms in the community. The person must have the capacity to function safely in the community with adequate supervision, often provided by family or friends. If the client fails to comply with outpatient treatment, a law enforcement officer may bring the client to the treatment center or a new civil commitment petition may be initiated (Hiday & Scheid-Cook, 1989). Current civil commitment procedures may not address the needs of the chronically mentally ill with a history of dangerousness to self or others who are not imminently a danger but may become dangerous if untreated.

Table 5–6
Criteria for Involuntary Commitment

Each state has specific statutes establishing criteria for involuntary commitment that usually contain the following elements:

- A person who is mentally ill, and because of that mental illness is in imminent danger of physically hurting himself or someone else based on something they did or a significant threat, *or*
- A person who is mentally ill, and because of that mental illness has demonstrated an inability to attend to basic physical needs such as food, clothing, and shelter that are needed to prevent serious harm, *or*
- A person who is mentally ill and considered gravely disabled, whose judgment is so impaired that he or she is unable to understand the need for treatment and whose behavior can reasonably be expected to result in significant physical harm to himself or someone else

Data from Weiner, B. A., & Wettstein, R. M. (1993). *Legal issues in mental health care.* New York: Plenum Press.

Emergency Hospitalization. In addition to the general commitment process, all states also have the authority to detain a person in an emergency situation for a limited time until a probable cause hearing is held. The same criterion of imminent danger to self or others or an inability to meet physical needs because of mental illness is used. The amount of time a person can be held varies from state to state but is usually 3 to 5 days. This allows time to provide life-saving treatment, evaluate, and determine the diagnosis to decide if commitment will be sought (Weiner & Wettstein, 1993). The following case study illustrates the application of the criterion for emergency hospitalization.

Case Study: Emergency Hospitalization

A 57-year-old woman with a history of bipolar disorder told her daughter over the phone that she wanted to kill herself. The daughter went to her mother's house and found her mother incoherent, with slurred speech, and locked in her bedroom. The mother threatened to take her whole bottle of lithium, and the daughter realized the lithium was missing from the bathroom medicine cabinet. The mother stated, "I don't see any reason to go on, and I'm not coming out of here alive." The daughter called the police for assistance with emergency hospitalization.

Temporary Involuntary Hospitalization (Observational Commitment). Following the emergency treatment period, the court will find that a small number of clients remain seriously mentally ill, and in some states additional treatment following emergency commitment may be sought. Some clients agree to voluntary treatment, others are discharged, and still others may be categorized as incompetent and guardianship may be sought. Temporary involuntary hospitalization is generally 2 to 6 weeks in length, and treatment focuses on stabilizing symptoms (Bloom & Asher, 1982; Weiner & Wettstein, 1993).

Extended Involuntary Hospitalization. Most people who are committed to treatment return quickly to the community. However, a few are mandated to extended hospitalization and are subjected to periodic review at least annually. The focus of treatment is to improve the ability of clients to live in the community (Bloom & Asher, 1982).

TRANSFER

Transfer may occur within an institution, such as between units or rooms, or it may be accomplished from institution to institution. The transfer may be initiated by the client or the institution. In the United States, citizens have the right to be treated in an emergency department for an emergency condition. The client can be transferred to another institution if the physician certifies that the person is stable and that there is no foreseeable risk to health (Annas, 1992).

ELOPEMENT (ESCAPE)

Elopement, *absconding*, and *absent without official leave* are terms used for hospitalized clients who are absent from a psychiatric facility without complying with the proper procedures for absence. Institutions have removed restrictions on client's liberties, which often includes having unlocked units, and this may add to the risk of elopement. Elopement can cause great anxiety to staff members who must assess the client's legal status and the risks involved with the client being out in the community. Clients often return to the hospital having been brought back by police or relatives or by returning on their own (Falkowski et al., 1990).

DISCHARGE

Discharge from a psychiatric hospital ideally occurs when the client has successfully met the treatment goals for that hospitalization, is no longer a danger to self or others, and is sufficiently stabilized to return to the community. Discharge requires a written order from a physician who is familiar with the client's condition. A person who is legally competent and does not meet the state's criteria for involuntary commitment may leave the hospital, and any attempt to restrict the person from leaving would be considered false imprisonment in a court of law. In the absence of a physician's order, a client may be asked to sign a form indicating that the discharge is **against medical advice** (Annas, 1992). Many states require that requests for discharge be in writing. By law, a client may not be released at the moment of request but within a short period, within 1 week in most states. This allows the providers to determine whether or not the client meets civil commitment criteria (Weiner & Wettstein, 1993).

Over the past decade, hospital lengths of stay have decreased dramatically, and admission and continued hospitalization are based on "medical necessity" of inpatient treatment (Freishtat, 1991). Many third-party payers of psychiatric treatment (such as insurance companies) employ utilization review practices to monitor the appropriateness of hospitalization for their subscribers. Often, this review is concurrent with hospitalization. The review is conducted with the treating physician or a designee (often a nurse) from the hospital by discussing the case on an ongoing basis with the third-party payer. Based on the review and the "medical necessity" criteria, the third-party payer will determine whether to certify the use of insurance benefits for continued treatment. The hospitalized client faced with no longer receiving insurance benefits for hospitalization may choose to be discharged despite the treatment team's objections (Freishtat, 1991).

Until recently, the physician bore sole legal responsibility for any improper or premature discharge when an untoward event occurred subsequently, for example, when a client committed suicide shortly after discharge. Recent legislation ruled that third-party payers are not immune from liability related to utilization review activities if their actions are a "substantial factor" in improper discharge (Freishtat, 1991).

Conditional Discharge. A person who has been civilly committed to treatment may be discharged with conditional requirements in most states. The conditions of release may include stipulations such as where the client will live, followup treatment requirements, or behavior that must be avoided. If clients violate the conditions of the release within a set period, they will be returned to inpatient hospitalization. If they disagree with a revocation of discharge, they may request a hearing (Weiner & Wettstein, 1993).

Absolute Discharge. An absolute or unconditional discharge often takes place after a hospitalized client has successfully completed a conditional release. *Absolute discharge* means that no further treatment is legally required after discharge and the client is no longer under court jurisdiction.

COMPETENCY VERSUS INCOMPETENCY

Competency refers to the ability to perform a specific act; it may vary over time and between particular tasks (Davis & Underwood, 1989). *Legal incompetency* refers to the status of persons who have been declared incompetent in a court of law and to minors. The legal criteria for competency include the ability to understand the proceedings of due process and to assist an attorney in preparing for a hearing. The competency evaluation is a separate process that involves persons who have already been determined to be mentally ill (Bloom & Faulkner, 1987). Mental illness does not necessarily mean incompetence (Weiss, 1990). Even a civilly committed client is assumed competent, and only when the court has declared the client incompetent may the nurse assume incompetence (Weiner & Wettstein, 1993).

FORENSIC PSYCHIATRY

Forensic psychiatry involves mental health issues that relate to the legal system. This includes both civil procedures, such as determining when a mentally ill person requires legal guardianship, and criminal procedures, such as determining when a defendant is competent to stand trial (National Institute of Mental Health, 1991).

Table 5–7
Assessing Intent to Harm

When assessing for serious intention to harm others, it is necessary to look for the characteristics that would increase the likelihood of harm, such as the following:

1. A definite plan
2. Resources to carry out the plan
3. Ability to carry out the plan (e.g., does the client know how to use a gun?)
4. History of violence
5. Impulsivity
6. Extreme emotional changes
7. Depression

All characteristics are not necessarily present, and if there is a question about the seriousness of the client's intent, the nurse should seek a collaborative consultation.

Data from Yorker, B. C. (1988). Confidentiality—an ethical dilemma: Balancing the "duty to warn" against the right to privacy. *AAOHN, 36*(8), 346–347.

INSANITY DEFENSE

For a person to be held legally accountable for a crime, the physical act of the crime and the mental state of intention both are necessary elements (Weiner & Wettstein, 1993). The insanity defense argues that a person by virtue of mental illness cannot know and appreciate the nature of a criminal act and cannot control his or her behavior because of the mental illness. Antisocial personality disorder and "voluntary insanity" produced by substance abuse are excluded (Vandenberg, 1993). The insanity defense is used in fewer than 1 percent of U.S. criminal cases (Missouri Department of Mental Health, 1993; Weiner & Wettstein, 1993).

DUTY TO WARN

Mental health care is not an exact science. A health care professional who is counseling a client is expected to use reasonable judgment when assessing, planning, and intervening. It is important to assess and inquire about signs and symptoms as well as to use available information to make sound treatment judgments (Knapp & Vandercreek, 1983). It is not always possible to know whether or not a client has serious intentions to hurt others.

Both the duty to warn and duty to protect are closely related. They are legal obligations based on the case of *Vitaly Tarasoff v. the Regents of the University of California,* which was brought to the California Supreme Court in 1976. In this case, the University and its psychotherapists were accused of being responsible for the murder of Tatiana Tarasoff by a psychiatric client (Vitaly Tarasoff, 1976). The death was reportedly due in part to Tatiana Tarasoff and her parents not being informed that the client planned to murder her when she returned from vacation (Smith, 1990). The court determined that if a professional believes that a client is a danger to others, then there is a legal responsibility of the professional to take necessary steps to protect the potential victim (Vitaly Tarasoff, 1976). Table 5–7 provides guidelines for assessing a client's intent to harm.

The Tarasoff case has been used to approve breaking confidentiality and protecting others (by warning possible victims). Although many states have laws similar to those based on the decision of the Tarasoff case, each individual state has its own laws, and these laws may vary from the Tarasoff decision (Knapp & Vandercreek, 1983). It is the nurse's responsibility to know the law and variations in his or her state. If the victim is not warned, based on reasonable judgment, this usually gains approval by the court, whereas lack of knowledge of the law is an unacceptable defense (Yorker, 1988).

The following are comments and suggestions for a nurse working with a client who is believed to be a danger to someone: The nurse does not necessarily track down the potential victim, but interventions include notifying the psychiatrist; notifying appropriate administrative personnel, possibly in writing; and documenting in the chart all details, including the nurse's interventions (Gaudinski, 1990).

DOCUMENTATION

Documentation is a record of occurrences, observations, and planning related to client care. Documentation includes not only charting on both the progress notes and medication sheets but also ongoing nursing care plans and multidisciplinary treatment plans (Sanders & DuPlessis, 1985). It is important that all significant situations, actions, and interventions, including any resolutions, be written in a factual, nonbiased manner. These inform and guide other nursing shifts and other health care workers outside the inpatient unit (such as outpatient therapists who are working with the client and family). It also provides important information that will aid in providing the rationale for treatment given. The following case study illustrates proper documentation.

Case Study: Applying Proper Documentation

A 34-year-old man was admitted involuntarily to the psychiatric unit due to an explosive personality. He began to threaten a fellow client, and the following chart entry was made:

The nurse, speaking in a soft, calm voice, approached the client and offered alternatives of moving away from the conflict or calming down in his room. The nurse then asked the client to walk to a quiet area of the unit to decrease the stimulation and offered to give the client a PRN medication. The client stood in the hall with his fists clenched and muscles rippling, assumed a fighting stance within 6 inches of a staff member's nose, and yelled, "I'm going to fight to the death." The nurse and two staff members placed the client in restraints, and the nurse administered a neuroleptic agent (haloperidol [Haldol]) intramuscularly in the left upper outer quadrant.

Table 5–8
Situations in Which the Nurse May Legally Breach Confidentiality

1. During an emergency involving an immediate danger of serious physical harm; for example, notifying a relative without consent about a client's suicide attempt
2. Protecting others from potential violence by client; for example, notifying an ex-spouse that a client has threatened bodily harm
3. Conforming to child abuse reporting requirements; for example, notifying the proper authorities of suspected sexual abuse of a minor
4. Conforming to other statutory reporting requirements; for example, notifying the proper authorities of reportable sexually transmitted diseases
5. Discussing the client with supervisors and other providers directly participating in care
6. Situations in which civil commitment is being sought; for example, providing information without consent explaining why civil commitment is warranted

Data from Weiner, B. A., & Wettstein, R. M. (1993). *Legal issues in mental health care.* New York: Plenum Press.

While a client is in restraints, documentation must continue to indicate the ongoing need for control in this manner with no other available option to ensure the safety of the client and others. The nurse must document that the client is observed constantly while in leather restraints and describe the client's behavior during this time.

Careless or partial documentation can make good care appear delinquent (Morgan, 1987). Objective documentation must be present to show evidence of proper procedures or facts on which decisions were made and to demonstrate that adequate professional care was given. This evidence may include items such as observations, assessments, treatments, and medications given. If the nurse delegates the documentation to other members of the health care team, the documentation should still reflect whether care that would be expected was completed. It can be assumed in court that only those things documented were done. Jakacki and Payson (1985) advised the following:

> *Document enough information to prove that you acted as any reasonable, prudent nurse would act under the same or similar circumstance. If, in your judgment, an emergency exists, document all observable facts plus the thinking you used in determining that immediate intervention was necessary.* (p. 1336)

Adequate documentation is a responsibility that nurses have for all clients in their care.

CONFIDENTIALITY

Confidentiality is an obligation of nurses that is necessary to foster a professional, trusting relationship between the nurse and the client (Melrose, 1990). Information that is shared verbally or in writing between the health team members should be kept confidential from those outside the health care team. Specific laws pertaining to confidentiality may vary; therefore, nurses must be aware of the laws in the state in which they practice. The nurse is challenged when the police, the family that plans to care for the client, the outpatient therapist, the employer, and others insist on obtaining confidential information related to the client. It is important to always elicit the client's preference in handling these situations and to request that a release-of-information permission form be signed by the client if necessary for the client's treatment (Puskar & Obus, 1989).

Even though information is not shared outside the hospital by the staff, the client's medical record may be subpoenaed by the court and used by the judicial system (Bender et al., 1989; Smith, 1990). Nurses should know the requirements of the law to avoid litigation and protect themselves if accused of breaking a client's confidentiality (Stern, 1990) (see Table 5–8).

REPORTING OF ABUSE

Child Abuse. Child abuse is any action by a caretaker that purposefully injures the child physically or emotionally. Abuse includes physical, emotional, and sexual types or neglect of a child younger than 18 years of age (Fiesta, 1992).

Nurses and physicians in all states are required to report child abuse (Fiesta, 1992). Nurses report child abuse to various agencies depending on the state in which the abuse occurs (Smith, 1989). The nurse has no responsibility to keep that information confidential (Smith, 1990), and the child's right to be protected takes precedence over laws of confidentiality (Smith, 1989). If the reporter acts in good faith, most states provide immunity for the health care worker. Failure to report child abuse may result in the health care worker being liable for abuse that occurred later owing to lack of previous intervention (Fiesta, 1992). These laws have contributed to an increasing number of reported child abuse cases (Smith, 1989). (See Chapter 19 for discussion on abuse throughout the life span.)

Elder Abuse. Most states have some type of reporting system that mandates reporting elder abuse. It is important to know the particular laws associated with elder abuse in the state in which the nurse works. Interventions vary and range from criminal prosecution of the abuser to guardianship of the victim (Haviland & O'Brien, 1989).

Hospitals or other health care institutions caring for elderly clients need explicit policies in compliance with state and nursing standards regarding abuse. Nurses must assess, document, and take actions associated with the requirements of the laws of the state. It is both a legal and an ethical duty to intervene when abuse occurs (Nursing practice, 1992). Janing (1992) stated the following:

> *It is not enough to be angered by the specific cases of abuse we see. . . . We must speak out as individuals and as a profession to both our state and federal legislatures. It is time to be an advocate.* (p. 58)

PRINCIPLE OF TORT LAWS

Christoffel and Teret (1991) defined **tort law** as when a person or a group "must pay compensation for civil, noncontractual wrongs caused to others" (p. 1661). Intentional tort occurs when one deliberately inflicts abuse on another person, such as in the case of assault, defamation of character, and invasion of another's privacy. For instance, nurses may be charged with assault after striking an out-of-control client in the process of protecting themselves. The inquiry regarding deliberately inflicting pain on a client in an environment expected to be safe and protected may be in question.

NEGLIGENCE

Christoffel and Teret (1991) defined **negligence** as injury that is unintentional due to failure to take the usual precautions expected in that instance. Tort law gives the client the opportunity to complain while being in an equal status. To win a lawsuit against a health care worker, the client must prove the nurse was obligated to act in a particular way, the nurse did not fulfill the professional duty, the client suffered harm, and the reason for the client's harm was because the nurse did not function as expected.

There has been some type of tort reform in every state in the United States. According to Morgan (1987), some of these reforms include the following:

- Reducing the length of time in which a suit can be filed
- Establishing attorney fees on a sliding scale dependent on the amount of settlement
- Setting up a pretrial screening panel to review the case and make recommendations to the court
- Sanctioning the ability to make the jury aware of any compensation received before the trial
- Limiting the amount of damages
- Allowing the defendant to pay a large award in installments

CLIENT RIGHTS

The 1970 case *Wyatt v. Stickney* sparked the proliferation of laws establishing the rights of hospitalized mentally ill clients. This case established a precedent in psychiatric facilities for staff–client ratios, nutritional requirements of hospital meals, and physical requirements such as the minimum number of showers, among other standards. Hospitalized mentally ill clients today maintain a number of rights that are mandated by law (Weiner & Wettstein, 1993). Client rights, however, are not self-executing, and the psychiatric nurse plays a significant role in defending these rights.

Rights of Children or Minors

In *Parham v. J. R.* (1979), the U.S. Supreme Court's majority decision was that the court would support the family unit as it had historically. The court stated that parents make decisions for the child when the child has not developed adequate cognitive ability. They further stated that the affection parents have for their children would result in parents making the best decision for the child with regard to psychiatric treatment. Due process for children did not necessarily mean judicial process, but the process that parents fulfill in their duty to assess the needs of their children. A balance in the process was that the admitting physician could deem whether admission was appropriate for a child (deLeon Siantz, 1988).

The nurse's relationship regarding the child's rights includes using interventions that protect the child, supporting the family's decision-making ability while supporting the child's best interests, and ensuring that the child is treated fairly (deLeon Siantz, 1988). Although minors may not legally refuse treatment, a method by which the nurse can acknowledge a minor's need to have control is the ethical means of asking the child to give informal assent or agreement to treatment. Information regarding treatment should be given to children on a level they can understand. Giving minors the opportunity for assent and choices when possible provides empowerment and results in fewer power struggles between the nursing staff and the client. This sets the stage for positive relationships with the nursing staff by providing the child with an opportunity to develop decision-making skills and increasing his or her openness to treatment (Erlen, 1987). Adolescents may be developmentally able to give consent to treatment and, if interested, should be given the opportunity to sign a consent form along with the parent or guardian.

Due Process

Due process is based on Section One of the Fourteenth Amendment to the Constitution, which states that no citizen may be denied life, liberty, or property without an impartial hearing and the same rights as all citizens (Jakacki & Payson, 1985). The client has the right to fair procedures, to be able to attend any hearings and present evidence, and to seek independent advice (Cichon, 1991).

Right to Treatment

The right to treatment is specifically mandated by the U.S. Supreme Court. A client must receive individualized care that is considered adequate for his or her needs (Sanders & DuPlessis, 1985). In a study by Wolpe et al. (1991), more than one fourth of the clients did not know they had a right to actively participate in their treatment plan. It is the nurse who must help safeguard the right of clients to obtain and participate in their treatment.

Least-Restrictive Alternatives

Psychiatric care may consist of various alternatives, including hospitalization, outpatient treatment, and other community-based options. The goal of treatment is to move the client to a productive life in the community as soon as possible. The level of treatment is determined by the client's particular needs, providing the maximum amount of liberty while protecting the client from danger (*Dixon v. Weinberger*, 1975). States are mandated to provide the least restrictive programs and services available; however, states do not always have a wide continuum of services (Cushing, 1988).

In dealing with situations involving violent or potentially violent clients, the nurse may use a variety of interventions, including the use of seclusion or restraints. Before seclusion or mechanical or chemical restraint are employed, though, less intrusive interventions must be attempted or at least considered. The nurse is legally bound to use the least-restrictive method necessary to minimize injury to self and others (Myers, 1990).

Informed Consent

Informed consent is based on the fundamental belief that clients should be able to have control over their own bodies (Grove, 1990). This not only legally provides **autonomy** for the client (in which no one should touch or treat the client without permission from the client) but also encourages the ethical aspect of the client's decision-making ability (Weiss, 1990).

There are four elements necessary for legal consent (Kjervik & Grove, 1988):

1. A person must be capable of consenting.
2. A person must have the ability to refuse consent.
3. A person must have adequate information for consent or have agreed to waive the right to information.
4. The consent must not be illegal.

The nurse has a vital role in aiding the client to understand the information in any case requiring informed consent (Grove, 1990). The nurse or physician should witness the client's or legal guardian's verbalization of understanding and observe the signature being placed on the consent form or, in an emergency, hear the telephone consent given (Davis & Underwood, 1989).

Informed consent for medication is an important responsibility in psychiatric nursing and involves informing the client about the indications and side effects before initiating medication. Often written material is included in the information provided. When a crisis occurs, informed consent may be waived at the discretion of the nurses and physicians if a true life-threatening emergency exists (Gaudinski, 1990; Puskar & Obus, 1989).

An ethical dilemma may emerge for the nurse if consent is needed for treatment for which the client is reluctant to sign. For instance, a client who has been unresponsive to treatment of depression may be hesitant to sign for electroconvulsive therapy (ECT). The nurse is faced with the dilemma of encouraging (not coercing), providing further information, or choosing to say little and respecting the decision of the client (Loubardias, 1991). The nurse may encourage a client to look at options, but if the client's decision is different from what the nurse believes to be best, the final decision should still be that of the client.

Right to Refuse Treatment

A client has the right to refuse treatment when he or she is considered competent (Carroll & Maher, 1990) or not imminently dangerous to self or others. The judicial system has the right to make a final clinical decision in circumstances in which there is a conflict of opinion between health care providers and the client. The legal system considers the autonomy of the client to be paramount without considering that the mental illness may have already robbed the client of autonomy (Schwartz et al., 1988). Thus, if unresolved conflict arises, the intervention must be postponed until the court decides the outcome. The following case study addresses the right to refuse treatment.

Case Study: Application of Right to Refuse Treatment

A 54-year-old woman refused to go to activity therapy, stating that her knee hurt. The physician had written specific orders to encourage activity therapy because this client often had "excuses" to avoid therapy. The nurse reported seeing the client limping, but the physician verified that the client should be urged to attend therapy. The client begged with tears in her eyes and stated, "I have so much pain." The nurse informed the client that her knee had been x-rayed and no fracture was apparent. The client did go to activity therapy; while she was there, she fell and broke her leg. This was because of pain and an inability to bear weight, later found to be related to infection in the synovial fluid of the knee. The nurse later believed that she had violated the client's right to refuse treatment and that the client's request should have been granted.

The client's desire or refusal to follow the treatment plan is a legal and ethical right, unless otherwise ordered by the judicial system. It is the nurse's responsibility to be an advocate and to protect client rights by being aware of the laws of the state (and eventually working to changes those laws if necessary), discussing with other professionals involved in the care and the hospital legal counsel to focus attention on questionable ethical and legal issues.

Right to Refuse Medication. The legal right to refuse antipsychotic medication was established more than 15 years ago, with differing interpretations and methods of enforcement depending on the jurisdiction. Weiss (1990) noted that "by the early 1980s, 45 of 51 state and territorial jurisdictions in the United States had implemented a variety of medication administration policies in their public treatment facilities" (p. 25). Even involuntarily committed clients have been allowed to refuse medication, although refusal may further delay discharge by prolonging symptoms and extending the length of hospitalization. The interesting aspect of this is that most clients who initially refuse medication eventually receive it anyway because of a court decision (Appelbaum, 1988) (see the accompanying Research Study: Do You Feel Powerless When a Patient Refuses Medication?).

The nurse may not forcibly give medication unless the client is seen as an imminent danger to self or others. If the nurse does not give PRN medication as ordered, owing to client refusal, and the client hurts himself or herself or others, the nurse's actions will be reviewed by the hospital and possibly by a court to see if the incident could have been prevented. If the nurse forcibly gives medication, the nurse's actions will also be reviewed to see if the nurse had the right to administer the medication. How does the nurse get out of this "double bind?" The nurse must document observations of the details surrounding the events, and the interventions attempted during the incident to indicate the basis for judgments made. The decision of the nurse must be supported in the documentation to substantiate that the nurse acted as any professional nurse would according to the legal standards of the state (Jakacki & Payson, 1985) (see the accompanying Research Study: Autonomy and the Right to Refuse Treatment: Patients' Attitudes After Involuntary Medication).

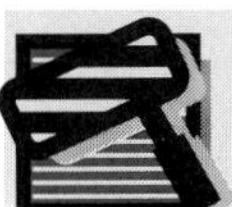

RESEARCH STUDY

Autonomy and the Right to Refuse Treatment: Patients' Attitudes After Involuntary Medication

Schwartz, H. I., Vingiano, W., & Perez, C. B. (1988). *Hospital and Community Psychiatry, 39*(10), 1049–1054.

This study examined the opinion of 24 involuntarily medicated clients whose wishes for treatment had been overridden by health professionals. More than 70% of the clients reported being glad that they had been forced into treatment and hoping this would be done again if necessary. Those who persisted in denying the need for treatment were clients described as having psychotic symptoms and responding poorly to treatment. The study concluded that those who refused medication were not necessarily making an autonomous decision.

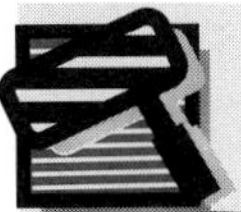

RESEARCH STUDY

Do You Feel Powerless When a Patient Refuses Medication?

Carey, N., Jones, S. L., & O'Toole, A. W. (1990). *Journal of Psychosocial Nursing and Mental Health Services, 28*(10), 19–25.

This study examined the relationship between client refusal of medication and resultant feelings reported by the nurse in a pilot study of 32 nurses. Because the nurse cannot force medication and can only advise, it was found that nurses reported indirect indicators of powerlessness elicited in a written questionnaire given. Nurses felt that they had not achieved their goal because of the client's refusal to take medication. The conflict over medication was perceived by the nurses to negatively influence nursing care, hurt the relationship with the client, and adversely affect client teaching.

Other Client Rights

All states have statutes that mandate the right of hospitalized clients to communicate with others outside the facility. Contact may include visitation, mail, and telephone contact. Most states allow institutions to employ reasonable restrictions, such as designated visitation hours. Some states require unrestricted access to clients' attorneys. These rights may be restricted if communication is harassing or harmful to someone. For example, if the nurse overhears a client using the phone to make threatening statements, the phone privileges may be suspended. The restriction as well as the rationale for the restriction should be documented in the client's record (Weiner & Wettstein, 1993).

Until the 1970s, hospitalized psychiatric clients frequently worked for the institution without compensation providing services such as housekeeping and grounds maintenance. The work was often of little therapeutic value. Today, about half of the states guarantee compensation for work such as employment in sheltered workshop programs that teach necessary skills. Clients may still be expected to perform chores such as making their own beds and doing their own laundry (Weiner & Wettstein, 1993).

About half of the states have laws guaranteeing clients the right to personal possessions while hospitalized. This includes the right to wear their own clothes and have grooming items. These rights may be restricted if the personal items are potentially harmful (such as razors and belts), stolen or damaged, expensive, or disruptive to the unit. For example, the nurse may restrict a client from bringing an expensive stereo to the unit. On admission to the hospital, psychiatric clients may be searched, including their clothing, belongings, and rooms. Clients may be searched at other times with reasonable cause for suspicion of the presence of contraband (Weiner & Wettstein, 1993).

SOMATIC THERAPIES

Electroconvulsive Therapy

ECT may be recommended for persons with endogenous depression that does not respond to other types of treatment (see Chapter 27). Serious complications are rare, and the benefits can be significant (Loubardias, 1991). A competent person has the right to agree to or refuse ECT. Injuries related to ECT that result from failure to obtain informed consent, unnecessary ECT, careless administration of ECT, and failure to administer medication to prevent injury caused by induced seizure may result in malpractice liability (Leong & Eth, 1991; Smith, 1991).

Psychosurgery

Psychosurgery, such as lobotomy conducted on sections of the brain, as therapy for psychiatric disorders may be considered effective in eliminating symptoms such as aggression. The use of this treatment has declined since the mid-1950s with the advent of other less-invasive treatments (Lesse, 1984). To prevent possible abuses, the practice of psychosurgery, although not banned, is subject to strict regulations (Smith, 1991) (see Chapter 27).

FUTURE ISSUES CHALLENGING PSYCHIATRIC NURSES

Psychiatric nursing is at a crossroads as it faces the future. Increased knowledge of the biological aspects of the brain and behavioral science needs to be incorporated into psychiatric nursing as it becomes available. It is important that psychiatric nursing have a research knowledge base for interventions (Betrus & Hoffman, 1992).

The United States faces financial deficits and hard questions related to health care now and in the future, and it faces the challenge of changing with the trends and needs of the nation. Psychiatric nursing has been a pacesetter historically. Psychiatric nurses have an urgency to move into the community to create and direct preventive as well as other treatment programs. It is time for psychiatric nursing to be proactive in meeting the legal and ethical challenges facing the citizens of our country, including opportunities related to

- The needs of our aging population, such as coping with the aging process, multiple grief issues, changes in living situations, and organic disorders
- Issues related to dysfunctional families, violence, addiction, and the impact of intrafamily and extrafamily relationships
- Ethical issues related to genetic counseling
- Preventive care for at-risk populations dealing with cultural, environmental, chemical dependence, and stress issues
- New creative approaches to intervene and work with chronic illnesses that presently involve much in health dollars, energy, and time
- The expanding definition of legal competence in relation to minors
- Access and availability of mental health services in a time of transition for the health care delivery system

These needs must be met by a variety of creative means in a diversity of settings.

Psychiatric nurses will test new roles and methods of providing care as they evaluate and shape the mental health system of the future (Betrus & Hoffman, 1992). The methods, knowledge base, and clinical settings used in teaching psychiatric nursing may be reshaped in response to the changing health care system. This is an exciting era to be at the forefront of psychiatric nursing. The future of psychiatric nursing depends in large part on active participation in decision making regarding legal and ethical issues that shape the roles that nursing will play and impact clients' treatment.

►CHAPTER SUMMARY

This chapter has addressed the complex legal and ethical issues that nurses are compelled to consider when intervening with clients. In cases requiring ethical or moral judgments, there are many subjective factors that influence nurses' decisions, and although they have tools and standards to guide them, there are few black-and-white answers. In legal matters as well, nurses must often rely on judgment that is grounded in the law but is often subject to interpretation.

Psychiatric clients are protected by a number of rights, some that are based in the U.S. Constitution (such as the right to due process), and others that stem from statutory law and case law (such as confidentiality). Still other more informal rights have been developed from a sense of ethical obligation to clients. Nurses play a key role in educating clients about these rights and protecting them from having their rights violated.

Nurses are held accountable to adhere to the standards and laws that govern their practice. They must be able to explain and defend the actions they take. Having a solid foundation in ethical and legal concepts, along with keeping abreast of changes in the law, can protect nurses from liability as well as enhance their ability to be advocates for their clients and safeguard their rights.

Suggestions for Clinical Conferences

1. Describe how you would use the areas of knowledge needed for ethical decision making presented in Table 5–4 to make a decision regarding the following incidents.
   a. A 16-year-old adolescent is scheduled for discharge at the end of the week. His parents are frustrated by his multiple hospitalizations and say they do not want him at home. The insurance company has stated that they will not certify any further hospital days. The client says that he will run away if he is sent home. What are the ethical issues involved in this case? What are the alternatives available, and what would be the consequences of each?
   b. A 25-year-old woman with anorexia nervosa has been hospitalized for a week. She is refusing to eat, and she continues to lose weight. The mental health team is concerned that the client is becoming dehydrated, so the physician orders tube feedings. The client states that she does not want the tube feedings. Using ethical principles, describe what actions the nurse should take.
   c. Someone you work with has had many stresses in his life during the last 6 months, including divorce, the death of his mother, and the hospitalization of his child with depression. You smell an odor that resembles alcohol on his breath. The coworker is not stumbling or having any apparent difficulty functioning. What should you do?
   d. A friend called who has just come into town and will be here only 4 hours. She sounds very sad, and you remember that she made a suicide attempt a couple of years ago. She says she is going through a crisis and *must* talk to you. You are scheduled for work and need to leave right away. What do you do? Look at your options and the various consequences.
   e. A 70-year-old psychotic client is delusional and actively hallucinating. She hears voices telling her that she is the ruler of the world. She refuses medication, and a coworker tells you to just go up to her and get right in her face so she will hit you. The coworker says that then you will have a reason to give medication forcibly, because the client really needs it anyway. What are the ethical issues involved in this situation? How might you respond to the coworker?
2. The Civil Rights movement is said to have affected the rights of the mentally ill. What are some of the changes in recent health care reforms, and how do you believe that this will alter future mental health treatment and laws?
3. What changes would you like to see take place in your community that would affect mental health care? What could you do directly or indirectly to influence or support these innovations?
4. If a neighbor called to ask your help in admitting a relative to a psychiatric facility:
   a. What information would you need?
   b. Where would you refer them for further information?
5. A good friend tells you that her husband has been beating her. She shows you large bruises on her body and you see that her arm is in a sling. She has just bought a gun and ammunition, which she says she will use to protect herself the next time her husband does this to her. What are your legal and ethical obligations?

References

Addington v. Texas, 441 U.S. 418 (1979) (Clearinghouse No. 17, 736).

American Nurses Association. (1985). *Code for nurses with interpretive statements*. Washington, DC: Author.

Annas, G. (1992). *The rights of patients*. Totowa, NJ: Humana Press.

Appelbaum, P. S. (1988). The right to refuse treatment with antipsychotic medications: Retrospect and prospect. *American Journal of Psychiatry*, *145*(4), 413–419.

Bender, B. M., Murphy, D. K., & Mark, B. A. (1989). Caring for clients with legal charges on a voluntary psychiatric unit. *Journal of Psychosocial Nursing and Mental Health Services*, *27*(3), 16–20.

Bennett, P. E. (1986). The meaning of "mental illness" under the Michigan mental health code. *Cooley Law Review*, *4*(65), 65–100.

Bernal, E. W. (1992). The nurse as patient advocate. *Hasting Center Report*, *22*(4), 18–23.

Betrus, P. A., & Hoffman, A. (1992). Psychiatric–mental health nursing: Career characteristics, professional activities, and client attributes of members of the American Nurses Association Council of Psychiatric Nurses. *Issues in Mental Health Nursing*, *13*(1), 39–50.

Bloom, B. L., & Asher, S. J. (Eds.). (1982). *Psychiatric patient rights and patient advocacy*. New York: Human Sciences Press.

Bloom, J. D., & Faulkner, L. R. (1987). Competency determinations in civil commitment. *American Journal of Psychiatry*, *144*(2), 193–196.

Carey, N., Jones, S. L., & O'Toole, A. W. (1990). Do you feel powerless when a patient refuses medication? *Journal of Psychosocial Nursing and Mental Health Services*, *28*(10), 19–25.

Carpenter, M. A. (1991). The process of ethical decision making in psychiatric nursing practice. *Issues in Mental Health Nursing*, *28*(10), 19–25.

Carroll, P., & Maher, V. F. (1990). Legal considerations for psychiatric patients. *Advancing Clinical Care*, *5*(6), 16–17.

Carty, L. A. (1992). The mental health law project's 20 years. *Clearinghouse Review*, *26*(1), 57–65.

Christoffel, T., & Teret, S. P. (1991). Epidemiology and the law: Courts and confidence intervals. *American Journal of Public Health*, *81*(12), 1661–1666.

Cichon, D. E. (1991). The potential impact of Harper v. Washington on South Dakota's statutory right to refuse psychiatric treatment. *South Dakota Law Review*, *36*(3), 478–498.

Cushing, M. (1988). *Nursing jurisprudence*. Norwalk, CT: Appleton & Lange.

Davis, A. J., & Aroskar, M. A. (1991). *Ethical dilemmas and nursing practice* (3rd ed.). Norwalk, CT: Appleton & Lange.

Davis, A. J., & Underwood, P. R. (1989). The competency quagmire: Clarification of the nursing perspective concerning the issues of competence and informed consent. *International Journal of Nursing Studies*, *26*(3), 271–279.

deLeon Siantz, M. L. (1988). Children's rights and parental rights. *Journal of Child and Adolescent Psychiatric and Mental Health Nursing*, *1*(1), 14–17.

Dice, M. R. (1987). The emerging constitutional rights of the mentally ill: 1787–1987. *Colorado Lawyer*, *16*(9), 1619–1623.

Dixon v. Weinberger, 405 F. Supp. 974 (D.D.C. 1975) (Clearinghouse No. 17, 175).
Erlen, J. A. (1987). The child's choice: An essential component in treatment decisions. *Children's Healthcare*, *15*(3), 156–160.
Eriksen, J. (1989). Steps to ethical reasoning. *Canadian Nurse*, *85*(7), 23–24.
Falkowski, J., Watts, V., Falkowski, W., & Dean, T. (1990). Patients leaving hospital without knowledge or permission of staff—absconding. *British Journal of Psychiatry*, *156*(4), 488–490.
Fiesta, J. (1992). Protecting children: A public duty to report. *Nursing Management*, *23*(7), 14–15, 17.
Freishtat, H. W. (1991). View from the Nation's Courts: Premature discharge due to utilization review—an emerging area of liability. *Journal of Clinical Psychopharmacology*, *11*(2), 133–134.
Freitas, L., & Pieranunzi, V. R. (1990). Ethical issues in the behavioral treatment of children and adolescents. *Journal of Child and Adolescent Psychiatric and Mental Health Nursing*, *3*(1), 3–8.
Garritson, S. H. (1988). Ethical decision-making patterns. *Journal of Psychosocial Nursing and Mental Health Services*, *26*(4), 22–29.
Gaudinski, M. A. (1990). The legal risks of psychiatric care. *RN*, *53*(8), 67–72.
Grove, K. (1990). Tardive dyskinesia: A key issue facing the psychiatric–mental health nurse. *Perspectives in Psychiatric Care*, *26*(3), 29–32.
Haviland, S., & O'Brien, J. (1989). Physical abuse and neglect of the elderly: Assessment and intervention. *Orthopaedic Nursing*, *8*(4), 11–18.
Hiday, V. A., & Scheid-Cook, T. L. (1989). A follow-up of chronic patients committed to outpatient treatment. *Hospital and Community Psychiatry*, *40*(1), 52–59.
Jakacki, M., & Payson, A. L. (1985). Out of control. *American Journal of Nursing*, *85*(12), 1335–1336.
Janing, J. (1992). Tarnis. . . the golden. *Emergency*, *24*(9), 40–43, 58.
Kentsmith, D. K., Salladay, S. A., & Miya, P. A. (Eds.). (1986). *Ethics in mental health practice*. Orlando: Grune & Stratton.
Kjervik, D. K., & Grove, S. J. (1988). The legal meaning of consent in unequal power relationships. *Journal of Professional Nursing*, *4*(3), 192–204.
Knapp, S., & Vandercreek, L. (1983). Malpractice risks with suicidal patients. *Psychotherapy: Theory, Research, and Practice*, *20*(3), 274–280.
Leong, G. B., & Eth, S. (1991). Legal and ethical issues in electroconvulsive therapy. *Psychiatric Clinics of North America*, *14*(4), 1007–1016.
Lesse, S. (1984). Psychosurgery. *American Journal of Psychotherapy*, *38*(2), 224–228.
Loubardias, S. (1991). Ethics of electroconvulsive therapy consent. *Rehabilitation Nursing*, *16*(2), 98–100.
McFadyen, J. A. (1989). Who will speak for me? *Nursing Times*, *8*(85), 45–48.
Melrose, N. H. (1990). "Duty to warn" vs. "patient confidentiality": The ethical dilemmas in caring for HIV-infected clients. *Nurse Practitioner*, *15*(2), 58–69.
Missouri Department of Mental Health. (1993). *Your rights and expectations as a forensic client*. Jefferson City, MO: Author.
Morgan, N. E. (1987). The current litigation crisis and tort reform. *Journal of American Medical Record Association*, *58*(1), 19–21.
Myers, S. (1990). Seclusion: A last-resort measure. *Perspectives in Psychiatric Care*, *26*(3), 24–28.
National Institute of Mental Health. (1991). *Law and mental health: Major developments and research needs* (DHHS Publication No. ADM 91–1875). Washington, DC: U.S. Government Printing Office.
Nixon, M. W. (1992). Mental health care rights of adolescents: What mental health nurses need to know. *Journal of Child and Adolescent Psychiatric and Mental Health Nursing*, *5*(2), 14–20.
Nursing practice: Issues and answers. (1992). *Ohio Nurses Review*, *67*(2), 16.
Parham v. J. L. & J. R. 442 U.S. 584 (1979).
Puskar, K. R., & Obus, N. L. (1989). Management of the psychiatric emergency. *Nurse Practitioner*, *14*(7), 9–24.
Sanders, J. B., & DuPlessis, D. (1985). An historical view of right to treatment. *Journal of Psychosocial Nursing and Mental Health Services*, *23*(9), 12–17.
Schwartz, H. I., Vingiano, W., & Perez, C. B. (1988). Autonomy and the right to refuse treatment: Patients' attitudes after involuntary medication. *Hospital and Community Psychiatry*, *39*(10), 1049–1054.
Smith, D. P. (1989). Child abuse and neglect: Legal and clinical implications for school nursing practice. *School Nurse*, *5*(4), 17–20, 25–26, 28.
Smith, J. (1990). Privileged communication: Psychiatric–mental health nurses and the law. *Perspectives in Psychiatric Care*, *26*(4), 26–29.
Smith, S. R. (1991). Mental health malpractice in the 1990's. *Houston Law Review*, *28*(1), 209–282.
Smoyak, S. A. (1986). Ethical perspectives. *Journal of Psychosocial Nursing and Mental Health Services*, *24*(11), 7.
Stern, S. B. (1990). Privileged communication: An ethical and legal right of psychiatric clients. *Perspectives in Psychiatric Care*, *26*(4), 22–25.
Valentine, N. M., Verhey, M., Hundert, E., & Kayne, P. (1990). A collaborative approach to clinical standards development. *Psychiatric Clinics of North America*, *13*(1), 171–185.
Vandenberg, G. H. (1993). *Court testimony in mental health: A guide for mental health professionals and attorneys*. Springfield, IL: Thomas Press.
Vitaly Tarasoff et al. Plaintiffs and appellants v. the regents of the University of California et al., defendants and respondent. SF 23042. (1976). *Pacific Reporter*, *551p.2d*, 334–362.
Wakefield, M. (1993). Contemporary issues in government. In D. J. Mason, S. W. Talbott, & J. K. Leavitt (Eds.), *Policy and politics for nursing: Action and change in the workplace, government, organizations, and community*. Philadelphia: W. B. Saunders.
Weiner, B. A. (1990). A general practitioner's guide to mental health law. *Illinois Bar Journal*, *78*(3), 153–155.
Weiner, B. A., & Wettstein, R. M. (1993). *Legal issues in mental health care*. New York: Plenum Press.
Weiss, J. (1990). The right to refuse: Informed consent and the psychosocial nurse. *Journal of Psychosocial Nursing and Mental Health Services*, *28*(8), 25–30.
Wilkinson, J. M. (1987). Moral distress in nursing practice: Experience and effect. *Nursing Forum*, *23*(1), 16–29.
Wolpe, P. R., Schwartz, S. L., & Sanford, B. (1991). Psychiatric inpatients' knowledge of their rights. *Hospital and Community Psychiatry*, *42*(11), 1168–1169.
Wyatt v. Stickney, 344, Fed. Supplement 373, 375, 1972.
Yorker, B. C. (1988). Confidentiality—an ethical dilemma: Balancing the "duty to warn" against the right to privacy. *AAOHN Journal*, *36*(8), 346–347.
Zinermon v. Burch, 108 L. Ed. 2d 115, 117 (1990).

CHAPTER

Therapeutic Communication

DEBORAH ANTAI-OTONG, M.S., R.N.,C.S.

OUTLINE

CHAPTER OBJECTIVES

Upon completion of this chapter, you will be able to:

1. Analyze the relationship between neurobiological, psychosocial, and developmental factors and communication.
2. Discuss the major communication theories.
3. Assess verbal and nonverbal communication.
4. List the major principles of therapeutic communication.
5. Describe the concepts of the nurse–client relationship.
6. Integrate Peplau's theory into the nursing process.

KEY TERMS

Active listening
Body language
Clarifying techniques
Communication
Confrontation
Focusing
Language
Nurse–client relationship
Personal space
Process recording
Self-concept
Self-esteem
Therapeutic communication
Therapeutic use of touch

People are social beings who use communication as the basis of all interactions. They convey feelings, attitudes, and emotions through speech, touch, facial expression, and various other modes. Communication is a dynamic process between people, used to influence, gain mutual support, and gather from others the essentials needed for well-being, growth, and survival (Howells, 1975).

Human beings depend on verbal and nonverbal communication to master their world. The infant learns to differentiate and relate to caregivers through feeding, crying, and touching. Early experiences lay the foundation of lifelong communication patterns and interpersonal relationships.

Establishing interpersonal relationships is an integral part of psychiatric–mental health nursing; it enables the nurse to appreciate the uniqueness of human behavior and establish healthy nurse–client interactions. *Interpersonal* refers to relations between persons. Clients experiencing distress benefit from therapeutic interactions with nurses.

Communication refers to the transmission of feelings, attitudes, ideas, and behaviors from one person to another. This process is generally classified as therapeutic or nontherapeutic.

Therapeutic communication refers to a healing or curative dialogue between people. This is particularly significant to the nurse because it is the basis of therapeutic relationships. Therapeutic communication fosters an active collaborative process that facilitates problem solving, change, learning, and growth. The **nurse–client relationship** is a dynamic partnership that defines, directs, and evaluates treatment outcomes.

The purpose of this chapter is to discuss the major communication theories and integrate them into psychiatric–mental health nursing practice.

CAUSATIVE FACTORS OF COMMUNICATION PATTERNS

Therapeutic communication is the matrix of psychiatric–mental health nursing. It involves an exchange of information between clients and nurses. Communication is conveyed through feelings, attitude, or thoughts. This reciprocal process enables the nurse to effect adaptive changes in the client (Travelbee, 1971).

The foundation of therapeutic communication is rapport. *Rapport* refers to harmony or accord between people. This initial alliance is vital to the formation of trust. As the therapeutic relationship evolves, so does the client's willingness to trust and share information. This relationship affords psychiatric–mental health nurses with opportunities to assess complex client needs, develop mutual outcome identification, and evaluate client responses. Evaluation is determined by the client's verbal and nonverbal communication patterns.

The nature of communication patterns is complex and involves several components. The major components of communication patterns relate to several neurobiological, psychosocial, and developmental issues.

NEUROBIOLOGICAL ISSUES

Information exchange occurs within the brain and the central nervous system. This process arises from biochemical processes that alter emotional and behavioral responses to higher brain levels, such as the cortex. Mediation of information throughout the nervous system is crucial to human survival and adaptation.

Adaptation models suggest that people constantly interact with internal and external environments. Appraisal of one's environment is determined by higher brain centers and is mediated by neuroendocrine processes. Stressors activate the hypothalamus directly or indirectly through the limbic system (see Fig. 11–1 in Chapter 11). The cerebrum, the hypothalamus, and the surrounding structures constitute the limbic system. The cerebrum is responsible for cognitive function, creativity, and intentional information, whereas the hypothalamus is the core of the limbic system. This area is only the size of a thumb tip, but its blood supply is one of the most abundant in the whole body. The hypothalamus is the locus of feelings of pleasure, rage, anger, sexual arousal, hunger, and thirst. The neural links of the cerebrum and the hypothalamus allow a constant circulation of biochemical processes that modulate human instinct and emotions. Emotional responses are located in these areas, and they evoke distress and other adaptive response to internal and external stimuli (Price, 1987).

Sensations and perceptions are used to experience internal and external stimuli. The senses enable people to acquire information through neural pathways and organs. What one hears, sees, feels, smells, and tastes influences one's perception of the world. *Perception* refers to the dynamic process of assimilating and organizing sensations.

People who are unable to communicate effectively for neurobiological or psychosocial reasons experience feelings of frustration, shame, and despair. Clients with aphasia or sensory deficits are vulnerable to psychological distress. Institutionalized elderly clients are particularly at risk for maladaptive responses to impaired communication. Assessing the needs of this population is vital to its socialization, self-care, and independence (Lubinski, 1981).

Buckwalter et al. (1988) described behavioral changes generated by a collaborative nursing and speech–language pathology intervention. Their subjects were elderly aphasic and dysarthric clients in a long-term care facility. Findings from this study suggested several interventions that minimize maladaptive responses in aphasic and dysarthric elderly clients, including the following:

- Assessment of client needs
- Increase in social interactions
- Establishment of one-on-one therapeutic relationships

The nursing implications from this study are that these easy, cost-effective interventions can reduce the need for various restraints and improve the quality of life for long-term care residents.

Findings from this study reinforce the need for nurses to appreciate sensory and perceptual deficits in various age groups and the mentally ill. The client experiencing auditory hallucinations and persecutory delusions is another example of how impaired sensory and perceptual processes affect communication. This client often communicates impaired verbal and nonverbal cues, such as incoherent speech, agitation, and aggressiveness. These behaviors suggest that neurobiological processes are largely responsible for impaired communication patterns.

Nurses need to assess impaired communication patterns and formulate interventions that reduce client distress. Establishing rapport and providing biological interventions, such as medication, can calm and reduce impaired sensory and perceptual responses.

The outcome of psychological distress is affected by accurate assessment and appropriate interventions that restore health. Psychiatric–mental health nurses can optimize this process by exploring the psychosocial and developmental factors that affect adaptation and communication.

PSYCHOSOCIAL ISSUES

People are social beings. Emotional ties foster a sense of identity, comfort, security, and support. From birth to death, relationships with others are central to human existence.

Early attachments lay the foundation of meaningful relationships. The quality of early attachments is influenced by the cultural, socioeconomic, and mental health status of the caregivers. Through various parental gestures and communication patterns, the infant learns about the world. Ideally, attentive parents convey safe and secure environments that nurture growth and facilitate congruent communication development.

In contrast, the person who grows up in an environment that lacks clear communication and uncertainty about the world is likely to have difficulty relating to others. Difficulty forming meaningful relationships interferes with expression of feelings, thoughts, and needs, further compromising optimal functioning.

Communication is critical to healthy human interactions. Integrating neurobiological and psychosocial factors into the communication process enhances the nurse–client relationship. Overall, it enables the psychiatric–mental health nurse to respond to complex client needs and facilitate health restoration.

DEVELOPMENTAL ISSUES

The third major factor that influences communication is developmental stage. Four stages have been identified in language development and communication:

1. The first stage and initial communication begins with the birth cry, which evolves into gurgles and variations in sounds and sucking rates that convey different needs.
2. The second stage involves cry vocalizations and variations in sounds and pitches.
3. The third stage is manifested by babbling, which varies with culture and is influenced by the intonation patterns and language of the primary caregivers.
4. The evolution of "true speech" begins in the fourth stage, which ends the first year and is described as prelinguistic vocabulary. These stages parallel cognitive and neurobiological development, which influences refinement of schemata and systematic growth of logical operations or understanding of self and the world. Sociological factors also play a major role in language and communication development. Learning takes place in the context of reciprocating motor gestures between the infant and the primary caregivers (Condon & Sander, 1974; Piaget, 1970).

Communication processes begin prenatally, at which time the stress level and coping abilities of the parents influence the fetus's neurobiological maturity. The fetus is also vulnerable to conditions that affect neurobiological development, such as genetics, rubella, and other teratogenic influences.

As the fetus moves from intrauterine life to the newborn stage, parents continue to provide basic survival needs. Bonding and attachment are essential aspects of infancy. Tactile stimulation promotes psychological and neurobiological growth. Early attachments and interactions with caregivers depend on how emotions, warmth, trust, and safety are conveyed. The sound and tone of the caregivers' voices, stroking, and facial expressions symbolize early messages about the world. Parents who transmit warmth and love foster trust and safety in the child (Ainsworth, 1985; Bowlby, 1969).

In comparison, parents who are unresponsive to the child's basic needs convey anger, distrust, and uncertainty about the world. A negative or indifferent portrayal of the world compromises neurobiological and psychosocial development. Delayed cognitive and motor development and, in severe cases, failure to thrive and death are potential outcomes for the neglected child. Delayed or impaired cognitive and motor development interferes with the child's ability to express feelings, thoughts, and ideas. Inability to communicate effectively affects the child's self-esteem, social skills, and growth. As the child moves into adolescence, these factors become more pronounced. The child who fails to develop trust, self-esteem, and autonomy is at risk for mental illness, particularly in adolescence.

Adolescence is a stage that exemplifies early childhood frustrations. The adolescent who fails to master previous developmental tasks is at risk for maladaptive responses, such as depression, substance abuse, and suicide. Several developmental issues that interfere with establishing therapeutic interactions in this age group include the following:

- Difficulty developing trust
- Frequent limit testing
- Need for immediate gratification
- Expressed hostility toward adults, such as parents and teachers
- Impatience
- Low tolerance to stress and frustration

The family who instills trust, self-esteem, and autonomy in the adolescent fosters growth, effective coping, and communication skills. The adolescent can form meaningful and lasting relationships and master future developmental tasks.

The relationship between early childhood interactions and adult behaviors is well documented. Adults can use competent communication skills to solve problems, meet basic needs, and form stable interpersonal relationships. Major adult developmental tasks are intimacy, generativity, and integrity.

Developmental issues are pertinent to understanding human behavior. Trust is crucial to human development because it influences how people relate to others. The complexity of therapeutic communication challenges nurses to understand factors that affect client behavior. Factors such as the client's ability to establish trust and the effects of neurobiological, psychosocial, and developmental issues are relevant to human responses (Table 6–1).

COMMUNICATION THEORIES

What is communication? The word *communicate* means to share, impart, and participate. Several theorists have defined communication.

DYADIC INTERPERSONAL COMMUNICATION MODEL

According to the dyadic interpersonal communication model described by Berlo in 1960, communication is a dynamic interaction that consists of a source, who has a purpose that is understandable to another person, and an encoder, who is able to understand the meaning of the message. The message is processed and decoded and understood by the recipient (decoder) (Berlo, 1960) (Fig. 6–1). In essence, people must convey clear messages if they expect the information to be understood.

BEHAVIOR AND COMMUNICATION

Walzlawick et al. (1967) contended that behavior is a form of communication and that messages convey information. They described this process as a message that is the basic communication unit; a series of messages is

TABLE 6–1

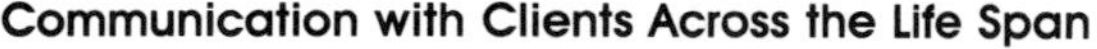

Communication with Clients Across the Life Span

	DEVELOPMENTAL INFLUENCES	AGE-SPECIFIC BEHAVIORS	AGE-SPECIFIC COMMUNICATION
Prenatal	Genetics, maternal health, damage during birth process		
Infancy	Mental retardation, fetal alcohol syndrome, sensory deprivation (aloof caregivers), impaired nutrition	Crying, cooing, poor eating, fretfulness, touching, eye contact, babbling (beginning of language at 6 months: putting sounds together)	Stroking; holding; feeding; eye contact (mirroring); soft, warm voice from caregivers
Childhood	Autism, mental retardation, sensory deprivation	Limited vocabulary that evolves using tones, inflections, tense	Concrete explanations; drawing a picture; warm, accepting approach
Adolescence	Psychosis, substance abuse, depression	Abstract thinking evolves, increased comprehension	Encourage participation in decision-making process; accepting and supportive approach; active listening
Adulthood	Medical conditions, substance abuse, psychosis, impaired nutrition	Cognitive function and abstract capabilities, adequate interpersonal skills	Establish rapport, genuine interest, empathy, active listening
Late adulthood	Medical conditions, aphasia, impaired cognitive/sensory function	Cognitive function intact, impaired hearing/vision, slowed thinking processes	Active listening; assess ability to speak, read, write; develop alternate way to communicate as needed; allow time to express feelings and respond to questions

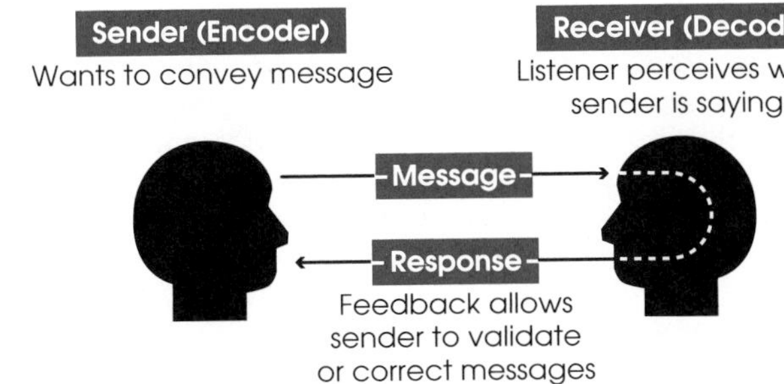

FIGURE 6-1
Berlo's (1960) dyadic interpersonal communication model.

called an *interaction*; and levels of communication are associated with specific patterns of interactions.

COMMUNICATION COMPETENCY

Virginia Satir (1967) surmised that the degree of communication competency represents how well people interact with others. The client with hallucinations or delusions is an example of how impaired communication affects social interactions. This client is distracted by internal and external stimuli that compromises interactions with the nurse.

In contrast, the politician who campaigns across the state uses effective communication skills to convey the political message to potential voters. This person's communication skills enable him or her to interact with constituents with little effort.

TRANSACTIONAL ANALYSIS AND COMMUNICATION

Eric Berne (1964) coined the term *transactional analysis* (TA). This theory incorporates four major themes necessary to understand human behavior: structural analysis (to assess what people are experiencing); TA (to assess what is going on between two people); racket and game analysis (to assess specific interactions that have negative payoffs); and script analysis (to assess individual life plans). For purposes of describing communication patterns, TA is discussed.

TA is based on the games people play to act out life scripts. A game is a set of behaviors and attitudes exhibited by a person interacting with another person. Berne (1964) asserted that everyone has three functional parts called *ego states*. Ego states depict feelings and relate sets of behavioral patterns. The three major ego states are the following:

Parent—comprises attitudes and behaviors from external sources, predominately primary caregivers such as parents
Adult—comprises rational processes that appraise reality; the main sources are information from internal and external environments
Child—comprises feelings, or emotions, and impulses that represent the natural or spontaneous part of the person

The fundamental element of TA is the appraisal of interactions between people. The healthy person puts the Adult in charge but allows the Child to emerge during fun times and dismisses early critical messages from the Parent ego stage.

THERAPEUTIC COMMUNICATION

Reusch (1961) described communication as a universal function that occurs everywhere. He enumerated the major components of therapeutic communication:

- It can occur anywhere.
- It can be used to promote independence and improve interactions with others.
- It is a natural part of human beings.
- It relies on spontaneous expression of feelings and thoughts.
- It enables clients to accept past experiences and integrate them into present-day perceptions.

SUMMARY

Overall, communication is a complex, dynamic process that involves a sender and a receiver. Messages are conveyed through various symbols and clues within a social context. The value of communication lies in the ability to use various symbols or ideas to convey a common understanding of the message (Peplau, 1952). Psychiatric–mental health nurses are confronted with deciphering verbal and nonverbal messages regarding client responses.

TYPES OF COMMUNICATION

NONVERBAL COMMUNICATION

Nonverbal communication refers to body language or transmission of messages without the use of words. It comprises behaviors such as crying, facial expression, physical appearance, eye contact, body movement, gestures, touch, and tone of voice. Nonverbal communication is a natural and spontaneous process that often occurs with verbal communication. Nonverbal behavior is a potent form of communication. Assessing the meaning of various client responses is an integral aspect of psychiatric–mental health nursing.

Nurse–client interactions consist of both verbal and nonverbal communication. *Nonverbal* refers to the process, whereas *verbal* refers to the content (Birdwhitsell, 1970). The goal of therapeutic interactions is congruency between nonverbal and verbal communications. The nursing student who tells the client that he is feeling well today, and his thoughts, mood, and facial expression reflect this message, conveys to the client that he indeed feels good today. In contrast, the client who tells the nursing student that she is not upset, but her facial expression is grimaced and her fists are clenched, conveys that she is upset. The client's verbal and nonverbal communications are incongruent.

Nonverbal communication has greater impact than verbal communication. The old adage, "action speaks louder than words," is relevant to understanding communication in any society. Birdwhitsell (1970) believed that 65 to 70 percent of communication is based on nonverbal cues and that 30 percent is spoken, or verbal. The impact of nonverbal communication on nurse–client interactions is noteworthy because it affects one's perception of clinical situations.

A major limitation of nonverbal communication is the inability to validate the meaning of feelings. Nonverbal expression such as screaming and shouting is easy to assess as anger. However, the meaning of a sad expression or inappropriate smiling is more difficult to assess unless the client validates its meaning. Nurses can validate perceptions through observations and verbal interactions with clients. Observing body language is a critical aspect of validating nonverbal communication.

Body language refers to the manifestation of feelings or thoughts by way of body gestures. The nurse's body language is just as significant as the client's. Clients observe nurse behaviors and can readily identify incongruent verbal and nonverbal communication. Gladstein (1987) described several nonverbal behaviors that convey warmth, caring, and calmness to clients as follows:

- Facing the client directly
- Maintaining eye contact (avoid staring)
- Nodding to convey validation, acceptance, and understanding
- Holding the arms in a manner that conveys openness, for example, arms resting on the chair (avoid crossing them)
- Presenting a natural, soft smile to communicate warmth

Body language is a powerful nonverbal communication tool. Recognizing its usefulness helps nurses understand their own behaviors and those of the client. Body language includes the following:

- Facial expression
- Physical appearance
- Eye contact
- Posture and gait
- Hand movements and gestures
- Tone of voice and rate of speech

Facial Expressions. Facial expressions reveal internal feelings and emotions. They convey a number of feelings that are reflected in the client's forehead, lips, mouth, and eyes. Intense messages are easier to assess than subtle responses. Expression of a flat, blunted, or incongruent affect often masks feelings and emotions.

Physical Appearance. Physical appearance (such as personal hygiene, posture, dress, appropriateness of clothes for season and weather, and coordination of color, patterns, and accessories) reveals the client's level of functioning, confidence, and self-worth. Clients with psychosis may present in a disheveled manner, suggesting that their ability to manage self-care is impaired. In addition to a disheveled appearance, these clients' clothes may be soiled, wrinkled, and smell of body odor. Mental status, emotional state, and current employment must be considered when assessing physical appearance.

Eye Contact. Eye contact provides a channel for nurses to connect with clients in a manner that conveys genuine concern and care. Inner feelings are often reflected through one's eyes. Eyes disclose important messages and communicate important information about the nurse and the client. Direct eye contact suggests involvement. In contrast, limited eye contact communicates a lack of interest or low self-esteem. Cultural and ethnic considerations must be made because the significance of eye contact varies among specific populations. Other factors that may influence the client's eye contact are alterations in mood or thought processes. The client with depression or schizophrenia may have poor eye contact, whereas the client with mania may be overly direct and intrusive.

Posture and Gait. Posture and gait communicate several nonverbal cues. Authority is communicated by the height from which one interacts with others. This can be seen when one person stands and the other sits, the former unconsciously places the self in a position of power. The client in a group session who jumps up to confront another client establishes power by this behavior.

The manner in which clients carry themselves often reflects self-concept, mood, and health. High self-esteem is reflected by an erect posture and active, purposeful stride. Low self-esteem or physical discomfort is exhibited by a slouched, slow, shuffling stride. Anxiety or anger are usually conveyed by rigid, tense, or rapid posture and gait. Pacing is indicative of agitation and restlessness in clients with psychotic disorders or those with potential for violence toward themselves or others.

Hand Movements and Gestures. Hand movements and gestures, like other body movements, are expressive. These gestures and others, such as pacing and speaking loudly, indicate agitation and potential violence. Nursing interventions include recognizing the meaning of these behaviors and reducing the risk of escalating the client's anger and agitation. Specific nonverbal communications that may be used in this situation include approaching the client in a calm, firm, and cautious manner; responding to eye contact; and maintaining a comfortable distance.

Clients with schizophrenia or paranoia tend to distance themselves and remain on guard. Guardedness and social withdrawal are shown when clients turn away from the nurse and present an invisible wall that shields them from external stimuli generated by interactions. In comparison, clients with a manic type of bipolar disorder are often intrusive and invade the personal space of others.

Tone of Voice and Rate of Speech. Voice tone and rate of speech are other nonverbal cues that mirror the client's emotional state. Manic or anxious clients often speak at a pressured or rapid rate. Angry or agitated clients may speak loudly, and depressed clients may speak in a low, passive tone.

VERBAL COMMUNICATION

Verbal communication, like nonverbal behavior, transmits feelings such as anger and happiness. This process involves an exchange of words, both spoken and written, between people. Nurses cannot assume that what is spoken means what is said. The effective use of verbal communication varies among individuals and is influenced by developmental stage, neurobiological components such as stress, cognitive function, and psychosocial and cultural factors.

What are the major principles of effective verbal communication? Rapport is the foundation of effective communication. It evolves as the client feels safe and at ease with the nurse. Specific techniques that encourage rapport are the following:

- A warm, caring approach
- Good eye contact
- A clear, firm voice
- Assertive but not aggressive posture
- Quiet, comfortable environment
- Simple, clear explanations based on education, developmental stage, and cognitive function
- Active listening

These techniques allay client anxiety, foster expression of feelings, resolve miscommunication, and provide a model for effective communication patterns.

Verbal communication is an integral part of nurse–client interactions. Nurses can use it to share thoughts, encourage expression of feelings, enhance problem-solving skills, and clarify miscommunication.

FACTORS AFFECTING THE COMMUNICATION PROCESS

Therapeutic communication is a complex process, and its effectiveness is influenced by various factors that direct the communication process, including

- Attitude
- Trust
- Empathy
- Language
- Culture
- Perceptions and observation
- Self-concept and self-esteem
- Anxiety and stress
- Personal space

ATTITUDE

The nurse's interest, acceptance, and attitude toward the client play major roles in therapeutic interactions. The nurse's **attitude** sets the mood of the nurse–client relationship. Clients need to feel valued and respected. The nurse conveys trust and empathy through verbal and nonverbal communication. The client needs to be approached in an unhurried manner, avoiding abrupt or indifferent responses. The client is more likely to be cooperative and participate in treatment when the nurse uses a calm, concerned approach.

TRUST

Trust is generated by the concerned and caring nurse. The client feels confident and safe in these environments. Building trust involves a number of conditions such as the following:

- Keeping promises
- Exhibiting consistency and reliability
- Expressing genuine interest and concern
- Accepting the client's feelings and concerns
- Providing safe client care
- Encouraging active participation in care
- Encouraging independence and growth through positive experiences
- Providing ongoing feedback regarding response to treatment

Therapeutic interactions foster feelings of closeness as each person maintains a sense of self, or separateness.

EMPATHY

Empathy communicates understanding and concern. It is defined as a critical aspect of therapeutic relationships. Ehmann (1971) defined empathy as a "means to share and experience the feelings of the patient" (pp. 75–76). This powerful communication tool conveys "I am with you and I have a sense of what you are experiencing" without totally losing one's identity. It promotes change, growth, and health restoration. This temporary sharing enables the nurse to appreciate the client's feelings and thoughts. The client can readily establish trust when the nurse conveys warmth and empathy. This can be communicated by nonverbal and verbal cues. Eye contact, an unhurried manner, and a simple touch are examples of nonverbal cues.

LANGUAGE

Verbal cues consist of using words to communicate ideas, thoughts, and feelings. The basis of verbal communication is **language.** Language is a complex phenomenon and the tool we use to communicate with each other. It activates higher cognitive processes such as understanding, thinking, remembering, and reasoning. Through language we learn, educate, socialize, create, and validate perceptions of ourselves and the world by sharing feelings and thoughts. Effective communication through language is linked with mental health.

Language is transmitted mainly through speech and is received through the senses. Communication relies on recognizable codes. Words are the central part of codes, and their meanings vary among people, cultures, states, and countries. Words alone do not convey feelings or thoughts. The interpretation of words is influenced by the recipient's perception of the message. The key to effective therapeutic communication is congruency between what the client says and the nurse's interpretation of the message. Effective communication is a reciprocal process. What the nurse says has an impact on this process along with the client's response. Unclear messages need to be validated through discussions with the client.

CULTURE

Culturally sensitive care is crucial to therapeutic communication. Psychiatric–mental health nurses must assess cultural congruency to minimize misunderstanding: Cultural influences may occur indirectly during client interactions and affect perception of client responses. When cultural incongruence is identified, the nurse needs to accept his or her limitations and seek ways to appreciate the client's uniqueness (Johnston, 1990). Clients need to feel accepted and treated with respect even though they are culturally different. Edward Hall (1966, 1989), a renowned anthropologist, recognized the significance of diversity and ethnicity as sources of strength. He described diversity as an invaluable asset to learn from others. Learning about others increases self-awareness. These processes are cornerstones to therapeutic interaction (see Chapter 3 for an in-depth discussion of cultural influences).

PERCEPTION AND OBSERVATION

Perception is the way events are interpreted through sensory stimulation. Perception is determined by past and present experiences and innate traits that validate or correct the receiver's interpretation. Thoughts are stimulated by perceptions, and feelings respond to thoughts. In the following example, the nurse's perception interferes with objective client care.

Nurse Brown may perceive clients who drink excessively as "bums." Her father was abusive when he drank excessively. Thoughts of her father generate negative feelings and anger toward the client abusing alcohol. Her ability to work with this type of client is compromised by her distorted perception of clients abusing alcohol.

Perceptions influence stereotyping and labeling of client responses. Historically, studies have shown that certain populations are more likely be diagnosed with chronic debilitating illnesses such as schizophrenia. Other groups are more likely to be diagnosed with less debilitating illnesses when their values and cultural and socioeconomic status are similar to those of the nurse.

Self-awareness is the key to understanding inaccurate perceptions and observations of client responses. Orlando (1961) asserted that nurses need to develop skills that enable them to explore the meaning of their perceptions of clients rather than making assumptions. Additionally, she surmised that this process is "crucial in understanding more fully what the patient is trying to communicate" (p. 45).

Accurate interpretation of data is crucial to therapeutic communication. It affects data collection, care planning, interventions, and the evaluation of client responses. Psychiatric–mental health nurses must strive to provide quality care using accurate perceptions and assessments of client needs.

SELF-CONCEPT AND SELF-ESTEEM

Self-concept refers to one's beliefs and feelings about self. It serves as a frame of reference for life experiences and perceptions about the world. It evolves over time and arises from interactions with others. Self-concept plays a major role in adaptation and the maturational process. Successful resolution of developmental tasks or stressors shapes a positive self-concept.

Smits and Kee (1992) investigated the relationship between self-concept and self-care among older adults residing in the community. The findings showed a significant relationship between self-care and self-concept scores.

Self-concept is relevant to psychiatric–mental health nurses because it determines how clients experience and manage stress. It affects the client's willingness to ask for and accept help. Clients with a poor self-concept are likely to feel unworthy of having their needs met. Their hesitancy to seek help often hinders the building of adaptive coping skills.

Self-esteem refers to self-worth and personal value. Maslow (1968, 1970) asserted that self-esteem is associated with having basic needs met. Basic needs are defined as physiological well-being, love, and safety. Self-esteem is closely related to self-concept.

Positive regard for self is comparable to high self-esteem. In contrast, negative self-regard suggests low self-esteem and associated feelings of worthlessness and inadequacy. These feelings can generate mood disorders such as depression and anxiety. These clients are also likely to use self-destructive behaviors such as substance abuse and suicide attempts to resolve stress.

Self-esteem and self-concept are dynamic and are largely shaped by interactions with significant others. Psychiatric–mental health nurses can use these concepts to understand certain communication patterns in clients experiencing distress. Clients with high self-esteem express and share their feelings with others. Conversely, those with low self-esteem are likely to be passive and hesitant to share their feelings. Assessing these behaviors helps nurses establish therapeutic interactions that increase self-worth.

ANXIETY AND STRESS

Client interactions normally produce anxiety in both the client and the nurse. Anxiety is described as a vague, uncomfortable feeling that manifests itself psychologically and biologically. Response to anxiety varies among people and can be both motivating and distressful. Lower levels of anxiety increase alertness and enhance problem-solving abilities. However, heightened levels of anxiety decrease cognitive processing, causing disruption and distress.

Sullivan (1954) described anxiety as the chief barrier to effective communication because it threatens self-esteem and self-respect. He also admitted that it is an inherent part of the human experience. As a natural part of human experiences, nurses need to take steps to help clients handle anxiety. Attempts to put the client at ease can be facilitated by using a calm, caring approach. A quiet, safe environment reduces distractions and facilitates expression of feelings and problem solving. Clients can control their feelings by using relaxation and stress-reducing exercises. Reducing anxiety and redirecting it into useful channels enhances communication.

PERSONAL SPACE

The concept of **personal space** in interpersonal relationships was introduced by Hall (1966). He believed that human beings are constantly changing positions and that social interactions are affected by space. He defined space or zone norms from a Western cultural perspective as the following:

1. Intimate distance: 6 to 18 in. (between people touching)
2. Personal distance: 1½ to 4 ft (arm's length)
3. Social distance: 4 to 12 ft (most frequently used in business activities)
4. Public distance: 12 to 25 ft (entertainer, public speaker)

Hall stressed the need to appreciate cultural differences as the basis of space and individual differences when interpreting the meaning of space. The role of space in the nurse–client interaction is significant because it is difficult to assess another's comfort zones. As a rule of thumb, personal distance is usually considered comfortable. However, some cultures define comfort zones as close as 6 to 8 inches (Hall, 1966).

THERAPEUTIC COMMUNICATION TECHNIQUES

A question often posed by students and nurses is, "What are therapeutic communication techniques?" A simple definition is that a therapeutic communication technique is one that facilitates therapeutic communication. In reality, the ability to communicate effectively is an art that uses basic listening and communication skills. The nurse can use this collaborative interaction to assess the client's needs, formulate client outcomes, and evaluate the effectiveness of interventions. Therapeutic techniques include the following:

- Active listening
- Questioning
- Clarifying techniques
- Therapeutic use of touch
- Therapeutic use of silence
- Humor
- Focusing
- Confrontation
- Summarizing

ACTIVE LISTENING

Active listening is the basis of all nurse–client interactions. Listening is more than just hearing. It is a dynamic process that requires enormous concentration and energy. It literally means using all the senses to assess verbal and nonverbal messages. The nurse listens for content as well as feelings. Active listening encourages clients to express feelings and thoughts.

Ceccio and Ceccio (1982) described the qualities of a good listener as the following:

- Maintains eye contact
- Gives client full attention, both mentally and physically (makes a conscious effort to inhibit sounds and screen distractions)
- Minimizes or eliminates barriers (see following)
- Avoids interruptions and interpretations
- Responds to content and feeling components of the message
- Listens for ideas (an essential aspect of interaction)
- Provides client with evidence that one is listening (i.e., reviews and restates in own words and reflects or plays back the message)
- Responds only to the content of the client's verbal message

Active listening demonstrates interest in the client. It fosters a trusting relationship that encourages the client to express feelings and share thoughts. Recognizing nursing behaviors that interfere with active listening is just as important as appreciating those that promote it.

Barriers to Active Listening. Barriers to active listening (Table 6–2) exist in all clinical situations. The psychiatric–mental health nurse plays an active role in reducing or eliminating them. Pluckman (1978) noted that most barriers are psychological rather than physical. Additional barriers include the following:

TABLE 6 – 2
Psychological Barriers to Active Listening

- Judgmental attitude (perception)
- Blaming
- Rigidity, dogmatic thinking (closed mindedness)
- Providing solutions rather than facilitating this process in clients
- Wrong vocabulary, cliches
- Introducing unrelated information
- Expressing disapproval
- Giving advice rather that options
- Discounting the client's feeling ("How can you be upset over something like that?")
- Interrupting, or changing the subject

- Lack of privacy
- Noises
- Seating arrangements
- Use of jargon
- Perceptual and sensory distortions in clients
- Countertransference
- Anxiety in the nurse
- Pain in the client

Other barriers include stereotyping the client by race, ethnic background, class, religion, or illness.

Students and nurse clinicians can enhance their communication skills by identifying barriers to active listening. The art of active listening requires perseverance and patience. Initially, the nurse enters the relationship with genuine interest and concern for the client. This puts the client at ease and enables the nurse to provide a safe, quiet, and private environment. Finally, the client experiences a sense of calmness, acceptance, and security and is able to verbalize feelings and thoughts.

QUESTIONING

Questioning is a valuable tool that nurses use to encourage the expression of feelings and self-disclosure and to gain insight into the meaning of present stressors. The basis of the client's response depends on his or her level of trust and security or in the comfort with the questions. Nurses can put their clients at ease by introducing themselves and calling them by name; making eye contact and shaking hands at the same time helps nurses connect with clients both verbally and nonverbally. This establishes a safe environment that promotes trust, care, and empathy. The nurse can use questioning as a tool to elicit pertinent information from the client.

Some examples of questions that elicit the most information from clients include the following:

- What major changes have you had during the past 6 months?
- How have they affected you or your lifestyle?
- What made you come in today?

Questions that begin with what, which, when, how, or who allow nurses to gather factual information and are defined as *open-ended questions*. They are direct, that is, they encourage clients to discuss and clarify their thoughts and feelings while passing the responsibility to the client to explore and understand these issues.

In contrast, *closed-ended questions* are less effective in collecting data than are open-ended ones. Closed-ended questions such as, "Would you like help with your problem today?" limit the client's responses to yes or no, thus minimizing the quality of information. A more efficient way to assess what the client wants may be asked in a question such as, "What can I help you with today, Mrs. Read?" This question allows the client to explain her needs while taking responsibility for problem identification. Closed-ended sentences are relevant at times when specific information is needed, such as marital and employment status.

Questions should be generated by client responses, both verbal and nonverbal. A raised eyebrow, nodding, and increased voice tone are examples of nonverbal cues to the client's thoughts or feelings.

As the relationship evolves, clients may feel comfortable or entitled to know about the nurse. Nurse clinicians or students may wonder how to respond to personal questions. It is essential to keep clients directed to their own issues. Questioning of the nurse may mean that the client is anxious, curious, or distracted. The nurse can use these situations to clarify what questioning means to the client.

CLARIFYING TECHNIQUES

Clarifying technique refers to the use of certain methods to clear up or make understandable. Communication is a complex, dynamic process that involves interaction between people. The likelihood of confusion exists in all human interactions. Clarifying communication patterns and exploring client responses are basic psychiatric–mental health nursing tools that reduce miscommunication and misunderstanding.

Specific clarifying techniques are paraphrasing or restatements. Paraphrasing involves listening to the client's basic messages and repeating them using similar words. This technique focuses on the content of the message. It affords the nurse with a clearer understanding of the client's distress. Client responses to paraphrasing validate or invalidate the nurse's perception of the client's message. Overall, the nurse's perception and observational skills are enhanced by clarifying techniques.

The following dialogue is an example of a nurse using clarifying techniques. The nurse begins the process by using a question to verify the meaning of a message. Note the use of this technique in the following situation.

Nurse–Client Dialogue 1

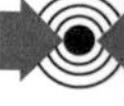

NURSE: [clarifying question] Mr. Key, what do you mean when you say your mind feels like scrambled eggs? [puzzled look on the nurse's face]

CLIENT: I don't know!

NURSE: [paraphrasing statement] It sounds like you are confused.

CLIENT: I am confused. Yes, I am very confused.

NURSE: What do you mean, "very confused?"

CLIENT: Well, my mind is playing tricks on me, and I feel like someone is watching me all the time.

NURSE: How long have you felt like this?

CLIENT: About 3 weeks.

NURSE: [paraphrasing statement] You have been feeling confused and afraid for the past 3 weeks.

CLIENT: Yes, that's it. I feel like I'm going out of my mind.

In this example, the nurse was unsure of what the client meant by saying his "mind felt like scrambled eggs." The nurse could have made assumptions about the meaning of these words, but the nurse chose to ask him to explain it. His explanation gave the nurse a clearer understanding of his distress. In addition to seeking clarification, the nurse communicated empathy and concern.

THERAPEUTIC USE OF TOUCH

Touching is another powerful, sometimes controversial, nonverbal communication. It is a critical aspect of human relationships throughout the life span. Touching is key to survival, particularly during infancy, because it conveys trust, safety, and love and it nurtures neurobiological and psychosocial development. As the child develops, touching becomes less important than other communication processes. Children tend to respond more favorably to touch than do adults.

Therapeutic use of touch refers to the healing powers of touch. The client experiences trust, reassurance, and acceptance from therapeutic touch. A trusting relationship is a prerequisite to the effective use of touch. Clients who are tearful and feeling sad usually find comfort from a touch on the shoulder or hand. Touching is mentally and physically comforting, especially to clients with hearing and visual impairments. Confused and regressed clients also value human contact.

Some clients have difficulty responding to touch favorably. The client may perceive it as an invasion of his or her personal space and react defensively. Clients who have difficulty trusting, such as children or adults who have been abused, may perceive touch as traumatic, invasive, frightening, or threatening. An inability to express feelings and warmth toward others undermines forming meaningful relationships.

Therapeutic use of touch, like other communication techniques, enables nurses to establish meaningful interactions with clients in distress. Its healing qualities foster growth, vitality, and health.

THERAPEUTIC USE OF SILENCE

Silence is a natural phenomenon; it is a deliberate restraint from expression. Silence is another effective communication technique.

Silence can be used to help clients explore the meaning of feelings and thoughts. An accepting, safe climate fosters self-awareness in both the nurse and the client. The depressed and tearful client needs silence to explore feelings and thoughts related to losing a dear friend. Silence may be uncomfortable to the nurse or the client, but it allows the nurse to explore his or her thoughts until the client resumes the interaction. The nurse needs to explore the meaning of feelings generated by silence.

HUMOR

Humor is associated with amusing and comical expressions. Is there a place for humor in psychiatric nursing? Of course there is, because of its healing nature. Humor helps clients express feelings, enables exploration of the humor, and reduces anxiety and tension (King et al., 1983; Lachman, 1983). Nurses can use humor to form meaningful relationships, to generate adaptive coping skills, and to build self-esteem.

Teaching clients to use humor helps them learn how to have fun. Developing hobbies and fun activities frees clients from fears and limitations. This coping process reduces tension and mobilizes client strengths and healing. Laughter stimulates biological and psychosocial processes that restore health. Humor, like other communication techniques, offers nurses and clients innovative strategies that enhance trust and acceptance.

FOCUSING

Focusing refers to clarifying a perception or spotlighting certain aspects of communication. This technique is useful when clients use vague communication. Focusing is useful when clients do not express their feelings and thoughts clearly, ramble, or discuss several issues at one time. Nurses can use it to assess relevant client needs by selecting certain aspects of the client's discussion. The following dialogue is an example of focusing.

Nurse–Client Dialogue 2

NURSE: You have looked concerned since returning from your leave.

CLIENT: My wife says she cannot pay the bills and take care of the children while I am looking for a job.

NURSE: It sounds like you are concerned about how she will manage things.

CLIENT: I am unsure. We have always had two incomes.

NURSE: It seems like you need to talk to her about your concerns.

This last statement asks for a specific response to a situation and provides a structure that helps the client organize his ideas and thoughts. The statement, "It sounds like you are concerned about how she will manage things," is an effort by the nurse to help the client focus on his feelings and concerns about his financial situation.

Focusing, like other communications, is used with other techniques to establish therapeutic interactions. Nurses use them to clarify and understand the meaning of client responses.

CONFRONTATION

Confrontation refers to an encounter or face-to-face meeting. Nurses often associate this term with conflict or angry discussions between opposing bodies. In reality, confrontation is a necessary aspect of nurse–client interactions. Like other techniques, it is an art that involves pointing out contradictions or incongruencies between feelings, thoughts, and behaviors. These discrepancies interfere with insight and self-exploration regarding specific conflicts.

Confrontation is a useful tool that enables clients to examine maladaptive behaviors. Nurses must employ patience and tact rather than a punitive approach to pointing out contradictory behaviors. The following is an example of confrontation.

Nurse–Client Dialogue 3

CLIENT: This is my third hospitalization, and I am still drinking.

NURSE: Mr. Lett, what does this mean to you?

CLIENT: You are the nurse; you tell me!

NURSE: Mr. Lett, I have worked with you for the past year, and I've noticed that when you are discharged from the hospital, you do not attend Alcoholics Anonymous meetings. It is difficult for you to stay sober if you do not participate in your 12-step program.

The nurse approaches the client in a warm but firm manner. This interaction encourages the client to appreciate certain behaviors, such as refusal to attend Alcoholics Anonymous meetings, that contribute to frequent relapses.

Confrontation is a dynamic, powerful interaction. Active empathetic listening is crucial to confrontation. Assessing verbal and nonverbal cues during this interaction enables the nurse to explore client strengths and maladaptive behaviors and to promote self-examination. Clients often respond in an angry or defensive manner when confronted. Acceptance of this behavior is essential to confrontation. Additionally, nurses must refrain from reacting in an angry or rejecting manner. These behaviors undermine the effectiveness of confrontation and interfere with objective client care.

SUMMARIZING

Summarizing is a communication tool that helps clients explore key points of a nurse–client interaction. This dynamic and collaborative process integrates perceptions of the nurse and the client. Major points are reviewed and used to generate future client outcomes.

The following interaction is an example of summarizing.

Nurse–Client Dialogue 4

NURSE: Mr. Effiong, I noticed that since your were diagnosed with diabetes 2 months ago, you have been stressed.

CLIENT: You are right. I have been unable to sleep and concentrate because I have never been sick before.

NURSE: What does it mean to have diabetes?

CLIENT: I don't know, but my uncle also had diabetes, and he eventually lost one of his legs.

NURSE: Tell me what you know about diabetes.

CLIENT: Well, I know that I have to take pills because my pancreas doesn't put out enough insulin. I am also on a special diet.

NURSE: How has this regimen affected your lifestyle?

CLIENT: Not bad, because I have always watched my diet, and taking one more pill in the morning doesn't bother me. Besides, my uncle had to take insulin shots. [The client sighs with relief, and his facial expression is more relaxed.]

NURSE: You look more relaxed. What does that mean?

CLIENT: I guess I am not as sick as my uncle, and as long as I watch my diet and take my medication, I will be fine.

NURSE: You were concerned about losing you leg.

CLIENT: You are right, and I realize that if I do as I'm told, the chances of this happening to me are slim.

NURSE: Well, now you know what was stressing you, which had to do with losing your leg. It sounds like you have decided that if you take your medication and stay on your diet, the chance of losing your leg is slim.

CLIENT: That's right.

The nurse and the client summarized major components of this interaction, and the nurse's comments reflected perceptions of the client's feelings, thoughts, and behaviors. The client validated these perceptions and helped the nurse understand his response to the situation. The client was an active participant in this process and was able to perceive his situation realistically. Verbalization of feelings and thoughts reduced his anxiety and helped him solve his problems more effectively.

NURSE–CLIENT INTERACTION: THE BASIS OF THE NURSING PROCESS

The nurse–client relationship is the basis of the nursing process. Therapeutic communication techniques are tools that are used to build and maintain these relationships. The effectiveness of these skills requires considerable thought and an understanding of the complexity of human behavior across the life span (see the Research Study display).

The importance of the nurse–client relationship was recognized as early as 1946 by a number of nurse theorists. Major contributors to the evolution of the one-on-one or nurse–client relationship are Peplau (1952), Mellow (1967), and Orlando (1961). These theorists established the foundation of psychiatric–mental health nursing. The heart of this specialty is therapeutic communication.

The communication process is complex and dynamic. Its breadth extends beyond talking and listening to clients. This nurse–client interaction is a powerful process that uncovers issues within the nurse and the client. These discoveries lay the foundation of adaptation and resolution of distress. Emphasis on this relationship is crucial to the psychiatric–mental health nurse and understanding complex human responses.

This discussion of the nurse–client interaction arises from the extensive contributions from Peplau. Her work has had profound impact on psychiatric–mental health nursing and the nurse–client relationship. Peplau's theory integrates major concepts from Sullivan's interpersonal theory. She delineated ways that the nurse uses the nurse–client relationship to appraise and formulate effective interventions. Interventions are used to reduce maladaptive responses and enhance interpersonal interactions.

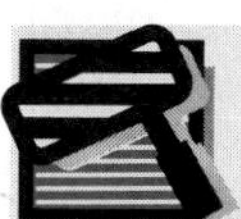

RESEARCH STUDY

Effect of Nurse–Client Transaction on Female Adolescents' Oral Contraception Adherence

Hanna, K. M. (1991). *Image, 25*(4), 285–290.

Study Problem/Purpose

The purpose of the study was to test the effect of a nurse–client transactional intervention on female adolescents' oral contraceptive adherence.

Method

The study consisted of 51 adolescent girls who were randomly assigned to either a control or an experimental group. All subjects experienced contraceptive education. Participants in the experimental group experienced a personalized interaction with a nurse, in which the nurse and the client focused together on perceived advantages and barriers associated with adherence to oral contraceptive use. The interaction included a group discussion and role playing, with a focus on responsibility and decision making. Perceptions of contraceptives were measured shortly postintervention and 3 months posttreatment.

Findings

The subjects in the experimental group had higher levels of oral contraceptive adherence than those in the other group.

Implications

The study results support the notion that effective communications or transactions can facilitate goal attainment.

NURSE–CLIENT RELATIONSHIP PHASES

Peplau's (1952) classic work, *Interpersonal Relations in Nursing,* described four phases of the nurse–client relationship. These phases are interlocking, and each outlines the task and role of the nurse and the client. The four phases are the following:

- Orientation
- Identification
- Exploitation
- Resolution

Orientation Phase

During the beginning, or orientation, phase, the client recognizes a need and seeks help. The orientation phase is the foundation of the nurse–client relationship. It establishes the basis of subsequent phases. The major nursing roles are "resource person, counseling relationship, surrogate for mother, and technical expert" (Peplau, 1952, p. 21). The resource person provides pertinent information that helps the client understand his or her personal problems. In the counseling relationship, the nurse uses active listening skills to assess the reasons for the client's present distress and the client's perception of it. The surrogate role allows the nurse to deal with transference issues. Finally, in the technical expert role, the nurse uses various health-promoting interventions to facilitate adaptation. Overall, this phase affords the client a caring and accepting environment that fosters the expression of feelings and thoughts. Client responses are assessed, and outcomes are identified (Fig. 6–2). Client outcomes need to be written in measurable and behavioral terms.

The following dialogue uses the nursing process to facilitate therapeutic interactions.

Text continued on page 114

Psychosocial Assessment Tool

Client's Name: ______________________ Date of Birth: ______________

Sex: M F Marital Status: ______________

Source of Information (client, relative, other—please specify):

1. Recent stressor(s) (i.e., loss, lifestyle changes, hospitalization)

> *Assess* the client's perception of the stressor(s).
>
> *Hospitalization* is a major source of stress for most clients because it places them in positions of powerlessness and loss of control. Hospitals have scheduled times to eat, bathe, and sleep.
>
> *Fears of the unknown,* such as tests, surgical procedures, pain, and separation from significant others, also increase anxiety and stress in clients.
>
> *Other areas of stress,* e.g., financial and familial, must be identified because they play pivotal roles in determining the client's responses to the present situation.
>
> *History of present signs and symptoms,* both emotional and physical, must be assessed because they are often chronic in nature. If a client complains of feeling depressed and this has persisted for many years, it is imperative to ask the client, "What made you decide to seek treatment at this time?"

2.. History of psychiatric treatment or counseling

Have you sought psychiatric treatment? No ______ Yes ______

What made you seek treatment?

Explain your response to treatment:

History of family psychiatric treatment or counseling: No ______ Yes ______

Explain:

3. Support systems (i.e., marital status, job, and relationships)

4. Suicidal or homicidal potential

Are you having thoughts of killing yourself or others at this time? No ______ Yes ______

If yes, describe:

How long have you had these thoughts? ______________

FIGURE 6–2
Example of a psychosocial assessment tool. (Form developed by Deborah Antai-Otong.)

Psychosocial Assessment Tool, page 2
Suicidal or homicidal potential, cont'd.

What has stopped you from acting on them?

History of attempt(s): No______ Yes______

Explain:

Dates: ________________________________

Circumstances:

Were you abusing drugs or alcohol during at the time of attempt(s)? No______ Yes______

Explain:

What kind of treatment did you receive?

Family history of suicide or attempts: No______ Yes______

Explain:

Question for family member:

What is your understanding of the reason(s) for the client's attempt(s)?:

Factors that increase the risk of suicidal behaviors:

- Age (adolescents and males >65 years of age; older adults usually see a physician 1 month or less before suicide)
- Race
- Previous attempts
- Family history
- Death or debilitating illness in spouse
- Substance abuse
- Lack of adequate support systems
- History of psychiatric disorders (i.e., psychosis, personaility disorders, and poor impulse control)
- Family turmoil, divorce, separation, death of a parent (adolescents)
- Depression
- Feelings of hopelessness, helplessness, or despair ("no options")

FIGURE 6–2 ***Continued***

Illustration continued on following page

Psychosocial Assessment Tool, page 3

5. *History of substance abuse:* No ______ Yes ______

Type:

Frequency:

Amount:

Last consumption:

Family history:

Treatment history:

Length of sobriety:

Legal history:

Blackouts: No ______ Yes ______

Explain:

Withdrawal seizures: No ______ Yes ______

Explain

Hallucinosis or delusions: No ______ Yes ______

Explain:

6. *Mental status examination*

Purpose:

1. To gather baseline information about the client's level of functioning, i.e., memory, appearance, behavior, and capacity for logical thought
2. To identify actual and potential problems
3. To assist the treatment team in making a medical diagnosis

The mental status examination must be done in an unhurried manner and in an environment that provides patients with privacy, safety, and acceptance.

FIGURE 6 – 2 *Continued*

Psychosocial Assessment Tool, page 4
Mental Status Examination, cont'd.

Level of consciousness: Alert______ Drowsy______ Other (describe):

Cooperative: No______ Yes ______

Describe:

Orientation: Person______ Place______ Date/Time______

Dress: Appropriate______ Neat______ Disheveled ______ Other________________

Eye contact (consider cultural aspects): Good______ Poor______

Affect: Congruent/appropriate______ Flat______ Blunted ______

Hallucinations: No______ Yes______ Auditory_________ Visual_________ Other_________

Describe:

Delusions: No______ Yes______ Persecutory_________ Grandiose _________

Describe:

Illusions: No______ Yes______

Describe:

Obsessions: No______ Yes______

Describe (Do you have habits that *bother* you?):

Compulsions: No______Yes ______

Describe (Do you have *special* ways that you do things?):

Phobias: No______ Yes______

Describe:

FIGURE 6–2 ***Continued***

Illustration continued on following page

Psychosocial Assessment Tool, page 5
Mental Status Examination, cont'd.

Speech: Clear____ Rapid____ Slurred____ Pressured____ Aphasic____ Mute____

Mood: Appropriate____ Anxious____ Agitated____ Elated____ Depressed____

Activity level: Appropriate____ Restless____ Psychomotor retarded____ Lethagric____ Restless____

Tremulous____ Changes positions often____

Explain:

Memory: Intact____; Difficulty with: Recent events____ Remote events____

Test recent memory with three objects in a 5-minute exercise (when needed)

Thought processes: Logical____ Relevant____ Coherent____

Does patient look stated age? Yes____ No____; Older____ Younger____

7. Medical History

During the past 3 to 6 months, have you had changes in the following:

Sleeping patterns? No____Yes____

Describe:

Appetite? No____Yes____

Describe:

Concentration patterns? No____ Yes____

Describe:

Energy level? No____ Yes____

Describe:

Libido? No____Yes____

Describe:

FIGURE 6–2 ***Continued***

Psychosocial Assessment Tool, page 6
Medical History, cont'd.

Current medical treatment: No _____ Yes _____

Explain:

Current medication(s): No _____ Yes _____

How long have you taken this medication?

Directions for taking:

What is your understanding of the reason(s) for taking this medication?

Are you taking your medications as ordered by your physician? Yes _____ No _____

Explain:

Surgical procedures during the past 12 months: No _____ Yes _____

Explain:

Allergies: No _____ Yes _____

Describe reaction:

FIGURE 6–2 ***Continued***

Nurse–Client Dialogue 5

NURSE: Mr. Lynn, I am Nurse Marshall, your nurse today. I understand that you were admitted several hours ago. I would like to know about your reasons for coming in today. [The nurse sits next to the client and on the same level. She has good eye contact, and her voice is clear and soft.]

CLIENT: My wife and kids say that I'm nuts! [The client's arms are folded, and he has poor eye contact.]

NURSE: Nuts? What do you mean?

CLIENT: Well I have been sleeping 12 hours a day, and I can't function at work.

NURSE: How long has this been going on?

CLIENT: Well, about a month this time.

NURSE: What made you come in today rather than 1 or 2 weeks ago?

CLIENT: Well, my boss is threatening to fire me. She's been through this too many times.

The nurse maintains a calm demeanor and uses good eye contact; her speech tone is unchanged. As a result, the clients sees the nurse as genuinely concerned about his well-being. He relaxes his arms and increases eye contact. He is less agitated and more cooperative.

The major nursing diagnoses (see Nursing Care Plan 6–1) based on this nurse–client interaction are

- High Risk for Violence, Self-Directed
- Ineffective Individual Coping
- Disturbance in Self-Concept related to low self-esteem

Identification Phase

The second phase, identification, emerges after the client clarifies and recognizes interventions that facilitate adaptive changes. The client becomes optimistic and ready for problem-solving as the nurse–client relationship evolves. The client begins to explore distressful feelings and thoughts, such as powerlessness, inadequacy, and helplessness. The nurse–client relationship nurtures initiative and learning (Peplau, 1952). This process encourages growth and adaptive coping patterns.

During the next few meetings, the client in the previous case begins to focus on his responsibilities in the treatment process. He discusses his feelings and thoughts and identifies maladaptive behaviors. This process generates behavioral changes and growth.

Nurse–Client Dialogue 6

NURSE: Mr. Lynn, what do you expect from this hospitalization?

CLIENT: I want to feel better about myself. I feel depressed all the time, and sometimes I wish I had never been born.

NURSE: What do you mean, you wish you had never been born?

CLIENT: I have disappointed my family, my boss, and myself. I just think they would be better off if I were dead.

NURSE: Mr. Lynn, are you saying that you want to kill yourself?

CLIENT: Not really, but there are times I wish I didn't wake up.

NURSE: I am concerned about your thoughts of dying and death. Have you ever tried to kill yourself?

CLIENT: No! I would never kill myself, but I feel very depressed at times.

NURSE: Have you had these thoughts before?

CLIENT: Yes, but not this bad.

NURSE: What was going on in your life when you had these thoughts in the past?

CLIENT: I was having marital problems, but we worked them out.

NURSE: How did you work things out?

CLIENT: We talked to a marriage counselor for about 6 months.

NURSE: What's your relationship like at this time?

CLIENT: It's fine. She just worries about me a lot.

NURSE: Tell me about recent changes or stressors in your life.

CLIENT: I really don't know of any, but I am concerned about my job. I feel worthless and helpless all the time.

NURSE: Tell me about these feelings, particularly about their duration.

CLIENT: I feel old. A young college boy was promoted to supervisor 2 months ago, and it didn't bother me at first. Then I began to think about it, and I realized that I have been an accountant for 25 years and I have reached my peak in promotions. This depresses me.

The nurse continues to encourage expression of feelings and provide an empathic response to his distress. She also recognizes that the client is experiencing a developmental crisis related to his career and concerns about his age.

Outcome Identification. Several client outcomes are identified by the nurse and the client:

- The client verbalizes his feelings rather than acting on them.
- The client makes a no-suicide contract with the nurse and other staff.
- The client identifies several positive self-attributes.
- The client develops enduring adaptive coping skills.

Nursing Care Plan 6-1 Therapeutic Interactions (Mr. Lynn)

▶ Nursing Diagnosis: High Risk for Violence: Self-Directed

OUTCOME IDENTIFICATION	NURSING ACTIONS	RATIONALES	EVALUATION
1. By [date], client will verbalize feelings rather than acting on them.	1a. Establish rapport. Encourage ventilation of feelings.	1a. Rapport is the basis of therapeutic interactions, conveying empathy, caring, and interest.	*Goal met:* Nurse forms therapeutic relationship. Client expresses feelings. Client is initially focused on death but is later able to look at other options.
	1b. Maintain safe environment. Assess level of dangerousness.	1b. Maintaining a safe environment provides control and decreases acting on thoughts of suicide.	
	1c. Observe for signs of mood change. Notify physician of changes.	1c. A change in mood increases level of dangerousness.	

▶ Nursing Diagnosis: Ineffective Individual Coping

OUTCOME IDENTIFICATION	NURSING ACTIONS	RATIONALES	EVALUATION
1. By [date], client will develop realistic perception of stressors and self.	1a. Explore reasons for present stressors.	1a. Exploring reasons for present stressors helps client understand self and present responses.	*Goal met:* Client returns to precrisis level of functioning. Client develops adaptive coping skills. Client's self-esteem increases.
	1b. Understand the meaning of present stressors.	1b. Understanding the meaning of present stressors validates client's responses.	
2. By [date], client will develop enduring adaptive coping skills.	2. Assist in identifying strengths and coping skills.	2. Identifying strengths and coping skills places focus on positive attributes that can be reinforced in treatment.	

▶ Nursing Diagnosis: Disturbance in Self-Concept Related to Low Self-Esteem

OUTCOME IDENTIFICATION	NURSING ACTIONS	RATIONALES	EVALUATION
1. By [date], client will verbalize positive attributes and increased self-esteem.	1a. Provide for successful experiences.	1a. Positive experiences increase confidence, sense of power and control, self-concept, and self-esteem.	*Goal met:* Client returns to precrisis level of functioning. Client develops adaptive coping skills. Client's self-esteem increases.
	1b. Communicate acceptance, and show genuine interest.	1b. Promotes development of nurse–client relationship.	
	1c. Encourage client to identify positive attributes.	1c. Increases self-esteem.	
	1d. Teach assertiveness skills.	1d. Promotes confidence and self-care.	
	1e. Encourage active participation in care.	1e. Enables client to feel powerful and in control.	

Exploitation Phase

The phase of exploitation emerges as the client appreciates the importance of the nurse–client relationship. The client learns how to get his or her needs met through these interactions. Anxiety emerges as the client struggles with dependence and independence issues in the relationship. The nurse must assess the client responses and formulate interactions that encourage self-care and independence.

Resolution Phase

The final phase of the nurse–client relationship is the resolution, or termination, phase. The success of this mutually planned stage is determined by previous ones. Resolution is influenced by the client's ability to use the nurse–client relationship to develop adaptive coping behaviors. The major themes in this phase include the exploration of feelings about termination and the summarization of major aspects of the relationship, including accomplishments and growth.

Peplau (1952) referred to this phase as a *freeing process*. Ideally, the client maintains independence and develops adaptive coping patterns. Appreciating the client's experience enhances the collaborative process and encourages empathy and the likelihood of education and growth.

The resolution phase is illustrated in the final part of the previous dialogue.

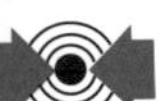

Nurse–Client Dialogue 7

NURSE: Mr. Lynn, how are you feeling today?

CLIENT: I am feeling a lot better, thanks to you and the others. I suddenly realized that there are more things in life than my job. My wife seems to think that we need a vacation.

NURSE: When was the last time you had a vacation?

CLIENT: It's been at least 10 years. I have always been too busy to do anything with my family.

NURSE: It sounds like you are long overdue for a vacation.

CLIENT: You are right, I have always looked at the negative side of things. I have to stop myself from thinking negative thoughts and focus on the brighter side of life. I am going home in 2 days. I am going to miss you and the other nurses.

NURSE: Mr. Lynn, it has been my pleasure to work with you, too. You have made a lot of progress over the past few weeks.

This phase of the relationship allowed the client and nurse to discuss areas of accomplishments and feedback regarding his progress. He developed adaptive coping skills and did not attempt to harm himself during hospitalization (see Nursing Care Plan 6–1 for an evaluation).

The nurse–client relationship is an invaluable process that integrates various theories to assess maladaptive behaviors and develop therapeutic interventions. Therapeutic interventions enable clients to assess maladaptive behaviors and replace them with adaptive ones that restore health.

TABLE 6–3
Instructions for Process Recordings

1. Establish rapport with client.
2. Determine the appropriateness of client and situation.
3. Select a portion of nurse–client interaction.
4. Write reports immediately after contact.
5. Answer the following questions:
   a. Were verbal and nonverbal cues identified?
   b. Were the nurse's verbal and nonverbal responses congruent?
   c. Were they therapeutic or nontherapeutic?
6. Discuss the evaluation with instructor, peers, and other nurses.

EVALUATING COMMUNICATION USING PROCESS RECORDING

The nurse–client interaction can be evaluated using feedback from clients, other health care providers, and the **process recording**. Process recordings are effective learning strategies that enhance learning affiliated with interpersonal communication. This process involves choosing a part of the nurse–client interaction, approximately 5 minutes, and recording a verbatim (word-for-word) account of the entire conversation (Table 6–3). Analysis of this teaching method is influenced by the process and the content.

The process recording is an in-depth evaluation of communication skills that can help students identify their strengths and weaknesses (Carpenito & Duespohl, 1985). The major shortcoming of this learning method is that it requires students to remember precisely what was said during the nurse–client interaction.

DEVELOPING SELF-AWARENESS OF COMMUNICATION PATTERNS

Self-awareness helps nurses recognize their strengths and limitations and adds dimension to the nurse–client relationship. This process is pertinent to understanding client responses and enables nurses to explore these issues in their clients. This growth-producing phenomenon involves recognition of anxiety-provoking circumstances. Understanding and exploring these issues are vital aspects of personal and professional growth.

Circumstances that generate anxiety or strong emotions interfere with objective, logical decision making. Factors such as past experiences, attitude, and responses to specific client populations or circumstances affect self-awareness. Nurses must recognize and explore the source of negative reactions, biases, and stereotyping.

Self-awareness helps nurses identify verbal and nonverbal communication patterns. Clients sense positive and negative reactions in nurses. Some clients may confront nurses to clarify their perception of a negative reaction. Frowns, abruptness, or unwarranted expression of fears are examples of negative nonverbal communication cues. The client's reactions and feedback must be explored because they represent the nurse's nonverbal communication cues.

Self-awareness encourages nurses and clients to analyze their reactions using therapeutic interactions. Healthy nurse–client interactions can use reality checks to maintain congruency. The capacity for total self-scrutiny is impossible, so nurses have to depend on others for validation. Furthermore, everyone has "blind spots" and unresolved issues from past experiences. Specific clients, situations, and issues arouse intense anxiety and defensiveness. These feelings usually interfere with objectivity and impede healthy client interactions. The term for these reactions is *countertransference*.

Countertransference is a psychoanalytical term that denotes unconscious conflict that results from unresolved developmental issues (Freud, 1958). Basch (1988) asserted that countertransference affects the nurse's capacity to assess client responses.

Clients diagnosed with borderline personality disorder stir up intense reactions in nurses. These clients are experts in evoking anger and negative responses in the nurse. Maladaptive patterns of manipulation and acting out help them recreate their own chaotic family dynamics. Chaotic relationships with nurses and other caregivers interfere with therapeutic interactions and the formation of effective interventions. For an in-depth discussion of countertransference, refer to Chapter 14.

Nurse–client relationships require enormous stamina, ingenuity, and commitment. Complex client problems challenge nurses to explore their own issues. Recognizing one's abilities and strengths also means assessing one's limitations and weaknesses. Self-awareness means growing personally and professionally.

DOCUMENTATION SYSTEMS

Communication among nurses and other health care providers is critical to quality client care. The client's progress is generally conveyed orally in morning rounds, shift reports, or informal meetings, or it is provided in documentation.

Documentation is the written form of communication that serves as a legal record with numerous purposes, including the following:

- Provides information needed for continuity of care
- Maximizes resources by using input from various health care providers to evaluate the treatment plan
- Indicates reimbursement needs
- Provides data for peer review
- Provides data for total quality improvement
- Presents an opportunity for research
- Offers opportunities for education and teaching

Documentation communicates information about the client's ongoing health status and current responses to interventions. Specific data may include medication administration, client interactions, mental status, and changes in behavioral patterns. Documentation is an account of the client's participation and response to treatment. Data are documented in progress notes, nursing care plans, and interdisciplinary treatment plans. The client's record can be used in a legal setting to elicit information that supports or disputes certain claims, such as malpractice. Client records belong to the respective facilities, but clients can obtain copies because of the Patient Bill of Rights.

Clients are usually concerned about the accuracy, reliability, and confidentiality of their records. The advent of computers threatens the security of client records, but institutions are responsible for maintaining confidentiality.

Documentation, like oral reporting, is a form of communication that involves clients, nurses, and other health care providers. Accurate accounts of client interventions, response, and behavioral patterns are vital elements of quality care.

▶CHAPTER SUMMARY

Communication is a complex, dynamic process that evolves throughout the life span. Primary caregivers provide the basis of socialization and communication. Early interactions, as well as neurobiological, psychosocial, and cultural factors, affect the quality of social interactions.

Communication is the foundation of survival and social interactions. Parents respond to the crying infant by providing nourishment and safety. The infant's survival depends on communicating the need to be fed (crying) and appropriate parental responses. Basic needs are met through communication that conveys information from one person to another.

Therapeutic nurse–client interactions are built on trust, empathy, and an understanding of human responses. Clients can get their needs met when they feel safe and secure. Therapeutic interactions afford the client with opportunities to express feelings and thoughts. Accurate assessment of client needs is the basis of effective interventions.

The psychiatric–mental health nurse is often challenged to form interpersonal relationships with clients who are using maladaptive coping patterns. These clients have difficulty trusting and forming meaningful interactions. Impaired sensory and perceptual responses, low self-esteem, and impaired social skills can interfere with this process. Nurses can use the nursing process to identify maladaptive behaviors and formulate interventions that promote health.

Effective communication enables the nurse to form therapeutic nurse–client relationships and to communicate with other health care providers through written documentation. Communication maximizes resources and facilitates health promotion.

Suggestions for Clinical Conferences

1. Role play and assess communication techniques.
2. Present process recording evaluation, and discuss therapeutic and nontherapeutic responses.
3. Invite a clinical specialist to discuss the principles and relevance of self-awareness to nurses.
4. Present a case history using Peplau's phases of the nurse–client relationship.

References

Ainsworth, M. D. (1985). Attachments across the life span. *Bulletin of the New York Academy of Medicine, 61*(9), 792–812.

Basch, M. F. (1988). *Understanding psychotherapy*. New York: Basic Books.

Berlo, D. K. (1960). *The process of communication*. New York: Holt, Rinehart, & Winston.

Berne, E. (1964). *Games people play*. New York: Grove Press.

Birdwhitsell, R. (1970). *Kinesics and content*. Philadelphia: University of Pennsylvania Press.

Bowlby, J. (1969). *Attachment and loss: Vol. 1. Attachment*. New York: Basic Books.

Buckwalter, K. C., Cusack, D., Beaver, M., Sidles, E. & Wadle, K. (1988). The behavioral consequences of a communication intervention on institutionalized residents with aphasia and dysarthria. *Archives of Psychiatric Nursing, 2*(5), 289–295.

Carpenito, L. J., & Duespohl, T. A. (1985). *A guide for effective clinical instruction* (2nd ed.). Rockville, MD: Aspen Publications.

Ceccio, J. F., & Ceccio, C. M. (1982). *Effective communication in nursing: Theory and practice*. New York: John Wiley & Sons.

Condon, W. S., & Sander, L. W. (1974). Neonate movement is synchronized with adult speech: Interactional participation and language acquisition. *Science, 183*, 99–101.

Ehmann, V. E. (1971). Empathy: Its origins, characteristics, and process. *Perspectives in Psychiatric Care, 9*(2), 72–80.

Freud, S. (1958). The dynamics of transference. In J. Strachey (Ed. and Trans.) The standard edition of the complete psychological works of Sigmund Freud (Vol. 19, pp. 97–108). London: Hogarth Press. (Original work published 1923)

Gladstein, G. A. (1987). *Empathy and counseling*. New York: Springer-Verlag.

Hall, E. T. (1966). *The hidden dimension*. Garden City, NJ: Doubleday.

Hall, E. T. (1989). *Beyond culture*. New York: Doubleday.

Howells, J. G. (1975). *Principles of family psychotherapy*. New York: Brunnel/Mazel.

Johnston, N. E. (1990). Culturally relevant care in mental health nursing. In A. Baumann, N. E. Johnston, & D. Antai-Otong (Eds.), *Decision making in psychiatric and psychosocial nursing* (pp. 4–5). Philadelphia: B. C. Decker.

King, M., Novik, L., & Citrenbaum, C. (1983). *Irresistible communication: Creative skills for the health professional*. Philadelphia: W. B. Saunders.

Lachman, V. D. (1983). *Stress management: A manual for nurses*. Orlando: Grune & Stratton.

Lubinski, R. (1981). Environmental language intervention. In R. Chapley (Ed.), *Language interventions in adult aphasia*. Baltimore: Williams & Wilkins.

Maslow, A. H. (1968). *Toward a psychology of being* (2nd ed.). New York: Van Nostrand Reinhold.

Maslow, A. H. (1970). *Motivation and personality* (2nd ed.). New York: Harper & Row.

Mellow, J. (1967). Evolution of nursing therapy through research. *Psychiatric Opinion, 4*(1), *15–21*.

Orlando, I. J. (1961). *The dynamic nurse–patient relationship*. New York: G. P. Putman.

Peplau, H. E. (1952). *Interpersonal relations in nursing*. New York: G. P. Putnam.

Piaget, J. (1970). Piaget's theory. In P. H. Mussen (Ed.), *Carmichael's manual of child psychology* (pp. 703–732). New York: John Wiley & Sons.

Pluckman, M. L. (1978). *Human communication: The matrix of nursing*. New York: McGraw-Hill.

Price, J. L. (1987). The amygdaloid complex. In G. Adelman (Ed.), *Encyclopedia of neuroscience* (Vol. 2; pp. 40–42). Boston: Birkhauser.

Reusch, J. (1961). *Therapeutic communication*. New York: W. W. Norton.

Satir, V. (1967). *Conjoint family therapy* (revised ed.). Palo Alto, CA: Science and Behavior Books.

Smits, M. W., & Kee, C. C. (1992). Correlates of self-care among the independent elderly. *Journal of Gerontological Nursing, 18*(9), 13–18.

Sullivan, H. S. (1954). *Psychiatric interview*. New York: W. W. Norton.

Travelbee, J. (1971). *Interpersonal aspects of nursing*. Philadelphia: F. A. Davis.

Walzlawick, P., Beavin, J. H., & Jackson, C. D. (1967). *Pragmatics of human communication: A study of interactional patterns, pathologies, and paradoxes*. New York: W. W. Norton.

CHAPTER

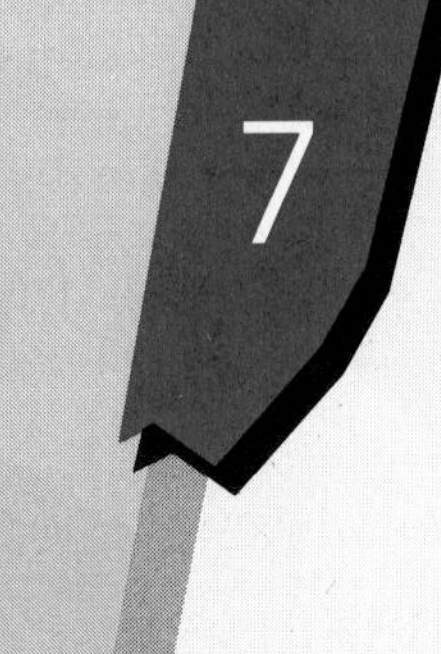

Stress, Coping, and Adaptation

DEBORAH ANTAI-OTONG, M.S., R.N.,C.S.

OUTLINE

CHAPTER OBJECTVES

Upon completion of this chapter, you will be able to:

1. Analyze the relationship between adaptive responses and stress throughout the life span.
2. Identify internal and external factors that influence coping ability.
3. Understand the mental health–illness continuum.
4. Define primary and secondary appraisals.
5. Understand the impact of stress on mental illness.
6. Identify the role of nursing in mental health promotion.

KEY TERMS

Adaptation
Coping
Defense mechanism
Ego function
Hardiness
Mental health
Mental illness
Primary appraisal
Secondary appraisal
Stress

Life is stressful and represents a constant, dynamic exchange of energy between people and their environment. The human organism uses innate processes to maintain and restore homeostasis under stressful conditions. The nature of stress is determined by one's repertoire of resources and coping mechanisms and response to internal and external demands (Cannon, 1914).

The complexity of adaptive processes results from an integration of the neurobiological, psychological, and sociocultural factors that enable people to change and minimize the injurious effects of stress.

- *Neurobiological factors* include developmental stage, nutritional status, genetic predisposition, and processes that affect temperament, immune responses to stress, and neuroendocrine activation and contribute to various illnesses, such as mood and schizophrenic disorders.
- *Psychological factors* include emotional maturity, ego function, coping skills, hardiness, and appraisal of stressors. As the person evolves throughout the life span, the ability to adapt to change is influenced by psychological factors.
- *Sociocultural factors* include social support systems and interpersonal relationships. These factors determine status, role, social norms, rituals, and belief systems.

Overall, stress is an inherent part of everyday living and is encountered throughout the life span. This chapter focuses on the complexity of the effect of stress and coping on adaptation and mental health. In addition, it defines the role of the nurse in prevention and health promotion throughout the life span.

DEFINITIONS

Daily interactions with internal and external demands contribute to stress in human beings, who constantly are changing and adapting to their environment. Stressful events normally generate feelings of impotency and a loss of control that activate both physiological and psychosocial responses. These responses are major components of coping. An inability to cope with internal and external stressors increases feelings of helplessness and vulnerability to illness or death (Glass, 1977; Seligman, 1975).

Stress. ***Stress*** refers to a stimulus (stressor) or situation that produces distress. Stress is defined as a condition or demand that arises from ineffective coping behaviors that fail to mobilize resources and maintain homeostasis (Antonovsky, 1979; Lazarus & Folkman, 1984).

Coping. ***Coping*** stems from the Latin word *colpus*, which means to alter. It is an effort to reduce tension by minimizing, replacing, and resolving uncomfortable feelings such as anxiety, anger, frustration, and guilt. The endeavors are defense mechanisms that act as buffers or protection against distress (Holroyd & Lazarus, 1982) (Table 7–1).

Adaptation. ***Adaptation*** is derived from the Latin word *adaptare*, which means to fit; it also refers to mobilizing resources and sustaining homeostasis.

Hardiness. ***Hardiness*** stems from the French word *hardi*, to make hard, and refers to a personality trait that enables one to maintain health and cope with stressful events. Its buffering qualities are associated with enhancement of adaptation and mediation between stress and illness. Based on this premise, hardiness parallels health and growth and buffers against illness. The degree of hardiness varies among people and depends on resilience, self-assuredness, and enthusiasm for life. Additionally, a hardiness personality consists of three tendencies, specifically *commitment* rather than distance, *control* rather than helplessness, and *challenge* rather than risk. These tendencies enable people to respond to stressful events using *transformational,* or adaptive, rather than *regressive,* or maladaptive, coping skills (Kobasa, 1979; Kobasa et al., 1985; Pollock, 1986; Pollock & Duffy, 1990).

Health and Mental Health. It is difficult to define health, but most describe it as physical, psychological, and social well-being. *Healthy People 2000* (U.S. Department of Health and Human Services, 1990), a statement of the National Health Promotion and Disease Prevention objectives, parallels health with people's sense of well-being. Additionally, it suggested the health results from

> *reducing unnecessary suffering, illness, and disability, . . . and improved quality of life.* (p. 6)

Mental health refers to the ability of people, couples, families, and communities to respond adaptively to external and internal stressors.

Selye's (1976) major contribution to defining mental health was his explanation of stress in terms of adaptation. He believed that stress compromises health when adaptive and coping patterns are unable to master the condition. Additionally, he concluded that stress responses occur whenever an organism encounters persistent stress. He described this phenomenon as *generalized adaptation syndrome*. Reactions that occur with generalized adaptation syndrome include the following:

- *Alarm reaction* (first phase): mobilizes the body's defenses and protective responses against the stressor; as the autonomic nervous system reacts to stress, large amounts of adrenaline and cortisone are activated and prepare the person for "fight or flight"
- *Stage of resistance* (second phase): adaptive responses attempt to lessen damage from the stressor by limiting its effects and resisting change
- *Stage of exhaustion* (third phase): final stage, which evolves after the body's attempts to adapt to change fail; in essence, the stressor may overwhelm existing adaptive reservoirs if interventions to relieve the stress are unsuccessful

Others depict mental health as successful adaptation that maintains homeostasis or equilibrium and the physiochemical state (Cannon, 1939; Menninger, 1963). Mental health has many definitions, but there is broad agreement that the key components include the following:

- The ability to respond effectively to stress
- The capacity to tolerate anxiety, stress, and frustration and to delay gratification of needs (impulse control)

TABLE 7–1
Major Defense Mechanisms

DEFENSE MECHANISM	DEFINITION	EXAMPLE
Displacement	Redirection of negative urges or feelings from an original object to a safer or neutral substitute	The man who is angry with his boss and returns home and becomes angry instead with his wife or children
Denial	Refusal to admit to a painful reality, which is treated as if it does not exist	The woman who miscarries denies that she has lost the baby and continues to wear maternity clothes
Intellectualization	Use of excessive reasoning rather than reacting or changing	A woman attending an Alcoholics Anonymous meeting reports that she is a nurse and has conducted many 12-step sessions
Introjection	Engulfment or incorporation of specific traits, behaviors, or qualities into self or ego structure	A depressed man who incorporates the negative feelings and hatred of his estranged wife, who recently filed for divorce
Projection	Blame of others or things for one's own feelings or thoughts	The client experiencing paranoia blames others for disliking him
Rationalization	An effort to replace or justify acceptable reasons for feelings, beliefs, thoughts, or behaviors for real ones	A woman with overextended credit cards rationalizes that she can use her savings to pay for a new dress she recently purchased
Reaction formation	Repression of painful or offensive attitudes or traits with unconscious opposite ones	The college student who feels angry and hostile toward her professor is overly friendly and agreeable in class
Regression	Retreat to an earlier developmental stage	The 3-year-old child who begins wetting his pants after the birth of a new sibling
Repression	Unconscious, purposeful forgetting of painful or dangerous thoughts (the most basic defense mechanism)	The married woman who expresses hostility toward a male coworker to avoid dealing with her sexual attraction to him
Sublimation	Normal form of dealing with undesirable feelings or thoughts by keeping them in an acceptable context	The woman who is unable to bear children begins working in a preschool
Suppression	Conscious and deliberate forgetfulness of painful or undesirable thoughts and ideas	A rape victim attempts to forget the incident and fails to report it to the proper authorities

- The capacity to realistically and objectively appraise events and situations in one's world

Ego Function and Mental Health. Caplan (1961) believed that the most essential factor that predicts mental health is **ego function**. *Ego* is defined as the major personality mechanism that mediates between the person and the environment. Major ego functions include adaptation to reality, modulation of anxiety, and problem solving. Menninger (1963) described the ego as the guardian of the vital balance

> *which recognizes, receives, stores, discriminates, integrates, and acts by restraining, modifying, and directing impulses.* (p. 104)

Ego function refers to the inherent ability to adapt to internal and external demands or stress of environments (Hartmann, 1958). Its foundation arises from early significant relationships that established trust and meaningful interactions. Ego function evolves over time and varies with personality structure and developmental stage.

Stress and Illness. A number of studies have shown a relationship between stress and disequilibrium or illness (Brown, 1993; Fristad et al., 1993; Holmes & Rahe, 1967; Yehuda et al., 1993). Holmes and Rahe (1967) developed a system for determining the degree of life stressors and predicting illness by placing a value on various life events that require change or adaptive responses. Their Readjustment Rating Scale was developed to measure a number of stressful events over a 12-month period, and they found an increased vulnerability to medical or psychiatric illness with increasing numbers of events over this period. If scores reached 300 on the scale, the chance of illness increased to 80 percent. The Readjustment Scale has been criticized because of its lack of relevancy to many ethnic groups and developmental stages.

Criticism of this scale led to the development of other tools that determine how people handle daily hassles. One such tool is the Jalowiec Coping Scale (Jalowiec, 1979) (Table 7–2), which determines how people cope with various life stressors. It consists of 40 coping behaviors that are rated on a 1-to-5 scale to indicate the

TABLE 7–2
Examples of Coping Behaviors from the Jalowiec Coping Scale

1. Hope for improvement
2. Maintain control
3. Information-seeking
4. Think through solutions
5. View problem objectively
6. Eat/smoke
7. Try out solutions
8. Make use of past experience
9. Find purpose/meaning
10. Pray
11. Get nervous
12. Worry
13. Handle problem in steps
14. Seek comfort/help from others
15. Set goals
16. Accept situation
17. Want to be alone
18. Laugh it off
19. Put problem aside
20. Daydream
21. Expect the worst
22. Discuss problem
23. Try to change situation
24. Get mad
25. Sleep
26. Don't worry
27. Withdraw from situation
28. Activity/exercise
29. Compromise
30. Take tensions out on others
31. Resign because it's hopeless
32. Try anything
33. Blame others
34. Let someone else solve the problem

Data from Jalowiec, A., & Powers, M. J. (1983). Stress and coping in hypertensive and emergency room patients. *Nursing Research, 30*(1), 10–15.

magnitude of use, with 1 indicating "never" and 5 "always." A checklist format is used to indicate the frequency each response is used to handle certain situations (Jalowiec, 1988; Jalowiec & Powers, 1983). The accompanying Research Study used the Jalowiec scale to assess coping in patients with myocardial infarction.

Stress and Anxiety. The phenomena of stress and anxiety are remarkably interrelated. Stress produces enormous human strain, which consequently leads to inner conflict or anxiety.

Response to Stress. Response to stressful situations is primarily biological, but psychosocial factors impact the perception of and number of stressors. Furthermore, coping skills, cultural factors, support systems, and ego function (i.e., defense mechanisms) affect reactions to stress.

Defense Mechanisms. The term ***defense mechanism*** refers to a predominantly unconscious self-protective process that seeks to shield the ego from intense feelings or affect and impulses. Additionally, these intrapsychic processes modify, nullify, or convey painful affects or tendencies so they can be tolerated consciously.

Mental Health–Illness Continuum. Mental health and adaptation are relative and lie on a continuum with mental illness and maladaptation. Disorganization or **mental illness** occurs as available coping and adaptive mechanisms fail to handle stress. Mental illness may be manifested in various ways, such as ineffective problem solving, poor reality testing, and impaired cognitive functioning.

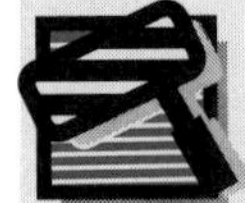

RESEARCH STUDY

Coping and Adjustment to Illness in the Acute Myocardial Infarction Patient.

Keckeisen, M. E., & Nyamathi, A. M. (1990). *Journal of Cardiovascular Nursing, 5*(1), 1–12.

Study Problem/Purpose

This study examined the coping mechanisms of patients experiencing acute myocardial infarction 1 month after discharge.

Method

The original Jalowiec Coping Scale (JCS) was used to assess problem- and emotional-focused coping mechanisms. The Psychological Adjustment to Illness Scale (PAIS-SR) was used to assess the intensity of psychologic and social adjustment 1 month after discharge.

Findings

The sample consisted of subjects ranging from 28 to 74 years of age (mean 58 years). The average hospital stay was 2 weeks. The results showed that patients with acute myocardial infarction who used more problem-focused coping strategies had better adjustment scores on PAIS-SR. These findings suggest that patients who used this form of coping had more positive outcomes than those who used emotion-focused coping patterns.

Implications

Nurses can use their knowledge of the coping process and possible outcomes to enhance coping strategies. Patient education, emotional support, collaboration, and encouragement of self-care are critical to positive outcomes in patients with acute myocardial infarctions.

CLASSIFICATION OF MENTAL ILLNESS AND DISORDERS

Classification of mental disorders flourished during the nineteenth century. Many symptoms were reported during earlier writings, but there was a lack of formal classification of mental disorders until the twentieth century.

Emil Kraepelin. Kraepelin, a German psychiatrist, was a pioneer in the classification of mental disorders. His description of dementia praecox, later referred to as schizophrenia, and manic depression fell short because he focused primarily on the course of mental illnesses rather than the etiology. In spite of major shortcomings, his work inspired others to create a formal classification of mental disorders (Deutsch, 1937).

Eugen Bleuler. Bleuler (1950), a Swiss psychiatrist, followed in Kraepelin's footsteps, but he ventured further than describing the symptoms and the syndrome. He explored specific responses generated by symptoms and presented the term *schizophrenia,* which replaced Kraepelin's *dementia praecox*. A major flaw in Bleuler's description of schizophrenia was its lack of precision, which led to numerous misdiagnoses. Bleuler's work also encouraged psychiatry to explore the underlying processes of mental illness.

Sigmund Freud, Adolf Meyer, and Franz Alexander. Other contributions to the systematization of mental disorder include the works of Freud (1953), who linked mental disorders with unconscious conflicts or neurosis. Meyer (1957) believed in the holistic personality theory, which comprised biological, psychosocial, and cultural factors; he also believed that mental disorders had psychobiological origins. Alexander (1939) also emphasized the interrelationship between emotions and biological processes, which suggested the influence of external and internal causes of disease.

DIAGNOSTIC AND STATISTICAL MANUAL OF MENTAL DISORDERS (DSM)

DSM-I (1952) and DSM-II (1968). In 1934, the American Psychiatric Association (APA) attempted to classify mental illnesses and identified 24 main groups with 82 subdivisions. This format produced upheaval within the profession and questionable treatment practices. Efforts to provide a useful and consistent classification were made in 1952, when the APA published the DSM-I; DSM-II was published in 1968. DSM-I and DSM-II presented a classification based on a hierarchical system with the following categories: organic mental disorders, followed by psychotic, neurotic, and personality disorders. This system also lacked consistency and clarity in defining psychosis and neurosis and led to a continued need to improve the differentiation of mental disorders.

TABLE 7–3
Organizational Framework for DSM-IV

AXIS	EXPLANATION
Axis I	Clinical syndromes and V codes Conditions not attributable to a mental disorder that are a focus of attention or treatment, e.g., marital problems or other family circumstances
Axis II	Personality disorders Specific developmental disorders
Axis III	Physical disorders and conditions
Axis IV	Severity of psychosocial stressors
Axis V	Highest level of adaptive functioning in the past year

The first three axes constitute the official diagnostic assessment. Axes IV and V are available for use in special clinical and research settings.
Data from American Psychiatric Association (1994). *Diagnostic and statistical manual of mental disorders* (4th ed.). Washington, DC: Author.

DSM-III (1980) and DSM-III-Revised (DSM-III-R) (1987). DSM-III (1980) and DSM-III-R (1987) differed from previous editions in that they formulated childhood mental disorder categories. Additionally, DSM-III deleted the psychosis and neurosis categories and replaced them with a new section that classified disorders based on psychopathology, such as mood, anxiety, and dissociative disorders. This new format allowed for multiple diagnoses on several axes (Table 7–3) and placed less emphasis on hierarchical exclusions and advanced experimental research.

There has been discussion among nursing educators and practitioners regarding the overall usefulness of the DSM-III-R, because it does not address issues associated with self-care or nursing's unique contribution to 24-hour care. Furthermore, around-the-clock monitoring has been described as the most significant effort to meet basic human needs, which include comfort, hygiene, nutrition, and social interaction (Morrison et al., 1985). However, there is consensus among other psychiatric–mental health nurses who contend that DSM-III-R is useful in several ways. First, it permits nurses to share roles and communicate effectively with members of the interdisciplinary team. Second, it provides opportunities to assess the client's biopsychosocial needs, identifying diagnostic data, current stressors, and overall level of adaptive functioning (APA, 1987). Third, it provides financial opportunities for nurses in advanced practice who use it to apply for third-party and medicare reimbursement. Finally, DSM-III-R can be used with nursing models integrating major concepts with nursing diagnoses to identify complex need of clients when planning nursing care.

DSM-IV (1994). DSM-IV (APA, 1994) is welcomed as an attempt to increase the proficiency of diagnosis and differential diagnosis among clinicians. This new edition is distinct from previous editions in several ways. First, diagnostic criteria are not bound by specific categories or mental disorders. This simply means that a set of symptoms may be listed under several categories, such as "Disorders Due to General Medical Condition." It takes into account general medical conditions that may contribute to or be the sole source of presenting psychiatric symptoms (e.g., anxiety disorder due to alcohol withdrawal or hyperthyroidism).

A second noticeable change in the DSM-IV is its strong emphasis on using clinical judgment and various measures to assess the client's condition other than diagnosis. A third change is the description of mental disorders as serious behavioral and psychological manifestations triggered by a stressful event that affects the level of function and increases the risk of disability (APA, 1994).

An outcry from various groups for cultural sensitivity and awareness contributed to the fourth major change in the DSM-IV. The importance of diversity, specifically ethnic and cultural considerations, is underscored as an integral part of client care. Amazingly, previous editions of the DSM regarded certain cultural practices, rituals, and beliefs as manifestations of mental illness. An appreciation of these behaviors as culture bound contributed to changes in the DSM-IV. Major features include a description of culture-bound syndromes that are not classified in the DSM-IV but are listed in the DSM-IV Appendix I along with a template of cultural frame of reference and a glossary. The usefulness of this information lies in helping clinicians appreciate and systematically assess the cultural needs of their clients.

The last major feature of the DSM-IV is its well-defined diagnostic criteria. Well-defined criteria improve communication between mental health professionals and help them identify patterns, individuality, and diversity among various populations. These data can be used to promote quality care through research endeavors.

Overall, the DSM-IV is strikingly different from and more useful than previous editions. Nurses can use it confidently alone or as an adjunct to other assessment tools to provide quality care. (See Table 7–4 for a comparison of the DSM-III-R and the DSM-IV).

TABLE 7–4
Comparison of DSM-III-R and DSM-IV

MAJOR FEATURES OF THE DSM-III-R (APA, 1987)	MAJOR FEATURES OF THE DSM-IV (APA, 1994)
1. Focuses on past improvement from previous diagnoses.	1. Focuses on presenting manifestations of biological behaviors and psychological patterns generated by a stressful event that interfere with optimal level of function (includes severity and specific course of mental disorders).
2. Diagnostic categories provide more criteria than previous editions, but there is still a need to use empirical research to improve the credibility of clinical judgment.	2. Minimal labeling is used, and more factual descriptions are used to define a condition, such as "the client experiencing delirium" rather than "the delirious client."
3. Diagnostic categories are not applicable to diverse populations (culture, gender, or age).	3. Distinct clarification of diagnostic criteria is based on considerable empirical research.
4. Axis III is the only category that considers the impact of a general medical condition on mental disorder.	4. Acknowledges the significance of diversity and provides a section on culture-bound syndromes (Appendix I: Outline for Cultural Formulation and Glossary of Culture-Bound Syndromes). Each diagnostic category suggests using clinical judgment to include the influence of the culture, age, and sex of the client.
5. Categorizes cognitive disorders under "organic mental syndromes and disorders."	5. Delineates the contrast between mental disorder and general medical condition and includes new criteria under major mental disorders and labeled "indicate general medical condition" (e.g., anxiety disorder due to: *indicate general medical condition*).
6. The Psychoactive Substance Use Disorders is described primarily in terms of a separate entity.	6. New category for cognitive disorders is "Delirium, Dementia, and Amnestic and Other Cognitive Disorders" (including dementia due to HIV disease and head trauma).
7. No discussion of medication-induced movement or adverse drug reactions. Abuse is not included in diagnostic categories.	7. "Substance-induced . . . disorder" is listed under major mental disorders/conditions, such as anxiety and delirium.
8. Appendix A lists several diagnostic criteria (limited number of cases) for research study.	8. New category labeled "Other Conditions that may be a Focus of Clinical Attention" includes a section on Medication-Induced Movement Disorders (e.g., neuroleptic malignant syndrome, neuroleptic-induced acute akathisia and tardive dyskinesia, and adverse effects of medication not otherwise specified). This section also includes "Problems Related to Abuse or Neglect" across the life span (e.g., physical abuse of a child, sexual abuse of a child, sexual abuse or rape of an adult).
	9. Appendix B list criteria sets and axes provided for further study: this section includes numerous diagnostic categories ranging from postconcussional disorder and medication-induced movement disorders. It also includes several research tools.

DSM, *Diagnostic and Statistical Manual of Mental Disorders.*

Data from American Psychiatric Association. (1987). *Diagnostical and statistical manual of mental disorders, third edition, revised.* Washington, DC: Author; and American Psychiatric Association. (1994). *Diagnostic and statistical manual of mental disorders* (4th ed.). Washington, DC: Author.

Table 7–5
Roy's Adaptation Model: Assumptions and Beliefs About the Human Organism

- Human beings are dynamic; they constantly interact with their environment
- Human behavior has meaning and purpose
- Emotions activate, orient, and organize adaptive processes
- Human beings are whole persons in action
- Human beings are biologically rooted but socially interactive
- The human body is sensitive to change and automatically adjusts to maintain homeostasis
- Human beings need to be free of overwhelming anxiety
- Foundations of adaptation and coping evolve and change throughout the life span
- Stress is part of life, and response to it varies from individual to individual, based on neurobiological, psychosocial, and cultural factors
- Self-care must be supported and maintained

Data from Dix, 1991; Nightingale, 1860; and Roy, 1976.

COPING AND ADAPTATION ACROSS THE LIFE SPAN

Roy (1976) conceptualized people as open and dynamic systems interchanging with their environments to sustain adaptation (Table 7–5). Furthermore, she surmised that instinctual and learned coping skills enable people to adapt to constant environmental changes. Coping skills are determined by biological, psychosocial, and cultural influences. These concepts can be applied throughout the life span based on the premise that people are adaptive systems. Goals for adaptation include survival, growth, reproduction, and mastery (Roy & McLeod, 1981).

The human organism is complex, and understanding the role of stress, coping, and adaptation throughout the life span involves appreciating the premise that all behavior has meaning and purpose. Additionally, neurobiological and psychosocial factors affect the appraisal of these encounters and determine the outcome.

Numerous studies suggest that individual coping and adaptive patterns begin to form during gestation and evolve throughout the life span. These patterns may change or adjust to given circumstances based on one's appraisal of stressors, access to resources, developmental stages, and level of vulnerability.

PRENATAL PERIOD

Studies conducted by Patterson et al. (1978) and Gabella (1976) associated genetics with maternal stress during the first 6 weeks of gestation, at which time the autonomic nervous system is undergoing differentiation. Additionally, these studies inferred that stress affects the chemical environment that regulates the development of the sympathetic nervous system and nerve growth and lays the foundation for adaptive processes. The major site of production of nerve growth is the placenta. The chemical composition of the placenta is determined by disease and stress (Sroufe & Rutter, 1984). The role of stress during gestation on future coping and adaptation must be appreciated. Implications from these findings emphasize the importance of promoting mental health in prospective parents through innovative interventions such as stress management, adequate rest and nutrition, and healthy parenting skills.

INFANCY

Other important processes are begun during early infancy, including neurobiological and perceptual growth of the central nervous system in the first few months of life. Infancy represents the most vulnerable stage of development because resources and coping abilities have not evolved. Vulnerability to trauma and disruption are influenced by external environments and primary caregivers. During this developmental stage, infants learn about the world and themselves through early interactions with primary caregivers. The infant receives pleasure through fulfillment of basic needs such as feeding, attachment or bonding, and nurturing (Dreyfus-Brisac, 1979).

Bowlby (1969) believed attachment or bonding to be an essential aspect of development that prepared the infant for defending against negative environmental stressors. He delineated four critical stages of early childhood as follows:

First stage (2 to 3 months): the infant has ambiguous social responsiveness; the infant has not bonded with primary caregivers and can only distinguish people from inanimate objects in the environment
Second stage (2 to 6 months): the infant learns to discern primary caregivers from others
Third stage (6 to 35 months): the infant begins to develop neuromuscular abilities that facilitate mobility and independence
Fourth stage (3 years): final stage of attachment, at which time the child understands the relationship with caregivers

Furthermore, Bowlby considered these stages of attachment as sources of stress for the infant and child.

Early influences, such as the infant's responses to discomfort and pain associated with hunger and a wet diaper, also produce stress. Reactions to these stressors include crying, fretfulness, and disturbances in eating and sleeping patterns. Lipsitt (1983) considered crying as a human response to distress and an adaptive mechanism that gets attention, produces comfort, and eases pain. Additionally, crying is considered the primary coping mechanism for responding to stress. Other coping mechanisms found during infancy include the startle response to loud noises, such as the Moro reflex. These early coping and defense mechanisms reflect basic undeveloped neurobiological adaptive processes. Overall, early developmental changes and experiences are related to complex processes, both psychosocial and neurobiological, and at any given stage of development adaptive or maladaptive responses may be used.

Caregivers' Influence on Coping and Adaptation in Infancy. The capacity of parents or early primary caregivers to effectively manage stress is vital to the development of adaptive responses in the infant. The quality of parenting is governed by the perception of stressors and the level of coping and adaptation. High stress levels in the parents usually parallel inconsistent or harsh discipline. Likewise, chronic and intense effects of stress in parents indicate dysfunction and distress and increase the risk of abuse and maladaptive developmental outcomes in children (Forehand et al., 1987; McLoyd, 1990).

In comparison, parents who handle stressful situations effectively are more likely to enhance adaptive coping skills in their children. Parents who are able to solve problems and resolve conflicts and who are caring and nurturing exhibit healthy parenting skills. Overall, parental competence and vulnerability to stress are influenced by early developmental experiences and genetic, psychosocial, and neurobiological factors, which are the basis of coping and adaptive mechanisms. The importance of parental competency and nurturing parallels optimal childhood functioning by fostering the child's ability to interact with peers, which determines adult responses to stress in later life. These processes are the basis for child development and adaptation (Belsky, 1981, 1984; Keitner & Miller, 1990; Swindle et al., 1989).

As the child becomes mobile and autonomous, stress arises from limit setting, early discipline, and prolonged separation from primary caregivers. Stress reactions include temper tantrums, withdrawal, and depression. The encounters allow the toddler to experience rewards and failures, further producing a sense of self-worth that is reinforced through primary caregivers. Major parental stressors include toilet training and learning how to maintain consistent limit setting with the mobile toddler.

CHILDHOOD

Early and late childhood responses to stress are influenced by the child's temperament, behavioral style, neurobiological and cultural factors, and psychosocial environment. As children mature, their coping and adaptive skills also change. Major stressors associated with exploration of self and others vary with social interactions. Specific determinants for social interactions include school, community, and religious affiliation, which facilitate learning how to compete and interact with peers, skills for sharing, and problem solving. Early social interactions with parents and later interaction with peers and other adults enhance coping and adaptive skills (Caplan, 1961; Erikson, 1963, 1968).

Caregivers' Influence on Coping and Adaptation in Childhood. Major parental tasks during this developmental stage include praising the child's efforts and accomplishments while preparing for the advent of puberty. Parents' interest in the child's academic and athletic activities enhances his or her self-worth and acceptance.

In summary, early and late childhood developmental tasks include achieving trust, attachment or bonding, autonomy, mastery, and self-esteem. As the person emerges from childhood, his or her life experiences continue to impact early life experience, which lays the foundation for adult responses. Understanding the adaptive level of parental function enables one to predict adaptation in children. Moreover, emotional and behavioral states of the parents and the child are interdependent and influence adaptation throughout the life span.

ADOLESCENCE

Adolescence is a time of profound neurobiological and psychosocial changes. The major developmental tasks are role and sexual identity, neurobiological adaptation, and demands associated with cultural and educational expectations. Each area represents turmoil, increased psychosocial stress, and the struggle to adapt to changes in body image, control of the environment, movement from dependence to independence within social contexts, and the formation of meaningful interpersonal relationships. Roles are tested with the need to integrate ideas, values, and norms with internal and external demands (Blos, 1962; Erikson, 1968; Mishne, 1986).

Stress in the adolescent is normally manifested by disagreements with authority figures, anxiety, and depression. Some adolescents may experience stress reactions and exhibit them through acting-out behaviors, such as misusing substances (alcohol, illicit drugs), practicing promiscuity, and carrying out antisocial behaviors (such as shoplifting). These latter behaviors may also be symptoms of psychiatric illnesses. Twenty percent of adolescents experience psychiatric disorders or mental illness, and the most common diagnoses include personality, affective, and conduct disorders (Borst et al., 1991; Kovacs et al., 1993; Pfeffer et al., 1988).

Healthy interpersonal relationships with family and peers reduce vulnerability to stress and promote high self-esteem and positive self-worth. Accomplishment of developmental tasks allows adolescents to deal with life experiences and stressors effectively, producing healthy separation from families and increasing independence. Additionally, healthy separation and independence allow the adolescent to make the transition into adulthood with adaptive coping skills.

EARLY AND MIDDLE ADULTHOOD

The young adult approaches life experiences with a sense of identity and integration of values and healthy personality traits. The major commitments during early adulthood include career goals and interpersonal relationships or intimacy. Stressors are often associated with relationship problems, job changes or pressures, unemployment, and parenthood.

As adults establish stable relationships and move into marriage and, later, parenthood, the major developmental tasks include generativity versus stagnation (Erikson, 1963), when people begin to examine their contributions to society that arise from creativity and productivity. The basis of these endeavors is making contributions to or influencing the next generation and may include activities such as rearing children, producing works of art, writing, or participating in projects that protect the environment.

Other stressors generated by middle adulthood include neurobiological and psychosocial changes, such as menopause and "empty nest syndrome." Adults using healthy coping mechanisms normally mobilize resources and adapt to these changes. Others using maladaptive coping skills may experience stagnation and feel they have not made any significant contribution in life and perceive the aging process as threatening and empty. Major stresses in adulthood manifest in many ways, including anger, irritability, substance abuse, dysfunctional family interactions, and poor social and occupational performance. Other symptoms of stress may include changes in appetite, sleeping, or concentration.

LATE ADULTHOOD

Adaptation in the older adult depends on defense mechanisms used throughout the life span. The major developmental task of older adults is integrity versus despair (Erikson, 1963). Adaptive coping mechanisms help older adults maintain mental and physical health. Loss is the predominant theme that characterizes stress in the elderly. Major losses include close relatives and friends, physical abilities, and financial status. The ability to resolve grief taxes the older adult's coping skills.

Nursing interventions during this last stage of development include crisis intervention, grief counseling, and support of adaptive coping mechanisms. Older adults are at risk for suicide if there are significant losses, such as chronic illness and the death of a spouse. Nurses must assess these clients for signs of depression, level of dangerousness, and ineffective coping patterns.

Responses to stress throughout the life span consist of coping, both action oriented and intrapsychic, to master, tolerate, curtail, and lessen environmental and internal demands. Coping focuses on altering behaviors and cognitions to promote a sense of well-being through neurobiological and psychological processes. Response to stress depends on the direct attempts to alter the threatening condition.

COPING MECHANISMS

Using coping mechanisms refers to overcoming or managing stress by mobilizing internal and external resources. Internal resources include one's repertoire of mechanisms such as ego function (intrapsychic) and neurobiological factors, whereas external resources include social support and cultural factors. Coping mechanisms serve to

- Influence overall morale, health, and well-being
- Promote growth and maturity
- Assist in problem solving
- Influence adaptation to stress

The concept of stress provides a means of understanding holistic responses to external and internal demands that unfold into important complex neurobiological or psychosocial processes. Examples of stressful events include a major automobile accident, reaction to a spider bite, and the death of a loved one. When a stressor is encountered, it is perceived as a challenge or threat and the fight-or-flight mechanism is triggered. Responses to stress are influenced by appraisal of the event. A person's perception of a stressor is decisive in determining the outcome of neurobiological responses. Appraisal and response are further influenced by the level of ego function, developmental stage, available resources, previous experiences, and the number of stressors. These reactions trigger metabolic and cellular responses. Additionally, emotional and biological responses are adaptive and pivotal to regulation of human behavior (Lazarus & Folkman, 1984; Selye, 1976).

Empirical studies suggest that cognitive appraisal of life events determines the response as expressed by emotions (Lazarus & Launier, 1978). Appraisal pertains to value or appreciation, and in terms of coping refers to the significance of internal and external events that are linked with health and adaptation. Events may be perceived as irrelevant, benign or nonthreatening, or threatening or harmful. Lazarus (1966) identified two forms of appraisals: primary and secondary.

PRIMARY APPRAISALS

Lazarus (1966) described the initial response to a stressor as **primary appraisal** and the ultimate goal of prevailing over the situation. Furthermore, he delineated three types of primary appraisal, including (1) irrelevant; (2) benign positive; and (3) stressful. *Irrelevant appraisals* take place when the person confronts external occurrences that do not pose a threat to his or her livelihood. *Benign appraisals* are events that have a genuinely positive appraisal, or they enhance adaptation or stimulate a sense of well-being. These events generate feelings of pleasure, joy, and happiness and may also be accompanied by guilt and anxiety.

Stress appraisals are regarded as (1) injurious; (2) hazardous; or (3) demanding or challenging (Lazarus, 1966). Life events that have negative connotations or cause damage, such as physical illness, injury to self-esteem, and loss of normal functioning, are defined as *injurious*. *Hazardous* threats are anticipated occurrences that encourage people to use coping skills to reduce anticipated risks. This form of appraisal normally arouses negative feelings and thoughts, such as anger, helplessness, anxiety, and fear. The potential for adaptive as well as maladaptive responses exists with hazards. The woman who discovers that her husband is having an affair with another woman perceives this situation as a threat to her marriage and livelihood. She is determined to keep her marriage together by seeking marital therapy. Initially, her husband is reluctant to seek treatment, but later he agrees and discovers the basis of marital discord and attempts to work things out. *Demanding* or *challenging* situations also provide opportunities for using and enhancing coping and adaptive responses, but responses differ from the hazardous form, because they generate positive feelings, such as enthusiasm, motivation, and excitement. The couple anticipating the birth of triplets is challenged to manage multiple births with enormous parenting responsibilities. A challenge form of appraisal normally produces positive thoughts, such as "We've been through worse times. We can make it on one income." The implication is that challenge appraisals represent healthier adaptive and coping skills that promote a sense of well-being.

SECONDARY APPRAISALS

Secondary appraisal emerges with any form of perceived threat or harm if primary appraisals are ineffective or maladaptive. The rationale of secondary appraisal is to assess coping resources, options, and choices. Lazarus (1966) emphasized the significance of secondary appraisals as follows:

- They are the basis of coping mechanisms.
- They enhance or promote a positive outcome of primary appraisals.
- They strengthen coping resources and options.

The outcome of the coping process depends on individual efforts to alter threatening events and attempts to change the person's appraisal of the stress to minimize the threat (Hansen & Johnson, 1979).

The impact of psychosocial factors and neurobiological processes has been demonstrated in illness, such as posttraumatic stress disorder, that produces morphological changes in the brain. These changes are generated by recurring stimulation from the client's environment that exceeds the cortex's ability to process events, such as a rape or act of violence, causing permanent synaptic changes. Even in this disorder, the client's perception of the event determines the extent of synaptic alterations (Gabbard, 1992).

The shared impact of neurobiological and psychosocial sciences on mental health reinforces the importance of holistic health care. Healthy adaptation is based on complex neurobiological and psychosocial factors that people mobilize during stressful events.

THE NURSE'S ROLE

Prevention and health promotion are major domains of nursing. Understanding the effects of stress, coping, and adaptation is crucial to health promotion. Furthermore, appreciating the impact of stress on human behavior enhances the assessment process and helps the nurse identify client strengths, resources, and interventions that can reduce the deleterious effects of stress across the life span. Assessing present and past coping behaviors and developmental and behavioral competencies is a vital component of the nursing process. Mastering stress across the life span is critical to the formation of adaptive coping skills and health. Healthy adaptation arises from mobilizing biological, psychological, and sociocultural resources during stressful periods.

Psychiatric–mental health nurses are challenged to integrate major neurobiological and psychosocial concepts to understand individual responses to stress. Appreciating the complexity of relationships between people and their environments is critical to understanding the causes of mental illness and health. Psychosocial stressors and individual appraisals correlate with neurochemical and neuroanatomical changes (Kandel, 1983, 1979). Nursing implications for this relationship between these concepts include understanding the client's perception of stressors, identifying available resources for coping, and teaching adaptive health practices. The nurse can identify clients at risk for mental illness or exacerbation and develop interventions that encourage a sense of well-being and mental health.

The stigma and prevalence of mental illness prevail as psychiatric–mental health nursing approaches the twenty-first century. Numerous forces impact social reactions to mental illness, including the media, which continue to portray people with mental illness as violent, unpredictable, and disruptive. The increased visibility of homeless mentally ill people also reinforces these stereotypes and beliefs.

Throughout history, the plight and perception of the mentally ill have been influenced by social, economic, and legislative conditions. Psychiatric–mental health nurses must take the lead in transforming the negative image of mental illness while promoting mental health throughout the life span. This process begins by defining mental health and mental illness.

THE NURSING PROCESS

The nursing process is defined as the diagnosis and treatment of human responses to actual or potential problems (American Nurses Association, 1980). It is a deliberate interactive problem-solving approach to effect change in the client. (The major phases of the nursing process are described in Chapter 4.) The effectiveness of the nursing process is influenced by the nurse's understanding and application of broad behavioral and neurobiological concepts of adaptation across the life span. Additionally, effective communication skills are needed to interact with clients, families, and members of the mental health team.

During this interaction process the client and nurse mutually determine a plan of care. Assessing the client's responses to internal and external demands, such as neurobiological and psychosocial factors, can be accomplished during this initial phase of the nursing process.

The following case study provides a useful framework in which to examine the nursing process.

Case Study: Mr. L.

Mr. L. is a 54-year-old man with a history of bipolar disorder, manic type. His wife is very supportive, and he has been compliant with treatment the past 2 years. He was recently laid off from his job in sales in which he had worked for the past 10 years. Accompanied by his wife, Mr. L. presented with complaints of increased social withdrawal and depression during the past few weeks. He is psychomotorly retarded and withdrawn and has poor eye contact. His appearance is unkempt, and his mood is depressed; his speech is monotone and clear; and he is alert and oriented to time, place, and person. Additionally, his thoughts are relevant, logical, and coherent. He denies having suicidal or homicidal ideations or making gestures in the past, but he admits feeling that his family would be better off if he were dead. His appetite is poor, and he reports a weight loss of 20 pounds over the past 3 weeks. He sleeps at least 10 hours a day and he still feels tired. He is presently taking lithium, which has stabilized his mood during the past 2 years. This is his first experience with major depression, but he has had several manic episodes.

Assessment (Data Collection)

Mood disorders are linked with a chemical imbalance or have a neurobiological basis. Psychosocial factors also play major roles in precipitating bipolar disorders (Ellicott, 1990). Mr. L.'s present psychosocial stressors include a recent job loss associated with feelings of low self-esteem and a sense of loss and helplessness regarding the prospect of finding employment because of his age and mental illness.

Nursing Diagnoses

- Ineffective Individual Coping
- Alterations in Mood, Depression
- Sleep Pattern Disturbance: Increased Sleep
- Altered Nutrition: Less than Body Requirements

Planning

Major planning and nursing interventions include enhancing Mr. L.'s present strengths and promoting adaptive and lasting coping skills that will enable him to appraise present and future crises realistically. Adaptive coping skills facilitate resumption of self-care, maintenance of adequate nutritional status, and revival of past interests and responsibilities. Normal sleeping patterns generally return with the formation of healthy coping skills and a resolution of the current crisis (see the accompanying Nursing Care Plan).

Implementation

Establishing and maintaining a caring, nonjudgmental, and supportive attitude enables nurses to assist clients in identifying the meaning of current stressors and recent lifestyle changes as well as present and past coping patterns. Maladaptive responses interfere with the successful resolution of a crisis. Nurses must assess the level of dangerous behavior such as suicidality, current nutritional status, self-care, and sleeping patterns to minimize maladaptive responses. Other nursing interventions include measures to reduce distress, enhance coping skills, and increase knowledge. Administering psychotropics, monitoring client responses to interventions, and collaborating with clients and families in discharge planning can facilitate successful resolution of crisis situation.

Evaluation

To evaluate the client's response to treatment, the nurse needs to determine whether the client has returned to the precrisis level of function. Manifestations of successful crisis resolution and formation of adaptive coping skills include minimal or absent depression; expression of hope and a will to live; a realistic, positive outlook on life; increased self-esteem; and resumption of meaningful relationships.

In the case study, Mr. L.'s chief stressors are identified, such as losing a job and poor self-esteem generated by the loss. His general appearance and mood and information from his wife facilitate problem identification or nursing diagnoses as alterations in perceptions, nutrition, and mood. Outcome identification provides opportunities to implement both medical and nursing interventions such as administering psychotropics, maintaining adequate nutrition, monitoring his responses (both desired and adverse), and providing emotional support that encourages restoration to previous level of functioning. Additionally, facilitating the wife's participation is an important nursing intervention in health promotion.

In addition to helping clients meet their basic needs, nurses continue to play pivotal roles in prevention, advocacy, and altering the negative image of mental illness. The process of changing attitudes requires commitment, education, and political savvy. To overcome the stigma of mental illness, nurses must examine these attitudes about the mentally ill to identify fears, myths, and stereotypes on which they might be based. Educating students is only part of this process: families and clients must be active participants in directing health care, and educating communities is an integral aspect. Political savvy is the final part of this process and involves psychiatric nurses playing active roles in assessing high-risk behaviors and voting on issues that affect the prevention and treatment of the mentally ill.

►CHAPTER SUMMARY

Stress and coping are natural aspects of developmental stages. One's ability to manage stress and cope effectively is influenced by a myriad of highly complex internal and external processes that begin prenatally and evolve throughout the life span. Early responses to

Nursing Care Plan 7–1 The Client with a Bipolar Disorder, Manic Type (Mr. L.)

Nursing Diagnosis: Ineffective Individual Coping

OUTCOME IDENTIFICATION	NURSING ACTIONS	RATIONALES	EVALUATION
1. By [date], client will develop adaptive and lasting coping skills.	1a. Establish and maintain a caring, nonjudgmental, and supportive attitude.	1a. Helps client feel less defensive and more comfortable sharing feelings.	*Goal met:* Client returns to a precrisis level of functioning. Client develops adaptive coping skills (i.e., improved problem solving). Client resumes meaningful relationships.
	1b. Assist client in identifying meaning of current stressors.	1b. Helps client understand self and present responses.	
	1c. Collaborate with client and wife to identify strengths and past and present coping skills.	1c. Places focus on positive attributes and increases self-esteem.	

Nursing Diagnosis: Sleep Pattern Disturbance

OUTCOME IDENTIFICATION	NURSING ACTIONS	RATIONALES	EVALUATION
1. By [date], client will resume normal sleeping patterns.	1a. Assess normal sleeping patterns.	1a. Determines baseline sleeping patterns.	*Goal met:* Client resumes normal sleeping patterns.

Nursing Diagnosis: Altered Nutrition: Less than Body Requirements

OUTCOME IDENTIFICATION	NURSING ACTIONS	RATIONALES	EVALUATION
1. By [date], client will maintain nutritional status to sustain body requirements.	1a. Assess client's nutritional status.	1a. Determines nutritional needs status.	*Goal met:* Client's normal eating patterns are reestablished and, before leaving the hospital, client is within 4 lb of normal weight.
	1b. Weigh as needed. Monitor intake and output.	1b. Assesses nutritional and hydration status.	
	1c. Encourage selection of favorite, appealing foods.	1c. Improves appetite and establishes eating patterns.	
	1d. Provide pleasant eating environment.	1d. Improves appetite.	
	1e. Encourage mouth care.	1e. Improves taste sensations and appetite.	

stress are influenced by internal factors, including genetic predisposition, neurobiological and psychosocial elements, and developmental stage. External factors include prenatal competency, support systems, and interpersonal interactions.

Nurses play a key role in assessing client responses to stress throughout the life span. Appreciating the impact of neurobiological and psychosocial processes on human behavior is critical to this process. Assessing the client's present and past coping skills is also an essential aspect of nursing care. A plan of care based on these data provides the basis for interventions such as teaching problem-solving or coping skills and reinforcing support systems in clients at risk. Strategies that minimize the client's feelings of helplessness and strengthen adaptive responses are important aspects of restoration and health.

Suggestions for Clinical Conferences

1. Develop case histories of clients at different developmental stages, focusing on the nursing process.
   a. Identify adaptive and maladaptive responses.
   b. Identify present and past coping strategies.
   c. Develop nursing interventions that enhance coping skills.
2. Encourage students to discuss their coping behaviors specifically during stressful periods.
3. Identify personal coping patterns.

References

Alexander, F. (1939). Psychological aspects of medicine. *Psychosomatic Medicine, 1*(1), 7–18.

American Nurses Association. (1980). *A social policy statement.* Kansas City, MO: Author.

American Psychiatric Association. (1952). *Diagnostic and statistical manual of mental disorders.* Washington, DC: Author.

American Psychiatric Association. (1968). *Diagnostic and statistical manual of mental disorders* (2nd ed.). Washington, DC: Author.

American Psychiatric Association. (1980). *Diagnostic and statistical manual of mental disorders* (3rd ed.). Washington, DC: Author.

American Psychiatric Association. (1987). *Diagnostic and statistical manual of mental disorders, third edition, revised.* Washington, DC: Author.

American Psychiatric Association. (1994). *Diagnostic and statistical manual of mental disorders* (4th ed.). Washington, DC: Author.

Antonovsky, A. (1979). *Health, stress, and coping.* San Francisco: Jossey-Bass.

Belsky, J. (1981). Early human experience: A family perspective. *Child Development, 17,* 3–23.

Belsky, J. (1984). The determinants of parenting: A process model. *Child Development, 55,* 83–96.

Bleuler, E. (1950). Dementia praecox or the group of schizophrenias (J. Zinkin, Trans.). New York: International Press (Original work published 1911).

Blos, P. (1962). On adolescence. New York: Free Press.

Borst, S. R., Noam, G. G., & Bartok, J. A. (1991). Adolescent suicidality: A clinical–developmental approach. *Journal of the American Academy of Child and Adolescent Psychiatry, 30,* 796–803.

Bowlby, J. (1969). *Attachment and loss* (Vol. 1). New York: Basic Books.

Brown, G. W. (1993). Life events and affective disorder: Replication and limitations. *Psychosomatic Medicine, 55*(3), 248–259.

Cannon, W. B. (1914). The emergency function of the adrenal medulla in pain and the major emotions. *American Journal of Physiology, 33*(3), 356–372.

Cannon, W. B. (1939). *The wisdom of the body* (2nd ed.). New York: W. W. Norton.

Caplan, G. (1961). *An approach to community mental health.* New York: Grune & Stratton.

Deutsch, A. (1937). *Mental illness in America.* New York: Doubleday.

Dix, T. (1991). The affective organization of parenting: Adaptive and maladaptive processes. *Psychological Bulletin, 110*(1), 3–25.

Dreyfus-Brisac, C. (1979). Ontogenesis of brain bio-electrical activity and sleep organization in neonates and infants. In F. Faulkner & J. M. Tanner (Eds.), *Human growth* (Vol. 3; pp. 157–182). New York: Plenum Press.

Ellicott, A., Hammen C., Gitlin M., Brown, G., & Jamison K. (1990). Life events and the course of bipolar disorder. *American Journal of Psychiatry, 147*(9), 1194–1198.

Erikson, E. (1963). *Childhood and society.* New York: W. W. Norton.

Erikson, E. (1968). *Identity: Youth and crisis.* New York: W. W. Norton.

Forehand, R., McCombs, A., & Brody, G. H. (1987). The relationship between parental depressive mood states and child functioning. *Advances in Behavior Research and Therapy, 9,* 1–20.

Freud, S. (1953). *The standard edition of the complete psychological works of Sigmund Freud.* New York: Macmillan.

Fristad, M. A., Jedel, R., Welles, R. A., & Welles, E. B. (1993). Psychosocial functioning in children after the death of a parent. *American Journal of Psychiatry, 150*(3), 511–513.

Gabbard, G. O. (1992). Psychodynamic psychiatry in the decade of the brain. *American Journal of Psychiatry, 149*(8), 991–998.

Gabella, G. (1976). Structure of the autonomic nervous system. London: Chapman & Hall.

Glass, D. C. (1977). Stress, behavior patterns, and coronary disease. *American Scientist, 65,* 177–187.

Hansen, D. A., & Johnson, V. A. (1979). Rethinking family stress theory: Definitional aspects. In W. R. Burr, R. Hill, F. I. Nye, & I. L. Reiss (Eds.), *Contemporary theories about the family: Research-based theories* (Vol. 1; pp. 582–603). New York: Free Press.

Hartmann, H. (1958). *Ego psychology and the problem of adaptation.* New York: International Universities Press.

Holmes, T. H., & Rahe, R. H. (1967). The social readjustment rating scale. *Journal of Psychosomatic Research, 11,* 213–218.

Holroyd, K. A., & Lazarus, R. S. (1982). Stress, coping, and somatic adaptation. In L. Goldberger & S. Breznitz (Eds.), *Handbook of stress* (pp. 21–35). New York: Free Press.

Jalowiec, A. (1979). *Stress and coping in hypertensive and emergency room patients.* Unpublished master's thesis, University of Illinois, Chicago.

Jalowiec, A. (1988). Confirmatory factor analysis of the Jalowiec Coping Scale. In C. F. Waltz & O. L. Strickland (Eds.), *Measurement of nursing outcomes,* Vol. 1. *Measuring client outcomes* (pp. 287–308). New York: Springer.

Jalowiec, A., & Powers, M. J. (1983). Stress and coping in hypertensive and emergency room patients. *Nursing Research, 30*(1), 10–15.

Kandel, E. R. (1979). Psychotherapy and the single synapse: The impact of psychiatric thought on neurobiologic research. *New England Journal of Medicine, 310*(10), 1028–1037.

Kandel, E. R. (1983). From metapsychology to molecular biology: Explorations into the nature of anxiety. *American Journal of Psychiatry, 140,* 1277–1293.

Keitner, G. I., & Miller, I. W. (1990). Family functioning and major depression: An overview. *American Journal of Psychiatry, 147,* 1128–1137.

Kobasa, S. C. (1979). Stressful life events, personality, and health: An inquiry into hardiness. *Journal of Personality and Social Psychology, 37,* 1–11.

Kobasa, S. C., Maddi, S. R., Puccetti, M. C., & Zola, M. A. (1985). Effectiveness of hardiness, exercise, and social support as resources against illness. *Journal of Psychosomatic Research, 29,* 525–533.

Kovacs, M., Goldston, D., & Gatsonis, C. (1993). Suicidal behaviors and childhood onset depressive disorders: A longitudinal investigation. *Journal of the American Academy of Child and Adolescent Psychiatry, 32,* 1–8.

Lazarus, R. S. (1966). *Psychological stress and the coping process.* New York: McGraw-Hill.

Lazarus, R. S., & Folkman, S. (1984). *Stress, appraisal, and coping.* New York: Springer.

Lazarus, R. S., & Launier, R. (1978). Stress-related transactions between personality and environment. In L. A. Pervin & M. Lewis (Eds.), *Perspectives in interactional psychology* (pp. 287–327). New York: Plenum.

Lipsitt, L. R. (1983). Stress in infancy: Towards understanding the origins of coping behavior. In N. Garmezy & M. Rutter (Eds.), *Stress, coping, and development in children* (pp. 161–190). New York: McGraw-Hill.

McLoyd, V. C. (1990). The impact of economic hardship in black families and children: Psychological distress, parenting, and socioemotional development. *Child Development, 61,* 311–346.

Menninger, K. (1963). *The vital balance.* New York: Viking Press.

Meyer, A. (1957). *Psychobiology: A science of man.* Springfield, IL: Charles C Thomas.

Mishne, J. M. (1986). *Clinical work with adolescents.* New York: Free Press.

Morrison, E., et al. (1985). Nursing adaptation evaluation. *Journal of Psychosocial Nursing and Mental Health Services, 8*(23), 10–13.

Nightingale, F. (1860). *Notes on nursing: What it is and is not*. London: Harrison.

Patterson, P. H., Potter, D. D., & Furshpan, E. J. (1978). The chemical differentiation of nerve cells. *Scientific American, 239*, 50–59.

Pfeffer, C. R., Plutchik, R., & Mizruchi, M. (1988). Normal children at risk for suicidal behaviors. A two-year followup study. *Journal of the American Academy of Child and Adolescent Psychiatry*, *27*, 34–41.

Pollock, S. E. (1986). Human responses to chronic illness: Physiologic and psychosocial adaptation. *Nursing Research*, *35*, 90–95.

Pollock, S. E., & Duffy, M. E. (1990). The health-related hardiness scale: Development and psychometric analysis. *Nursing Research*, *39*, 218–222.

Roy, C. (1976). *Introduction to nursing: An adaptation model*. Englewood Cliffs, NJ: Prentice-Hall.

Roy, C., & McLeod, D. (1981). Theory of person as an adaptive person. In C. Roy & S. L. Roberts (Eds.), *Theory construction in nursing: An adaptation model*. Englewood Cliffs, NJ: Prentice-Hall.

Seligman, M. E. D. (1975). *Learned helplessness: On depression and development*. San Francisco: W. H. Freeman.

Selye, H. (1976). *The stress of life*. New York: McGraw-Hill.

Sroufe, L. A., & Rutter, M. (1984). The domain of developmental psychopathology. *Child Development, 55*, 17–29.

Swindle, R. W. Jr., Cronkite, R. C., & Moos, R. H. (1989). Life stressors, social resources, coping, and the four-year course of unipolar depression. *Journal of Abnormal Psychology, 98*(4), 468–477.

U.S. Department of Health and Human Services. (1990). Healthy people 2000: National health promotion and disease prevention (DHHS Publication No. PHS 91-50212). Washington, DC: U.S. Government Printing Office.

Yehuda, R., Resnick, H., Kahuna, B., & Gillen, E. L. (1993). Long-lasting hormonal alterations to extreme stress in humans: Normative or maladaptive? *Psychosomatic Medicine, 55*(3), 287–297.

CHAPTER

8

Crisis Intervention and Management: The Role of Adaptation

DEBORAH ANTAI-OTONG, M.S., R.N.,C.S.

OUTLINE

CHAPTER OBJECTIVES

Upon completion of this chapter, you will be able to:
1. Analyze the major concepts of crisis theory.
2. Differentiate between normal and abnormal grief reactions.
3. Use the nursing process in crisis intervention.
4. Compare maturational and situational crises.
5. Analyze factors that affect the outcome of crisis situations.

KEY TERMS

Cathexis
Crisis intervention
Crisis
Disaster
Grief
Maturational crisis
Support system

Crisis is an integral aspect of human growth and development. Successful resolution of a crisis is a complex process shaped by one's repertoire of adaptive coping behaviors. The core of coping behaviors parallels ego function, developmental stage, and neurobiological and psychosocial factors.

TERMINOLOGY

The terms ***crisis*** and *stress* are often used interchangeably and are related to the term *adaptation*. Delineating the meaning of these terms is important to understanding the concept of crisis.

Crisis. The concept of crisis is often associated with the potential for adaptive responses and is usually not akin to illness. In contrast, the concept of stress is often associated with negative connotations or high risk for illness (Rapoport, 1965). People are constantly adapting to internal and external changes that are critical to survival, health, and growth. Adaptation to these demands depends on mobilization of psychological and physiological resources.

What is a crisis? How is it different from stress? Caplan (1961, p. 18) defined a crisis as a situation

> *when a person faces an obstacle to important life goals that is, for a time, insurmountable through the utilization of customary methods of problem solving. A period of disorganization ensues, a period of upset, during which many abortive attempts at solutions are made.*

In other words, crisis refers to acute emotional turmoil that stems from developmental, biological, situational, or psychosocial stressors that momentarily render the person's normal coping mechanisms inadequate.

Successful resolution of crisis is a complex process and represents adaptive responses to stressful encounters. Crises evolve when normal coping mechanisms fail to abate anxiety. Failure to reduce stress using normal coping behaviors results in an increase in anxiety and tension and feelings of helplessness, unfolding into a state of turmoil. A crisis situation is also a time in which individual ego defenses are amenable to growth and adaptive change (Caplan, 1961, 1964; Davanloo, 1978).

Stress. *Stress* refers to the reaction to a stressful event and circumstances that precipitated it. No two people respond to stressors in the same manner. A stressor can be psychological or physiological, and its source can be both internal and external. Selye (1976) described stress as the body's nonspecific response to demands in terms of potential illness or disequilibrium. Stressful events are potential sources of crises if they are not handled effectively.

Lazarus (1966) disputed the notion that stress depicts only illness or the potential for maladaptation. He suggested that stress is a complex phenomenon that influences adaptation and is associated with stimulus or response. In simple terms, stress is a relationship between the person and the environment that is appraised as taxing or surpassing available resources and threatening one's well-being (Lazarus & Folkman, 1984).

Other investigators minimize the impact of stress and refer to it as meaningless and insignificant. They contend that this term is outdated and its uses should be limited to catastrophes or disasters (Hinkle, 1977; Pasnau & Fauzy, 1989; Weiner, 1985). The role of stress in adaptation and health continues to be debated, but understanding its effect on human behavior remains a significant aspect of psychiatric–mental health nursing.

Adaptation. The term *adaptation* stems from the Latin word *adaptare,* which means to adjust, and is defined as a turning point in which adaptive coping responses are used to manage stressful situations. Adaptive responses are those that maintain homeostasis or health, such as survival, maturity, procreation, and mastery of developmental tasks (Andrews & Roy, 1986).

This chapter discusses the historical aspects of crisis theory, analyzes major concepts of crisis management, and defines the role of the psychiatric–mental health nurse in helping clients who are experiencing crises across the life span.

PERSPECTIVES AND THEORIES

LEGISLATIVE INFLUENCES: THE COMMUNITY MENTAL HEALTH MOVEMENT

Modern concepts of the community mental health delivery services were introduced by the Joint Commission on Mental Illness and Mental Health in 1961. President Kennedy's communication to the U.S. Congress and the passage of the Mental Health Act of 1963 underscored the prevention, treatment, and rehabilitation of mental illness. The President stressed the community's responsibility in providing care for this population. As a result of Kennedy's messages, major changes in American psychiatry emerged (Caplan, 1964), and the new principles became the basis of a comprehensive community and preventive approach to mental health care. The U.S. Congress responded to this need by decreeing that each mental health center have a minimum of five essential services, including

1. Twenty-four-hour emergency care
2. Outpatient services
3. Partial hospitalization
4. Inpatient services
5. Consultation and education

Subsequent legislation stipulated additional services for children and the elderly, screening prior to hospitalization, aftercare, transitional housing, substance abuse treatment, and victim programs. Crisis centers were crucial to the community mental health model. Efforts to expend energy on removing conditions that contribute to mental illness became a major focus of community mental health care. The levels of preventive care that are provided through these centers include primary (health promotion), secondary (early case finding), and tertiary (rehabilitation).

Overall, the major objectives of the community mental health centers are to maximize resources, provide for various levels of prevention, and evaluate interventions and research. However, recent legislative and socioeconomic factors have curtailed funding and interest in supporting community mental health programs. New health care reforms promise to further positively impact the community mental health services because of the growing trend of community-based preventive care.

CRISIS THEORY

Historically, crisis theory stems from various concepts of human growth and development. The commonality of these theories lies in their relationship to adaptive and maladaptive responses to stress. Adaptive behaviors are shaped by neurobiological and psychosocial factors that contribute to ego and personality development. Early theorists, such as Freud, Erikson, Lindemann, and Caplan, contributed to the evolution of the crisis theory.

Crisis intervention is a relatively new approach to preventing mental illness. Its primary focus is early case finding and the assessment and prevention of the deleterious effects of stress (Caplan, 1961). Its interdisciplinary roots highlight the significant role of psychiatric–mental health nurses in prevention and health promotion.

PSYCHOANALYTICAL THEORIES

Sigmund Freud

Freud's (1961) theory of psychosexual development emphasized the influence of conscious and unconscious conflicts on adaptation. These developmental periods are marked by normal neurobiological and psychosocial stresses. The capacity to master these tasks depends on a person's developmental stage, ego function, and personality traits. These influences represent one's repertoire of coping skills.

Freud and other psychoanalytical theorists stressed the importance of early childhood experiences on adaptive and maladaptive coping responses throughout the life span. They also postulated the impact of these experiences on the progression of growth and development and coping patterns during normal and maturational crises. An in-depth discussion of ego and personality development is found in Chapter 14.

Erik Erikson

Erikson's theory of **maturational crisis** (1963) concurred with that of Freud and other psychoanalysts, paralleling its stages of psychosocial growth and development with Freud's psychosexual tasks. Erikson's theory stressed the relevance of the individual's ability to master normal developmental tasks. He surmised that "psychosocial survival is safeguarded only by vital virtues which develop in the interplay of successive and overlapping generations" (Erikson, 1964, p. 114). Additionally, he clarified the notion that "life cycle is an integrated psychosocial phenomenon" based on early childhood milestones (Erikson, 1964, p. 114).

Early childhood experiences are the basis of ego function or strength. Healthy ego function is determined by mastering the initial task of trust, which fosters a sense of self-worth (Erikson, 1964). These beginnings serve as the foundation for confronting subsequent developmental tasks. In other words, the person's ability to adapt to crisis effectively begins at birth and progresses throughout the life span. The ego governs this entire process.

Erikson's (1963) eight stages of development encompass specific tasks or maturational crises. Resolution of each stage is determined by resolution of the previous developmental task. These stages are discussed in detail in "Life Span Issues: Maturational Crises" in this chapter and are displayed in Table 8–1.

Maturational or developmental crises are predictable and anticipated responses to developmental tasks. People with healthy ego function tend to respond to developmental crises effectively using adaptive coping skills. In contrast, people with poor or inadequate ego function tend to become overwhelmed by stress and are vulnerable to developmental arrest. Developmental arrest increases the risk of illness and other maladaptive responses.

Individual responses to crisis are influenced by internal and external coping resources. Internal coping resources are composed of innate and acquired processes. Innate processes are influenced by genetic, ego function, and neurobiological factors; they are presumed to be unconscious. Acquired processes evolve through life experiences (Roy & Andrews, 1991). External resources involve psychosocial and cultural factors, such as the number and meaning of stressors, and available

TABLE 8–1

Maturational Crises: Erikson's Eight Stages of Development

	PRIMARY DEVELOPMENTAL TASK	SOURCES OF MALADAPTIVE RESPONSE TO CRISES
Infancy	Basic trust vs. mistrust	Birth ("the most radical change of all"); unreliable provision of basic needs by caregiver
Toddler Period	Autonomy vs. shame and doubt	Overcontrolling, smothering, neglectful, or rejecting parents
Preschool Period	Initiative vs. guilt	Failure to develop trust; impaired self-esteem
Middle Childhood	Industry vs. inferiority	Entering school: dealing with criticism, authority figures, working with others
Adolescence	Identity vs. role confusion	Endocrine changes; social pressures; divorce; lack of empathy and consistent limit setting from family; acceptance of own inadequacies ("apt to suffer more deeply" than at any other stage)
Early Adulthood	Intimacy vs. isolation	Formation of intense interpersonal relationships; clarifying sexuality; lack of validation from early caregivers
Middle Adulthood	Generativity vs. stagnation	Divorce; empty nest syndrome; aging/menopause; major illness; retirement; self-absorption; isolation
Late Adulthood	Integrity vs. despair	Prospect of death

Adapted from THE LIFE CYCLE COMPLETED: A Review by Erik H. Erikson, with the permission of W. W. Norton & Company, Inc.

support systems. External resources allow people to adapt and cope with stress effectively.

Erikson's (1963) delineation of adaptive and maladaptive responses to developmental tasks provides nurses with parameters for assessing healthy coping behaviors. Psychiatric–mental health nurses can support and reinforce adaptive behaviors by recognizing normal and abnormal responses to developmental tasks.

GRIEF THEORY

Erich Lindemann

Lindemann's (1944) contribution to crisis theory arises from his classic grief and bereavement study with loved ones of the victims of the Boston Coconut Grove Club fire in 1942 that killed 491 people. His studies focused on the phenomenon of the mourning process and its impact on health. He delineated the normal bereavement process and described predictable stages that people go through after emotional disturbances. He surmised that this process takes 4 to 6 weeks and involves a progression of psychological stages. Caplan (1964) contended that Lindemann's work provided the foundation of the crisis theory as a conceptual framework for preventive psychiatry.

In his studies, Lindemann found that most people who were mourning resolved their grief effectively and recovered from emotional and biological distress within 4 to 6 weeks. Additionally, he found a smaller group of mourners who did not resolve their grief as well as the former group; people in the smaller group exhibited severe psychiatric and psychosomatic disturbances, including depression and gastrointestinal problems. He then compared characteristics of people in each group and found that those who were able to work through their grief tended to manifest several reactions, such as withdrawal from daily activities, emotional pain and loneliness, crying spells, and loss of appetite. They focused primarily on the loss and the memories of their loved one. Lindemann believed that the latter symptoms were the basis of the phenomenon of mourning. Additionally, he noted that reliving memories of lost ones allowed people to gain a sense of reality of their loss.

Lindemann (1944) stated that the time frame of healthy grief reaction rests on the mastery of grief work, particularly freedom from intense emotional ties with the deceased, adaptation to loss of the loved one, and establishment of new meaningful relationships. Furthermore, he postulated a relationship between the absence of mourning and the formation of maladaptive responses, and he noted the following characteristics of those who fail to mourn:

- They continue to live their lives as usual.
- They fail to cry or express emotional pain.
- They complain of feeling numb.
- They do not become preoccupied with the loved one.
- They deny feelings regarding their loss.
- They experience alterations in their social interactions.

These people are likely to develop illness and express anger or resentment toward health professionals. Lindemann stressed the need for health care professionals to facilitate the grief process by recognizing adaptive and maladaptive behaviors in the mourning client (see Chapter 9 for a discussion of normal and abnormal grief reactions).

Appreciation of the grief process involves understanding the meaning of grief, bereavement, and mourning (see Table 8–2 for the *Diagnostic and Statistical Manual of Mental Disorders* description of bereavement). The term ***grief*** arises from the Latin word *gravis* and is a normal profound emotional response to loss. It promotes mental health by allowing the client to work through and cope with loss and accept its reality. Additionally, it facilitates social processing and sharing of

TABLE 8–2
DSM-IV Concepts on Bereavement

- Focus of clinical attention is a "normal" response to the loss of a loved one and includes the following:
  1. Individuals who present with symptoms illustrative of major depressive disorder, such as alterations in sleep, appetite, and cognitive function.
  2. Individuals who perceive symptoms as a natural part of the grief process.
  3. Individuals who seek professional treatment for relief of associated appetite and sleep disturbances.
- Symptoms may vary among various culture groups.
- If symptoms persist longer than 2 months, a diagnosis of Major Depressive Disorder may be considered.

Data from American Psychiatric Association. (1994). *Diagnostic and statistical manual of mental disorders* (4th ed.). Washington, DC: Author.

feelings and emotional pain generated by loss. Grief reactions are actual, anticipatory, unresolved, or pathological.

Anticipatory grief refers to experiencing grief before it occurs. For example, an 18-year-old student who knows he has to leave home to live on a college campus may grieve the loss of his youth and the security of his parents' taking care of his major needs. Another example is the young woman who is diagnosed with acquired immunodeficiency syndrome (AIDS). She and her family grieve over her eventual death.

People experiencing anticipatory or actual grief may feel angry, sad, or guilty. Unresolved or pathological grief reaction has been discussed earlier. Depression and perceptual disturbances are possible negative or maladaptive outcomes of grief reactions. Bereavement occurs when loss is inevitable. Mourning is the process by which grief is resolved.

Management of Grief Reactions

The aim of grief management is to prevent chronic and deleterious reactions to loss. The impact of loss leaves the client bewildered and experiencing immense emotional pain. Grief work is a process that helps the client accept and resolve the pain of sorrow. This process begins when clients free or release themselves from the bondage of their loved one; readjust to living without the deceased; and form new meaningful relationships. Grief work can be enhanced by

- Coping with painful experiences
- Reliving experiences and times with the loved one
- Experiencing and trying out rewarding relationships

Eventually, the intensity of emotional pain dissipates and becomes more tolerable as the client masters and embraces the loss of a loved one (Lindemann, 1944, 1979).

Grief work is strengthened by spiritual beliefs that often provide emotional comfort, promote healthy discussions of life, and reduce guilt. Nurses play a critical role in assessing spiritual needs and mobilizing resources that provide emotional support during stressful periods. Some clients may feel uncomfortable asking for spiritual support. Nurses can minimize that discomfort by asking the client about any interest or preference he or she may have for spiritual support. Approaching the client in a caring and nonjudgmental manner allows the nurse to assess spiritual needs. Furthermore, understanding the meaning of one's own personal spiritual beliefs and grief reactions enhances understanding those of the client.

PREVENTIVE PSYCHIATRY

Caplan's early work with Lindemann in 1946 at the Harvard-Wellesley Project established early crisis intervention concepts. Numerous so-called suicide prevention centers were established in this country in the 1960s. The quality of services provided varied with each center's role and function and paralleled the national mental health movement, which included suicide prevention and crisis intervention (McGee, 1974).

Gerald Caplan

Caplan's (1964) renowned work, *Principles of Preventive Psychiatry,* was the foundation of most literature and research associated with crisis theory. A number of nurse theorists have modified his work and made notable contributions to nursing practice, but the principal nurse contributors have been Aguilera (1978, 1990, 1994) and Hoff (1989).

Caplan's (1964) definition of preventive psychiatry referred to a comprehensive perspective that integrated theoretical and clinical concepts used to decrease the prevalence of mental illness (primary prevention), the duration of symptoms (secondary prevention); and the deleterious effects of disorders (tertiary prevention).

Caplan described primary prevention from a life span perspective, noting that people have various basic needs that parallel the developmental stages. He sorted these needs into three groups: biological, psychosocial, and sociocultural. Biological needs include nourishment, safety, sensory stimulation, and exercise. Psychosocial needs refer to interactions with significant others that promote cognitive and affective maturation. Sociocultural needs arise from customs, rituals, values, and social structure that influence personality maturity and ego function. Social norms and expectations have a profound effect on behavior and feelings about one's self and role in the world. Furthermore, culture influences language, values, traditions, and behaviors.

Caplan (1961) also linked mental health, or successful crisis resolution, with ego function. He listed three criteria used to assess ego function during crisis situations. The first criterion is the capacity to modulate affect, such as anger, anxiety, and frustration, during stressful periods. People with healthy ego function tend to mobilize internal and external resources to maintain health or homeostasis. The second criterion is the use of adaptive problem solving. Does the person cope effectively with stress, or does the person become ill or use maladaptive problem solving to reduce the overwhelming effects of stress?

The third criterion is the ability to maintain reality

testing. People who use adaptive coping behaviors have a repertoire of internal and external resources that maintain reality testing. In face of a threat or loss, the person handles the crisis effectively. People with inadequate coping skills tend to regress when faced with a crisis situation in which internal and external resources are overtaxed. Regression is a primitive defense mechanism used to revert to an earlier stage of development or childlike thinking to deal with crisis. Impaired reality testing ranges from severe anxiety reactions to psychosis (Caplan, 1961). The impact of a crisis is based on complex processes that determine how anxiety is modulated, problem-solving skills are mobilized, and reality testing is maintained.

ORIGINS OF CRISIS

People constantly interact with their environment. The daily stress of living forces people to maintain a steady-state or equilibrium using a repertoire of innate and acquired coping skills. An array of habitual problem-solving mechanisms is constantly called on to minimize the effects of uncomfortable feelings and thoughts. These mechanisms are primarily unconscious. A crisis evolves when the usual coping behaviors fail to maintain integrity (Caplan, 1961). What conditions contribute to crisis situations?

Parad and Caplan (1965) described three interrelated conditions that produce a state of crisis as follows:

1. A hazardous event that poses a threat
2. An emotional need that denotes earlier threats and increased vulnerability
3. An inability to respond adaptively

Understanding the human response to crisis requires clarifying its origins and meaning to the individual (Hoff, 1989). Crises originate from various sources and complex processes, such as life events (situational) and developmental or maturational events.

Situational Crisis

Situational or unexpected crises originate from the following three sources (Hoff, 1989):

1. Environmental, such as tornadoes, fires, riots, and outbreak of disease
2. Physical or personal, such as amputations and debilitating or terminal illness
3. Interpersonal or psychosocial, such as the death of a loved one or a divorce

Maturational Crisis

Maturational, or developmental, crises are described as normal crises because they are expected in association with normal growth and development. These periods are marked by biological, psychosocial, and social transitions that generate characteristic disturbances in behavior and emotional responses. The basis of maturational crises is depicted in Freud's psychosexual theory and Erikson's eight developmental tasks, which delineate human development and associated biological and cognitive behaviors evolving throughout the life span. Each state generates enormous stress and the need to master developmental crises. Erikson (1968) believed that each developmental stage was a turning point that provided opportunities for both adaptation and maladaptation.

MANIFESTATIONS OF CRISIS

Caplan (1964) listed the major characteristics of crisis as the following:

- A state of increased tension and feelings of helplessness are present.
- Emergency coping or problem-solving mechanisms are needed.
- A state of disorganization may ensue.
- The situation is self-limiting and usually lasts 1 to 6 weeks.

Crisis situations frequently render people more dependent on external resources than at other times in their lives. This has been depicted as situational dependency or an adaptive response. Clients are responsive to the possibility of constructive changes during this period, and nurses are in pivotal positions to facilitate a higher level of function.

CRISIS: THE ROLE OF ADAPTATION

COPING MECHANISMS

Crisis situations confront people with novel experiences that frequently exhaust their usual coping mechanisms. Crisis resolution is a complex process that is affected by appraisal of the event or stressor, available support systems, sociocultural and neurobiological factors, and ego function. Coping mechanisms are both conscious and unconscious and determine how one adapts to environmental demands. The aim of coping is homeostasis or adaptation. Internal and external resources are the basis of adaptation.

Lazarus and Folkman (1984, p. 141) defined coping as

> *constantly changing cognitive and behavioral efforts to manage specific external and/or internal demands that are appraised as taxing or exceeding the resources of the person.*

Additionally, they defined coping as a dynamic process that is mobilized by continuous appraisal and reappraisals of environmental transactions.

Cognitive appraisal underscores the perception of stressful events and threats to one's well-being. Stressful encounters force people to use coping mechanisms to either alter, reduce, or eliminate danger or change its meaning. Successful crisis resolution usually generates positive emotions, whereas unsuccessful or inadequate resolution generates negative responses, such as anger, grief, and helplessness (Zegans, 1983). This premise suggests that there are no universal stressors and that danger and threats are determined by individual perception of situations (Barnard, 1985). The reaction of an adolescent who has lost her home in a hurricane disaster is an example of how people appraise situations. She can perceive the situation as hopeless because her parents were underinsured, or she can see it as a challenge to pull together as a family.

Lazarus and Folkman (1984) delineated three types of appraisal: primary appraisal, secondary appraisal, and reappraisal. (For a discussion of appraisals, see Chapter 7.)

Clinical Example

An example of secondary appraisal of coping options is seen in the adolescent who became angry with his parents after he was grounded for failing a class. He expressed anger to his parents, and he later got into a heated argument with his sister. He shouted and reminded her of a recent breakup with her boyfriend, who is now dating someone else. The boy felt guilty because his sister began to cry. He realized that he was responsible for the argument and for being grounded. He later apologized to his sister and parents for yelling and arguing when he realized that this was not the best way to handle his frustration and anger. His self-esteem had been threatened because of poor grades and being grounded.

Overall, the three forms of appraisal—primary, secondary, and reappraisal—determine the scope of stress and emotional reactions to stressful situations. Cognitive appraisal is an evaluation of the environment, perception of stress, and use of coping mechanisms. Stressful events or crises provide opportunities to improve adaptation and coping skills (Lazarus & Folkman, 1984).

SUPPORT SYSTEMS

Social support is crucial to everyday living, because it affords people a sense of value, security, and self-esteem. Studies show that people with an adequate **support system** develop a sense of well-being and respond more adaptively to stressful events. Furthermore, social networking provides a feedback mechanism that maintains social identity, security, a sense of belonging, and validation (Spaniol & Zipple, 1988; Spaniol et al., 1992; Weidl, 1992). Typically, support systems comprise families and friends, who feel their needs are addressed during crises. Crisis situations can present people with distressful experiences, and families are the most significant resource promoting effective coping mechanisms. Families validate members' feelings and facilitate the mourning process.

In contrast, people with inadequate support systems are more likely to use maladaptive responses during crises. These clients are vulnerable to the deleterious effects of a crisis. In this situation, crisis intervention is useful in assessing client needs, promoting a sense of well-being, reinforcing adaptive coping behaviors, and mobilizing resources through feedback and validation of feelings.

In summary, social support is vital to effective coping. Close, caring relationships provide a protective buffer during crisis situations. Furthermore, social networking fosters a sense of sharing, validates feelings, and provides reassurance and acceptance. People experiencing crises often isolate themselves when they most need to turn to others for support (Cowen, 1982). Isolation or inadequacy of support systems increases the likelihood of deleterious effects of crisis and mental illness. Crisis intervention is a useful strategy that helps clients mobilize resources, enhances support systems, and facilitates the formation of adaptive coping mechanisms.

SOCIOCULTURAL FACTORS

As previously discussed, people normally do not face a crisis alone but within a social network composed of a spouse, family, friend, community, or religious affiliation. Social systems typically comprise common bonds such as values, traditions, and beliefs systems. Close ties afford people resources that support and reinforce adaptive problem-solving skills.

Social systems determine the perception of crisis and one's ability to master it. Social functioning is related to individual roles, relationships, and cultural factors. An example of the impact of sociocultural factors is seen in the family faced with coping with an unmarried pregnant adolescent. One family may perceive this situation as devastating and insist that the daughter consider having an abortion, whereas another family may perceive the same situation as being undesirable but they may decide to keep the child within the family. Each family resolves crisis situations based on its common beliefs, values, and traditions. The outcome really depends on the family members' ability to express feelings and receive support during the crisis.

The concept of coping involves a host of factors, including sociocultural influences (see Chapter 3). Psychiatric–mental health nurses need to assess client needs, incorporating their uniqueness into interventions that facilitate adaptive coping responses to stressful events.

EGO FUNCTION

The ego is the core of the personality, and it modulates the social function of cognition (perceptions), behavior, anxiety, problem solving, and reality testing. Its role in adaptation arises from its ability to mediate between the person and reality through the use of defense mechanisms (internal and external environments). The ego uses defense mechanisms to protect itself against impulses and affects such as guilt, anxiety, and shame. *Ego strength* refers to the ability to modulate these functions in the face of numerous stimuli or stress. The principal goal of ego function is to maintain equilibrium or adaptation (Caplan, 1961).

NEUROBIOLOGICAL FACTORS

Neurobiological responses to emotions or stress are a critical part of coping, stress, and adaptation because they influence all other types of responses to stressful situations. This premise has been well documented by researchers such as Cannon and Selye. Cannon (1914) coined the term *fight-or-flight response*. This response activates physiological processes in the form of anger or fear, arousing the sympathetic nervous system (Brooks, 1987). Cannon studied the role of the adrenal medulla in mediating the biological response generated by strong emotions and pain.

Selye's studies (1946) supported Cannon's theory; he referred to the physical reaction to stress as the *general adaptation syndrome* (Selye, 1946) and, later, *stress response* (Selye, 1956). Both theorists surmised that strong emotions, such as anxiety and fear, activate the release of cortisol from the adrenal cortex.

Selye (1976) also postulated that disorders such as allergies and collagen diseases arise from abnormal or prolonged stress responses. Others supported this notion and linked life events to illness (Holmes & Rahe, 1967; Squire, 1987) (see Chapters 7 and 11).

Stein (1986) noted that four decades have failed to produce evidence to support the premise that prolonged stress destroys any tissues. In fact, recent studies have disputed this premise (Connolly, 1985; Stein, 1986), whereas others contend that stress affects health (e.g., the immune system) and places people at risk for illness (Melnechuk, 1988). Researchers continue to assert that neurobiological and psychosocial factors represent complex nonspecific aspects of stress response and that specific components involve external (control and anticipation) and internal resources (coping mechanisms, perception of stressor).

The neurobiological basis of coping has been linked with the immune response, neurotransmitters, neuroendocrine systems, and genetics. Recent studies have found that a number of neuroendocrine patterns are activated and that there is no normal response to all stress. (These factors are discussed in Chapters 7 and 11.)

Adaptation to stress and healthy outcomes are based on an integration of the appraisal process, available support systems, sociocultural factors, ego function, and neurobiological factors. Assessing coping patterns, reinforcing adaptive responses, and mobilizing resources are critical nursing interventions that facilitate adaptation to crisis situations.

DISASTERS: RESPONSE TO MASSIVE STRESS

Disasters have been described as calamities or adversities that create vast stress. These are stressful events that generate feelings of profound fear, panic, horror, and doom. Disasters disrupt normal patterns of living and force people to respond to crisis situations without the use of their normal coping mechanisms. When entire communities are ravaged, people also lose their roots or frame of reference and their sense of safety, control, and closeness (McCann & Pearlman, 1990).

Disasters occur in varied forms and include both natural and man-made types, war atrocities, childhood abuse, and life-threatening illnesses such as AIDS and cholera.

RESEARCH ON PSYCHOLOGICAL RESPONSES TO DISASTERS

The 1972 flood disaster of Buffalo Creek, West Virginia, left 125 people dead and nearly 5000 homeless. Everyone exposed to this disaster experienced some form of the psychological manifestations of the survivors described by Lifton and Olson (1976). Psychological impact included the following five constellations:

1. *Death imprint* and *death anxiety*—consists of vivid memories and images of the disaster and its destructiveness. People experienced sleeplessness, a fear of crowds, and recurrent nightmares.
2. *Death guilt* (survivor's guilt)—manifests by preoccupation with persistent thoughts of dead relatives or friends. These feelings were frequently part of their nightmares. Survivors often had problems forgiving themselves for surviving.
3. *Psychic numbing*—refers to an impaired capacity to feel, and this was shown by distancing, social withdrawal, aloofness, and limited interpersonal relationships. Survivors of the Buffalo Creek flood exhibited apathy, confusion, and indifference. Numbing is a defense mechanism used to deny or to protect the survivor from confronting or reliving the horrible experience. Biological aspects of numbing are associated with an activation of endorphins that results in "emotional numbing" (Van der Kolk, 1988).
4. *Impaired interpersonal relationships*—refers to the enormous need for survivors to seek love and affection while being unable to accept available resources. Survivors tend to be suspicious of closeness and affection during times that they really need them. Anger and unexpressed rage often emerge, putting more distance in relationships. These responses tend to disperse and increase when survivors fail to adequately externalize rage and anger.
5. *Struggle for significance*—refers to efforts to make sense of almost dying from and then surviving a traumatic experience.

Other disasters stem from war atrocities and traumatic experiences. Several investigators have demonstrated a relationship between the intensity of combat exposure and the evolution of posttraumatic stress disorder (PTSD) (Kuch & Cox, 1992; Yehuda et al., 1992). These studies explored the severity of psychopathology, both PTSD and depression, and level of function in clients exposed to war atrocities and traumatic combat. A number of survivors of the Nazi Holocaust experience symptoms of PTSD and exhibit symptoms similar to those of the Vietnam War veterans (Behar, 1987; Kuch & Cox, 1992) (see Chapter 10).

Historically, studies exploring the meaning of and responses to disasters date back to Lindemann's renowned study of the Coconut Grove fire of 1944. Clinical and empirical research was also generated by the Buffalo Creek flood disaster, which destroyed an entire community (Erikson, 1976). Major findings from these studies suggest that survivors have widespread and persistent personality and behavioral changes, such as maladaptation and bereavement (Green et al., 1985).

FACTORS INFLUENCING RESPONSE TO DISASTERS

Disasters place immense stress on people, families, and communities, taxing resources and compromising adaptive responses. Sarason and Sarason (1984) surmised that the outcome of disasters is influenced by several factors, such as predictability, duration, intensity, locus of control, and state of self-concept.

Predictability. Predictability affects stress reactions, which may be of low or high intensity. It affects the ability of the person and the community to cope or prepare for the disaster.

Duration. Recent examples of disasters are Hurricane Andrew in Florida and Louisiana in 1992 and severe flooding in the midwestern states in 1993. Victims of these disasters lost their homes, property, and sense of well-being. In spite of the destruction of the hurricane and floods, communities were able to deal with their immediate needs by banding together to seek shelter, food, water, and safety. The disasters were forecast in advance, but their intensity and duration were so profound that victims attempted to cope with their losses for an extended period after the disaster had occurred.

Intensity. Intensity or severity varies with the degree of loss, the type of injury, the repertoire of coping mechanisms, and the appraisal of the event.

Locus of Control. The nature of disasters makes it difficult to predict or have control of their impact on the lives of people and communities. Recent disasters of the hurricane and severe flooding left many victims feeling helpless, with little control over recovering their losses or finding temporary food and living quarters. Loss of control frequently generates feelings of powerlessness, helplessness, frustration, and depression.

State of Self-Concept. Impaired self-confidence or low self-esteem results in feelings of inadequacy or ineffectiveness in handling stressful situations. For example, in a natural disaster in which families have lost their homes and possessions, a man may feel that his family relies on him for shelter, food, and safety. The man who feels confident is likely to maintain calm within himself and his family by seeking support from other victims and other community resources. Even though he is unable to locate immediate shelter, his confident response promotes a sense of safety and security in his family. In contrast, the man who is fearful and uncertain about himself and his family members will lack confidence in managing the situation and will not cope as well.

THE NURSE'S ROLE IN DISASTERS AND CRISES

Disasters and crises have a profound and unpredictable effect on people, families, and communities (see Research Study display on p. 142). Nurses are challenged to assess the impact of disaster and crisis on survivors and to recognize both adaptive and maladaptive responses. Survivors show the resilience of the human spirit and survival instinct. Nurses play a major role in mobilizing internal and external resources that facilitate a sense of control and confidence and that reinforce support systems. Restoration and maintenance of health and adaptation are basic to survivors' well-being. Lifton and Olson (1976) suggested that psychological health can be improved in survivors by the following:

- Recognizing their profound agony
- Identifying causes of the disaster or trauma
- Encouraging the desire to live and rebuild
- Educating people about the meaning of disaster and strength as a survivor

Psychiatric triage is often an initial intervention that prioritizes care and enables survivors to receive immediate emotional support through crisis intervention. Crisis intervention is used to mobilize resources by identifying viable options, such as shelter, food, water, and safety, during the early stages of emotional, social, and physical turmoil. Several treatment modalities, such as crisis intervention, family therapy (see Chapter 22), and psychotherapy (see Chapter 21), can facilitate health promotion.

LIFE SPAN ISSUES: MATURATIONAL CRISES

The human experience is stressful. Everyday living presents people with potential crises, and their ability to mobilize internal and external resources determines the impact of stressful encounters. This process begins in utero and continues until death. Life span crises include moving through developmental stages and events such as becoming a parent, getting married, being a victim of violence, and developing a terminal illness.

Erikson's (1963) eight developmental stages (see Table 8–1) represent maturational crises. As previously mentioned, these stages are anticipated and present people with normal disturbances or crises. Each stage challenges people to master specific tasks that are based on successful resolution of previous stages. Erikson described each stage as a crisis state generated by radical changes that provides the potential for growth. Addi-

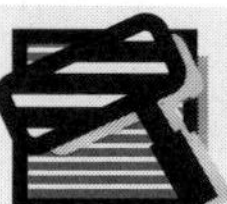

RESEARCH STUDY

Psychosocial Effects of a Catastrophic Botulism Outbreak

Hardin, S. B., & Cohen, F. L. (1988). *Archives of Psychiatric Nursing*, *2*(3), 173–184.

Study Problem/Purpose

A 3-year longitudinal, descriptive study of the psychosocial responses of 22 patients and 51 family members affected by the 1983 Peoria, Illinois, botulism outbreak.

Methods

Repeated-measures descriptive design data were collected over a 3-year period. A team of nurse psychotherapists and medical-surgical clinical specialists conducted home visits and nursing clinics to assess physiological and psychosocial responses. Structured audiotaped and videotaped interviews using crisis intervention principles were employed.

Sample

Twenty-two botulism victims participated in the study, ranging in age from 20 to 73 years, with a mean of 42.4 years.

Findings

Major findings showed that 100 percent of participants and families perceived the botulism attack as a crisis. Additionally, the findings supported the occurrence of anxiety, depression, and long-term anger as major features of psychological consequences of this outbreak.

Implications

Psychiatric nurses can use home visits and community services to understand psychosocial responses to traumatic illnesses such as botulism. Furthermore, crisis intervention can alleviate or minimize the deleterious effects of a crisis and improve client and family coping.

tionally, developmental crises are turning points, manifested by increased vulnerability, and are a source of "generational strength" and maladaptation (Erikson, 1968).

INFANCY: TRUST VERSUS MISTRUST

Erikson (1968) asserted that the most radical change of all begins with the birth experience, as the infant evolves from intrauterine to extrauterine existence. This period represents a crisis not only for the newborn but also for the new parents. Interactions with primary caregivers serve as the basis for the child's emotional and biological well-being.

Bowlby's attachment theory (1969) emphasized the importance of bonding and its effects on the child's sense of trust and validation. The role of primary caregivers in this process involves accessibility and responsiveness to the infant's needs (e.g., nurturance, nutrition, and protection). Bowlby further believed that attachment behaviors or affectional bonds are vital to survival and the ability to form meaningful relationships throughout the life span.

The primary developmental task during this period is trust versus mistrust. Trust emerges as the primary caregivers meet the infant's basic need through consistent, affectionate, and caring environments. Early trusting interactions provide the foundation of personality development and self-concept. (The attentive mother who responds to a crying infant by holding and feeding the infant provides an example of a positive bonding experience. In contrast, the mother who ignores the cries of the infant provides an example of an abusive and neglectful experience.) Bonding enables parents to communicate love, warmth, safety, and validation to the infant. When the infant develops and gains a sense of well-being and trust, anxiety and sadness are generated by the normal separation-individuation process (Erikson, 1963).

In contrast, impaired early affectional bonding compromises healthy parent–child interactions, increasing the likelihood of mistrust. Mistrust usually evolves when the infant is unable to rely on primary caregivers for having his or her basic needs met. Events that affect early bonding process include serious illnesses, socioeconomic concerns, and impaired family interactions. Disturbances in this process contribute to the formation of maladaptive behaviors throughout the life span (Erikson, 1963).

Early interactions with primary caregivers affect how the child adapts to subsequent developmental stages. Newly found mobility and the need for autonomy challenge the child and parents to master the stress of the second stage: autonomy versus shame and doubt.

TODDLER PERIOD: AUTONOMY VERSUS SHAME AND DOUBT

The second year is marked by accelerated motor and intellectual growth. The child experiences a newly found sense of mobility, autonomy, and early speech. The major developmental task is autonomy versus shame and doubt (Erikson, 1963). The toddler develops a sense of mastery over self and impulses. Major sensorimotor developments during this stage are feeding one's self; controlling the anal sphincter (toilet training); tolerating delays; variable reasoning, listening, and concentrating (Piaget, 1952, 1969); and exploring the environment.

Successful resolution and mastery of autonomy and

independence depend on the primary caregivers' parenting skills. Parents who encourage, reward, and set consistent limits regarding acceptable behaviors provide environments that promote autonomy, independence, and self-esteem in the toddler. The toddler continues to separate and individuate from caregivers who support this newly found independence. Parents continue to provide safety and assist with encounters that the child is unable to handle. The child learns that even with newly found freedom, the parents are accessible for emotional "refueling."

In comparison, parents who are overcontrolling, smothering, neglectful, or rejecting provide climates that discourage autonomy and separateness. Feelings of shame and self-doubt arise, laying the foundation for maladaptation manifested by poor self-concept, depression, and self-destructive behaviors in adolescence and adulthood.

PRESCHOOL PERIOD: INITIATIVE VERSUS GUILT

The child with a sense of self-worth and independence has the capacity to initiate motor and intellectual activity. Children who are 3 to 5 years old begin to play with peers and interact with others. An understanding of right or wrong (moral sense or superego) evolves during this stage. The child who successfully resolves the task of initiative is conscientious and dependable and exhibits some self-discipline. These attributes emerge as part of the child's personality.

The child who fails to develop a sense of trust often feels shame and experiences doubt about himself or herself. Impaired self-esteem interferes with the confidence needed to endure independence and initiative. As a result, guilt and feelings of inadequacy arise as symptoms of unsuccessful resolution of this developmental stage.

MIDDLE CHILDHOOD: INDUSTRY VERSUS INFERIORITY

Entering school is a crisis for the youngster and family. School places customary demands for academic performance associated with learning and proficiency. Additionally, school provides socialization that involves dealing with acceptance, criticism, authority figures, and effective working with others. The child with a positive self-concept is challenged by these demands, participates in traditional learning, and masters and fulfills goals. Active parental participation in school and home endeavors plays a critical role in enhancing the child's well-being and self-esteem.

Furthermore, physical and cognitive development enable the child to perform complex motor tasks such as ballet, gymnastics, and soccer. Concrete thought processes become more organized and logical (Piaget, 1969). Successful resolution of industry permits the child to actively share and interact with others while experiencing a sense of companionship.

In contrast, children with a negative self-concept who feel socially alienated may find school overwhelming. These children tend to feel lonely, depressed, or extremely anxious. These responses often reflect impaired family–child relationships that are overprotective, indifferent, or rejecting.

ADOLESCENCE: IDENTITY VERSUS ROLE CONFUSION

Adolescence is a critical stage of development in that it represents a time of turmoil that places the youth at risk for crisis. Kaplan (1984) described adolescence as "an inner emotional upheaval, a struggle between the eternal human wish to cling to the past and the equally powerful wish to get on with the future" (p. 19). Erikson (1968) noted that the pressures of adolescence are associated with the "final stage of identity formation" and that the youth is "apt to suffer more deeply" (p. 163) than at any previous stage or any stage thereafter. Resolution of this developmental crisis is built on successful resolution of previous stages. The major developmental task of adolescence is identity versus role confusion (Erikson, 1963).

Early Adolescence

Early adolescence challenges the youth to master drastic role changes precipitated by tremendous neurobiological and psychosocial demands. Neurobiological demands are activated by endocrine changes connected with maturation of the cells of the hypothalamus and stimulation of gonadal hormones. These endocrine changes affect the mood and behavior of the adolescent and produce the major physical changes of secondary sex characteristics (Hamburg, 1974).

Psychosocial demands include negotiating the transition from elementary school to middle school. Academic demand is clearly increased, with an emphasis on achievement. Biological and psychosocial demands or puberty changes affect the adolescent's self-image, contributing to fears of insecurity and failure.

Early adolescence also represents a period when peers are important because they facilitate the process of separating from parents (Mishne, 1986). Parents continue to play vital roles in the adolescent's life, but separation from them increases **cathexis** (concentration of psychic energy on self) (Mishne, 1986). Parent–child relationships validate the youth through emotional support and acceptance. Parental coalitions also buffer the youth against negative feelings, behaviors, and choices. Furthermore, parents are challenged to deal with the youth's mood swings and defiance against them. Adolescents can benefit from healthy parental alliances that respond to these behaviors with love, understanding, and consistent limit setting. Healthy and predictable parental behaviors are critical to successful resolution of crisis during adolescence. Family turmoil, marital discord, or divorce can be devastating to adolescents (Mishne, 1986).

Middle Adolescence

Middle adolescence finds the youth constantly seeking and forming new relationships apart from the family to displace early close family ties (Blos, 1962). Additionally, this stage denotes maturation of sexual identity. Self-absorption and self-awareness impart self-reliance and separateness from significant others, which are the basis of identity. Adolescents attempt to individuate in terms of sexual changes and societal demands as adults. Heterosexual relationships become important and lay the foundation for dealing with the challenges of early adulthood.

Adolescent confusion frequently arises from struggles with independence versus dependence, separation issues, and gaining a sense of who one is. The term *identity* is used to describe the ability to experience one's uniqueness and relevance. Successful resolution of this task is confirmed during subsequent developmental stages.

Late Adolescence

Integration of the personality to promote stable work and intimate relationships and a personal value system are aspects of crisis resolution in late adolescence. The older adolescent often experiences a sense of mourning coupled with depression or anxiety connected with acceptance of his or her limitations and inadequacies (Erikson, 1963; Mishne, 1986).

The adolescent who unsuccessfully resolves the crisis of this state develops role confusion. This person is unable to form an adult identity and has difficulty responding to societal expectations. This adolescent has failed to resolve crises related to trust, autonomy, initiative, and industry, which are the foundation of identity. Families that lack empathy or consistency and predictable limit setting produce chaotic environments that increase vulnerability to maladaptive responses in their members.

EARLY ADULTHOOD: INTIMACY VERSUS ISOLATION

The young adult comes of age representing another generation in a family system. The ability to define an identity of self and form intense interpersonal relationships provides the basis of this developmental crisis. *Identity* in this life stage refers to the capacity to make adult decisions and manage adult stress. Resolution of previous developmental crises prepares the young adult to embark on the path of defining his or her place in society. The crisis of this stage is intimacy versus isolation (Erikson, 1963).

Intimacy refers to the capacity to form close, meaningful relationships with others and to clarify one's sexuality. Basic qualities of intimacy are a proficiency in the sharing of feelings, mutual understanding, commitment, responsibility, and love. Erikson (1968) defined love as the most vital human quality and the basis of trust and successful resolution of all developmental tasks.

A lack of love or validation by early caregivers interferes with the capacity to form close, warm, intimate relationships. The young adult with this experience is often distrustful or interacts with others superficially. Moreover, this person has a heightened sense of self-absorption that interferes with self-awareness that is gained through feedback and perceptions from others (Erikson, 1963). The withdrawn and isolated person is likely to use maladaptive responses to cope with crisis situations.

Endeavors that facilitate resolution of this stage include the pursuit of career and jobs and the formation of meaningful relationships. Career and jobs are pursued through higher academic institutions or technical or other training programs. Proficient social skills are essential aspects of this process that help young adults make realistic adult decisions.

Marrying or forming other long-term relationships affects sexuality, fidelity, and loyalty, which impact the capacity to master shared identity or intimacy. Intimate relationships and careers lay the foundation for future crises and resolution of developmental tasks. An inability to establish intimacy interferes with self-understanding and self-actualization. Parenthood ushers in a new generation and enhances further growth and maturity in the young adult.

MIDDLE ADULTHOOD: GENERATIVITY VERSUS STAGNATION

The developmental crisis for middle adulthood is generativity versus stagnation. Generativity is concerned with "establishing and guiding" (Erikson, 1968, p. 138), enhancing productivity and creativity, and contributing to the next generation. Bearing and raising children, establishing pastimes outside the family, and sustaining meaningful relationships are examples of generativity. Generativity arises from the need to promote continuity and a heritage for subsequent generations. Caring for others and one's self is the basis of this developmental task. People begin to look over their lives and examine family, community, and social accomplishments and contributions.

Successful resolution of this challenge arises from adaptive responses to previous developmental crises. Various crises affect the middle-aged adult, including divorce, empty nest syndrome, biological changes related to aging and menopause, major medical illnesses, and retirement. Factors such as a positive self-concept and the capacity to form meaningful relationships promote effective resolution of this developmental crisis.

In contrast, people concerned about themselves rather than others are less likely to function interdependently. They tend to experience boredom and a sense of emptiness and lack the capacity to contribute to subsequent generations. A sense of stagnation compromises the ability to feel needed or loved. Self-absorption and increased isolation pose threats to self-concept and create a vulnerability to maladaptation.

LATE ADULTHOOD: INTEGRITY VERSUS DESPAIR

The final developmental crisis is integrity versus despair (Erikson, 1963). Successful resolution of this crisis, as in other stages, depends on a sense of trust, autonomy, initiative, industry, identity, intimacy, and generativity. Each generation is responsible for maintaining wisdom and mature judgment. The members sustain and share the integrity of experience while fostering the needs of the next generation. Vigor, productivity, and stamina wane with aging, but the gifts of wisdom and knowledge provide the new generation with a sense of closure, connectedness, and appreciation of life.

Integrity refers to soundness and completeness. It fosters a sense of wholeness and acceptance that minimizes the despair and disgust of completing the life cycle and experiencing a sense of powerlessness generated by the prospect of death. The person who unsuccessfully resolves this crisis often feels life has been too short and finds it difficult to accept psychosocial and biological changes. Death is not perceived as life's finite boundary (Erikson, 1968).

In summary, Erikson (1963) delineated developmental tasks in terms of the whole life cycle process, including the sequence of generations and interactions with society. Developmental stage or maturational crises are anticipated, and predictable responses evolve throughout the life cycle; each stage lays the foundation for subsequent adaptation. Factors such as the characteristics of early caregivers, sociocultural considerations, and neurobiology play major roles in the formation of self-concept and the capacity to adapt to crises. Crisis situations provide opportunities to form adaptive coping behaviors and to promote growth

THE NURSE'S ROLE IN CRISIS INTERVENTION

Crisis intervention is an effective treatment modality that facilitates adaptation and health restoration. Psychiatric–mental health nurses can use crisis intervention in all clinical settings in which clients experience distress or crises. Client situations may range from disasters, such as a hurricane, to the developmental-related task of parenthood. The primary goal of the generalist psychiatric–mental health nurse in crisis intervention is to collaborate with other members of the crisis team to resolve the immediate crisis or emergency. The generalist uses interventions that foster health, enhance coping skills, and decrease disability (American Nurses Association, 1994).

In comparison, the advanced-practice nurse incorporates basic crisis intervention techniques with various other approaches, such as psychotherapy and prescriptive authority, to strengthen coping skills and minimize the deleterious effects of crisis. Additionally, the advanced-practice nurse provides direct and independent clinical care to assess and manage complex client problems.

FAMILIES IN CRISIS

The present socioeconomic climate of this country places people and families at risk for crises. Tremendous stress on families stems from responses to psychosocial factors such as deterioration of family systems, variable employment rates, and violence. Other societal stressors include an epidemic of sexually transmitted diseases and AIDS, an increasing incidence of substance misuse, and a soaring rate of teenage pregnancies.

Families seeking help are often referred for treatment after a member exhibits symptoms of self-destructive behavior, such as attempting suicide and running away from home. A crisis occurs when people or families encounter stressful situations and normal coping mechanisms fail to resolve the disruption (Caplan, 1964). Additionally, families in crisis experience impaired or ineffectual interactional patterns that generate disruptive coping responses.

What factors determine how families handle crisis situations? Caplan (1961) described the following five interpersonal requisites for the maintenance of well-being or health in individuals and families:

1. *Love* (unconditional)—the need to love and be loved
2. *Support*—related to the need to "depend" on others
3. *Impulse control*—psychological and biological control of gratification of needs
4. *Feeling part of a group*—a sense of security, belonging, and identity
5. *Personal achievement and recognition* (culturally determined)—the need to feel content about personal accomplishments and validation

Families who integrate these attributes provide environments that foster trust, independence, initiative, and industry. Each crisis challenges children and families to use previously successful and resourceful coping behaviors to grow and sustain their health and well-being.

Healthy families take care of the needs of their members and support each other during crises (Caplan, 1964). Additional adaptive qualities of healthy families include strong parental leadership qualities, effective communication patterns, clear boundaries and roles, and flexibility. Healthy family interactions facilitate the formation of close, meaningful relationships within and outside of the family system. Family activities are directed toward helping members master problems rather than avoiding or restricting activities to relieve tension. Specific behaviors, such as the child who easily expresses feelings and relates to others effectively, often mirror the parents' sense of well-being and health.

In comparison, unhealthy families fail to integrate Caplan's attributes and create climates of inconsistency in leadership, sometimes placing children in adult roles during crises. These families also tend to use impaired communication patterns and unclear, blurred, or rigid boundaries and roles. Children are often scapegoated and experience various forms of abuse. Children and adolescents exhibiting maladaptive behaviors such as substance abuse, depression, and suicide attempts must be assessed as soon as possible to reduce the deleterious effects of stressful events. Maladaptive behaviors in the young often arise from chaotic family systems and reflect inner feelings of helplessness, low self-esteem, and frustration.

Family responses to crisis situations are time limited and increase responsiveness to external influences to facilitate adaptive responses. Theories on crisis intervention with families surmise that the family is the core of the crisis and that it has the greatest influence on maintaining or resolving the situation. Crisis intervention needs to focus on the child's behavior as a symptom of family disruption (Caplan, 1961).

The Nursing Process: Crisis Intervention

The following case history points out areas that must be assessed and addressed when a family presents with a crisis.

Case Study: The Family Experiencing a Crisis

Ten-year-old Johnny was seen in the emergency department (ED) after he sustained several dog bites from the neighbor's pet. Johnny was quiet and withdrawn. He refused to discuss the incident and stated that he wished he were dead. His mother was disturbed by his statement. She informed the nurse that her son had been behaving differently for several months (he had begun to sleep in class, and his grades had been falling the past 6 weeks) and that she was concerned about his safety. Additionally, she commented that she was unsure if the child let the dog bite him on purpose. Later, Johnny's father came to the ED after parking the car, and his mother discussed her concerns with the father. The child and his parents were referred to the psychiatric liaison consultant nurse for evaluation and crisis intervention. The nurse discovered that the family had been experiencing major financial problems since the father was laid off his $100,000-a-year job. He had been unable to find gainful employment over the past 6 months. He is a 49-year-old aerospace engineer who feels pessimistic about finding a comparably paying job because of his age and reduced government spending on defense. He and Johnny's mother admitted that this had been devastating to the family, particularly since they have two older children in college. They also admitted that they had been ignoring their 10-year-old son. Other family stressors included the parents' concerns about maintaining their current lifestyle and frequent arguments that have created a distance in their relationship. Johnny stated that he feels responsible for the family problems and that he cries a lot during the night. Furthermore, he is frightened by the arguments between his parents, and he feels that no one cares about him.

How can this family be helped? Crisis intervention is a useful strategy in which parents and children can find relief from overwhelming circumstances such as those in the case study. It is a mechanism that furnishes immediate emotional support, feedback, and clarification of incongruencies.

Family crises usually occur when a couple's usual coping and problem-solving skills fail to adapt to major lifestyle changes. Langsley and Kaplan (1968) pointed out that family crisis intervention has several advantages. It enhances self-awareness, clarifies the roles of members in sustaining it, develops fresh coping skills, and provides the family with a sense of competency to manage the situation. Some families may benefit from family therapy (see Chapter 22 for an in-depth discussion of family therapy).

Assessment

The assessment process begins with establishing rapport and assessing members with a here-and-now and present crisis to determine present stressors and reasons for seeking treatment at this time. The following questions are useful in eliciting information regarding the nature of the family crisis:

- What specific event or circumstances brought you in today?
- How did this occur?
- How has the family dealt with it?
- What has made it difficult for you to deal with it at this time?

Inquiring about present and past coping patterns provides invaluable information about the family's level of function, communication patterns, developmental stage, and problem-solving skills. When there is a high risk for injury, levels of danger must be assessed and dealt with immediately. In the case of Johnny, it is imperative to resolve the following questions:

- How long has he had thoughts of dying?
- What does dying mean to him?
- What has stopped him from acting on his thoughts?
- Does he have a plan or the means to kill himself?
- Has he made attempts in the past?

Additionally, Johnny's parents must be assessed for potential for injury to themselves or others, including their present and past behaviors.

Nursing Diagnoses

The major nursing diagnoses of family crisis are

- Ineffective Family Coping: Disabling
- Anxiety
- Altered Family Processes

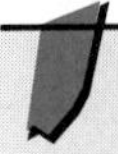

Nursing Care Plan 8–1 The Family Experiencing a Crisis Situation (Johnny, Mother, Father)

OUTCOME IDENTIFICATION	NURSING ACTIONS	RATIONALES	EVALUATION
► Nursing Diagnosis: Ineffective Family Coping, Disabling			
1. By [date], family will identify realistic perception of stressors or crisis.	1a. Assist family in identifying precipitating event.	1a. Identifying precipitating event facilitates identification of the problem (crisis situation).	*Goal met:* Family members are able to identify recent changes or stressors.
	1b. Explore and assess meaning of major lifestyle change or stressor.	1b. Assessing the meaning of lifestyle changes and stress helps the family gain insight into the present crisis.	
2. By [date], family will develop adaptive coping patterns.	2. Assess family's current and past coping skills.	2. Assessing the family's past coping skills assists in identifying the present level of functioning and coping skills.	
► Nursing Diagnosis: Anxiety			
1. By [date], family will learn how to decrease anxiety effectively.	1a. Assess level of anxiety.	1a. Family gains an understanding of present level of anxiety.	*Goal met:* Family gains an understanding of ineffective problem solving. Anxiety is reduced by effective communication skills.
	1b. Teach members adaptive stress-reducing measures.	1b–d. Problem solving mobilizes resources and reduces stress and decreased feelings of helplessness.	
	1c. Encourage problem solving.		
	1d. Confront self-defeating behaviors.		
	1e. Teach effective communication skills.	1e. Effective communication of feelings promotes understanding and insight into the family's response to stress.	
► Nursing Diagnosis: Altered Family Processes			
1. By [date], family will express and share their feelings regarding present crisis.	1. Encourage sharing of feelings.	1. Sharing feelings allows members to support each other and to clarify the crisis situation.	*Goal met:* Family develops effective coping skills and resolves crisis effectively.
2. By [date], family will maintain functional system.	2a. Identify the family's strengths and weakness.	2a–c. Identifying strengths and options and reorganizing roles decrease feelings of powerlessness and problem areas.	
	2b. Provide and offer the family options and resources.		
	2c. Assist the family in reorganizing their roles around decisive concerns.		

The family is at least temporarily unable to mobilize adequate resources and effective problem solving to resolve a crisis situation.

Planning

Nursing Care Plan 8–1 identifies the desired outcomes for the nursing diagnoses listed earlier and delineates the nursing actions needed to achieve these outcomes, along with the rationales for these actions.

Implementation

Nursing interventions are based on the assumption that a family crisis is time limited and susceptible to adaptive changes. This process begins when the nurse suggests several options for handling the crisis. The nurse–client relationship is used to focus on the reasons for the present crisis, to identify recent coping responses and strengths, and to explore ways to reduce the symptoms and the distress. Encouraging family participation reduces their feelings of helplessness and encourages problem solving.

Evaluation

In this case study, it is important for Johnny's parents to take charge of the present situation by providing safety for the child. Their concerns for his safety and their willingness to seek help promote a sense of security in the child—children often feel frightened and confused when sudden life changes occur. Johnny's parents also had difficulty handling their fears and uncertainty about the situation, and this heightened his feelings of helplessness. Johnny's expression of wanting to die symbolized these feelings. In consultation with the nurse, the parents expressed their feelings and identified the reasons for the present crisis. This discussion clarified and dispelled the notion that the child was responsible for his parents' present crisis. His parents were encouraged to tell the child how important he was and to spend quality time with him.

►CHAPTER SUMMARY

A crisis is a turning point that stems from an imbalance between a stressful event and an inability to mobilize resources to adapt to it. A period of disorganization often ensues, providing an opportunity for the formation of improved coping skills and potential growth. Ideally, people emerge from a crisis situation at a precrisis or higher level of functioning.

Caplan's and Lindemann's contributions to the crisis theory and crisis management have prevailed for almost half a century, providing nurses with a practical and effective approach to helping clients in crises. Crisis intervention mobilizes internal and external resources that promote adaptive coping responses.

Suggestions for Clinical Conferences

1. Invite a psychiatric–mental health clinical specialist to discuss general principles associated with crisis intervention in a psychiatric triage emergency unit.
2. Present several disaster scenarios, and encourage students to role play using crisis intervention.
3. Present case histories of clients experiencing grief reactions, and assess normal and abnormal behaviors.
4. Discuss attitudes of students regarding death and dying.

References

Aguilera, D. C. (1990). *Crisis intervention: Theory and methodology* (6th ed.). St. Louis: C. V. Mosby.

Aguilera, D. C. (1994). *Crisis intervention: Theory and methodology* (7th ed.). St. Louis: Mosby-Year Book.

Aquilera, D. C. & Messick, J. M. (1978). *Crisis intervention: Theory and methodology* (3rd ed.). St. Louis: C. V. Mosby.

American Nurses Association (1994). *A statement on psychiatric–mental health clinical nursing practice and standards of psychiatric–mental health clinical nursing practice.* Washington, DC: Author.

American Psychiatric Association. (1994). *Diagnostic and statistical manual of mental disorders* (4th ed.). Washington, DC: Author

Andrews, H., & Roy, C., Sr. (1986). *Essentials of the Roy adaptation model.* Norwalk, CT: Appleton-Century-Crofts.

Barnard, D. (1985). Psychosomatic medicine and the problem of meaning. *Bulletin of the Menninger Clinic, 29*, 10–28.

Behar, D. (1987). Flashbacks and posttraumatic stress symptoms in combat veterans. *Comprehensive Psychiatry, 28*, 459–466.

Blos, P. (1962). *On adolescence.* New York: Free Press.

Bowlby, J. (1969). *Attachment and loss: Vol. 1. Attachment.* New York: Basic Books.

Brooks, C. M. (1987). Autonomic nervous system: Nature and functional role. In G. Adelman (Ed.), *Encyclopedia of neuroscience* (Vol. 2, pp. 96–98). Boston: Birkhaeuser.

Cannon, W. B. (1914). The function of the adrenal medulla. *American Journal of Physiology, 33*(3), 356–377.

Caplan, G. (1961). *An approach to community mental health.* New York: Grune & Stratton.

Caplan, G. (1964). *Principles of preventive psychiatry.* New York: Basic Books.

Connolly, J. (1985). Life happenings and organic disease. *British Journal of Hospital Medicine, 33*, 24–27.

Cowen, E. L. (1982). Help is where you find it: Four helping groups. *American Psychologist, 37*, 385–395.

Davanloo, H. (1978). *Basic principles and techniques of short-term psychotherapy.* New York: Spectrum Publications.

Erikson, E. (1963). *Childhood and society* (rev. ed.). New York: W. W. Norton.

Erikson, E. (1964). *Insight and responsibility.* New York: W. W. Norton.

Erikson, E. (1968). *Identity: Youth and crisis.* New York: W. W. Norton.

Erikson, K. T. (1976). Loss of community at Buffalo Creek. *American Journal of Psychiatry, 133*(3), 302–325.

Freud, S. (1961). The ego and the id. In J. Strachey (Ed. and Trans.). *The standard edition of the complete psychological works of Sigmund Freud* (Vol. 19, pp. 3–66). London: Hogarth Press. (Original work published 1923)

Green, B. L., Grace, M. C., & Gleser, G. C. (1985). Identifying survivors at risk: Long-term impairment following the Beverly Hills Supper Club fire. *Journal of Consulting and Clinical Psychology, 53*(5), 672–678.

Hamburg, B. (1974). Early adolescence: A specific and stressful stage of the life cycle. In I. G. Coelho, D. Hambury, & J. Adams (Eds.), *Coping and adaptation* (pp. 101–124). New York: Basic Books.

Hardin, S. B., & Cohen, F. L. (1988). Psychosocial effects of a catastrophic botulism outbreak. *Archives of Psychiatric Nursing, 2*(2), 173–184.

Hinkle, L. E. (1977). The concept of stress in the biological and social sciences. In Z. J. Lipowski, D. C. Lipsitt, & P. C Whybron (Eds.), *Psychosomatic medicine: Current trends and clinical applications* (p. 27). New York: Oxford Press.

Hoff, L. A. (1989). *People in crisis* (3rd ed.). Redding, MA: Addison-Wesley.

Holmes, T. H., & Rahe, R. H. (1967). The social readjustment rating scale. *Journal of Psychosomatic Research, 11,* 213–218.

Joint Commission on Mental Health and Mental Illness. (1961). *Action for mental health science edition.* New York: Basic Books.

Kaplan, L. J. (1984). *Adolescence: The farewell to childhood.* New York: Simon & Schuster.

Kuch, K., & Cox, B. J. (1992). Symptoms of PTSD in 124 survivors of the Holocaust. *American Journal of Psychiatry, 149*(3), 337–340.

Langsley, D., & Kaplan, D. (1968). *Treatment of families in crisis.* New York: Grune & Stratton.

Lazarus, R. S. (1966). *Psychological stress and the coping process.* New York: McGraw-Hill.

Lazarus, R. S., & Folkman, R. (1984). *Stress, appraisal, and coping.* New York: Springer Publications.

Lifton, R. J. (1968). *Death in life.* New York: Random House.

Lifton, R. J., & Olson, E. (1976). The human meaning of total disaster: The Buffalo Creek experience. *Psychiatry, 39*(1), 1–18.

Lindemann, E. (1944). Symptomatology and management of acute grief. *American Journal of Psychiatry, 101,* 141–148.

Lindemann, E. (1979). *Beyond grief: Studies in crisis intervention.* New York: Jason Aronson.

McCann, I. J., & Pearlman, L. A. (1990). *Psychological trauma and the adult survivor.* New York: Brunner/Mazel.

McGee, R. K. (1974). *Crisis intervention in the community.* Baltimore: University Park Press.

Melnechuk, T. (1988). Emotions, brain, and immunity and health: A review. In M. Clynes & J. Panksepp (Eds.), *Emotions and psychopathology* (pp. 181–247). New York: Plenum Press.

Mishne, J. M. (1986). *Clinical work with adolescents.* New York: Free Press.

Parad, H. J., & Caplan, G. (1965). Framework for studying families in crisis. In H. J. Parad (Ed.), *Crisis intervention: Selected readings* (pp. 53–72). New York: Family Service Association of America.

Pasnau, R. O., & Fawzy, F. I. (1989). Stress and psychiatry. In H. I. Kaplan & B. J. Sadock (Eds.), *Comprehensive textbook of psychiatry* (Vol. 2, 5th ed., pp. 1231–1239). Baltimore: Williams & Wilkins.

Piaget, J. (1952). *The origins of intelligence in children.* New York: International Universities Press.

Piaget, J. (1969). *The early growth of logic in the child.* New York: W. W. Norton.

Rapoport, L. (1965). The state of crisis: Some theoretical considerations. In H. J. Parad (Ed.), *Crisis intervention: Selected readings* (pp. 22–31). New York: Family Service Association of America.

Roy, C., Sr., & Andrews, H. (1991). *The Roy adaptation model: The definitive statement.* Norwalk, CT: Appleton-Century-Crofts.

Sarason, I. G., & Sarason, B. (1984). *Abnormal psychology* (4th ed.). Englewood Cliffs, NJ: Prentice-Hall.

Selye, H. (1946). The general adaptation syndrome and the diseases of adaptation. *Journal of Clinical Endocrinology, 6,* 117–196.

Selye, H. (1956). *The stress of life.* New York: McGraw-Hill.

Selye, H. (1976). *The stress of life* (rev. ed.). New York: McGraw-Hill.

Spaniol, L., & Zipple, A. M. (1988). Families and professional perceptions of family needs and coping strengths. *Rehabilitative Psychology, 33,* 37–45.

Spaniol, L., Zipple, A. M., & Lockwood, D. (1992). The role of family in psychiatric rehabilitation. *Schizophrenia Bulletin, 18*(3), 341–348.

Squire, L. R. (1987). *Memory and the brain.* New York: Oxford Press.

Stein, M. (1986). A reconsideration of specificity in psychosomatic medicine: From olfaction to the lymphocyte. *Psychosomatic Medicine, 48*(1/2), 3–22.

Weidl, K. H. (1992). Assessment of coping with schizophrenia: Stressors, appraisals, and coping behaviors. *British Journal of Psychiatry, 161*(Suppl. 518), 114–122.

Weiner, H. (1985). The concept of stress in light of studies on disasters, unemployment, and loss: A critical analysis. In M. R. Zales (Ed.), *Stress in health and disease* (pp. 24–94). New York: Brunner/Mazel.

van der Kolk, B. A. (1988). The biological response to psyche pain. In F. M. Ochberg (Ed.), *Post-traumatic therapy and victims of violence* (pp. 25–38). New York: Brunner/Mazel.

Yehuda, R., Southwick, S. M., & Giller, E. L., Jr. (1992). Exposure to atrocities and severity of chronic posttraumatic stress disorder in Vietnam combat veterans. *American Journal of Psychiatry, 149*(3), 333–336.

Zegans, L. S. (1983). Emotions in health and illness: An attempt at integration. In L. Temoshok, C. Van Dyke, & L. S. Zegans (Eds.), *Emotions in health and illness* (pp. 235–256). New York: Grune & Stratton.

Unit 1 Study Questions

See Appendix I for answers.

CHAPTER 1

1. During the early ages, insanity was associated with which of the following?
   a. The plight of the poor.
   b. Demonic possession and sin.
   c. High curability rate.
   d. Heredity.

2. Historically, treatment for the mentally ill was
   a. Inhumane and brutal.
   b. Sensitive and humane.
   c. Administered by concerned citizens.
   d. Administered by people who were not family members.

3. In the Middle Ages, "bedlam" referred to
   a. A clean and safe haven.
   b. The first mental asylum.
   c. A refuge of tranquility.
   d. A poorhouse.

4. Hildegard Peplau's major contributions to psychiatric–mental health nursing include all of the following *except*
   a. The book *Interpersonal Relations in Nursing*.
   b. A theory of nursing based on interpersonal concepts from Harry Stack Sullivan.
   c. Integration of earlier psychiatric nursing concepts.
   d. Promotion of healthy adaptation to stress.

5. The "father" of American psychiatry is
   a. Clifford Beers.
   b. Sigmund Freud.
   c. Benjamin Rush.
   d. William Tuke.

CHAPTER 2

1. The structure of personality that maintains reality orientation and mediates conflict is the
   a. Id.
   b. Ego.
   c. Eros.
   d. Superego.

2. According to psychoanalytical theory, the personality's first line of defense to keep unwanted thoughts out of awareness is
   a. Sublimation.
   b. Anxiety.
   c. Suppression.
   d. Repression.

3. According to psychoanalytical theory, problems of excessive orderliness and neatness arise in which of the following developmental stages?
   a. Oral.
   b. Anal.
   c. Phallic.
   d. Genital.

4. Carl Jung termed the public personality, or the aspects of the self that one reveals to others, the
   a. Persona.
   b. Anima.
   c. Animus.
   d. Shadow.

5. The concept of "good-me," "bad-me," "not-me" was explicated by which of the following theorists?
   a. Freud.
   b. Horney.
   c. Sullivan.
   d. Adler.

6. Reinforcement occurs before the response in which of the following behavioral theories?
   a. Operant conditioning.
   b. Classic conditioning.
   c. Modeling.
   d. Respondent conditioning.

7. The concept from cognitive theory that refers to applying a rule, drawn from one or more isolated incidents, across the board to unrelated situations is
   a. Arbitrary inference.
   b. Selective abstraction.
   c. Overgeneralization.
   d. Personalization.

8. Distorting the significance of an event is
   a. Magnification.
   b. Dichotomous thinking.
   c. Selective abstraction.
   d. Overgeneralization.

9. The theorist who defined nursing as a significant, therapeutic, interpersonal process is
   a. Roy.
   b. Neuman.
   c. Orem.
   d. Peplau.

10. Attributing one's own unacknowledged thoughts and feelings to others is
    a. Intellectualization.
    b. Displacement.
    c. Denial.
    d. Projection.

11. Which of the following did Vaillant call a mature defense?
    a. Sublimation.
    b. Denial.
    c. Repression.
    d. Reaction formation.

CHAPTER 3

1. The fact that psychiatric symptoms are perceived, evaluated, and acted on differently by people from different cultures is the result of
   a. Cultural conditioning.
   b. Illness behavior.
   c. Cultural patterns.
   d. Ethnic behavior.

2. Groups of symptoms that indicate a specific illness in non-Western cultures but are not found in Western cultures are
   a. Culture-bound disorders.
   b. Psychosomatic disorders.
   c. Idiopathic disorders.
   d. Somatic disorders.

3. Psychiatric nurses who are unclear about their own values and beliefs tend to be
   a. Assertive.
   b. Inconsistent.
   c. Apathetic.
   d. Reliable.

4. Second- and third-generation Asian Americans may experience stress-engendered conflict between
   a. Yin and yang.
   b. Extended family and nuclear family.
   c. Ethnic ideology and American ideology.
   d. None of the above.

5. An adaptive response of some clients from non-Western cultures is
   a. Extended future perspective.
   b. Fatalistic perspective.
   c. Individualism.
   d. Egalitarianism.

CHAPTER 4

1. S. J. is admitted to the hospital for detoxification. For the past 3 years, she has used 2 mg of alprazolam (Xanax) three times a day for treatment of panic attacks. She is tired of taking the medication, but she is afraid that if she discontinues it she will have a grand mal seizure. What type of prevention is needed in this situation?
   a. Primary.
   b. Secondary.
   c. Tertiary.
   d. All of the above.

2. Case management is
   a. A new approach in psychiatric–mental health nursing.
   b. A comprehensive and outcome-directed approach.
   c. Advanced education preparation.
   d. A fragmented approach to health care.

3. During morning report, the social worker criticizes the night nurse because the client complained of receiving his pill late. The most effective way for the nurse to deal with this situation is to
   a. Tell the social worker she is out of line.
   b. Leave morning report and look at the medication record.
   c. Talk to the social worker after morning report.
   d. Express anger over the social worker's criticism.

4. The chief role of the mental health team is to
   a. Provide continuous and comprehensive care.
   b. Reduce conflict between various disciplines.
   c. Help clients understand the role of mental health professionals.
   d. Provide a forum for health care providers.

5. Psychiatric–mental health nurses have a unique role in helping clients in distress. This process is facilitated by
   a. The therapeutic use of self.
   b. Self-disclosure.
   c. Effective use of sympathy.
   d. Explaining the meaning of maladaptive behavior.

CHAPTER 5

1. J. B. is a 21-year-old bank teller who is admitted to the hospital with major depression. He refuses to take his medication and states he has a right to make his own decisions. After analyzing the issues, S. S., R.N., believes that the client has the right to refuse treatment in this instance. On which ethical principle is S. S. basing her decision?
   a. Beneficence.
   b. Autonomy.
   c. Justice.
   d. Fidelity.

2. Under what circumstances would S. S., R.N., have the right to force J. B. to take his medication against his will?
   a. If J. B.'s physician states, "If he doesn't take his medication I will discharge him, and I expect you to get him to take his medication."
   b. If J. B. is constantly asking for attention from S. S., R.N., and is irritating her.
   c. If J. B. is actively attempting suicide.
   d. If J. B. is taking up too much staff time and it is difficult to attend adequately to other clients.

3. If J. B. asks to be discharged, the health care team's decision will be based on
   a. Whether the insurance company will support payment of further treatment.
   b. Whether J. B. is smiling and appears energized.
   c. Whether J. B.'s family says they will take responsibility.
   d. Whether J. B. is an imminent danger to himself or others.

4. J. B. states that he has homicidal thoughts toward his wife. When assessing for serious intent to harm others, S. S., R.N., considers which of the following factors the most significant indicator of likelihood of harm?

a. J. B. has a history of violence with a definite plan and a resource to carry out the plan.
b. He sees many people who might irritate him in his work as a bank teller.
c. He gets angry driving home in rush-hour traffic.
d. J. B.'s wife nags him and is unsupportive of his treatment.

5. J. B. asks S. S., R.N., to keep a secret and states that he was only angry when he said he wanted to kill his wife and doesn't really want to do so. He also says that his wife is filing for divorce and he doesn't want her to learn of his homicidal statements in court. What should S. S., R.N., do?
a. Realize that J. B. was just blowing off steam and that documenting his homicidal statement could harm him.
b. Tell staff of the homicidal statement only by word of mouth and not document it in the medical record.
c. Document facts and observations without including her opinion.
d. Realize that J. B. is developing trust in her, because he is able to share his personal secrets.

CHAPTER 6

1. R. L. is paranoid and suspicious. Which of the following techniques should be avoided?
a. Direct eye contact.
b. Silence.
c. Therapeutic touch.
d. Encouragement of expression of feelings.

2. R. L. begins to pace and clench his fist. What should the nurse do in this instance?
a. Leave the room.
b. Offer an injection of haloperidol (Haldol).
c. Explore the meaning of the behavior.
d. Call security services.

3. The major purpose of the process recording is to
a. Evaluate the client's responses.
b. Evaluate the nurse's response.
c. Evaluate the nurse–client interaction.
d. Evaluate the client's verbal cues.

4. Which of the following statements reflects self-awareness?
a. "I am very angry at A. J. because she is so irritable."
b. "J. T., you can stay up later than the other clients tonight."
c. "I do not want to be assigned to B. P. tonight."
d. "The client in Room 10 is an alcoholic."

CHAPTER 7

1. M. L., a 10-year-old girl, is brought to the clinic by her parents, who report that she has become isolative and severely depressed since the death of her close friend several weeks ago. They have attempted to engage her in various family activities, but her depression has worsened over the past week. What is the most important determinant of a child's coping patterns?
a. His or her early social interactions with parents.
b. The quality of his or her peer relationships.
c. The child's problem-solving capacity.
d. The child's sense of self.

2. A major nursing intervention for M. L. would be to
a. Encourage her to verbalize her feelings.
b. Reinforce her peer relationships.
c. Teach her parents how to talk to her.
d. Encourage her to depend on her parents.

3. After several weeks, M. L.'s parents report that she is more outgoing and is relating to them and to her peers. An important message to convey to the parents is that
a. They are doing a good job.
b. This is temporary and she may regress.
c. They need to encourage M. L. to become more independent.
d. M. L.'s condition is unpredictable.

4. A major nursing implication of hardiness is that it
a. Parallels illness and interferes with health.
b. Is associated with life-threatening situations.
c. Can be enhanced by adaptive health practices.
d. Is decreased by stressful events.

5. Overall, adaptation and coping are influenced by a number of factors. Which of the following factors has the *least* influence on adaptation and coping?
a. Developmental level.
b. Neurobiological factors.
c. Cultural background.
d. Social development.

CHAPTER 8

1. Several members of a family are brought to the emergency department with severe burns and smoke inhalation due to a neighborhood fire. The mother is found crying in the waiting area with her 6-year-old son. As a member of the psychiatric triage unit, what is your initial response to this family?
a. Approaching them in a calm, reassuring manner.

b. Inquiring about the events surrounding the fire.
c. Encouraging the mother to express her feelings about the fire.
d. Letting the mother know that her crying will only upset her son.

2. After spending time with her son, the mother leaves the room and continues to cry. The *best* nursing intervention at this time is to
a. Leave her alone until she seeks your assistance.
b. Assess her thoughts and feelings about the situation.
c. Acknowledge her pain and provide emotional support.
d. Encourage her to stay strong for the family.

3. Crisis intervention may be used in this situation to
a. Identify and mobilize resources.
b. Identify past psychiatric treatment.
c. Assess past responses to stress.
d. Recognize the impact of early childhood traumas.

4. T. L. recently lost his wife of 45 years. His family brings him to the emergency department, stating that he has become increasingly despondent and isolative over the past few weeks and cries all the time. He denies needing psychiatric help, but he admits missing his wife. T. L.'s symptoms suggest that he is experiencing
a. A normal grief reaction.
b. An abnormal grief reaction.
c. Physical problems that need attention.
d. Major depressive symptoms.

5. T. L. may benefit from grief work. The major goals of grief work include all of the following except
a. Establishment of a therapeutic alliance.
b. Mobilization of resources.
c. Assessment of coping patterns.
d. Provision of psychotropic medications.

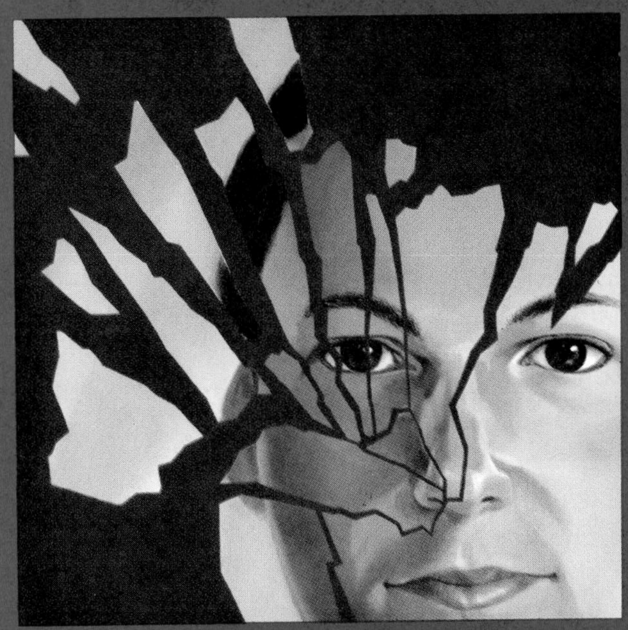

UNIT 2

Response to Stressors Across the Life Span

CHAPTER 9

The Client with a Mood Disorder (Depression)

NANCY R. TOMMASINI, M.S.N., R.N.,C.S.

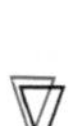

OUTLINE

CHAPTER OBJECTIVES

Upon completion of this chapter, you will be able to:

1. Define six types of depression according to their DSM-IV diagnostic criteria.
2. Explain the neurobiological and psychosocial theories of the cause of depression.
3. Describe and differentiate the types of depression on the basis of prevalence, clinical picture, course, and complications across the life span.
4. Differentiate between depression and dementia in the elderly.
5. Describe the manifestations of normal grief across the life span.
6. Distinguish normal from pathological grief.
7. Discuss the major somatic and psychotherapeutic approaches used to treat depression.
8. Explain the nurse's role in the treatment of depression.
9. Apply the nursing process to the care of the depressed client.

KEY TERMS

Affect
Anhedonia
Dysphoria
Hypersomnia
Hyperphagia
Insomnia
Libido
Mood
Neurotransmitter
Neurovegetative symptoms
Psychomotor retardation
Self-deprecatory ideas
Somatic preoccupation

Depression affects the lives of millions of Americans and costs billions of dollars. In the United States, nearly 10 million people experience a depressive illness during any 6-month period. Depressive illnesses cause grief and pain, interfere with people's ability to function, may disrupt the family's functioning, and may contribute to premature death. Although it is impossible to apply a price tag to human suffering, the economic costs of depression have been estimated at $16 billion annually, of which $10 billion is due to time lost from work. Of all the mental disorders, depressive illnesses are the most treatable. With appropriate intervention, approximately 80 percent of even serious depressions can be alleviated (Sargent, 1989).

Bipolar disorder, also called *manic–depressive illness*, is a serious mental illness involving episodes of mania and depression. The person's mood usually swings from overly high and irritable to sad and hopeless and then back again, with periods of normal mood in between. Bipolar disorder typically begins in adolescence or early adulthood and continues throughout life. It is often not recognized as an illness, and people who have it may suffer needlessly for years or even decades. Nearly 2 million Americans have bipolar disorder. Treatments are available that greatly alleviate the suffering caused by this disorder and can usually prevent its devastating complications, which include alcohol and drug abuse, job loss, divorce, and suicide. Although some information on bipolar disorder is presented in this chapter, a more detailed discussion can be found in Chapter 12. This chapter focuses on the various forms of depression.

DEFINITIONS OF DEPRESSION

Everyone experiences transient feelings of sadness and depression, usually in response to unhappy events or failures. Intense grief and sadness are also normal responses, brought about by the loss of a loved one. People with a depressive illness, however, experience their depressive symptoms for months and sometimes years.

Depression comes in several forms and is referred to by various terms, including *major*, *melancholic*, *unipolar*, and *dysthymia*. *Major depression* refers to a clinical depression that meets specific diagnostic criteria as to duration, impairment in functioning, and presence of a cluster of physiological and psychological symptoms. *Melancholic depression* is a severe form of major depression believed to be particularly responsive to antidepressant medications or electroconvulsive therapy. *Unipolar depression* means that the person suffers from major depression but not from manic–depressive illness, which is called *bipolar disorder* (Sargent, 1989). *Dysthymia* is a less severe, but more chronic, form of depressive illness. These forms of depression are sometimes referred to as "primary" because a specific cause cannot be identified. "Secondary" depressions refer to depressive symptoms that occur in response to a specific event (adjustment disorder with depressed mood) or that are caused by a specific organic factor such as hypothyroidism (organic mood syndrome). Accurate diagnosis of mood disorders has important implications for management and treatment.

CAUSATIVE FACTORS: PERSPECTIVES AND THEORIES

The exact causes of most forms of depression and bipolar disorder remain a mystery at this time. Sorting out the environmental, psychological, biological, and genetic influences in the development of affective illness is extremely complex. Much of what is known about affective disorders has been derived from increased understanding of the pharmacological actions of drugs that are known to cause or improve depressed mood (Hale, 1993; Leonard, 1993). It is generally accepted that some combination of neurobiological and psychosocial factors is usually involved.

NEUROBIOLOGICAL FACTORS

Investigative neurobiological research involving neurotransmitter activity supports the theory that neurotransmitter responses are altered in mood disorders (Fig. 9–1). Clues to the altered response lie in genetic transference, neuroendocrine studies, and circadian rhythms as well as altered neurotransmitter circulation. The influence of each of these factors is reviewed in the following sections.

Genetic Factors

Studies of unipolar and bipolar disorders in families consistently show that these illnesses have significant familial concordance. First-degree adult relatives (parents, siblings, children) of persons with mood disorders are two to three times more likely than the general population to be affected by a mood disorder themselves. The most common affective disorder in relatives of people with bipolar disorder is unipolar illness, whereas bipolar illness is the next most common. Among relatives of people with unipolar disorder, there is a tendency for bipolar disorder to appear more often than in control groups (Beck, 1993; Goodwin & Jamison, 1990).

Adoption and twin studies also support the hypothesis of an underlying genetic component for unipolar and bipolar disorder. Twin studies show that 76 percent of monozygotic (identical) twins are concordant for mood disorders compared with only 19 percent of dizygotic (fraternal) twins. The fact that monozygotic twins do not have 100 percent concordance suggests that nongenetic factors play a role in the etiology (Akiskal & Weller, 1989). Also, concordance is less pronounced in the unipolar group members who experience fewer than three episodes of depression, which suggests that genetic factors are more relevant to recurring affective disorders.

Neurotransmitter Hypothesis

Much of what is understood about neurotransmitter involvement in affective disorders is based on the hypothesized actions of psychopharmacologic agents that affect mood. The major neurotransmitters that have been studied in relation to mood disorders are outlined in Table 9–1.

Catecholamine Hypotheses. Catecholamines (norepinephrine, acetylcholine, and dopamine) are important excitatory neurochemicals that initiate neuronal responses to demands for higher brain function. It has been postulated that depression results from a deficit of norepinephrine at important receptor sites in the brain, whereas mania results from an excess of this amine (see Chapter 10). The deficit component of this theory is based on the serendipitous observation that depressive symptoms developed in approximately 15 percent of hypertensive clients treated with reserpine, a catecholamine-depleting agent (Bunny & Davis, 1965). Many other medications used to treat other medical illnesses deplete catecholamines as a treatment mechanism and have the reported side effect of depression.

In contrast with reserpine, monoamine oxidase (MAO) inhibitors and tricyclic antidepressants (TCAs) increase the availability of catecholamines, specifically norepinephrine, at the postsynaptic receptor sites. Both classes of drugs are found to be effective in treating depression. MAO inhibitors presumably inhibit the normal breakdown of norepinephrine by MAO, whereas TCAs block the reuptake of norepinephrine into the presynaptic neuron (Bunny & Davis, 1965; Schildkraut, 1965, 1978). The treatment response to MAO inhibitors and TCAs is immediate increased amounts of norepinephrine; however, clinical improvement lags 2 to 4 weeks, suggesting that the release and availability to the postsynaptic neuron is delayed. Subsequent investigations attempting to address this discrepancy have suggested that presynaptic receptor mechanisms exist that are capable of modulating transmitter release (Heninger, et al., 1990).

Lithium's effects on norepinephrine are less clear. Lithium has not been found to have a direct stimulatory or inhibitory effect, although it does alter postsynaptic membrane receptors for norepinephrine. This may explain the clinical observations that lithium precipitates neither mania nor depression (in contrast with MAO inhibitors and TCAs, which can precipitate mania in persons with bipolar illness). Lithium is prescribed for treatment of both bipolar phases and acts slowly, with greatest effect in the prevention of manic episodes (Goodwin & Jamison, 1990).

Fluctuation in mood states may represent a relative imbalance between norepinephrine and acetylcholine (see Chapter 13). More specifically, it is possible that a greater proportion of acetylcholine to norepinephrine activity may lead to clinical depression, whereas a greater amount of norepinephrine may contribute to mania (Janowsky et al. 1972). Evidence to support this is grounded in observations of the depressive effects of the cholinesterase inhibitor neostigmine, which prolongs cholinergic activity by delaying acetylcholine breakdown (Golden & Janowsky, 1990). In addition, it has been observed that exposure to compounds that prevent acetylcholine production induced or intensified depressive symptoms (Bowers et al., 1964; Gershon & Shaw, 1961) and switched manic clients toward depressed states (Janowsky et al., 1974).

Serotonin Hypothesis. Although the norepinephrine hypothesis was important to the early understanding of mood disorders and their treatment, it soon became evident that imbalances of other neurotransmitters also contributed to depression. For example, research has linked serotonin deficit to depression (Golden & Janowsky, 1990). The original indolamine hypothesis suggested that a deficiency in serotonin could lead to the emergence of depressive illness (Coppen et al., 1965). As with the catecholamine hypothesis, this was supported by findings that the first clinically effective antidepressants (MAO inhibitors and TCAs) increased the availability of serotonin, as well as norepinephrine, in the brain. When tryptophan, the amino acid precursor for serotonin formation, was observed to be effective in treating mania, the indolamine hypothesis was revised. This "permissive hypothesis" suggests that a deficit in serotonergic neurotransmission permits the emergence of affective illness. When a deficit in serotonin is coupled with decreased norepinephrine, depression may develop; an increase in norepinephrine in the context of decreased serotonin may lead to mania (Prange et al., 1974).

Other Neurotransmitters. Gamma-aminobutyric acid (GABA) is the major inhibitory neurotransmitter, and its functions include a general inhibitory role on brain excitability (Goodwin & Jamison, 1990). GABA-ergic transmission is enhanced by drugs that reduce mania, such as lithium, carbamazepine, valproate, and pro-

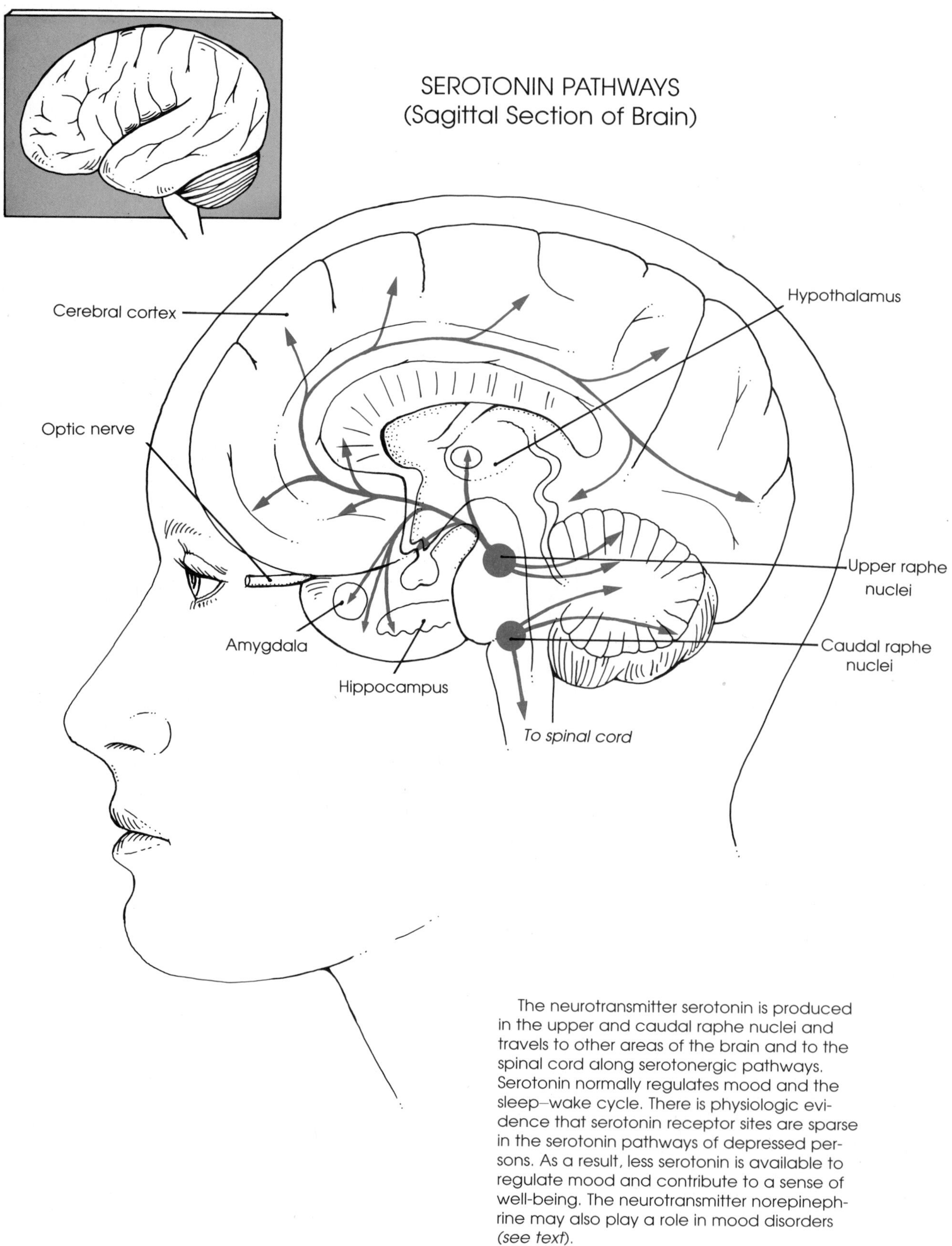
SEROTONIN PATHWAYS
(Sagittal Section of Brain)
Cerebral cortex
Hypothalamus
Optic nerve
Upper raphe nuclei
Caudal raphe nuclei
Amygdala
Hippocampus
To spinal cord
The neurotransmitter serotonin is produced in the upper and caudal raphe nuclei and travels to other areas of the brain and to the spinal cord along serotonergic pathways. Serotonin normally regulates mood and the sleep–wake cycle. There is physiologic evidence that serotonin receptor sites are sparse in the serotonin pathways of depressed persons. As a result, less serotonin is available to regulate mood and contribute to a sense of well-being. The neurotransmitter norepinephrine may also play a role in mood disorders (see text).

FIGURE 9–1
The serotonin hypothesis in relation to mood disorders. (Illustration concept: Gail Kongable, M.S.N., C.N.R.N., C.C.R.N., Department of Neurosurgery, University of Virginia Health Sciences Center. Illustration by Marie T. Dauenheimer.)

SEROTONIN AND THE LIMBIC SYSTEM

The limbic system is a network of neuronal clusters connected by neurotransmitter pathways. This subdivision of the cortex overlying the brain stem plays a primary role in behavioral responses, mood, memory, and learning.

A deficit in the amount of serotonin available to the limbic system has a number of physiologic and emotional effects. A decrease in serotonin available to the **amygdala**, the emotional center of the brain, can cause sadness, a decreased libido, and a general lack of motivation. A serotonin deficit also affects the **hypothalamus**, which is responsible for appetite control; the depressed person may have little appetite or may overeat. The **pituitary gland** may react to serotonin deficit by releasing an excess of pituitary hormones that can cause gastric distress, menstrual irregularities, and sleep disturbances.

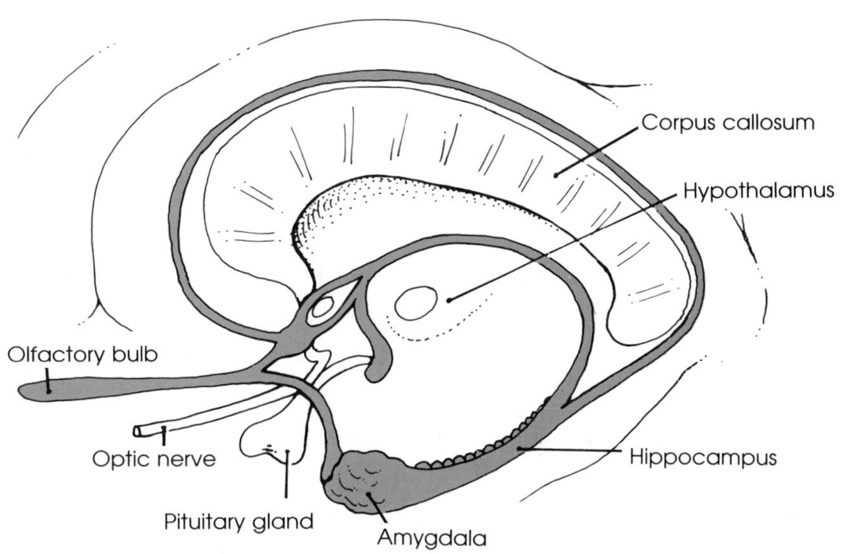

HOW DRUGS AFFECT THE SEROTONERGIC SYNAPSES

Some depressed clients are treated with medications that affect the breakdown of serotonin or block or inhibit its reuptake. These drugs act to increase the amount of serotonin available for transmission. On the other hand, drugs used to treat certain medical conditions can cause or exacerbate depression as a side effect because they decrease the level of serotonin at the serotonergic synapses. *(See Fig. 2-4 for an explanation of synaptic structures.)*

1. Serotonin is synthesized from tryptophan, a basic amino acid.
2. Serotonin is stored in synaptic vesicles. *Some antihypertensive drugs can cause depression because they interfere with the uptake and storage of serotonin.*
3. Vesicles migrate to the presynaptic membrane and release serotonin.
4. Stimulation of the postsynaptic receptor sites initiates an impulse in the dendrite of the next neuron. *Most antidepressants work by prolonging exposure of the postsynaptic membrane to serotonin.*

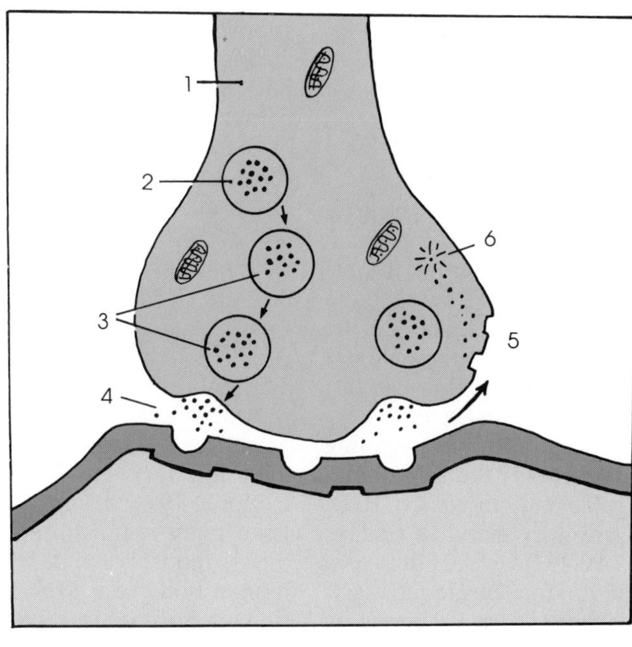

5. Serotonin action is stopped by resorption into the presynaptic terminal. *Fluoxetine (Prozac) and most tricyclic antidepressants probably work by acutely blocking serotonin reuptake. Serotonin reuptake inhibitors (SRIs) work in a similar way.*
6. Serotonin present in a free state within the presynaptic terminal can be broken down by the enzyme monoamine oxidase (MAO). *MAO inhibitors (MAOIs), used to treat some forms of depression, prevent the breakdown of serotonin.*

TABLE 9–1
Neurotransmitters Theoretically Involved in Mood Disorders

Monoamine neurotransmitters
- Catecholamines
  - Epinephrine
  - Norepinephrine (noradrenergic)
  - Dopamine
- Indoleamines
  - Serotonin

Cholinergic neurotransmitter
- Acetylcholine

Amino acid neurotransmitter
- Gamma-aminobutyric acid

pranolol. This finding has led to the proposal that a deficiency of GABA may be involved in the etiology of manic syndromes (Bernasconi, 1982). The role of GABA is also being investigated in relation to depressive illness.

The development of new antidepressants that have significant effects on dopamine has led to interest in the possible role of this neurotransmitter in affective illness. The dopamine hypothesis of mood disorders proposes that mania is associated with increased dopaminergic neuronal activity, whereas depression, especially depression with **psychomotor retardation,** is associated with decreased dopaminergic activity (Willner, 1985).

Neuroendocrine Hypothesis

The hypothalamic–pituitary–adrenal (HPA) axis and the hypothalamic–pituitary–thyroid (HPT) axis are also relevant to the study of mood disorders. These axes can be conceptualized as paths of biochemical communication that affect mood-related behavior (McEnany, 1990). Although abnormalities in these neuroendocrine systems have been found in clients with unipolar and bipolar disorders, it remains unclear whether these changes represent markers of dysfunction or are themselves directly responsible for pathophysiological changes (Grebb et al., 1988).

Hypothalamic–Pituitary–Adrenal Axis. Research has consistently shown that clients with major depression (especially the melancholic type) secrete abnormally large amounts of cortisol. Bipolar clients have also been found to have elevated cortisol levels during the depressed, but not the manic, phase of their illness (Gold, 1988; Goodwin & Jamison, 1990; Rubinow et al., 1984). When psychological or physiological stress is experienced, the HPA axis is activated, ultimately leading to the secretion of cortisol. Specifically, the hypothalamus secretes corticotropin-releasing factor (CRH), which stimulates the anterior pituitary gland to release adrenocorticotropic hormone (ACTH). ACTH acts as a messenger to the adrenal glands to secrete cortisol. Normally, cortisol then shuts off the stress response by acting on the hypothalamus to stop its secretion of CRH (Tirrell & DeForest, 1987). In the depressed person, this process goes awry: the body's response to stress does not shut off (Gold et al., 1988b). Further research is needed to identify the exact mechanism involved in this process.

The clinical picture of depression supports the notion of hypothalamic dysfunction. Hypothalamic centers govern food intake, libido, and circadian rhythms. Depressed persons can exhibit anorexia or **hyperphagia** (overeating), **hypersomnia** or **insomnia**, decreased libido, and disturbances in rapid eye movement (REM) sleep and body temperature rhythms. Findings that the neurohormones that are responsive to stress play a prominent role in the pathophysiology of depression are also consistent with clinical observations that the onset and natural history of major depression are influenced by psychological conflict, counterproductive methods of coping, and external stressors (Altemus & Gold, 1990).

Hypothalamic–Pituitary–Thyroid Axis. Disorders of thyroid function have been frequently observed to accompany changes in mood (Prange et al., 1974; Gewirtz & Maspina, 1988). Regulation of thyroid hormone secretion begins in the hypothalamus, from which thyrotropin-releasing hormone (TRH) is released. TRH then binds to specific cells in the pituitary that release thyroid-stimulating hormone (TSH). This hormone is then released into the general circulation and stimulates the thyroid gland to synthesize and release thyroid hormones, which have widespread effects in the central and peripheral nervous systems (Goodwin & Jamison, 1990).

Significant abnormalities of HPT axis functioning have been found in many clients with bipolar disorder, especially those with rapid cycles. Specifically, a blunted TSH response has been found in manic clients. Examination of HPT functioning at different phases of illness in the same bipolar client revealed that TSH response was increased during depression and blunted during mania (Extein et al., 1980; Gold et al., 1977; Kirkegaard et al., 1978). Interestingly, lithium and carbamazepine, both effective in treating bipolar disorder, have been shown to alter HPT function (Goodwin & Jamison, 1990). Furthermore, thyroid hormone in combination with standard mood-stabilizing medications can attenuate cycles in bipolar clients (Bauer & Whybrow, 1988; Goodwin, 1986).

Circadian Rhythm Hypotheses

Throughout their lives, humans are surrounded by the rhythmic cycles of nature and the universe—the temperature, the seasons of the year, and the alternations of light and darkness that occur every 24 hours (Betrus & Elmore, 1991; Elmore, 1991; Moore-Ede et al., 1983). Like plants and animals, humans exhibit daily (circadian), monthly, and seasonal cycles. Functions of the human body (e.g., the sleep–wake cycle and the secretion of hormones) appear to have characteristic daily rhythms that are endogenous and self-sustained. It is hypothesized that circadian rhythms are generated in the hypothalamus in the brain by at least two oscillators, or biological clocks (Ryan et al., 1987). Research has been conducted to test the theory that mood disorders involve disturbances in the regulation of biological rhythms that synchronize body functions (Simmons-Alling, 1987). Several features of depressive illness suggest abnormalities in biological rhythms. These features include the inherent cyclicity of depression (in many cases, episodes of depression recur and remit spontaneously); abnormalities in the rest–activity cycle; and abnormalities in sleep architecture, that is, the length and timing of sleep stages (Gold et al., 1988a).

One avenue of research in this area has suggested that the timing or phase of circadian rhythms is disturbed relative to the timing of sleep onset. Specifically, people with endogenous depression appear to have circadian rhythms (e.g., REM sleep) that are phase advanced relative to their sleep onset, meaning that they occur earlier than usual after sleep onset. For example, depressed persons demonstrate an earlier onset and increased amount of REM sleep than do nondepressed persons. This observation has become known as the phase-advance hypothesis of depression. Interestingly, antidepressant medications delay the onset of REM sleep (Elmore, 1991). More systematic study of this model is needed to gain a better understanding of its applicability to depression.

Seasonal affective disorder (SAD) is the cyclical mood fluctuation associated with change of season. This circadian-related mood disorder is believed to be related to the length of daylight, with depressed mood occurring during the winter months in susceptible people. One treatment currently under investigation is prolonged exposure to sunlight or natural light during the winter months.

PSYCHOSOCIAL FACTORS

Psychosocial theories of the etiology of depression come from psychoanalytical theory, cognitive–behavioral theories, and research on coping and adaptation.

Psychoanalytical Theory

Early psychoanalytical theorists sought to understand pathological depression by analyzing it in relationship to grief and mourning. Abraham (1960a, 1960b) stated that in mourning, the individual grieves over the loss of the person, whereas in depression, feelings of loss, guilt, and inadequacy result from unconscious hostility toward the lost person. A vulnerability to depression is viewed as stemming from problems (e.g., withdrawal of maternal love and support) during the oral phase of psychosexual development. When a person who had problems during the oral phase of psychosexual development later experiences loss (real, threatened, or perceived), depression results.

Freud (1957) expanded on the work of Abraham in "Mourning and Melancholia." Freud stated that the normal grieving process after a loss involves the working through of ambivalent feelings (love and anger) toward the lost person through recalling and expressing past experiences and feelings related to this person. In the depressed, or, as Freud described, melancholic, person, this process does not occur. Instead, anger toward the lost person is turned inward, leading to dysphoria, guilt, and loss of self-esteem. This anger is focused not on the self but rather on the lost person, who is unconsciously identified with the self. Similar to Abraham, Freud suggested that traumatic experiences in early childhood, such as loss, result in vulnerability to depression when future losses occur (Hirschfeld & Goodwin, 1988).

Although subsequent writers have presented views different from those of Abraham and Freud, all psychoanalytical formulations are essentially similar in terms of how depression is understood. That is, disturbances in interpersonal relationships in early childhood, usually involving a loss or disappointment, impair later relationships. People who experience traumas in interpersonal relationships in childhood are particularly vulnerable to later disappointments and losses, which may lead to depression (Hirschfeld & Shea, 1989).

Cognitive–Behavioral Theories

In the early 1970s, a concerted effort to apply learning models to the phenomena of depression began. Behavioral models (e.g., reinforcement theory) were the first learning approaches to be applied. In recent years, the psychology of learning has gone through a cognitive revolution. The earlier behavioral theories of depression have evolved in a cognitive direction (e.g., learned helplessness theory), and new theories have developed from a cognitive perspective (e.g., Beck's cognitive theory) (Rehm, 1990).

Reinforcement Theory. The application of a behavioral model to depression has been most extensively developed by Lewinsohn (1974). In essence, depression is viewed as resulting from losses of important sources of positive reinforcement, a high rate of aversive experiences, or both. In addition to depressed mood, a reduction in behavior occurs. Other symptoms, such as low self-esteem and hopelessness, are believed to stem from the reduced level of functioning. For example, a man experiences a depressed mood after a breakup with his girlfriend (an important source of reinforcement). Before the breakup, much of the man's behavior was probably organized around his relationship with his girlfriend; for example, going to the movies with her was a pleasurable activity and was thus reinforcing. Reinforcement theory proposes that if as part of his depression this man no longer goes to the movies, it is because he went with his girlfriend in the past and now that source of reinforcement is no longer present.

According to this theory, there are two other ways in which insufficient reinforcement may occur. In addition to the loss of reinforcement, as in the preceding example, the person may (1) lack the necessary skills to obtain reinforcement even though reinforcement is potentially available (e.g., poor interpersonal skills could preclude the development of satisfying social relationships) or (2) lack the ability to enjoy available reinforcers because of interfering anxiety.

Finally, reinforcement theory asserts that once a depressive syndrome has occurred, it is maintained through the reinforcing concern and sympathy as well as the negative responses that depressive behaviors elicit from others (Coyne, 1976).

Learned Helplessness Theory. The term *learned helplessness* was originally used by Seligman (1975) and his colleagues to describe the helpless behavior dogs developed when they were exposed to uncontrollable shocks in the laboratory. Many analogies to human depression were seen in the behavior of these animals, leading to the adoption of the learned helplessness paradigm as an explanation of human helplessness and depression. The inescapable shock was viewed as analogous to the traumatic loss that may precipitate depression. Other symptom parallels included passivity, weight loss, and lack of appetite (Rehm, 1990).

Subsequent revisions to the model have been important in attempting to explain key symptoms of depression, such as guilt and loss of self-esteem, that were not addressed in the original formulation. In its revised form, the theory suggests that a person's *attributions*, or interpretation of negative events, determine whether the occurrence of such events will make the person feel depressed. Three types of attributions, or causal explanations, after negative events are hypothesized to result in depression (Hirschfeld & Goodwin, 1988)

- Perceiving the cause of the event as internal (oneself is to blame for the event) rather than external (the event was caused by the situation)
- Perceiving the cause as a stable factor (persistent or unchangeable) rather than unstable factor (transitory and able to be changed)
- Perceiving the cause as global (affecting many areas of living) rather than specific (limited to a particular event)

The learned helplessness model of depression can be summarized as follows: Individuals develop consistent attributional styles, or ways of understanding the causes of events in their lives. A particular attributional style consists of habitually attributing negative outcomes to internal, stable, global causes and ascribing positive events to external, unstable, specific causes. Mild to severe depression results when this attributional style is coupled with uncontrollable, aversive events (Rehm, 1990). The following example of a depressed woman illustrates this process.

Case Study: Learned Helplessness Leading to Depression (Ms. T.)

Ms. T. is a 27-year-old woman who was admitted to the psychiatric inpatient unit for depression and suicidal ideation. Her boyfriend of 5 years had recently left her and was dating another woman. Ms. T. viewed herself as completely to blame for the breakup, even in the face of evidence to the contrary (*internal attribution*). She described herself as pitiful and worthless and believed that this would always be so (*stable attribution*). Furthermore, Ms. T. saw herself as a failure not only in her relationship with her boyfriend but also in her job and at school (*global attribution*).

Cognitive Theory. Beck (1963, 1964, 1967) developed the cognitive theory of depression. He proposed that depression in its various forms (major, melancholic, dysthymic, and bipolar) results from a negative cognitive triad, specific schemas, and cognitive errors (i.e., faulty information processing).

The *cognitive triad* is made up of (1) a negative view of the self (e.g., seeing oneself as defective, inadequate, worthless, and undesirable), (2) a negative view of the world (e.g., experiencing the world as a demanding and defeating place in which failure and punishment are to be expected), and (3) a negative view of the future (e.g., expecting ongoing hardship, suffering, deprivation, and failure).

Schemas are the stable cognitive patterns through which people interpret or understand their experience. In depression, schemas are analogous to viewing the world through dark glasses (Hirschfeld & Shea, 1989). The theory proposes that schemas are activated by negative life events (e.g., a loss) that are psychologically similar to the early life experiences in which the schemas developed (Wright & Beck, 1983).

Cognitive errors, or distortions, are automatic errors in thinking that stem from the activation of negative schemas. They are referred to as automatic because they occur rapidly and are not subjected to systematic, logical analysis. Although depressed persons are usually not aware that these thoughts are occurring, they are conscious thoughts and can be retrieved with careful questioning (Wright & Beck, 1983).

Several types of cognitive distortions have been identified in depressed persons. *Selective abstraction* involves coming to a conclusion based on a single detail, while ignoring other, more important aspects of a situation. For example, while congratulating an employee on a promotion an employer says, "Don't underestimate your future with this company." The depressive employee concludes, "She thinks I have no self-confidence." *Magnification* and *minimization* are cognitive distortions in which negatives are overemphasized and positives are underemphasized. Applying a distorted label to an event and then reacting to the label rather than the event is termed *inexact labeling*. In the preceding example with the boss, the employee would label the conversation a "criticism session" and expect to be fired (Rehm, 1990).

The cognitive theory of depression suggests that disturbances in thinking are the core of depression and that other symptoms associated with depression (e.g., sad mood, an inability to experience pleasure, and decreased motivation) are reinforced by the cognitive disturbances. The cognitive model does not posit a cause-and-effect relationship between cognitive dysfunction and depression; rather, the cognitive distortions are viewed as one component of the depressive syndrome (Wright & Beck, 1983).

THE ROLE OF COPING AND ADAPTATION

Coping has been defined as "constantly changing cognitive and behavioral efforts to manage specific external and/or internal demands that are appraised as taxing or exceeding the resources of the person" (Lazarus & Folkman, 1984, p. 141). The possible role of coping style in the etiology of clinical depression has only recently been the focus of empirical research. Depressed persons' coping styles have been found to differ from those of nondepressed persons.

Depressed people use more emotion-focused coping strategies (e.g., emotional release, elicitation of emotional support, hostile confrontation, and wishful thinking) than do nondepressed people (Billings, et al., 1983; Coyne et al., 1981; Folkman & Lazarus, 1986). Depression has also been associated with the use of fewer active coping strategies (e.g., problem solving) and with avoidance (Mitchell & Hodson, 1983). It remains unclear, however, whether these coping strategies contribute to the development of depression or are the result of the illness.

DEPRESSION ACROSS THE LIFE SPAN

Although certain characteristics of depression are consistently seen across the life span, developmental stage is important in influencing how this disorder is manifested. Table 9–2 lists characteristics that distinguish depression in various age groups.

CHILDHOOD

Depression is relatively uncommon in preschoolers, although it does occur at a prevalence rate of 0.3 percent. This rate increases in school-age children to 2 percent and is greater in school-age boys than in school-age girls (Akiskal & Weller, 1989). The risk of depression during childhood is increased by chronic physical conditions; physical abuse; homelessness; poverty; parental separation, divorce, or death; and parental psychiatric illness (Austin, 1990; Damrosch et al., 1988; Kazdin et al., 1985; Pothier, 1988).

Depressed children as young as 4 years describe self-destructive wishes. Under the age of 12, boys more often than girls develop suicidal behavior. Methods that are used by young children are easily mistaken for accidents and include jumping out of windows, running in front of cars, stabbing themselves, and ingesting pills (Akiskal & Weller, 1989).

Children with a depressive disorder are at high risk for future recurrence and the development of bipolar disorder.

TABLE 9–2

Characteristics of Depression Across the Life Span

CHILDHOOD	
Infants and Preschoolers	**Prepubertal Children**
Insidious onset Apathy, fatigue, withdrawal Poor appetite, weight loss Agitation, sleeplessness Rarely, spontaneous disclosure of feeling sad	Possible disclosure of sadness, suicidal thoughts Irritability, self-criticism, weepiness Decreased initiative and responsiveness to stimulation, apathy Fatigue, sleep disturbance Enuresis, encopresis Weight loss, anorexia Somatic complaints Poor school performance Social withdrawal, increased aggressiveness
ADOLESCENCE	
Feelings of sadness less frequent than in other age groups Unhappy restlessness, boredom, irritability Intense, labile affects Low self-esteem, hopelessness, worthlessness Associated anxiety Feelings of loneliness and being unloved Pessimism about the future Loss of interest in friends and activities, apathy Low frustration tolerance	Poor school performance Argumentativeness Increased conflict with peers Acting-out behavior, e.g., running away, stealing, physical violence Sexual activity Substance abuse Complaints of headaches, abdominal pain Hypersomnia
EARLY AND MIDDLE ADULTHOOD	
Depressed mood Anhedonia Feelings of worthlessness, hopelessness, guilt Reduced energy, fatigue Sleep disturbance, especially early morning awakening and multiple nighttime awakenings	Decreased sexual interest and activity Psychomotor retardation Anxiety Decreased appetite and weight loss or increased appetite and weight gain
LATER ADULTHOOD	
Unlikely to complain of depressed mood or present with tearful affect Feelings of helplessness Pessimism about the future Ruminating about problems Critical and envious of others Loss of self-esteem Guilt feelings	Longer and more severe depressions than in middle adulthood Perceived cognitive deficits Somatic complaints Constipation Social withdrawal Loss of motivation Change of appetite
CORE SYMPTOMS ACROSS AGE GROUPS	
Suicidal ideation Diminished concentration Sleep disturbance	

ADOLESCENCE

There is a significant increase in the rate of depression from childhood to adolescence. The prevalence rate for depression in adolescence is 5 percent and is similar for girls and boys (Kaplan & Sadock, 1991). Because adolescence is a time of enormous changes in physical appearance, family and peer relationships, cognitive development, and endocrine functioning, mood swings and transient feelings of depression are to be expected (Sadler, 1991). Depression becomes pathological when the symptoms associated with it are prolonged.

Depressive disorders in adolescence are associated with physical, sexual, and emotional abuse as well as parental chronic illness, especially psychiatric illness and illness requiring hospitalization (Beardslee et al., 1983; Friedman et al., 1984; Rosen et al., 1990). Adolescents whose parents have a history of major depression are at increased risk for depressive illness (Weissman et al., 1984). It appears that adolescents from a lower socioeconomic status and minority ethnic groups are at greater risk for depression; however, research results are not consistent (Kandel & Davies, 1982; Kaplan et al., 1984; Schoenbach et al., 1982).

Suicide is the third most common cause of death in adolescent boys and the fourth most common cause of death in adolescent girls. Although teenage girls attempt suicide more often, boys more frequently succeed in killing themselves. Successful suicides increase with age during this developmental period, with 15- to 19-year-olds being 10 times more likely to commit suicide than 10- to 14-year-olds. Methods commonly used by adolescents are drug and alcohol ingestion, shooting, hanging, and carbon monoxide poisoning from automobile exhaust. Although one in three depressed adolescents admits to suicidal ideation and 5 percent of depressed teens present with a history of a suicide attempt, the prevalence of mood disorders as a contribution to suicide remains unclear (Akiskal & Weller, 1989). Other factors hypothesized to contribute to adolescent suicidal behavior are discussed in Chapter 16.

Like children, adolescents with a depressive disorder are at high risk for future recurrence as well as the development of bipolar illness. With the onset of adolescence, many depressed children cycle into hypomania or mania (Akiskal & Weller, 1989).

ADULTHOOD

Half of all persons with a depressive disorder have an onset of the disorder between the ages of 20 and 50—the average age of onset is 40 years. The 6-month prevalence rate for a mood disorder in adulthood is 5.8 percent (Weissman, 1987). Throughout the world, depression is twice as common in women than men. It tends to occur more frequently in those who are divorced or separated or who have no close interpersonal relationships. Rates in adults are not dependent on socioeconomic status and do not differ according to race. There is a tendency, however, for clinicians to underdiagnose mood disorders and overdiagnose schizophrenia in clients whose racial or cultural backgrounds are different from their own. Depression appears to be more common in rural than in urban areas (Kaplan & Sadock, 1991).

Two thirds of depressed adults think about ending their lives. Approximately 10 to 15 percent actually do (Kaplan & Sadock, 1991). In an early study, it was found that a large number of depressed people who committed suicide had communicated their intent to others before doing so, often with a direct statement (Robins et al., 1959). Relatively few risk factors for suicide in the adult with clinical depression have been consistently identified across studies. Those that have been identified include experiencing early parental loss, having a family history of suicide, living alone, being foreign born, and having a history of attempted suicide (Barraclough et al., 1974; Egeland & Sussex, 1985; Murphy & Robins, 1967; Roy, 1983). For all depressed patients, the 1- to 2-year period after psychiatric hospitalization is one of high risk for suicide, especially in the first few months (Black et al., 1985).

OLDER ADULTHOOD

Depressive disorders and depressive symptoms are common in the elderly. The 6-month prevalence rate for major depression has been reported at 0.8 percent, although significant depressive symptoms occur with a frequency of 20 percent (Blazer et al., 1987). The rate of major depression in nursing homes increases to 12.6 percent (Rovner et al., 1991), and 20 to 50 percent of the medically ill hospitalized elderly are depressed (Blazer & Williams, 1980).

Biological, psychological, and social variables appear to increase the risk for depression in the elderly. Central nervous system changes that occur with normal aging (e.g., increased MAO activity) possibly predispose the older adult to clinical depression (Robinson et al., 1971). Poor physical health has frequently been associated with a high level of depressive symptoms (Cadoret & Widmer, 1988; Kennedy et al., 1989; Phifer & Murrell, 1986), and chronic financial strain may raise the elderly's risk for depression (Krause, 1987).

Although the elderly may occasionally present with a picture of depression similar to that presented by people in early and middle adulthood, a different constellation of symptoms often exists (see Table 9–2). A depressive disorder in the elderly can be easily missed because of this different symptomatology and because the older adult with depression frequently does not complain of depressed mood (Dreyfus, 1988). Depression in the elderly may also be confused with and misdiagnosed as dementia. This is a potentially tragic situation in that a severe depression may be left untreated and a person inappropriately institutionalized. Differentiating characteristics of depression and dementia are presented in Table 9–3.

Suicide is a significant risk in the depressed older

TABLE 9–3
Differentiating Characteristics of Depression and Dementia

CLINICAL FEATURE	DEPRESSION	DEMENTIA
Onset	Relatively rapid	Insidious
Precursors	Usually a recent history of a stressful event	No clear precursor
Psychiatric history	History of depression	No history of depression
Cognitive impairment	Fluctuating	Constant
Orientation	Orientation in all spheres	Impaired orientation
Memory	Equal or no impairment in recent and remote memory	Greater impairment in recent than in remote memory
Learning capacity	Usually intact	Impaired
Mental status results	Usually "don't know" answers, emphasis on impairments	Usually errors, minimization or concealment of impairments
Sense of distress (feels depressed)	Yes	No
Affect	Irritable, constricted	Shallow and labile
Behavior	Little effort to perform even simple tasks	Struggle to perform tasks
Response to treatment	Improvement with antidepressants or electroconvulsive therapy	Lack of response

Data from Ban, T. (1984). Chronic disease and depression in the geriatric population. *Journal of Clinical Psychiatry, 45*(3), 18–24; Dreyfus, J. (1988). Depression assessment and interventions in the medically ill frail elderly. *Journal of Gerontological Nursing, 14*(9), 27–36; and Wells, C. E. (1979). Pseudodementia. *American Journal of Psychiatry, 136*, 895–900.

adult. The suicide rate is highest among the elderly (50 percent higher than among the young), and the majority of these suicides occur within the context of a depressive disorder (Katz et al., 1988; Osgood & Thielman, 1990). Caucasian males and the very old (75+) are at highest risk. Feelings of hopelessness and helplessness are especially characteristic of depression and suicide in the elderly (Farber, 1968; Farberow & Shneidman, 1970). The period after the loss of a spouse, especially in men, is a time of high risk (Helsing et al., 1982; Kaprio et al., 1987).

LOSS AND GRIEF ACROSS THE LIFE SPAN

THE STRESS OF BEREAVEMENT

Every year, an estimated 8 million Americans experience the death of an immediate family member. Numerous others grieve the loss of significant people in their lives (Osterweis et al., 1987). Bereavement is an extreme stressor that has physiological, psychological, and social consequences. As with other stressors, the consequences of bereavement are variable and are influenced by the bereaved person's constitutional makeup and personality, the nature of the bereaved person's relationship with the deceased, and the circumstances of the death.

Certain facts about bereavement are clear. First, grief is associated with measurable distress in virtually everyone. Second, although the intensity of the distress and its effect on functioning vary, the distress is long-standing, anywhere from 1 to 3 years. Furthermore, although patterns of bereavement have been identified, reactions to the death of another are highly individualistic and do not fit neatly into well-defined stages. Finally, some bereaved people are at increased risk for illness as well as death (Osterweis et al., 1987).

Research on the potential complications of bereavement has revealed the following:

- Young and middle-aged widowed men are about 1 1/2 times more likely to die than are young and middle-aged married men. This risk is greatest during the first year of widowhood; however, in the absence of remarriage, the risk continues for many years (Helsing & Szklo, 1981).
- The higher mortality rate in men than in women is related to death by suicide, accidents, cardiovascular disease, and some infectious diseases (Osterweis et al., 1987).
- Women have an increased mortality rate in the second year after the death of a spouse and are at increased risk of death from cirrhosis (Burnell & Burnell, 1989).
- Bereaved adults have increased rates of alcohol consumption, smoking, and tranquilizer use. This is especially true among those who used these substances prior to the loss (Osterweis et al., 1987).
- Clinically diagnosable depressions have been found in 10 to 20 percent of widows and widowers a year or more after their loss (Clayton & Darvish, 1979). The rates of depression after other types of bereavement, such as bereavement over the death of a child, sibling, or parent, are unknown.
- The risk for suicide is relatively high for older widowed men and for single men who have lost their mothers (Burnell & Burnell, 1989).
- Bereaved children are at greater risk than nonbereaved children for depression and suicide in adult life, although this is not as widespread or inevitable as previously thought (Bowlby, 1980; Elizur & Kaffman, 1982; Osterweis et al., 1987).
- A perceived lack of social support is one of the most significant predictors of poor outcome among bereaved persons (Burnell & Burnell, 1989). The presence of a consistent, dependable caretaker appears to be especially important in determining outcome in children who have lost a parent or sibling (Osterweis et al., 1987).

THE TASKS OF MOURNING

Disequilibrium occurs after a loss, and certain tasks need to be accomplished to work through the loss and regain equilibrium. These four tasks of mourning are outlined in the following sections.

1. Accepting the Reality of Loss. The bereaved must accept the fact on both an intellectual and emotional level that the person is dead and will not return. Rituals such as the funeral are often helpful in this process. Disbelief and denial are common early in the grieving process and then appear intermittently as the loss is worked through. Ongoing denial indicates maladaptation.

2. Working Through to the Pain of Grief. Physical and emotional pain are experienced with loss, and it is important that the grieving person allow himself or herself to feel this pain. Cutting off or denying feelings may be achieved through avoiding painful thoughts or any reminders of the deceased, as well as through the use of alcohol or drugs. However, avoiding painful feelings at the time of loss increases the risk of a depressive disorder in the future.

3. Adjusting to an Environment in Which the Deceased Is Missing. The various roles filled by the deceased (e.g., household manager, child caretaker, or finance handler) will influence the extent to which the bereaved person needs to develop new skills and take on new roles. The bereaved person's sense of the world may also require adjustment; loss through death often challenges fundamental life values and philosophical beliefs.

4. Relocating the Deceased Emotionally and Moving on with Life. This last task can be the most difficult to accomplish, because it requires that the bereaved person let go of his or her attachments to the deceased and form new attachments. This does not mean that thoughts and memories of the lost loved one are abandoned but rather that they are relocated in one's emotional life in a way that allows for going on with life (Worden, 1991).

MANIFESTATIONS OF NORMAL GRIEF

A wide range of feelings and behaviors are experienced after a loss. Table 9–4 outlines how these are manifested during different periods of a person's life.

Although children have many of the same feelings of grief that adults experience, their reactions are at the same time unique. This is due to their immaturity and lack of well-developed coping skills. Rather than expressing their feelings of sadness, anger, and fear directly, they may manifest them in misbehavior or temper tantrums that can arise for many years after the loss (Osterweis et al., 1987). Because a child's capacity to experience intense emotions is more limited than an adult's, emotional and behavioral manifestations of grief are intermittent rather than continuous (Burnell & Burnell, 1989).

"What did I do to cause this to happen?", "Will this happen to me too?", and "Who will take care of me now?" are three common concerns of children who have lost a parent. Children should be repeatedly reassured as to the answers to these questions, even if they go unasked. A more favorable outcome can be expected for the child who is able to talk freely about the dead parent in either positive or negative terms (Burnell & Burnell, 1989). Factors that may increase a child's risk of psychological or behavioral problems after the death of a parent or sibling are (1) a troubled relationship with the deceased before the death; (2) unstable, inconsistent caregiving; and (3) a troubled surviving parent who depends excessively on the bereaved child (American Academy of Pediatrics, Committee on Psychosocial Aspects of Child and Family Health, 1992).

Adolescents tend to show less outward manifestation

TABLE 9–4

Manifestations of Normal Grief Across the Life Span

	FEELINGS	PHYSICAL SENSATIONS	BEHAVIORS	COGNITIONS
Childhood	Sadness, fearfulness	Bowel and bladder disturbances	Angry outbursts, eating disturbance, speech disturbances, withdrawal or excessive caregiving, deterioration of school behavior and academic achievement	
Adolescence	Guilt, denial		Sexual promiscuity, alcohol and drug use	Worry about future, preservation of family, and new responsibilities
Adulthood	Sadness, anger, guilt and self-reproach, anxiety, loneliness, fatigue, helplessness, shock, yearning, emancipation, relief, numbness	Hollowness in stomach, tightness in chest and throat, oversensitivity to noise, depersonalization, breathlessness, muscle weakness, dry mouth	Sleep disturbance, appetite disturbance, absent-minded behavior, social withdrawal, dreams of deceased, calling out for deceased, sighing, restless overactivity, crying	Disbelief, confusion, preoccupation, sense of presence, hallucinations
Late Adulthood	Similar to adult	More pronounced physical sensations than in adulthood, possibly imitating the symptoms of the deceased	Similar to those in adulthood, plus marked irritability	Similar to those in adulthood, plus negativistic thinking

of their grief than do bereaved in other age groups. This may stem from a fear of appearing different or abnormal during an already turbulent developmental period (Burnell & Burnell, 1989; Kuntz, 1991).

Manifestations of grief have been most extensively described for the adult. Although not all of the characteristics listed in Table 9–4 will be experienced by one person, they are all normal after the loss of a loved one. Sadness is the most common feeling. A sense of relief is typical if the death followed a lengthy or painful illness. Anxiety, ranging from a sense of insecurity to panic, stems from a heightened sense of the survivor's own mortality and a fear of being unable to manage without the deceased. A preoccupation with the deceased is common and often includes obsessive thoughts about how to recover the lost person. The grieving adult frequently senses that the deceased is still present and will describe seeing the loved one or hearing his or her voice (Worden, 1991).

In 1984, there were 7.8 million widowed elderly (65 years of age and older) women and 1.5 million widowed elderly men in the United States. Complicating the grieving process in the elderly are the multiple losses that occur during this stage of life (Worden, 1991).

The relationship of the bereaved to the deceased influences both how grief is manifested and subsequent adjustment. The loss of a spouse through death typically occurs in later adulthood; when it is experienced at a younger age, it is particularly stressful, because major lifestyle adjustments are required. The loss of a child is likely the most traumatic experience a parent can undergo. Feelings of guilt, self-blame, and anger are more prominent and intense than in other types of losses. The course of grief is lengthy, lasting 2 to 5 years. Marital stress is common, and the estimated rate of divorce after the death of a child is 50 to 70 percent. Parents' ability to meet the needs of surviving siblings may also be impaired. Because it is generally accepted that as people age they are more likely to die, the loss of a parent during adulthood is generally less traumatic than the loss of a child (Burnell & Burnell, 1989).

The manifestations of grief normally diminish in frequency and intensity over time. It is not uncommon or abnormal, however, for the feelings and behaviors associated with mourning to recur at various points throughout a person's life. Anniversary dates of the birth and death of the deceased, holidays, or other occasions that

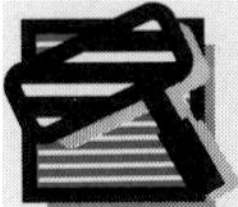

RESEARCH STUDY

Hiding and Healing: Resolving the Suicide of a Parent or Sibling

Demi, A. S., & Howell, C. (1991). *Archives of Psychiatric Nursing*, 5, 350–356.

Study Problem/Purpose. The purpose of this study was to describe the long-term effects of the suicide of a parent or sibling on children and young adults.

Methods. A grounded-theory approach was used to determine survivors' perceptions of the suicide and the effect it had on their lives. Interviews of 1 to 1 1/2 hours' duration were conducted with 17 subjects, ages 26 to 50 years. Five were men, and 12 were women; 15 were Caucasian, and 2 were African Americans. The mean length of time since the suicide was 17 years, with a range of 2 to 40 years. At the time of the suicide, 6 of the subjects had been children, 6 had been adolescents, and 5 had been young adults. Eleven had experienced the suicide of a parent; 6, the suicide of a sibling. Transcripts of the tape-recorded interviews were analyzed through comparing and coding of the data until categories emerged. Common themes were then identified.

Findings. Three major themes emerged from the data: *experiencing the pain, hiding the pain, and healing the pain.* Experiencing the pain involved anger; a sense of family disintegration; feelings of stigma, loneliness, sadness, and lowered self-esteem; blaming; and worries about one's own mental health. The findings also revealed that a great deal of energy was devoted to hiding the pain. Subjects hid their pain through denial, avoidance, secrecy, fleeing, work, and addictive behavior. The majority reported that there was no shared expression of grief in the family at the time of the suicide, and for many subjects there was never any shared grieving. Healing of the pain typically occurred many years after the suicide, through therapy that was sought for a work or interpersonal problem. In addition, healing of the pain was effected through expressing and sharing thoughts and feelings.

Implications. The results of this study point to a need for (1) family education on ways the needs of the child or young adult survivor of suicide can be met and (2) early identification of unresolved grief, with appropriate referrals for counseling. The authors recommended that educational efforts be directed toward destigmatizing suicide, teaching healthy patterns of coping with grief, and mobilizing support systems for suicide survivors.

DSM-IV CRITERIA FOR MAJOR DEPRESSIVE EPISODE

A. Five (or more) of the following symptoms have been present during the same 2-week period and represent a change from previous functioning; at least one of the symptoms is either (1) depressed mood or (2) loss of interest or pleasure.

Note: Do not include symptoms that are clearly due to a general medical condition, or mood-incongruent delusions or hallucinations.

(1) depressed mood most of the day, nearly every day, as indicated by either subjective report (e.g., feels sad or empty) or observation made by others (e.g., appears tearful). **Note:** In children and adolescents, can be irritable mood.
(2) markedly diminished interest or pleasure in all, or almost all, activities most of the day, nearly every day (as indicated by either subjective account or observation made by others)
(3) significant weight loss when not dieting or weight gain (e.g., a change of more than 5% of body weight in a month), or decrease or increase in appetite nearly every day. **Note:** In children, consider failure to make expected weight gains.
(4) insomnia or hypersomnia nearly every day
(5) psychomotor agitation or retardation nearly every day (observable by others, not merely subjective feelings of restlessness or being slowed down)
(6) fatigue or loss of energy nearly every day
(7) feelings of worthlessness or excessive or inappropriate guilt (which may be delusional) nearly every day (not merely self-reproach or guilt about being sick)
(8) diminished ability to think or concentrate, or indecisiveness, nearly every day (either by subjective account or as observed by others)
(9) recurrent thoughts of death (not just fear of dying), recurrent suicidal ideation without a specific plan, or a suicide attempt or a specific plan for committing suicide

B. The symptoms do not meet criteria for a Mixed Episode.

C. The symptoms cause clinically significant distress or impairment in social, occupational, or other important areas of functioning.

D. The symptoms are not due to the direct physiological effects of a substance (e.g., a drug of abuse, a medication) or a general medical condition (e.g., hypothyroidism).

E. The symptoms are not better accounted for by Bereavement, i.e., after the loss of a loved one, the symptoms persist for longer than 2 months or are characterized by marked functional impairment, morbid preoccupation with worthlessness, suicidal ideation, psychotic symptoms, or psychomotor retardation.

From American Psychiatric Association. (1994). *Diagnostic and statistical manual of mental disorders, fourth edition*. Washington, DC: Author.

remind the survivor of the deceased typically provoke a recurrence of mourning.

DISTINGUISHING BETWEEN GRIEF AND DEPRESSION

Grief is often indistinguishable from depression, and so in assessing a person with symptoms of depression, it is important that the nurse question the presence of recent loss. Certain characteristics of the two states do differ, however. The bereaved regard their feelings of depression as normal rather than abnormal. There is usually not a loss of self-esteem in the depressed grieving person, and feelings of guilt are typically associated with some specific aspect of the loss rather than being more pervasive. Whereas the bereaved person views the world as poor and empty (Freud, 1957), the depressed person *feels* poor and empty (Worden, 1991).

The Research Study display on page 169 demonstrates how 17 subjects dealt with depression and grief after the suicide of a parent or sibling.

SPECIFIC MOOD DISORDERS

Several forms of depression have been defined in the fourth edition of the *Diagnostic and Statistical Manual of Mental Disorders* (DSM-IV; American Psychiatric Association [APA], 1994). This section provides an overview of these forms of depression, including their diagnostic criteria, onset, course, and complications.

THE CLIENT WITH MAJOR DEPRESSION

The DSM-IV diagnostic criteria for a major depressive episode are outlined in the accompanying display, "Criteria for Major Depressive Episodes." The average age of onset for this disorder is the later 20s, although it can occur at any age, including infancy. Onset frequently occurs after a major psychosocial stressor, such as divorce. Although some people with major depression experience a single episode in their lifetime, this disorder tends to be cyclical, characterized by periods of illness and periods of health. Approximately 50 to 85 percent of all clients have a second episode, often 4 to 6 months after the first one (Kaplan & Sadock, 1991). A subgroup of people experience a chronic course of depression, with symptoms lasting as long as 2 years (APA, 1994).

Major depressive illness is always associated with impairment in functioning. This may range from difficulty concentrating and completing tasks at school or work to the inability to feed or clothe oneself. Psychotic symptoms may or may not be present during a major depressive episode. When delusions or hallucinations are present, their content is usually consistent with the person's mood. Hallucinatory voices may tell the person that he or she is bad and worthless. The delusional belief that one has cancer or one's insides are rotting away is not uncommon.

Particular subtypes of major depression have been identified and include melancholic type and seasonal pattern depressions (see displays, "Criteria for Melancholic Features Specifier" and "Criteria for Seasonal Pattern Specifier"). The presence of symptoms of melancholia suggests a more severe form of major depression believed to be especially responsive to antidepressant medications. The seasonal pattern subtype, also known as seasonal affective disorder (SAD), is typically characterized by depression, psychomotor slowing, hypersomnia, and hyperphagia that appear in autumn or winter and recede in spring and summer. SAD appears to be responsive to treatment with sleep deprivation or high-intensity light therapy (Kaplan & Sadock, 1991).

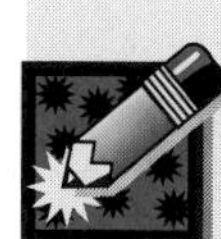

DSM-IV CRITERIA FOR MELANCHOLIC FEATURES SPECIFIER

Specify if:

With Melancholic Features (can be applied to the current or most recent Major Depressive Episode in Major Depressive Disorder and to a Major Depressive Episode in Bipolar I or Bipolar II Disorder only if it is the most recent type of mood episode)

A. Either of the following, occurring during the most severe period of the current episode:
- (1) loss of pleasure in all, or almost all, activities
- (2) lack of reactivity to usually pleasurable stimuli (does not feel much better, even temporarily, when something good happens)

B. Three (or more) of the following
- (1) distinct quality of depressed mood (i.e., the depressed mood is experienced as distinctly different from the kind of feeling experienced after the death of a loved one)
- (2) depression regularly worse in the morning
- (3) early morning awakening (at least 2 hours before usual time of awakening)
- (4) marked psychomotor retardation or agitation
- (5) significant anorexia or weight loss
- (6) excessive or inappropriate guilt

From American Psychiatric Association. (1994). *Diagnostic and statistical manual of mental disorders, fourth edition.* Washington, DC: Author.

THE CLIENT WITH BIPOLAR DISORDER (DEPRESSED)

The difference between the client with unipolar depression and the client with bipolar depression is that the latter has a history of one or more manic episodes (see the display, "Criteria for Manic Episode"). The diagnostic criteria for depression in the person with bipolar illness are the same as those for major depression. However, clients with bipolar depression have been found to experience more psychomotor retardation, lethargy, delusions, and hallucinations than clients with unipolar depression (Goodwin & Jamison, 1990).

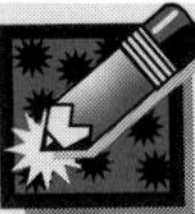

DSM-IV CRITERIA FOR SEASONAL PATTERN SPECIFIER

Specify if:

With Seasonal Pattern (can be applied to the pattern of Major Depressive Episodes in Bipolar I Disorder, Bipolar II Disorder, or Major Depressive Disorder, Recurrent)

A. There has been a regular temporal relationship between the onset of Major Depressive Episodes in Bipolar I or Bipolar II Disorder or Major Depressive Disorder, Recurrent, and a particular time of the year (e.g., regular appearance of the Major Depressive Episode in the fall or winter).

Note: Do not include cases in which there is an obvious effect of seasonal-related psychosocial stressors (e.g., regularly being unemployed every winter).

B. Full remissions (or a change from depression to mania or hypomania) also occur at a characteristic time of the year (e.g., depression disappears in the spring).

C. In the last 2 years, two Major Depressive Episodes have occurred that demonstrate the temporal seasonal relationships defined in Criteria A and B, and no nonseasonal Major Depressive Episodes have occurred during that same period.

D. Seasonal Major Depressive Episodes (as described above) substantially outnumber the nonseasonal Major Depressive Episodes that may have occurred over the individual's lifetime.

From American Psychiatric Association. (1994). *Diagnostic and statistical manual of mental disorders, fourth edition*. Washington, DC: Author.

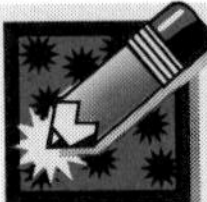

DSM-IV CRITERIA FOR MANIC EPISODE

A. A distinct period of abnormally and persistently elevated, expansive, or irritable mood, lasting at least 1 week (or any duration if hospitalization is necessary).

B. During the period of mood disturbance, three (or more) of the following symptoms have persisted (four if the mood is only irritable) and have been present to a significant degree:

(1) inflated self-esteem or grandiosity
(2) decreased need for sleep (e.g., feels rested after only 3 hours of sleep)
(3) more talkative than usual or pressure to keep talking
(4) flight of ideas or subjective experience that thoughts are racing
(5) distractibility (i.e., attention too easily drawn to unimportant or irrelevant external stimuli)
(6) increase in goal-directed activity (either socially, at work or school, or sexually) or psychomotor agitation
(7) excessive involvement in pleasurable activities that have a high potential for painful consequences (e.g., engaging in unrestrained buying sprees, sexual indiscretions, or foolish business investments)

C. The symptoms do not meet criteria for a Mixed Episode.

D. The mood disturbance is sufficiently severe to cause marked impairment in occupational functioning or in usual social activities or relationships with others, or to necessitate hospitalization to prevent harm to self or others, or there are psychotic features.

E. The symptoms are not due to the direct physiological effects of a substance (e.g., a drug of abuse, a medication, or other treatment) or a general medical condition (e.g., hyperthyroidism).

Note: Manic-like episodes that are clearly caused by somatic antidepressant treatment (e.g., medication, electroconvulsive therapy, light therapy) should not count toward a diagnosis of Bipolar I Disorder.

From American Psychiatric Association. (1994). *Diagnostic and statistical manual of mental disorders, fourth edition*. Washington, DC: Author.

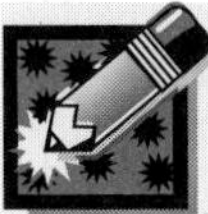

DSM-IV DIAGNOSTIC CRITERIA FOR DYSTHYMIC DISORDER

A. Depressed mood for most of the day, for more days than not, as indicated either by subjective account or observation by others, for at least 2 years. **Note:** In children and adolescents, mood can be irritable and duration must be at least 1 year.

B. Presence, while depressed, of two (or more) of the following:
(1) poor appetite or overeating
(2) insomnia or hypersomnia
(3) low energy or fatigue
(4) low self-esteem
(5) poor concentration or difficulty making decisions
(6) feelings of hopelessness

C. During the 2-year period (1 year for children or adolescents) of the disturbance, the person has never been without the symptoms in Criteria A and B for more than 2 months at a time.

D. No Major Depressive Episode has been present during the first 2 years of the disturbance (1 year for children and adolescents); i.e., the disturbance is not better accounted for by chronic Major Depressive Disorder, or Major Depressive Disorder, In Partial Remission.

Note: There may have been a previous Major Depressive Episode provided there was a full remission (no significant signs or symptoms for 2 months) before development of the Dysthymic Disorder. In addition, after the initial 2 years (1 year in children or adolescents) of Dysthymic Disorder, there may be superimposed episodes of Major Depressive Disorder, in which case both diagnoses may be given when the criteria are met for a Major Depressive Episode.

E. There has never been a Manic Episode, a Mixed Episode, or a Hypomanic Episode, and criteria have never been met for Cyclothymic Disorder.

F. The disturbance does not occur exclusively during the course of a chronic Psychotic Disorder, such as Schizophrenia or Delusional Disorder.

G. The symptoms are not due to the direct physiological effects of a substance (e.g., a drug of abuse, a medication) or a general medical condition (e.g., hypothyroidism).

H. The symptoms cause clinically significant distress or impairment in social, occupational, or other important areas of functioning.

Specify if:
Early Onset: if onset is before age 21 years
Late Onset: if onset is age 21 years or older

Specify (for most recent 2 years of Dysthymic Disorder):
With Atypical Features

From American Psychiatric Association. (1994). *Diagnostic and statistical manual of mental disorders, fourth edition.* Washington, DC: Author.

Because mania is rare before the onset of puberty, this diagnosis is not typically seen in children (Kaplan & Sadock, 1991). In terms of course of illness, both the manic and major depressive episodes in bipolar disorder are more frequent than depressive episodes in unipolar depression without a history of mania (APA, 1994).

THE CLIENT WITH DYSTHYMIA

Dysthymia is a relatively common form of depression, with an estimated lifetime prevalence ranging from 2.9 to 5.4 percent. The signs and symptoms of dysthymia are chronic and are less severe than those of major depression (see Diagnostic Criteria display, "Diagnostic Criteria for Dysthymia"). Onset is typically insidious and occurs during childhood, adolescence, or early adulthood. When asked how long they've been depressed, these people commonly reply, "All my life." People with dysthymia often appear introverted, morose, and self-deprecating. They may be chronically complaining, demanding, brooding, and sarcastic. Because of their chronic difficulties in concentrating, social withdrawal, and difficulty sustaining emotional intimacy in relationships, these people commonly experience school failure, unemployment, and divorce. Other complications of dysthymia are alcohol and drug abuse, as well as episodes of major depression.

Individual insight-oriented psychotherapy is the most common form of treatment and is recommended as the treatment of choice by many clinicians. Psychotherapy is sometimes combined with antidepressant medication (Kaplan & Sadock, 1991).

THE CLIENT WITH CYCLOTHYMIA

Cyclothymia is a chronic mood disturbance considered to be a mild form of bipolar disorder. It is characterized by numerous periods of abnormally elevated, expansive, or irritable mood (hypomania), alternating with numerous periods of depressed mood or a mixture of symptoms from both states (see Diagnostic Criteria display, "Diagnostic Criteria for Cyclothymia"). Approximately 50 percent of people with this disorder have depression as their major symptom and are most likely to seek professional help when depressed.

The lives of these people are difficult, because changes in mood are irregular and abrupt, sometimes occurring within hours. Marital difficulties, unstable relationships, impaired school and work performance, and alcohol and drug abuse are common. Lithium is the treatment of choice for cyclothymia (Kaplan & Sadock, 1991).

THE CLIENT WITH MOOD DISORDER DUE TO A GENERAL MEDICAL CONDITION (DEPRESSED)

Numerous general medical conditions, both physical disorders and associated drug therapy, are capable of causing depressive symptoms. A mood with depressive features resembles a major depressive episode but is due to a specific physiological disturbance (APA, 1994).

Medical illnesses commonly associated with depression include acquired immunodeficiency syndrome, endocrine disorders such as Cushing's and Addison's syndromes, and diabetes; metabolic disturbances such as hyperthyroidism, hypothyroidism, and hypoxia; vitamin deficiences including thiamine, niacin, and B_{12}; vascular disturbances such as cerebral arteriosclerosis, hypertensive encephalopathy, and systemic lupus erythematosus; neoplastic processes such as space-occupying lesions in the brain or cancer of the pancreas; and neurological diseases such as stroke, Parkinson's and Alzheimer's diseases, and Huntington's chorea. The most common drugs associated with depressive syndromes are antihypertensives, oral contraceptives, steroids, barbiturates, benzodiazepines, cimetidine, beta-blockers, and cocaine (Cassem, 1987).

When possible, the underlying general medical condition responsible for the depression is corrected. In the case of medications, lowering the dose, switching to an alternative drug, or discontinuing the drug altogether should result in the resolution of depressive symptoms. When the underlying cause cannot be eradicated, the depressive illness needs to be treated actively. Antidepressant medications, psychostimulants, and electroconvulsive therapy all have been found to be effective in treating medically ill persons who have a depressive syndrome.

THE CLIENT WITH ADJUSTMENT DISORDER WITH DEPRESSED MOOD

An adjustment disorder may occur at any age. The characteristic feature of this disorder is a maladaptive reac-

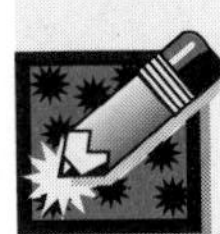

DSM-IV DIAGNOSTIC CRITERIA FOR CYCLOTHYMIC DISORDER

A. For at least 2 years, the presence of numerous periods with hypomanic symptoms and numerous periods with depressive symptoms that do not meet criteria for a Major Depressive Episode. **Note:** In children and adolescents, the duration must be at least 1 year.

B. During the above 2-year period (1 year in children and adolescents), the person has not been without the symptoms in Criterion A for more than 2 months at a time.

C. No Major Depressive Episode, Manic Episode, or Mixed Episode has been present during the first 2 years of the disturbance.

Note: After the initial 2 years (1 year in children and adolescents) of Cyclothymic Disorder, there may be superimposed Manic or Mixed Episodes (in which case both Bipolar I Disorder and Cyclothymic Disorder may be diagnosed) or Major Depressive Episodes (in which case both Bipolar II Disorder and Cyclothymic Disorder may be diagnosed).

D. The symptoms in Criterion A are not better accounted for by Schizoaffective Disorder and are not superimposed on Schizophrenia, Schizophreniform Disorder, Delusional Disorder, or Psychotic Disorder Not Otherwise Specified.

E. The symptoms are not due to the direct physiological effects of a substance (e.g., a drug of abuse, a medication) or a general medical condition (e.g., hyperthyroidism).

F. The symptoms cause clinically significant distress or impairment in social, occupational, or other important areas of functioning.

From American Psychiatric Association. (1994). *Diagnostic and statistical manual of mental disorders, fourth edition*. Washington, DC: Author.

tion to one or more psychosocial stressors (see Diagnostic Criteria display, "Diagnostic Criteria for Adjustment Disorders."). Examples of stressors that may lead to an adjustment disorder with depressive symptoms include physical illness, marital discord, divorce, getting married, leaving home for college, and natural disasters. The disorder generally resolves after the stressor ceases or, if the stressor persists, when a new level of adaptation is achieved (APA, 1994).

DSM-IV DIAGNOSTIC CRITERIA FOR ADJUSTMENT DISORDERS

A. The development of emotional or behavioral symptoms in response to an identifiable stressor(s) occurring within 3 months of the onset of the stressor(s).

B. These symptoms or behaviors are clinically significant as evidenced by either of the following:
(1) marked distress that is in excess of what would be expected from exposure to the stressor
(2) significant impairment in social or occupational (academic) functioning

C. The stress-related disturbance does not meet the criteria for another specific Axis I disorder and is not merely an exacerbation of a preexisting Axis I or Axis II disorder.

D. The symptoms do not represent Bereavement.

E. Once the stressor (or its consequences) has terminated, the symptoms do not persist for more than an additional 6 months.

Specify if:
Acute: if the disturbance lasts less than 6 months
Chronic: if the disturbance lasts for 6 months or longer

From American Psychiatric Association. (1994). *Diagnostic and statistical manual of mental disorders, fourth edition.* Washington, DC: Author.

THE CLIENT WITH PATHOLOGICAL GRIEF

Pathological grief, also called *complicated bereavement* and *unresolved grief,* may be manifested in several ways. Worden (1991) identified four categories of pathological grief: (1) chronic grief reactions, (2) delayed grief reactions, (3) exaggerated grief reactions, and (4) masked grief reactions.

Chronic grief is excessive in duration and never comes to a satisfactory conclusion. People experiencing chronic grief are generally aware of the problem and may describe their distress by saying, "I'm not getting back to living" or "This thing is not ending for me."

In delayed grief, the person did not sufficiently experience his or her emotional reactions at the time of the loss. Subsequently, when another loss occurs, the person experiences symptoms of grief that seem excessive.

Exaggerated grief response refers to situations in which a normal grief reaction is intensified to the extent of becoming disabling. A depressive syndrome is a normal reaction to the loss of a loved one, but when the bereavement is associated with suicidal ideation, severe functional impairment, and morbid preoccupation with worthlessness, it is considered to be complicated by a major depression (APA, 1994). Severe alcoholism or other substance abuse that develops in response to the death is another example of exaggerated grief (Worden, 1991).

People with a masked grief reaction do not recognize that their symptoms are related to a loss. Grief may be disguised as a physical symptom or some type of maladaptive behavior. The physical symptoms that develop may be similar to those of the deceased.

Factors that may predispose a person to a pathological grief reaction include the circumstances surrounding the loss, the person's relationship to the deceased, and social and personal variables. Table 9–5 provides an outline of these risk factors.

TABLE 9–5
Risk Factors for Pathological Grief Reactions

CIRCUMSTANCES SURROUNDING THE LOSS
- Uncertainty over the loss (e.g., a soldier missing in action)
- Multiple losses (e.g., resulting from a fire or airplane crash)

RELATIONSHIP TO THE DECEASED
- Ambivalent relationship with unexpressed hostility
- Highly dependent relationship
- History of sexual abuse by the deceased

SOCIAL VARIABLES
- Absence of social support network
- Death not socially accepted as a loss (e.g., abortion)
- Socially unacceptable death (e.g., suicide)

PERSONAL VARIABLES
- Personal history of depressive illness
- Self-concept includes the role of the "strong one"
- Inability to tolerate severe emotional distress

Data from Worden, J. W. (1991). *Grief counseling and grief therapy: A handbook for the mental health practitioner* (2nd ed.) New York: Springer Publishing; and Lazare, A. (1979). *Outpatient psychiatry: Diagnosis and treatment.* Baltimore: Williams & Wilkins.

THERAPEUTIC INTERVENTIONS

SOMATIC TREATMENTS

Pharmacological Treatment

Tricyclic antidepressants (TCAs) continue to be a frequently used treatment for unipolar depression. The improvement rate ranges from 50 to 85 percent and averages 65 percent (Hirschfeld & Goodwin, 1988). Researchers who have attempted to identify which depressed clients will respond best to TCAs have found the following factors to be predictive of a positive outcome: (1) a diagnosis of major depression, melancholic type; (2) the absence of significant personality disturbance prior to the depressive episode; (3) one or more previous episodes of depression that were followed by complete or nearly complete recovery; (4) a prior positive response to antidepressant treatment; (5) a positive family history of depression; and (6) a past history of multiple depressive episodes. The subgroup of clients diagnosed with dysthymia have also been found to respond favorably to TCAs. When psychotic features (e.g., delusions) are present in a major depression, the combination of a neuroleptic and a TCA provides the best results (Simpson & Singh, 1990). The improvement rate for childhood depression with the administration of TCAs appears to be similar to that of adults. Adolescents, however, have been found to have a less favorable overall response (40 to 50 percent) (Akiskal & Weller, 1989).

The monoamine oxidase inhibitors (MAOIs) are effective alternatives to the TCAs. These drugs tend to be used less frequently though, because of the risk of hypertensive crisis associated with the ingestion of tyramine-containing foods and beverages (see Fig. 9–2 in Nursing Process section later in the chapter). Although MAOIs and TCAs are similarly efficacious in treating endogenous depression, the MAOIs appear to be superior for depressions that are described as atypical. Differing from clients with typical endogenous depression, these clients present with symptoms of overeating, oversleeping, lethargy, and high levels of anxiety (Kurtz, 1990). Studies are now being conducted on the use of MAOIs in adolescents.

For a number of depressed persons who do not respond to a TCA or MAOI, the addition of lithium carbonate has been found to augment the response. Once remission of overt symptoms has occurred, antidepressant drugs are continued for 6 to 12 months to prevent relapse (Hirschfeld & Goodwin, 1988).

Because clients with bipolar disorder may become manic or hypomanic when given antidepressants, those with moderate or moderately severe depression are generally treated with lithium alone. With severe bipolar depressions, treatment is begun with lithium and an antidepressant together (Hirschfeld & Goodwin, 1988). Ongoing treatment, or maintenance therapy, with lithium has been found to reduce the severity and frequency of depressive episodes in clients with bipolar and unipolar disorder (Jefferson & Greist, 1990).

Lithium carbonate is being used more frequently in children and adolescents, especially those with bipolar illness or those whose illness does not respond to TCAs. Lithium is more likely than TCAs to be effective in depressed adolescents with a family history of bipolar disorder, even in the absence of a personal history of hypomania or mania. Because the long-term effects of lithium on growing children are unknown, treatment needs to be carefully monitored (Akiskal & Weller, 1989). Monitoring the client's response to the pharmacological treatment of depression is an important nursing function. The nurse can expect that the first symptoms to improve are poor sleep and appetite patterns, followed by agitation, anxiety, depressed mood, and hopelessness. Additional target symptoms for the antidepressants include low energy, poor concentration, helplessness, and decreased libido (Kaplan & Sadock, 1991). Assessment of suicide risk should be repeated during the period in which the client is experiencing greater energy in response to the pharmacological treatment. Continuing suicidal ideation in the presence of increased energy can lead to acting out of self-destructive thoughts. The monitoring of unpleasant side effects as well as more serious untoward reactions, such as urinary retention in the case of TCAs, is also critical. Finally, nurses have an important role in ensuring that the client and family understand the purpose, actions, and effects of these medications.

Electroconvulsive Therapy

Electroconvulsive therapy (ECT) is the electrical induction of modified grand mal seizures for the purpose of producing therapeutic change. It is an accepted, safe, and efficacious form of treatment for major depression, although the exact mechanism of action remains unclear. Generally, ECT is used only after a trial of antidepressant medication has failed; however, in certain situations (e.g., history of poor antidepressant drug response or good ECT response or a high risk of suicidal behavior), it might be chosen as an initial treatment. Although there are no conditions under which ECT is absolutely contraindicated, certain circumstances are associated with a higher risk of mortality or significant morbidity. These include increased intracranial pressure, such as caused by space-occupying intracerebral lesions; recent myocardial infarction; unstable vascular aneurysm or malformation; retinal detachment; and pheochromocytoma. The use of ECT in children is extremely rare and should be reserved for extreme cases of depression that are clearly unresponsive to all other available treatments (Weiner & Coffey, 1990).

ECT should always be a voluntary procedure, and the client should be fully informed of the reasons for and nature of the procedure, alternative treatment options, the probable number of ECT treatments, and the major potential risks. A formal consent document should be signed by the client.

In addition to a complete medical and psychiatric history and examination, a pre-ECT evaluation should include a review of the case by the anesthesia provider and results from the following laboratory tests: serum electrolyte levels, hemoglobin or hematocrit, and electrocardiogram. It is generally recommended that psychotropic medications be discontinued (Weiner & Coffey, 1990).

ECT is generally conducted in a treatment room set up especially for this purpose. The treatment team includes a psychiatrist experienced in administering ECT, an anesthesia provider, an ECT nurse, and post anesthesia nurses. Treatments are given three times per week until a plateau is reached in terms of clinical improvement. This usually occurs after 6 to 12 treatments. Prior to each treatment, the patient remains NPO for at least 8 hours to avoid the risk of vomiting and aspiration. An anticholinergic premedication such as atropine is administered within 30 minutes of the treatment to prevent bradycardia or asystole. After positive-pressure ventilation with 100 percent oxygen is begun, general anesthesia, as well as a muscle relaxant such as succinylcholine, is administered. While the client is asleep, either unilateral or bilateral electrodes are placed on the frontotemporal regions of the head. Unilateral ECT is often as effective as bilateral ECT and produces less memory loss. Because of the pronounced, although transient and usually benign, increases in heart rate and blood pressure that occur with ECT, vital sign and electrocardiographic monitoring is carried out throughout the procedure (Weiner & Coffey, 1990).

After each ECT treatment, nursing staff monitor vital signs and neurological status every 5 minutes until the client is awake and then every 15 minutes until the client is alert (Sands et al., 1987). Confusion is common after ECT, and the client needs to be reoriented to person, time, and place as necessary. A nurse remains with the client until he or she is reoriented and reassures the client that any memory loss is temporary. Over the course of ECT, nursing observations of the client's response in terms of mood and behavior are critical in determining the need for additional treatments.

See Chapter 27 for an in-depth discussion of ECT.

Sleep Manipulation

Manipulation of the sleep–wake cycle has been attempted as a treatment for depression on the basis of findings indicating disturbed circadian rhythms in depressed persons. Studies being conducted at the National Institutes of Health are finding that in most endogenously depressed clients, a single night of sleep deprivation brings about a temporary remission in symptoms. Rapid-cycling manic–depressive clients are especially responsive to sleep deprivation during their depressive phase, often switching out of depression after 24 hours without sleep. Partial sleep deprivation, during the second half of the night (e.g., staying awake from 3:00 A.M. to 11:00 A.M.), has been found to be as effective as total sleep deprivation in some depressed clients. However, most who respond to either approach awaken depressed after their next night of sleep (Ryan et al., 1987). Possible explanations for recent findings related to sleep manipulation and ways of sustaining the antidepressant effect are the subject of current investigations.

High-Intensity Light Therapy

SAD, also known as *winter depression*, appears to be causally related to seasonal change in the amount of light in the environment and has been shown to be responsive to treatment with high-intensity light or phototherapy. The exact mechanism of action is as yet unclear. In the few studies done thus far, this form of treatment has been found to be ineffective in other forms of depression.

Current research indicates morning phototherapy as the treatment of choice for the typical winter-depressive client with hypersomnia and difficulty awakening in the morning. One to two hours of 2500-lux light should be administered immediately upon awakening. This is approximately five times the intensity of light found in a well-lit office. Clients sit about 3 feet away from the phototherapy unit with the light source at eye level. It is generally recommended that clients look at the light source directly for a few seconds every few minutes. Otherwise they are free to engage in an activity such as reading, watching television, or exercising.

An antidepressant response to treatment can be expected within 2 to 4 days and is usually complete by the end of 2 weeks. Daily phototherapy of 30 minutes' duration is generally effective in maintaining improvement. Side effects have thus far been uncommon, although they may include irritability, eye strain, headaches, and insomnia. Decreasing the duration of therapy or sitting farther from the light source may serve to reverse these effects (Elmore, 1991).

The nurse working with the client receiving high-intensity light therapy plays an important role in ensuring its proper implementation so that potential beneficial effects are maximized and untoward effects minimized. Because of the amount of time light therapy entails, clients may need help reorganizing their daily schedules to fit the therapy into their routine. It is important that nurses working with depressed clients strongly discourage self-administration of phototherapy as well as the use of unapproved light sources, such as sun or heat lamps, because clients may inadvertently harm themselves.

PSYCHOTHERAPEUTIC INTERVENTIONS

Several forms of psychotherapy are available for the treatment of depression that may or may not be used in conjunction with somatic interventions. The therapies described in this section are most appropriately used by those with advanced training. However, the psychiatric staff nurse may usefully apply certain aspects of the therapies in individual and group work with hospitalized clients. More detailed discussions of psychotherapy, differentiating the role of the generalist staff nurse from that of the advanced specialist, are provided in Chapters 21 and 23.

Psychoanalytical Psychotherapy

The primary goal of psychoanalytical psychotherapy is to effect change in the personality structure rather than simply alleviate symptoms. Therapy is aimed at improving the capacity for interpersonal trust and intimacy, strengthening coping mechanisms, increasing the range of emotions that can be experienced, and enhancing the capacity to grieve. Therapy often continues for many years, although in recent decades several short-term psychoanalytical approaches have been developed.

Psychoanalytical psychotherapy differs from the other psychotherapeutic approaches in its focus on the transference relationship developed between the client and therapist. This relationship is used to examine and reexperience important past and present relationships that may be contributing to the client's depression (Hirschfeld & Shea, 1989).

Clients most suitable for psychoanalytical psychotherapy are those who (1) are highly motivated to change; (2) have the capacity for introspection and the ability to see connections among thoughts, feelings, and behaviors; and (3) are able to tolerate anxiety and frustration. A psychodynamic treatment approach is most commonly used to treat depressions that are chronic and of mild severity (Hirschfeld & Goodwin, 1988).

Interpersonal Therapy

Interpersonal therapy was developed by Klerman and Weissman (Klerman et al., 1984) and is based on the theoretical work of Meyer (1948–1952) and Sullivan (1953). The primary goals of interpersonal therapy are the alleviation of depressive symptoms, the improvement of self-esteem, and the development of more effective skills for dealing with social and interpersonal relationships. The therapeutic focus is on current situations in the person's life, and the course of treatment is relatively short (e.g., 12 to 16 weekly sessions). This approach was specifically developed to treat nonpsychotic and nonbipolar depressions.

In interpersonal therapy, the client is educated about depression, with emphasis placed on its good prognosis. One or two major problem areas are then defined and become the focus of treatment. Problem areas commonly addressed include abnormal grief reactions, interpersonal role disputes (e.g., marital conflict), role transitions (e.g., divorce), and interpersonal deficits (e.g., lack of social skills). Medications are often used as an adjunct to reduce depressive symptoms (Hirschfeld & Shea, 1989).

Behavioral Therapy

Which behavioral theory of depression is followed guides the treatment approach used. Regardless of the interventions used, the primary goals of therapy are to increase the number of positively reinforcing interactions with the environment and to decrease the number of negative interactions in the depressed person's life. Treatment is usually short term (4 to 12 weeks) and highly structured.

Strategies used in behavioral therapy include having the client keep a daily record of his or her moods and activities. Based on these records the therapist encourages increased involvement in activities associated with positive moods and avoidance of situations that trigger feelings of depression. In addition, the client is taught how to manage reactions to negative events better, that is, through preparation for such events and substitution of positive for negative thoughts about them. Time management is used to increase the client's participation in enjoyable events. Assertiveness training and role playing may be used to address social skills deficits and problematic interaction patterns. Relaxation training is used to produce a mood state incompatible with depression. Detailed manuals that outline specific behavioral treatment approaches for unipolar, nonpsychotic depression have been developed (Hirschfeld & Shea, 1989).

Cognitive–Behavioral Therapy

Cognitive–behavioral therapy was developed by Beck (1979) specifically for the treatment of nonpsychotic, unipolar depression. It is a short-term therapy, typically lasting from 12 to 20 sessions. The primary goals are to alleviate depression and decrease the likelihood of its recurrence through helping clients change their way of thinking.

The following are the three overall components to cognitive–behavioral therapy:

- Didactic teaching, in which the cognitive–behavioral view of depression is explained
- Cognitive techniques, involving the elicitation and testing of negative automatic thoughts and identification and analysis of the maladaptive assumptions on which they are based
- Behavioral techniques, such as scheduling of pleasurable activities, role playing, and graded task assignments

The premise behind these techniques is that identifying and changing maladaptive cognitions and relevant behaviors will reverse the symptoms of depression (Wright & Beck, 1983).

The psychiatric staff nurse can use many of the strategies of behavioral and cognitive–behavioral therapy with the hospitalized depressed client. The daily activity schedule, testing of negative automatic thoughts, and graded task assignments, as discussed in the following sections, are a few of them.

Daily Activity Schedule. A written daily activity schedule can be created in the form of a chart that specifies each waking hour with blank spaces next to it. Using the chart, the nurse works with the client to list all daily activities as they take place and to record how much enjoyment was experienced for each activity. A scale of 1 to 5 can be used, with 1 equal to very little enjoyment and 5 indicating a lot of enjoyment. After looking back over their daily activity schedule, depressed clients are often surprised to see how much they can do and what they are still able to enjoy. This activity record can also serve as a tool to help clients increase their involvement in activities associated with positive moods (Dreyfus, 1988).

Testing of Negative Automatic Thoughts. The identification and testing of negative automatic thoughts have been likened to a scientific investigation, in which data are collected to test the stated hypothesis (Manderino & Bzdek, 1989). For example, consider the common situation of the depressed client refusing to get out of bed and protesting with statements such as, "I'm too tired and weak," "I can't get up," "It won't make me feel any better," and "I'll only feel worse." To intervene, the nurse begins by identifying aloud the client's negative thinking and gently questioning the validity of the assumption that getting out of bed will have no positive effect. This by itself may serve to disprove the client's self-defeating thinking and lead to a change in behavior. If not, the nurse moves to the next step—having the client test the truth of the negative assumption. The nurse engages the client in an "experiment" involving getting out of bed and experiencing what this feels like. Often, the effort is experienced positively by the client. At this stage, the nurse helps the client recognize that the favorable outcome contradicts his or her negative predictions (Manderino & Bzdek, 1989).

Graded Task Assignment. Another easily applied behavioral technique is the graded task assignment, in which what seems like an overwhelmingly large task to the depressed client is broken down into small, manageable steps. For example, for the client who has become isolated and withdrawn from others, the nurse and client might develop the following graded tasks:

- *Assignment 1:* Eat lunch in the dining room with other clients present. Do not feel obligated to interact with the others.
- *Assignment 2:* Watch television in the day room and discuss some aspect of the program with one other client present.
- *Assignment 3:* Respond to the comments of another client during a group psychotherapy session.
- *Assignment 4:* Initiate a game of cards with another client on the unit.

It is important that the assignments be designed to maximize the possibility of the client's success. The series of assignments should begin with a fairly simple task, with additional tasks gradually becoming more complex. As the client experiences success, self-confidence will likely increase (Manderino & Bzdek, 1989).

Family Therapy

Although family therapy is not viewed as a primary treatment for depression, it is indicated for situations in which a client's depression appears to be maintained by marital and family interactions or when the depression negatively influences the person's functioning in the family. Episodes of depression have been associated with family dysfunction. Studies have found that depressed persons have a high rate of divorce, and approximately 50 percent of spouses report they would not have married the person or had children had they known that the person was going to have a mood disorder (Kaplan & Sadock, 1991). Furthermore, children with a depressed parent are at increased risk of psychiatric disorder. The psychiatric clinical nurse specialist is best prepared to provide family therapy; however, the psychiatric staff nurse can fulfill the important role of educating family members about mood disorders and their treatment. Such education can improve the client's compliance with treatment as well as the family's ability to provide a supportive environment (Goldwyn, 1988).

THE NURSE'S ROLE

In working with the depressed client, the nurse applies one or more of the etiological theories of depression described earlier. Theory provides the nurse with a basis for understanding the client's experience and guides the interventions chosen as well as the evaluation of these interventions. In addition to the etiological theories of depression, several nursing theories are relevant to working with the depressed client, for example, Orem's (1971) theory of self-care and Peplau's (1952, 1962) writings on the therapeutic nurse–client relationship. Knowledge of milieu and group theory helps the nurse provide a therapeutic environment for the depressed client.

THE NURSING PROCESS

The professional practice standards of psychiatric–mental health nursing developed by the American Nurses Association serve as the framework for the application of the nursing process to depression (American Nurses Association, 1994).

Assessment

Collecting data from the severely depressed client can be a long and tedious process. Thinking is slowed, and responses to questions may be in monosyllables; both of these characteristics are symptoms of the illness. An empathic and patient approach is especially important with the depressed person who already suffers from low self-esteem. Seeking data from other sources such as family and previous health care providers can be invaluable.

Predisposing risk factors for depression are often found in the client's social and developmental history. The nurse should always ask the client about problems and stresses during childhood, such as separations, family deaths or illnesses, and sexual or physical abuse. School, work, and social histories provide important information on the client's level of functioning over time, potential strengths, and possible areas of stress.

Physical appearance is a useful indicator of the severity of depression. For example, an emaciated, disheveled presentation may indicate a severe lack of appetite and an inability to care for oneself. Depressed persons are at high risk for self-harm, and so details of past and present suicidal ideation need to be carefully assessed. See Chapters 8 and 16 for a full discussion of the nursing assessment of the potential for suicide.

The following case study of Mary M. illustrates a useful framework for gathering and documenting an initial assessment (see also Nursing Care Plan 9–1). Documentation of how the depression developed, including onset, precipitating events, and progression, makes up the history of the present problem. **Neurovegetative symptoms**, including disturbances in sleep, appetite, weight, **libido**, energy level, and interests, are compared with the client's baseline in these areas. A past psychiatric history, including prior episodes of depression or mania, is important for an accurate diagnosis of the current problem. Previous treatment for depression and the outcome of the treatment have implications for which treatment approach will be used for the current problem. For example, people who responded well to a particular antidepressant medication in the past are likely to do so again. It is important to take a thorough medical history, including a list of prescribed medications, to rule out an organic basis for depression. Family medical and psychiatric histories can also contribute to an understanding of the client's problems not only because depression is a familial illness but also because the family history can reveal stressors that exacerbate the client's depression. Also, if a depressed family member has responded favorably to a particular somatic treatment, it is more likely that the present client also will respond to this treatment.

Case Study: The Client with Major Depression (Mary)

Identifying Information. Mary M. is a 61-year-old married woman referred to the inpatient psychiatric unit by her internist. She is a practicing Roman Catholic and has worked as a secretary for 18 years at a school for emotionally disturbed children. Mary lives with her husband, Ron, and a 24-year-old daughter, Gail, in their own home.

Presenting Complaint. Mary states, "My husband is tired of me crying all of the time, and so am I."

History of Present Problem. Mary states that over the past 3 months, she has experienced increasing **dysphoria, anhedonia**, feelings of guilt and worthlessness, intense crying, social isolation, and inadequate work performance.

Mary sleeps 10 to 15 hours per night, experiencing no difficulty falling asleep or middle-of-the-night or early-morning awakening. Her appetite has diminished during the past month, with a reported weight loss of 12 pounds. She eats erratically, usually snacks, and meals are prepared by her husband and daughter. She has not been able to work, cook, sew, or do household chores and generally spends the day in bed. She has had no sexual interest or activity for the past year. Mary describes no interests or involvements outside the home, except for weekly attendance at church.

Mornings are the most difficult for Mary—she feels increased anxiety, has difficulty breathing, and crys a lot. She admits to occasional suicidal ideation in the form of a passive wish to be dead in hopes of relieving her emotional pain. She denies a history of suicide attempts or current suicidal plan. She denies alcohol or drug abuse.

Current life stressors reported by Mary include

- Her brother's death 6 months ago. Mary had not seen him in 15 years and expresses guilt that they were not close.
- Her sister's surgery for cancer 5 months earlier. Mary is fearful that she will die in the near future.
- Her daughter Gail's plans to leave home to marry. Mary fears that she will be even more lonely when her daughter leaves.
- Impending retirement from her job. Marry worries about how she will use so much free time.

Past Psychiatric History. Mary has had no prior hospitalizations or outpatient psychiatric treatment. She denies previous episodes of depression. There is no history of mania or hypomania.

Medical History. Mary's only physical ailment is borderline hypertension, not treated by medication.

Family History. Mary's mother died from a myocardial infarction at the age of 72, 20 years ago. Her father died from a myocardial infarction at the age of 80, 10 years ago. Mary's brother, who died 6 months ago of a stroke, was 62 years old. Her sister is 59 years old and is divorced with two daughters, ages 31 and 34; she was recently diagnosed with cervical cancer. Mary believes her maternal grandmother was depressed but knows no details about this.

Social and Developmental History. Mary is the middle child of three siblings. Her mother's labor and delivery with her were normal, and developmental milestones (talking, walking, etc.) were reached at an early age. She denies any maladaptive behaviors or experiencing unusual stresses as a child. Academically, Mary was an A student throughout her educational experience. She had friends at school and in the community and did not date until after high school. She completed 2 years of business school via night courses while working as a secretary. Mary has held three secretarial jobs. Her present job is a lower status position than those previously held.

Mary was raised in Vermont and lived there until she was 22, at which time she moved to New York to marry Ron. They remained childless for 12 years before adopting Gail at the age of 3 months. Gail, now 24 years old, is a legal secretary and is planning to marry soon. Mary describes her own 39-year marriage as good but states they both take it for granted. She and Ron have not engaged in sexual activity for 1 1/2 years, which Mary attributes to her present emotional distress.

Mary is a practicing Roman Catholic, attending

weekly mass and occasional confession. Despite her husband's encouragement, she does not attend church social groups or participate in any other outside activity.

Mental Status Examination

General Appearance. Mary is an underweight woman who is appropriately dressed, although with a disheveled appearance. She presents with a downcast, averted gaze.

Speech. Mary speaks slowly and quietly. Her responses to questions are delayed, but her thinking is goal directed.

Thought Content. Themes of worthlessness, helplessness, guilt, hopelessness, and somatic concerns predominate.

Affect and Mood. **Affect** is constricted, with **mood** sad and depressed. Mary frequently engages in intense bouts of crying.

Motor Behavior. Posture is rigid, slumped slightly forward, with few spontaneous movements.

Perceptions. There is no evidence of delusions or hallucinations.

Suicide Potential. The wish for death is present, but there is no active suicidal intent or plan.

Orientation. Mary is oriented to person, place, and time.

Concentration. Concentration is impaired, as evidenced by an inability to do Serial 7s accurately and a digit span of 4 forward, none backward.

Recent and Remote Memory. Mary's recent memory is intact, with three of three objects recalled after 5 minutes. She is able to describe accurately events from the past.

Insight and Judgment. Mary has insight into her illness. Her judgment is intact.

Formulation of Impression

Mary presents with a 3-month history of depressed mood; anhedonia; feelings of worthlessness, guilt, hopelessness, and helplessness; suicidal ideation; withdrawn behavior and impaired functioning; decreased concentration; **somatic preoccupations;** and decreased appetite and weight loss. Symptoms are consistent with that of a major depression with melancholia. Mary's preoccupation with worthlessness, her suicidal ideation, and her marked functional impairment, all occurring in the context of multiple losses, are suggestive of bereavement complicated by major depression.

Nursing Diagnoses

The following nursing diagnoses for Mary M. are derived from the assessment data gathered:

- Mood Disturbance
- Dysfunctional Grieving
- Risk for Self-Directed Violence
- Self-Esteem Disturbance
- Self-Care Deficit
- Social Isolation
- Altered Nutrition

Additional nursing diagnoses that may apply to the person with depression include Altered Thought Processes, Sleep Pattern Disturbance, Anxiety, and Sensory-Perceptual Alterations.

The DSM-IV multiaxial diagnoses for Mary M. are as follows:

Axis I: 296.2x Major Depressive Disorder, Single Episode, With Melancholic Features
Axis II: V71.09 No Diagnosis
Axis III: Hypertension
Axis IV: Psychosocial and Environmental Problems: death of brother, serious illness of sister, anticipated retirement, daughter's impending marriage and move from parental home
Axis V: Current Global Assessment of Functioning (GAF) score: 31; highest GAF score in the past year: 7

Planning

Nursing Care Plan 9–1 for Mary M. illustrates how nursing diagnoses guide the development of goals and therapeutic interventions. Ideally, the nurse collaborates with the client in planning care. This can be difficult to do with the depressed person who is feeling hopeless, helpless, and unmotivated. The nurse's communication of the firm belief that the client will feel better with time can often be enough to engage the client in at least going along with the care plan. Setting small, short-term goals that the client can accomplish without much difficulty is important in fostering a sense of hope and improved self-esteem. The nurse should expect that with the immobilized depressed client, early interventions may need to be aimed at "doing for" the client, but the expectation should be that the client will gradually assume more independent functioning.

Implementation

Nursing interventions are guided by the nursing care plan. For the depressed client, priority needs to be given to preventing self-harm through ongoing assessment of suicide potential and maintenance of a safe environment. In addition, improving and maintaining physical health are important foci of care for the depressed client, who is likely to have an altered nutritional status and disturbed sleeping pattern. Monitoring for side effects of somatic treatments for depression is equally important to maintain biological integrity.

The depressed client is often socially isolated and withdrawn. Involving the client in individual and group interactions in the hospital unit will decrease his or her isolation and foster a sense of self-worth.

As the client's symptoms of depression respond to the psychotherapeutic and somatic interventions implemented, psychoeducation becomes feasible. Clients should be educated about the type of depression they have, as well as its possible causes. Specifically, the contribution of both neurobiological and psychosocial factors to the onset of depressive illness should be discussed. Informing the client of the signs and symptoms of depression is important so that recurrence can be

Nursing Care Plan 9–1 The Client with Major Depression (Mary M.)

► Nursing Diagnosis: Mood Disturbance

OUTCOME IDENTIFICATION	NURSING ACTIONS	RATIONALES	EVALUATION
1. By [date], Mary will recognize her mood disturbance and need for treatment.	1. Provide education about major depression and its treatment to Mary and her family.	1. Knowledge about their illness and its treatment gives clients a sense of control and increases the likelihood that they will comply with treatment.	*Goals met:* Mary has recognized her mood disturbance and the need for treatment.
2. By [date], Mary will accept the need for the somatic treatment prescribed.	2a. Observe and document Mary's response to somatic treatment. 2b. Observe for side effects, untoward reactions.	2a. Accurate evaluation of response to treatment is important in ongoing planning of treatment. Pointing out symptom improvements to client will facilitate continued acceptance of somatic treatment. 2b. Early observation of side effects decreases the possibility that they will become more severe with appropriate intervention. Decreasing discomfort from side effects increases the probability of the client's acceptance of treatment.	Mary's response to treatment has been good, as evidenced by a broad range of affect, decreased tearfulness, increased eye contact, and improved mood.
3. By [date], Mary will evidence change in mood by displaying a broader range of affect, decreased tearfulness, and increased eye contact and subjectively reporting improved mood.	3a. Document Mary's mood and affect through observation and subjective assessment. 3b. Administer psychotropics as prescribed.	3a. Although certain symptoms of major depression can be observed, the primary mood disturbance needs to be evaluated via client report. 3b. Antidepressant medication is usually an important part of the treatment of major depression and is highly effective.	

► Nursing Diagnosis: Dysfunctional Grieving

OUTCOME IDENTIFICATION	NURSING ACTIONS	RATIONALES	EVALUATION
1. By [date], Mary will identify recent and impending losses.	1. Assist Mary in the identification of losses.	1. Clients often do not identify certain events as losses. Being aware of losses facilitates the grieving process.	*Goals met:* Mary is able to identify her recent and impending losses.
2. By [date], Mary will express her thoughts and feelings related to her multiple losses.	2a. Encourage Mary to verbalize her thoughts and feelings and be available simply to listen. 2b. Foster communication between Mary and her family related to developmental life changes (e.g., daughter's marriage, Mary's retirement).	2a. Verbalizing thoughts and feelings related to losses serves to decrease the client's sense of isolation, allows for unrealistic blame and guilt to be challenged, and permits an exploration of the meaning of the losses to the client. 2b. Open communication among family members can lead to individual members' supporting each other and thus can strengthen the unit as a whole.	Mary is able to express her thoughts and feelings related to these losses with her nurse and family members.

Nursing Care Plan 9–1 The Client with Major Depression (Mary M.) (Continued)

OUTCOME IDENTIFICATION	NURSING ACTIONS	RATIONALES	EVALUATION
Nursing Diagnosis: Risk for Self-Directed Violence			
1. Mary will not harm herself.	1a. Maintain a safe environment. 1b. Assess for suicidal ideation on an ongoing basis.	1a. Easy access to means of harming themselves increases clients' likelihood of acting on suicidal ideation. 1b. Ongoing assessment is crucial, because clients with depression are at higher risk of acting on suicidal ideation when their energy level increases in response to treatment.	*Goal met:* Mary has been able to discuss her wish to be dead, rather than act on it. Her wish to be dead is no longer present.
2. By [date], Mary will discuss her wishes to be dead, rather than act on them.	2. Encourage nondestructive ventilation of feelings.	2. Describing and analyzing thoughts and feelings reduces the potential for acting on them destructively.	
Nursing Diagnosis: Self-Esteem Disturbance			
1. By [date], Mary will evidence a decrease in verbalizations of self-deprecatory ideas and will verbalize feelings of self-worth.	1a. Encourage Mary to get involved in tasks that can be accomplished with success. 1b. Provide praise for Mary's accomplishments. 1c. Assist Mary in identifying her strengths.	1a. Experiences of success lead to feelings of self-worth. 1b. Praise from others reinforces sense of self-worth. 1c. Clients with depression have a distorted cognitive view of themselves and need help identifying their strengths.	*Goal met:* Mary is able to express feelings of self-worth in relation to tasks accomplished and expresses fewer negative comments about herself.
Nursing Diagnosis: Self-Care Deficit			
1. By [date], Mary will resume self-care behaviors.	1a. Gradually increase the expectation that Mary will assume responsibility for hygiene and grooming. 1b. Provide Mary with positive feedback on her self-care behaviors.	1a. The expectations of those in a person's environment can significantly influence the person's behavior. 1b. Positive feedback increases the likelihood that desired behavior will recur.	*Goal met:* Mary has resumed self-care activities; her hygiene is good, and her appearance is no longer disheveled.
Nursing Diagnosis: Social Isolation			
1. By [date], Mary will become integrated into the unit milieu.	1. Encourage Mary to participate in groups, meetings, and social activities.	1. Participation with others on the unit decreases clients' social isolation, which not only stems from, but contributes to, depression.	*Goal met:* Mary has become an active participant within the unit milieu. She has taken on a leadership role in groups,

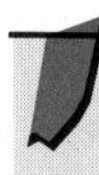

Nursing Care Plan 9–1 The Client with Major Depression (Mary M.) (Continued)

OUTCOME IDENTIFICATION	NURSING ACTIONS	RATIONALES	EVALUATION
2. By [date], Mary will initiate interactions with others.	2. Provide Mary with constructive feedback on her style of interactions with staff and others.	2. Depressed clients are often unaware that they tend to push others away through their negative style of interacting.	encouraging the involvement of others.

Nursing Diagnosis: Altered Nutrition

OUTCOME IDENTIFICATION	NURSING ACTIONS	RATIONALES	EVALUATION
1. By [date], Mary will achieve adequate nutritional status, and this will be maintained.	1a. Obtain Mary's diet history to determine her food preferences and eating habits.	1a. Clients are more likely to eat foods they previously enjoyed and if their eating habits are taken into consideration.	*Goal met:* Mary has achieved adequate nutritional status through eating regular meals, as evidenced by return to her baseline weight.
	1b. Consult with the nutritionist.	1b. The nutritionist can determine the client's nutritional needs and recommend how they can best be met.	
	1c. Monitor Mary's intake and weight.	1c. Information on the client's progress is important for ongoing planning.	
	1d. Physically feed Mary, if necessary.	1d. Severe depression can leave clients unable to feed themselves. As the illness improves with treatment, clients are actively encouraged to take responsibility for feeding.	
	1e. Sit with Mary during meals and encourage eating and drinking.	1e. Because eating tends to be a social experience, it can be helpful to be with the client during meals.	

identified early. Education regarding the maintenance of medication regimens should be conducted and supplemented with written materials (Fig. 9–2). See Appendix II at the end of the book for sources of additional information on depression.

Evaluation

Evaluation of the client's responses to nursing interventions should be ongoing. Questions the nurse might ask to evaluate the effectiveness of the nursing process with the depressed client include the following:

Does the client describe an improvement in mood and energy level?
Is there any evidence of suicidal ideation?
Has the client learned new, more effective ways of expressing feelings?
Has the verbalization of **self-deprecatory** ideas diminished?
Is the client initiating interactions with others?
Has the client's appetite improved? Has he or she gained weight?

In asking these and other questions, the nurse reflects on his or her own observations; on the observations of

FIGURE 9–2
An example of a handout that may be given to a client for whom a monoamine oxidase (MAO) inhibitor is prescribed for the treatment of depression. Instructions for foods, beverages, and drugs to avoid while taking MAO inhibitors are shown. (Adapted from McGlynn, T. J., & Metcalf, H. L. [Eds.]. [1989]. *Diagnosis and treatment of anxiety disorders: A physician's handbook* [p. 114]. Washington, DC: American Psychiatric Press.)

The following foods, beverages, and drugs must be avoided while you are taking MAO inhibitors **and for two weeks after discontinuing use:**

Meat and fish

- ⊘ Meats prepared with tenderizers
- ⊘ Meat extracts
- ⊘ Smoked or pickled fish
- ⊘ Beef or chicken liver
- ⊘ Dry sausage (Genoa salami, hard salami, pepperoni, bologna)

Fruits and vegetables

- ⊘ Canned figs
- ⊘ Broad bean (fava bean) pods
- ⊘ Bananas and avacodos (especiallly if overripe)

Dairy products

- ⊘ Cheese and foods containing cheese, such as cheese crackers and pizza (cottage cheese and cream cheese are allowed)
- ⊘ Yogurt and sour cream

Beverages

- ⊘ Beer, red wine, and other alcoholic beverages

Miscellaneous

- ⊘ Soy sauce
- ⊘ Yeast extract (including brewer's yeast in large quantities)
- ⊘ Excessive amounts of chocolate and caffeine
- ⊘ Spoiled or improperly refrigerated, handled, or stored protein-rich foods such as meats, fish, and dairy products
- ⊘ Foods that have undergone protein changes by aging, pickling, fermentation, or smoking

Drugs

- ⊘ Cold, hay fever, or sinus tablets or liquids
- ⊘ Nasal decongestants (tablets, drops, or spray)
- ⊘ Asthma inhalant medications
- ⊘ Anti-appetite or weight-reducing preparation
- ⊘ "Pep" pills or stimulants
- ⊘ Narcotics, including cocaine

other team members and the client's family; and, of utmost importance, on the client's description of his or her own experience.

▶CHAPTER SUMMARY

Depression is a significant mental health problem in the United States, resulting in tremendous costs to individuals, families, and society. There are several forms of depression, including major depression, bipolar depression, dysthymia, cyclothymia, organic mood syndrome, and adjustment disorder with depressed mood. Depression affects people of all ages and differs in its presentation at various developmental stages across the life span. Depression is a normal response to loss, but it becomes pathological when the tasks associated with mourning remain unresolved.

Multiple theories have been posited to explain the etiology of depression. As yet, no one theory fully explains this illness. Rather, most forms of depression likely result from complex interactions between neurobiological and psychosocial factors.

Several therapies, both somatic and psychotherapeutic, are available for the treatment of depressive disorders. The type of therapeutic approach used depends on a number of variables, including the type and severity of depression, the client's prior response to treatment, and the nurse therapist's theoretical orientation. A combination of somatic and psychotherapeutic interventions is commonly used.

The nurse working with the depressed client in a psychiatric setting plays an important role in (1) educating the client and his or her family about depression and its treatments, (2) conducting initial and ongoing assessment of the client's depressive symptoms, (3) monitoring the effects of treatment, and (4) providing a safe and therapeutic environment.

Suggestions for Clinical Conference

1. As an empathy-enhancing exercise, read William Styron's (1990) book about his own depression: *Darkness Visible.* Discuss your reactions to the book with your group.
2. Role-play an interview between a nurse and a grieving person who recently lost a loved one. Using the section on loss and grief, discuss and evaluate the findings of the interview, taking into account the client's phase in the life span.
3. Obtain case studies that portray examples of the six types of depression described in this chapter. A good source of these case studies is *DSM-IV Casebook* (Spitzer et al., 1994). As a group, evaluate each case study, apply a DSM-IV diagnosis and nursing diagnoses, and develop a nursing care plan.

References

Abraham, K. (1960a). A short study on the development of the libido. In *Selected papers on psychoanalysis* (pp. 418–501). New York: Basic Books. (Original work published 1924)

Abraham, K. (1960b). Notes on the psychoanalytic investigation and treatment of manic-depressive insanity and allied conditions. In *Selected papers on psychoanalysis* (pp. 137–156). New York: Basic Books. (Original work published 1911)

Akiskal, H. S., & Weller, E. B. (1989). Mood disorders and suicide in children and adolescents. In H. I. Kaplan & B. J. Sadock (Eds.), *Comprehensive textbook of psychiatry IV* (Vol. 2, pp. 1981–1994). Baltimore: Williams & Wilkins.

Altemus, M., & Gold, R. W. (1990). Neuroendocrinology and psychiatric illness. *Frontiers in Neuroendocrinology, 11*, 238–265.

American Academy of Pediatrics, Committee on Psychosocial Aspects of Child and Family Health. (1992) The pediatrician and childhood bereavement. *Pediatrics, 89*, 516–518.

American Nurses Association. (1994). *Statement on psychiatric–mental health nursing practice and standards of psychiatric–mental health clinical nursing practice.* Washington, DC: Author.

American Psychiatric Association. (1994). *Diagnostic and statistical manual of mental disorders* (4th ed.). Washington, DC: Author.

Austin, J. (1990). Assessment of coping mechanisms used by parents and children with chronic illness. *Maternal–Child Nursing, 15*, 98–102.

Ban, T. (1984). Chronic disease and depression in the geriatric population. *Journal of Clinical Psychiatry, 45*(3), 18–24.

Barraclough, B., Bunch, J., Nelson, B., & Sainsbury, P. (1974). A hundred cases of suicide: Clinical aspects. *British Journal of Psychiatry, 125*, 355–373.

Bauer, M. S., & Whybrow, P. C. (1988). Thyroid hormones and the central nervous system in affective illness: Interactions that may have clinical significance. *Integrated Psychiatry, 6*, 75–100.

Beardslee, W., Keller, M., Lavori, P., et al. (1983). Children of parents with major affective disorder: A review. *American Journal of Psychiatry, 140*, 825–833.

Beck, A. T. (1963) Thinking and depression, I: Idiosyncratic content and cognitive distortions. *Archives of General Psychiatry, 9*, 36–45.

Beck, A. T. (1964). Thinking and depression, II: Theory and therapy. *Archives of General Psychiatry, 10*, 561–571.

Beck, A. T. (1967). *Depression: Clinical, experimental, and theoretical aspects.* New York: Harper & Row.

Beck, A. T., Rush, A. J., Shaw, B. F., & Emery, G. (1979). *Cognitive theory of depression.* New York: Guilford Press.

Bernasconi, R. (1982). The GABA hypothesis of affective illness: Influence of clinically effective antimanic drugs on GABA turnover. In H. M. Emrich, J. B. Aldenhoff, & H. D. Lux (Eds.), *Basic mechanisms in the action of lithium* (pp. 183–192). Amsterdam: Excerpta Medica.

Betrus, P. A., & Elmore, S. K. (1991). Seasonal affective disorder, Part I: A review of the neural mechanisms for psychosocial nurses. *Archives of Psychiatric Nursing, 5*, 357–364.

Billings, A. G., Cronkite, R. C., & Moos, R. H. (1983). Social-environmental factors in unipolar depression: Comparisons of depressed patients and nondepressed controls. *Journal of Abnormal Psychology, 92*, 119–133.

Black, D. W., Warrack, G., & Winokur, G. (1985). The Iowa record linkage study, I. Suicide and accidental death among psychiatric patients. *Archives of General Psychiatry, 42*, 71–75.

Blazer, D., Hughes, D. C., & George, L. K. (1987). The epidemiology of depression in an elderly community population. *Gerontologist, 27*, 281–287.

Blazer, D., & Williams, G. (1980). Epidemiology of dysphoria and depression in elderly population. *American Journal of Psychiatry, 137*, 439–444.

Bowers, M. B., Goodman, E., & Sim, V. M. (1964). Some behavioral changes in man following anticholinesterase administration. *Journal of Nervous and Mental Disease, 138*, 383.

Bowlby, J. (1980). *Attachment and loss* (Vol. 3). New York: Basic Books.

Bunny, W. E., & Davis, J. M. (1965). Norepinephrine in depressive reactions: A review. *Archives of General Psychiatry, 13*, 483–494.

Burnell, G. M., & Burnell, A. L. (1989). *Clinical management of bereavement: A handbook for healthcare professionals*. New York: Human Sciences Press.

Cadoret, R. J., & Widmer, R. B. (1988). The development of depressive symptoms in elderly following onset of severe physical illness. *Journal of Family Practice*, *27*, 71–76.

Cassem, E. H. (1987). Depression secondary to medical illness. In A. J. Francis & R. E. Hales (Eds.), *American Psychiatric Press review of psychiatry* (Vol. 7, pp. 256–273). Washington, DC: American Psychiatric Press.

Clayton, R. J., & Darvish, J. S. (1979). Course of depressive symptoms following the stress of bereavement. In J. E. Barrett (Ed.), *Stress and mental disorder*. New York: Raven Press.

Coppen, A., Shaw, D. M., Malleson, A., Eccleston, E., & Gundy, G. (1965). Tryptamine metabolism in depression. *British Journal of Psychiatry*, *111*, 993–998.

Coyle, J. T. (1988). Neuroscience and psychiatry. In J. A. Talbott, R. E. Hales, & S. C. Yudofsky (Eds.), *The American Psychiatric Press textbook of psychiatry* (pp. 3–32). Washington, DC: American Psychiatric Press.

Coyne, J. C. (1976). Toward an interactional description of depression. *Psychiatry*, *39*, 28–40.

Coyne, J. C., Aldwin, C., & Lazarus, R. S. (1981). Depression and coping in stressful episodes. *Journal of Abnormal Psychology*, *90*, 439–447.

Damrosch, S., Sullivan, P., & Scholler, P. (1988). On behalf of homeless families. *Maternal–Child Nursing*, *13*, 259–263.

Demi, A. S., & Howell, C. (1991). Hiding and healing: Resolving the suicide of a parent or sibling. *Archives of Psychiatric Nursing*, *5*, 350–356.

Dreyfus, J. K. (1988). Depression assessment and interventions in the medically ill frail elderly. *Journal of Gerontological Nursing*, *14*(9), 27–36.

Egeland, J. A., & Sussex, J. N. (1985). Suicide and family loading for affective disorders. *Journal of the American Medical Association*, *254*, 915–918.

Elizur, E., & Kaffman, M. (1982). Children's bereavement reactions following death of the father. *Journal of the American Academy of Child Psychiatry*, *21*, 474–480.

Elmore, S. K. (1991). Seasonal affective disorder, Part II: Phototherapy, an expanded role of the psychosocial nurse. *Archives of Psychiatric Nursing*, *5*, 365–372.

Extein, I., Pottash, A. L., Gold, M. S., & Martin, D. M. (1980). Differentiating mania from schizophrenia by the TRH test. *American Journal of Psychiatry*, *137*, 981–982.

Farber, M. L. (1968) *Theory of suicide*. New York: Funk & Wagnalls.

Farberow, N. L., & Shneidman, E. S. (1970). Suicide and age. In E. S. Shneidman, N. L. Farberow, & R. E. Litman (Eds.), *The psychology of suicide* (pp. 164–174). New York: Science House.

Folkman, S., & Lazarus, R. S. (1986). Stress processes and depressive symptomatology. *Journal of Abnormal Psychology*, *95*, 107–113.

Freud, S. (1957). Mourning and melancholia. In J. Strachey (Ed. & Trans.), *The standard edition of the complete psychological works of Sigmund Freud* (Vol. 14, pp. 243–258). London: Hogarth Press. (Original work published 1917)

Friedman, R., Corn, R., Hurt, S., Fibel, B., Schulick, J., & Swirsky, S. (1984). Family history of illness in the seriously suicidal adolescent: A life cycle approach. *American Journal of Orthopsychiatry*, *54*, 390–397.

Gershon, S., & Shaw, F. H. (1961). Psychiatric sequelae of chronic exposure to organophosphorus insecticides. *Lancet*, *1*, 1371–1374.

Gewirtz, G., Malaspina, D., Hatterer, J. A., Feurelsen, S., Klein, D., & Gorman, J. M. (1988). Occult thyroid dysfunction in patients with refractory depression. *American Journal of Psychiatry, 145*(8), 1012–1014.

Gold, J. R. (1990). Levels of depression. In B. B. Wolman & G. Stricker (Eds.), *Depressive disorders: Facts, theories, and treatment methods* (pp. 203–228). New York: Wiley.

Gold, P. W., Goodwin, F. K., Wehr, T., & Rebar, R. (1977). Pituitary thyrotropin response to thyrotropin-releasing hormone in affective illness: Relationship to spinal fluid amine metabolites. *American Journal of Psychiatry*, *134*, 1028–1031.

Gold, P. W., Goodwin, F. K., & Chrousos, G. P. (1988a). Clinical and biochemical manifestations of depression: Relation to the neurobiology of stress: I. *New England Journal of Medicine*, *319*, 348–353.

Gold, P. W., Goodwin, F. K., & Chrousos, G. P. (1988b). Clinical and biochemical manifestations of depression: Relation to the neurobiology of stress: II. *New England Journal of Medicine*, *319*, 413–420.

Gold, P. W., et al. (1988c). The clinical implications of corticotropin-releasing hormone. In G. P. Chrousos, D. L. Loriaux, & P. W. Gold (Eds.), *Mechanisms of physical and emotional stress* (pp. 507–519). New York: Plenum.

Golden, R. N., & Janowsky, D. S. (1990). Biological theories of depression. In B. Wolman & G. Stricker (Eds.), *Depressive disorders: Facts, theories, and treatment methods* (pp. 3–21) New York: Wiley.

Goldwyn, R. M. (1988). Educating the patient and family about depression. *Medical Clinics of North America*, *72*, 887–896.

Goodwin, F. K. (1986). Pharmacological consultation in major depressive disorders. In D. C. Jimerson & J. P. Docherty (Eds.), *Psychopharmacology consultation* (pp. 2–17). Washington, DC: American Psychiatric Press.

Goodwin, F. K., & Jamison, K. R. (1990). *Manic–depressive illness*. New York: Oxford University Press.

Grebb, J. A., Reus, V. I., & Freimer, N. B. (1988). Neurobehavioral chemistry and physiology. In H. H. Goldman (Ed.), *Review of general psychiatry* (2nd ed., pp. 121–135). Norwalk, CT: Appleton & Lange.

Hale, A. S. (1993). New antidepressants: Use in high-risk patients. *Journal of Clinical Psychiatry, 54* (8, suppl.), 61–70.

Helsing, K. J., Comstock, G. W., & Szklo, M. (1982). Causes of death in a widowed population. *American Journal of Epidemiology*, *116*, 524–532.

Helsing, K. J., & Szklo, M. (1981). Mortality after bereavement. *American Journal of Epidemiology*, *114*, 41–52.

Heninger, G. R., Charney, D. S., & Delgado, P. L. (1990). Neurobiology of treatments for refractory depression. In A. Tasman, S. M. Goldfinger, & C. A. Kaufman (Eds.), *American Psychiatric Press review of psychiatry* (Vol. 9, pp. 33–59). Washington, DC: American Psychiatric Press.

Hirschfeld, R. M., & Goodwin, F. K. (1988). Mood disorders. In J. A. Talbott, R. E. Hales, & S. C. Yudofsky (Eds.), *The American Psychiatric Press textbook of psychiatry* (pp. 403–441). Washington, DC: American Psychiatric Press.

Hirschfeld, R. M. A., & Shea, M. T. (1989). Mood disorders: Psychosocial treatments. In H. I. Kaplan & B. J. Sadock (Eds.), *Comprehensive textbook of psychiatry IV* (Vol. 1, pp. 933–944). Baltimore: Williams & Wilkins.

Janowsky, D. S., El-Yousef, M. K., Davis, J. M., & Sererke, H. J. (1972). A cholinergic-adrenergic hypothesis of mania and depression. *Lancet*, *2*, 6732–6735.

Janowsky, D. S., El-Yousef, M. K., Davis, J. M., & Sererke, H. J. (1973). Parasympathetic suppression of manic symptoms by physostigmine. *Archives of General Psychiatry*, *28*, 542–547.

Janowsky, D. S., David, J. M., El-Yousef, M. K., & Davis, J. M. (1974). Acetylcholine and depression. *Psychosomatic Medicine*, *36*, 248–257.

Jefferson, J. W., & Greist, J. H. (1990). The clinical application of lithium. In J. D. Amsterdam (Ed.), *Pharmacotherapy of depression: Applications for the outpatient practitioner* (pp. 111–127). New York: Marcel Dekker.

Kandel, D. B., & Davies, M. (1982). Epidemiology of depressive mood in adolescents: An empirical study. *Archives of General Psychiatry*, *39*, 1205–1212.

Kaplan, H. I., & Sadock, B. J. (1991). *Synopsis of psychiatry* (6th ed.). Baltimore: Williams & Wilkins.

Kaplan, S. L., Hong, G., & Weinhold, C. (1984). Epidemiology of depressive symptomatology in adolescents. *Journal of the American Academy of Child Psychiatry*, *23*, 91–98.

Kaprio, J., Koskenvuo, M., & Rita, H. (1987). Mortality after bereavement: A prospective study of 95,647 widowed persons. *American Journal of Public Health*, *77*, 283–287.

Katz, I. R., Curlik, S., Nemetz, P., et al. (1988). Functional psychiatric disorders in the elderly. In L. W. Lazarus (Ed.), *Essentials of geriatric psychiatry*. New York: Springer Publishing.

Kazdin, A., Moser, J., Colbus, D., & Bell, R. (1985). Depressive symptoms among physically abused and psychiatrically disturbed children. *Journal of Abnormal Psychology*, *94*, 298–307.

Kennedy, G. J., Kelman, H. R., Thomas C., Wishiewski, W., Metz,

H., & Bijur, P. E. (1989). Hierarchy of characteristics associated with depressive symptoms in an urban elderly sample. *American Journal of Psychiatry, 146*, 220–225.

Kirkegaard, C., Bjorum, N., Cohn, D., & Lauridsen, U. B. (1978). Thyrotropin-releasing hormone (TRH) stimulation test in manic-depressive illness. *Archives of General Psychiatry, 35*, 1017–1021.

Klerman, G. L., Weissman, M. M., Rounsaville, B. J., & Chevron, S. (1984). *Interpersonal psychotherapy of depression*. New York: Basic Books.

Krause, N. (1987). Chronic financial strain, social support, and depressive symptoms among older adults. *Psychology of Aging, 2*, 185–192.

Kuntz, B. (1991). Exploring the grief of adolescents after the death of a parent. *Journal of Child Psychiatric Nursing, 4*(3), 105–109.

Kurtz, N. M. (1990). Monoamine oxidase inhibiting drugs. In J. D. Amsterdam (Ed.), *Pharmacotherapy of depression: Applications for the outpatient practitioner* (pp. 93–109). New York: Marcel Dekker.

Lazare, A. (1979). Unresolved grief. In A. Lazare (Ed.), *Outpatient psychiatry: Diagnosis and treatment*. Baltimore: Williams & Wilkins.

Lazarus, R. & Folkman, S. (1984). *Stress, appraisal, and coping*. New York: Springer Publishing.

Leonard, B. E. (1993). The comparative pharmacology of new antidepressants. *Journal of Clinical Psychiatry, 54* (8, suppl.), 3–15.

Lewinsohn, P. M. (1974). A behavioral approach to depression. In R. Friedman & M. Katz (Eds.), *The psychology of depression: Contemporary theory and research* (pp. 157–185). New York: Wiley.

Manderino, M., & Bzdek, V. M. (1989). Mobilizing depressed clients. In L. Beeber (Ed.), *Depression: Old problems, new perspectives in nursing care* (pp. 91–99). Thorofare, NJ: Slack.

McEnany, G. W. (1990). Psychobiological indices of bipolar mood disorder: Future trends in nursing care. *Archives of Psychiatric Nursing, 4*, 29–38.

Meyer, A. (1948–1952). *Collected papers of Adolf Meyer* (Vols. 1–4). Baltimore: Johns Hopkins University Press.

Mitchell, R. E., & Hodson, C. A. (1983). Coping with domestic violence: Social support and psychological health among battered women. *American Journal of Community Psychology, 11*, 629–654.

Moore-Ede, M. C., Czeisler, C. A., & Richardson, G. S. (1983). Circadian timekeeping in health and disease; Part 1: Basic properties of circadian pacemakers. *New England Journal of Medicine, 309* (8), 469–476.

Murphy, G. E., & Robins, E. (1967). Social factors in suicide. *Journal of the American Medical Association, 199*, 303–308.

Orem, D. E. (1971). *Nursing: Concepts of practice*. New York: McGraw-Hill.

Osgood, N. J., & Thielman, S. (1990). Geriatric suicidal behavior: Assessment and treatment. In S. J. Blumenthal & D. J. Kupfer (Eds.), *Suicide over the life cycle: Risk factors, assessment, and treatment of suicidal patients* (pp. 341–379). Washington, DC: American Psychiatric Press.

Osterweis, M., Solomon, F., & Green, M. (1987). Bereavement reactions, consequences, and care. In S. Zisook (Ed.), *Biopsychosocial aspects of bereavement* (pp. 3–19). Washington, DC: American Psychiatric Press.

Peplau, H. E. (1952). *Interpersonal relations in nursing*. New York: G. P. Putnam's Sons.

Peplau, H. E. (1962). Interpersonal techniques: The crux of psychiatric nursing. *American Journal of Nursing, 62*(6), 50–54.

Phifer, J. F., & Murrell, S. A. (1986). Etiologic factors in the onset of depressive symptoms in older adults. *Journal of Abnormal Psychology, 95*, 282–291.

Pothier, P. (1988). Child mental health problems and policy. *Archives of Psychiatric Nursing, 11*, 165–169.

Prange, A. J., Jr., Wilson, I. C., Lynn, C. W., Alltop, L. B., & Stikeleather, R. A. (1974). L-Tryptophan in mania: Contribution to a permissive hypothesis of affective disorders. *Archives of General Psychiatry, 30*, 56–62.

Rehm, L. P. (1990). Cognitive and behavioral theories. In B. B. Wolman & G. Stricker (Eds.), *Depressive disorders: Facts, theories, and treatment methods* (pp. 64–91). New York: Wiley.

Robins, E., Murphy, G. E., Wilkinson, J. R., et al. (1959). Some clinical considerations in the prevention of suicide based on a study of 134 successful suicides. *American Journal of Public Health, 49*, 888–899.

Robinson, D. S., Davis, J. M., Nies, A., Ravarif, C. L., & Sylvester, D. (1971). Relation of sex and aging to monoamine oxidase activity of human brain, plasma, and platelets. *Archives of General Psychiatry, 24*, 536–539.

Rosen, D., Xiangdong, M., & Blum, R. (1990). Adolescent health: Current trends and critical issues. *Adolescent Medicine: State of the Art Review, 1*, 15–31.

Rovner, B. W., German, P. S., Brant, L. J., Clark, R., Burton, L., & Folstein, M. F. (1991). Depression and mortality in nursing homes. *Journal of the American Medical Association, 265*, 993–996.

Rowntree, D. W., Neven, S., & Wilson, A. (1950). The effects of diisopropylfluorophosphonate in schizophrenia and manic depressive psychosis. *Journal of Neurology, Neurosurgery and Psychiatry, 13*, 47–62.

Roy, A. (1983). Suicide in depressives. *Comprehensive Psychiatry, 24*, 487–491.

Roy, A. (1984). Suicide in recurrent affective disorder patients. *Canadian Journal of Psychiatry, 29*, 319–321.

Rubinow, D. R., Post, R. M., Gold, P. W., Ballenger, J. C., & Wolff, E. A. (1984). The relationship between cortisol and clinical phenomenology of affective illness. In R. M. Post & J. C. Ballenger (Eds.), *Neurobiology of mood disorders* (pp. 271–289). Baltimore: Williams & Wilkins.

Ryan, L., Montgomery, A., & Meyers, S. (1987). Impact of circadian rhythm research on approaches to affective illness. *Archives of Psychiatric Nursing, 1*, 236–240.

Sadler, L. S. (1991). Depression in adolescents: Context, manifestations, and clinical management. *Nursing Clinics of North America, 26*, 559–572.

Sands, D., McCary, R. C., Bigler, E. D., Becker, H. A., & Waller, T. R. (1987). Understanding ECT. *Journal of Psychosocial Nursing, 25*(8), 27–30.

Sargent, M. (1989). *Depressive illnesses: Treatments bring new hope* (Department of Health and Human Services Publication No. ADM 89-1491). Washington, DC: U.S. Government Printing Office.

Schildkraut, J. J. (1965). The catecholamine hypothesis of affective disorders: A review of supporting evidence. *American Journal of Psychiatry, 122*, 509–522.

Schildkraut, J. J. (1978). Current status of the catecholamine hypothesis of affective disorders. In M. A. Lipton, A. DiMascio, & K. F. Kellam (Eds.), *Psychopharmacology: A generation of progress* (pp. 1223–1234). New York: Raven Press.

Schoenbach, V. J., Kaplan B. H., Grimson, R. C., & Wagner, E. H. (1982). Use of a symptom scale to study the prevalence of a depressive syndrome in young adolescents. *American Journal of Epidemiology, 116*, 791–800.

Seligman, M. E. P. (1975). *Helplessness: On depression, development, and death*. San Francisco: Freeman.

Simmons-Alling, S. (1987). New approaches to managing affective disorders. *Archives of Psychiatric Nursing, 1*, 219–224.

Simpson, G. M., & Singh, H. (1990). Tricyclic antidepressants. In J. D. Amsterdam (Ed.), *Pharmacotherapy of depression: Applications for the outpatient practitioner* (pp. 75–91). New York: Marcel Dekker.

Snyder, S. H. (1986). *Drugs and the brain*. New York: Scientific American Books.

Spitzer, R. L., Gibbon, M., Skodal, A. E., Williams, J. B., & First, M. B. (1994). *DSM-IV casebook* (4th ed). Washington, DC: American Psychiatric Press.

Styron, W. (1990). *Darkness visible*. New York: Random House.

Sullivan, H. S. (1953). *The interpersonal theory of psychiatry*. New York: W. W. Norton.

Tirrell, C., & DeForest, D. (1987). Neuroendocrine factors in affective disorders. *Archives of Psychiatric Nursing, 1*, 225–229.

Weiner, R. D., & Coffey, C. E. (1990). Electroconvulsive therapy. In J. D. Amsterdam (Ed.), *Pharmacotherapy of depression: Applications for the outpatient practitioner* (pp. 201–224). New York: Marcel Dekker.

Weissman, M. M. (1987). Advances in psychiatric epidemiology: Rates and risks for major depression. *American Journal of Public Health, 77*, 445–451.

Weissman, M. M., Leckman, J. F., Merikangas, K. R., Gammon,

G. D., & Prusoff, B. A. (1984). Depression and anxiety disorders in parents and children. *Archives of General Psychiatry, 41*, 845–852.

Wells, C. E. (1979). Pseudodementia. *American Journal of Psychiatry, 136*, 895–900.

Willner, P. (1985). Dopamine and depression: A review of recent evidence, I. Empirical studies. *Brain Research Review, 6*, 211.

Worden, J. W. (1991). *Grief counseling and grief therapy: A handbook for the mental health practitioner* (2nd ed.). New York: Springer Publishing.

Wright, J. H., & Beck, A. T. (1983). Cognitive therapy of depression: Theory and practice. *Hospital and Community Psychiatry, 34*, 1119–1127.

CHAPTER 10

The Client Experiencing Anxiety

DEBORAH ANTAI-OTONG, M.S., R.N.,C.S.

OUTLINE

CHAPTER OBJECTIVES

Upon completion of this chapter, you will be able to:

1. Identify symptoms of the most prevalent anxiety disorders.
2. Explain the relationship between cognitive processes and anxiety.
3. Explain the role of neurobiological and psychosocial factors in anxiety disorders.
4. Develop a plan of care for the client experiencing an anxiety disorder.
5. Recognize symptoms of anxiety throughout the life span.

KEY TERMS

Adaptation
Anxiety
Arousal
Attachment theory
Avoidant behaviors
Cognitive processes
Comorbidity
Compulsions
Depersonalization
Desensitization
Dissociation
Homeostasis
Neurotransmitter
Obsessions
Paresthesias
Phobia
Progressive relaxation
Separation anxiety
Visual imagery

The word ***anxiety*** stems from the Latin word *anxietas*, which means "to vex or trouble." Anxiety represents uneasiness and is an integral aspect of human nature, because it plays a major role in adaptation and homeostasis. It often extends beyond adaptive importance for the individual. Anxiety is a state that is produced by stress or change and is often associated with fear. However, anxiety differs from fear in that it is a diffuse, anticipatory reaction to danger when there is no real danger, whereas fear stems from real or potential threats of danger. The continuum of anxiety ranges from a mild form that produces little effect to a severe form that disrupts homeostasis by activating maladaptive responses, such as avoidance or **phobias** (Rosenbaum & Gelenberg, 1991). Anxiety may be thought of as a protective, innate form of communication that the body uses to mobilize its coping resources to maintain homeostasis, and failure to respond adaptively further compromises homeostasis (Basch, 1988).

Anxiety generates an array of autonomic, behavioral, motor, and cognitive responses. Autonomic, or neurobiological, responses include increased respiration, tachycardia, paresthesias, diaphoresis, and dizziness. Behavioral responses include rituals, avoidance, help seeking, and increased dependency. Motor reaction often presents as muscle tension, tremors, stuttering, and restlessness. Cognitive, or psychological, symptoms include a sense of doom or powerlessness, vigilance, rumination, helplessness, dissociation, distortions, and confusion (Table 10–1).

Throughout history, people have faced tremendous socioeconomic and technological changes and demands. Various anxiety reactions stem from individual responses to stressful situations. Anxiety disorders are the most common psychological illnesses, affecting approximately 15 percent of the general population at some point during their lifetime. In addition, anxiety is one of the most common reasons for seeking medical and psychiatric treatment (Regier et al., 1990a).

A person's reaction to stress is influenced by the adaptive coping skills available to him or her. When these resources fail, anxiety disorganization often ensues, with the potential to become overwhelming and chronic. Gaining control over anxiety reactions requires understanding the circumstances that precipitated them (Basch, 1988).

The aim of this chapter is to discuss major anxiety disorders listed in the fourth edition of the *Diagnostic and Statistical Manual of Mental Disorders,* (DSM-IV) (American Psychiatric Association [APA], 1994), various factors associated with anxiety disorders, and the role of psychiatric nursing in the evaluation of clients with anxiety disorders and the prevention and treatment of these disorders.

CAUSATIVE FACTORS: PERSPECTIVES AND THEORIES

Various theories have been posited to explain anxiety's causes, complexity, and relevance to **adaptation** and **homeostasis**. Psychodynamic, cognitive–behavioralist, existentialist, developmental, neurobiological, and psychosocial theories strengthen the premise that anxiety is an integral aspect of human nature.

PSYCHODYNAMIC THEORIES

The foundation of psychoanalytical theory is the premise that various factors, such as conflict, pleasure, morality, and fantasies, are the basis of symptoms and neurosis. Neurobiological, behavioral, and psychosocial expansions have replaced or been added to psychodynamic theories as the sole basis of mental illness. In spite of these expansions, an appreciation of the major psychodynamic concepts of anxiety is vital to understanding the significance of anxiety and human responses.

Sigmund Freud (1936) believed that anxiety occurs when the ego attempts to deal with psychic conflict or emotional tension. He defined anxiety as "the reaction to danger" and that the birth process is the initial response to danger that varies throughout the life span. This initial trauma originates from separation from the mother, and its severity depends on the person's ability to overcome it. Lifelong adaptive responses to anxiety

TABLE 10–1
Common Global Anxiety Responses

AUTONOMIC/ NEUROBIOLOGICAL	BEHAVIORAL	MOTOR	COGNITIVE OR PSYCHOLOGICAL
Increased respirations	Rituals	Motor tension	Sense of doom
Shortness of breath	Avoidance	Tremors	Powerlessness
Tachycardia	Help seeking	Stuttering	Intense fear
Diaphoresis	Increased dependence	Restlessness	Vigilance
Dizziness	Clinging		Rumination
Paresthesias	Following (infant)		Helplessness
	Crying (infant)		Dissociation
			Distortions
			Confusion
			Overgeneralization

arise from this early developmental task, and as the ego matures the person becomes more adept at managing internal and external stress (S. Freud, 1936). Thus, a child is less able than an adult to cope with traumatic experiences.

Freud's daughter, Anna Freud (1936), produced a classic work, *The Ego and the Mechanisms of Defense*, that also contributed to the understanding of the psychodynamics of anxiety. She contended that everyone uses various defense mechanisms to defend against and reduce discomfort that arises from internal and external demands. Major coping processes include unconscious defense mechanisms such as repression, sublimation, denial, projection, and reaction formation, the purposes of which are to control, reduce, and protect the ego from intense anxiety reactions. In addition, psychodynamic theories suggest that if repression fails to protect the ego from overwhelming anxiety, other primitive defense mechanisms, such as **dissociation**, displacement, or regression, may evolve, thus increasing the risk of mental illness (Breuer & Freud, 1957).

EXISTENTIALIST THEORY

Rollo May (1977) defined anxiety as a reaction to a threat to survival. Existentialists also surmise that anxiety enables people to preserve their existence and that it stems from the empty feeling that results when people view their lives as unimportant.

COGNITIVE–BEHAVIORAL THEORIES

Beck and Emery (1985) defined anxiety from a **cognitive processes** perspective and asserted that it occurs when a threat or danger is perceived. (*Cognitive* refers to thought processes related to judgment, reasoning, comprehension, attitude, and perception of the self and the world.) Anxious persons often exaggerate the threat of danger by using faulty cognitions. Faulty or distorted cognitions are characterized by overgeneralization; "awfulizing;" and "all or none" perception of self, others, and the world. These thoughts often generate intense anxiety and impaired social functioning (e.g., avoidant behaviors), which cause them to feel powerless and helpless. Public speaking is an example of an event that often generates anxiety. The businessperson preparing a talk may experience severe anxiety generated by the fear of "losing it" and looking foolish during the presentation. If this lack of confidence is sensed by the audience, their negative reaction may increase the person's anxiety about speaking in public.

Behavioralists propose that intense or disabling anxiety is a learned maladaptive response to stress. Families and other psychosocial factors shape various personality traits and the ability to cope and to respond to stress effectively. Specific family qualities, such as a lack of warmth and nurturance or overprotectiveness, increase the likelihood of maladaptive responses in children (Andrews & Crino, 1991; Leon & Leon, 1990).

DEVELOPMENTAL THEORIES

Bowlby's (1969) **attachment theory** asserted that anxiety initially occurs with separation from early primary caregivers. He described **separation anxiety** as a predictable process involving several stages:

1. Protest (separation anxiety): the child cries and often looks and calls for caregiver(s)
2. Despair (grief and mourning): the child fears that the caregivers will not return
3. Detachment (coping/defense mechanism): the child emotionally separates from caregivers

The infant's attachment behaviors, such as smiling, clinging, crying, and following, activate a response from the primary caregivers and facilitate closeness. The infant uses these behaviors often during the first 4 months of life and continues to do so until age 3. Throughout infancy and childhood, behavioral patterns change from clinging and sucking to using words and playing alone. By the age of 3, the child is able to tolerate the short-term absence of the primary caregivers and feel secure with surrogate attachment figures, such as a relative or babysitter. Bowlby believed that the child's ability to cope successfully with separation anxiety depends on the quality of attachment or bonding during early infancy.

Ainsworth (1985) supported and clarified Bowlby's theory, emphasizing the importance of attachment and its anxiety-reducing qualities in helping children to separate successfully from primary caregivers and adapt to external and internal stressors. Furthermore, she asserted that accomplishment of this developmental task is the basis of lifelong adaptive and coping ability. In contrast, children who leave infancy with disturbed or inadequate attachment or bonding tend to experience developmental incompetencies manifested by impaired socialization and problem solving and a lack of emotional stability.

NEUROBIOLOGICAL THEORIES

Many of the neurobiological theories of anxiety disorders have come from examination of behavior and adaptation to internal and external stimuli that may be positive or negative (Cannon, 1914; Cloninger, 1986; Eysenck, 1981; Pavlov, 1927). A combination of neurochemicals and neurohormones affects a network of brain regions whenever a person experiences anxiety. A prominent study conducted by Hans Eysenck (1981) revealed that anxiety results from activation of the autonomic nervous system (ANS) and arousal of the limbic system to prepare for increased mental and physical demands to confront the threat. Two clusters of specialized neurons of the ANS in the brain stem—the locus

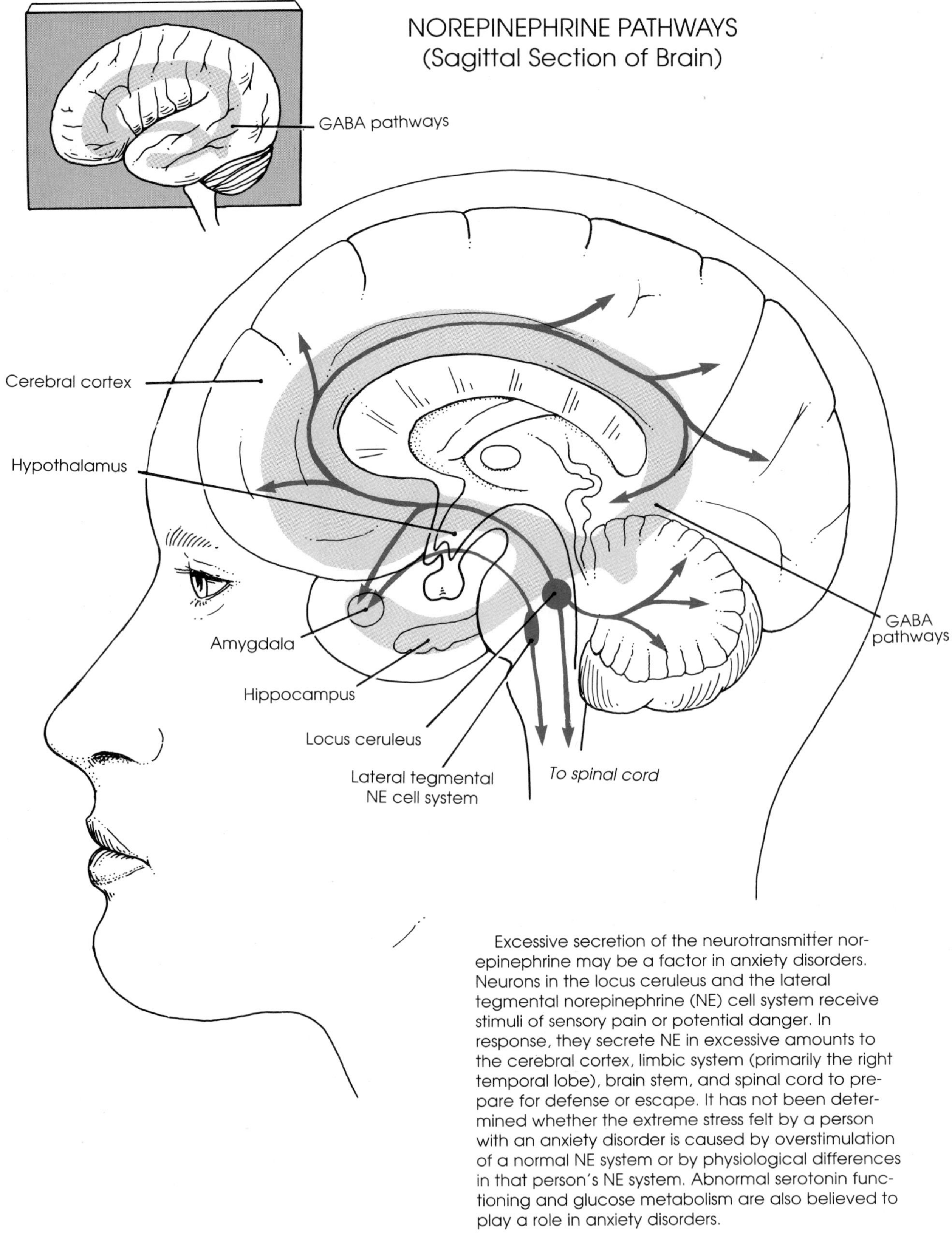

Excessive secretion of the neurotransmitter norepinephrine may be a factor in anxiety disorders. Neurons in the locus ceruleus and the lateral tegmental norepinephrine (NE) cell system receive stimuli of sensory pain or potential danger. In response, they secrete NE in excessive amounts to the cerebral cortex, limbic system (primarily the right temporal lobe), brain stem, and spinal cord to prepare for defense or escape. It has not been determined whether the extreme stress felt by a person with an anxiety disorder is caused by overstimulation of a normal NE system or by physiological differences in that person's NE system. Abnormal serotonin functioning and glucose metabolism are also believed to play a role in anxiety disorders.

FIGURE 10–1
The role of norepinephrine and gamma-aminobutyric acid in anxiety disorders. (Illustration concept: Gail Kongable, M.S.N., C.N.R.N., C.C.R.N., Department of Neurosurgery, University of Virginia Health Sciences Center. Illustration by Marie T. Dauenheimer.)

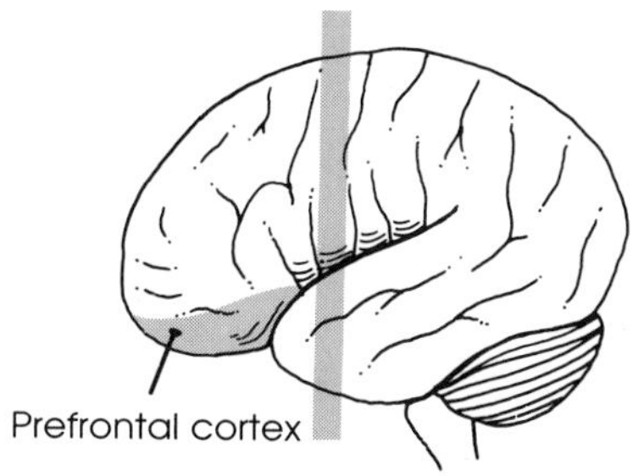

Gamma-aminobutyric acid (GABA), an amino acid that serves as the brain's modulator, is an important inhibitory neurotransmitter. Without adequate GABA biosynthesis, release, and activity, the brain would react to the continuous bombardment of even the smallest external and internal stimuli. GABA receptors throughout the brain counteract the effects of the excitatory neurotransmitters norepinephrine and dopamine, preventing disorganized and frenzied responses to continual stimuli and dampening emotional arousal. A person with low levels of GABA or fewer GABA receptors is theoretically more susceptible to anxiety disorders.

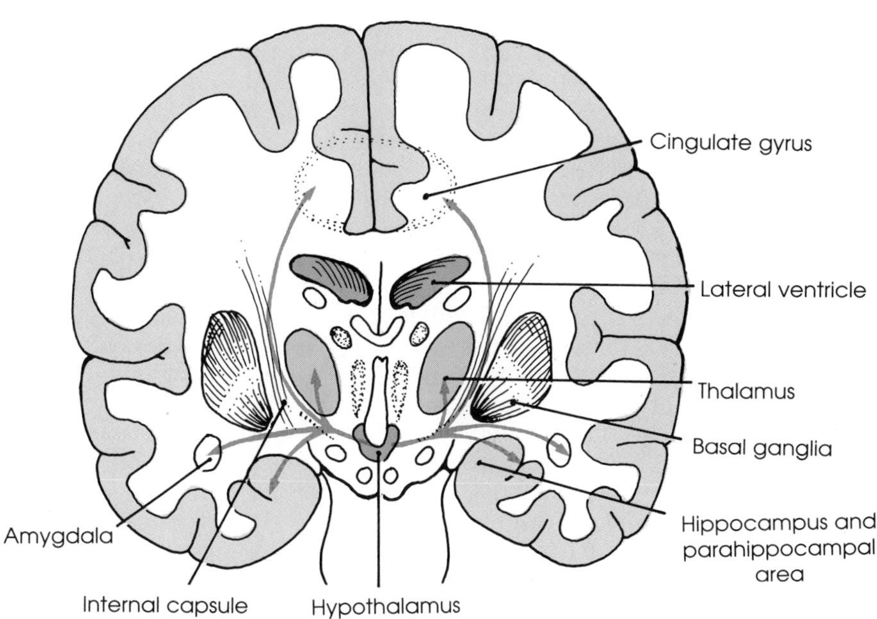

HOW DRUGS WORK IN ANXIETY DISORDERS

Uncontrolled anxiety results from unsuccessful defense against anxiety-provoking stimuli. Sometimes anxiety may be related to chronic depression; in such cases treatment with tricyclic antidepressants or monoamine oxidase inhibitors can cause the anxiety to resolve. Drugs that enhance the action of GABA can also be effective in treating anxiety. *(See Fig. 2-4 for an explanation of synaptic structures.)*

1. Norepinephrine (NE) is synthesized from a dopamine and tyrosine hydroxylase reaction. GABA is synthesized from glutamate, a common amino acid.
2. NE and GABA are stored in synaptic vesicles. *Some antihypertensive drugs interfere with the uptake and storage of NE and deplete NE stores. Although they are prescribed for other reasons, these drugs may have the side effect of alleviating anxiety.*
3. Vesicles migrate to the presynaptic membrane and release NE and GABA into the synaptic cleft. *Because amphetamines stimulate the release of NE and block its reuptake, they can contribute to anxiety (see Figure 17-1).*
4. Stimulation of GABA receptor sites makes the target neuron less sensitive to stimulation by NE and other neurotransmitters. *Benzodiazepines such as chlordiazepoxide (Librium) and diazepam (Valium) are effective in treating anxiety because they enhance the binding of GABA to its receptor sites.*

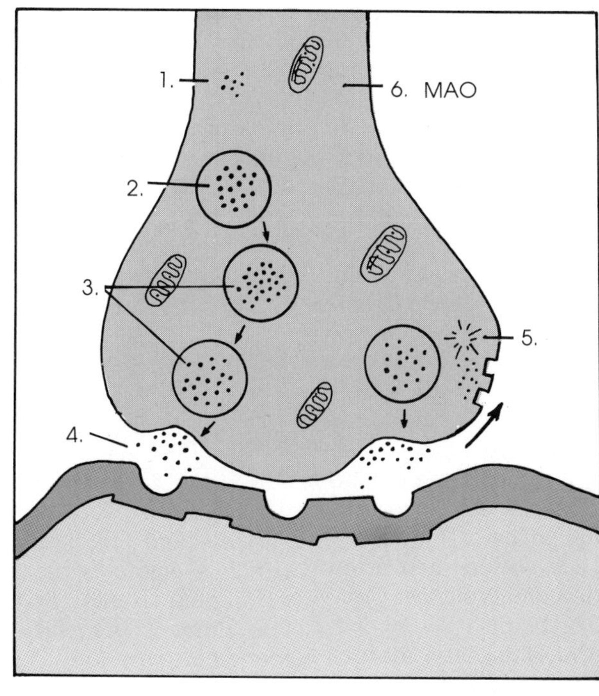

5. The action of NE is stopped by its resorption into the presynaptic terminal. *The tricyclic drug desipramine (Norpramin), used to treat posttraumatic stress disorder, inhibits the resorption of NE, resulting in larger available amounts that may cause increased anxiety.*
6. NE present in the free state within the presynaptic terminal can be broken down by the enzyme monoamine oxidase (MAO). *MAO inhibitors (MAOIs), sometimes used to treat anxiety disorders caused by underlying depression, prevent the breakdown of NE in the presynaptic terminal.*

ceruleus and the lateral tegmental NE cell system—receive the stimuli of impending danger or sensory pain and secrete norepinephrine, a stimulating neurotransmitter, which floods the limbic system and hypothalamic-pituitary-adrenal (HPA) axis (Charney et al., 1993; Somson & Weiss, 1988) (Fig. 10–1). Physiological arousal is reflected in increased heart rate, breathing rate, and hyperalertness that are tied to release of the hormone corticotropin-releasing factor from the hypothalamus and adrenocorticotropin from the pituitary (see Chapter 11 and Fig. 11–1). The release of cortisol and adrenalin from the adrenal glands maintains the level of readiness.

A number of neuroendocrine studies suggest increased cortisol levels in acute stress and related symptoms are comparable to what happens in anxiety disorders. Suppression of cortisol through administration of dexamethasone has been associated with posttraumatic stress disorder (PTSD), suggesting an underlying heightened glucocorticoid feedback sensitivity of the HPA axis in these patients (Yehuda et al., 1991, 1993). However, investigations have failed to support the notion that all anxiety disorders consistently result from activation of the HPA, and stress and anxiety are generally considered separate phenomena (Unde, 1994; Unde et al., 1988).

Rosenbaum (1990) referred to this arousal as "limbic alert." The limbic system, an area in the forebrain encircling the brain stem, plays a major role in formation of abnormal responses such as anxiety reactions. Its association with the brain stem aids in sustaining emotional steadiness and alertness but also activates the locus ceruleus to release the **neurotransmitter** norepinephrine (de Montigny, 1989; Redmond et al., 1976) (see Fig. 10–1). Stimulation of this region is thought to arouse feelings of doom and fear and is the potential site of maladaptive anxiety disorders (Kashani et al., 1991).

In addition, the raphe nuclei, as described in Chapter 9, release serotonin to inspire depressed mood and motivation. The improved response of persons with the type of anxiety disorder characterized by obsessive–compulsive activity to serotonin reuptake blockers, such as clomipramine, fluvoxamine, and fluoxetine, suggests that this disorder is caused by abnormal serotonin function (Murphy et al., 1989; Pigott et al., 1990).

It has not been determined whether the extreme stress felt by persons with anxiety disorders is caused by overstimulation of normal norepinephrine circulation or by an abnormal norepinephrine system in those persons. Panic attacks, characterized by acute uncontrollable anxiety symptoms, can be evoked with sodium lactate and yohimbine, an adrenergic antagonist (Liebowitz et al., 1986; Rainey et al., 1987; Southwick et al., 1993), suggesting a norepinephrine genesis. Injection of sodium lactate supposedly increases carbon dioxide levels, which induces hyperventilation and enhances locus ceruleus activity (Liebowitz et al., 1986).

Gray (1982) proposed that the affective and motivational systems influence the sensation and experience of anxiety, and genetic predisposition and personality traits have been linked to neurotransmitter release and function during the anxiety state (Cloninger, 1986). Anxiety for persons with these characteristics becomes a maladaptive response: heightened anxiety or chronic anxiety generates intense cognitive, neurobiological, and emotional activation (Rosenbaum, 1990). This chronic anxiety state related to anticipated threat serves to reinforce avoidance activities, as well as to potentially limit pleasant or new positive experiences (Cloninger, 1986).

Dysregulation of gamma-aminobutyric acid (GABA) has also been proposed as a component of anxiety disorders. GABA is a regulatory neurotransmitter normally released in the brain to dampen the response to norepinephrine. A person with low levels of GABA or fewer GABA receptors may not be physiologically capable of overriding the effects of excessive norepinephrine secretion.

Neuroanatomical studies using positron emission tomography and computed tomography have shown abnormalities in glucose metabolism in the frontal and prefrontal cortex and the basal ganglia of the brain in clients with panic disorders. In addition, magnetic resonance imaging tests have shown cortical atrophy in the right temporal lobe of clients experiencing panic attacks (Cowley & Arana, 1990; Nordahl et al., 1989; Swedo et al., 1989). Although these findings are not definitive, they support the premise that panic attacks and anxiety disorders arise from specific brain areas (Redmond, 1987).

GENETIC FACTORS

Genetic studies suggest familial patterns of anxiety disorders, such as generalized anxiety disorder and phobias (Kendler et al., 1992a, 1992b). A study by Lenane et al. (1990) supports this premise: approximately 25 percent of the children and adolescents in the sample had a first-degree relative with obsessive disorder. Perhaps one of the most exhaustive twin studies linking genetics to familial transmission of panic disorder was conducted by Torgersen (1983). Evidence from this study showed that monozygotic (identical) twins were five times more likely to develop panic disorder than dizygotic (fraternal) twins.

ANXIETY ACROSS THE LIFE SPAN

CHILDHOOD AND ADOLESCENT ANXIETY DISORDERS

Anxiety and fear are common childhood experiences, being associated with various aspects of growth and development (Bauer, 1976). For example, during infancy, fear induces the startle reflex in response to sudden movements or loud noises, and strangers elicit a fear response during the latter part of the first year. Jean Piaget's (1954, 1958) research on human growth and development has shown that children's level of logical and cognitive function differs from that of adults, and they have trouble understanding that while primary caregivers may be out of sight, they still exist. The child's immature logic is the basis of this fear and anxiety when the primary caregivers leave the room. Normally, the child's cognitive processes mature, enabling him or her to recognize and escape danger. Separation anxiety is a normal response to estrangement from primary caregivers and adaptive coping in the child. As the cognitive processes mature and the child masters various developmental tasks, separation anxiety abates.

As their cognitive abilities mature, children's imaginations become vivid, and they fear monsters and other imaginary characters. The evolving ego and cognitive function enable children to think about the past and anticipate the future, consequently transforming their responses to fear (Graziano et al., 1979).

During late childhood and early adolescence, cognitive and ego function continue to mature, enabling the youth to deal more realistically with fear and anxiety. Anxiety tends to vary with age, and fears of strangers and separation decline with age. Early fears and anxiety are replaced with concerns about one's appearance, interactions with peers, and self-confidence (Kashani & Orvaschel, 1990).

The APA (1994) lists separation anxiety under childhood and adolescent anxiety disorders in the DSM-IV. Other anxiety disorders, such as PTSD, obsessive–compulsive disorder, overanxious disorder, and social phobia are found in this age group.

Separation Anxiety Disorder

Separation anxiety is associated with psychosocial, learning, and genetic factors. Children with separation anxiety experience panic when their primary caregiver temporarily leaves them or extreme fear of losing the primary caregiver. A number of children may even ruminate about losing their parents, getting lost, or having accidents. Professional help is often sought when the child is unable to adapt socially and cope with the environment (Silverman et al., 1988). Other behavioral responses include the fear of being harmed, poor self-esteem, frequent crying when primary caregivers leave the room, and refusal to attend school. Some children may even complain of somatic problems, such as nausea, headaches, or stomach pain (APA, 1994).

Social Phobia

Avoidant behaviors in children and adolescents are manifested as persistent or extremely constricted social interaction with unfamiliar people, to the point of intense social impairment or interaction with peers. These behaviors may occur as early as 2½ years of age and endure for at least 6 months, and they tend to be associated with a desire to be involved with others. If this disorder continues into adulthood, it is linked with avoidant personality disorder (APA, 1994).

Factors that increase the risk of social phobia in children and adolescents include modeling of shy, aloof behaviors by the primary caregivers, child abuse, early traumatic childhood losses, chronic medical problems, and impaired social skills (Andrews & Crino, 1991; Leon & Leon, 1990).

Overanxious Disorder

The essential features of overanxious disorder are unwarranted distress over the future or the appropriateness of past behavior, somatic complaints, and the inability to relax or settle down, all occurring for at least a 6-month period (APA, 1994). Children suffering from this disorder are extremely sensitive, and their overanxious behavior is exaggerated during stressful periods; they need enormous consolation during times of stress. These children tend to be overly concerned about their social performance and competency.

Posttraumatic Stress Disorder

The relationship between grief and traumatic occurrences in children is a matter that has long been overlooked. Eth and Pynoos (1984) explained this lack of attention as stemming from clinicians' difficulty describing children's grief and trauma, because of their immature ego and cognitive functioning, which makes them less able to experience grief without suffering immense emotional pain. The effects of childhood traumas are influenced by several factors, such as the nature of the stressor (e.g., sudden versus foreseen death of a loved one or sexual or physical abuse), available support systems, and the child's ability to work through their pain (Everstine & Everstine, 1993; Pynoos & Eth, 1985). Children who have adequate emotional support and nurturing families are more likely to express feelings about the trauma than are those from chaotic, blaming, and nonsupportive families. Furthermore, there is growing evidence that parents of anxious children may also have an anxiety or other mental disorder that interferes with keeping the child in treatment and providing positive reinforcement (Burgess et al., 1987; Kendall et al., 1992).

The following are suggestions for helping the child experiencing severe trauma to express his or her feelings:

- Establish a trusting relationship
- Engage the child by asking him or her to draw a picture or inviting the child to play with puppets and other toys
- Tell a story

In addition, Pynoos and Eth (1985) asserted that projective approaches link intrusive thoughts of the trauma to grief issues that can be explored through assessment of the child's overt and covert behavior and expressions. There is no standardized test to assess trauma in children and adolescents, because each experiences trauma differently (Everstine & Everstine, 1993).

Major manifestations of PTSD in the child or adolescent include the following:

- Rejection of closeness
- Child's sense of a loss of the vigor and magic of youth
- Cognitive impairment or forgetfulness

- Sleep disturbances (e.g., nightmares) that persist more than several days
- Dependency behaviors manifested by clinging, separation anxiety, and reluctance to attend school
- Extreme fear or distress associated with events that remind the child of the trauma
- Behavioral or emotional changes
- Dissociation (an unconscious defense mechanism used to detach from painful memories and emotions that arise from a traumatic event)
- Regression to previous developmental stage
- Questions about self-worth and expression of need for solitude
- In profound cases, personality development arrest (Everstine & Everstine, 1993; Pynoos & Eth, 1985)

Often, intrusive thoughts that arise from memories of the violent traumatic event interfere with various developmental tasks, increasing the risk of poor school or work performance. Traumatic childhood events include the death of a parent or sibling; child abuse; witnessing violent acts such as murder; and natural disasters, such as tornados, floods, or earthquakes. See Table 10–2 for the symptoms of PTSD in childhood.

Obsessive–Compulsive Disorder

Childhood-onset obsessive–compulsive disorder was thought to be rare until recent studies of 5596 high school students revealed a lifetime prevalence of this disorder of 1 percent (Berg et al., 1989; Flament et al., 1988). In these studies, children with obsessive–compulsive disorder manifested the following symptoms:

- Obsessive thoughts
- Rituals, such as washing and checking
- Repeatedly rewriting a letter or number until it was perfect

Major treatment modalities for these children are consistent with adult treatment modalities and include cognitive–behavioral, family, and group therapy and psychopharmacology. Interventions are determined by developmental stage, severity of symptoms, and parental involvement. Cognitive–behavioral therapy is useful for stopping ruminating thoughts. It also fosters independence and adaptive behavioral change. Family therapy is vital to decreasing the family's involvement in the child's rituals and dealing with dysfunctional family dynamics. Group therapy is effective in reducing anxiety, improving social skills, and assessing the meaning of symptoms or behaviors (Kendall, 1993; Lenane, 1991).

Psychopharmacological interventions have been used successfully to treat obsessive–compulsive disorder in children. Major psychotropics, such as those used in adults (selective serotonin reuptake inhibitors [SSRIs] and clomipramine) have been among these agents (Leonard et al., 1989).

Comorbidity Issues

A major problem associated with childhood and adolescent anxiety disorders is the **comorbidity** of anxiety with other psychiatric disorders, such as depression, substance misuse, and personality disorders. Comorbidity tends to impede the assessment process in children presenting with anxiety reaction. Several diagnostic tools may be used to make a differential diagnosis, such as the Revised Children's Manifest Anxiety Scale (Reynolds & Richmond, 1987) and the Child Assessment Schedule (Hodges et al., 1987), which diagnose developmental anxiety. These assessment tools have corresponding forms that parents complete regarding their children's behaviors, enabling mental health professionals to assess children's maladaptive coping.

Summary

In summary, childhood and adolescent anxiety disorders tend to become adult anxiety disorders, such as agoraphobia, generalized anxiety disorder, and panic disorder. Furthermore, family studies and retrospective reports support the notion that the anxiety disorders form a continuum that evolve from childhood through adulthood (Gittelman & Klein, 1984; van der Molen et al., 1989).

Like adults with anxiety disorders, children with anxiety disorders may experience feelings of powerlessness, increased dependency, and poor self-esteem and have impaired social skills. These problems compromise the youth's ability to cope, increasing the risk of chronicity and persistent avoidance behaviors that impede growth and development (see the Research Study display). Psychoeducation is a critical aspect of treatment and involves teaching healthy parenting skills in terms of providing positive reinforcement and celebrating small accomplishments, while minimizing feelings of guilt, helplessness, and inadequacy in the parent dealing with the child's illness. Table 10–3 lists the major treatment goals for youth experiencing anxiety disorders.

TABLE 10–2 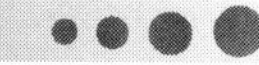

Symptoms of Posttraumatic Stress Disorder Across the Life Span

CHILDHOOD/ADOLESCENCE

Short-Term Effects

- Sleep disturbances
- Persistent thoughts of trauma
- Fear that another traumatic event will occur
- Hyperalertness
- Regression in young children (i.e., to thumb-sucking, bed-wetting, and dependent behaviors)

Long-Term Effects

- Antisocial behaviors
- Vandalism
- Psychosomatic illness (e.g., peptic ulcer disease)
- Truancy and conduct disorders
- Mood disorders
- Eating disorders

ADULTHOOD

- Persistent, recurrent, and intrusive thoughts or dreams of the trauma
- Avoidance behaviors or depersonalization
- Neurobiological responses, such as emotional numbing, hypervigilance and arousal of the sympathetic nervous system

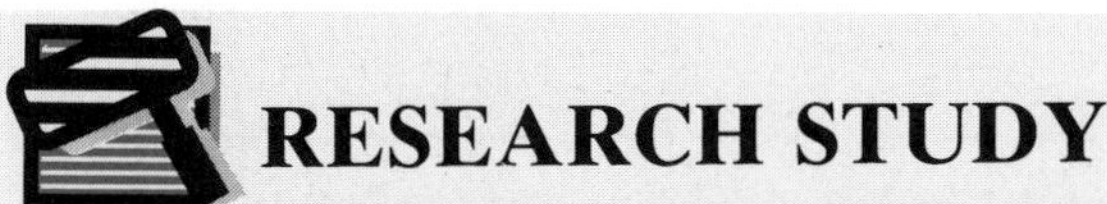

RESEARCH STUDY

Abused to Abuser: Antecedents of Socially Deviant Behaviors

Burgess, A. W., Hartman, C. R., & McCormack, A. (1987) *American Journal of Psychiatry, 144*, 1431–1436.

Study Problem/Purpose

This study explored the impact of childhood physical abuse on later socially deviant behaviors.

Method

Thirty-four youngsters with a history of sexual abuse as children 6 or 8 years after the abuse occurred were compared with 34 control subjects who had not been abused. These children were divided into Study 1 and Study 2. Study 1 was an 8-year followup of 17 sexually abused students, ages 14 to 20, with histories of participation in a sex ring. Study 2 was a 6-year followup of 17 sexually abused students, ages 17 to 21, also used in a sex ring. The researchers used a semistructured interview comprising three parts. The first part elicited descriptions of the nature of sexual abuse, sexual contacts, and background of perpetrators; reports of abuse; and involvement of legal system. The second part consisted of data from the family interview, such as family structure, demographics, frequency of new abuse, and the impact of disclosure. The third part was the child's interview and consisted of the Harris Children's Self-Concept Scale, the Moos Family Environment Scale, the Life Events Scale, the Impact of Event Scale, a coping checklist, a behavior checklist, and assessment of present sexual behavior.

The control group participated in separate semistructured interviews that included questions regarding any sexual abuse history and exploitation.

In addition, the researchers compared youngsters who had been sexually abused less than a year with those who had been abused more than a year.

Findings

The findings suggested a relationship between childhood sexual abuse and socially deviant behaviors later in life. Abused children who came from home environments that lacked support, blamed the child for participation in sexual activities, and openly displayed hostility and disharmony (Study 2) tended to have difficulty forming close, meaningful relationships, and engaged in aggressive behaviors. In contrast, those abused children whose families were supportive and nonblaming for taking part in sexual activities (Study 1) tended not to exhibit these behaviors. Furthermore, Study 1 showed no significant differences in deviant and delinquent behaviors from their control group. However, Study 2 exhibited deviant and delinquent behaviors more than their control group.

Nursing Implications

These findings suggest the influence of early childhood sexual abuse on formation of maladaptive or deviant behaviors. Nurses need to assess children and families at risk and use various interventions, such as stress management, parenting classes, and crisis intervention.

ADULT ANXIETY DISORDERS

Anxiety is a striking feature of most mental disorders and continues to be one of the most common mental disorders, with an estimated 15 percent of the population experiencing it at some time during their lifetime (Regier et al., 1990a). Nearly 25 years ago, anxiety disorders were classified as anxiety neuroses and delineated into panic and generalized disorders. The DSM-IV (APA, 1994) defines a number of disorders, including generalized anxiety disorder (GAD), panic disorder, agoraphobia, obsessive–compulsive disorder, stress disorder, substance-induced anxiety disorder, acute anxiety due to general medical condition (Table 10–4), and PTSD.

TABLE 10–3
Major Treatment Goals for Youth Experiencing Anxiety

- Overcome fear of threat
- Differentiate among various feelings
- Become familiar with feelings
- Understand the links among feelings, thoughts, and behaviors
- Understand that arousal is a symptom of fear
- Enhance problem-solving skills
- Gain a sense of mastery
- Develop adaptive coping behaviors

Data from Ollendick, T. H., & Francis, G. (1988). Behavioral assessment and treatment of childhood phobias. *Behavior Modification, 12*, 165–204.

Generalized Anxiety Disorder

The major symptoms of GAD include nervousness, irritability, apprehension, agitation, tension, tachycardia, diaphoresis, shortness of breath, difficulty falling and staying asleep, and edginess (APA, 1994). Symptoms of GAD tend to overlap those of panic and depressive disorders. Generalized anxiety disorder differs from panic

TABLE 10–4
DSM-IV Criteria for Specific Anxiety Disorders

ANXIETY DISORDER/CONDITION	DSM-IV CRITERIA
Acute Stress Disorder	A. Person exposed to a traumatic event that posed threat to self or others' physical integrity; impact on person involves profound fear, powerlessness, or terror B. During exposure or after exposure to trauma event, *three* or more of the following dissociative manifestations are present: ► numbness, void of emotional responsiveness ► "being in a daze" ► derealization ► depersonalization ► dissociative amnesia C. The traumatic event is persistently reexperienced in one of the following: recurrent vivid memories, nightmares, flashbacks, and distress (neurobiological arousal) arising from memory of the event D. Marked avoidance of stimuli behaviors E. Profound anxiety or autonomic arousal F. Interference with optimal level of function G. Duration of symptoms persists for at least 2 days and no longer than a month and occurs within a month of traumatic exposure H. Not due to a substance or medical condition ► Differs from posttraumatic stress disorder because manifestations of this disorder must evolve within 1 month and resolve within this 1-month period
Anxiety due to a General Medical Condition	A. Pronounced anxiety, specific anxiety disorder (e.g., panic attacks) is chief complaint B. Physiological symptoms directly parallel a general medical condition (e.g., hypoglycemia, hyperthyroidism) C. Symptoms are not associated with another mental disorder D. Symptoms are not part of the course of delirium E. Symptoms interfere with optimal level of functioning
Substance-Induced Anxiety Disorder	A. Pronounced anxiety, specific anxiety disorder (e.g., panic attacks) is chief complaint B. Anxiety symptoms evolved during or within the past month of substance intoxication or withdrawal; medication use is directly associated with presenting symptoms C. Symptoms are not directly caused by a specific anxiety disorder D. Manifestations are not part of the course of delirium E. Symptoms interfere with optimal level of function

Data from American Psychiatric Association. (1994). *Diagnostic and statistical manual of mental disorders* (4th ed.). Washington, DC: Author.

disorder in that it never really remits and its onset is in earlier developmental stages, with an absence of sympathetic arousal. The course of GAD tends to begin during the second decade of life and has a chronic episodic course (Appenheimer & Noyes, 1987). Depression is estimated to accompany at least 50 percent of cases of GAD at some time during the course of illness (Brawman-Mintzer et al., 1993). Table 10–5 presents the prevalence and primary symptoms of the major anxiety disorders. See Chapter 9 for an in-depth discussion of depression.

Panic Disorder

The term *panic* stems from the Greek work *panikos*, meaning "fear." The major symptoms of panic disorder include a sudden onset of unanticipated intense anxiety generated by arousal of the sympathetic nervous system, such as tachycardia, lightheadedness, diaphoresis, **paresthesias**, and a sense of doom. Profound fear may also accompany panic disorder and underlie symptoms of agoraphobia.

Panic attacks rarely occur before the age of 12 or after the age of 49, and their prevalence is less than 50 percent in people over age 65, compared with those between the ages of 25 and 44 (Robins et al., 1984). In a large epidemiological study from the National Comorbidity Survey (n = 8098), the first of its kind to comprise the entire United States, Eaton et al. (1994) found that 15.6 percent of participants reported lifetime occurrence of panic attack and 3.8 percent experienced an attack the previous month. Fifty percent of participants denied symptoms of agoraphobia. Other major findings from this study showed that women were two to three times more likely to have this disorder than men. The peak age for women with panic attacks is between the ages of 35 to 44 years of age. Other factors that impact the incidence of panic disorders include sociodemographic factors. People who were employed, married, and living with others were less likely to experience panic disorders than their counterparts. Furthermore, people living in the northeastern part of the country experienced higher rates of panic attacks, panic disorder, and panic attack with agoraphobia. The lifetime prevalence of panic attacks was higher in this study than a previous study conducted by Eaton et al. (1991).

TABLE 10–5
Symptoms and Prevalence of the Major Anxiety Disorders

	PRIMARY SYMPTOMS	PREVALENCE
Panic Disorder (with or without agoraphobia)	► Shortness of breath ► Dizziness ► Diaphoresis ► Palpitations ► Depersonalization ► Chest pain ► Feelings of doom ► Concern of having another attack ► Avoidance behaviors ► Fear of being in open places	► Isolated recurrent attacks: 10% of adult population. ► Full criteria for panic attacks: 3.6% of adult population ► Full-blown attack: 1.6% of population (Weissman & Merikangas, 1986) ► Thirty percent to 50% of population with panic attacks have agoraphobia (APA, 1994)
Specific Phobia (formerly called Simple Phobia)	► Arousal of anxiety in and avoidance of specific circumstances: natural, environmental type (e.g., snake or spider phobia) or situational (e.g., fear of heights or flying)	► Lifetime prevalence: 10–11.3% (APA, 1994)
Social Phobia	► Persistent fear and avoidance of circumstances that expose one to embarrassment or humiliation (e.g., public speaking or eating in restaurants)	► Lifetime prevalence in men: 1.7% ► Lifetime prevalence in women: 2.8% (Regier et al., 1990a)
Obsessive–Compulsive Disorder	► Thoughts or images of excessive worries regarding life situations (obsessions) ► Ritualistic behaviors such as handwashing, counting, or hoarding (compulsions)	► Lifetime prevalence in U.S.: 1.2–2.4% (Karno et al., 1988)
Posttraumatic Stress Disorder	► Recurrent nightmares ► Hypervigilant behavior ► Intrusive thoughts of traumatic event ► Autonomic arousal generated by nightmares, thoughts, or images ► Acute or delayed symptoms	► Lifetime prevalence in men: 0.5% ► Lifetime prevalence in women: 1.2% (Epstein, 1989)
Generalized Anxiety Disorder	► Restlessness ► Tension ► Arousal of autonomic nervous system ► Agitation/irritability ► Free-floating anxiety	► Lifetime prevalence of general population: 5%

Data from American Psychiatric Association. (1994). *Diagnostic and statistical manual of mental disorders* (4th ed.). Washington, DC: Author.

Panic attacks result in serious emotional and psychosocial impairment, particularly when accompanied by agoraphobia. A number of clients also suffer marital discord and depression, and the suicide rate among persons with panic disorder is high (Johnson et al., 1990; Markowitz et al., 1989).

Sheehan (1986) delineated the possible progression of panic attacks as follows:

Stage 1: Insignificant symptoms
Stage 2: Panic attacks
Stage 3: Hypochondriasis
Stage 4: Minimal avoidance phobic behavior
Stage 5: Severe avoidance behavior
Stage 6: Secondary depression

Panic disorder is primarily treated with alprazolam (Xanax), a benzodiazepine. It is the only drug approved by the Food and Drug Administration for panic disorder. Major benefits of alprazolam include its rapid effectiveness and the fact that it is well tolerated. It has recently been introduced as a once-a-day, sustained-release preparation that is highly effective in the acute treatment of panic disorder (Cross-National Collaborative Panic Study, Second Phase Investigators, 1992; Schweizer et al., 1993). Other treatment modalities include tricyclic antidepressants and monoamine oxidase inhibitors. Clients suffering from panic disorder with or without agoraphobia have shown marked improvement with 1-year maintenance of imipramine (Tofranil), a tricyclic antidepressant (Mavissakalian & Perel, 1992). (See Chapter 26 for an in-depth discussion of benzodiazepines and other antianxiety agents.) Nonpharmacological interventions such as behavioral and cognitive therapies have been reported to enhance antipanic agents. Progressive relaxation, guided imagery, and deep muscle relaxation are examples of these therapies (Andrews & Crino, 1991; Beck & Emery, 1985; Beck et al., 1992).

Agoraphobia

Clients suffering from agoraphobia with or without panic attacks are generally incapacitated by their avoidance behaviors, which impair their emotional and psychosocial functioning. The disabling quality of agoraphobia increases the likelihood of maladaptive behaviors such as substance abuse. In addition, clients with agoraphobia often find it difficult to seek help in spite of feeling like they are "going crazy." Symptoms of panic attacks and agoraphobia are very frightening, and clients really feel like they are dying and may often present in emergency departments with symptoms of hyperventilation, chest pains, and flushing. They must be assessed for medical conditions such as myocardial infarction, mitral valve prolapse, endocrine disorders such as hypoglycemia, and respiratory distress. Medical examination may consist of an electrocardiogram and laboratory studies, such as electrolytes and cardiac enzymes. Approaching these clients in a calm, reassuring, and nonjudgmental manner can allay their fear and sense of doom or feeling of going crazy.

Obsessive–Compulsive Disorder

The term *obsession* stems from the Latin *obsesus*, meaning "to besiege," and *compulsion* from *compulsus*, meaning "to compel." **Obsessions** are intrusive, recurrent, and persistent thoughts, impulses, or images. Examples of these are thoughts of stealing or harming others, sexual impulses, and somatic concerns (APA, 1994). **Compulsions** are behaviors that seem purposeful but are enacted in a stereotypical and repetitive manner. Examples of compulsions are repetitive handwashing, counting, checking, touching, cleaning, or hoarding. The client with obsessive–compulsive disorder often attempts to alleviate the anxiety that arises from his or her obsessions by performing various rituals, or compulsions.

This potentially disabling disorder is estimated to affect up to 4 percent of inpatients and 2 percent of outpatients (Karno et al., 1988; Rasmussen & Tsuang, 1984).

Major pharmacological interventions for obsessive–compulsive disorder include SSRIs such as clomipramine (Anafranil), a tricyclic. Its efficacy in treating obsessive–compulsive disorder has surpassed other SSRIs (Clomipramine Collaborative Study Group, 1991; Jenike et al., 1989). Nonpharmacological interventions for obsessive–compulsive disorder include cognitive and behavioral therapies (Beck & Emery, 1985). See Tables 10–6 and 10–7 for the nonpharmacological and pharmacological interventions used to treat anxiety disorders.

Posttraumatic Stress Disorder

In the past century, PTSD has appeared in the literature under several names: hysteria, war neurosis, shell shock, and battle fatigue. Regardless of the terminology used, this disorder comprises a complex constellation of symptoms that evolve in survivors of traumatic or stressful events. Symptoms often arise from the occurrence of a traumatic event or circumstance that is beyond the breadth of normal human experience and would be considered stressful to anyone. Psychic trauma is precipitated by exposure to an overpowering event, "resulting in helplessness in the face of intolerable danger, anxiety, and instinctual arousal" (Eth & Pynoos 1984, p. 173). Traumatic events such as natural disasters, rape, incest, combat experiences, and catastrophic accidents are likely to generate symptoms of PTSD.

Symptoms of PTSD may be experienced immediately after the event or later. Acute PTSD symptoms may occur within 6 months; after this time, symptoms are referred to as delayed. A preexisting emotional problem or mental illness tends to increase the risk of maladaptive response to traumatic experiences. The major symptoms of PTSD in adults fall into three major groups:

- Persistent recurrent and intrusive thoughts or dreams of the trauma
- Avoidance behaviors or **depersonalization**
- Neurobiological responses, such as emotional numbing, hypervigilance, and arousal of the sympathetic nervous system (APA, 1994; Glover, 1992; van der Kolk et al., 1985)

Summary

See Table 10–4 for a summary of the DSM-IV criteria for specific anxiety disorders.

THE NURSE'S ROLE

THE GENERALIST'S ROLE

Understanding the basis of anxiety disorders and the interventions used to treat them enables the generalist psychiatric–mental health nurse to identify the mental health needs of the anxious client and intervene to reduce the frequency and severity of the symptoms of anxiety. Major nursing interventions include enhancing present coping skills, assessing maladaptive responses, and minimizing the deleterious effects of anxiety. Case management and psychoeducation can be used to

- Enhance coping skills and self-care
- Identify physical and cognitive symptoms that suggest an impending panic attack and administer medications that minimize the severity and frequency of attacks
- Monitor the client's responses to medication and other treatment modalities
- Coordinate and mobilize various resources
- Teach progressive relaxation, cognitive techniques, and other anxiety-reducing measures
- Provide crisis intervention
- Participate in comprehensive care planning (American Nurses Association [ANA], 1994)

ROLE OF THE ADVANCED-PRACTICE NURSE

The advanced psychiatric–mental health nurse incorporates the role of the generalist and autonomously applies advanced clinical skills, knowledge, and experience to complex client needs (ANA, 1994). Psychotherapy, prescription of medication, case management, and researching the effectiveness of treatment are major measures used by the advanced nurse. Psychotherapy enables the nurse to assess the impact of underlying psychodynamic issues, such as early childhood traumas and abuse, on current symptoms and behaviors. Understanding pharmacokinetics and pharmacodynamics and the neurobiological aspects of anxiety disorders permits the nurse to prescribe psychotropic medication that reduces the deleterious effects of anxiety disorders and to monitor the client's responses to the medication. Case management and research enable the advanced nurse to collaborate with the client to develop a comprehensive plan of care. A comprehensive plan of care facilitates identification of positive and negative outcomes and continuous monitoring of the client's complex needs.

Regardless of the nurse's level of practice, clients can expect a comprehensive plan of care that promotes health and minimizes the deleterious effects of anxiety disorders.

THE NURSING PROCESS

Anxiety disorder represents a continuum of symptoms that affect psychosocial, biological, and vocational well-being. Its comorbidity with other disorders such as depression underscores the need for health care professionals to understand the complexity of the human response to internal and external demands and develop effective interventions. The nursing process has critical roles in the assessment, intervention, and evaluation of clients' responses to stressful and traumatic situations. Establishing rapport, facilitating adaptive coping behaviors, individualizing teaching, encouraging active client participation, and administering psychotropics are major treatment strategies for various anxiety disorders.

Case Study: A Client Experiencing Panic Disorder (Jennie L.)

Jennie is a 25-year-old who presents in the emergency department complaining of chest pains, shortness of breath, and the fear of dying. Her husband reports that she has had these symptoms episodically over the past 6 months and says he decided to bring her in because he feared she was having a heart attack.

The physician on call orders an electrocardiogram and laboratory studies, including cardiac enzymes and a toxicology screen. Her physical examination and diagnostic studies are negative. The physician informs Jennie and her husband that there is no physical basis for Jennie's presenting symptoms and says that it sounds like she is having panic attacks. She refers Jennie for a psychiatric consultation. The couple expresses anger, stating that her symptoms are real and she is not crazy.

Assessment

The psychiatric clinical specialist approaches Jennie in a calm and caring manner, seeking to elicit more information regarding present symptoms. Jennie and her husband reluctantly follow the nurse into a quiet private area. During the initial assessment, the nurse reassures Jennie that her symptoms are real and distressful, even though she feels like she is losing touch with reality. The sense of losing touch with reality is associated with depersonalization, paresthesias, lightheadedness, and a negative physical examination.

The following information is gathered during the interview and assessment:

- Jennie has a history of shortness of breath, intense anxiety, lightheadedness, and chest pain episodically over the past 4 to 6 months, usually once or twice per week.
- These symptoms "come out of the blue."
- Jennie says she is presently experiencing no stressors, except for the fear of having an attack while driving or on the job.
- Jennie fears she is losing control over her life.
- There is increased tension between Jennie and her husband because of these fears.
- Jennie is unable to concentrate at work, and her boss has expressed concern about her job performance.
- She has no history of psychiatric treatment or substance abuse.

Nursing Diagnoses

Jennie's DSM-IV diagnosis is panic disorder with possible agoraphobia, and the following are her major nursing diagnoses:

- Ineffective Individual Coping related to perceived lack of control over self and environment
- Anxiety related to perception of powerlessness
- Altered Thought Processes related to negative, irrational, and self-defeating thoughts
- Self-Esteem Disturbance related to personal and professional role performance

Planning

Nursing Care Plan 10–1 identifies the desired outcomes for Jennie's nursing diagnoses and delineates the nursing actions needed to achieve these outcomes, along with the rationales for these actions.

Implementation

The initial intervention is the establishment of a therapeutic relationship with the client and spouse. A sound teaching program then begins, with the nurse teaching the client that anxiety is a disorder that arises from external and internal stimuli that trigger an arousal of the autonomic nervous system to protect the body. Coping with anxiety is a two-part endeavor that consists of the client's assessing his or her perception of threat and using specific coping behaviors to reduce or eliminate distorted cognitions (Andrews & Crino, 1991).

Facilitating adaptive coping behaviors through client

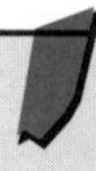

Nursing Care Plan 10–1 The Client Experiencing Anxiety (Jennie)

OUTCOME IDENTIFICATION	NURSING ACTIONS	RATIONALES	EVALUATION
Nursing Diagnosis: Ineffective Individual Coping related to perceived lack of control over self and environment			
1. By [date], Jennie will develop adaptive coping behaviors.	1a. Provide a safe, caring environment.	1a. Providing a safe, caring environment encourages clients to express their feelings and thoughts.	*Goal met:* Jennie is able to express her feelings and consider adaptive coping options.
	1b. Assess Jennie's present and past coping patterns.	1b. Maladaptive coping patterns are revealed.	
	1c. Discuss coping options.	1c. Viable coping alternatives identified.	
2. By [date], Jennie will be able to identify feelings that precede an anxiety attack.	2a. Encourage Jennie to identify anxiety-provoking stimuli and her thoughts associated with the stimuli.	2a. Enables client to understand the meaning of cognitive distortions or erroneous belief systems and gain self-understanding.	*Goal met:* Jennie is able to understand the feeling's and thoughts generated by stimuli and develop adaptive coping behaviors.
	2b. Teach Jennie anxiety-reducing techniques and provide feedback.	2b. Use of anxiety-reducing techniques reduces the number of anxiety experiences.	
Nursing Diagnosis: Anxiety related to perception of powerlessness			
1. By [date], Jennie will experience minimal emotional and biological discomfort.	1a. Help Jennie recognize the relationships among her thoughts, feelings, and biological responses.	1a. Recognizing the relationship between thoughts and feelings and biological responses increases understanding of the disease process and aspects client can control.	*Goal met:* Jennie attempts to control the number of panic attacks she experiences.
	1b. Teach Jennie breathing and relaxation techniques. 1c. Administer anxiolytics.	1b–c. Relaxation techniques and anxiolytics promote behavioral, emotional, and biological comfort.	
Nursing Diagnosis: Altered Thought Processes related to negative, irrational, and self-defeating thoughts			
1. By [date], Jennie will perceive her fears realistically.	1a. Point out Jennie's self-defeating or negative self-talk. 1b. Explore the basis of Jennie's negative thinking. 1c. Teach Jennie cognitive–behavioral techniques (e.g., positive self-talk). 1d. Provide positive reinforcement.	1a–d. Challenging of self-defeating and negative talk changes impaired cognitions and helps clients assess fears realistically.	*Goal met:* Jennie practices positive self-talk and perceives fears realistically. Her anxiety attacks decrease over time.

Nursing Care Plan 10–1 The Client Experiencing Anxiety (Jennie) (Continued)

OUTCOME IDENTIFICATION	NURSING ACTIONS	RATIONALES	EVALUATION
Nursing Diagnosis: Self-Esteem Disturbance related to personal and professional role performance			
1. By [date], Jennie will verbalize several positive self-attributes.	1. Provide successful experiences paralleling Jennie's level of function.	1. Successful experiences enhance/increase self-esteem.	*Goal met:* Jennie identifies her strengths and positive attributes.
2. By [date], Jennie will demonstrate interest in self-care.	2. Provide positive feedback on accomplishments.	2. Feedback validates positive attributes and strengths.	Jennie begins to function at precrisis level.
3. By [date], Jennie will complete tasks.	3. Explore with Jennie her current strengths.	3. Completing tasks enhances self-confidence and self-image.	Jennie directs self-care.

education is critical to reducing cognitive distortions and empowering the client and family. Teaching strategies need to focus on **progressive relaxation** or deep breathing techniques, which enable the client to control some aspects of anxiety attacks by aborting or reducing emotional and physiological responses to them (Andrews & Crino, 1991). Furthermore, cognitive and behavioral approaches facilitate a sense of control and can increase self-esteem. Teaching the client to recognize adaptive and maladaptive responses to stress is an important aspect of client education. Adaptive responses include interruption of self-defeating or negative self-talk, deep breathing, and relaxation techniques. Maladaptive responses include substance abuse and avoidance behaviors (Gelder, 1991). Table 10–6 lists a number of anxiety-reducing techniques that the nurse can recommend or teach to the client.

Behavioral therapy focuses on corrective learning experiences that enhance coping behaviors and effective communication and provide opportunities to reduce self-defeating behaviors and thoughts. The basis of the use of cognitive therapy to treat anxiety disorders is the notion that anxiety increases with thoughts or images of social or physical danger. The effectiveness of cognitive–behavioral approaches depends on the completion of structured activities (e.g., homework assignments) that teach clients to recognize and target irrational thoughts or cognitions and replace them with positive self-talk. The client may find behavioral strategies such as meditation and **visual imagery** useful ways to reduce anxiety or enhance cognitive techniques (Beck & Emery, 1985; Ellis, 1962). Furthermore, the active participation of significant others in helping the client maintain adaptive coping behaviors is vital to the success of cognitive–behavioral techniques (Lazarus, 1971). Psychotherapy and psychotropics can also enhance cognitive–behavioral techniques. See Chapter 21 for discussions of various cognitive–behavioral techniques and psychotherapy.

The overall treatment outcomes for anxiety disorders depend on the client's ability to

- Acknowledge his or her anxiety and verbalize associated feelings and thoughts
- Develop adaptive coping skills, such as relaxation and deep-breathing techniques and positive self-talk
- Avoid maladaptive responses
- Reduce the emotional and physiological discomforts of anxiety by using anxiety-reducing techniques such as thought blocking and positive self-talk and by taking prescribed anti-anxiety agents
- Perform at an optimal level of functioning
- Mobilize support systems

Psychopharmacology. The psychosocial and neurobiological bases of anxiety disorders have been well documented in this chapter. Nursing implications in the treatment of anxiety disorders include assessing the effectiveness of pyschotropics. Administration of psychotropics depends on the severity of presenting symptoms, the client's specific anxiety disorder, the client's motivation, whether there is a history of substance abuse, and the client's previous responses to medication and other interventions (McGlynn & Metcalf, 1989). Table 10–7 lists the major anxiolytic agents.

Other nursing implications of the psychopharmacological approach to treating anxiety disorders include client education regarding the desired and adverse actions of anxiolytic agents; observation and documentation of the client's reactions to these agents; and assessment of psychological and physiological dependence, particularly in the case of benzodiazepines. Clients experiencing anxiety are at risk for substance abuse and must be continuously assessed for maladaptive responses to minimize the risk of relapse and the development of chronic ineffective coping patterns. Medications are usually given as an adjunct to behavioral–cognitive therapy to maximize the effectiveness of the nonpharmacological interventions.

TABLE 10–6
Anxiety-Reducing Techniques

COGNITIVE–BEHAVIORAL TECHNIQUES

Cognitive Therapy

Therapy is based on principle of internal dialogue or self-talk and its impact on thoughts and feelings or emotions and behaviors. Major goals are to

- Assess the client's belief systems and cognitive distortions
- Challenge and alter the client's distorted/negative thoughts and self-defeating behaviors
- Enhance the client's coping skills

Homework assignments are used to test cognitions (e.g., stimulus → thoughts → feelings). Various behavioral techniques can be used.

Behavioral Role Rehearsal

The client role-plays anticipated stressful situations. The therapist assesses the client's reactions and provides feedback to the client as a teaching modality. The client can use modeling to shape behavior.

SYSTEMATIC DESENSITIZATION

The client is taught to maintain relaxation while imaging various stages of ranked anxiety-evoking situations. For example, for an agoraphobic client, situations that evoke an anxiety reaction are ranked from least to most:

1. Going outside
2. Being alone
3. Driving
4. Going to a shopping mall

The client neutralizes anxiety by using deep-muscle relaxation techniques and visual imagery, while the nurse assesses the client's subjective response.

PROGRESSIVE RELAXATION

Visual imagery is the basis of this technique. Directions to the client are as follows:

- Choose a dark, quiet area.
- Close your eyes.
- Focus on all muscle groups from scalp to tips of toes.
- Tense each group of muscles and maintain tension for 4 to 8 seconds.
- Tell yourself to relax and immediately release tension.
- Progress until you have tensed and relaxed all muscles.

Progressive relaxation can also be done using deep-breathing exercises: The client lies on his or her back and inhales through the nose and exhales through the mouth.

Data from Beck, A. T., & Emery, G. (1985). *Anxiety disorders and phobias: A cognitive perspective.* New York: Basic Books; and Wolpe, J. (1973). *The practice of behavioral therapy.* New York: Pergamon Press.

Evaluation

The evaluation process begins with the initial assessment and continues throughout treatment. Criteria for effectiveness are based on outcome identification, the client's feedback, and the observations of the nurse and other mental health professionals regarding the client's response to interventions.

TABLE 10–7
Major Anxiolytic Agents Used to Manage Anxiety Disorders

Benzodiazepines (Diazepam, Alprazolam, Lorazepam, and Clonazepam)

Generalized anxiety disorder
Panic disorder

Nonbenzodiazepines (Buspirone)

Generalized anxiety disorder

Serotonin Reuptake Inhibitors/Antidepressants (Fluoxetine and Clomipramine)

Obsessive–compulsive disorder

Tricyclic Antidepressants (Imipramine and Desipramine)

Panic disorders
Posttraumatic stress disorder
Phobic disorders

Monoamine Oxidase Inhibitors (Phenelzine)

Panic disorders
Posttraumatic stress disorder
Phobic disorders

Beta-Blockers (Propranolol)

Panic disorder
Generalized anxiety disorder

Data from Rosenbaum, J. F., & Gelenberg, A. J. (1991). Anxiety. In A. G. Gelenberg, et al. *The practitioner's guide to psychoactive drugs* (3rd ed., pp. 179–218). New York: Plenum Press.

CHAPTER SUMMARY

Anxiety is an integral aspect of the human experience. It is associated with arousal, the body's mobilization of its neurobiological resources. Clients tend to seek treatment when their anxiety becomes overwhelming and interferes with their psychosocial and biological functioning. Symptoms of anxiety range from mild to severe forms of distress.

Psychiatric nurses are challenged to assess clients' adaptive and maladaptive responses and to provide them with adequate and effective treatment. The nursing process is an effective mechanism that identifies disabling symptoms and effective interventions that promote adaptive responses. In addition, education of the client and his or her significant others regarding anxiety and their active participation in treatment are critical to successful treatment outcomes.

Suggestions for Clinical Conference

1. Present case histories of clients experiencing anxiety disorders. For each case, identify the (a) psychosocial issues, (b) neurobiological factors, (c) treatment modalities, (d) life span issues, and (e) client/family teaching needs.
2. Discuss several treatment modalities for clients experiencing anxiety disorders, such as progressive relaxation, visual imagery, and psychopharmacological interventions.

References

Ainsworth, M. D. (1985). Attachments across the life span. *Bulletin of the New York Academy of Medicine, 61*, 792–812.

American Nurses Association. (1994). *Statement on psychiatric–mental health nursing practice and standards of psychiatric–mental health clinical nursing practice*. Washington, DC: Author.

American Psychiatric Association. (1994). *Diagnostic and statistical manual of mental disorders* (4th ed.). Washington, DC: Author.

Andrews, G., & Crino, R. (1991). Behavioral therapy of anxiety disorders. *Psychiatric Annals, 21*, 358–367.

Appenheimer, T., & Noyes, R. (1987). Generalized anxiety disorder. *Primary Care, 14*, 635–648.

Basch, M. F. (1988). *Understanding psychotherapy*. New York: Basic Books.

Bauer, D. H. (1976). An exploratory study of developmental changes in children's fears. *Journal of Child Psychology and Psychiatry, 17*, 69–74.

Beck, A. T., & Emery, G. (1985). *Anxiety disorders and phobias: A cognitive perspective*. New York: Basic Books.

Beck, A. T., Skodol, L., Clark, D. A., Berchick, R., & Wright, F. (1992). A crossover study of focused cognitive therapy for panic disorders. *American Journal of Psychiatry, 149*, 778–783.

Berg, C. Z., et al. (1989). Childhood obsessive compulsive disorder: A two-year prospective follow-up of a community sample. *Journal of the American Academy of Child and Adolescent Psychiatry, 28*, 528–533.

Bowlby, J. (1969). *Attachment and loss* (Vol. 1). New York: Basic Books.

Brawman-Mintzer, O., et al. (1993). Psychiatric comorbidity in patients with generalized anxiety disorder. *American Journal of Psychiatry, 150*, 1216–1218.

Breuer, J., & Freud, S. (1957). Studies in hysteria (J. Strachey, Trans.). New York: Basic Books. (Original work published 1895)

Burgess, A. W., Hartman, C. R., & McCormack, A. (1987). Abused to abuser: Antecedents of socially deviant behaviors. *American Journal of Psychiatry, 144*, 1431–1436.

Cannon W. B. (1914). The emergency function of the adrenal medulla in pain and the major emotions. *American Journal of Physiology, 33*, 356–372.

Charney, D. S., et al. (1993). Psychobiological mechanisms of post-traumatic stress disorder. *Archives of General Psychiatry, 50*, 294–305.

Clomipramine Collaborative Study Group. (1991). Efficacy of clomipramine in OCD: Results of a multicenter double-blind trial. *Archives of Psychiatry, 48*, 730–738.

Cloninger, C. R. (1986). A unified biosocial theory of personality and its role in the development of anxiety states. *Psychiatric Development, 5*, 167–226.

Cowley, D. S., & Arana, G. W. (1990). The diagnostic utility of lactate sensitivity in panic disorder. *Archives of General Psychiatry, 47*, 277–287.

Cross-National Collaborative Panic Study, Second Phase Investigators. (1992). Drug treatment of panic disorder: The comparative efficacy of alprazolam, imipramine, and placebo. *British Journal of Psychiatry, 160*, 191–202.

de Montigny, C. (1989). Cholecystokinin tetrapeptide induces panic-like attacks in health volunteers: Preliminary findings. *Archives of General Psychiatry, 46*, 511–517.

Eaton, W. W, Dryman, A, & Weissman, M. M. (1991). Panic and phobia. In L. N. Robins & D. A. Regier (Eds.), *Psychiatric disorders in America: The epidemiological catchment area study*. New York: Free Press.

Ellis, A. (1962). *Reason and emotion in psychotherapy*. New York: Lyle Stuart.

Epstein, R. S. (1989). Post traumatic stress disorder: A review of diagnostic and treatment issues. *Psychiatric Annals, 19*, 556–563.

Eth, S. & Pynoos, R. (1984). *Post-traumatic stress disorder in children*. Washington, DC: American Psychiatric Press.

Everstine, D. S., & Everstine, L. (1993). *The trauma response*. New York: W. W. Norton.

Eysenck, H. J. (1981). *A model for personality*. New York: Springer-Verlag.

Flament, M. F., et al. (1988). Obsessive compulsive disorder: An epidemiological study. Journal of the American Academy of Child and Adolescent Psychiatry, 27, 764–771.

Freud, A. (1936). *The ego and the mechanisms of defense*. New York: International University Press.

Freud, S. (1936). *The problem of anxiety* (H. A. Bunker, Trans.). New York: Psychoanalytic Quarterly Press. (Original work published (1926)

Gelder, M. S. (1991). Psychological treatment of agoraphobia. *Psychiatric Annals, 21*, 354–357.

Gittelman, R., & Klein, D. F. (1984). Relationship between separation anxiety and panic and agoraphobia. *Psychopathology, 17*(Suppl. 1), 56–65.

Glover, H. (1992). Emotional numbing: A possible endorphin-mediated phenomenon associated with post traumatic disorders and other allied psychopathologic states. *Journal of Traumatic Stress, 5*, 643–675.

Gray, J. A. (1982). *The neuropsychology of anxiety*. New York: Oxford University Press.

Graziano, A. M., DeGiorani, I., & Garcia, K. (1979). Behavioral treatment of child's fear. *Psychological Bulletin 56*, 804–830.

Hodge, K. K., McKnew, D., & Burbach, D. J. (1987). Diagnostic concordance between two structured child interviews, using lay examiners: The child assessment schedule and the Kiddie-SADS. *Journal of the Academy of Child and Adolescent Psychiatry, 26*, 654–661.

Jenike, M. A., Baer, L., Summergrad, P., Weilburg, J. B., Hollrho, A., & Seymour, R. (1989). Obsessive-compulsive disorder: A double-blind, placebo-controlled trial of clomipramine in 27 patients. *American Journal of Psychiatry, 146*, 1328–1330.

Johnson, J., Weissman, M. M., & Klerman, G. L. (1990). Panic disorders, comorbidity, and suicide attempts. *Archives of General Psychiatry, 47*, 805–808.

Karno, M., Golding, J. M., Sorenson, S. B., & Burnam, M. A. (1988). Epidemiology of obsessive-compulsive disorder in five U.S. communities. *Archives of General Psychiatry, 45*, 1094–1099.

Kashani, J. J., Dandoy, A. C., & Orvaschel, H. (1991). Current perspectives on anxiety disorders in children and adolescents: An overview. *Comprehensive Psychiatry 32*, 481–495.

Kashani, J. J., & Orvaschel, H. (1990). A community study of anxiety disorders in children and adolescents. *American Journal of Psychiatry, 147*, 313–318.

Kendall, P. C. (1993). Cognitive behavioral therapies with youth: Guiding theory, current status, and emerging developments. *Journal of Consulting and Clinical Psychology, 61*, 235–247.

Kendall, P. C., Kortlander, E., Chansky, T. E., & Brady, E. U. (1992). Comorbidity of anxiety and depression in youth: Treatment implications. *Journal of Consulting and Clinical Psychology, 60*, 869–880.

Kendler, K. S., Neal, M. C., Kessler, R. C., Heath, A. C., & Eaves, L. J. (1992a). Generalized anxiety disorder in women. *Archives of General Psychiatry, 49*, 267–272.

Kendler, K. S., Neale, M. C., Kessler, R. C., Heath, A. C., & Eaves, L. J. (1992b). The genetic epidemiology of phobias in women: The interrelationship of agoraphobia, social phobia, situational phobia, and simple phobia. *Archives of General Psychiatry, 49*, 273–281.

Lazarus, A. A. (1971). *Behavior therapy and beyond*. New York: McGraw-Hill.

Lenane, M. C. (1991). Family therapy for children with obsessive-compulsive disorder. In M. S. Paton & J. Zohar (Eds.), *Current treatment of obsessive-compulsive disorder* (pp. 103–113). Washington, DC: American Psychiatric Press.

Lenane, M. C., Swedo, S. E., Leonard, H., Pauls, D. L., Sceery, W., & Rapaport, J. (1990). Psychiatric disorders in first-degree relatives of children and adolescents with obsessive-compulsive disorder. *Journal of the American Academy of Child and Adolescent Psychiatry, 29*, 407–412.

Leon, C. A., & Leon, A. (1990). Panic disorder and parental bonding. *Psychiatric Annals, 20*, 503–508.

Leonard, H. L., Swedo, S. E., Rapoport, J. L., Koby, E. V., Lenane, M. C., Cheslow, D. L., & Hamburger, S. D. (1989). Treatment of childhood obsessive compulsive disorder with clomipramine and desipramine: A double-blind crossover comparison. *Archives of General Psychiatry, 46*, 1088–1092.

Liebowitz, M. R., Gorman, J. M., Fryer, A., et al. (1986). Possible mechanism for lactate's induction of panic. *American Journal of Psychiatry, 143*, 646–648.

Markowitz, J. S., Weismann, M. M., Ouelette, R., Lish, J. D., &

Klerman, G. L. (1989). Quality of life in panic disorder. *Archives of General Psychiatry, 46*, 984–992.

Mavissakalian, M., & Perel, J. M. (1992). Protective effects of imipramine maintenance treatment in panic disorder with agoraphobia. *American Journal of Psychiatry, 149*, 1053–1057.

May, R. (1977). *The meaning of anxiety* (2nd ed.) New York: W. W. Norton.

McGlynn, T. J., & Metcalf, H. L. (1989). *Diagnosis and treatment of anxiety disorders*. Washington, DC: American Psychiatric Press.

Murphy, D. L., Mueller, E. A., Hill, J. L., Tolliver, T. J., & Jacobsen, F. M. (1989). Comparative anxiogenic, neuroendocrine, and other physiologic effects of *m*-chlorophenylpiperazine given intravenously or orally to healthy volunteers. *Psychopharmacology, 98*, 275–282.

Nordahl, T., et al. (1989). Cerebral glucose metabolic rates in obsessive-compulsive disorder. *Neuro-Psychopharmacology, 2*, 23–28.

Ollendick, T. H., & Francis, G. (1988). Behavioral assessment and treatment of childhood phobias. *Behavior Modification, 12*, 165–204.

Pavlov, I. P. (1927). *Conditioned reflexes: An investigation of the physiological activity of the cerebral cortex* (G. C. Andrep, Trans. and Ed.). London: Oxford University Press.

Piaget, J. (1954). *The construction of reality in the child.* New York: Basic Books.

Piaget, J. (1958). *The growth of logical thinking from childhood to adolescence*. New York: Basic Books.

Pigott, T. A., Pato, M. T., Bernstein, S. E., Grover, G. N., Hill, J. L., Tolliver, T. J., & Murphy, D. L. (1990). Controlled comparison of clomipramine and fluoxetine in the treatment of obsessive-compulsive disorder: Behavioral and biological results. *Archives of General Psychiatry, 47*, 926–934.

Pynoos, R. S., & Eth, S. (1985). Children traumatized by witnessing acts of personal violence: Homicide, rape, or suicide behavior. In S. Eth & R. S. Pynoos (Eds.), *Post-traumatic stress disorders in children* (pp. 19–43). Washington, DC: American Psychiatric Press.

Rasmussen, S. A., & Tsuang, M. T. (1984). The epidemiology of obsessive-compulsive disorder. *Journal of Clinical Psychiatry, 45*, 450–457.

Redmond, D. E., Jr. (1987). Studies of the nucleus locus coeruleus in monkeys and hypothesis for neuropharmacology. In H. Y. Meltzer (Ed.), *Psychopharmacology* (pp. 967–975). New York: Raven Press.

Redmond, D. E., et al. (1976). Behavioral effects of stimulation of the nucleus locus coeruleus in the stump-tailed monkey, *Macaca arctoides. Brain Research, 116*, 502–510.

Regier, D. A., Burke, J. D., & Burke, K. C. (1990a). Comorbidity of affective and anxiety disorders in the NIMH Epidemiologic Catchment Area Program. In J. D. Maser & C. R. Cloninger (Eds.), *Comorbidity of mood and anxiety disorders* (pp. 113–122). Washington, DC: American Psychiatric Press.

Regier, D. A., Farmer, M. E., Rae, R. S., Locke, B. Z., Keith, S. J., Judd, L. L., & Goodwin, F. K. (1990b). Comorbidity of mental disorders with alcohol and other drug abuse: Results from the Epidemiological Catchment Area (ECA) Study. *Journal of the American Medical Association, 264*, 2511–2518.

Reynolds, C. R. & Richmond, B. D. (1978). What I think and feel: A revised measure of children's manifest anxiety. *Journal of Abnormal Child Psychology, 6*, 271–280.

Robins, L. N., Heltzer, J. E., Weismann, M. M., Orvaschel, H., Gruenberg, E., Burke, J. D., & Regier, D. A. (1984). Lifetime prevalence of specific psychiatric disorders in three sites. *Archives of General Psychiatry, 41*, 949–958.

Rosenbaum, J. F. (1990). A psychopharmacologist's perspective on panic disorder. *Bulletin of the Menninger Clinic, 54*, 184–196.

Rosenbaum, J. F., & Gelenberg, A. J. (1991). Anxiety. In A. G. Gelenberg, et al. (Eds.), *The practitioner's guide to psychoactive drugs* (3rd ed., pp. 179–218). New York: Plenum.

Schweizer, E., et al. (1993). Double-blind, placebo-controlled study of a once-a-day, sustained-release preparation of alprazolam for the treatment of panic disorder. *American Journal of Psychiatry, 150*, 1210–1215.

Sheehan, D. V. (1986). *The anxiety disease* (2nd ed.). New York: Bantam Books.

Silverman, W. K., Cerny, J. A., Nelles, W. B., & Burke, A. E. (1988). Behavior problems in children of parents with anxiety disorders. *Journal of the American Academy of Child and Adolescent Psychiatry, 27*, 779–784.

Simson, P. E., & Weiss, J. M. (1988). Responsiveness of locus coeruleus neurons to excitatory stimulation is uniquely regulated by alpha-2 receptors. *Psychopharmacology Bulletin, 24*, 349–354.

Swedo, S. E., Schapiro, M. B., Grady, C. L., Cheslow, D. L., Leonard, H. L., Kumar, A., Friedland, R., Rapoport, S. I., & Rapoport, J. L. (1989). Cerebral glucose metabolism in childhood-onset obsessive-compulsive disorders. *Archives of General Psychiatry, 46*, 518–523.

Torgersen, S. (1983). Genetic factors in anxiety disorders. *Archives of General Psychiatry, 40*, 1085–1089.

Uhde, T. W., Jaffee, R. T., Jimerson, D. C., et al. (1988). Normal urinary free cortisol and plasma MHPG in panic disorder: Clinical and theoretical implications. *Biological Psychiatry, 23*, 565–585.

Uhde, T. W. (1994). Anxiety and growth disturbance: Is there a connection? A review of biological studies in social phobia. *Journal of Clinical Psychiatry, 55* (Suppl. 6), 17–27.

van der Kolk, B. A., Greenberg, M., Boyd, H., & Krystal, J. (1985). Inescapable shock, neurotransmitters and addiction to trauma: Towards a psychobiology of post-traumatic stress. *Biological Psychiatry, 20*, 314–325.

van der Molen, G. M., van der Hout, A. C., van Dieren, A. C., & Greiz, E. (1989). Childhood separation anxiety and adult onset panic disorders. *Journal of Anxiety, 3*, 97–106.

Weissman, M. M., & Merikangas, A. S. (1986). The epidemiology of anxiety and panic disorders: An update. *Journal of Clinical Psychiatry, 47* (Suppl. 6), 11–17.

Wolpe, J. (1973). *The practice of behavioral therapy*. New York: Pergamon Press.

Yehuda, R., Lowy, M. T., Southwick, S. M., Shaffer, D., & Giller, E. L. Jr. (1991). Lymphocyte glucocorticoid receptor number in posttraumatic stress disorder. *American Journal of Psychiatry, 148*, 499–504.

Yehuda, R., Southwick, S. M., Krystal, J. H., Bremmer, D., Charney, D. S., & Mason, J.M. (1993). Enhanced suppression of cortisol following dexamethasone administration in posttraumatic stress disorder. *American Journal of Psychiatry, 150*, 83–86.

CHAPTER

11

The Client with Stress-Related Illness (Psychophysiological Disorders)

DEBORAH ANTAI-OTONG, M.S., R.N.,C.S.

OUTLINE

CHAPTER OBJECTIVES

Upon completion of this chapter, you will be able to:

1. Analyze the effects of stress in mental and physical illnesses.
2. Discuss psychosocial and biological responses to stress.
3. Develop nursing care plans for clients experiencing psychophysiological disorders.
4. Recognize the impact of psychophysiological disorders on the client and the client's family.

KEY TERMS

Adaptation
Catecholamine
Disease-prone behaviors
Psychophysiological disorders
Self-healing behaviors
Sick role
Stress
T cells
Type A personality
Type B personality

The interrelationship between the body and the mind is well documented. Emotions and physiological responses are elicited by internal and external environments. Franz Alexander (1950) believed that intense or prolonged emotions trigger physiological responses. For example, he hypothesized that underlying anger or rage contributes to heart disease and that helplessness produces gastrointestinal disease. Alexander's premise suggests that humans respond to stressful situations by using both neurobiological and psychological resources to maintain and restore homeostasis. Humans are holistic beings, and when stress affects one system, all other systems are influenced. Circumstances that threaten homeostasis activate complex neurobiological and psychosocial coping processes that arise from the autonomic nervous system.

Anger is an example of an intense emotion that triggers the sympathetic nervous system, which in turn stimulates adrenaline production and the flight-or-fight response. Neurobiological responses usually return to normal levels when anger abates. When people internalize anger or fail to manage it effectively, their bodies keep producing biological responses to stress. The sustained stimulation of the autonomic nervous system in these people results in continual production of catecholamines, which are potent vasopressors. Major catecholamines are norepinephrine and epinephrine. These substances affect all body systems, including the cardiovascular, gastrointestinal, and immunological systems, and chronic production can damage tissues regardless of their origin (Alexander, 1939).

A holistic approach to client care is a major goal of nursing, and it requires assessing complex client needs that relate to emotional and biological responses to stress. Furthermore, nurses teach clients strategies that enhance their coping skills and reduce stress, and they educate clients and their families about the long-term effects of stress, noncompliance, and ineffective coping patterns.

This chapter focuses on the behavioral and psychological factors that affect nonpsychiatric medical conditions. Nonpsychiatric medical conditions that are caused by behavioral or psychological factors are called *psychophysiological disorders*. The role of the psychiatric–mental health nurse in identifying clients' high-risk behaviors, reducing stress, and facilitating clients' adaptive coping skills is discussed.

DEFINITION

Historically, the term *psychosomatic* was used to describe a physical problem that was caused by an emotional state. The fourth edition of the *Diagnostic and Statistical Manual of Mental Disorders* (DSM-IV) (American Psychiatric Association [APA], 1994) uses the term *psychological factors affecting medical conditions*. To be considered psychophysiological, a disorder must present with a medical condition on Axis III (e.g., hypertension). Other criteria include one of the following:

1. The course of the general medical condition is worsened or triggered by psychological factors (e.g., intense stress)
2. Psychological factors or emotional states unfavorably impact the course or outcome of treatment (e.g., client forgets to take hypertension medication or misses followup appointments)
3. Psychological factors or emotional states place the client at greater risk for health problems (e.g., increased risk of stroke or renal failure)
4. Psychological factors hasten stress-related physiological processes that worsen the general medical condition (e.g., hypertension persists in spite of adherence to medication regimen and later the client suffers a stroke or renal failure)

Prior to the DSM-IV, psychophysiological disorders were referred to as "psychological factors affecting physical conditions" (DSM-III, DSM-III-R) and "psychosomatic disorders" (DSM-I, DSM-II).

CAUSATIVE FACTORS: PERSPECTIVES AND THEORIES

Human responses to stress involve psychosocial and neurobiological processes. In stressful situations, the body switches on its autonomic nervous system and neurobiological processes in an attempt to maintain homeostasis. Psychosocial adaptive processes are mobilized and sustained by temperament and personality traits that help the person cope with stressful situations.

PSYCHODYNAMIC THEORIES

Alexander (1939), a prominent pioneer of psychosomatic medicine and research, described "organ neurosis" or "functional disturbance" as a biological response to psychological stressors. He suggested that every emotional reaction corresponds with biological changes hastened by sympathetic adrenal arousal. Acute stress reactions were perceived as normal everyday responses that generally produced few injurious effects, in comparison with persistent sympathetic nervous system activation, which produced anatomical changes or physiological disorders.

Later, Alexander (1950) delineated seven psychosomatic disorders: essential hypertension, skin disorders, rheumatoid arthritis, hyperthyroidism, ulcerative colitis, peptic ulcer diseases, and asthma. He believed that visceral or organ dysfunction arose from primarily unconscious personality traits or inadequate coping behaviors that interfered with reduction of intense emotions, such as anger, or repressed sustained fears, anxiety, and aggression.

Freud (1958) hypothesized that unreleased psychological tension was converted into symptoms such as paralysis or blindness. He termed this reaction *conversion hysteria* and suggested that it stemmed from the inability to express feelings.

A contemporary term for conversion hysteria is *conversion disorder*. The DSM-IV categorizes these disorders as somatoform disorders and lists several criteria:

- The loss or change in physical function is initially associated with a physical cause.
- Later, psychological components, such as intense stress and anxiety, are linked to the physical symptoms.
- The phenomenon is unintentional and unconscious.
- The symptom is not part of cultural mores, general medical condition, or substance misuse.
- The symptom is not associated with pain or disturbance in sexual performance.
- The symptom interferes with the client's optimal level of function.

NEUROBIOLOGICAL THEORIES

Stress is an integral part of living. Highly complex neurobiological and psychosocial processes are activated by stress, and they determine how internal and external demands are handled. Prolonged stimulation of the autonomic nervous system produces neurobiological changes and affects brain activity. A person's inability to manage stress effectively increases his or her vulnerability to illness (Selye, 1976).

The premise of Selye's general adaptation syndrome is that there is a relationship between stress and neurobiological changes that arise from stimulation of the hypothalamic–pituitary–adrenal axis (Fig. 11–1). Effective mastery of stress restores homeostasis and allows **adaptation**.

Stress can also alter various immunological processes. The immune system mediates intricate neurobiological processes and behavior to maintain homeostasis. The exact role it plays in adaptation remains unclear (Ader et al., 1987, 1991). However, several studies suggest a relationship between stress and a reduction in natural killer (NK) cell activity. NK cells are believed to be instrumental in fighting certain viruses and tumors (Glaser et al., 1987, 1990). Other stress-related alterations include decreased white blood cell, gamma interferon, and T-cell production. Transitory stress-induced change in the immune system is generally considered adaptive, but chronic stress reactions are believed to compromise the immune system and increase the risk of certain viral conditions and cancer (Ader et al., 1987, 1991).

Neuroendocrine processes are surmised to parallel dysregulation of the immune system. Prolonged stress is also associated with increased cortisol levels and epinephrine and norepinephrine production, which may alter the immune system (Ader et al., 1987, 1991; Brosschot et al., 1994).

More recent studies link immunological suppression with depression; maladaptive coping behaviors and social interactions; and substance abuse, cancer, and other physical disorders (Eysenck, 1991; H. S. Friedman & VandenBos, 1992). Inappropriate and chronic release of stress hormones (adrenocorticotropic hormone and cortisol) eventually damages the normal neural and physiological mechanisms that maintain physical and mental adaptation. Long exposure to cortisol has been shown to contribute to systems diseases such as hypertension, atherosclerosis, and myocardial infarction. Perpetual stress has also been shown to destroy brain regions that normally shut down the stress response (i.e., gamma-aminobutyric acid pathways), allowing the response to continue unchecked to the point of exhaustion.

The additional biological factor that is influenced by stress and adaptation is temperament. Temperament incorporates inherited behavioral and genetic factors that make some people vulnerable to allergic reactions and hay fever. The basis of this relationship is that emotional responses affect the sympathetic nervous system, which in turn causes nasal epithelium to react (Kagan et al., 1991) (see Chapter 8).

COGNITIVE AND BEHAVIORAL FACTORS: PERSONALITY (COPING) STYLES

Cognitive and behavioral factors that derive from personality styles also affect responses to stress. There is a relationship between personality or coping style and predisposition to certain illnesses. The **Type A personality** and **Type B personality** were introduced by M. Friedman and R. H. Rosenman (1974) more than 20 years ago; these researchers suggested that there was a positive relationship between Type A personality and

THE STRESS RESPONSE

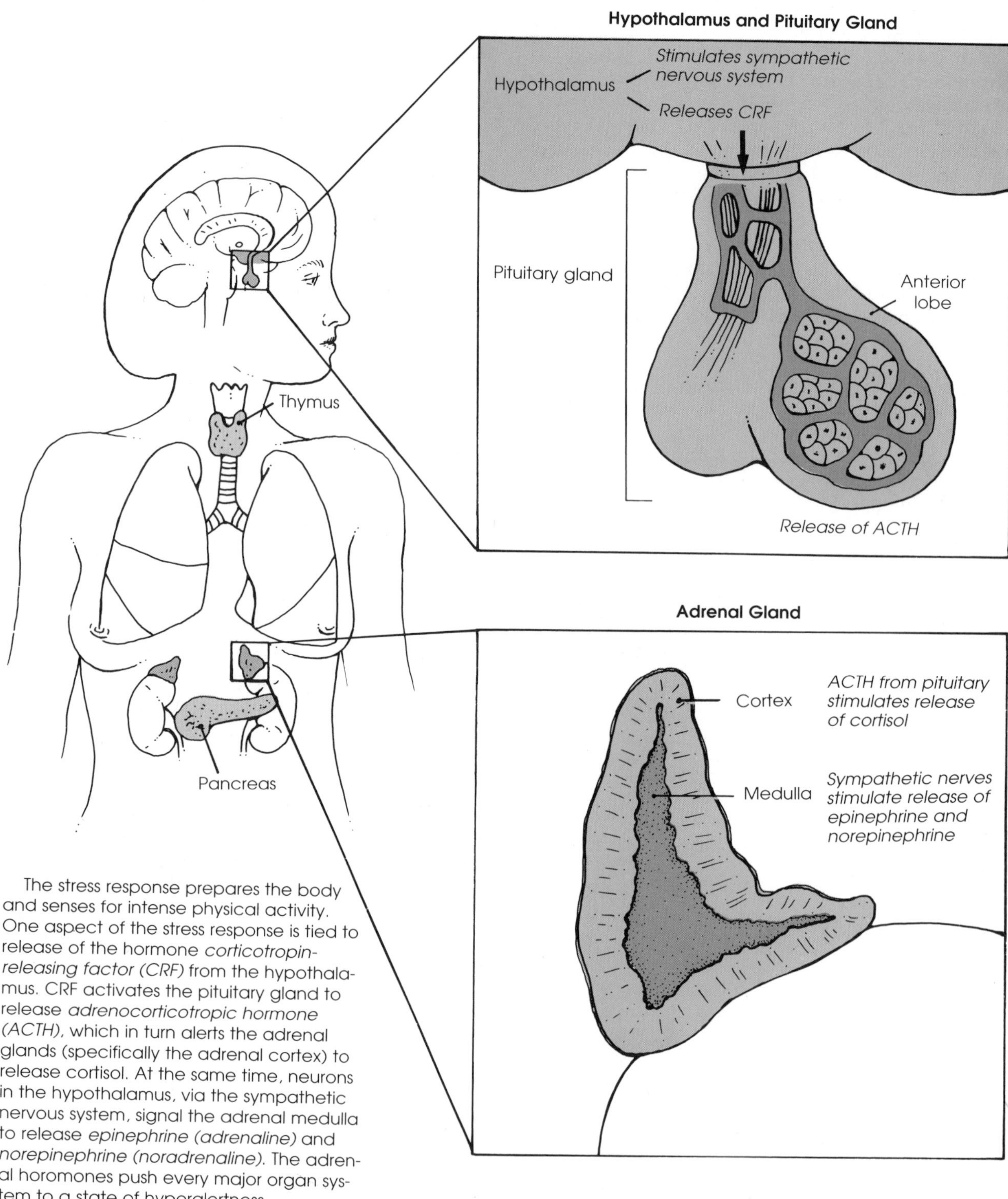

The stress response prepares the body and senses for intense physical activity. One aspect of the stress response is tied to release of the hormone *corticotropin-releasing factor (CRF)* from the hypothalamus. CRF activates the pituitary gland to release *adrenocorticotropic hormone (ACTH)*, which in turn alerts the adrenal glands (specifically the adrenal cortex) to release cortisol. At the same time, neurons in the hypothalamus, via the sympathetic nervous system, signal the adrenal medulla to release *epinephrine (adrenaline)* and *norepinephrine (noradrenaline)*. The adrenal horomones push every major organ system to a state of hyperalertness.

Chronic stress can affect body organ function as well as the immune system. Inappropriate and chronic release of cortisol, epinephrine, and norepinephrine eventually exhausts normal mechanisms for maintaining homeostasis, and destroys brain regions (GABA pathways) that normally shut down the stress response. *(See Fig. 10–1 for a discussion of norepinephrine and GABA pathways.)* Benzodiazepines (Valium, Librium) are sometimes prescribed for persons vulnerable to chronic stress reactions; these tranquilizers enhance GABA production and uptake, and dampen emotional response.

FIGURE 11–1
The stress response: the role of hormones and the physical and emotional effects of chronic stress. (Illustration concept: Gail Kongable, M.S.N., C.N.R.N., C.C.R.N., Department of Neurosurgery, University of Virginia Health Sciences Center. Illustration by Marie T. Dauenheimer.)

PHYSICAL AND EMOTIONAL EFFECTS OF STRESS

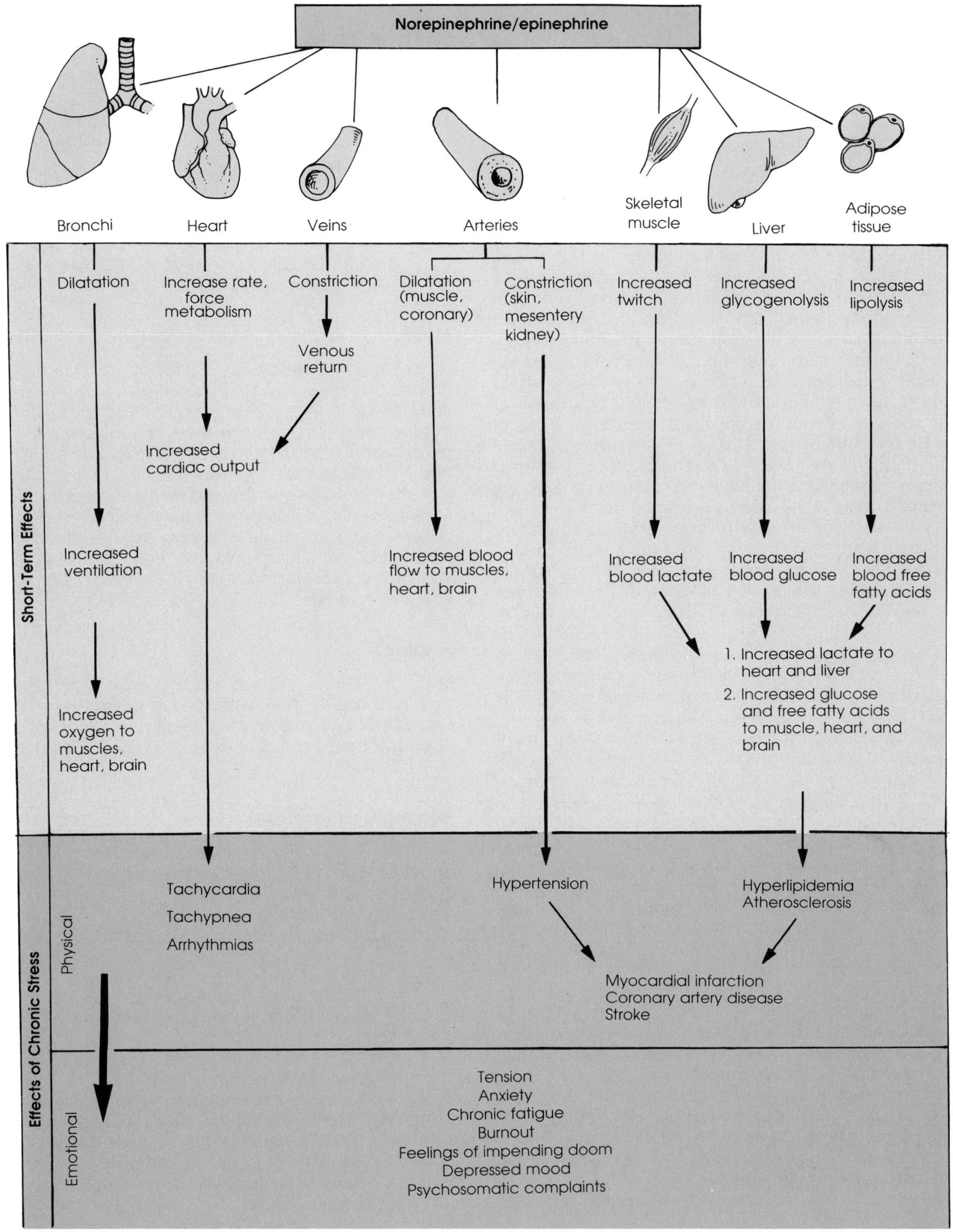

heart disease. The Type A personality includes the following characteristics:

- Rapid speech
- Rapid walking
- Irritability
- Time consciousness
- Difficulty relaxing
- Persistent need to stay busy
- Attempts to do more than one thing at a time

According to Friedman and Rosenman, Type A people are extremely competitive and aggressively strive for success and achievement. They frequently have high-pressure jobs and are referred to as workaholics, perfectionists, and overachievers. Underlying deficits in self-worth, self-esteem, and self-acceptance and excessive dependence on the approval of others are pervasive characteristics in these people. They are driven, constantly on the run, and tend to internalize their feelings. Psychological and biological needs are frequently ignored, further increasing the risk of stress-related illnesses (Friedman & Rosenman, 1974). Coping styles tend to include appraisal of events and perception of control. The Research Study display describes a recent study that showed that Type A personality was linked with higher blood pressure and cholesterol levels in African American women. However, there is controversy regarding Type A personality traits and the risk of coronary disease (see the Controversy display on p. 215).

People with Type B personalities are less driven than these with Type A personalities. They are generally more easygoing, laid back, and reposed. Their lifestyles are relaxed and goal directed (Friedman & Rosenman, 1974).

Research suggests that some people are more vulnerable to stress than others. Risk factors include personality traits, genetics, diet, and environmental stressors. A lifestyle of chronic negative emotions, such as hostility, seems to produce neurobiological changes that increase a person's vulnerability to stress. People who chronically experience these negative emotions tend to repress their feelings and are likely to abuse substances, which further compromises their well-being. The inability to express feelings is manifested by closed body language, such as folded arms and poor eye contact, an overly appeasing attitude, and an anxious mood. Inability or unwillingness to express feelings has been associated with sustained arousal of the sympathetic nervous system. The behaviors of chronically negative persons have been labeled **disease-prone behaviors**, and they include distance, guarded social interactions, pessimism, repression, and despair (Barefoot, 1992; Friedman & VandenBos, 1992; Pennebacker, 1992). Conversely, clients with **self-healing behaviors** are generally described as emotionally balanced. They tend to be excited, energetic, questioning, spontaneous, humorous, and inspirational and to have healthy interpersonal skills. They tend to generate enthusiasm and motivation in others. Table 11–1 compares the behaviors of disease-prone and self-healing personalities.

Prolonged stress has deleterious effects on neurobiological processes, which are understood as the basis of psychophysiological disorders. Responses to stress vary across the life span and depend on mobilization of internal and external resources, which are the basis of adaptation. Nursing implications include identifying high-risk behaviors and formulating interventions that strengthen coping skills and reduce the deleterious effects of stress reactions.

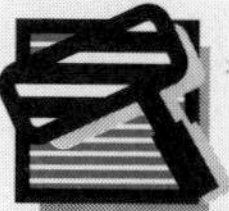

RESEARCH STUDY

A Path Model of Type A and Type B Responses to Coping and Stress in Employed Black Women

Smyth, K. A., & Yarandi, H. N. (1992). *Nursing Research, 41*, 260–264.

Study Problem/Purpose

The researchers tested the conceptual model of the effects of age, weight, personality type (A or B), cholesterol level, systolic blood pressure, and coping on the stress response of southern African American women.

Method

A convenience sample of 280 employed African American women ages 20 to 65 years (M = 38.76) living in the southeastern United States was studied. Several tools were used to measure hypercholesterolemia (the Reflotron was used to analyze various blood chemicals), and coping was measured by the Revised Ways of Coping Scale. Structured interviews were audiotaped and analyzed. Blood pressures were measured every minute before, during, and after a stress-evoking interview conducted to determine whether participants had Type A or Type B personalities.

Findings

Findings showed that subjects with Type A personality traits had higher resting blood pressures, cholesterol levels, and stress levels and lower coping scores than did those with Type B personality traits.

Nursing Implications

Major nursing implications include opportunities to assess individual teaching and health-promoting needs and help clients assess their adaptive and maladaptive coping skills.

CONTROVERSY

Is the Type A Personality a Predictor of Coronary Artery Disease?

Despite numerous studies linking Type A personality traits with increased risk of coronary artery disease, controversy prevails. Some researchers posit that people with Type A personalities have twice the risk of coronary artery disease that people with Type B personalities have (Williams, 1985). Other researchers suggest that Type A personality traits may not be a predictor of coronary artery disease and that other risk factors such as angina and depression have a greater impact (Light et al., 1991).

SPECIFIC PSYCHOPHYSIOLOGICAL DISORDERS AND TREATMENT MODALITIES

The **psychophysiological disorders** are divided into several categories: cardiovascular, pulmonary, immunological, gastrointestinal (GI), skin, and chronic pain.

CARDIOVASCULAR DISORDERS

The cardiovascular system is composed of the heart and blood vessels, which circulate blood and use oxygen, various nutrients, and intricate neurobiological processes to supply cells and deport waste and impurities. Cardiovascular disorders refer to impairments of the heart and blood vessels.

TABLE 11–1
Characteristics of Disease-Prone and Self-Healing Personality Styles

DISEASE-PRONE CHARACTERISTICS	SELF-HEALING CHARACTERISTICS
► Chronic negative emotions ► Chronic emotional tension ► Chronic animosity ► Dominance and argumentativeness ► Competitiveness and irritability ► Tension and aggression ► Impaired interpersonal relationships ► Repressed feelings, holding back of thoughts and feelings	► Enthusiasm ► Emotional security ► Responsiveness and energeticness ► Spontaneity ► Adaptability ► Ability to relax ► Problem solving, diligence ► Positive interpersonal relationships

Data from Friedman, H. S., & VandenBos, G. R. (1992). Disease-prone and self-healing personalities. *Hospital and Community Psychiatry, 43*, 1177–1179.

Coronary Heart Disease. Coronary heart disease continues to be the leading cause of death in the United States. It results from blockage of coronary arteries, which interferes with perfusion of blood to the heart and general circulation. The lack of adequate oxygen perfusion and removal of waste products creates hypoxia and angina pectoris (chest pain). Coronary heart disease is linked with a number of high-risk behaviors, including personality traits (e.g., Type A behaviors), elevated cholesterol levels, smoking, lack of regular exercise, and uncontrolled high blood pressure.

Persistent and chronic activation of the sympathetic nervous system has been linked with physiological cardiovascular changes (M. Friedman & Rosenman, 1974; Kasl & Cooper, 1987). However, there is disagreement regarding the impact of Type A behaviors on heart disease (Williams et al., 1991). In addition, a 10-year followup study of 248 men conducted by Shekelle et al. (1991) dispelled the notion that chronic distressful complaints increased the risk of coronary artery disease; however, it did demonstrate an increased incidence of a nonartherosclerotic form of angina in these subjects.

Hypertension. Hypertension is another major cardiovascular disease linked with stress. Stress activates the autonomic nervous system, which activates the release of **catecholamines** (epinephrine and norepinephrine). These biochemicals produce profound changes in the cardiovascular system by raising the blood pressure and heart rate and causing other physiological changes that produce the flight-or-fight response. Persistent sympathetic stimulation produces vasoconstriction, increasing the risk of hypertension.

Who is at risk for hypertension? Persons at risk for this disorder are those with family histories of heart disease, diabetes, and maladaptive personality or coping styles. Psychosocial stressors, such as impoverished living conditions, high-pressure jobs, and strained interpersonal relationships, also play key roles in the development of hypertension.

Treatment Modalities. Prevention is critical to the treatment of hypertension and other cardiovascular disorders. By assessing the client's present stressors and coping styles and developing an individualized teaching plan, the nurse can help the client recognize the maladaptive nature and consequences of his or her disease-prone behaviors and explore adaptive ways to manage stress. An interdisciplinary approach is critical to the success of health education and restoration. Major interventions include smoking cessation, weight loss, administration of cardiovascular agents and compliance with the medication regimen, diet restrictions and healthy eating habits, a regular exercise program, and stress management. Stress management, psychoeducation, and cognitive–behavioral and other forms of psychotherapy help clients express their feelings and develop effective coping skills. Progressive relaxation exercises teach clients how to relax (see Chapter 10 for specific techniques). See Table 11–2 for a description of stress-reducing techniques.

TABLE 11–2
Therapeutic Measures for Stress-Related Illness

BIOFEEDBACK

Biofeedback is an electronic indication of a person's stress level that is provided by instrumentation that registers the person's psychophysiological responses. A tone or signal provides the client with immediate feedback. The goal is to keep the tone below a certain threshold for 15 seconds on four occasions. The client learns to observe and control subtle internal body responses (blood pressure, temperature, and muscle tension). This intervention enables clients to play an active role in the promotion of their own health.
Indications: Migraine headaches, hypertension, Raynaud's disease, chronic pain, gastrointestinal disorders.

DEEP MUSCLE RELAXATION

The client is taught how to achieve deep muscle relaxation, which is basic to all behavioral stress reduction techniques. The following instructions are given to the client:

- Find a quiet area away from distraction.
- If desired, use a relaxation tape.
- Get into a comfortable position, such as lying on your back.
- Close your eyes and inhale deeply through your nose, allowing your lungs to fill with air and feeling your chest expand. Then slowly exhale.
- Repeat.

The success of deep relaxation depends on daily practice. The goal is to decrease respirations, reduce blood pressure, and reduce peripheral vasodilation.
Indications: Tension headaches, muscle tension, hypertension.

VISUAL IMAGERY

Deep muscle relaxation is imperative during visual imagery. A pleasant, quiet, peaceful place is visualized to reduce stress or pain and to enhance relaxation. As with deep muscle relaxation, ongoing practice is necessary for successful use of this technique.
Indications: Childbirth, gastrointestinal disorders, chronic pain, cancer.

SELF-TALK

In this form of cognitive therapy, clients provide themselves with evaluative statements and suggestions to reduce stress and promote relaxation.
Indications: To reduce anxiety, stress, and faulty cognitions.

Definitions are from Benson (1975) and Fuller (1977).

PULMONARY DISORDERS

Breathing patterns reveal emotions. Rapid breathing or hyperventilation is a common sign of anxiety attacks or intense fears. In contrast, shallow breathing or sighs may also indicate distress. Lung tissue is innervated by the parasympathetic (vagal) and sympathetic nervous systems. Stimulation of the parasympathetic nervous system, which may be precipitated by dust, cold air, or emotions, causes bronchospasm.

Asthma. *Asthma* is a Greek term that means panting, or labored breathing. It is a common respiratory disorder that has numerous causes and is associated with bronchoconstriction, which is the pervasive narrowing of air passages that results from vagal stimulation that is caused by stress, allergic reactions, cold, dust, or infections. Major manifestations of asthma include coughing, wheezing, shortness of breath, and intense anxiety and fear.

Treatment Modalities. Asthma attacks are distressful and, regardless of the cause, require immediate medical attention. Other interventions include approaching the client in a nonjudgmental manner; identifying the precipitants of the attacks, such as stress, infections, or allergies; and developing teaching plans that incorporate stress reduction and strengthen coping skills.

IMMUNOLOGICAL DISORDERS

As previously mentioned, stress alters people's immunological processes and resistance to illness. Inadequate cellular immune response or alteration in tumor and viral-fighting **T cells** compromises the immune system, increasing vulnerability to illnesses such as acquired immunodeficiency syndrome; cancer; and the common cold, flu, herpes simplex Type I, and Epstein-Barr viruses (Glaser et al., 1991; Kiecolt-Glaser, et al., 1985).

GASTROINTESTINAL DISORDERS

GI disorders have long been associated with emotions. The GI tract is innervated by the autonomic nervous system and, like other major organs, is affected by stress and tension. Stress and other emotional reactions create tension in the gut and can produce nausea, vomiting, or diarrhea. Overproduction of gastric secretions and disturbance in motility are major symptoms of GI disorders (Clouse, 1992).

The relationship between emotions and the GI tract can be traced to the works of Hippocrates and Alexander, who related illness to prolonged stress. The GI tract has been referred to as the "little brain" and associated with expressions such as "gut reactions" and "gut feelings" (Wingate, 1985). Researchers have linked early sexual and child abuse in women with gastrointestinal disorders (Drossman, 1992; Walker et al., 1990). In addition, anxiety and other mood disorders have been found in clients experiencing GI disorders. Mood disorders and activation of the GI system are both surmised to result from activation of the autonomic nervous system, particularly the locus coeruleus, which plays a major role in mediating intense feelings and arousal states (Lydiard et al., 1993; Walker et al., 1990).

Major GI disorders include irritable bowel syndrome, peptic ulcer disease, ulcerative colitis, and Crohn's disease. The following discussion of irritable bowel syndrome is an example of a psychophysiological GI disorder.

Irritable Bowel Syndrome. Clients with irritable bowel syndrome and other GI disturbances need to be approached in a calm, caring manner so that their concerns and fears are reduced. Identification of their present stressors, coping styles, support systems, and patterns of physical and emotional response is a major aspect of the assessment process. The long-term effects of irritable bowel syndrome are potentially life-threatening and debilitating and affect numerous body systems. In addition to complying with strict medical regimens, the client and family have enormous emotional needs and intense psychosocial stress that stem from feelings of helplessness and a lack of control over their bodies and lives.

Treatment Modalities. Irritable bowel syndrome has been aligned with several mood disorders, including panic, agoraphobia, and depression. People with this syndrome tend to be tense, anxious, depressed, and irritable and to internalize their feelings. Major interventions for irritable bowel syndrome are relaxation techniques, stress reduction, assertiveness training, and biofeedback. Psychotherapy and psychopharmacology (e.g., anxiolytics or antidepressants) may be indicated for some clients. Major treatment goals are strengthening and improving clients' coping behavior and communication skills and reducing psychological and biological stress.

SKIN DISORDERS

The skin, like other major systems, responds to the environment and is responsive to various emotions, such as anger, embarrassment, and terror. The condition of the skin often reflects health status. Clammy, cool skin may indicate a serious medical problem or intense fear and anxiety. A generalized rash suggests an allergic reaction or an intense emotional response. Regardless of the cause, skin disorders need to be evaluated and treated immediately to ensure clients' psychological and physiological well-being.

Treatment Modalities. Skin disorders considered to be psychophysiological conditions include alopecia, pruritus (itching), psoriasis, and urticaria (hives). Psychosocial stress tends to aggravate skin disorders. Nursing implications include identifying stressors and developing interventions that reduce the intensity of stressors and strengthen and develop effective coping skills. In addition, stress reduction interventions, such as cognitive–behavioral techniques and desensitization, provide relief for some clients suffering from stress-induced illnesses (Wise, 1992). The chronic nature of some skin disorders creates intense emotional stress arising from feelings of helplessness and decreased self-esteem.

CHRONIC PAIN DISORDERS

The psychophysiological basis of pain is complex. Perman (1954) described pain as a friend because of its life-saving value. Pain signals both psychological and physiological response. Emotions generated by pain include rage, fear, and humiliation, and they serve as a force to resolve the situation (Thompson, 1988). Chronic recurrent pain can be emotionally and physically incapacitating and create feelings of guilt, low self-esteem, and discouragement (Menninger, 1963). Psychosocial stress can exaggerate pain and mask depression, hypochondriasis, malingering, and other conditions that provide secondary gains (Bouckoms & Hackett, 1991).

Treatment Modalities. Major nursing interventions for chronic pain begin with approaching the client in a caring and nonjudgmental manner. This approach is critical to allaying the client's fears that the pain is all in his or her head. Major therapeutic measures include hydrotherapy, massage, physiotherapy, and analgesics. Additional major interventions include cognitive–behavioral techniques, humor, biofeedback, progressive relaxation, and imagery (Lachman, 1983; Wise, 1992). Table 11–2 describes some of the therapeutic measures recommended for clients with stress-related illnesses (see Chapters 9 and 10 for an in-depth discussion of cognitive–behavioral techniques).

STRESS-RELATED ILLNESSES ACROSS THE LIFE SPAN

CHILDHOOD

Childhood psychophysiological disorders have been linked with the need for protection and attachment to primary caregivers. Separation anxiety plays a key role in the formation and exacerbation of physical symptoms. Immature cognitive function and an inability to express feelings often compel the child to communicate anxiety and stress through physical symptoms (Garralda, 1992; Lloyd, 1986). Other childhood stressors include disabling disorders, abuse, family chaos, and unstable living conditions.

Family dynamics play a major role in formation of childhood psychophysiological disorders. Common family dynamics include overresponsiveness, limited autonomy, rigidity, overprotectiveness, and rejection. Many parents of children with psychophysiological disorders are difficult to work with because they lack insight into their role in their children's illness (Liebman et al., 1974).

Clinical Example

Baby Judy was an unplanned birth. Her mother was in the process of a divorce when she discovered her pregnancy. Since her birth, Judy's mother has spent little time with her. Several months later, Judy developed symptoms of respiratory distress. She has been diagnosed with asthma. Her mother is forced to spend time with her, and Judy experiences respiratory distress when she is ignored or left alone for long intervals.

Research has shown a positive correlation between childhood asthma symptoms and intense separation anxiety, suggesting that childhood emotional distress affects complex neurobiological responses. This is especially true in children with chronic, severe, and frequent asthma attacks that occur in spite of comprehensive medical management (Pinkerton, 1969; Pinkerton & Weaver, 1970).

What role do the child's symptoms play in family dynamics? Minuchin et al. (1975) suggested that the child's psychophysiological symptoms serve as a "homeostatic mechanism regulating family interactions" (p. 1032). This premise suggests that the child's symptoms maintain family "stability." They identified three factors as playing major roles in the formation of the child's symptoms:

1. Vulnerability (neurobiological predisposition)
2. Specific family dynamics—enmeshment, overprotectiveness, rigidity, and ineffective conflict resolution (Minuchin, 1974)
3. The usefulness of the **sick role** in sustaining homeostasis, which serves to reinforce illness

Dysfunctional family interactions tend to create an environment of control and tension. See Chapter 22 for an in-depth discussion of family dynamics and interventions.

ADOLESCENCE

The psychological and neurobiological maturation of the adolescent is very perplexing. Adolescence is a period of intense biological and psychosocial turmoil as the youth searches for a sense of identity and strives to separate from primary caregivers. Other psychosocial stressors are tremendous academic demands and interpersonal relationships, which emerge as important developmental tasks preparing the youth for adulthood.

Healthy family interactions serve as a buffer for the youth, providing emotional support and validating the youth's struggle and need for self-identity and independence. In contrast, dysfunctional family interactions increase the likelihood and maintenance of psychophysiological disorders in the adolescent. Adolescents often respond to impaired family interactions with sadness, anxiety, internalized anger, feelings of inadequacy, and maladaptive behavior, and they fail to master identity and separation (Mishne, 1986).

ADULTHOOD

The long-term effects of biological response to chronic stress have been well documented. Certain people seem to be at risk for developing psychophysiological disorders or they are disease prone. Disease-prone behaviors include certain personality traits, chronic tension, and internalized emotions. Table 11–3 lists psychophysiological disorders that may be experienced in adulthood.

TABLE 11–3
Selected Psychophysiological Disorders in Adulthood by Body System

CARDIOVASCULAR DISORDERS
Hypertension
Mitral valve prolapse
Myocardial infarction
Coronary heart disease
PULMONARY DISORDERS
Hyperventilation
Asthma
Allergies
IMMUNOLOGICAL DISORDERS
Certain cancers
Autoimmune disease
Herpes zoster
Herpes simplex
Rheumatoid arthritis
Acquired immunodeficiency syndrome
GASTROINTESTINAL DISORDERS
Peptic ulcer disease
Crohn's disease
Ulcerative colitis
Irritable bowel syndrome
SKIN DISORDERS
Rashes
Urticaria
Psoriasis
Alopecia
Warts
ENDOCRINE DISORDERS
Diabetes
Thyroid disorders

THE NURSE'S ROLE

THE GENERALIST'S ROLE

The primary roles of the psychiatric–mental health nurse are to assess clients' current and past coping behaviors, help clients resolve crisis situations, minimize exacerbation of symptoms, and strengthen and promote adaptive coping behaviors. Hospitalized clients experiencing acute exacerbation of symptoms require close monitoring so that homeostasis is maintained. Interventions such as adequate dietary intake and hydration and control of pain involve assessing client response and promotion of self-care. Psychoeducation, crisis intervention, and stress-reducing activities are major nursing interventions for clients experiencing psychophysiological disorders. As members of the health team, generalist nurses play a major role in helping clients and their families reduce the deleterious effects of stress in various community settings.

THE ROLE OF THE ADVANCED-PRACTICE NURSE

Nurses in the advanced-practice role also work with clients and families to minimize exacerbation of symptoms and promote self-care and adaptive coping skills. In addition, the advanced-practice nurse identifies complex problems and collaborates with clients to modify behavior and coping patterns. Major interventions include various psychotherapies, such as cognitive–behavioral and psychodynamic approaches. Furthermore, prescriptive authority enables the advanced-practice nurse to prescribe various psychotropics that enhance other treatment modalities. Assessing client responses and participating in comprehensive planning in inpatient, community, or home health care settings are critical roles of the advanced-practice nurse.

THE NURSING PROCESS

The following case study is an example of the impact of stress on the GI tract, and it illustrates the nursing care of a client with a psychophysiological disorder.

Case Study: The Client with Irritable Bowel Syndrome (Mr. Ekpe)

A 33-year-old man, Mr. Ekpe, is referred to psychiatric triage for evaluation of a recent exacerbation of irritable bowel syndrome. His presenting symptoms—a sudden onset of fear and anxiety, abdominal pain, diarrhea, and nausea—began a week prior to his visit. His current treatment regimen consists of dietary modifications (e.g., fiber and bulk use) and education about the nature of irritable bowel syndrome (Drossman, 1987).

Mr. Ekpe, recently moved to the United States and has experienced great demands from his job and family in the past 18 months. He has recently made several visits to the emergency department complaining of abdominal cramps and diarrhea.

Assessment

In treating the client with a psychophysiological disorder, the nurse is challenged to integrate biological concepts to assess the client's symptoms, identify nursing outcomes, develop effective interventions, and evaluate responses. This process first requires establishing rapport by approaching the client in a caring and nonjudgmental manner; encouraging client–family participation in treatment; and gathering data on current stressors, substance misuse and psychiatric and medical history, present and past symptoms, and coping behaviors. Many clients presenting with psychophysiological disorders have experienced rejection of and skepticism toward their symptoms. In addition, their being referred to psychiatry gives them the feeling that their symptoms are "all in their head." This premise needs to be dispelled quickly to get beyond suspiciousness and anger and focus on building adaptive coping skills.

These feelings can be reduced by inquiring about reasons for seeking treatment and about past treatments and whether they were helpful. When past treatment has been unsuccessful, the client's perception of the reasons for the lack of success needs to be assessed. Clients with chronic pain disorders are often sensitive to criticism of their illness and may become defensive or argumentative when questioned about pain medication.

Complete physical and mental status examinations are critical components of the assessment process. Age-appropriate tools can elicit information on life span factors.

Children and adolescents must be assessed both individually and in the context of the family to determine the significance of the sick role and its impact on homeostasis. Family organization may be tied to the development and maintenance of the child's illness. Assessment of the family's developmental stage and interaction, especially those associated with overprotectiveness, rigidity, and poor problem-solving skills, indicates the family's level of function. Data on the history of symptoms; precipitating stressors, both biological and psychosocial; and symptom maintenance can help the nurse surmise the child's role within the family (Minuchin et al., 1975).

Nursing Diagnoses

- Altered Nutrition: Less Than Body Requirements
- Ineffective Individual Coping
- Knowledge Deficit regarding the role of stress and irritable bowel syndrome

Planning

Nursing Care Plan 11–1 identifies the desired outcomes for the nursing diagnoses listed above, the nursing actions needed to achieve these outcomes, and the rationales for these actions. In general, major outcomes for clients with stress-related disorders include the following:

1. Development of adaptive coping behaviors
2. Crisis resolution
3. Strengthening and mobilization of support systems
4. Minimization of exacerbation of symptoms
5. Promotion of self-esteem

Implementation

Major nursing interventions have been identified earlier in this chapter, in the discussions of specific disorders. Interventions are based on the client's presenting symptoms, developmental stage, motivation to modify behavior and coping patterns, and access to internal and external resources. Major treatment goals include the development of adaptive stress reduction methods that affect biological processes. Role playing, various psychotherapies, and psychoeducation regarding the effect

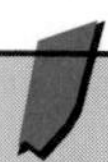

Nursing Care Plan 11–1 The Client with Irritable Bowel Syndrome (Mr. Ekpe)

OUTCOME IDENTIFICATION	NURSING ACTIONS	RATIONALES	EVALUATION
Nursing Diagnosis: Altered Nutrition: Less Than Body Requirements			
1. By [date], Mr. Ekpe will maintain adequate caloric intake.	1a. Assess Mr. Ekpe's nutritional status. 1b. Decrease environmental stress. 1c. Provide Mr. Ekpe with dietary instructions. 1d. Administer prescribed medications.	1a. Assessing clients' nutritional status determines baseline information. 1b. Stress increases gastrointestinal motility. 1c. Providing instructions allows clients to control some aspects of their care (e.g., their diet). 1d. Medications can reduce physical distress.	*Goal met:* Mr. Ekpe and his family cooperate in providing baseline information. Mr. Ekpe's GI disturbances are minimal and he no longer requires medication.
Nursing Diagnosis: Ineffective Individual Coping			
1. By [date], Mr. Ekpe will develop adaptive coping behaviors.	1a. Assess Mr. Ekpe's coping patterns. 1b. Discuss alternative coping strategies with Mr. Ekpe. 1c. Encourage Mr. Ekpe to ventilate his feelings and identify current stressors.	1a–b. Assessing coping patterns and discussing alternatives helps the nurse identify the client's present and past coping patterns. 1c. Ventilation of feelings decreases the client's tension and facilitates the development of adaptive coping skills.	*Goal met:* Mr. Ekpe verbalizes his feelings and is willing to interact and form meaningful relationships with nursing staff. Mr. Ekpe's coping patterns improve.
Nursing Diagnosis: Knowledge Deficit regarding the role of stress and irritable bowel syndrome			
1. By [date], Mr. Ekpe will understand the relationship between stress and physical symptoms.	1. Develop an individualized teaching plan to teach Mr. Ekpe the following: • The role of stress in biological response • Stress reduction techniques • Maximization of coping skills • Symptoms that need to be reported	1. An individualized teaching plan meets the client's unique needs, increases the client's understanding of the disease process and role of stress, reduces sympathetic nervous system arousal, and promotes healing.	*Goal met:* Mr. Ekpe and his family participate in the teaching process and understand the relationship between stress and irritable bowel syndrome.

of emotions and ineffective coping behaviors on biological processes can enhance clients' coping skills.

Psychophysiological disorders place tremendous demands on clients and families. Family involvement is crucial to the success of interventions. Family members may feel helpless or angry about the client's immense emotional and physical needs, which affect the quality of their lives. Family life tends to center on the client's symptoms, interfering with intimacy and healthy family interactions. Involving the family in the client's treatment decreases feelings of inadequacy, helplessness, and promotes a sense of control and well-being.

Evaluation

Evaluating the client's responses to interventions is a dynamic process based on outcome identification and includes feedback from the client, his or her family, and other members of the health team. Adaptive behaviors must be strengthened throughout treatment. Changing or eliminating maladaptive behaviors requires patience and understanding, because clients with stress-related disorders tend to be demanding, perfectionist, hostile, and sensitive to criticism (Friedman, 1992; Ganster et al., 1991; Price, 1982, 1988). Staff support groups can help the nurse in evaluating his or her feelings and thoughts generated by client behaviors.

►CHAPTER SUMMARY

The relationship between the body and the mind has been well documented. There is a positive correlation between stress and alterations in various neurobiological processes. Certain illnesses, such as heart disease, asthma, and skin disorders, have been associated with stress.

Nurses play major roles in identifying clients' high-risk behaviors; developing effective, innovative interventions that reduce clients' stress; and promoting effective coping patterns. Major techniques include psychoeducation, relaxation techniques, assertiveness training, and psychotherapy.

Suggestions for Clinical Conference

1. Present a case history of a client with a psychophysiological disorder, and identify the psychosocial and biological interface.
2. Role-play assertiveness techniques and progressive relaxation exercises.
3. Discuss the role of the nurse and interdisciplinary team in managing the client experiencing chronic pain.
4. Discuss personal feelings generated by working with clients with chronic stress-related illnesses.

References

Ader, R., Cohen, N., & Felton, D. L. (1987). Editorial. *Brain, Behavior, and Immunity, 1*, 1–6.

Ader, R., Felton, D. L., & Cohen, N. (1991). *Psychoimmunology*. San Diego, CA: Academic Press.

Alexander, F. (1939). Psychological aspects of medicine. *Psychosomatic Medicine, 1*, 7–18.

Alexander, F. (1950) *Psychosomatic medicine: Its principles and applications*. New York: W. W. Norton.

American Psychiatric Association. (1994). *Diagnostic and statistical Manual of Mental Disorders* (4th ed.). Washington, DC: Author.

Barefoot, J. C. (1992). Developments in the measurement of hostility. In H. S. Friedman (Ed.), *Hostility, coping, and health* (pp. 13–31). Washington, DC: American Psychological Association.

Benson, H. (1975). *The relaxation response*. New York: William Morrow.

Bouckoms, A., & Hackett, T. P. (1991). The pain patient: Evaluation and treatment. In N. H. Cassem (Ed.), *Massachusetts General Hospital handbook of general psychiatry* (3rd ed., pp. 39–68). St Louis: Mosby-Year Book.

Brosschot, J. F., Benschop, R. J., Godaert, G. L. R., Olff, M., De Smet, M., Heijen, C. J., & Ballieux, R. E. (1994). Influence of life stress on immunological reactivity to mild psychological stress. *Psychosomatic Medicine, 56*, 216–224.

Clouse, R. E. (1992). Psychiatric interaction with the esophagus. *Psychiatric Annals, 22*, 598–605.

Drossman, D. A. (1987). Psychosocial treatment of the refracting patient with irritable bowel syndrome. *Journal of Clinical Gastroenterology, 9*, 253–255.

Drossman, D. A. (1992). Sexual abuse and physical abuse and GI disorders in women: What is the link? *Emergency Medicine Clinics of North America, 24*, 171–175.

Eysenck, H. J. (1991). Personality, stress, and disease: An interactional perspective. *Psychological Inquiry, 2*, 221–232.

Freud, S. (1958). On psycho-analysis. In J. Strachney (Ed. and Trans.), *The Standard edition of the complete psychological works of Sigmund Freud* (Vol. 12, pp. 207–211). London: Hogarth Press. (Original work published 1911)

Friedman, H. S. (1992). *Hostility, coping, and health*. Washington, DC: American Psychological Association.

Friedman, H. S., & VandenBos, G. R. (1992). Disease-prone and self-healing personalities. *Hospital and Community Psychiatry, 43*, 1177–1179.

Friedman, M., & Rosenman, R. H. (1974). *Type A behavior and your heart*. New York: Knopf.

Fuller, G. D. (1977). *Biofeedback: Methods and procedures in clinical practice*. San Francisco: Biofeedback Press.

Ganster, D. C., Schaubroeck, J., Sime, W. E., & Mayes, B. T. (1991). The nomological validity of the type A personality among employed adults. *Journal of Applied Psychology, 76*, 143–168.

Garralda, M. E. (1992). A selective review of child psychiatric syndromes with a somatic presentation. *British Journal of Psychiatry, 161*, 759–773.

Glaser, R., et al. (1987). Stress-related immune suppression: Health implications. *Brain, Behavior, and Immunity, 1*, 7–20.

Glaser, R., Rice, J., Sheridan, J., Fertel, R., Stout, J., Speicher, C., Pinsky, D., et al. (1990). Psychological stress modulation of IL-2 production of peripheral leukocytes. *Archives of General Psychiatry, 47*, 707–712.

Glaser, R., Pearson, G. R., Jones, J. F., Hillhouse, J., Kennedy, S., Mao, H. Y., & Kiccolt-Glaser, J. K. (1991). Stress-related activation of Epstein-Barr virus. *Brain, Behavior, and Immunity, 5*, 219–232.

Kagan, J., Snidman, N., Julia-Sellers, M., & Johnson, M. O. (1991). Temperament and allergic symptoms. *Psychosomatic Medicine, 53*, 332–340.

Kasl, S., & Cooper, C. L. (1987). *Stress and health: Issues in research methodology*. New York: John Wiley & Sons.

Kiecolt-Glaser, J. K., Glaser, R., Willinger, D., Stout, J., Messick, G., Sheppard, S., Ricker, D., Romisher, S. C., Briner, W., Bonnel, G., et al. (1985). Psychosocial enhancement of immunocompetence in a geriatric population. *Health Psychology, 4*, 25–41.

Lachman, V. D. (1983). *Stress management: A manual for nurses*. Orlando, FL: Grune & Stratton.

Liebman, R., Minuchin, S., & Baker, L. (1974). The use of structural family therapy in treatment of intractable asthma. *American Journal of Psychiatry, 131*, 535–540.

Light, K. C. Herbst, M. C., Braydon, E. E., Hinderliten, A. L., Koch, G. C., Davis, M. R., & Sheps, D. S. (1991). Depression and type A behavior pattern in patients with coronary artery disease: Relationships to painful versus silent myocardial ischemia and β-endorphin response during exercise. *Psychosomatic Medicine, 53*, 669–683.

Lloyd, G. G. (1986). Psychiatric syndromes with a somatic presentation. *Journal of Psychosomatic Research, 30*, 113–120.

Lydiard, R. B., Fossey, M. D., Marsh, W., & Ballenger, J. C. (1993). Prevalence of psychiatric disorders in patients with irritable bowel syndrome. *Psychosomatics, 34*, 229–234.

Menninger, K. (1963). *The vital balance*. New York: Viking Press.

Minuchin, S. (1974). *Families and family therapy: A structural approach*. Cambridge, MA: Harvard University Press.

Minuchin, S., Baker, L., Rosman, B. L., et al. (1975). A conceptual model of psychosomatic illness in children. *Archives of General Psychiatry*, *32*, 1031–1038.

Mishne, J. M. (1986). Clinical work with adolescents. New York: Free Press.

Pennebacker, J. W. (1992). Inhibition as the linchpin of health. In H. S. Friedman (Ed.), *Hostility, coping, and health* (pp. 127–139). Washington, DC: American Psychological Association.

Perman, J. (1954). Pain as an old friend. *Lancet*, *1*, 633–635.

Pinkerton, P. (1969). Patho-physiology and psychopathology as co-determinants of pharmacotherapeutic response in childhood asthma. In A. Pletscher & A. Marino (Eds.), *Psychotropic drugs in internal medicine* (pp. 115–127). Amsterdam: Excepta Medica.

Pinkerton, P., & Weaver, C. M. (1970). Childhood asthma. In O. Hill (Ed.), *Modern trends in psychosomatic medicine* (pp. 81–104). London: Butterworths.

Price, V. A. (1982). *Type A behavior pattern: A model for research and practice*. San Diego, CA: Academic Press.

Price, V. A. (1988). Research and clinical issues in treating type A behavior. In B. K. Houston & C. R. Snyder (Eds.), *Type A behavior pattern: Research, theory, and intervention* (pp. 275–311). New York: Wiley.

Selye, H. (1976). *Stress in health and disease*. New York: McGraw-Hill.

Shekelle, R. B., Vernon, S. W., & Ostfeld, A.M. (1991). Personality and coronary heart disease. *Psychosomatic Medicine*, *53*, 176–184.

Thompson, T. L. (1988). Psychosomatic disorders. In J. A. Talbott, R. E. Hales, S. C. Yudofsky (Eds.), *Textbook of psychiatry* (pp. 493–532). Washington, DC: American Psychiatric Press.

Walker, E. A., Roy-Byrne, P. P., Katon, W. J., Li, L., Amos, D., & Jiranek, G. (1990). Psychiatric illness and irritable bowel syndrome: A comparison with inflammatory bowel disease. *American Journal of Psychiatry*, *147*, 1656–1661.

Williams, R. B., Jr., Suarez, E. C., Kuhn, C. M., Zimmerman, E. A., & Schanberg, S. M. (1991). Biobehavioral basis of coronary-prone behavior in middle-aged men: I. Evidence for chronic SNS activation in type As. *Psychosomatic Medicine*, *53*, 517–527.

Wingate, D. L. (1985). The brain-gut link. *Viewpoints of Digestive Disease*, *17*, 17–20.

Wise, T. N. (1992). Psychiatric management of functional gastrointestinal disorders. *Psychiatric Annals*, *22*, 606–611.

CHAPTER 12

The Client with Altered Sensory Perception: Schizophrenia and Other Psychotic Disorders

KAY PERRY, M.S.N., R.N.,C.S., A.R.N.P.
DEBORAH ANTAI-OTONG, M.S., R.N.,C.S.

OUTLINE

CHAPTER OBJECTIVES

Upon completion of this chapter, you will be able to:

1. Analyze the relationship between neurobiological and psychosocial factors of schizophrenia.
2. Interact effectively with the client experiencing psychosis.
3. Develop a plan of care for the client with schizophrenia.
4. Assess the major signs and symptoms of schizophrenia.
5. Recognize life span issues associated with schizophrenia and other psychotic disorders.

KEY TERMS

Autism	Hallucinations	Psychoeducation
Basal ganglia	Negative symptoms	Schizophrenia
Delusions	Neuroleptic agent	Tardive dyskinesia
Dopamine	Positive symptoms	

One in 100 people in the world has the illness of **schizophrenia** (Torrey, 1988). Thus, about 40 million families worldwide have a family member with the disorder (Walsh, 1985). In the United States, the prevalence of schizophrenia ranges from 1 to 1.9 percent of the population (Andreasen & Black, 1991). It is estimated that by 2000, about 2.6 million Americans will be victims of this illness. These data, coupled with the prevalence of substance abuse and homelessness among this population, contribute significantly to the social and economic impact of chronic mental illness. Half of all beds for the mentally ill and one fourth of the total hospital beds are occupied by clients with schizophrenia. This disorder accounts for approximately 40 percent of all long-term patient care days, compared with 27 percent for cardiovascular disorders (North, 1991). Research indicates that approximately 250,000 people diagnosed each year with this illness will return to live with their families after hospitalization (Torrey, 1988).

Schizophrenia is one of the most costly and inadequately treated mental illnesses. Its prevalence across the life span and a lack of comprehensive and effective treatment expand its maximal morbidity. The emotional and physical losses clients and families experience are tragic. Personal costs arise from the long-term consequences of schizophrenia associated with social, vocational, and emotional impairment, which increase the risk of life-time dependency on families and society and the incidence of substance abuse (Andreasen, 1991; Mueser et al., 1992).

Historically, schizophrenia has been described as a chronic, debilitating, incurable mental illness, but now this is changing. This neurobehavioral disorder challenges nurses to appreciate the link between neurobiological factors and behaviors seen in schizophrenia and other psychotic disorders. Linking these factors enables nurses to use the nursing process to assess, plan, intervene, and evaluate client responses to treatment modalities. Even in this day of immense neurobiological expansion and technological advances, its cause remains unknown. In spite of its enigma, there is increasing evidence suggesting that schizophrenia is a complex system disorder with mediating biological and behavioral processes that are influenced by stress. Schizophrenia, along with other chronic mental illnesses, must be treated effectively, and efforts to prevent its onset must be aggressively pursued (Ciompi, 1989; Strauss, 1989).

Our knowledge or understanding of the complexity of schizophrenia is expanding at a phenomenal rate. Additionally, psychiatric–mental health nurses must evaluate recent scientific findings and apply them to everyday nursing situations to bridge the gap between research and clinical practice (Malone, 1990). By identifying stressors and assisting clients in developing coping skills, the nurse can help relieve the symptoms that may have necessitated hospitalization.

Psychotic disorders other than schizophrenia include brief reactive psychosis, schizoaffective disorder, and drug-induced psychotic disorders (American Psychiatric Association [APA], 1994). This chapter discusses complex biological and behavioral processes associated with schizophrenia and other psychotic disorders. Additionally, it provides an in-depth perspective on the nurse's role in helping clients and families cope with a chronic, potentially debilitating mental illness.

CAUSATIVE FACTORS: PERSPECTIVES AND THEORIES

During the past decade, considerable knowledge has accumulated about the nature of schizophrenia, yet its exact cause is unknown. Hypotheses about the etiology of schizophrenia are multifaceted and include genetic, neurobiological, psychosocial, stress-related, and psychodynamic factors.

GENETIC FACTORS

Even before birth, a child may have genetic characteristics that predispose him or her to schizophrenia. The evidence from classic clinical studies for a genetic contribution to schizophrenia is well documented. Studies of families, twins, and adopted children have shown a familial risk for schizophrenia and nonaffective psychosis (Cloninger, 1989). According to these studies, first-degree relatives (i.e., mother, father, sister, brother, or child) of a person with schizophrenia have approximately a 10 percent chance of developing the illness as compared with a 1 percent chance for the general population. Second-degree relatives (e.g., granddaughter or niece) have a 2 to 4 percent chance (Costa, 1992). Nonaffective disorders, including schizoaffective and paranoid disorder and chronic atypical cases, are also associated with a higher risk factor (7.8 percent) for relatives than for nonrelatives (Cloninger, 1989).

Twin studies have consistently demonstrated a high rate of concordance for schizophrenia. If one monozygotic (genetically identical) twin has schizophrenia, studies have found that 46 to 48 percent of the co-twins are likely to have the illness, compared with a concordance rate of only 14 to 17 percent for dizygotic twins who share about half of their genes (Andreasen & Black, 1991; Bracha et al., 1992). There is some evidence for genetic cause, yet the results are not 100 percent in monozygotic twins (Table 12–1). Murray and Harvey (1989) indicated a correlation in liability in first-degree relatives when they compared the estimate of likelihood for schizophrenia (0.37 to 0.43) with that for diabetes (0.27 to 0.40), coronary artery disease (0.33), and hypertension (0.24). These data place the risk factors for schizophrenia into a better perspective with other diseases. Kety's adoptive studies in Denmark were intended to separate the effects of rearing from those of genetics. These studies showed that the risk for schizophrenia is higher in biological relatives than in adoptive relatives (Gottesman, 1991).

Other genetic hypotheses are under investigation. Genes involved in the immune process, such as human leukocyte antigen complex chromosome 6, have been considered (Cloninger, 1989) because of repeated observations that rheumatoid arthritis and paranoid schizophrenia seldom occur in the same person. A recent study reported that children of mothers exposed to an influenza epidemic during the second trimester of pregnancy were at increased risk for developing schizophrenia (Mednick et al., 1988); however, there is no direct evidence that such viral infections alone are sufficient to cause schizophrenia. Bruton et al. (1990) presented the possibility of a defect in cell proliferation in the developing brain, particularly affecting hippocampal formation (see Fig. 12–1). This theory is supported by computed tomography (CT) scan evidence of a decreased number of cells in the hippocampus in some people with schizophrenia. Another factor in understanding the genetics of schizophrenia is the possibility that there is no gene to code negative symptoms. Instead, researchers may find a defective neurodevelopmental pattern that results in a set of structural changes that predispose a person to schizophrenia.

TABLE 12–1
Genetic Risk Factors for Schizophrenia

STATUS	RISK (%)
First-degree relatives (mother, father, sister, brother, child)	10
Second-degree relatives (granddaughter, niece, nephew)	2–4
Monozygotic twins (genetically identical)	46–48
Dizygotic twins (share half their genes)	14–17

Data from Kaplan, H. I., & Sadock, B. J. (eds.). (1989). *Comprehensive textbook of psychiatry* (Vol. 1, 5th ed.). Baltimore: Williams & Wilkins; and Costa, P. (1992). A conversation with Philip Holzman. *Menninger Perspective, 23*(3), 19–23.

NEUROBIOLOGICAL FACTORS

Historically, psychiatry has searched for causes of mental illness within the realm of neurobiology. Attempts to understand brain abnormality began when Emil Kraepelin and others used post mortem studies of brain tissue to identify specific neuropathological abnormalities. Kraepelin focused on the frontal lobes as a pathological site possibly important in causing schizophrenia. Biochemical and genetic factors continue to be the major focus of research studies on schizophrenia. These studies also play critical roles in understanding this illness and searching for medications that decrease symptoms with few adverse reactions.

The complexity of schizophrenia requires that nurses understand the biological–behavioral interface of this mental illness and collaborate with families and other mental health professionals to identify effective treatment outcomes. Knowledge of neurobiological processes and theoretical inferences as to the cause of schizophrenia enhances nursing practice (Thompson, 1990).

Psychiatric nurses should be familiar with the various systems within the brain that represent disturbed functions in mental illness. Andreasen and Black (1991) divided these brain functions into five systems: prefrontal, limbic, basal ganglia, language, and memory. They further divided the brain into anatomic, functional, and neurochemical systems. The three anatomic systems (prefrontal, limbic, and basal ganglia) all are interconnected and work interactively. The two functional system (memory and language) are highly dependent on each other and on the anatomic systems. The neurochemical system provides the "fuel" that permits the other two systems to run (Andreasen & Black, 1991).

Anatomical System

Prefrontal System. The *prefrontal system* (prefrontal cortex) mediates a variety of functions, such as abstract thought, problem solving, social interrelatedness, and responsibility. Other functions include attention and perception, affect, and emotions. The prefrontal cortex has been suggested to have information about integrating functions that connect various parts of the brain, including areas that involve auditory, visual, and somatic functions. It also plays a role in learning and memory located in these areas. Another major task is regulation of the limbic functions via direct connections with the hypothalamus. The direct connection to the basal ganglia appears to be excitatory, in that the dopamine-rich basal ganglia may be the mechanism by which the prefrontal cortex mediates symptoms of psychosis.

During the past decade, new technologies have developed that provide evidence supporting structural and other brain abnormalities in schizophrenia, specifically in the prefrontal area and the ventricles. CT scans produce images of the living brain showing that the fluid-filled cavities known as *ventricles,* specifically the third ventricle on the left side, are sometimes larger than average in the brains of people with schizophrenia (Lieberman et al., 1992a, 1992b). Magnetic resonance imaging (MRI) studies suggest that the frontal lobes of persons with schizophrenia are usually smaller than average (Andreasen & Black, 1991; Jernigan et al., 1991). Regional blood flow studies also suggest that people with schizophrenia have a relatively small frontal lobe (Andreasen, 1986, 1991). Furthermore, positron emission tomography (PET) studies have shown decreased glucose utilization in the frontal lobes in schizophrenia. Both MRI and CT scans indicate the possibility of a developmental or degenerative process (see Fig. 12–1).

Limbic System. The *limbic system* is a circular ring of nuclei that connects with the prefrontal, parietal, and occipital areas of the brain. It is often referred to as the *visceral* brain because cognitions affect emotional and neurobiological responses. The limbic system plays a significant role in emotions, motivation, and cognitive functioning and governs the amygdala and hippocampus, which serve as memory and learning centers. Therefore, references to past experiences also occur within the limbic system. Furthermore, lesions in the amygdala region lead to fearfulness and suspiciousness, which suggests a role in the development of paranoia (Kandel et al., 1991).

Basal Ganglia. The primary role of the ***basal ganglia***, five subcortical nuclei located in the midbrain area, has been identified as regulating and mediating motor activity. This area is believed to be the site of the development of side effects of long-term neuroleptic treatment, such as **tardive dyskinesia**. Furthermore, the basal ganglia may play a pivotal role in the expression and regulation of emotion and cognition. Recent studies suggest that the basal ganglia, which are rich in dopamine receptors, may be the only areas that contain dopamine type 2 (D_2) receptors. Antipsychotic medications, which decrease positive symptoms of schizophrenia, such as **hallucinations** and **delusions**, are highly correlated with D_2 receptors, suggesting that this region may somehow mediate psychotic symptoms (Andreasen & Black, 1991).

Functional System

The functions of learning and memory are integrated primarily in the regions of the hippocampus and the amygdala. Some researchers speculate that neural mechanisms of psychotic phenomena such as delusions and hallucinations may be partially based on either abnormal excitability or abnormal "wiring" in brain subregions dedicated to the storage and interpretation of memories (i.e., the amygdala and the hippocampus).

Language System. The *language system* is localized almost completely in the left hemisphere, where there are three regions that mediate the capacity to communicate: Broca's area, Wernicke's area, and the auditory cortex. Broca's area, where speech is produced, contains information about words that connect the thought content. Wernicke's area, which is referred to as the *auditory association cortex,* encodes the information in a meaningful way (Andreasen & Black, 1991). Neural signals are received in the auditory cortex, and the meaning of words is achieved through comparison in Wernicke's area.

Wernicke's aphasia and Broca's aphasia are sometimes found in people with schizophrenia, suggesting that left-hemispheric dysfunction may be a component of schizophrenia. Wernicke's aphasia produces disorganized speech sometimes described as "word salad." Broca's aphasia produces improverished speech and decreased verbal-cognitive functions, such as a verbal intelligence quotient (IQ) measuring lower than the performance IQ and impairment as determined by language tests.

Memory System. The findings of Saykin et al. (1991) in their neuropsychological studies of schizophrenia are consistent with temporolimbic dysfunction. Measures of verbal memory and learning suggested left medial–temporal involvement congruent with a hypothesis of left-hemispheric dysfunction in schizophrenia. This also supports recent anatomic and physiological data that show temporohippocampal abnormalities on morphometric pathological examination and MRI, CT, and electrophysiological studies. Crow's (1990) studies suggest that the development of asymmetry is genetically determined via a Mendelian dominant gene and that there is close relationship between the disease process and those genes.

Neurochemical System

In addition to the anatomic and functional systems, Andreasen (1986) described the neurochemical system that enables the other two systems to communicate. Clusters of neurons release neurotransmitters that initiate a series of responses. The neurotransmitters hypothesized to be involved in the neurochemistry of schizophrenia are **dopamine**, norepinephrine, serotonin, and gamma-aminobutyric acid (GABA) (Table 12–2).

The most common pathophysiological explanation for schizophrenia is the dopamine hypothesis, which suggests that symptoms are caused by hyperactivity in the dopamine system (Heritch, 1990; Thompson, 1990) (Fig. 12–1). Evidence to support this view includes the action of antipsychotic or **neuroleptic agents**, which are believed to block dopamine receptors. This blocking limits dopamine activity and decreases symptoms of schizophrenia. Stimulants such as amphetamines, which increase production of dopamine, are known to exacerbate the symptoms of schizophrenia.

Crow (1990) reported that "the most reproducible neuropathological finding in schizophrenia is that of increased numbers of D_2 receptors in the basal ganglia region." Some studies using PET to assess D_2 receptors in drug-naive persons (those who have not taken drugs) have been published, with contradictory results. However, researchers have identified five dopamine receptors and hypothesize that within the next few years probably 10 more will be identified (Leonard, 1992), which will lend more evidence to the association of dopamine with schizophrenia.

The other major neurotransmitters are norepinephrine, serotonin, and GABA. Norepinephrine is most highly concentrated in the hypothalamus, the limbic system, and the cerebellum. It plays a pivotal role in learning, memory, reinforcement, the sleep–wake cycle, anxiety, and the regulation of blood flow and metabolism. Wise and Stein (1973) proposed that schizophrenia may be related to a defect in the selective norepinephrine neuron degeneration, producing the anhedonia, or the lack of self-initiated, goal-directed behavior characteristic of a number of people with schizophrenia. Studies thus far have not provided sufficient evidence indicating that norepinephrine is a primary factor in the development of schizophrenia.

The serotonin hypothesis is based on the similarities of serotonin and the hallucinogen lysergic acid diethylamide (LSD). Earlier reports involving the administration of reserpine, which were found to alleviate some symptoms of schizophrenia, led researchers to postulate that an increase in serotonin levels may cause schizophrenia. Studies of peripheral measurements of serotonin and its principal metabolite, 5-hydroxyindoleacetic acid have been inconsistent (Kandel, 1991; Losonczy et al., 1987).

GABA is widely distributed in the brain. Thirty percent of all brain synapses are believed to interact in some way with GABA. It is likely that decreased amounts of GABA inhibit dopamine activity. This is consistent with the hypothesis that an excessive level of dopamine is a contributing cause of schizophrenia.

TABLE 12–2
Neurotransmitters Hypothesized to Be Involved in Schizophrenia

CAUSE	PROPOSED MECHANISMS OR EVIDENCE
Dopamine system hyperactivity	► Antipsychotic agents decrease symptoms of schizophrenia, possibly by blocking dopamine receptors, thus limiting dopamine activity ► Stimulants and amphetamines increase production of dopamine and are known to exacerbate symptoms of schizophrenia
Norepinephrine elevation	► Norepinephrine plays a major role in learning and memory; in schizophrenia, there is diminished learning and memory ► Anhedonia (lack of self-initiated, goal-directed behavior) is characteristic of schizophrenia, and this may be related to norepinephrine neuron degeneration
Serotonin elevation	► There are similarities between serotonin and LSD. (Serotonin receptor sites are sensitive to LSD.) Because LSD causes hallucinations, excess serotonin may also have that effect. ► Reserpine alleviates some symptoms of schizophrenia
Diminished levels of gamma-aminobutyric acid (GABA)	► Because 30% of all brain synapses are believed to interact in some way with GABA, decreased amounts of this neurotransmitter may inhibit dopamine activity.
Decreased co-enzyme for conversion of phenylalanine to tyrosine	► Higher fasting serum phenylketonuria in schizophrenics

LSD, lysergic acid diethylamide.
Data from Kaplan, H. I., & Sadock, B. J. (Eds.). (1989). *Comprehensive textbook of psychiatry* (Vol. 1, 5th ed.) Baltimore: Williams & Wilkins; Iqbal, N., Goldsamt, L. A., Weltzler, S., et al. (1993). Serotonin and Schizophrenia. *Psychiatric Annals, 23,* 186–192; and Pickar, D., Owen, R. R., Litman, R. E., et al. (1992). Clinical and biologic response to clozapine in patients with schizophrenia: Crossover with fluphenazine. *Archives of General Psychiatry, 49,* 345–353.

NEUROBEHAVIORAL FACTORS

Linking neurobiological processes and behaviors of schizophrenia is critical to understanding the complexity of this disorder and developing effective treatment.

Behavioral Manifestations of Frontal Lobe Alterations. Cognitive and psychomotor disturbances have been linked to frontal lobe damage and disturbances in regional cerebral metabolism. Major behavioral manifestations of frontal lobe impairment include difficulties in problem-solving and in initiating goal-directed behaviors. Additionally, persons with schizophrenia have alterations in abstract thinking and disturbances of attention. Psychomotor disturbances include slow response and alterations in smooth-pursuit eye movement and purposeful motor responses (Goldberg & Weinberger, 1988; Merriam et al., 1990, 1993).

Behavioral Manifestations of Disturbances in the Basal Ganglia. Movement disorders, such as dystonia and tremors, are associated with neuroleptic exposure and disturbances in the basal ganglia wherein dopamine levels become too low.

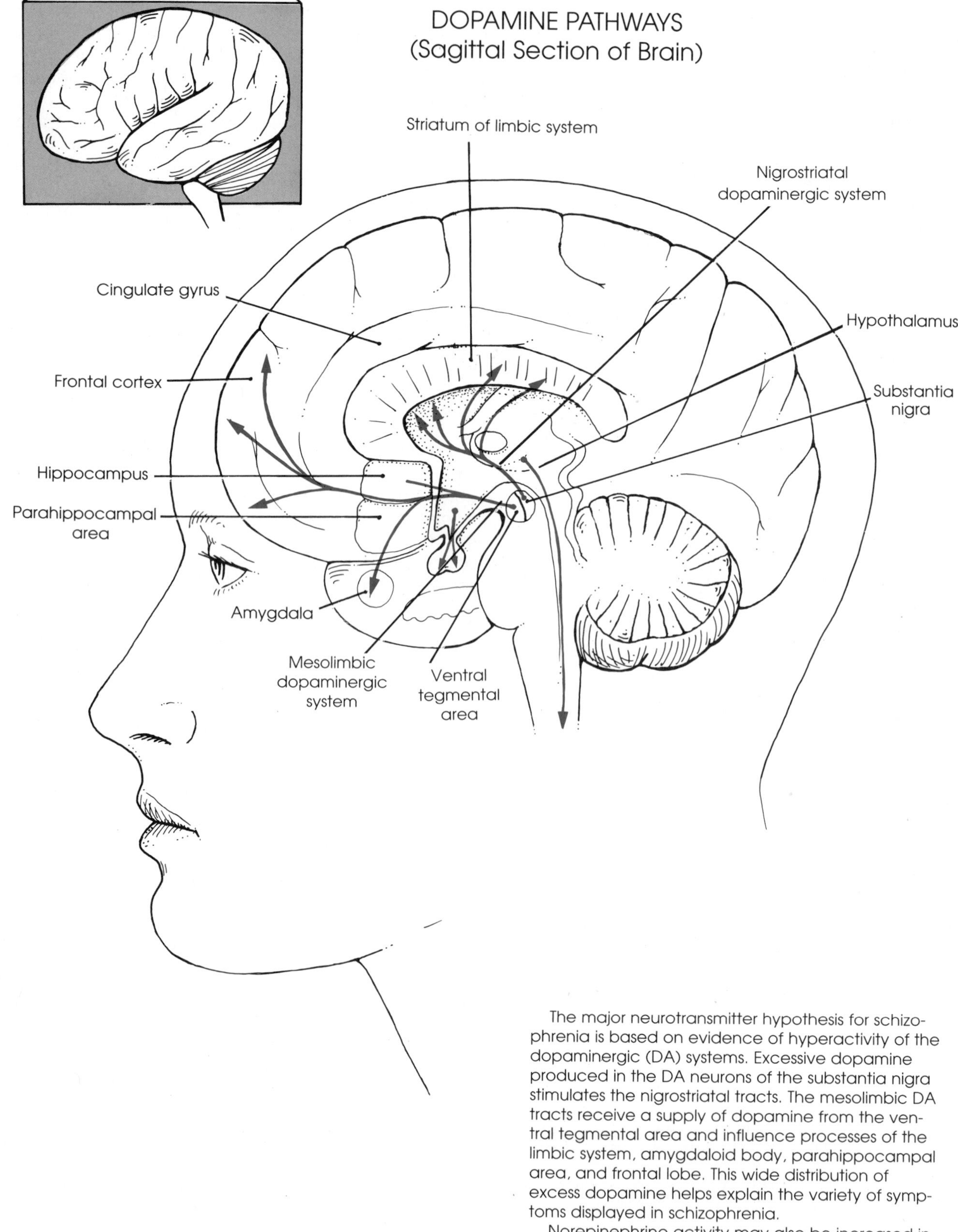

The major neurotransmitter hypothesis for schizophrenia is based on evidence of hyperactivity of the dopaminergic (DA) systems. Excessive dopamine produced in the DA neurons of the substantia nigra stimulates the nigrostriatal tracts. The mesolimbic DA tracts receive a supply of dopamine from the ventral tegmental area and influence processes of the limbic system, amygdaloid body, parahippocampal area, and frontal lobe. This wide distribution of excess dopamine helps explain the variety of symptoms displayed in schizophrenia.

Norepinephrine activity may also be increased in schizophrenia and may lend a paranoid component to the clinical picture *(see text)*.

FIGURE 12–1
Neurobiological aspects of schizophrenia: the dopamine hypothesis, limbic system degeneration, and the use of psychopharmacological agents. (Illustration concept: Gail Kongable, M.S.N., C.N.,R.N., C.C.,R.N., Department of Neurosurgery, University of Virginia Health Sciences Center. Illustration by Marie T. Dauenheimer, M.A.)

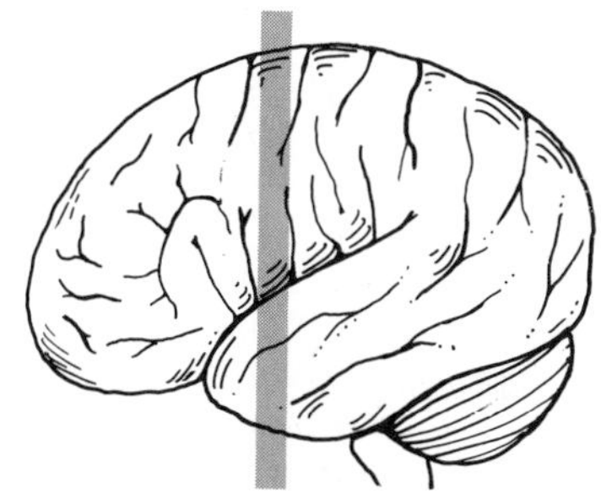

Much is still unknown about the cause of schizophrenia. Biological, genetic, and psychosocial factors combine to make certain people — about 1 in 100 — more vulnerable to this disorder. One proposed biological explanation for schizophrenia is that an event during prenatal development of the brain destroyed a significant amount of the neurons of the limbic system. There is radiographic evidence of degeneration in the medial temporal lobe, the cingulate gyrus, the amygdala, the hippocampus, and the basal ganglia that supports the hypothesis of abnormal neurotransmitter activity and response. *(Arrows in drawing indicate dopamine pathways.)*

LIMBIC SYSTEM DEGENERATION (Coronal Section)

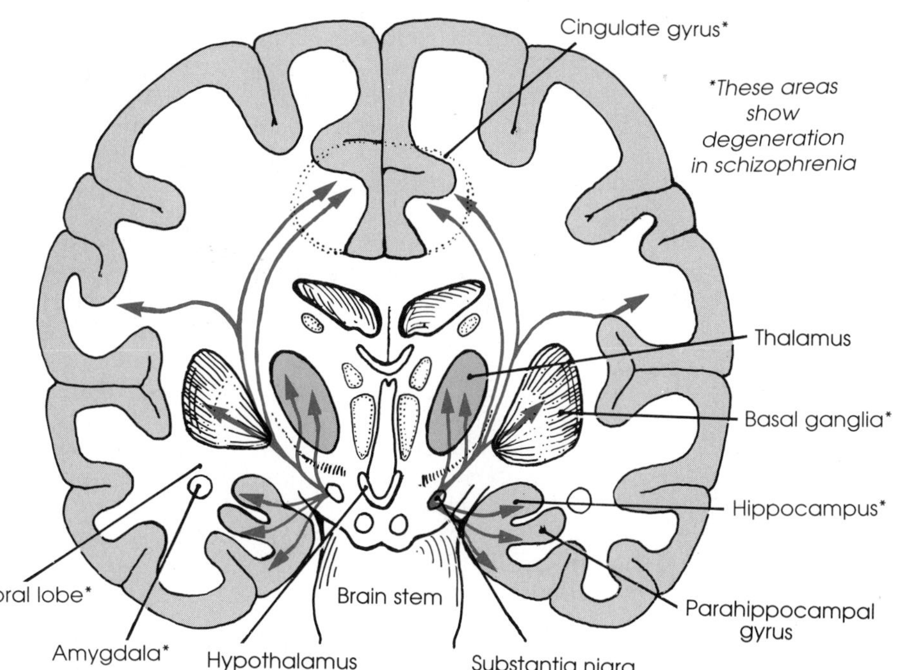

HOW DRUGS AFFECT THE DOPAMINERGIC SYNAPSES

Most of the medications used to treat symptoms of schizophrenia act by blocking dopamine receptor sites. Other medications work by blocking dopamine synthesis or by preventing the breakdown of dopamine. Hallucinogens, amphetamines and certain prescribed drugs can initiate or exacerbate psychotic episodes by increasing the amount of available dopamine. *(See Fig. 2-4 for an explanation of synaptic structures.)*

1. Dopamine is synthesized from tyrosine, a basic amino acid.
2. Dopamine is stored in synaptic vesicles.
3. Vesicles migrate to the presynaptic membrane and release dopamine into the synaptic cleft. *Because amphetamines and some antihypertensive drugs stimulate release of dopamine and effectively block reuptake at the presynaptic membrane, they can exacerbate symptoms of schizophrenia and related psychosis.*
4. Receptor stimulation of the postsynaptic membrane initiates an impulse in the dendrite of the next neuron. *Antipsychotic drugs such as perphenazine (Trilafon) and haloperidol (Haldol) block receptor sites to prevent stimulation, alleviating symptoms of schizophrenia.*
5. Dopamine activity stops when dopamine is resorbed into the presynaptic membrane. *Benztropine (Cogentin), used to treat the extrapyramidal side effects of antipsychotics, inhibits this reuptake mechanism. In larger doses, Cogentin can precipitate psychosis.*
6. Dopamine is broken down by monoamine oxidase (MAO). *MAO inhibitors prevent the breakdown of dopamine and are used to treat extrapyramidal effects.*

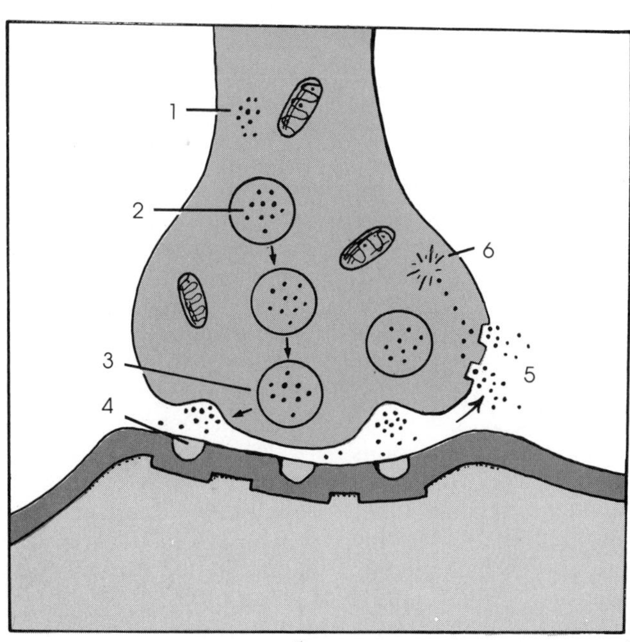

Behavioral Manifestations of Temporal Lobe Alterations. Studies suggest a relationship between cognitive and behavioral disturbances and temporolimbic alterations. Attention, memory (especially relaying of information to the hippocampus), and affect arise from the limbic system. Major manifestations of temporolimbic alterations include hyperarousal, increased alertness, distractibility, and short-term memory disturbances. Disorganization of thought processes and speech, such as thought insertion and auditory hallucinations, is surmised to arise from disturbances in the temporolimbic regions (Frith & Done, 1988; Merriam et al., 1993).

The complexity of brain function and its impact on human behavior continues to perplex researchers and challenge them to develop effective therapy for schizophrenia and other mental disorders that may have biological and biochemical components.

THE ROLE OF STRESSORS

Historically, the "diathesis-stress" model was first described by Meehl (1962), who proposed a combination of constitutional and environmental influences on the cause and course of schizophrenia. Aspects of vulnerability involve genetic and biological factors, including intrauterine, birth, and postnatal complications. Psychosocial and developmental stressors are linked with the emergence of psychotic symptoms. The outcome is determined by the amount of vulnerability and stress and by the person's strengths and environmental supports. Symptoms can progress in a downward spiral to a full-blown episode.

Various external stress factors can affect the course of schizophrenia, including poverty, ignorance, unemployment, social isolation, poor nutrition, and marginal health status. Significant losses caused by death, acute illness, and relocation are examples of major stressors, especially if they are unanticipated, undesired, and uncontrolled (Leff, 1987). Such major stressful life events also play a pivotal role in psychotic relapse (Nuechterlein et al., 1992). Psychotic relapse, or acute exacerbation, is manifested by returning or worsening symptoms of psychosis, such as hallucinations, disorganization of thoughts, social withdrawal, delusions, irritability, and agitation. A major factor contributing to relapses is that the stressors, including the psychotic symptoms, were not under the person's control (Nuechterlein et al., 1992). The study by Nuechterlein et al. included individuals who took their medication as prescribed (compliant) and those who did not. Furthermore, the study showed that independent life events that were out of the person's control clustered in 3 weeks before the first onset or relapse of illness.

"Personally influenced" events include expansions of life experiences, such as returning to work, receiving a promotion, beginning to date, and experiencing major disappointment (Nuechterlein et al., 1992). Moving away to college and experimenting with hallucinogic drugs were also considered stressors. Moller (1991) identified several personal life events that cause stress in seriously mentally ill clients, including any change that affects structured daily activities, for example, a change in residence, finances, family relationships, holidays, vacations, and hospitalizations.

Historically, studies of schizophrenia paralleled relapse with high expressed emotion, which is delineated as fault-finding, hostility, or emotional overinvolvement of one or more family members. This theory surmised that relapse in the client with schizophrenia was caused solely by the family's behaviors. This concept has been misused in the past.

Furthermore, relapse in clients with schizophrenia has been associated with either certain emotional attitudes in the relatives or the occurrence of independent life events. However, these studies did not suggest that all expression of emotions parallels higher relapse rates. Nuechterlein et al. (1992) showed that high expressed emotion may occur, in part, through direct exposure to the mentally ill client during the time prior to hospitalization, which is more common in the early onset of illness. Recent advocate movements for the mentally ill, along with biological advances, suggest that social environments have only a partial role in the formation of mental illness and that the exact cause of schizophrenia remains unknown (Hartfield et al., 1987; Kanter et al., 1987).

THE ROLE OF SUBSTANCE ABUSE

The high incidence of substance abuse in clients with schizophrenia is a major health care problem because it further complicates the treatment and course of schizophrenia. The prevalence of substance abuse in this population is estimated to range between 10 and 65 percent and to occur more often in young men with chronic mental illness (Ananth et al., 1989; Mueser et al., 1990; Safer, 1987). Substance abuse is linked to poor medication compliance; increased incidence of acute, severe, and chronic symptoms; suicide attempts; and hospitalizations (Cohen et al., 1990). Repeated relapses and hospitalizations and erratic lifestyles increase the likelihood of homelessness, legal problems, and subsequent social, financial, and vocational impairment.

The global distress and impairment associated with schizophrenia increases the risk of using maladaptive coping behaviors such as substance abuse. Major substances used include central nervous system (CNS) stimulants and depressants. CNS stimulants such as cocaine and amphetamines are often used to alleviate negative symptoms of schizophrenia (such as depression and apathy). Alcohol and cannabis are also often used to decrease symptoms of delusions, hallucinations, and boredom (Mueser et al., 1992). Other reasons include "self-medication" to reduce the distress of anxiety and depression that often accompany schizophrenia. Some researchers question the notion of self-medication as the basis of substance abuse and negate its value in explaining its prevalence in clients with schizophrenia (Dixon et al., 1991; Mueser, 1990).

PSYCHODYNAMIC FACTORS

Historical Background

Modern history credits Kraepelin, a prominent nineteenth century German psychiatrist, with the identification of schizophrenia. He introduced the term *dementia praecox* to describe this condition: *dementia* emphasized the chronic, deteriorating course and *praecox* indicated the early age of onset, usually in adolescence. Kraepelin also differentiated clients with dementia praecox from those with manic-depressive psychosis. He provided detailed descriptions of symptoms such as hallucination, delusions, and negativism.

Eugen Bleuler, a Swiss psychiatrist, renamed the illness *schizophrenia* (a term that meant "splitting of the mind"). Bleuler's theory, based largely on the work of Sigmund Freud, reflected the belief that the cause of the illness was disharmony in the person's psychic function versus a deteriorating course. Bleuler divided the symptoms into characteristics of thought disorders and affective emotional disturbances. Bleuler and Kraepelin both assumed that there was an underlying biological basis for this disorder (Campbell, 1958).

Major Psychodynamic Concepts

Psychodynamic theorists believe that schizophrenia results in part from early interactions with primary caregivers who fail to provide warm emotional ties. Early adaptive difficulties may generate developmental disturbances and affect the infant's sense of trust and security. Freud (1950) believed that family relationships were the basis of schizophrenia and other maladaptive responses. A lack of early meaningful relationships generates profound frustration, conflict, fear, and distrust of the world. Maladaptive parental responses to disturbances in the child often increases stress, and this interaction in turn generates symptoms in the child (Allen, 1991). Intense frustration and distrust eventually culminate into regression that is often accompanied by a withdrawal of emotional investment or expectation of warmth or support from others. Thus, by the time of adolescence, the youth has developed maladaptive coping behaviors, such as social isolation, suspiciousness, a tendency to retreat into a fantasy world, and excessive dependence on others. These protective mechanisms severely impair the youth's capacity to accomplish developmental tasks and cope with reality and life in general.

Any person is extremely sensitive to separation and loss associated with various changes, such as leaving home, attending college, and seeking employment. The vulnerable person continues to experience a profound sense of failure as reality becomes too painful, and psychosis evolves as a defensive effort to protect oneself. Examples are thoughts of "someone is putting thoughts into my head" or "my parents cannot survive without me" rather than "I may not be able to find a job or complete a college course." Attributing the cause of failure to something or someone helps one avoid facing the pain of failure and anxiety about the future. Additionally, confusion impedes successful resolution of various stressful situations. As psychosis evolves, the person creates distorted perceptions that further diminish self-esteem.

ROLE OF THE FAMILY IN SCHIZOPHRENIA

THE FAMILY AS A CAUSE OF SCHIZOPHRENIA

Historically, the proposition that family was the cause of a child's developing schizophrenia was based primarily on the concepts developed by Bateson et al. (1956) on the "double bind," Lidz (1973) on "marital skew," and Wynne and Singer (1963) on "pseudomutuality." These concepts created an extremely nontherapeutic and destructive atmosphere between hospitalized clients and their family members and mental health professionals.

Although early concepts about the family as a cause of schizophrenia are now viewed as nontherapeutic, family studies over the years have been beneficial to mental health professionals. For instance, the knowledge of how a family adjusts to or copes with a member's illness may assist the nurse in understanding the needs of the family during a time of crisis and facilitate adaptive responses in family members (Perry, 1983).

COPING WITH SCHIZOPHRENIA

Family Systems Theory

Family systems theory characterizes a healthy family as one that adapts to situational and developmental stressors. In schizophrenia the first psychotic episode usually occurs during late adolescence or early adulthood, so this timing presents situational and developmental crises occurring simultaneously in the family.

Buckley (1967) described the family system as a complex, open, adaptive, organizational, and information-processing system. A family's openness is measured by the interchange with its environment. This interchange is an essential factor underlying the family system's ability to adapt to change. Bowen (1976), a renowned family therapist, defined an *open communication system* as one in which people can freely communicate their inner thoughts and feelings to others who respond accordingly. In contrast, Bowen described a *closed communication system* as an automatic emotional reflex to protect oneself from anxiety found in the other person.

Two significant factors influence family openness around a family member with schizophrenia. First, there is a "stigma" attached to mental illness, especially schizophrenia, that often inhibits a family's willingness to talk about their thoughts and feelings. Second, as previously discussed, complex biological factors of the illness interfere with the memory and language system, which in turn affects the process of sharing information by the ill family member.

Family Stress Theories

Historically, sociologists studying families have suggested a set of resources that, by their presence or absence, keep the family from crisis (Hill & Hansen, 1964: McCubbin, 1979; Olson et al., 1979). Two primary concepts were *family integration* and *family adaptation*. *Adaptability* was defined as the capacity to meet obstacles and change course as a family. Components of adjustment to crisis are crisis, disorganization, recovery, and reorganization, which parallel the recovery process of bereavement. Families of persons experiencing schizophrenia often experience the grief process (Hyland, 1990; Walsh, 1985).

Grief Stages in Families of Clients with Schizophrenia

The personal impact of schizophrenia on families is often tragic and includes financial, social, and productive losses. The severity of schizophrenia symptoms affects the quality of life for clients and families. Watching a family member experience hallucinations and delusions and have difficulty speaking or thinking is devastating. Furthermore, families observe a gradual or abrupt change in personality or hygiene of a son or daughter. Feelings of helplessness and grief reactions arise in family members who witness these behaviors for seemingly a lifetime. The loss of a child or sibling to schizophrenia is the basis of most grief reactions, which are manifested initially by disbelief and denial and subsequently by noncompliance with the treatment regimen. Admitting that a family member has a chronic debilitating mental illness often challenges one's self-esteem and increases feelings of shame and self-blame. Severe symptoms and numerous acute psychiatric hospitalizations often convince families that the client is ill and in need of long-term treatment. Additionally, realization often generates feelings of anger and, later, depression. Working with nurses and other mental health professionals facilitates the resolution and acceptance of mental illness.

Miller et al.'s (1990) study of family members' initial and present feelings about their relative's loss of mental health indicated low levels of grief at the time the client was diagnosed but higher levels of grief during the follow-up interviews years later. (The median length of schizophrenia was 2 to 5 years.) This study included family members with schizophrenia and bipolar disorders. The results suggested that there is measurable grief among family members of severely mentally ill persons and that such grief may be comparable in magnitude with that experienced by families suffering a death (Miller et al., 1990; Perry, 1983). Implications from these findings indicate a need for nurses to conceptualize family members' suffering as a grief response. Encouraging family members to talk about the potential impact of the child's illness on his or her optimal level of function is important. This intervention permits the nurse objectively to assess the family's reaction to the child's illness and facilitate the grief process.

McCubbin (1979) suggested that families experience two major stressors during crisis situations. The initial stressor is followed by later "pile ups" of family life changes. McCubbin identified the following six strains on the family:

1. Stressful event or change
2. Role and boundary ambiguity
3. Family transition
4. Additional life changes
5. Increased energy required to cope
6. Social and medical ambiguity

During the initial nursing assessment, it is important to obtain information regarding the number of perceived stressors and to evaluate their effects on family function.

Wahl and Harmon's (1989) survey indicated that both family members and the mentally ill client were stigmatized by mental illness. Families of persons with psychotic disorders have been stigmatized and blamed by mental health professionals, including nurses. Many respondents could describe some of the specific harmful effects, including damage to self-esteem and difficulty getting and maintaining employment (McCubbin, 1979). Adaptive family responses are strengthened by the following:

1. Self-reliance and self-esteem
2. Family integration
3. Social support
4. Social action
5. Collective group support

This study showed that 487 family members believed that factual information about the illness, socialization, building support inside the family, and increased understanding and awareness of the biological basis of mental illness reduced the stigma of mental illness (Seeley, 1992).

Self-help groups are a significant social support mechanism. They instill hope and empower families through educational programs that enhance problem-solving and communication skills. Family alliance support groups enable members to cope successfully with the effect of schizophrenia on their lives. Major support groups include the National Alliance for the Mentally Ill, the American Schizophrenia Association, and the National Alliance for Research on Schizophrenia and Depression.*

* National Alliance for the Mentally Ill (NAMI), 2101 Wilson Blvd., Ste. 302, Arlington, VA 22201—(703) 524-7600; American Schizophrenia Association, 900 N. Federal Hwy, Ste. 330, Boca Raton, FL 33432—(407) 393-6167; National Alliance for Research on Schizophrenia and Depression, 60 Cutter Mill Road, Ste. 200, Great Neck, NY 11021—(516) 829-0091.

SCHIZOPHRENIA ACROSS THE LIFE SPAN

COURSE OF THE ILLNESS

Premorbid Course

A general overview of the course of schizophrenia begins with onset, which usually occurs during adolescence or early adulthood. As many as two thirds of people who experience an initial psychotic episode never regain their premorbid level of function. They also may fail to attain age-appropriate social and vocational functions. One fifth of people with schizophrenia require continuous monitoring (Lieberman et al., 1992a, 1992b). Deterioration generally occurs early and within the first 5 years of onset. As the illness progresses, its severity seems to level off, with signs of improvement becoming evident during middle adulthood (Bilder et al., 1992; Harding et al., 1987a, 1987b).

Subchronic Course

The American Psychiatric Association, in its *Diagnostic and Statistical Manual of Mental Disorders* (DSM), has moved toward more objective and less theoretical defining criteria for the subchronic course of schizophrenia (see DSM-IV Diagnostic Criteria display). DSM-IV (1994) places more emphasis on negative symptoms of schizophrenia, as well as on enhancing educational efforts. DSM IV delineates the subchronic course of schizophrenia into three phases: (1) prodromal, (2) active, and (3) residual (Table 12–3).

Prodromal Phase. The *prodromal phase* is defined as a clear deterioration in functioning that occurs before the active phase. It usually develops over a 1-year period. The minimum duration of this phase is 6 months. The 6-month period must include an active phase of continuous disturbances lasting at least 1 week or 1 month. Multiple symptoms occur during this phase. Major symptoms of this phase include a substantial deterioration in self-care deficit and academic, occupational, and social function, and the emergence of unusual behavior, thoughts, and perceptual experiences (APA, 1994).

Active Phase. The *active phase* involves psychotic symptoms that require medical intervention or hospitalization. To meet the DSM-IV criteria for schizophrenia, the duration of this phase must be 1 month (as compared with 1 week, as previously defined). Crow (1990) presented a hypothesis differentiating positive and **negative symptoms** and believed that positive symptoms were associated with adequate premorbid functioning, an acute onset, normal cognition, and a positive responses to treatment, specifically neuroleptics. Additionally, Crow delineated the psychotic symptoms of the active phase, which he termed ***positive symptoms***, as hallucinations, delusions, disorganized thinking and speech, and gross behavioral disturbances. Furthermore, he surmised that the basis of positive symptoms was unrelated to structural brain abnormality, such as ventricular enlargement. Most studies support the notion that positive symptoms arise from a neurochemical abnormality, particularly when there is a positive response to neuroleptics.

TABLE 12–3
Schizophrenia: Course of the Illness

ACUTE (ACTIVE) PHASE	PRODROMAL AND RESIDUAL PHASES
Definition Active Phase: presence of psychotic symptoms—at least one from the list of positive symptoms (DSM-IV Option AI) **Symptoms** Positive symptoms ► Delusion ► Hallucination ► Disorganized speech ► Bizarre or disorganized behavior Negative symptoms ► Flat affect ► Avolition ► Alogia ► Anhedonia ► Attention impairment Impairment in functioning (one or more major areas) ► Work ► Interpersonal relations ► Self-care ► Failure to achieve expected levels of interpersonal, academic or occupational development **Minimum Duration** One month	**Definitions** Prodromal phase—clear deterioration in functioning occurring prior to active phase involving minimum of two symptoms listed below. Residual phase—persistence of minimum of two symptoms following active phase. **Symptoms** ► Marked social isolation and withdrawal ► Marked impairment in role functioning as wage earner, student, or homemaker ► Markedly peculiar behavior ► Marked disturbance in speech Circumstantial Poverty of speech and content Vague Overelaborate ► Odd beliefs ► Unusual perceptual experiences ► Marked lack of initiative, interests, energy **Minimum Duration** Continuous signs persisting a minimum of 6 months Must include active-phase period lasting 1 week to 1 month

Data from American Psychiatric Association Task Force on DSM-IV. (1991). *DSM-IV options book: Work in progress.* Washington, DC: Author.

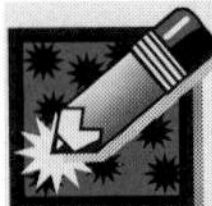

DSM-IV DIAGNOSTIC CRITERIA FOR SCHIZOPHRENIA

A. *Characteristic symptoms:* Two (or more) of the following, each present for a significant portion of time during a 1-month period (or less if successfully treated):

(1) delusions
(2) hallucinations
(3) disorganized speech (e.g., frequent derailment or incoherence)
(4) grossly disorganized or catatonic behavior
(5) negative symptoms, i.e., affective flattening, alogia, or avolition

NOTE: Only one Criterion A symptom is required if delusions are bizarre or hallucinations consist of a voice keeping up a running commentary on the person's behavior or thoughts, or two or more voices conversing with each other.

B. *Social/occupational dysfunction:* For a significant portion of the time since the onset of the disturbance, one or more major areas of functioning such as work, interpersonal relations, or self-care are markedly below the level achieved prior to the onset (or when the onset is in childhood or adolescence, failure to achieve expected level of interpersonal, academic, or occupational achievement).

C. *Duration:* Continuous signs of the disturbance persist for at least 6 months. This 6-month period must include at least 1 month of symptoms (or less if successfully treated) that meet Criterion A (i.e., active-phase symptoms) and may include periods of prodromal or residual symptoms. During these prodromal or residual periods, the signs of the disturbance may be manifested by only negative symptoms or two or more symptoms listed in Criterion A present in an attenuated form (e.g., odd beliefs, unusual perceptual experiences).

D. *Schizoaffective and Mood Disorder exclusion:* Schizoaffective Disorder and Mood Disorder With Psychotic Features have been ruled out because either (1) no Major Depressive, Manic, or Mixed episodes have occurred concurrently with the active-phase symptoms; or (2) if mood episodes have occurred during active-phase symptoms, their total duration has been brief relative to the duration of the active and residual periods.

E. *Substance/general medical condition exclusion:* The disturbance is not due to the direct physiological effects of a substance (e.g., a drug of abuse, a medication) or a general medical condition.

F. *Relationship to a Pervasive Developmental Disorder.* If there is a history of Autistic Disorder or another Pervasive Developmental Disorder, the additional diagnosis of Schizophrenia is made only if prominent delusions or hallucinations are also present for at least a month (or less if successfully treated).

From American Psychiatric Association. (1994). *Diagnostic and statistical manual of mental disorders, fourth edition.* Washington, DC: Author.

Crow (1990) described negative symptoms of schizophrenia, which include affective blunting, poverty of speech (alogia), anhedonia (inability to experience pleasure), apathy or a lack of feeling, and attention impairment. These symptoms usually begin insidiously, and affected persons have a longer history of premorbid functioning or state of health prior to onset of the illness. The course tends to be more chronic, and studies show higher rates of structural brain abnormalities. Clients with negative symptoms tend to show greater impairment on neuropsychological testing and lower educational achievement. Additionally, their past response to neuroleptics is poor. The person with schizophrenia may experience a minimum of two of these symptoms, with one being positive. Additional changes in the DSM-IV include the classification of the course of schizophrenia as follows:

- Continuous—persistent psychotic symptoms throughout the observational period
- Episodic—progressive emergence of negative symptoms between psychotic periods
- Episodic—enduring but "nonprogressive" negative symptoms between psychotic episodes
- Episodic—periods of remission between psychotic episodes
- Partial remission after a lone episode
- Full remission after a lone psychotic episode

During the active or acute-symptom phase of schizophrenia, the person is usually treated in acute care settings, and during initial interviews they may make characteristic statements such as, "I always knew I was different from other people. As a child in school, I often daydreamed because it was difficult to concentrate. I had few friends and spent a lot of time playing alone." Some parents may describe the child as quiet and well behaved, a loner with few dates or social activities who is interested in listening to music or watching television by himself or herself.

Residual Phase. The *residual phase* is similar to the prodromal phase, and the person must continue to experience at least two symptoms of schizophrenia. However, the person's affect may be more flattened, and he or she may experience role impairment. Relapses may follow. Initially, there may be increased positive symptoms and, later, an emergence of increased negative symptoms. The classification of a chronic course requires the same criteria as a subchronic course, but symptoms must last longer than 2 years.

Prognosis

What is the prognosis of schizophrenia? A review of outcome studies indicates that recovery from schizophrenia varies from 10 to 74 percent. Types of recovery range from no rehabilitation (an ability to live a relatively normal life; 20 to 30 percent), to moderate symptoms (20 to 40 percent), to significant impairments (40 to 60 percent) (Kaplan & Sadock, 1989). The last group is characterized by a progressive decline, more negative symptoms, and a higher prevalence in males.

Several research studies indicate a poor outcome for clients experiencing negative symptoms. These symptoms, particularly emotional blunting and disorganized thoughts, are associated with an insidious and progressive decline. Clients who present with positive affective symptoms, particularly prominent depressive features, anxiety, subjective distress, or confusion, have a better prognosis (Table 12–4).

Negative symptoms of schizophrenia are also associated with poor premorbid functioning, including poor cognitive function, scholastic achievement, and social adaptation (Andreasen, 1990). Mastery of age-appropriate social, academic, and occupational development prior to the first psychotic episode is evidence of a nondeteriorating form of the illness and a good outcome (Haas & Sweeney, 1992).

Researchers report that the longer the client has symptoms of schizophrenia before receiving treatment, the greater the likelihood of a poor outcome. Furthermore, if the client is untreated during the acute phase, lasting effects may prevent an effective response to future treatment. A person who does not receive treatment may experience frequent unsuccessful periods of employment and conflictual relationships, which reinforce a deteriorating course of schizophrenia. Furthermore, clients with a family history of an affective disorder have a better outcome than those with a family history of schizophrenia (Andreasen, 1991). A major distinction between these two family histories is that those with schizophrenia fail to return to baseline functioning following relapse, whereas those with affective disorders usually return to a previous level of functioning.

Recent studies suggest that the course of illness and predictors of outcome in chronic schizophrenia parallel the severity and course of illness and allocation of community-based resources versus hospital-based resources. There is general agreement that the initial phase of schizophrenia, which lasts approximately 5 years, constitutes the most deterioration from premorbid levels of function. Additionally, recent studies show that this illness does not have a lifelong course of deterioration. Current speculations are based on neurobiological factors, such as brain structure, response to neuroleptics, gender, and premorbid level of function (Breier et al, 1991, 1992; Carpenter & Strauss, 1991; Carpenter et al., 1988).

TABLE 12–4
Schizophrenia: Prognostic Indicators

POOR OUTCOME	GOOD OUTCOME
Negative symptoms	Positive symptoms
► Insidious or progressive decline	► Acute onset
► Absent depressive symptoms	► Affective symptoms—depression, anxiety, confusion
► Emotional blunting	► Neurochemical abnormality
► Disorganized thoughts	Good premorbid functioning
► Structural brain abnormality	Age-appropriate development
Poor premorbid functioning	► Social
► Poor cognitive function	► Academic
► Poor scholastic achievement	► Occupational
► Poor social adaptation	Early treatment
Delayed treatment	Family history, mood disorder
Family history of schizophrenia	

Data from Andreasen, N. C., & Black, D. W. (1991). *Introductory textbook of psychiatry.* Washington, DC: American Psychiatric Press; and Kaplan, H. I., & Sadock, B. J. (Eds.). (1989). *Comprehensive textbook of psychiatry* (Vol. 1, 5th ed.). Baltimore: Williams & Wilkins.

CHILDHOOD

Major childhood mental disorders include pervasive developmental disorders (autism), schizophrenia with childhood onset, Rett's disorder, childhood disintegrative disorder, and Asperger's disorder. These disorders are often manifested by behaviors or responses that deviate from normal growth and developmental patterns. A major task of psychiatric nurses and mental health professionals is assessment to make an accurate diagnosis.

A process for eliciting data to establish a differential diagnosis includes the following criteria (Lewis, 1989):

- Distinction between normal and abnormal age-appropriate childhood behaviors
- Duration and frequency of symptoms
- Presenting symptoms
- Social adaptation
- Endurance of inappropriate or maladaptive behaviors

Assessment of children is similar to that of adults and focuses on determining maladaptive responses and their origins, including data collection, which can be facilitated by clinical interviews, diagnostic instruments, and structured diagnostic interviews (Lewis, 1989). Researchers continue to search for consistent diagnostic tools to evaluate disturbed behavior in infants and young children.

The diagnostic process needs to involve primary caregivers in the initial interviews, which are arranged in a manner that allows the couple and family, with the child and individually. It includes the following:

- Collection of demographic data
- Assessment of critical developmental tasks (e.g., talking, walking), parenting skills, familial interactions and structure, and the child's coping skills and mental status
- Physical and neurological examination (Kaplan & Sadock, 1991; Mishne, 1986; Pfeffer, 1986)

Physical examinations, including neurological aspects, are crucial when neurobiological disorders are suspected (Table 12–5). Major childhood neurobiological disorders include mental retardation, chronic brain syndromes, failure to thrive, and sensory impairment, such as auditory and visual disturbances. These disorders tend to exaggerate the child's responses to stress, contribute to learning or social disabilities, and interfere with role performance (Mishne, 1986).

Psychosocial factors, such as emotional and social deprivation, may also contribute to the formation of childhood symptoms that resemble infantile autism, brain damage, schizoid personality, and childhood schizophrenia. Emotionally or socially deprived children often lack social, motor, and sensory skills associated with normal growth and development. Historically, children with psychotic disorders were identified as schizophrenics. Criticism of this form of classification arose from its generalization of severely emotionally disturbed children. The DSM-III (APA, 1980) responded to the challenge by establishing another category of childhood psychiatric illnesses called *pervasive developmental disorder*. Later, the DSM-III-R (APA, 1987) refined the definition of this disorder, creating three groups: (1) autistic disorders; (2) pervasive developmental disorders not otherwise specified; and (3) schizophrenia with childhood onset.

The DSM-IV (APA, 1994) also uses the pervasive developmental disorders category to define several childhood disorders, including the previous autistic disorder and pervasive developmental disorder not otherwise specified. Additional disorders include Rett's disorder, childhood disintegrative disorder, and Asperger's disorder (Table 12–6).

TABLE 12–5
Diagnostic Tests: Children and Adolescents with a Suspected Psychotic Disorder

	TESTS AND EXAMINATIONS	RATIONALE
Physical	Configuration and size of head Circumference of head Facial signs, e.g., nose, mouth, brows Handprinting or dermatoglyphics	To assess for microcephaly, hydrocephalus, Down's syndrome
Neurological	Skull radiographs CT scan, MRI Electroencephalogram	Disturbances in motor areas, e.g., spasticity or hypotonia Sensory impairments, e.g., hearing, visual cranial defects, central nervous system abnormalities, and seizure disorders, to assess for Down's syndrome
Laboratory	Urinalysis and serum Hearing and speech evaluations	Metabolic disorders Enzymatic abnormalities (chromosomal disorders, such as Down's syndrome) Hearing and speech development, to assess for mental retardation
Psychological	Screening tests such as Gesell, Catell, Bayley (for infants) Stanford-Binet, Wechsler Intelligence Scale for Children–Revised (WISC-R), Bender-Gestalt, Benton Visual Retention tests	Developmental assessment Detection of brain damage

Autistic Disorders

Leo Kanner, a child psychiatrist, first used the term *infantile* ***autism*** in 1943 in his famous paper, "Autistic Disturbance of Affective Contact." Typical manifestations of autistic disorder are emotional aloofness, solitariness, inability to perform speech, highly repetitive play, and stereotypical movements such as rocking, rolling, and twirling (APA, 1994).

The prevalence of autism is 0.04 to 0.05 percent in children younger than 12 to 15 years of age, and symptoms tend to emerge before the child is 3 years old. This disorder is three to five times more likely to occur in boys than in girls, but symptoms are more pronounced in the latter. An estimated 75 percent of these children are mentally retarded, and 25 percent have seizure disorders. Additionally, the incidence of autistic disorder increases directly with socioeconomic status (Institute of Medicine, 1989; Kaplan & Sadock, 1991).

Other contributing factors in autistic disorders include psychosocial and neurobiological variables. Family dynamics are surmised to play a role in the formation of autistic disorders. A number of researchers emphasize the significance of parent–child interactions. Kanner's (1943) study supported the notion that parents of these children were distant and emotionally cold. However, studies over the past 45 years have failed to support this premise.

Probably the most consistent factor associated with autistic disorders is the neurobiological one. Several causes are associated with defects in the CNS that may arise from prenatal complications such as rubella and phenylketonuria. Other environmental factors, such as high maternal stress levels during the first trimester of

TABLE 12–6
Pervasive Developmental Disorders According to the DSM-IV

DISORDER	MAJOR DSM-IV CRITERIA	OTHER FEATURES
Rett's Disorder	The emergence of a regressive developmental course manifested by multiple deficits that occur after a seemingly normal psychomotor development after birth ► Head size decreases between the ages of 5 and 48 months ► Loss of previously acquired psychomotor development ► Decreased social interaction ► Emergence of incoordination in gait and trunk movements ► Impaired language development with profound psychomotor retardation	Onset before 4 years of age Lifelong course Occurs only in females
Childhood Disintegrative Disorder	The emergence of symptoms after at least a 2-year course after birth of normal growth and development Loss of previously age-appropriate developmental mastery of ► Expressive or receptive language ► Social or coping skills ► Control over bowel and bladder ► Play ► Psychomotor skills Regressive functioning in ► Social interactions ► Language/communication skills ► Repetitive and stereotyped behavioral patterns, mannerisms, and motor skills	Associated with mental retardation More common in males Can only be diagnosed if symptoms occur after the child has at least 2 years of normal growth and develoipment and the onset is before the age of 10 years Course may be insidious or abrupt Lifelong course
Asperger's Disorder	Profound social interaction manifested by (2) of the following: ► Striking alterations in age-appropriate nonverbal communication skills ► Impaired socialization skills ► Apathy ► Lack of emotional relatedness Repetitive and stereotypical behavioral patterns, interests, and social interactions in at least (1) of the following areas: ► Preoccupation with one or more of these repetitive, stereotyped manifestation(s) ► Rigid adherence to insignificant rituals ► Repetitive, stereotyped psychomotor activities, such as finger or hand flapping ► Intense attention on object pieces Global impairment (such as, social and academic) No clinical language impairment	Onset later than autistic disorder Motor delays may occur during preschool age Obvious social impairment more likely to be observed during school age Possible familial pattern More common in males

Data from American Psychiatric Association. (1994). *Diagnostic and statistical manual of mental disorders* (4th ed.). Washington, DC: Author.

pregnancy (Cook, 1990), immunological factors such as incompatible tissue between the mother and fetus (Warren et al., 1990), and genetic factors (Payton et al., 1989) appear to play a role in the development of autism.

Diagnostic studies show that these children have neurobiological lesions that may stem from prenatal complications. Furthermore, electroencephalographic studies suggest that autistic children have failed cerebral lateralization, which refers to linguistic dominance and handedness (Kandel et al., 1991). MRI studies reveal hypoplasia of cerebellar vermal lobules VI and VII and cortical abnormalities (Courchesne et al., 1988; Piven et al., 1990).

Clinical Signs and Symptoms. Symptoms of autism often occur between the ages of 1 and 2 years. Parents describe early symptoms as delayed language development and loss of previous conversational language (Rogers & DiLalla, 1990; Short & Schopler, 1988). Major clinical signs and symptoms are manifested by physical, social, and behavioral impairments.

Children with autism tend to be physically shorter than other children and may be ambidextrous due to failed cerebral lateralization. They may also have an increased incidence of upper respiratory infections and febrile seizures due to autonomic nervous system abnormalities.

Behavioral symptoms of autistic disorders include the following:

- A lack of relatedness
- Impaired communication and language patterns
- Ritualistic and stereotypical movements
- Impaired intellectual function with mild to severe mental retardation

Socially, a lack of relatedness is manifested by the absence of social smiling in infancy, abnormal eye contact, a lack of separation anxiety, and impaired social interactions with peers and social incompetence. Impaired communication is exhibited in language deficits and babbling, clicking, and other sounds. Ritualistic movements, such as rocking, banging, and spinning, suggest either an overreaction or a lack of reaction to sensory stimuli and change (Kaplan & Sadock, 1991).

Major Interventions. Major treatment goals include developing a comprehensive plan of care that minimizes maladaptive behavior and maximizes the child's full developmental potential through a collaborative effort between the mental health team and the parents. Care also consists of regular mental, physical, and developmental screening and identification of potential problems. Parents must be active participants in this process and must be trained in behavioral modification and problem solving. Children with autistic disorders have immense emotional, psychosocial, and biological needs that place enormous stress on the family system. The child and the family can benefit from education that includes parenting skills, stress-reducing activities, child-centered family preservation services, crisis intervention, and supportive therapy. Nurses skilled in family education can teach using learning principles that prepare parents for long-term caregiving.

Another treatment strategy is psychopharmacology. Anderson et al. (1989) found haloperidol (Haldol) to be an effective treatment of hyperactivity, stereotypical movements, irritability, and other childhood behavioral disturbances. Psychoeducation is a critical aspect of psychopharmacological interventions (see Chapter 26). The prognosis for clients with infantile autism is guarded because of the disorder's multifaceted causes and abnormal neurobiological findings.

Evaluating the effectiveness of these strategies is an ongoing process that challenges nurses to employ patience, persistence, and humility in dealing with parents and their need to handle the child's complex needs and demands effectively. The nurse's attitude can have enormous consequences on the parents' self-esteem.

Schizophrenia with Childhood Onset

Several problems interfere with making a definitive diagnosis of childhood schizophrenia. First, there are few standardized diagnostically reliable instruments. Second, there are relatively few descriptive or phenomenological studies of childhood or preadolescent schizophrenia. Finally, there is sparse research that focuses on childhood schizophrenia, and most studies examine a spectrum of psychotic disorders (Russell et al., 1989).

Several studies suggest a small percentage of children with autism eventually develop schizophrenia (Petty et al., 1984; Watkins et al., 1988). Major differences between infantile autism and childhood schizophrenia are the following:

- Autistic children have global maladaptive functioning, beginning early in life and always before 3 years of age.
- The onset of schizophrenia is usually during adolescence or young adulthood and not earlier than 5 years of age.
- Autism is associated with an increased incidence of mental retardation, and schizophrenia is not associated with changes in intelligence.

Childhood schizophrenia is rare. Children exhibiting bizarre or abnormal behavior must be thoroughly evaluated to determine the basis of psychotic symptoms. Children with childhood schizophrenia have severe cognitive and behavioral disturbances, such as social withdrawal and impaired communication. Their immense emotional and physical needs place tremendous stress on their families.

ADOLESCENCE

Adolescence normally is associated with tremendous developmental stress and turmoil. Complex biological, academic, and psychosocial factors place immense demands on the youth at a time of undue vulnerability to maladaptation. The psychosis of schizophrenia often occurs during this developmental stage. Initial symptoms of adolescent schizophrenia often emerge as extreme change in behavior, such as social isolation, peculiar mannerisms, lowered academic performance, and acting out (Mishne, 1986). Because of the prevalence of substance-induced psychosis in the adolescent, differential diagnosis is critical to appropriate and effective treatment. Psychosis is later manifested by chronic patterns of indifference, social withdrawal, hallucinations, delusions, and disorganized thought patterns (Holzman & Grinkler, 1977).

Other influences that impact the outcome of adolescent-onset schizophrenia include the onset of symptoms, family support, developmental crisis, and premorbid history. The outcome is more promising with a history of adaptive developmental mastery, anxiety, and depression (Arieti, 1974). A comprehensive plan of care is critical to positive outcomes from adolescent-onset schizophrenia, and major interventions include **psychoeducation** and regular mental, physical, and developmental screening to identify current and potential responses. Additionally, child-centered family preservation is necessary to maintain the youth in the home and help families cope effectively.

EARLY AND MIDDLE ADULTHOOD

The normal course of schizophrenia often expands from adolescence through middle adulthood and consists of remissions and relapses. Major adult types of schizophrenia include catatonic, disorganized, paranoid, undifferentiated, and residual, as defined in Table 12–7. Schizophrenia is a chronic mental illness; periods of acute exacerbation of psychotic symptoms may occur in subchronic and chronic courses. Treatment consists of inpatient hospitalization to manage acute symptoms and

TABLE 12–7
Major Types of Adult Schizophrenia

Catatonic—marked by a catatonic state or stupor in which the client is unresponsive to his or her surroundings and displays a lack of spontaneous psychomotor activity (rigid posture or bizarre) or mutism
Disorganized—major symptoms include confusion or loose association, disorganized thoughts, and blunt or inappropriate affect
Paranoid—marked by one or more systematic persecutory delusions, auditory hallucinations with a single theme
Undifferentiated—manifested by pronounced delusions, hallucinations, and disorganized thought processes and behavior
Residual—generally there is an absence of pronounced delusions, hallucinations, confusion, or disorganized thoughts or behaviors

Data from American Psychiatric Association. (1994). *Diagnostic and statistical manual of mental disorders* (4th ed.) Washington, DC: Author.

community-based services for medication maintenance, social skills training, and various psychotherapies. Major treatment outcomes depend on the type and course of the illness, the client's compliance with treatment, the presence of negative or positive symptoms, family support, and coping skills. In spite of recent neurobiological and psychosocial discoveries in schizophrenia, most clients experience a limited existence, although a limited number maintain stable employment and living conditions. Others are homeless and untreated or dependent on family members to assist in their care.

Nursing care of the client with schizophrenia consists of managing acute symptoms associated with the illness and substance abuse, administering medications, assessing client responses to treatment, providing psychoeducation, dealing with crisis intervention, and collaborating with clients, families, and other mental health professionals to develop a comprehensive plan of care.

LATE ADULTHOOD

Historically, schizophrenia has been described as an unremitting disorder with a progressively deteriorating course. Contemporary studies suggest the opposite, noting that the schizophrenic process varies and that there is a possibility of improvement with age. Some data suggest improvement occurs in older clients; however, most research tracking the course of schizophrenia has been limited to 20 years from the onset of symptoms. In other words, the studies showed that most symptoms of psychosis, such as delusions, confusion, and auditory hallucinations, seen during initial hospitalization had abated in the clients studied, and only a small percentage of older clients had worsened symptoms. Enduring symptoms of schizophrenia found in older clients included memory difficulties, blunted affect, and decreased speech. These data suggest that older clients have more positive symptoms but more problems with negative symptoms of schizophrenia. Improvement may arise from decreased positive symptoms, whereas others recover regardless of age group (Ciompi, 1985; Harding et al., 1987a, 1987b; Keefe et al., 1987).

Breier et al. (1992) described three phases of schizophrenia: early, middle, and last. The *early,* or acute, *phase* is manifested by deterioration from the client's previous level of functioning. Years ago, Kraepelin surmised that this initial course of illness was unrelenting, with a persistent downhill course. However, recent studies dispute this premise, suggesting that early deleterious effects often end within the first 5 years of onset (Carpenter & Strauss, 1991; McGlashan, 1988). The *middle phase* is described as a sustained period of stability for some clients who experience few changes in level of functioning. This phase may persist for years. The *last phase* is described as the improving stage. Long-term outcome studies propose that later stages of schizophrenia demonstrate minimal changes and some improvement in some clients (Harding et al., 1987a, 1987b).

A number of neurobiological and psychosocial factors influence the long-term course of schizophrenia. Brain morphology and long-term responses to neuroleptics are included in the neurobiological factors that determine negative and positive symptoms of schizophrenia (Breier et al., 1991; Pearlson et al., 1985). Breier et al.'s (1992) study of chronic schizophrenia was unable to support the premise that premorbid negative and positive symptoms were predictors of outcome in elderly clients with schizophrenia. Elderly clients 65 years of age and older are at a greater risk for developing tardive dyskinesia than are other clients taking neuroleptics. When these agents were introduced in the 1950s, large doses were given to control aggressive behavior, but they also increased the likelihood of tardive dyskinesia. In a study by Toenniessen et al., (1985) 50 percent of elderly clients were found to have tardive dyskinesia.

Aging in the U.S. population parallels an increase in the number of elderly clients with schizophrenia. What happens to these clients? An increasing number of them reside in nursing homes. Several researchers assert that only a small percentage, 1 to 2.5 percent, remain in the community (Blazer, 1980; Robins et al., 1984). These findings are attributed to the fact that a large number of these clients reside in county or state institutions. Despite the lower number of acute psychiatric hospitalizations in this population, older clients with schizophrenia consume a large portion of mental health services because of their other age-related health needs.

Nurses caring for elderly clients with schizophrenia must be cognizant of the era in which this diagnosis was established. Several decades ago, anyone with a psychotic-like illness was given this label. However, other psychiatric illnesses, such as bipolar disorder, or physical disorders, such as endocrine and infectious disease processes, could have accounted for the symptoms that would had led to the diagnosis of schizophrenia. Each client must have a complete physical and neuropsychological examination during the initial assessment to determine the cause of bizarre or abnormal behavior.

DIFFERENTIAL DIAGNOSIS

MEDICAL AND NEUROLOGICAL DISEASES

Many medical and psychiatric disorders mimic the symptoms of schizophrenia (Andreasen, 1990; Keshavan & Schooler, 1992; Neuchterlein et al., 1992). Much of the diagnostic decision depends on the client's history and present clinical information, and the differential diagnosis can be facilitated by carefully obtaining individual and family history of neurological and psychiatric disorders (Table 12–8). Complete physical and neurological examinations are critical to making a definitive diagnosis and in ruling out organic or physical causes for presenting symptoms that resemble schizophrenia. Additionally, various laboratory tests and procedures (such as tests for thyroid, liver, and renal function, human immunodeficiency viral infection, complete blood count, and urinalysis) may be useful in ruling out other organic causes. CT and MRI scans are also helpful in the evaluation process.

TABLE 12–8
Medical, Neurological, and Psychiatric Diseases That May Mimic Symptoms of Schizophrenia

MEDICAL AND NEUROLOGICAL DISEASES

- Temporal lobe epilepsy, parkinsonism
- Tumor, stroke, brain trauma
- Endocrine/metabolic disorders
  Porphyria
  Cushing's disease
  Thyroid disorder
- Vitamin deficiency (e.g., B_{12})
- Infectious (e.g., herpes encephalitis, neurosyphilis, acquired immunodeficiency syndrome)
- Autoimune (e.g., systemic lupus erythematosus)
- Toxic (e.g., heavy metal poisoning—mercury, arsenic)
- Alzheimer's, Huntington's, and Wilson's disease
- Drug induced
  Stimulants—amphetamine, cocaine
  Hallucinogens—phencyclidine
  Withdrawal from alcohol, barbiturates, and anticholinergics

PSYCHIATRIC DISEASES

Mood Disorder
- Major depressive with psychotic features
- Bipolar disorder, manic episode
- Schizoaffective disorder

Delusional Disorders
Personality Disorders
- Paranoid
- Schizotypal
- Borderline

Data from Andreasen, N. C., & Black, D. W. (1991). *Introductory textbook of psychiatry.* Washington, DC: American Psychiatric Press; and Kaplan, H. I., and Sadock, B. J. (Eds.). (1989). *Comprehensive textbook of psychiatry* (Vol. 1, 5th ed.). Baltimore: Williams & Wilkins.

PSYCHIATRIC DISEASES RESEMBLING SCHIZOPHRENIA: OTHER PSYCHOTIC DISORDERS

Psychiatric disorders that resemble schizophrenia include delusional, personality, and mood disorders (Andreasen, 1986, 1990; Kaplan & Sadock, 1989) (see Table 12–8). Major mood disorders with psychotic features are bipolar disorder during a manic episode and schizoaffective disorder. Other psychotic disorders include brief reactive psychosis and those due to medical and substance-induced conditions (APA, 1994).

Delusional Disorders

Major symptoms of delusional disorder include nonbizzare delusions consisting primarily of real-life occurrences, such as being watched or followed, having a medical disease, and being cheated on by a spouse, for at least 1 month. Major types of delusional disorders include grandiose, jealous, persecutory, or somatic.

Personality Disorders

These disorders often present with symptoms similar to schizophrenia, yet they usually are evidenced by longstanding patterns of behavior and do not have a specific date of onset. Clients with an "eccentric cluster" in their personality disorder manifest indifference to social relationships and bizarre ideation, yet they are not psychotic.

Mood Disorders

Bipolar Disorder (Manic Episode). Manifestations of a manic episode include a definite period of peculiar and persistent increased, expansive, or irritated mood. Other symptoms include ideas of grandeur, decreased need for sleep, talkativeness, flight of ideas, distractibility, hallucinations, and persecutory delusions (APA, 1994).

Schizoaffective Disorder. Major disturbances of schizoaffective disorder include either a major depression or manic episode paralleling major symptoms of schizophrenia, such as delusions, hallucinations, flat or inappropriate affect, and disturbances in thought processes, and the diagnosis of schizophrenia has been ruled out.

The most differentiating characteristic is that the affective component of schizophrenia is brief compared with the duration of mood disorders, indicating primary symptoms. Additionally, schizophrenia tends to include more negative symptoms, which, as indicated earlier, portend a deteriorating course. In contrast, depressed clients usually recover from negative and positive symptoms. Those experiencing a manic episode recover from thought disorders.

Other Psychiatric Disorders

Brief Reactive Psychosis. Major symptoms of brief reactive psychosis include a brief duration of impaired reality testing, such as delusions, hallucinations, and disorganized and impaired thought processes, lasting from a few hours to 1 month, at which time a return to previous level of function occurs. This disorder occurs concurrently with intense emotional turmoil.

Psychotic Disorder due to a General Medical Condition. Major symptoms of this psychotic disorder include marked delusions or hallucinations and a history of a physical assessment or laboratory results of a medical condition judged to be the basis of presenting psychotic symptoms (APA, 1994).

Substance-Induced Psychotic Disorder. Prominent symptoms of substance-induced psychosis include hallucinations or delusions and a history, physical examination, or laboratory results of substance intoxication or withdrawal and symptoms occurring within 1 month of major substance intoxication or withdrawal. Major types are determined by specific substances, such as alcohol, amphetamine, and cocaine (APA, 1994). Schizophrenia is characterized by bizarre delusions, whereas a delusional disorder involves persecutory delusions. Unlike a delusional disorder, schizophrenia commonly has positive symptoms (i.e., hallucinations).

IMPAIRED PERCEPTIONS AND SENSORY FUNCTIONING: HALLUCINATIONS AND DELUSIONS

What is it like in the world of the client with schizophrenia? What is it like to have a psychotic episode? Hallucinations and delusions are probably the most frightening symptoms of the psychotic process (see the Client Experience display below).

Hallucinations are defined as false sensory perceptions from one or more of the following senses when there is no external stimulus:

- Auditory (voices, sounds, or music)
- Visual (images)
- Gustatory (unpleasant taste)
- Tactile (touch)
- Olfactory (unpleasant smells)

Delusions relate to thought processes. They are defined as fixed false beliefs unchanged by logic. Types of delusions include paranoid ("The FBI is watching me"), religious ("I am God"), grandiose ("I have special power and ability"), and nihilistic ("I feel like part of me is dead"). Delusions can include thought broadcasting (thinking that others hear one's thoughts), thought insertion (thinking that someone can put

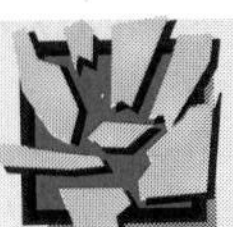

MY EXPERIENCES WITH PSYCHOSIS

A person who has struggled with hallucinations and delusions shares some thoughts about her experiences.

I have sought treatment for the last 25 years for a condition now diagnosed as schizoaffective disorder; that is, I have suffered from mood swings and schizophrenic symptoms, such as hearing voices and having delusions.

I began to hear voices when I was 16 years old. These audio hallucinations were not only very friendly and humorous but they also caused me to feel quite euphoric. They convinced me to stop taking my medication. They also informed me that I was not psychotic, that everyone else hears them, and that I was to keep this psychic phenomenon to myself. The big secret.

I was given an antipsychotic medication and my hallucinations stopped. However, soon thereafter, I began smoking marijuana regularly again, and the voices returned. (My withdrawal from reality was characterized by my thinking that I was telepathic or that I was a very famous person). I worked and went to school between frequent hospitalizations, as I was constantly up and down and hallucinating. Even though I stopped using street drugs, the hallucinations persisted and became very negative and hateful. This led to the delusion that even loved friends and family hated me. Hence, I became alienated and isolative.

Three years ago I entered a long-term inpatient unit on the East Coast and was taken off all my medication so I could see how I was affected by Clozaril. Since taking the new medication, the hallucinations have been reduced substantially. In addition to the very new medication, therapy and daily activities have really helped me reenter reality.

I have been afflicted by what my treaters and I call "the connective symptom." The messages I get from this "connection" are often misleading, seemingly attempting to make me feel suicidally disappointed, or at least testing my patience and temper. Most often, these messages (what I call "plants"—short for "implanted thoughts"—) are from a boy I dated and was very fond of who died 20 years ago. My treaters explain this experience as my subconscious manifesting my loneliness and grief by creating the imaginary company of a boy I cared about. I read the messages by paying attention to my own and other people's involuntary motions and what they seem to say.

I've been on Clozaril for about 28 months now. While I've had to deal with depression over the lack of my imaginary company in the form of audio hallucinations, I have been outside the hospital during that time. I have stopped feeling suicidal, I know my friends and family love me, and I'm working on maintaining and developing real relationships. I have improved my concentration and retention regarding what I perceive to an incredible degree.

My coordination has been also impressively improved. I have no craving for street drugs. I have cut down on my consumption of caffeine and nicotine. I have been exercising regularly and eating better and have lost 50 to 60 pounds. All this improvement has led to much better self-esteem and basic relationships with myself and others. Also, I've been getting much more rest and am, in my opinion and according to the observations of treaters, much more consistent and level in my moods.

In closing, I will just say that I feel my treatment and Clozaril have improved the quality of my life, and my life is just getting better and better.

thoughts into another's mind), and thought withdrawal (thinking one's thoughts are being extracted from the mind).

What are the causes of hallucinations and delusions? There is a substantial body of knowledge that points toward multiple causes of hallucinations. Hallucinations and delusions represent a complex interplay among (1) brain physiology, (2) current environmental stimuli, and (3) the person's frame of reference (earlier life experiences). Several theorists (Asaad & Shapiro, 1986) take the *psychophysiological* approach and believe that

- There is an abnormal brain excitability.
- There is a greater glucose uptake by auditory areas.
- Dreams and hallucinations lie on a continuum, with an inhibitory factor preventing their emergence into the waking state (as suggested by sleep studies).

Biochemical theorists believe messengers in the brain called *neurotransmitters,* especially dopamine and serotonin, influence hallucinations. Neuroleptics or antipsychotic medications are thought to interact with these neurotransmitters to inhibit hallucination symptoms. Hallucinations may occur because current environmental stimulation is either too little or too much. Certain stressful situations, such as imprisonment, space flights, and high altitudes, have been known to precipitate hallucinations in people who do not have a mental disorder.

Finally, *psychodynamic* theorists suggest that hallucinations develop as an adaptive response to anxiety. Hallucinations are thought to represent a breakthrough of unconscious feelings and thoughts coming into awareness. The content of hallucinations is thought to have significant meaning to the individual. For instance, a person experiencing guilt may hear critical voices. Someone who cannot directly express intense anger may have visual images of someone being aggressive (Asaad & Shapiro, 1986).

STAGES OF HALLUCINATIONS AND DELUSIONS

Hallucinations and delusions often emerge over time. Hildegarde Peplau first outlined the four states of the hallucinatory process in the 1950s as comforting, condemning, controlling, and conquering. Janice Clack expanded these concepts in 1962, based on clinical reports and observations. Different levels of anxiety are associated with each state. Clack describes these stages as follows.

Stage I: Comforting. This stage correlates with mild anxiety. The person experiences anxiety, loneliness, or guilt and focuses on relieving anxiety with comforting thoughts. An example is the child who frequently plays alone and creates an imaginary friend to play with. Persons in this stage realize that the thoughts are their own, and they can control them.

Stage II: Condemning. This stage parallels moderate anxiety. If anxiety increases, the client places himself or herself into a state of listening for the hallucination that begins with this process. At this time, the person becomes afraid that others hear the voices, which are negative, and, consequently, socially withdraws. Furthermore, the person's attention span begins to narrow, and vital sign changes may parallel the intensity of anxiety.

Stage III: Controlling. This stage correlates with severe anxiety. In this stage the person gives up trying to fight the voices. The voices become omnipotent, and the client follows their directions. The person's attention span is so constricted that he or she is unable to relate to others. At this time, if the voices cease, the person feels extremely lonely. For example, one person experienced grandiose delusions for 7 years. She talked about how she would experience depression when her delusions were gone. Sometimes, she was reluctant to fight the delusions or take her medication because she knew that without her symptoms she would experience depression and loneliness.

Stage IV: Conquering. This stage correlates with panic anxiety. The voices become threatening if the person does not follow their commands. The hallucinations often become interwoven with delusions. During this stage the client may even become suicidal or violent. Voices are real to the client and can generate feelings that range from pleasure to terror. The latter response may result in a suicide attempt—out of despair, 20 percent of people experiencing this stage will attempt suicide, and 10 percent will succeed. Half of the people who attempt suicide are doing what the auditory commands tell them to do.

INTERRUPTING THE HALLUCINATION OR DELUSIONAL PROCESS

How can the hallucination or delusional process be interrupted? The goal in working with a client who experiences hallucinations and delusions is to help the client become aware that these are aspects of the illness that can be controlled. The initial step in interrupting hallucinations is the establishment of rapport. For example, one client was more open about his self-destructive voices when he understood that his mental health therapist would not automatically recommend hospitalization or an increase in medication dosage.

Nurses can teach various strategies to facilitate control of hallucinations or delusions, as follows:

- Clients can participate in activities that require verbal responses.
- During the first stage of hallucinations, clients can command the voices to go away and leave them alone.
- Clients can become more reality oriented by learning about what is happening in their environment.
- Clients can learn to identify psychosocial factors and link behavior to anxiety.

- Clients can discover the purpose of the hallucination (the underlying need) and learn alternative ways to satisfy this need.

The nurse and family need to determine whether the source of hallucinations is the person's emotions or an external toxin, such as alcohol and other drugs. Several strategies, such as the following, are useful in facilitating this process:

1. The nurse needs to assess if the client is using alcohol or other drugs. The client and the family need to understand the dangers of using these agents, especially in combination with prescribed medications. It is also important to know that hallucinations have also been reported as side effects from various prescribed and over-the-counter medications, including antidepressants, digoxin, propranolol (Inderal), atropine, and diphenhydramine (Benadryl).
2. There may be a physical basis for hallucinations such as neurological disorders (e.g., systemic lupus erythematosus). Additionally, there may be frontal lobe seizures, an organic mental disorder, such as Alzheimer's disease and brain trauma, or ear and eye diseases. Regardless of the cause, clients experiencing hallucinations or delusions may need protection from injury to self or others.
3. Clients experiencing hallucinations or delusions often state that it is helpful to hear nurses tell them to separate symptoms of the illness from who they are as a person.

The client with schizophrenia has an episodic illness in which anxiety plays a role in escalating hallucinations. Nurses can help these clients manage hallucinations and delusions so they can live a quality life.

TREATMENT MODALITIES

Schizophrenia is a complex disorder that requires a diverse approach and therapies that vary depending on the phase of illness and the quality of social support and other resources. Treatment approaches derive from the therapeutic relationship, which enables the nurse to assess, intervene, and collaborate with clients and families and other health professionals to develop a comprehensive treatment plan. Major goals include reducing the severity of symptoms and stress, mobilizing resources, and enhancing the client's and family's coping skills and strengths. Major interventions include psychopharmacology, supportive psychotherapy, psychoeducation, social skills training, and stress management.

PSYCHOPHARMACOLOGY

Neuroleptics or antipsychotic agents are currently the most widely used drugs for treating schizophrenia during the acute and maintenance stages. Nurses must have a broad understanding of desired and adverse effects of these agents and the relevancy of low potency, medium potency, and high potency. Low-potency agents, such as chlorpromazine (Thorazine), thioridazine (Mellaril), and clozapine (Clozaril), are helpful because of their sedative and anxiolytic properties. Furthermore, these agents tend to have fewer extrapyramidal side effects than do high-potency agents such as haloperidol, thiothixene (Navane), and fluphenazine (Prolixin) (Maggliozzi & Schaff, 1988). Additionally, low-potency drugs are more likely to cause more anticholinergic effects and orthostatic hypotension than are high-potency agents (Breslin, 1992). Side effects from medium-potency agents, such as perphenazine (Trilafon) and loxapine (Loxitane), tend to fall between the low-potency and high-potency agents. High-potency agents have been used primarily for acute and maintenance treatment of schizophrenia since the mid 1970s.

Figure 12–1 explains how some of these agents affect the dopaminergic synapses. Acute and long-term side effects are discussed in depth in Chapter 26.

Medication Compliance. Compliance is a major concern for clients with schizophrenia and other psychotic disorders. Noncompliance has been linked with experiencing medication-induced side effects, dosing of neuroleptics, and a lack of insight into the illness (Kane, 1990).

SUPPORTIVE PSYCHOTHERAPY

Clients with schizophrenia cope with a spectrum of impairments that consist of disordered thoughts and corresponding behavior, reality testing, impaired social and coping skills, low self-esteem, and fluctuation in feelings or affect. Various treatment strategies have enabled these clients to effectively cope with these impairments. One such treatment is supportive psychotherapy. Supportive psychotherapy can facilitate enduring, constructive changes. Positive changes can arise from formation of a therapeutic relationship in which the client learns social and interpersonal skills, psychoeducation, management of behaviors or symptoms, and a sense of well-being (McGlashan, 1986; McGlashan & Nayfack, 1988).

Before the advent of psychotropic medications, psychotherapy was not the treatment of choice for clients with schizophrenia. Currently, however, supportive psychotherapy is considered the most effective form of psychotherapy when used as an adjunct to psychotropics (Muller et al., 1992; Sarti & Courous, 1990). The success of this approach depends on several components: (1) a therapeutic relationship; (2) individual needs and vulnerability as a basis of therapy; (3) a reality-oriented approach that focuses on behaviors rather than their meaning; and (4) client education.

Treating clients with schizophrenia is a challenging process that enables nurses to identify and address complex needs. Collaboration with the client, the family, and other mental health professionals is critical to developing effective treatment modalities.

PSYCHOEDUCATION

The treatment of clients with schizophrenia has evolved since the 1950s from its initial focus on ways to control agitation and other behaviors arising from psychosis. There has been a shift toward treatment that centers on assessing the client's personality, communication patterns, and ability to cope effectively with the debilitating effects of psychosis (Boker, 1992).

Boker (1992) identified the four major coping strategies clients use to manage problem areas and patterns of their illness as the following:

1. Clients compensate for prodromal symptoms of psychosis.
2. Clients lessen disturbing positive symptoms.
3. Clients cope with the debilitating effects of their illness.
4. Clients develop and improve their social and coping skills.

Boker (1992) also surmised that the client's ability to develop adaptive skills played a major role in managing psychotic symptoms, minimizing relapse, and altering the long-term debilitating effects of schizophrenia. Furthermore, he believed that this is a learning process based on a therapeutic relationship that provides the structure necessary to educate the client about his or her responsibility in managing medication side effects and the course of illness.

Nurses and other mental health professionals need to collaborate with clients and families to educate and assist them in understanding and coping effectively with mental illness. Few families are prepared to meet the enormous needs of clients with schizophrenia. A number of families experience feelings of helplessness, self-blame, embarrassment, anger, and a sense of loss when faced with a mentally ill family member. Clients with schizophrenia often mirror these feelings. Additionally, the client experiences pervasive feelings of low self-esteem, ineffective coping skills, cognitive impairment, and a lack of social support. Families often look to nurses for answers and empathy in dealing with these issues.

How can nurses assist these clients? Spaniol et al. (1992) delineated several components that are useful in developing psychoeducational programs for families. They include

- Clarifying roles of family members, the client, and the health care professional
- Working collaboratively with families and clients
- Developing individualized educational strategies
- Including families in the planning stage
- Responding effectively to the family's intense feelings and needs
- Meeting with local client advocate and support groups
- Maximizing family strengths
- Taking care of oneself

Psychoeducational programs have emerged over the past decade as a mechanism for providing emotional support, social skills training, crisis intervention, and increased sensitivity among nurses and other mental health professionals to meet the needs of clients and their families (Hartfield & Lefley, 1987; Zipple & Spaniol, 1987).

SOCIAL SKILLS TRAINING

Social skills training involves teaching those behaviors that allow people to accurately communicate their feelings, thoughts, and needs to facilitate interpersonal goals. Successful interactions involve effective use of both verbal and nonverbal communication skills. Liberman et al. (1989) defined social interactions in terms of a three-stage process that involves mastering well-defined skills at each level, referred to as *receiving, processing,* and *sending*.

The initial stage of social skills training involves using receiving skills. These skills are determined by the ability to accurately perceive input from internal and external environments and respond to them appropriately. Clients with schizophrenia may initially have difficulty interpreting environmental cues because of altered thought processes and sensoriperceptual abilities. Ideas of reference (a thought disorder in which a person believes that a conversation or grinning from others is directed at one's ideas, such as, "everybody is laughing at me") interfere with the ability to approach people in a group and respond appropriately. A typical response may be, "Why are you looking at me like that?" or " I don't like the way you said that." Additionally, clients with schizophrenia are often irritable and agitated, further compromising the ability to relate to others effectively and increasing social isolation. These behaviors and reactions reflect an inability to determine reality. Nursing intervention, such as administration of neuroleptic medications, can reduce psychotic symptoms. In addition, establishing a one-to-one therapeutic relationship rather than using a group approach minimizes external stimuli and anxiety and increases a sense of reality.

The second stage of this communication process requires processing skills, which enable the client to choose the most effective short-term and long-term goals. Problem solving is basic to this stage, and it entails identifying options and evaluating solutions and consequences. The client with a sense of reality is able to size up a situation with help from nurses, family members, and other mental health professionals. Assignments must be based on the client's level of functioning, strengths, and motivation. A client should start from simple but challenging tasks and eventually progress to more complex ones. Successful experiences provide a sense of accomplishment and improve self-esteem.

The last stage in this communication process is based on the client's ability to accurately understand and perceive the environment and learn pertinent skills for appropriate interaction. This stages requires sending skills. Overall, these skills involve actual appropriate social interactions between the client and the staff, using both verbal and nonverbal communication. Communication tools pertinent to using these skills effectively include selecting and using the right words to convey what one means (Liberman et al., 1989).

The client with schizophrenia is challenged to participate in social skills groups as a way of improving communication patterns. Effective communication skills enable the client to establish meaningful relationships, express feelings, and cope with illness. Furthermore, the nurse is confronted with forming a relationship with a client who lacks social competence and has difficulty establishing trust. Forming a meaningful relationship with the client with schizophrenia requires patience, commitment, and a willingness to deal with rejection. These behaviors convey caring and empathy to the client and family members.

STRESS MANAGEMENT

Liberman et al. (1989) asserted that a lack of social competence and difficulty expressing feelings interfere with establishing meaningful relationship and threaten the quality of life. They suggest that regardless of the cause of social incompetence, social skills training can be a useful treatment intervention that improves the client's level of functioning and overall health (see the Research Study display). Major components of social skills training include improving coping behavior, learning stress management, and understanding the nature of illness.

Assessing baseline coping skills is pivotal to understanding psychoeducational needs. Asking clients and family members about past symptoms and crises and how they were handled, available support systems, substance abuse history, and medication compliance is a critical aspect of identifying coping patterns. The ability to cope with stressors is influenced by several factors, including neurobiological and psychosocial factors. Schizophrenia increases vulnerability to stress that may be related to internal and external stimuli.

Because relapse is associated with high stress levels (Zubin et al., 1992), nursing intervention needs to be based on early detection, with an emphasis on reducing and minimizing the noxious effects of stress. Hogarty et al. (1991) surmised that the most effective relapse prevention strategies included those that combined family interventions, social skills training, and medication regimens. Their 2-year study showed that 75 percent of clients did not relapse during followup. Relapse is often associated with ineffective coping abilities in both clients and their families.

Nursing implications from these findings suggest the need to develop innovative strategies that improve coping behaviors, stress management, and compliance. These endeavors can be enhanced by actively involving the client and family members in the treatment process, beginning with admission to the acute inpatient and outpatient settings. Specific stress management strategies include the following:

- *Crisis intervention*—provides immediate emotional and social support while it assists in identifying adaptive options and understanding the relevance of precipitating stressors (Aguilera, 1990, 1994)
- *Addressing of medication and compliance issues in medication groups or supportive therapy*—enables nurses to teach clients and families about the importance of medication and control of symptoms, including desired and adverse effects. Other issues that can be discussed in these groups include

RESEARCH STUDY

Technique for Training Schizophrenic Patients in Illness Self-Management: A Controlled Trial

Eckman, T. A., Wirshing, W. C., Marder, S. R., Liberman, R. P., Johnston-Cronk, K., Zimmerman, K., & Mintz, J. (1992). *American Journal of Psychiatry, 149*(11), 1549–1555.

Purpose of Study

The purpose of the study was to determine if schizophrenic outpatients receiving low-dose antipsychotic agents could learn self-management skills based on cognitive and behavioral approaches devised to compensate for learning disabilities associated with schizophrenia.

Methods

Forty-one patients diagnosed with schizophrenia receiving low-dose drug treatment were randomly selected to participate in structured, modulated skills training or in supportive group psychotherapy. This 18-month study consisted of weekly visits, case management, and intramuscular injections of fluphenazine decanoate. Modular training consisted of social skills training (medication and symptom management) twice weekly over a 6-month period. Other strategies included homework assignments and vivo exercises.

The supportive group participants employed an insight-oriented and supportive group process focusing on an unstructured psychoeducational curricula.

Findings

Participants who received modular training retained more information than those in the supportive group training.

Nursing Implications

Modular psychoeducational training enables some clients to control their symptoms and illness while promoting a sense of mastery and self-care. This approach can enhance the treatment of persons with schizophrenia.

dealing with feelings and thoughts about the long-term effects of a chronic illness and gaining emotional and social support from peers (Antai-Otong, 1989)

- *Providing clear directions for adaptive, desired behaviors*—can be facilitated by role playing or rehearsal of adaptive behaviors, praise and reinforcement of these behaviors, and encouragement in self-evaluation regarding successes (Liberman et al., 1989). Providing ongoing positive reinforcement of adaptive coping behaviors can assist the client in assessing areas that need improvement.

THE NURSE'S ROLE

GENERALIST ROLE

To develop a comprehensive treatment plan for the client with schizophrenia, the generalist nurse collaborates with other members of the health care team, including the client and the family. The generalist nurse also administers medication, monitors response to interventions, and provides psychoeducation for the client and the family.

ADVANCED-PRACTICE ROLE

The advanced-practice nurse acts as a case manager, forming a collaborative relationship with the client during hospitalization and in the community group home. Other important functions include providing family and supportive therapy and working with other members of the team to maximize community resources. In many states, the advanced-practice nurse has prescriptive authority.

MANAGING ACUTE AND CHRONIC SYMPTOMS OF SCHIZOPHRENIA

The chronically mentally ill have a high rate of recidivism, and many of these clients do receive inadequate aftercare, which results in homelessness and problems accessing mental and health care services and are at risk for substance abuse and violence. Furthermore, a lack of effective coping skills, poor support systems, and fragmented health care and social services contribute to high relapse rates and staggering health care costs and the descent of persons with chronic mental illness into homelessness and poverty (Lamb et al., 1993). Proposed health care reforms are focusing on increasing the quality of care and reducing health care costs.

One solution to this problem is comprehensive, continuous health care. This interdisciplinary approach evolves over time in various clinical settings. Studies show that comprehensive, continuous treatment is clinically and fiscally effective, specifically those methods using psychopharmacological and social skills training (Vaccaro et al., 1992). Treatment is based on a functional assessment that encompasses identifying client life goals, behavioral impairments, and disability, such as altered thought processes, to specific interventions. Other components of this assessment include identifying the client's level of function, strengths, resources, and self-care skills (Vacarro et al., 1993). Goal setting is the basis of success in comprehensive treatment planning. The client plays a major role in identifying goals and strengths, resources, and behavioral impairments.

Major treatment goals include enabling clients to

- Reach their highest level of function
- Adapt and meet their environmental needs through mobilization of social and physical resources
- Employ their strength, and increase competency levels
- Restore hope
- Increase autonomy through vocational goals
- Facilitate a sense of accomplishment and mastery, and increase self-esteem
- Experience resocialization
- Enhance and direct their self-care using their experiences, ideas, and needs (Bachrach, 1992; Liberman, 1992).

THE NURSING PROCESS

The following case history provides an example of how the nurse's role in comprehensive care can be used to move the client through various phases in acute inpatient to community-based settings.

Case Study 1: The Client with Schizophrenia (Mr. Livingston)

Acute Phase

Mr. Livingston is a 28-year-old man diagnosed with chronic schizophrenia, paranoid type, with acute exacerbation. He was brought to the emergency department by his sister, who reported that she found him wandering on the streets talking to himself in a state of confusion. He was speaking in a loud voice, his appearance was disheveled, his mood was agitated, and he was repeatedly looking around the room, questioning the reasons for the interview, and not making eye contact. His sister reported that he had disappeared a week ago and no one knew where he was. His history reveals that he has been hospitalized at least several times a year because of his refusal to take medication and abuse of marijuana. Additionally, he has no acute medical problems, except that he has lost about 10 pounds in the past week. He was observed to be incoherent, acting suspicious, and smiling often during the assessment process. He was uncooperative and refused to talk to the nurse.

Assessment

Reducing environmental stimuli and assessing the nature of Mr. Livingston's hallucinations and delusions, present medications, substance abuse, and psychiatric history are major components of this initial interview.

Nursing Diagnoses

Major nursing diagnoses identified during this initial assessment include the following:

- Altered Thought Processes
- Anxiety
- Knowledge Deficit: Client and Significant Others
- Ineffective Individual Coping related to substance abuse

Planning and Implementation

Major goals during the acute period include identifying measures to reduce harm, managing disordered behavior and symptoms, facilitating a rapid return to the highest level of function, and forming an alliance with the client and the family to develop a comprehensive and coordinated plan of care. Psychopharmacological interventions include administering neuroleptics and monitoring client response to treatment. Providing a therapeutic milieu also involves reducing environment stimuli and providing a nonthreatening and empathic relationship (McGlashan, 1986) (see Chapter 24).

Nurses participate in a broad spectrum of activities during the acute, stabilization, and rehabilitation phases. Input into the functional assessment is based on clinical observations, client responses, and individual needs and abilities.

This client, Mr. Livingston, is overtly psychotic, and major nursing intervention indications from this initial interview include establishing rapport, conveying empathy, asking direct questions, reducing hallucinations and delusions, and promoting comfort.

The emergency department physician ordered oral lorazepam (Ativan) and haloperidol (Haldol) to reduce psychotic symptoms. Initially, Mr. Livingston was uncooperative, but his sister talked him into taking the medication orally. The action of neuroleptic or antipsychotic agents is potentiated by benzodiazepines (such as lorazepam), which lower the risk of side effects and rapidly reduce agitation and irritability while reducing hallucinations and delusions. After a short period, Mr. Livingston was calmer and more cooperative. He allowed the nurse to take his vital signs, and he assisted in the completion of his physical and psychiatric examination.

Subacute Phase

Mr. Livingston was admitted to an acute inpatient unit for medication stabilization and referral to a community home. He was hospitalized for 1 week, and he rapidly responded to the milieu and medication regimen.

Major goals during this period include reducing the risk of relapse and preparing the client for discharge and community-based interventions. The generalist nurse collaborates with other members of the mental health team, the client, and the family to develop a comprehensive treatment plan. The clinical specialist was assigned to be case manager for Mr. Livingston and was also an active participant on the mental health team. Major roles of the generalist include medication administration, monitoring his response to interventions, and participating in psychoeducation of the client and family members.

Stabilization Phase: Psychiatric Rehabilitation

Mr. Livingston was ready for referral to a community home. During previous admissions, his family was not actively involved in his care. His sister had recently moved to the area and was anxious to participate in helping the client.

Major goals after stabilization include preventing relapse and promoting health and a sense of well-being using various interventions, such as medication, psychoeducation, and supportive, family, or group therapy. Twelve-step groups are an essential part of helping clients maintain abstinence and learning ways to reduce and manage stress effectively.

Evaluation

Evaluation is determined by identification of outcomes; observation of the client's response to treatment such as absence of hallucinations, delusions, and increased self-care; and feedback from the client, the family, and members of the mental helath team. Mr. Livingston no longer experiences psychotic symptoms, and he is gaining insight into his role in reducing relapse and maintaining a state of health. His family also continues to play an active role.

Summary

The advanced-practice, or clinical specialist, role of the psychiatric–mental health nurse involves identifying complex needs of the client based on functional assessments and forming a collaborative relationship with the client during hospitalization and in the community group home. As case manager, the advanced-practice nurse provides family and supportive therapy to maintain present coping behaviors and assist family members in dealing with stress associated with caring for the client. The advanced-practice nurse also works with the staff in the community group home, the client, and the family to maximize community resources, enhance family involvement, and develop effective, comprehensive, and coordinated treatment. The advanced-practice nurse also has prescriptive authority and is involved in monitoring compliance and response to various interventions.

Case management is a part of the continuous comprehensive care that involves providing interventions to reduce the risk of exacerbation of illness, enhance coping skills, provide psychoeducation, and ally with other social services. The success of case management depends on several factors, including integrating, coordinating, and advocating for resources for clients, families, and communities. This holistic approach enables nurses to ally with other community social services, provide direct care, evaluate responses, and support new and complex initiatives consisting of adequate housing, antipoverty programs, better health services, and vocational training projects. Evaluating the effectiveness of pharmacological and psychosocial interventions is a vital part of comprehensive, coordinated treatment. The overall goal of comprehensive, coordinated treatment is to increase the client's and family's level of functioning and sense of well-being by increasing self-care and symptom management (Bower, 1992; Cohen & Thompson 1992; Krauss, 1993).

THE NURSING PROCESS

The following case study provides a useful framework for examining the nursing process in the acute care setting.

Case Study 2: The Client with Schizophrenia (Johnny)

Johnny is an 18-year-old admitted to an acute psychiatric unit with a diagnosis of schizophrenia, acute, paranoid type. His parents reported that his grades have dropped from As to Cs, and he has been getting failing grades in school the past 12 months. He has also become increasingly withdrawn, agitated, and irritable during this period. He has been overheard talking and arguing in his room during the day and night. Initially, his parents thought that he was taking drugs and they sought medical treatment. His physical examination and drug screening results were negative. During the past 2 weeks, Johnny has refused to eat and has expressed fears that his mother has been trying to poison him. Additionally, he has refused to attend school or to come out of his room. His parents became concerned about his deteriorating mental and physical condition and brought him to the emergency department. His appearance was disheveled—his hair was uncombed and his clothes were wrinkled. Johnny was pacing, and his mood was irritable and agitated. His eye contact was poor and his thoughts were irrelevant, incoherent, and illogical. He was thinly built, 6 feet tall, and weighed about 137 pounds. He was easily distracted, and his responses were inappropriate. His parents were the chief informants.

Assessment

Johnny is thinly built (disproportionate weight for height), with a weight loss of 25 to 35 pounds over several months. He demonstrates a disorganized thought process (i.e., disturbances in sensory and perceptual functioning) as well as moderate agitation and irritability.

Nursing Diagnoses

- Altered Nutrition, Less Than Body Requirements
- High Risk for Injury; High Risk for Self-Mutilation
- Altered Thought Processes
- Self-Care Deficit
- Anxiety
- Knowledge Deficit related to lack of information about the illness

Planning and Implementation

Nursing Care Plan 12–1 identifies the desired outcomes for the nursing diagnoses listed earlier and delineates the nursing actions needed to achieve these outcomes, along with the rationales for these actions.

Evaluation

Evaluation is based on identification of outcomes and feedback from the client, the family, and other mental health professionals. In the case history, Johnny was hospitalized for several weeks and responded rapidly to psychotropics. He was discharged to a partial hospital setting, and his parents continued to play active roles in psychoeducation and provide emotional and psychosocial support during this stressful ordeal.

► CHAPTER SUMMARY

The term *schizophrenia* was coined almost a century ago, and since then numerous researchers have attempted to understand the complexity of this chronic, debilitating mental disorder. Its prevalence continues to impact various aspects of society, ranging from mental health facilities to families and communities.

The impact of schizophrenia on families and clients is phenomenal. Grief and stigma issues can affect the family's response to the client and their participation in the treatment process. Client advocacy groups and the advent of studies that link schizophrenia with neurobiological factors have alleviated some of these feelings, enabling families to work with nurses and other mental health professionals to maximize resources and promote self-care.

Historically, causative factors have focused on psychodynamic theories that related schizophrenia to dysfunctional family interactions. These theories are outdated, but they represented creative thinking by various mental health professionals, such as psychiatrists, psychologists, social scientists, and nurses. These were sincere attempts to explain a phenomenon before technological advances brought new insights into neurobiological and behavioral responses in a social context.

Furthermore, recently, mental health advocacy groups and families collaborated to dispel this premise by educating the public and legislature through publications and community meetings. However, in spite of expansion of neuroscientific information and knowledge, the exact cause of schizophrenia remains unknown.

Nursing Care Plan 12–1 The Client with Schizophrenia (Johnny)

OUTCOME IDENTIFICATION	NURSING ACTIONS	RATIONALES	EVALUATION
Nursing Diagnosis: Altered Nutrition: Less Than Body Requirements			
1. By [date], Johnny will maintain adequate nutritional status to meet body requirements.	1a. Assess nutritional status. 1b. Decrease environmental stimuli. 1c. Provide adequate nutrition.	1a. To determine baseline information. 1b. Decreased stimuli minimize anxiety/stress. 1c. Helps ensure adequate intake.	*Goal met:* With parental encouragement, Johnny begins to take in adequate nutrition and demonstrates gradual weight gain.
Nursing Diagnosis: High Risk for Injury; High Risk for Self-Mutilation			
1. Johnny will refrain from harming himself or others during the treatment process.	1a. Assess level of dangerousness (previous attempts, means, and thoughts). 1b. Remove dangerous items from the environment. 1c. Assess for changes in mood, affect, and thoughts (e.g., pacing, agitation). 1d. Administer neuroleptic/antianxiety agents. 1e. Encourage Johnny to express feelings rather than acting on thoughts.	1a. Provides baseline information. 1b. Removal of dangerous items decreases risk of harm to self or others. 1c. Changes in these areas may indicate imminent danger. 1d. Medication promotes reality testing and decreases agitation and level of dangerousness. 1e. Expression of feelings enables nurse to assess response to medication.	*Goal met:* Johnny does not harm himself or others. Johnny experiences less agitation and fewer hallucinations and delusions after administration of medication. Only side effect of medication is sedation.
Nursing Diagnosis: Altered Thought Processes			
1. By [date], Johnny experiences improved reality testing (decreased or alleviated psychotic symptoms).	1a. Administer neuroleptics or antianxiety agents, and assess desired and adverse responses. 1b. Reduce environmental stimuli. 1c. Assess and support reality. 1d. Introduce self to Johnny, and state intentions in simple, short sentences. 1e. Assess nature of Johnny's hallucinations, delusions (verbal and nonverbal cues). 1f. Avoid laughing or whispering in front of Johnny.	1a. Administration of medication promotes reality testing and decreases agitation and level of dangerousness. 1b. Promotes reality testing and reduces agitation. 1c. Enables nurse to assess mental status and response to interventions. 1d. Promotes reality testing. 1e. Important to know what voices are saying to client and the effectiveness of interventions. 1f. These behaviors increase suspiciousness and distrust.	*Goal met:* Johnny's hallucinations and delusions are gradually reduced. Johnny demonstrates a calm mood and increased trust of the nurse.

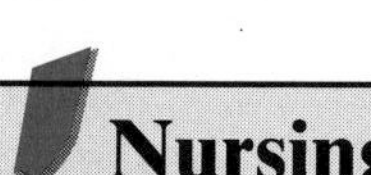

Nursing Care Plan 12–1 The Client with Schizophrenia (Johnny) (Continued)

OUTCOME IDENTIFICATION	NURSING ACTIONS	RATIONALES	EVALUATION
▶ Nursing Diagnosis: Self-Care Deficit			
1. By [date], Johnny participates in and initiates self-care activities.	1a. Assess self-care needs.	1a. To determine client's needs.	*Goal met:*
	1b. Assist Johnny in self-care activities.	1b. Promotes a sense of caring and concern.	Johnny increases self-care activities.
	1c. Encourage Johnny to participate in self-care as soon as possible.	1c. Encourages autonomy, self-worth, and confidence.	Johnny is able to socialize in one-to-one interactions but still has difficulty with group socializing.
	1d. Increase socialization and provide positive reinforcement for accomplishments	1d. Promotes a sense of mastery and reality testing.	Johnny initiates self-care activities prior to discharge.
▶ Nursing Diagnosis: Anxiety			
1. By [date], Johnny will display ability to concentrate and cope effectively with immediate environmental stimuli.	1a. Approach Johnny in a nonthreatening and calm manner.	1a–b. Reduces anxiety and increases calmness.	*Goal met:*
	1b. Listen to Johnny in an unhurried manner.		Johnny is able to handle anxiety more effectively.
	1c. Assist Johnny in identifying basis of stress.	1c. Enables and teaches sources of stress.	Antianxiety agents effectively reduce moderate to severe anxiety.
	1d. Administer antianxiety agents as needed.	1d. Decreases anxiety, agitation, and environmental stimuli.	Johnny participates in activities that reduce tension and anxiety.
	1e. Encourage participation in stress-reducing activities, such as exercise, reading, and listening to music.	1e. Promotes independence and reduces anxiety and stress.	There is a reduced need for antianxiety agents prior to discharge.
▶ Nursing Diagnosis: Knowledge Deficit related to lack of information about the illness			
1. By [date], Johnny will understand the nature of the illness and the need for active participation in comprehensive treatment planning.	1a. Throughout treatment, provide Johnny with information on symptom management.	1a. Encourages active participation in treatment process, and promotes mastery and competency.	*Goal met:*
			Johnny and his family are active participants in comprehensive treatment plan.
	1b. Provide information on how to cope with enduring symptoms of illness.	1b. Dealing with a chronic illness can be traumatic; adaptive coping skills are vital to this process.	Although Johnny is unsure of how his illness will affect his peer relationships, his family is very supportive and plans to participate in family support groups and followup with other community treatment for their son.
	1c. Provide information about medication (dosing, desired and adverse effects, side effects to report).	1c. Medication is a critical part of treatment. Encouraging active self-regulation increases independence and self-esteem.	

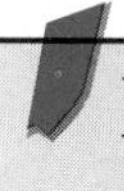

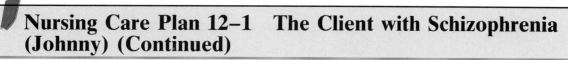

Nursing Care Plan 12–1 The Client with Schizophrenia (Johnny) (Continued)

OUTCOME IDENTIFICATION	NURSING ACTIONS	RATIONALES	EVALUATION
	1d. Provide information on community-based activities that enhance social, academic, and problem-solving skills.	1d. Increases independence and self-esteem.	
	1e. Counsel Johnny to avoid substance abuse.	1e. Increased awareness is associated with prevention.	
	1f. Educate Johnny about stress-reducing activities.	1f. Enhances coping skills and reduces tension/anxiety.	

The soaring cost of caring for the chronically mentally ill is being addressed in health care reforms. Efforts to identify high-risk populations, establish institutions of early interventions, and develop comprehensive health care are major endeavors of mental health professionals. Nurses play a pivotal role in treating clients with schizophrenia. Innovative strategies and collaboration with the client, families, and other mental health professionals are the basis of successful treatment modalities that promote health and minimize relapse.

Suggestions for Clinical Conferences

1. Present case histories of clients with psychotic symptoms.
2. Role-play an interview between a client with schizophrenia and the nurse.
3. Discuss the components of psychoeducation in the context of a case history.
4. Invite a nurse researcher to the class to discuss schizophrenia studies currently in progress and the role of nursing in those studies.
5. Discuss the biological and psychosocial factors associated with psychotic disorders using a typical case history.

References

Aguilera, D. C. (1990). *Crisis intervention: Theory and methodology* (6th ed). St. Louis: C. V. Mosby.

Aguilera, D. C. (1994). *Crisis intervention: Theory and methodology* (7th ed.). St. Louis: Mosby.

Allen, J. G. (1991). Development of schizophrenia. *Menninger Perspective, 22*(1), 9–13.

American Psychiatric Association. (1980). *Diagnostic and statistical manual of mental disorders* (3rd ed.). Washington, DC: Author.

American Psychiatric Association. (1987). *Diagnostic and statistical manual of mental disorder, 3rd edition, revised.* Washington, DC: Author.

American Psychiatric Association. (1994). *Diagnostic and statistical manual of mental disorders* (4th ed.). Washington, DC: Author.

Ananth, J., Vandewater, S., Kamal, M., Brodsky, A., Gamal, R., & Miller, M. (1989). Mixed diagnosis of substance abuse in psychiatric patients. *Hospital and Community Psychiatry, 40*, 297–299.

Anderson, L. T., Campbell, M., Adams, P., Small, A. M., Perry, R., & Shell, J. (1989). The effects of haloperidol on discrimination learning and behavioral symptoms in autistic children. *Journal of Autism and Developmental Disorders, 19*, 227–239.

Andreasen, N. C. (1986). Can schizophrenia be localized in the brain? Washington, DC: American Psychiatric Press.

Andreasen, N. C. (1990). *Schizophrenia: Positive and negative symptoms and syndromes*. Basel, Switzerland: Karger.

Andreasen, N. C. (1991). Assessment issues and the cost of schizophrenia. *Schizophrenia Bulletin, 17*, 475–481.

Andreasen, N. C., & Black, D. W. (1991). *Introductory textbook of psychiatry*. Washington, DC: American Psychiatric Press.

Antai-Otong, D. (1989). Concerns of the hospitalized and community psychiatric client. *Nursing Clinics of North America, 24*(3), 665–673.

Arieti, S. (1974). *Interpretation of schizophrenia* (2nd ed.). New York: Basic Books.

Asaad, G., & Shapiro, B. (1986). Hallucinations: Theoretical and clinical overview. *American Journal of Psychiatry, 143*(9), 1088–1097.

Bachrach, L. L. (1992). Psychosocial rehabilitation and psychiatry in the care of long-term patients. *American Journal of Psychiatry, 149*(11), 1455–1463.

Bateson, G., Jackson, D. D., Haley, J., & Weakland, J. H. (1956). Toward a theory of schizophrenia. *Behavioral Science, 1*, 251–264.

Bilder, R., Lipschultz-Brock, L., Reiter, G., Geisler, S. H., Mayerhoff, D. I., & Lieberman, J. A. (1992). Intellectual deficits in first-episode schizophrenia: Evidence for progressive deterioration. *Schizophrenia Bulletin, 18*(3), 437–448.

Blazer, D. (1980). The epidemiology of mental illness in late life. In E. W. Busse & D. G. Blazer (Eds.), *Handbook of geriatric psychiatry* (pp. 249–271). New York: Nostrand Reinhold.

Boker, W. (1992). A call for partnership between schizophrenic patients, relatives, and professionals. *British Journal of Psychiatry, 16*(Suppl.), 10–12.

Bowen, M. (1976). Family reaction to death. In P. J. Guerin (Ed.), *Family therapy: Theory and practice* (pp. 335–348). New York: Gardner Press.

Bower, K. (1992). *Case management by nurses*. Washington, DC: American Nurses Publishing

Bracha, H. S., Torrey, E. F., Gottesman, I. I., Bigelow, L. B., & Cuniff, C. (1992). Second-trimester markers of fetal size in schizophrenia: A study of monozygotic twins. *American Journal of Psychiatry, 149*(10), 1355–1361.

Breslin, A., (1992). Treatment of schizophrenia: Current and future promise. *Hospital and Community Psychiatry, 43*(9), 877–885.

Breier, A., Schreiber, J. L., Dyer, J., & Pickar, D. (1991). National Institute of Mental Health longitudinal study of chronic schizophrenia: Prognosis and predictors of outcome. *Archives of General Psychiatry, 48*(3), 239–246.

Breier, A., Schreiber, J. L., Dyer, J., & Pickan, D. (1992). Course of illness and predictors of outcomes in chronic schizophrenia: Implications for pathophysiology. *British Journal of Psychiatry, 161*(Suppl. 18), 38–43.

Bruton, C., Crow, T. J., Frith, C. D., Johnstone, E. C., Owens, D. G., & Roberts, G. W. (1990). Schizophrenia and the brain: A prospective clinico-neuropathological study. *Psychological Medicine, 20*, 285–304.

Buckley, W. (1967). *Sociology and modern systems theory*. Englewood Cliffs, NJ: Prentice-Hall.

Carpenter, W. T., & Strauss, J. S. (1991). The prediction of outcome in schizophrenia: IV. Eleven-year follow-up of the Washington IPPS cohort. *Journal of Nervous and Mental Disorders, 179*, 517–525.

Carpenter, W. T., Heinrichs, D. W., Wagman, A. M. (1988). Deficit and nondeficit forms of schizophrenia: The concept. *American Journal of Psychiatry, 145*, 660–669.

Campbell, R. J. (1958). The schizophrenias—current views: A report of Second International Congress for Psychiatry. *Psychiatric Quarterly, 32*, 318–334.

Ciompi, L. (1985). Aging and schizophrenia psychosis. *Acta Psychiatrica Scandinavica 71*(Suppl. 319), 93–105.

Ciompi, L. (1989). The dynamics of complex biological-psychological symptoms: Four fundamental psychobiological mediators in the long-term evolution of schizophrenia. *British Journal of Psychiatry, 155*(Suppl. 5), 15–21.

Clack, J. (1962). Nursing care of the disoriented patient: An interpersonal technique for handling hallucinations. In *Monograph of the American Nurses Association, 13*. Kansas City, MO: American Nurses Association.

Cloninger, C. R. (1989). Schizophrenia: Genetic etiological factors. In H. I. Kaplan & B. J. Sadock, (Eds.), *Comprehensive textbook of psychiatry* (Vol. 1, 5th ed., pp. 732–744). Baltimore: Williams & Wilkins.

Cohen, C. I., & Thompson, K. S. (1992). Homeless mentally ill or mentally ill homeless? *American Journal of Psychiatry, 149*(6), 816–823.

Cohen, L. J., Test, M. A., & Brown, R. L. (1990). Suicide and schizophrenia: Data from a prospective community treatment study. *American Journal of Psychiatry, 147*, 602–607.

Cook, E. H. (1990). Autism: Review of neurochemical investigation. *Synapse, 6*, 292–308.

Costa, P. (1992). A conversation with Philip Holzman. *Menninger Perspective, 23*(3), 19–23.

Courchesne, E., Yeung-Courchesne, R., Press, G. A., Hesselink, J. R., & Jernigan, T. L. (1988). Hypoplasia of cerebellar vermal lobules VI and VII in autism. *New England Journal of Medicine, 318*, 1349–1354.

Crow, T. J. (1990). Temporal lobe asymmetries as the key to the etiology of schizophrenia. *Schizophrenia Bulletin, 16*(3), 433–443.

Dixon, L., Haas, G., Weiden, P. J., Sweeney, J., & Frances, A. J. (1991). Drug abuse in schizophrenic patients: Clinical correlates and reasons for use. *American Journal of Psychiatry, 148*, 224–230.

Freud, S. (1950). Selected papers. In J. Strachey (Ed. and Trans.), *The standard edition of the complete psychological works of Sigmund Freud* (Vol. 3). London: Hogarth Press. (Original work published 1909)

Frith, C. D., & Done, D. J. (1988). Towards a neuropsychology of schizophrenia. *British Journal of Psychiatry, 153*, 437–443.

Goldberg, T. E., & Weinberger, D. R. (1988). Probing prefrontal function in schizophrenia with neuropsychological paradigms. *Schizophrenia Bulletin, 14*(2), 179–183.

Gottesman, I. (1991). *Schizophrenia genesis*. New York: W. H. Freeman.

Haas, G. L., & Sweeney, J. A. (1992). Premorbid and onset features of first-episode schizophrenia. *Schizophrenia Bulletin, 18*(3), 373–386.

Harding, C. M., Brooks, G. W., Ashikaga, T., Strauss, J. S., & Breier, A. (1987a). The Vermont longitudinal study of persons with severe mental illness: I. Methodology, study samples, and overall status 32 years later. *American Journal of Psychiatry, 144*(6), 718–726.

Harding, C. M., Brooks, G. W., Ashikaga, T., Strauss, J. S., & Breier, A. (1987b). The Vermont longitudinal study of persons with severe mental illness: II. Long-term outcome of subjects who retrospectively met the DSM III criteria for schizophrenia. *American Journal of Psychiatry, 144*(6), 727–735.

Hartfield, A. B., & Lefley, H. P. (1987). *Families of the mentally ill: Coping and adaptation*. New York: Guilford Press.

Hartfield, A. B., Spaniol, L., & Zipple, A. M. (1987). Expressed emotion: A family perspective. *Schizophrenia Bulletin, 13*(2), 221–226.

Heritch, A. J. (1990). Evidence for reduced and dysregulated turnover of dopamine in schizophrenia. *Schizophrenia Bulletin, 16*(4), 605–615.

Hill, R., & Hansen, D. A. (1964). Families under stress. In H. T. Christensen (Ed.), *Handbook of marriage and the family* (pp. 782–819). Chicago: Rand McNally.

Hogarty, G. E., Anderson, C. M., Reiss, D. J., Kornblith, S. J., Greenwald, D. P., Ulrich, R. F., & Carter, M. (1991). Family psychoeducation, social skills training, and maintenance chemotherapy in the aftercare treatment of schizophrenia. *Archives of General Psychiatry, 48*(4), 340–347.

Holzman, P., & Grinkler, R. (1977). Schizophrenia in adolescence. In S. Feinstein & P. Giovacchini (Eds.), *Adolescent psychiatry: Vol. 5. Developmental and clinical studies* (pp. 276–290). New York: Jason Aronson.

Hyland, P. A. (1990). *The stages family members experience while coping with mental illness of one of its members*. Presentation at a Family Enrichment Workshop, Menninger Clinic, Topeka, Kansas.

Institute of Medicine. (1989). *Research on children and adolescents with mental, behavioral, and developmental disorders: Mobilizing a national initiative*. Washington, DC: National Academy Press.

Jernigan, T. L., Zisook, S., Heaton, R. K., Moranville, J. T., Hesselink, J. R., & Braff, D. L. (1991). Magnetic resonance imaging abnormalities in lenticular nuclei and cerebral cortex in schizophrenia. *Archives of General Psychiatry, 48*(10), 881–890.

Kandel, E. R. (1991). Disorders of thought: Schizophrenia. In E. R. Kandel, J. Schwartz, & T. Jessell (Eds.), *Principles of neural science* (3rd ed., pp. 853–868). Norwalk: CT: Appleton & Lange.

Kandel, E. R., Schwartz, J. H., & Jessel, T. M. (1991). *Principles of neural science* (3rd ed.). Norwalk, CT: Appleton & Lange.

Kane, J. M. (1990). Treatment programme and long-term outcome of chronic schizophrenia. *Acta Psychiatrica Scandinavica, 82*(Suppl. 358), 151–157.

Kanner, L. (1943). Autistic disturbances of affective contact. *Nervous Child, 2*, 217–250.

Kanter, J., Lamb, H. R., & Loeper, C. (1987). Expressed emotion in families: A critical review. *Hospital and Community Psychiatry, 38*(4), 374–380.

Kaplan, H. I., & Sadock, B. J. (1989). *Comprehensive textbook of psychiatry* (Vol. 1, 5th ed.). Baltimore: Williams & Wilkins.

Kaplan, H. I., & Sadock, B. J. (1991). *Synopsis of psychiatry* (6th ed.). Baltimore: Williams & Wilkins.

Keefe, R. S., Mohs, R. C., Losonczy, M. F., Davidson, M., Silverman, J. M., Kendler, K. S., Horvath, T. B., Nora, R., & Davis, K. L. (1987). Characteristics of very poor outcome schizophrenia. *American Journal of Psychiatry, 144*(7), 889–895.

Keshavan, M. S., & Schooler, N. R. (1992). First-episode studies in schizophrenia: Criteria and characterization. *Schizophrenia Bulletin, 18*(3), 491–513.

Krauss, J. B. (1993). *Health care reform: Essential mental health services*. Washington, DC: American Nurses Publishing.

Lamb, H. R., Goldfinger, S. M., Greenfield, D., Minkoff, K., Nemiah, J. L., Schwab, J. J., et al. (1993). Ensuring services for persons with chronic mental illness under national health care reform. *Hospital and Community Psychiatry, 44*(6), 545–546.

Leff, J. P. (1987). A model of schizophrenia vulnerability environmental factors. In H. Hafner, W. F. Gattoz, & W. Janzarik (Eds.), *Search for the causes of schizophrenia* (pp. 317–330). Heidelberg: Springer-Verlag.

Leonard, B. E. (1992). *Fundamentals of psychopharmacology*. New York: John Wiley & Sons.

Lewis, M. (1989). Psychiatric examination of the infant, child, and adolescent. In H. I. Kaplan & B. J. Sadock (Eds.), *Comprehensive textbook of psychiatry* (Vol. 2, 5th ed., pp. 1716–1727). Baltimore: Williams & Wilkins.

Liberman, R. P. (1992). *Handbook of psychiatric rehabilitation*. New York: Macmillan.

Liberman, R. P., DeRisi, W. J., & Mueser, K. T. (1989). *Social skills training for psychiatric patients*. New York: Pergamon Press.

Lidz, T. (1973). The origin and treatment of schizophrenic disorders. New York: Basic Books.

Lieberman, J. A., Alvir, J. M., Woerner, M., DeGreef, G., Bilder, R. M., Ashtari, M., et al. (1992a). Prospective study of psychobiology in first-episode schizophrenia at Hillside Hospital. *Schizophrenia Bulletin, 18*(3), 351–371.

Lieberman, J. A., Bogerts, B., Degreef, G., Ashtari, M., Lantos, G., & Alvir, J. (1992b). Qualitative assessment of brain morphology in acute and chronic schizophrenia. *American Journal of Psychiatry, 149*(6), 784–794.

Losonczy, M., Davidson, M., & Davis, K. (1987). The dopamine hypothesis of schizophrenia. In H. Meltzer (Ed.), *Psychopharmacology: The third generation of progress* (pp. 715–726). New York: Raven Press.

Magliozzi, J. R., & Schaff, C. B. (1988). Psychosis. In J. P. Turpin, R. I. Shader, & D. S. Harnett (Eds.), *Handbook of clinical psychopharmacology* (2nd ed., pp. 1–48). Northvale, NJ: Jason Aronson.

Malone, J. (1990). Schizophrenia research update: Implications for nursing. *Journal of Psychosocial Nursing and Mental Health Services, 28*(8), 4–9, 31–32.

McCubbin, H. I. (1979). Integrating coping behavior in family stress theory. *Journal of Marriage and the Family, 41*, 237–244.

McGlashan, T. H. (1986). Schizophrenia: Psychosocial treatments and the role of psychosocial factors in its etiology and pathogenesis. In A. J. Frances & R. E. Hales (Eds.), *Psychiatric review* (pp. 96–111). Washington, DC: American Psychiatric Press.

McGlashan, T. H. (1988). A selective review of recent North American long-term follow-up studies of schizophrenia. *Schizophrenia Bulletin, 14*(4), 515–542.

McGlashan, T. H., & Nayfack, B. (1988). Psychotherapeutic models and the treatment of schizophrenia: The records of three successive psychotherapists with one patient at Chestnut Lodge for 18 years. *Psychiatry, 51*, 340–362.

Mednick, S. A., Machon, R. A., Huttunen, M. O., & Bonett, D. (1988). Adult schizophrenia following prenatal exposure to an influenza epidemic. *Archives of General Psychiatry, 45*(2), 189–192.

Meehl, P. E. (1962). Schizotaxia, schizotypy, schizophrenia. *American Psychologist, 17*, 827–838.

Merriam, A. E., Kay, S. R., Opler, L. A., Kushner, S. F., & van Praag, H. M. (1990). Neurological signs and the positive–negative dimension in schizophrenia. *Biological Psychiatry, 28*(3), 181–192.

Merriam, A. E., Medalia, A. A., & Wyszynski, B. (1993). Schizophrenia as a neurobehavioral disorder. *Psychiatric Annals, 23*(4), 171–178.

Miller, F., Dworkin, J., Ward, M., & Barone, D. (1990). A preliminary study of unresolved grief in families of seriously mentally ill patients. *Hospital and Community Psychiatry, 41*, 1321–1325.

Mishne, J. M. (1986). *Clinical work with adolescents*. New York: Free Press.

Moller, M. (1991). *Understanding relapse: Managing the symptoms of schizophrenia* [video]. Omaho, NE: NurSeminars, Inc.

Mueser, K. T., Yarnold, P. R., & Bellack, A. S. (1992). Diagnostic and demographic correlates of substance abuse in schizophrenia and major affective disorder. *Acta Psychiatrica Scandinavica, 85*, 48–55.

Mueser, K. T., Yarnold, P. R., Levinson, D. F., Singh, H., Bellack, A. S., Kee, K., Morrison, R. L., & Yadalam, K. G. (1990). Prevalence of substance abuse in schizophrenia: Demographic and clinical correlates. *Schizophrenia Bulletin, 16*, 31–56.

Muller, P., Bandelow, B., Gaebel, W., Kopche, W., Linden, M., Muller-Spahn, F., et al. (1992). Intermittent medication, coping, and psychotherapy. *British Journal of Psychiatry, 161*(Suppl. 18), 140–144.

Murray, R. M., & Harvey, I. (1989). The congenital origins of schizophrenia. *Psychiatric Annals, 19*(10), 525–529.

North, E. E., Jr. (1991). Psychiatry's unresolved riddle. *Menninger Perspective, 22*, 5–8.

Nuechterlein, K. H., Dawson, M. E., Gitlin, M., Venture, J., Goldstein, M. J., Snyder, K. S., et al. (1992). Developmental processes in schizophrenia disorders: Longitudinal studies of vulnerability and stress. *Schizophrenia Bulletin, 18*(3), 387–425.

Olson, D. H., Sprenkle, D. H., & Russell, C. S. (1979). Circumplex model of marital and family systems: I. Cohesion and adaptability dimensions, family types, and clinical applications. *Family Process, 18*(1), 3–28.

Payton, J. B., Steele, M. W., Wenger, S. L., & Minshaw, N. J. (1989). The fragile X marker and autism in perspective. *Journal of the American Academy of Child and Adolescent Psychiatry, 28*, 417–421.

Pearlson, C. G., Garbacz, D. J., Moberg, P. J., Ahn, H. S., & DePaulo, J. R. (1985). Symptomatic, familial, perinatal, and social correlates of computerized axial tomography (CAT) changes in schizophrenics and bipolars. *Journal of Nervous and Mental Disorders, 173*, 42–50.

Perry, K. (1983). *Family adaptability and emotional symptoms in bereaved parents following the sudden accidental death of a child.* Unpublished master's thesis, University of Kansas, School of Nursing, Kansas City.

Petty, L. K., Ornitz, E. M., Michelman, J. D., & Zimmerman, E. G. (1984). Autistic children who become schizophrenic. *Archives of General Psychiatry, 41*(1), 129–135.

Pfeffer, C. R. (1986). *The suicidal child*. New York: Guilford Press.

Piven, J., Berthier, M. L., Starkstein, S. E., Hehme, E., Pearlson, G., & Folstein, S. (1990). Magnetic resonance imaging evidence for defect of cerebral cortical development in autism. *American Journal of Psychiatry, 147*(6), 734–739.

Robins, L. N., Helzer, J. E., Weissman, M. M., Orvaschel, H., Gruenberg, E., Burke, J. D., Jr., & Regier, D. A. (1984). Lifetime prevalence of specific psychiatric disorders in three sites. *Archives of General Psychiatry, 41*, 949–958.

Rogers, S. J., & DiLalla, D. L. (1990). Age of symptom onset in young children with pervasive developmental disorders. *Journal of the American Academy of Child and Adolescent Psychiatry, 29*(6), 863–872.

Russell, A. T., Bott, L., & Sammons, C. (1989). The phenomenology of schizophrenia occurring in childhood. *Journal of the American Academy of Child and Adolescent Psychiatry, 28*(3), 399–407.

Safer, D. J. (1987). Substance abuse by young adult chronic patients. *Hospital and Community Psychiatry, 38*, 511–514.

Sarti, P., & Cournos, F. (1990). Medication and psychotherapy in the treatment of chronic schizophrenia. *Psychiatric Clinics of North America, 13*(2), 215–228.

Saykin, A. J., Gur, R. C., Gur, R. E., Mozley, P. D., Mozley, L. H., Resnick, S. M., Kester, D. B., & Stafiniak, P. (1991). Neuropsychological function in schizophrenia: Selective impairment in memory and learning. *Archives of General Psychiatry, 48*(7), 618–624.

Seeley, M. (1992). Menninger newsnotes for former patients and families, 2. Topeka, KS: Menningers.

Short, A. B., & Schopler, E. (1988). Factors relating to age of onset of autism. *Journal of Autism and Developmental Disorders, 18*, 207–216.

Spaniol, L., Zipple, A. M., & Lockwood, D. (1992). The role of family in psychiatric rehabilitation. *Schizophrenia Bulletin, 18*(3), 341–348.

Strauss, J. S. (1989). Mediating processes in schizophrenia: Towards a new dynamic psychiatry. *British Journal of Psychiatry, 155*(Suppl. 5), 22–28.

Thompson, L. W. (1990). The dopamine hypothesis of schizophrenia. *Perspectives in Psychiatric Care, 26*(3), 18–23.

Toenniessen, L. M., Casey, D. E., & McFarland, B. H. (1985). Tardive dyskinesia in the aged: Duration of treatment relationships. *Archives of General Psychiatry, 42*(3), 278–284.

Torrey, E. F. (1988). *Surviving schizophrenia: A family manual* (rev. ed.). New York: Harper & Row.

Vacarro, J., Cousino, I., & Vatcher, R. (1992). The growth of supported employment from horticulture therapy in the veterans' garden. In R. Linerman (Ed.), *Effective psychiatric rehabilitation: New directions for mental health services* (pp. 97–102). San Francisco: Jossey-Bass.

Vacarro, J. V., Young, A. S., & Glynn, S. (1993). Community-based care of individuals with schizophrenia. *Psychiatric Clinics of North America, 16*(2), 387–399.

Wahl, O. F., & Harmon, C. R. (1989). Family views of stigma. *Schizophrenia Bulletin, 15*(1), 131–139.

Walsh, M. (1985). *Schizophrenia: Straight talk for families and friends*. New York: Morrow.

Warren, R. P., Cole, P., Odell, J. D., Pingree, C. B., Warren, W. L., White, E., Yonk, J., & Singh, V. K. (1990). Detection of maternal antibodies in infantile autism. *Journal of the American Academy of Child and Adolescent Psychiatry, 29*(6), 873–877.

Watkins, J. M., Asarnow, R. F., & Tanguay, P. E. (1988). Symptom development in childhood-onset schizophrenia. *Journal of Child Psychological Psychiatry, 29*, 865–878.

Wise, C., & Stein, L. (1973). Dopamine-beta-hydroxylase deficiency in the brains of schizophrenic patients. *Science, 181*, 344–347.

Wynne, L., & Singer, M. (1963). Thought disorder and family relations of schizophrenics: I and II. *Archives of General Psychiatry 9*, 191–206.

Zipple, A. M., & Spaniol, L. (1987). *Families that include a mental illness: What they need and how to provide for it* [Trainer's Manual]. Boston: Center for Psychiatric Rehabilitation.

Zubin, J., Steinbauer, S. R., & Condray, R. (1992). Vulnerability to relapse in schizophrenia. *British Journal of Psychiatry, 161*(Suppl. 18), 13–18.

CHAPTER 13

Clients with Delirium, Dementia, Amnestic Disorders, and Other Cognitive Disorders

Jacqueline M. Stolley, M.A., R.N.,C.
Linda Garand, M.S., R.N.,C.S.
Christine McCormick Pries, M.A., A.R.N.P., C.S.
Kathleen C. Buckwalter, Ph.D., R.N.
Geri Richards Hall, M.A., A.R.N.P., C.S.

OUTLINE

CHAPTER OBJECTIVES

Upon completion of this chapter, you will be able to:

1. Explain the difference between cognitive disorders and inorganic mental syndromes and disorders.
2. Understand potentially reversible versus probable irreversible cognitive disorders.
3. Assess, plan, intervene, and evaluate care for persons with a cognitive disorder.
4. Explain the appropriateness of the use of medications to treat the symptoms of cognitive disorders.
5. Differential clients with an acute process from those with a chronic process.
6. Implement appropriate plans of care for clients with potentially reversible conditions and those with probable irreversible conditions.
7. Apply knowledge of both acute and chronic processes to the diagnosis and treatment of all persons who present with cognitive loss.

KEY TERMS

Alzheimer's disease
Asterixis
Astrocyte
Brain lesion
Chorea
Choreiform
Creutzfeldt-Jakob disease
Decerebrate
Decorticate
Delirium
Dementia
Focal neurological signs
Huntington's disease
Lewy bodies
Korsakoff's disease
Life expectancy
Life span
Myoclonus
Neuritic plaques
Neurofibrillary tangles
Normal pressure hydrocephalus
Parkinson's disease
Pick's disease
Potentially reversible disorders
Probable irreversible disorders
Pseudodementia
Status spongiosus
Vascular dementia

DEFINITIONS

In the third edition of the *Diagnostic and Statistical Manual of Mental Disorders* (DSM-III; American Psychiatric Association [APA], 1980), the essential feature of a mental disorder was "cognitive impairment." In the revised third edition (DSM-III-R), the essential feature of all organic mental disorders was "a psychological or behavioral abnormality associated with transient or permanent dysfunction in the brain" (APA, 1987, p. 98). The concept of organicity is no longer synonymous with the presence of cognitive impairment. In addition, in an attempt to take the emphasis off acute illness and cures in psychiatry, cognitive disorders are no longer divided into acute and chronic subtypes, because this division forced the classification of the client's condition as either reversible or irreversible. Throughout this chapter, the words *reversible* (acute) and *irreversible* (chronic) are used to indicate the foci of nursing interventions. When a client's condition is reversible, every effort is made to identify and treat the etiology, while nursing interventions are directed toward symptom management and promotion of safety. When a patient's condition is irreversible, nursing interventions are directed toward promotion of optimal functioning and adaptive responses to stress.

SYNDROME VERSUS DISORDER

Historically, the DSM-III-R distinguished between organic mental syndromes and organic mental disorders. "Organic mental syndrome" was used to refer to a constellation of psychological or behavioral signs and symptoms without reference to etiology (e.g., organic anxiety syndrome and dementia). "Organic mental disorder" designated a particular organic mental disorder in which the etiology is known or presumed (e.g., alcohol withdrawal delirium and vascular dementia). In the DSM-IV, the term *disorder* is used when an organic mental disorder is associated with an Axis III physical disorder or condition, as in organic delusional disorder due to a brain tumor. Because the etiology is identical with an Axis III physical disorder or condition, the term *disorder* is used in most cases in this chapter.

Organic mental disorders and syndromes were considered heterogeneous; no single description could characterize them all. The different clinical presentations of organic mental disorders and syndromes reflected differences in the localization, mode of onset, progression, duration, and nature of the underlying pathophysiological process.

COGNITIVE DISORDERS ARISING FROM GENERAL MEDICAL CONDITIONS VERSUS PSYCHIATRIC DISORDERS

The DSM-IV no longer refers to "organic mental syndromes" or "organic mental disorders." It focuses primarily on the degree of cognitive impairment and the underlying causes of the impairment, for example, substance abuse or degenerative changes such as those found in Alzheimer's disease (AD) and Huntington's disorders.

Cognitive disorders are categorized as either reversible and treatable or irreversible and untreatable. Examples of reversible cognitive disorders are delirium or dementia arising from substance abuse or from medical conditions such as hypoglycemia and hypoxia. Irreversible cognitive disorders include AD and Huntington's disease.

The DSM-IV omits the distinction between "organic" and "inorganic" mental disease because it suggests a mind–body duality. There is now a general consensus in modern psychiatry that for all major mental disorders, "there is not something biologically right" ("Medical News & Perspectives," 1993). In the DSM-IV, when a mental disorder is known to be due to physical causes, it is placed in the same category in which it is placed when it has no known medical etiology; for example, a mood disorder induced by substance abuse is listed as a mood disorder. Delirium, dementia, and amnestic disorders are categorized as "other cognitive disorders." Thus, cognitive disorders are conditions that are due to physiological processes, and the mind–body duality is lessened.

COMMON COGNITIVE DISORDERS

The most common cognitive disorders are delirium, dementia, intoxication, and withdrawal (APA, 1994). These disorders are highly variable; they differ from person to person and over time in the same person. In addition, more than one cognitive disorder may be present in a person simultaneously (e.g., delirium superimposed on dementia), and one organic mental disorder may succeed another (e.g., thiamine-deficiency delirium [Wernicke's encephalopathy] followed by alcohol amnestic disorder [Korsakoff's disease]).

NURSING IMPLICATIONS

The cognitive disorders are the only category of disorders in the DSM-IV for which the clinician must make an etiological diagnosis. A therapeutic consequence of this is that the clinician may overlook nonbiological factors contributing to illness, such as early life experiences, family history, medication history, and recent psychosocial stressors. The nurse who is devoted to the psychological, social, and spiritual, as well as the biological, care of clients must search for contributing factors to organic mental disorders in an effort to identify the full array of nursing interventions required.

COGNITIVE DISORDERS ACROSS THE LIFE SPAN

DEVELOPMENT OF THE BRAIN

Life begins as a single cell, but by the time of birth, billions of neurons in the brain are differentiated and ready for fine tuning. After birth, the most significant occurrences in the brain are growth in neuron size and axon length, and the development of efficient nerve conduction.

Although approximately 75 percent of brain growth (as shown by weight) occurs by the age of 2 years, the process of differentiation continues at a decelerating rate until adulthood, and axonal and dendritic growth continues until the onset of old age, or senescence (Carmichael, 1990). During intrauterine life, the developing brain is exquisitely sensitive to changes in the biochemical environment and the supply of essential nutrients, especially glucose and oxygen. Disruption of the supply of nutrients can result in temporary or permanent impairment. In addition, injury and localized brain disease can result in the direct loss of nervous tissue (Fig. 13–1). Obviously, if disruptions or insults occur early in fetal life, they often have catastrophic results, such as congenital malformations and severe mental retardation. The birth process itself can be a difficult transition with periods of anoxia (oxygen deficiency). The effects of anoxia are worse in premature newborns. Neurons do not multiply, and once injured, do not regenerate.

CHILDHOOD AND ADOLESCENCE

It is not the purpose of this chapter to review in detail all prevailing theories of growth and development in children and adolescents as they relate to cognitive disorders. Discussion within this chapter is limited to general concepts and principles that are germane to the understanding of the relationship between the brain and behavior that the psychiatric–mental health nurse must have. In addition, certain general issues must be remembered:

First, child and adolescent psychiatric–mental health nursing is concerned with *developing* behavior and biology. Although growth is a continuous process throughout the life span, it will never occur at this rapid rate again.

Second, there is still a wide gap between theory and practice and disagreement about how some theories should be applied. This often leads to polarized approaches to the same problem behavior.

Finally, it is not difficult to see that in some areas, such as etiological breakthroughs (such as genetic and pharmacological developments) that will affect clinical practice are imminent—the psychiatric nurse must stay

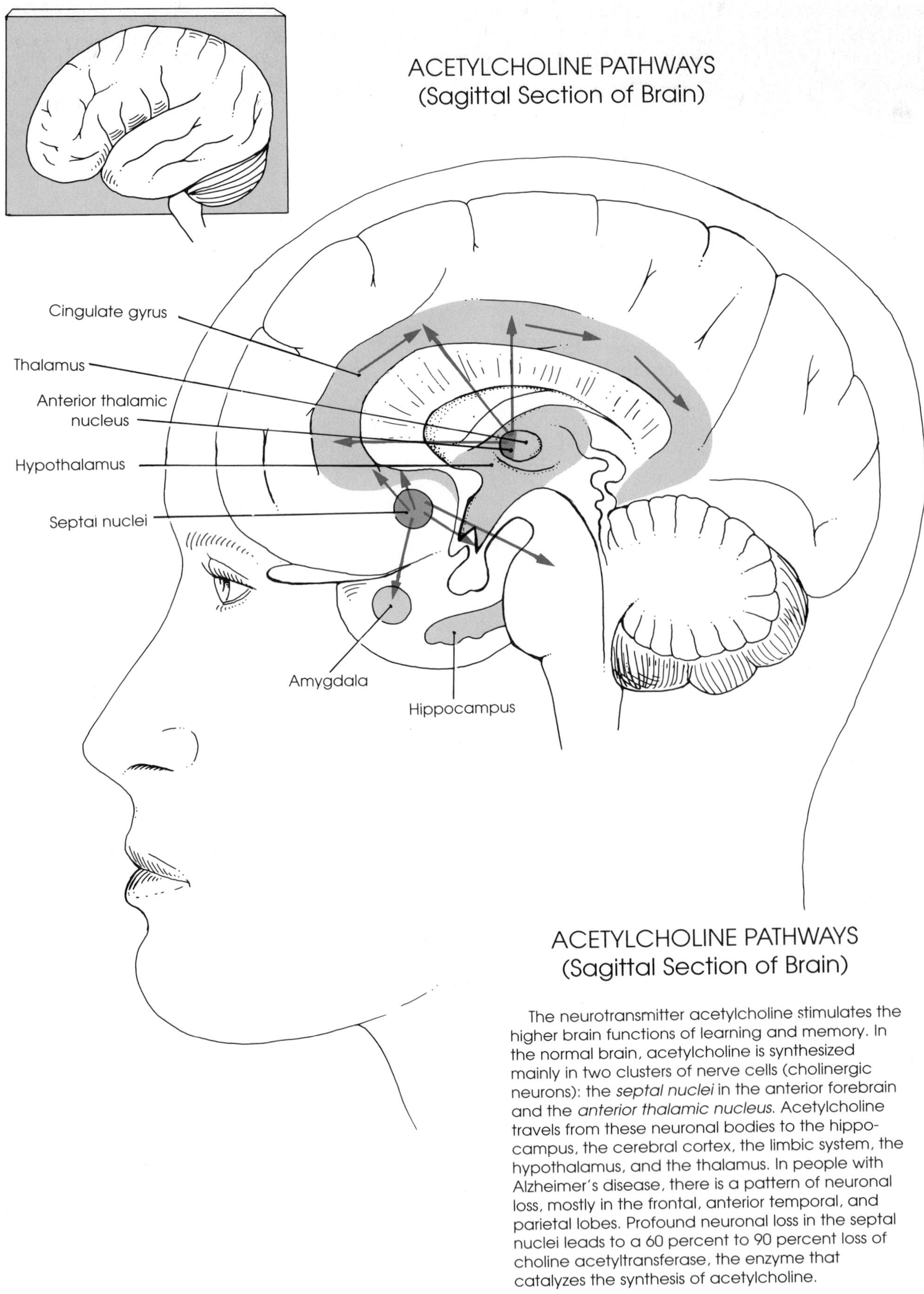

ACETYLCHOLINE PATHWAYS
(Sagittal Section of Brain)
Cingulate gyrus
Thalamus
Anterior thalamic nucleus
Hypothalamus
Septal nuclei
Amygdala
Hippocampus
ACETYLCHOLINE PATHWAYS
(Sagittal Section of Brain)
The neurotransmitter acetylcholine stimulates the higher brain functions of learning and memory. In the normal brain, acetylcholine is synthesized mainly in two clusters of nerve cells (cholinergic neurons): the *septal nuclei* in the anterior forebrain and the *anterior thalamic nucleus*. Acetylcholine travels from these neuronal bodies to the hippocampus, the cerebral cortex, the limbic system, the hypothalamus, and the thalamus. In people with Alzheimer's disease, there is a pattern of neuronal loss, mostly in the frontal, anterior temporal, and parietal lobes. Profound neuronal loss in the septal nuclei leads to a 60 percent to 90 percent loss of choline acetyltransferase, the enzyme that catalyzes the synthesis of acetylcholine.

FIGURE 13–1
The role of neuronal loss in cognitive disorders. (Illustration concept: Gail Kongable, M.S.N., C.N.R.N., C.C.R.N., Department of Neurosurgery, University of Virginia Health Sciences Center. Illustration by Marie T. Dauenheimer.)

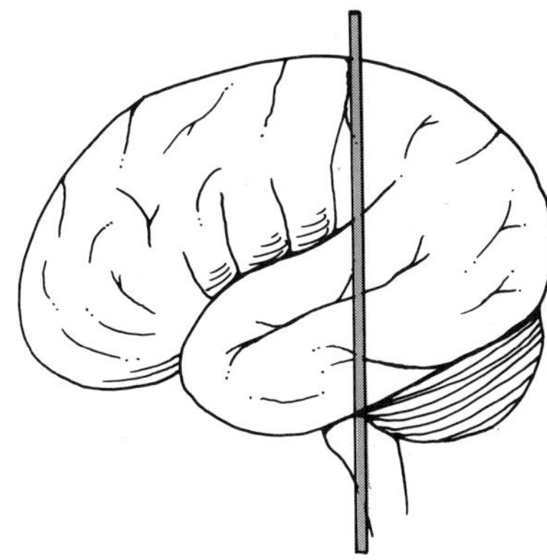

NEURONAL LOSS ACROSS THE LIFE SPAN (Coronal Section)

From fetal life through older adulthood, the brain is vulnerable to a number of physiological disruptions that can cause neuronal loss leading to cognitive disorders. Before birth, changes in the biochemical environment, including disruptions in the supply of essential nutrients, can cause neuronal loss that can result in mental retardation. Throughout life neuronal loss can occur from trauma, infection, endocrine and metabolic imbalances, various disease processes, environmental toxins, medications, and dietary insufficiency. Although reaching older adulthood is not a reason *per se* for intellectual decline, physiological changes that occur during aging can make the elderly more vulnerable to cognitive disorders.

White matter decay:
- Alzheimer's disease
- Creutzfeldt-Jakob disease
- Acquired immunodeficiency syndrome (AIDS)

Infectious agents

Cardiac causes:
- Atherosclerosis
- Hypertension
- Emboli/thrombi

Hypoxic injury:
- Epilepsy
- Ischemia due to low flow rate
- Near drowning

Global neuronal loss in all lobes due to aging

Abnormal cell growth (tumor)

Dietary insufficiency of essential vitamins, carbohydrates, protein, and minerals

Metabolic causes:
- Hypoglycemia
- Electrolyte imbalance

Trauma:
- Sheering of white matter/tracts

Cortical contusion

Medications to treat medical illnesses

Toxins:
- Alcohol
- Aluminum
- Lead
- Carbon monoxide

Endocrine causes:
- Hyper- or hypothyroidism
- Adrenocorticalism

Fetal and birth defects:
- Mental retardation
- Phenylketonuria (PKU)
- Down's syndrome
- Cerebral palsy

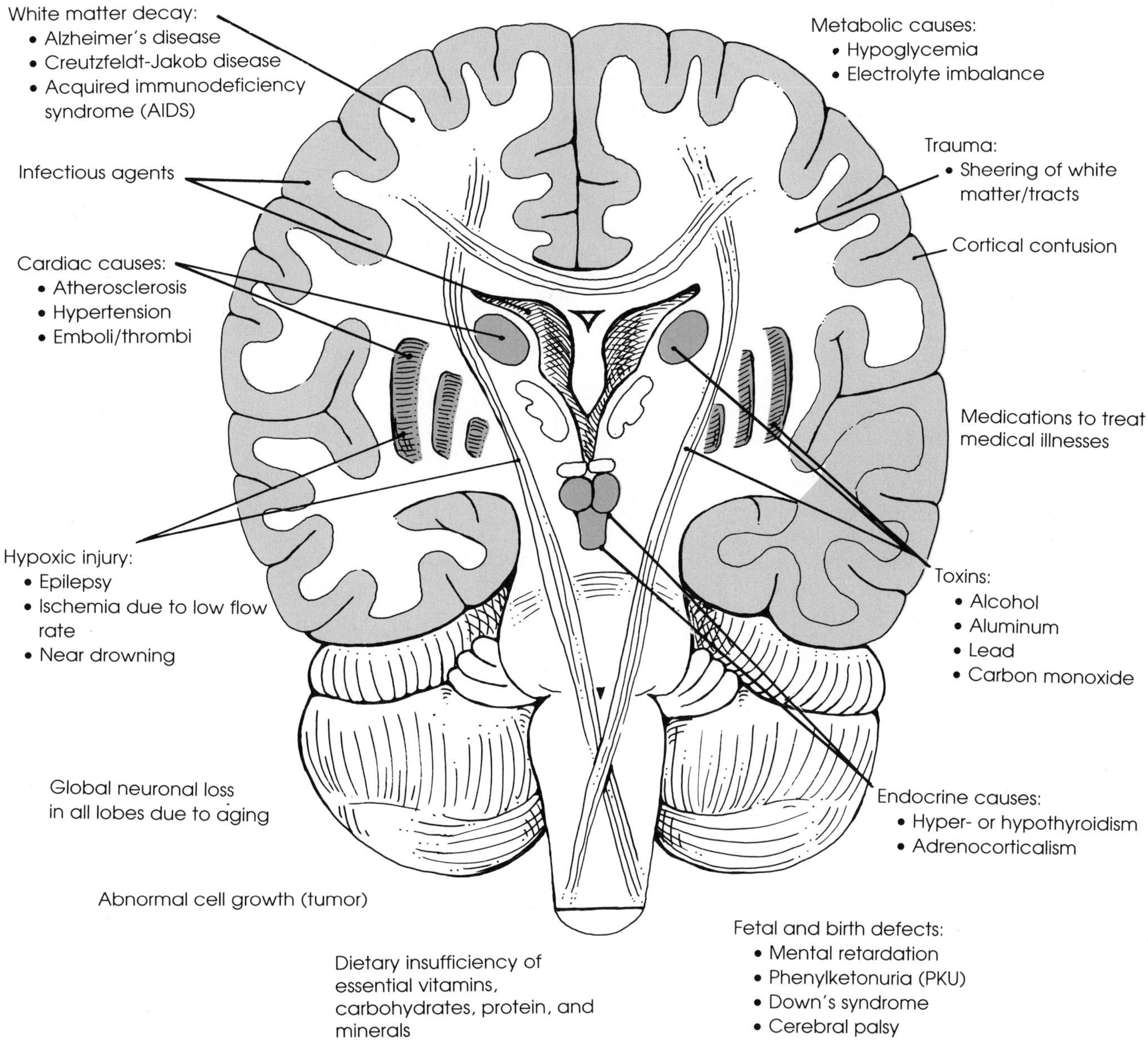

abreast of developing theories and research in these areas.

EARLY AND MIDDLE ADULTHOOD

Brain function is relatively stable throughout adulthood. Interruption of brain functioning through physiological processes (e.g., brain tumor) can occur. However, most cognitive disorders surface in older adulthood (60 years of age and older). There may be a gradual slowing of physiological functioning, and regeneration of tissues diminishes during middle and late middle adulthood. The primary physical changes during middle adulthood are in the reproductive system, in which reproductive organs atrophy.

OLDER ADULTHOOD

Gerontology is a relatively new field, having become the focus of research in only the last 15 years. The **life expectancy** at birth is now 75.5, compared with 47.3 in 1900, and it is projected to increase to 81.2 by 2080 (Greene et al., 1992). The reasons for the increase in life expectancy include better standards of living, a reduced death rate in children, control of infectious disease, and medical advances that are capable of extending the quantity and quality of life (Ferri, 1992; Greene et al., 1992).

Contrary to popular opinion, intellectual decline is not a normal part of aging. There are changes in reaction time and recall, slight changes in short-term memory, and an increased cautiousness that leads one to believe that the elderly person is unsure. However, there are increases in intelligence in normal elderly people that are not found in younger persons, and these are related to life experience and wisdom.

Physiological Changes. Many physiological changes occur in the elderly that can potentially affect memory function. There are also changes in the fat-to-lean body mass ratio and water balance that make medication prescription and maintenance of electrolyte balance challenging. Changes in liver and kidney function occur that can also affect these areas, and the nurse must keep them in mind when prescribing or administering medication for or diagnosing an elderly client who presents with "confusion."

Different species have different average life spans. Several physiological theories have been offered to explain human aging and the human **life span**, ranging from genetics, to biological clocks, to wear and tear. The physiological changes related to aging and the biological theories of aging are summarized in Tables 13–1 and 13–2.

Psychosocial Changes. Sociologists have presented several theories to explain human aging. These include the disengagement theory, activity theory, and continuity theory. Thus far, no theory of aging, whether biological or sociological, has been definitively proven.

As people age, they often experience psychosocial changes that affect their coping ability and general health. Losses that occur with aging and affect psychosocial activity include reductions in all five physical senses and loss of optimal body functioning. In addition, elders frequently experience the loss of a spouse, friends, siblings, occupation, home, and possibly children. These losses can present extraordinary burdens on the older person and must be kept in mind by the nurse caring for a geriatric client. Tables 13–3 and 13–4 summarize the psychosocial theories of aging and the life span. Textbooks on geriatrics or gerontology can provide in-depth information regarding these theories.

TABLE 13–1
Physiological Changes Associated with Age

	CHANGE NOTED	AGE SPAN (YEARS)
Total Body Water		
Men	Declines from 60% to 54%	20–80
Women	Declines from 54% to 46%	20–80
Muscle Mass	30% decrease	30–70
Taste Buds	70% decrease	30–70
Renal Perfusion	Reduced 50%	30–80
Brain Weight	Reduced 7%	20–80
Cardiac Reserve	Decreases from 4.6 to 3.3 times the resting cardiac output	25–70
Cerebral Blood Flow	Reduced 20%	30–70
Reproductive System	Menopause	50+
Liver	Loses mass	50+
Immune System	Declines	50+

TABLE 13–2
Biological Theories of Aging

FACTOR	HYPOTHESIS
Free-radical structure	Free radicals alter cellular structure; they are thought to be caused by environmental pollutants.
Cross-link of collagen	With age, collagen becomes more insoluble and rigid.
Cell programming	Biological clock triggers events (e.g., onset of puberty, menopause).
Autoimmune reactions	The body forms antibodies against itself. Autoimmunity plays a role in the development of infections, cancer, diabetes mellitus, atherosclerosis, hypertension, and rheumatic heart disease.
Lipofuscin	As age increases, the amount of accumulated lipofuscin also increases.
Somatic mutation	With age, defective cells multipiy and lead to organ abnormalities, and system dysfunction.
Stress	Wear and tear impairs the efficiency of cellular function, leading to physical decline.
Radiation	Exposure to ultraviolet light decreases life span.
Nutrition	The quality and quantity of diet is thought to influence life span.

TABLE 13–3
Psychosocial Theories of Aging

FACTOR	HYPOTHESIS
Disengagement (Cummings & Henry, 1961)	Aging individuals and society gradually withdraw from each other for mutual benefit. Theory's popularity was undermined by the recognition that each individual has a different aging pattern and the process often damages both society and the aged.
Activity (Havinghurst & Albrecht, 1953	Aging individuals should be expected to maintain norms of middle-aged adults, e.g., employment, activity, replacement of lost relationships. Universality of theory is reduced by fact that age-related physical, mental, and socioeconomic losses may present legitimate obstacles to maintaining activity.
Development/ continuity (Neugarten, 1968)	Basic personality, attitude, and behaviors remain constant throughout the life span. Theory allows multiple options for aging and recognizes the individuality of the aging process.

SPECIFIC COGNITIVE DISORDERS

Cognitive disorders are classified as potentially reversible or probable irreversible. Potentially reversible cognitive disorders are common and frequently unrecognized by health care professionals. If a potentially reversible condition is not recognized, however, the condition may develop into an irreversible condition and may even result in death.

TABLE 13–4 

Losses and Changes Across the Life Span

	AGE (YEARS)	TASK
Young Adulthood	20–28	Development of life dream Separation from nuclear family Erikson: intimacy vs. isolation
Adulthood	29–39	Changing commitments Childbearing and child rearing Self-identity Erikson: generativity vs. stagnation
Middle Adulthood	40–65 or 70	Reintegration of self-identity Launching of family Acceptance of physical aging Redefined attitudes about money, religion, and death Erikson: generativity vs. stagnation
Late Adulthood	65 or 70 to death	Capacity to feel whole in spite of diminishing health Adjustment to decreased physical strength and health, retirement, reduced income, and death of spouse Feeling of enduring significance Adjustment to and adoption of social roles Maintenance of maximum independence Erikson: ego integrity vs. despair

POTENTIALLY REVERSIBLE DISORDERS

It is important that a differential diagnosis be established for a client with cognitive impairment so that the appropriate treatment can be instituted. Similarly, the psychiatric nurse must remember that a potentially reversible disorder can be superimposed on a probable irreversible disorder, causing excess disability (Dawson et al., 1986). Excess disability can be defined as "a reversible deficit that is more disabling than the primary disability, existing when the magnitude of the disturbance in functioning is greater than might be accounted for by basic physical illness or cerebral pathology" (Dawson et al., 1986, p. 299). When the stressors that are causing excess disability are removed, cognitive and physical functioning may improve. If functioning does not improve, the client becomes more stressed, resulting in further disability and possibly death. The most common potentially reversible cognitive impairment is delirium.

Delirium

Delirium is a cognitive disorder characterized by acute onset and impairment in cognition, perception, and behavior (Beresin, 1988). The word *delirium* derives from the Latin words *de* (meaning "from or out of") and *lira* (meaning "furrow or track"). Thus, the word *delirium* implies a deviation from the usual state (Wells, 1985b).

Delirium is the most common cognitive disorder encountered by health care personnel. Wells (1985b) noted that 10 percent of all clients admitted to acute hospitals have delirium. He stated that the incidence of delirium would be even higher if every client admitted to a hospital were rigorously screened with repeated psychiatric evaluations. The incidence of delirium may be as high as 80 percent on acute geriatric hospital units (Wells, 1985b).

Lipowski (1980) described delirium as the most common and important form of psychopathology in later life. More than 20 terms have been used to describe delirium, including *organic brain syndrome*, *acute confusional state*, *acute brain failure*, and others. From a clinical standpoint, it is crucial that delirium be recognized and an etiological factor determined promptly. In the elderly, delirium is often the first sign of an underlying medical problem (e.g., acute infection, fecal impaction, or myocardial infarction) that may result in death if it is not diagnosed and properly treated (Rabins & Folstein, 1982).

The essential features of delirium are (1) reduced ability to maintain attention to external stimuli and to shift attention to new external stimuli and (2) disorganized thinking, as manifested by rambling, irrelevant, or incoherent speech. The disorder also presents with altered

DSM-IV DIAGNOSTIC CRITERIA FOR DELIRIUM DUE TO . . . [*Indicate the General Medical Condition**]

A. Disturbance of consciousness (i.e., reduced clarity of awareness of the environment) with reduced ability to focus, sustain, or shift attention.

B. A change in cognition (such as memory deficit, disorientation, language disturbance) or the development of a perceptual disturbance that is not better accounted for by a preexisting, established, or evolving dementia.

C. The disturbance develops over a short period of time (usually hours to days) and tends to fluctuate during the course of the day.

D. There is evidence from the history, physical examination, or laboratory findings that the disturbance is caused by the direct physiological consequences of a general medical condition.

*Associated General Medical Conditions: Etiological general medical conditions for delirium include systemic infections, metabolic disorders (e.g., hypoxia, hypercarbia, hypoglycemia), fluid or electrolyte imbalances, hepatic or renal disease, thiamine deficiency, postoperative states, hypertensive encephalopathy, postictal states, and sequelae of head trauma. Certain focal lesions of the right parietal lobe and inferomedial surface of the occipital lobe also may lead to a delirium.

Adapted from American Psychiatric Association. [1994]. *Diagnostic and statistical manual of mental disorders, fourth edition* (p. 129). Washington, DC: Author.

or clouded consciousness including sensory misperceptions (hallucinations, delusions, and/or illusions); disturbances in the sleep–wake cycle and level of psychomotor activity (agitation or stupor); disorientation to person, place, or time; and memory impairment. The onset of delirium is rapid, and the course typically fluctuates throughout the day and night. The duration is typically brief, and death may ensue if the underlying pathological processes are not resolved (APA, 1994).

Associated features of delirium include anxiety, fear, depression, irritability, anger, euphoria, and apathy. Emotional disturbances are common and quite variable. Some persons experience rapid and unpredictable changes from one emotional state to another. Fear is commonly experienced as a response to threatening hallucinations or delusions (APA, 1994). Delirium can occur at any age, but it is especially common in children and those over the age of 60.

Causative factors can be categorized into psychosocial influences and neurobiological factors. By definition, a biological stressor must be present for delirium to occur, but psychological or environmental factors are often involved. In one study (Purdie et al., 1981), 17 percent of reported cases of delirium were attributed to a change in the environment.

The neurobiological mechanisms underlying delirium remain a mystery. The organic causes of delirium are extensive and have been reviewed by Lipowski (1980) and Beresin (1988); a partial list is provided in Table 13–5. Delirium is often difficult to distinguish from other cognitive disorders and is frequently superimposed on a chronic dementing illness (e.g., AD). As a general rule, any rapid cognitive deterioration in a person known to have dementia is considered a delirium, unless proved otherwise, and necessitates a thorough search for causes (Beresin, 1985; Lipowski, 1980).

Wells (1985b) noted that the common feature in delirium is that it results from an abnormality of the nervous system at the level of cellular metabolism, although neurological signs are relatively uncommon. An important exception is the presence of abnormal movements. Both asterixis and multifocal myoclonus are abnormal movements largely limited to delirium. **Asterixis** is the inability of a person to maintain a fixed posture in space. Multifocal **myoclonus** is observed best while the client is at rest. It consists of quick, brief, irregular, asymmetrical contractions of muscles or groups of muscles. Although any area of the body may be involved, the muscles of the face and shoulders are usually affected. These contractions may or may not produce displacement of the body part, depending on the number and location of the muscles involved. Multifocal myoclonus is usually seen in the client with severe delirium (Wells, 1985b).

Autonomic signs—tachycardia, sweating, flushed face, dilated pupils, and elevated blood pressure—commonly occur in delirium. There may be a disruption of higher cortical functions, such as the inability to name objects (dysnomia) and inability to write (dysgraphia).

From the foregoing clinical features, it should be evident that, in severe delirium, nervous system metabolism is impaired at multiple levels—cerebral hemisphere, cerebellum, reticular activating system, peripheral nervous system, and autonomic nervous system (Wells, 1985b).

Brain tumors, subdural hematomas, strokes, transient ischemic attacks, and seizure disorders can all produce delirium. However, systemic causes of delirium are numerous. Cardiac disorders, including congestive heart failure, myocardial infarctions, arrhythmias, and postural hypotension (Beresin, 1986; Fine, 1978), contribute to reduced cerebral blood flow and neuronal hypoxia.

A fever not associated with an infection must be ruled out as an etiological factor for delirium in the elderly population. Also, any minor infections, such as a urinary tract infection, can dramatically worsen cognitive functioning in a client with a diagnosis of dementia (i.e., vascular dementia or Alzheimer's disease), because the delirium is superimposed on the symptoms of dementia.

TABLE 13–5
Medical Causes of Delirium

Intoxication
- Medications
  - Anticholinergics, tricyclic antidepressants, lithium, sedative-hypnotics, antihypertensive agents, antiarrhythmic drugs, Digitalis, anticonvulsants, antiparkinsonian agents, steroids and anti-inflammatory drugs, analgesics (opiates and nonnarcotic analgesics), disulfiram, antibiotics, antineoplastic drugs, and cimetidine
- Drugs of abuse
  - Alcohol, phencyclidine, and hallucinogenic agents
- Poisons
  - Heavy metals, organic solvents, methyl alcohol, ethylene glycol, insecticides, and carbon monoxide
- Withdrawal syndromes
  - Alcohol and sedative-hypnotics

Metabolic Causes
- Hypoxia
- Hypoglycemia
- Acid–base imbalance: acidosis or alkalosis
- Electrolyte imbalance: elevated or decreased sodium, potassium, calcium, or magnesium
- Water imbalance: dehydration, water intoxication, or inappropriate antidiuretic hormone
- Failure of vital organs: liver, kidney, or lung
- Inborn errors of metabolism: porphyria or Wilson's disease
- Remote effects of carcinoma, carcinoid syndrome
- Vitamin deficiency: thiamine (Wernicke's encephalopathy), nicotinic acid, or folate deficiency or cyanocobalamin

Endocrine Causes
- Thyroid: thyrotoxicosis and myxedema
- Parathyroid: hypoparathyroidism and hyperparathyroidism
- Adrenal: Addison's disease and Cushing's syndrome
- Pancreas: hyperinsulinism and diabetes
- Pituitary hypofunction

Cardiovascular Causes
- Congestive heart failure
- Cardiac arrhythmia
- Myocardial infarction

Neurologic Causes
- Head trauma
- Space-occupying lesions: tumor, subdural hematoma, abscess, and aneurysm
- Cerebrovascular disease: thrombosis, embolism, arteritis, hemorrhage, and hypertensive encephalopathy
- Degenerative disorders: Alzheimer's disease and multiple sclerosis
- Epilepsy

Infection
- Intracranial: encephalitis and meningitis (viral, bacterial, fungal, protozoal)
- Systemic: pneumonia, septicemia, subacute bacterial endocarditis, influenza, typhoid, typhus, infectious mononucleosis, infectious hepatitis, acute rheumatic fever, malaria, mumps, diphtheria, and acquired immune deficiency syndrome

Hematological Causes
- Pernicious anemia
- Bleeding diatheses
- Polycythemia

Hypersensitivity
- Serum sickness
- Food allergy

Physical Injury
- Heat: hyperthermia and hypothermia
- Electricity
- Burns

From Berensin, E. V. (1988). Delirium in the elderly. *Journal of Geriatric Psychiatry and Neurology, 1,* 132–133.

TABLE 13–6
Commonly Used Drugs Causing Delirium

GROUP	EXAMPLES
Analgesics	Opiates, salicylates
Antiarrhythmics	Lidocaine, procainamide
Antibiotics	Cephalexin, gentamicin, penicillin
Anticonvulsants	Phenytoin
Antihypertensives	Methyldopa
Anti-inflammatories	Indomethacin, steroids
Antineoplastics	5-fluorouracil, methotrexate
Antiparkinsonians	Levodopa, bromocriptine
Gastrointestinal	Cimetidine
Psychotropics	Antidepressants, barbiturates, benzodiazepines, lithium, neuroleptics
Sympathomimetics	Amphetamines, phenylephrine
Miscellaneous	Drug withdrawal (alcohol, barbiturates, benzodiazepines), bromides, disulfiram, timolol eyedrops, theophylline

Delirium is commonly caused by such systemic infections as pulmonary and urinary tract infections, cholecystitis, and diverticulitis (Beresin, 1986).

The elderly are very sensitive to drug-induced delirium. The major classes of medications that are associated with cognitive change in the elderly are listed in Table 13–6. Jenike (1989) noted that the low-potency antipsychotics (chlorpromazine and thioridazine) are much more likely than the high-potency antipsychotics (haloperidol, fluphenazine, and thiothixene) to cause delirium. Portnoi (1979) found 20 percent of the patients to have digitalis toxicity.

Many metabolic disorders can lead to delirium. Hypoxia from pulmonary, cardiovascular, and hematological disorders frequently presents as delirium (Beresin, 1988). Table 13–5 presents a partial list of the metabolic causes of delirium. Withdrawal disorders may contribute to episodes of delirium. When a person suddenly discontinues use of a sedative-hypnotic or alcohol, a withdrawal delirium can result.

The elderly may be intrinsically more vulnerable to delirium secondary to changes associated with normal aging, such as vision and hearing impairments, sensory deprivation, sleep deprivation, immobilization, metabolic changes, the presence of multiple medical conditions, and use of multiple medications. Age-related cell loss occurs in many brain centers, such as the hypothalamic nuclei, frontal cortex, hippocampus, and locus ceruleus (Jenike, 1989). This age-related cell loss, coupled with other age-related physiological changes, such as decreased acetylcholine synthesis, cerebral blood flow, and glucose metabolism, predisposes the vulnerable elderly to delirium.

Nursing Implications. Attention to the environment of the delirious client is important. The person's ability to respond appropriately to the environment can be influenced by even minor environmental manipulations such as using clocks, calendars, and night lights to improve orientation. Richeimer (1987, cited by Conn, 1991) described four types of interventions that may help the cognitively impaired delirious client:

- Clarification of perceptions
- Verification and validation of perceptions that are accurate
- Explanation of events and why they are difficult to understand
- Repetition of all important and helpful information

Further interventions that will reduce stress and support adaptive coping are (1) acknowledgment of feelings, (2) provision of a consistent routine (familiarity), (3) alleviation of isolation, (4) fostering of a sense of control, and (5) response to the client's need for hope as well as realistic information (Conn, 1991).

Jenike (1989) noted that delirium is most prevalent among clients on surgical and cardiac intensive care units and burn units, among clients undergoing open heart surgery, and among clients with multiple medical problems. The elderly and the very young are very susceptible to the development of delirium, and if they do develop delirium, it is a grave prognostic sign. Liston (1982) noted that in as many as 15 to 30 percent of cases of delirium, clients progress to stupor, coma, and death.

It is important to remember that common medical conditions in the elderly, such as fecal impaction or urinary retention, can have profound physiological and cognitive effects, such as delirium. It is also important to differentiate delirium from dementia, because the latter is not life threatening, and inappropriately labeling a delirious client as demented may delay the diagnosis of serious and treatable conditions. See Table 13–7 for a comparison of the symptoms of delirium and dementia. See also the DSM-IV Diagnostic Criteria displays for delirium and dementia.

TABLE 13–7
Comparison of the Symptoms of Delirium and Dementia

	DELIRIUM	DEMENTIA
Onset	Develops rapidly Precise time known	Gradual deterioration Uncertain date of onset
Course	Fluctuates sharply Nonprogressive	Fluctuates somewhat* Progressive loss of ability
Duration	Short	Present for many months/years
Mood (affect)	Fluctuates	Lability early; apathy late
Memory	Impaired memory for recent events	Impaired memory for recent events in early stages and remote events in later stages.
Consciousness	Clouded	Normal
Perception	Illusions common Visual hallucinations	Illusions possible Hallucinations possible
Thinking	Disordered Delusions possible	Disordered (progressive) Delusions common: simple to paranoid
Speech	Incoherent, rambling	Progressive loss of language
Sleep–Wake Cycle	Disturbed	May be disturbed*
Behavior	Agitated, restless Wandering possible Apathy possible	May be agitated* Wandering common Apathy common later
Mental Status	Poor performance—improves with recovery	Poor performance—consistent
Prognosis	Full recovery if treated	No return to previous level

*Most commonly the result of excess disability.
From Berensin, E. V. (1988). Delirium in the elderly. *Journal of Geriatric Psychiatry and Neurology, 1,* 138.

Mood Disorders Due to a General Medical Condition

Compared with delirium, other cognitive disorders occur much less frequently in children and adolescence and do not have as predictable a clinical course. These disorders are as follows:

Psychotic Disorder Due to a General Medical Condition with Delusions. This disorder is defined by the presence of predominant delusions that are due to a specific general medical condition. In children, this syndrome is usually seen after drug ingestion. In adults, drug ingestion and electrolyte imbalance are associated with this syndrome.

Psychotic Disorder Due to a General Medical Condition with Hallucinations. This disorder is characterized by the predominance of persistent or recurrent hallucinations that are due to a specific general medical condition (APA, 1994). In children and adolescents, this syndrome is usually precipitated by drug abuse or by an adverse reaction to medication.

Mood Disorder Due to a General Medical Condition. A predominant and persistent depressed, elevated, or expansive mood that is due to a specific physiological result of a general medical condition is characteristic of this disorder (APA, 1994). The most common causes include toxic or metabolic factors, endocrine disorders (hyperthyroidism or hypothyroidism and hyperadrenocorticalism or hypoadrenocorticalism), carcinomas, and viral illnesses. It is interesting to note that one of the earliest signs of pancreatic cancer is depression. For further discussion of depression, see Chapter 9.

Anxiety Disorder Due to a General Medical Condition. Prominent, recurrent, panic attacks or generalized anxiety caused by specific general medical conditions are characteristic of this anxiety disorder (APA, 1994). The most common etiological factors are intoxication from stimulants (caffeine, amphetamines, or cocaine) and endocrine disorders. See Chapter 10 for a discussion of anxiety.

Treatable Brain Lesions

Most **brain lesions** can be detected with computerized tomography (CT) or magnetic resonance imaging. Vascular occlusion and cerebral infarction, subarachnoid hemorrhage, and cerebral hemorrhage are acute lesions. Primary or metastatic brain tumors, subdural hematomas, or brain abscesses can also lead to delirium or confusional states, but they develop over a longer period of time. Rapid and careful differentiation is imperative, because the therapeutic approach to each of these lesions can differ.

The clinical picture is varied, and rapid changes are often seen. The most prominent manifestation is a clouding of consciousness, with an attendant disorientation to time, place, or person. Lesions are most common in elderly persons, particularly those with baseline cognitive impairment, but they can appear at any age. Except for meningiomas, primary brain tumors are less common in very old age than in earlier in life (Ham, 1992). Frontal lobe tumors may present a dementia-like picture. Personality and affect disturbances occur frequently, with symptoms of giddiness; irritability; inappropriate behavior; fearfulness; excessive energy; and possibly psychotic features, such as hallucinations or paranoia. Contradictory emotions are often displayed within a short time span. Disordered speech with prominent slurring is often observed, along with rapidity, neologisms, aphasic errors, or chaotic patterns.

Confusion regarding day-to-day events and daily routine, as well as roles, is common in persons with a brain lesion. Normal patterns of sleeping and eating are usually grossly distorted. Physical restlessness is often seen in the form of pacing, but apathy can also be a manifestation of acute processes. In fact, the severity and progression of each of these symptoms vary widely among clients and time periods. Family members and friends may report that the recent changes in behavior are alarming and out of character for the client. The time course for these changes is rarely more than hours or days, and they almost always precipitate a medical emergency.

Confusional states, which are milder cases of this cascade of symptoms, develop more slowly and persist for weeks or even months before being detected. The symptoms of confusional states may resemble those of delirium, but they may be less obvious and are less likely to require an emergency consultation.

Nursing Implications. Rapid evaluation of the client in a confusional state is imperative, because the underlying condition often changes acutely and is sometimes reversible. In the absence of a known cause, a thorough evaluation should include a detailed history (including information from as many relatives or caregivers as possible), physical examination, and mental status examination. Etiological diagnosis is based on the causes described earlier.

Many symptoms are treatable when the underlying cause is identified quickly and managed properly. Several general principles can assist management. Adequate fluids and nutrition must be administered. The environment should be as quiet and calm as possible; lighting should be low, with total darkness avoided. Staff and family members should offer reassurance as well as reinforce orientation and explain current proceedings at every opportunity. Because agitation can occur, clients must sometimes be treated symptomatically, especially when the well-being of the client, caregiver, or staff members is threatened. Additional drugs should be avoided unless they are relevant to the reversal of the underlying condition.

If the lesion is treatable, a neurosurgeon will perform a craniotomy to remove the lesion or create burr-holes to relieve pressure. Return of function may be slow or rapid, depending on the location and size of the lesion.

Elderly people are particularly susceptible to hematomas because the danger of falling increases with age (Stolley, 1992). Because the normal elderly person experiences some cerebral atrophy, the brain can shift inside the skull more easily, causing subarachnoid or subdural hematomas. Subarachnoid hematomas develop relatively quickly, but subdural hematomas may develop over a period as long as 3 months. The neurologist or neurosurgeon may elect to observe the client with a subdural hematoma, to determine if it will be resorbed by the body.

Normal Pressure Hydrocephalus

Chronic, communicating **normal pressure hydrocephalus** can cause an insidiously developing dementia in middle to late middle age. This condition is rare but potentially correctable, and it affects men more than women (Ham, 1992). Therefore, it must always be considered when dementia is suspected. Clients with dementia resulting from normal pressure hydrocephalus are slow and slovenly, in contrast to persons with AD, who are alert. Unsteady, slow, and shuffling gait and episodes of urinary incontinence are common. Gait changes include difficulty initiating the gait and reduced step height. This results in a type of shuffling in which the feet appear to be stuck to the floor. It is important to remember that the triad of shuffling gait, mental impairment, and incontinence is a hallmark of this disease, but gait impairments may occur in the absence of incontinence or mental changes. Pathogenesis is based on an impeded cerebrospinal fluid (CSF) circulation and absorption. There may have been a previous attack of meningitis, encephalitis, or head injury, and a few patients have tumors, particularly of the midbrain. CT scans show large dilated ventricles with little or no cortical atrophy. The CSF pressure is normal or high normal. Some improvement may follow the introduction of a ventriculoatrial shunt, especially when gait disorders precede or outweigh mental decline. Thus, this disorder is considered potentially reversible, but untreated, it may become irreversible.

Pseudodementia

Pseudodementia refers to severe depression that may be misdiagnosed as dementia, hence, the term *pseudo*, meaning "false." Because of poor concentration, the client appears to have short-term memory loss. However, with careful examination, a differential diagnosis can be made. The onset of dementia is usually gradual, with the client attempting to hide memory losses and remain independent. With depression, the change in behavior may be more abrupt, with the client's major complaint being memory loss and prior history of depression, despondency, and somatic complaints. Dependency is more apparent in depression than in dementia (Ronsman, 1988). Differentiating characteristics of depression and dementia are presented in Chapter 9.

PROBABLE IRREVERSIBLE DISORDERS

There are more than 70 different kinds of irreversible dementia that occur in the middle and late years (Blass, 1982; Katzman, 1986). **Dementia** is a global impairment of cognitive functioning, memory, and personality that occurs without a disturbance in consciousness or level of alertness. Unlike mental retardation, which is usually congenital, dementias are acquired. Although dementia is found predominantly in the elderly, some neuropsychiatric disorders (epilepsy, brain tumors, traumatic head injury, and acquired immunodeficiency syndrome [AIDS]) may cause dementia in childhood and adolescence. Other irreversible cognitive disorders are included in this section.

The diagnosis of dementia may be made at any time after the IQ is fairly stable, usually by age 3 or 4 (APA, 1994). It is important for the psychiatric nurse to remember that the onset, course, and clinical management of dementia in children, adolescents, and adults depend heavily on the underlying etiology.

The most common probable untreatable disorders seen in children are mental retardation, attention deficit hyperactivity disorder (ADHD), and epilepsy.

At 60 percent of cases of dementia, AD is the most prevalent form of dementia in adults, followed by vascular dementia (10 percent); mixed AD and vascular dementia (17 percent); and rare disorders (13 percent) of adults and children, some of which are discussed briefly in this section. Because mental retardation and AD are the most common of the irreversible cognitive disorders, this section focuses on these four diseases.

Mental Retardation

Significantly subaverage intellectual functioning that originates during the developmental period and is accompanied by deficits in adaptive functioning is defined as *mental retardation* (Grossman, 1973). The etiology of mental retardation is often unknown, but causes of mental retardation are categorized as either genetic or acquired. Table 13–8 summarizes the causes of mental retardation.

TABLE 13–8
Causes of Mental Retardation

GENETIC
Down's syndrome
Klinefelter's syndrome
Phenylketonuria
Hypothyroidism
Tay-Sachs disease
ACQUIRED
Rubella and prenatal viruses
Toxins
Placental insufficiency
Blood type incompatability
Anoxia
Birth injury
Prematurity
Infection—meningitis, encephalitis
Poisons—lead, medicine
Poor nutrition
Central nervous system insult
Sociocultural factors, such as extreme and prolonged physical and emotional deprivation

Standardized IQ tests are used to determine mental retardation. The person whose performance on these tests is similar to that of others of the same age is considered to have average intelligence (a score of 100). The IQ score expresses the relationship of mental age to chronological age. The basic formula is as follows:

$$\frac{\text{Mental age}}{\text{Chronological age}} \times 100 = \text{IQ}$$

The specific IQ cutoff point used to define mental retardation is 70. Mental retardation is divided into four broad categories: mild (IQ = 50 to 70), moderate (IQ = 35 to 50), severe (IQ = 20 to 35), and profound (IQ = below 20). The person with mild retardation is educable.

The long-term outcome of mental retardation is variable. People with severe or profound mental retardation often experience progressive deterioration and premature death, as early as the teens or early 20s. Many persons with moderate retardation also experience a somewhat reduced life expectancy (Andreasen & Black, 1991). Typically, mentally retarded children progress through the same sequence of developmental milestones that nonretarded children do, but they do so at a slower rate.

Nursing Implications. The differential diagnosis of mental retardation is important, but it is complex because of the frequent comorbidity of other childhood disorders. Differential diagnosis includes ADHD, academic skills disorder, autism, and childhood psychosis. The psychiatric nurse must also remember that seizure disorders are common in children with mental retardation.

The Epilepsies

Epilepsy is a condition characterized by sudden, recurrent, and transient disturbances of mental functioning or body movements that result from excessive discharging of groups of brain cells (Forster & Booker, 1988). On the basis of this definition, the psychiatric nurse should recognize that epilepsy is not a specific disease, but rather comprises a group of symptoms that have different causes in different people.

Grand Mal Seizures. A grand mal seizure is a tonic–clonic attack with a loss of consciousness. It is the most common form of generalized seizures. Many persons who experience grand mal seizures feel vague warning symptoms before a seizure, including a sense of discomfort; anxiety; mood changes; or physical discomfort such as headache, upset stomach, sweating, or a change in body temperature. An aura often immediately precedes a full-blown seizure. Dizziness, fainting, and sensory phenomena (lights, dots, sounds, odors, and tastes) are the more frequent kinds of auras.

The tonic phase is a dramatic stiffening of the muscles throughout the body. The head and neck are thrown back, the back is arched, and the extremities are in maximum extension. Respiration is halted, sometimes for as long as a minute, and the individual may appear cyanotic. Often, the force of the seizure and the rigid body position place the person at risk for injury. Repetitive jerking of all body muscles indicates the beginning of the clonic phase of the seizure. The person may bite his or her tongue or lose bladder and bowel control. The clonic phase ends with the person appearing to be in a deep coma, with the eyes turned upward and pupils dilated and nonreactive to light.

A postictal phase follows. The person awakens from the seizure dazed and sometimes confused. Amnesia for the seizure, headache, and sleepiness are common occurrences, which diminish over the following 1 to 4 hours.

Petit Mal Seizures. The petit mal seizure is common and often begins in childhood. There are three types of petit mal seizures: (1) a brief lapse of consciousness for 15 to 30 seconds, with very little twitching, a blank stare, and amnesia for the seizure; (2) a similar lapse of consciousness, with some twitches; and (3) sudden loss of muscle tone and consciousness.

The term *psychomotor epilepsy* is often used to refer to epileptic disturbances of the temporal lobe. The term is used very broadly and refers to increased tonicity of the muscles and movements of the head and neck and gulping or swallowing movements. There may be automatic or fixed behaviors (*automatisms*) of various degrees of complexity, such as buttoning/unbuttoning movements, endless talking, and hyperreligiosity.

Psychic Seizures. Psychic seizures, as the name implies, consist of perceptual or affective symptoms. These may include cognitive alterations such as flashbacks or déjà vu experiences, depersonalization, and derealization. The diagnosis is confirmed with clinical data and electroencephalogram results.

Focal Discharge Seizures. Focal discharge seizures are classified according to the location of the seizure. Usually, consciousness is not impaired. These seizures may present motor, sensory, or autonomic symptoms.

Causative Factors. The causes of the epilepsies are still unknown, but current research is investigating the importance of perinatal factors, trauma, nutrition, stress, stimulation, and genetic factors.

Attention Deficit Hyperactivity Disorder

ADHD is characterized by developmentally inappropriate degrees of inattention, impulsiveness, and hyperactivity (APA, 1994; see accompanying display). People with this disorder generally display some disturbance in each of these areas but to varying degrees.

ADHD has held the attention of researchers and clinicians for 30 years and is currently one of the most studied and controversial syndromes in child psychiatry. Although children, adolescents, and adults experiencing ADHD vary significantly in their clinical presentation, there is general agreement among practitioners that the following are the core difficulties of the syndrome:

- Restlessness or excessive activity
- Poor sustained attention
- Impulsiveness
- Difficulty getting along with others; noncompliance
- Underachievement
- Coexisting difficulties
- Poor self-esteem, secondary to the foregoing (Weiss, 1991)

Differential Diagnosis. The differential diagnosis of ADHD depends on accurate, descriptive information gathered from a history, a school report, behavior observations, and interviews with parents and teachers. Sometimes, parents and teachers are unsure of the level of activity appropriate for a particular age and confuse activity or energetic behavior with ADHD. The restlessness in ADHD takes the form of not only overactivity, but also activity off task that is often disruptive to those in the vicinity. Disorders often confused with ADHD include conduct disorder, adjustment disorder, anxiety disorders, and some behaviors associated with medication use (e.g., theophyllin).

Causative Factors. The definitive etiology of ADHD is unknown, and data suggest no single etiological factor. If there is a uniform central nervous system (CNS) dysfunction, its nature has not yet been determined. The expression of the syndrome, however, can be seen as difficulty regulating focal, sensory, social, motor, behavioral, and affective controls (Levine, 1987).

Genetic influences have been postulated as an etiological factor. One study suggests that a significant minority of fathers of ADHD children (without comorbidity) experience the same syndrome of ADHD currently or experienced it in their childhood (August & Stewart, 1983).

Lead poisoning in early childhood can produce behavior and cognitive disorders similar to ADHD symptoms in some children (Weiss, 1991). Diet, food additives, dyes, and sugars have been blamed by many laypersons, including parents of ADHD children, as a cause of the behaviors associated with this syndrome. In general, results from carefully controlled studies do not support this hypothesis, with the exception of one study, in which a small minority of hyperactive preschool children reacted with negative behaviors to food additives (Weiss, 1991).

Psychosocial factors continue to be examined in the study of ADHD. The association of family stress and economic factors cannot be underrated. Children who have a vulnerability to ADHD and experience the stresses of family disharmony, single parenting, blended families, the full-time employment of both parents, or

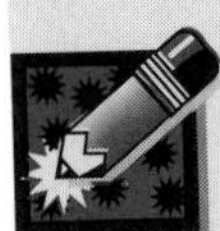

DSM-IV DIAGNOSTIC CRITERIA FOR ATTENTION DEFICIT/HYPERACTIVITY DISORDER

A. Either (1) or (2):

(1) six (or more) of the following symptoms of **inattention** have persisted for at least 6 months to a degree that is maladaptive and inconsistent with developmental level:

Inattention

(a) often fails to give close attention to details or makes careless mistakes in schoolwork, work, or other activities
(b) often has difficulty sustaining attention in tasks or play activities
(c) often does not seem to listen when spoken to directly
(d) often does not follow through on instructions and fails to finish schoolwork, chores, or duties in the workplace (not due to oppositional behavior or failure to understand instructions)
(e) often has difficulty organizing tasks and activities
(f) often avoids, dislikes, or is reluctant to engage in tasks that require sustained mental effort (such as schoolwork or homework)
(g) often loses things necessary for tasks or activities (e.g., toys, school assignments, pencils, books, or tools)
(h) is often easily distracted by extraneous stimuli
(i) is often forgetful in daily activities

(2) six (or more) of the following symptoms of **hyperactivity-impulsivity** have persisted for at least 6 months to a degree that is maladaptive and inconsistent with developmental level:

Hyperactivity

(a) often fidgets with hands or feet or squirms in seat
(b) often leaves seat in classroom or in other situations in which remaining seated is expected
(c) often runs about or climbs excessively in situations in which it is inappropriate (in adolescents or adults, may be limited to subjective feelings of restlessness)
(d) often has difficulty playing or engaging in leisure activities quietly
(e) is often "on the go" or often acts as if "driven by a motor"
(f) often talks excessively

Impulsivity

(g) often blurts out answers before questions have been completed
(h) often has difficulty awaiting turn
(i) often interrupts or intrudes on others (e.g., butts into conversations or games)

B. Some hyperactive-impulsive or inattentive symptoms that caused impairment were present before age 7 years.

C. Some impairment from the symptoms is present in two or more settings (e.g., at school [or work] and at home).

D. There must be clear evidence of clinically significant impairment in social, academic, or occupational functioning.

E. The symptoms do not occur exclusively during the course of a Pervasive Developmental Disorder, Schizophrenia, or other Psychotic Disorder and are not better accounted for by another mental disorder (e.g., Mood Disorder, Anxiety Disorder, Dissociative Disorder, or a Personality Disorder).

From American Psychiatric Association. (1994). *Diagnostic and statistical manual of mental disorders, fourth edition.* (pp. 83–85). Washington, DC: Author.

the forced unemployment of either parent often find themselves emotionally unsupported.

Alzheimer's Disease

Alois Alzheimer first documented the neuropathology of **Alzheimer's disease** in 1907, describing **neurofibrillary tangles** and **neuritic plaques** in the brain of a 55-year-old woman (Fig. 13–2). This neurological disorder occurs primarily in middle or late life, but it may occur earlier, depending on the cause. Several causes have been postulated, but except for the genetic causes of some types of AD, no definitive cause has been found. AD is characterized by progressive loss of memory, especially short-term memory; language impairments; poor impulse control; and poor judgment. The course of the disease lasts anywhere from 2 to 20 years, with 10 years being the average. Experts have staged the disease in three stages (Matteson, 1988), four stages (Hall & Buckwalter, 1987), and seven stages (Reisburg et al., 1982). In this chapter, the four-stage measurement is used.

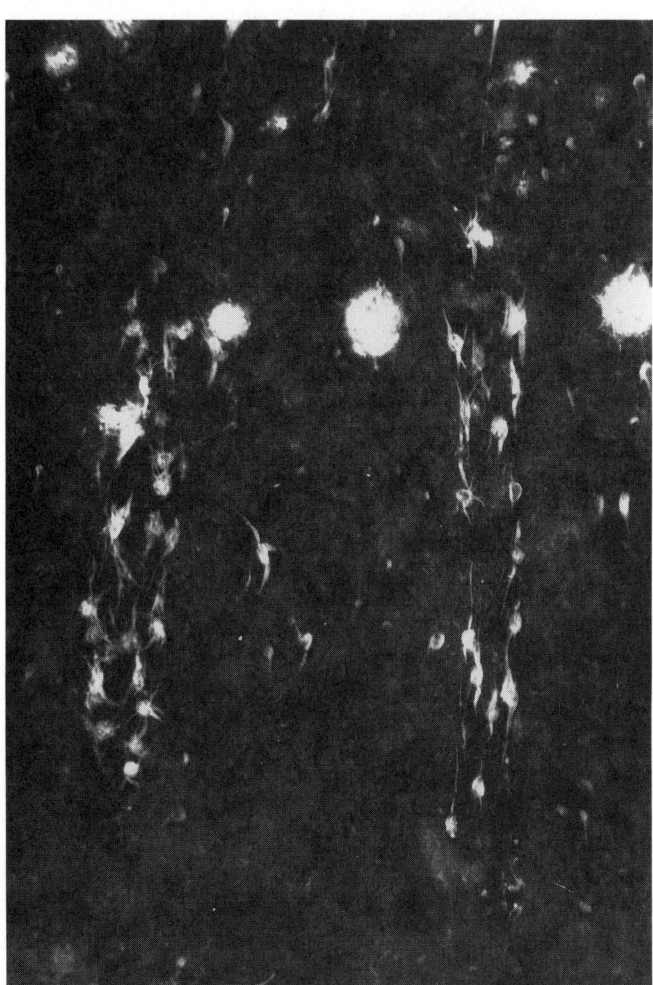

FIGURE 13–2
Photomicrograph of thioflavine S–stained neurofibrillar tangles and neuritic plaques from the cerebral cortex of a patient with Alzheimer's disease. The circular areas are abnormal neuritic plaques; the elongated areas are tangles, which are also abnormal. (Courtesy of Gary W. Von Hoesen, University of Iowa, Iowa City, IA.)

TABLE 13–9
Stages of Alzheimer's Disease

FORGETFULNESS
1. Short-term memory loss is experienced: Client misplaces, forgets, loses things
2. Client compensates with memory aides: lists, routine, organization
3. Client expresses awareness of problem; is concerned about abilities
4. Client may become depressed; makes symptoms worse
5. Illness is not diagnosable at this stage
CONFUSION
1. Memory decline progresses, interfering with all abilities: short-term memory is most impaired; long-term memory follows later
2. Client is disoriented for time, place, person, thing
3. Instrumental activities of daily living: deficits in money management, legal affairs, transportation difficulties, housekeeping, cooking
4. Denial is common, but client hints at fear of losing his or her mind
5. Depression is more common; client is aware of deficits and is frightened
6. Confabulation and stereotyped words are used to cover up for memory losses
7. More problems occur when client is stressed, fatigued, out of own environment, ill
8. Day care and in-home assistance are commonly needed
AMBULATORY DEMENTIA
1. Functional losses occur in activities of daily living (in approximate order): willingness and ability to bathe, grooming, choosing among clothing, dressing, gait and mobility, toileting, communication, reading, and writing skills
2. Client loses ability to reason, to plan for safety, and to communicate verbally
3. Frustration is common
4. Client becomes more withdrawn and self-absorbed
5. Depression resolves, as client's awareness of memory loss and disability decreases
6. Client becomes less accessible to others—is unable to retain information or use past experiences to guide his or her behavior
7. Communication becomes more and more difficult; language is lost
8. There is behavioral evidence of reduced stress threshold: client is up at night, wandering, pacing; is confused, agitated, belligerent, combative, withdrawn
9. Institutional care is usually needed
ENDSTAGE
1. Client doesn't recognize family members or even own image in a mirror
2. Client can no longer walk; there is little purposeful activity
3. Client is often mute but may yell or scream spontaneously
4. Client forgets how to eat, to swallow, and to chew; weight loss is common, and client may become emaciated
5. Problems associated with immobility arise: pneumonia, pressure ulcers, urinary tract infections, and contractures
6. Incontinence is common; client may have seizures
7. Client is most certainly institutionalized at this point

The four stages of AD and the symptoms associated with each are listed in Table 13–9. The DSM-IV diagnostic criteria for dementia of the Alzheimer's type are provided in the accompanying display.

Causative Factors. Presenile dementia is thought to be caused by a genetic error. Researchers have identified genes on the 14th, 19th, and 21st chromosomes. The

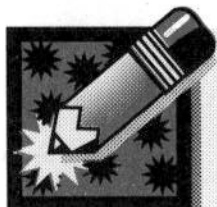

DSM-IV DIAGNOSTIC CRITERIA FOR DEMENTIA OF THE ALZHEIMER'S TYPE

A. The development of multiple cognitive deficits manifested by both
(1) memory impairment (impaired ability to learn new information or to recall previously learned information)
(2) one (or more) of the following cognitive disturbances:
(a) aphasia (language disturbance)
(b) apraxia (impaired ability to carry out motor activities despite intact motor function)
(c) agnosia (failure to recognize or identify objects despite intact sensory function)
(d) disturbance in executive functioning (i.e., planning, organizing, sequencing, abstracting)

B. The cognitive deficits in Criteria A1 and A2 each cause significant impairment in social or occupational functioning and represent a significant decline from a previous level of functioning.

C. The course is characterized by gradual onset and continuing cognitive decline.

D. The cognitive deficits in Criteria A1 and A2 are not due to any of the following:
(1) other central nervous system conditions that cause progressive deficits in memory and cognition (e.g., cerebrovascular disease, Parkinson's disease, Huntington's disease, subdural hematoma, normal-pressure hydrocephalus, brain tumor)
(2) systemic conditions that are known to cause dementia (e.g., hypothyroidism, vitamin B_{12} or folic acid deficiency, niacin deficiency, hypercalcemia, neurosyphilis, HIV infection)
(3) substance-induced conditions

E. The deficits do not occur exclusively during the course of a delirium.

F. The disturbance is not better accounted for by another Axis I disorder (e.g., Major Depressive Disorder, Schizophrenia).

From American Psychiatric Association. (1994) *Diagnostic and statistical manual of mental disorders, fourth edition.* (pp. 142–143.) Washington, DC: Author.

specific factor noted on the 19th chromosome is the ApoE gene, implicated in late-onset AD. It is speculated that ApoE-ε4 places persons at risk for developing AD (Strittmatter et al., 1993). It is interesting to note that the genetic anomaly associated with Down's syndrome is located on the 21st chromosome and persons with Down's syndrome who survive to age 40 almost always develop symptoms of AD. Early-onset familial AD is associated with an anomaly on the 14th chromosome, discovered in 1992 (Mullan et al., 1992; Schellenberg et al., 1992; St. George-Hyslop et al., 1992; Van Broeckhoven et al., 1992). Late-onset familial AD is associated with chromosome 19 (Mahley, 1988; Pericak-Vance et al., 1991; Strittmatter et al., 1993). Persons with AD who have at least one other relative affected are categorized as having familial AD. Clients with AD and no known family history for it are classified as having sporadic AD.

The slow-virus theory has also been offered to explain the cause of AD. Three degenerative diseases of the CNS—kuru, Creutzfeldt-Jacob disease (CJD), and Gerstmann's syndrome—have been transmitted to animals. These findings indicate a possible infectious agent. The incubation period is roughly one fourth of the affected person's normal life span; hence the label "slow-virus" (Prusiner, 1984; Wurtman, 1985). However, attempts to transmit AD have been unsuccessful for three reasons:

1. The infectious agent does not replicate in animals.
2. The agent is not transmissible to animals within the incubation times studied.
3. The infectious agent is not involved in the pathogenesis of AD.

Aluminum has also been considered as a causative factor in the development of AD. Injection of aluminum salts can generate neurofibrillary tangles in the brains of certain animals (Deary & Whalley, 1988; Terry & Pena, 1965). Aluminum has also been known to accumulate in the neurofibrillary tangles of persons with AD. Still, these findings are inconclusive. It is unclear whether the association is causative or a result of brain damage. It is postulated that although aluminum itself may not cause AD, its presence may contribute to the development of the disease in people with a predisposition to it.

A clear biochemical abnormality was discovered to be associated with AD in 1976. The level of this chemical, choline acetyltransferase, was reduced 90 percent in the hippocampus and cerebral cortex of AD clients (see Fig. 13–1). Choline acetyltransferase is a catalyst for the neurotransmitter acetylcholine, which is responsible for the functioning of the hippocampus, which is paramount in the formation of memory. Other neurotransmitters, such as norepinephrine, serotonin, and somatostatin, have been found to be deficient in the brains of persons with AD. Attempts to treat clients with purified lecithin, a precurser of acetylcholine, have thus far been unsuccessful (Wurtman, 1985), but the drug tacrine (tacrine hydrochloride or Cognex) has shown promise in slowing the progression of the disease (Farlow et al., 1992; Small, 1992). Tacrine has recently been recommended for approval by the Food and Drug Administration for the treatment of AD.

Abnormal protein structures are clearly associated with AD, leading to an autoimmunity theory. Genetic studies suggest that some persons carry an increased liability for selective degeneration of chromosomes, with the result that in later life, regulation of vital substances such as protein in brain cells may fail (Wurtman, 1985).

Researchers have investigated the relationship between trauma and the development of dementia (French et al., 1985; Heyman et al., 1984; Mortimer et al., 1985). Boxers develop a form of dementia known as *dementia pugilistica*, and researchers have reported a higher incidence of AD in persons with a history of head trauma resulting in loss of consciousness. It is possible that the trauma may cause microscopic damage to the blood–brain barrier, leaving the person vulnerable to penetration by either a slow virus or environmental toxins. Further study is needed to determine whether trauma with loss of consciousness is related to the development of AD.

Symptoms. Although the symptoms of AD are usually categorized by stages, the course of the disease is insidious, with one stage running into another. Progression is gradual, and staging is done for the benefit of professionals caring for or researching persons with AD. Table 13–9 lists symptoms associated with the four stages of AD.

Losses are associated with AD. These losses include cognitive (intellectual) losses, affective (personality) losses, and conative (planning) losses. By reviewing the behaviors associated with each state, the psychiatric nurse can determine the progression of the disease. In addition to these three clusters of loss, Hall and Buckwalter (1987) have postulated a fourth cluster of losses, the progressive inability to handle stress. On the basis of her theoretical framework and research, Hall has developed a conceptual model for the care of persons with AD and related dementias (including those discussed in the following sections), termed the *progressively lowered stress threshold* (PLST) model of care. This model of care is incorporated into the nursing process section of this chapter and can usually be used for irreversible dementias of all types, excluding Pick's disease and Korsakoff's disease.

Hall and Buckwalter (1987) postulated that persons with AD have three possible behavioral responses: baseline, anxious, and dysfunctional.

Baseline. Baseline behaviors include a basic awareness of the environment and the ability to interact and function, limited only by the amount of neurological deficits. The client remains cognitively and socially accessible and can communicate and respond.

Anxious. When the client becomes anxious, he or she is beginning to feel stress. The client may complain of feeling uneasy. Eye contact is poor or absent, and an increase in psychomotor activity may appear in response to noxious stimuli. However, the client remains intact.

Dysfunctional. If stress continues or increases, the client becomes dysfunctional. He or she becomes catastrophic and cognitively and socially inaccessible. Communication is impaired, and the person is unable to interpret environmental stimuli appropriately. The person may actively avoid what he or she perceives as noxious stimuli and become fearful and panic stricken. The result is increased confusion, purposeful wandering, night awakening, "sundowner's syndrome" (increased confusion and agitation during the late afternoon or early evening), agitation, fearfulness, panic, combativeness, and sudden withdrawal. The person may experience these symptoms at times early in the disease, but with disease progression they increase in frequency and intensity.

Nursing Implications. Five factors can contribute to anxious and dysfunctional behavior in the client with AD. The purpose of nursing intervention is to control these factors and provide a safe environment. The five factors are as follows:

1. Fatigue
2. Change in routine, caregiver, or environment
3. Multiple competing stimuli
4. Demands to achieve beyond capabilities
5. Physiological causes such as elimination problems (urinary retention or constipation), pain, infection, medication, and electrolyte imbalances (see discussion of delirium)

The assumptions underlying the PLST model were derived from psychological theories of coping and adaptation. In addition, concepts of rhythmicity and self-esteem were incorporated. These assumptions are basic principles of nursing care for all clients and should be applied in the care of all demented patients. They are as follows:

- All people require some control over their person and their environment and need some degree of unconditional positive regard.
- All behavior is rooted and has meaning; therefore, all catastrophic and stress-related behaviors have a cause.
- The confused or agitated client is not comfortable and should be regarded as frightened. All clients have the right to be comfortable.
- The client exists in a 24-hour continuum. Care cannot be planned or evaluated on an 8-hour shift basis. If the client has a problem during the night, some changes need to be implemented during the day (Hall & Buckwalter, 1987).

The accompanying Research Study display demonstrates that quality of life can be improved for AD clients using the PLST model.

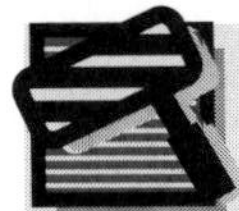

RESEARCH STUDY

Sheltered Freedom: An Alzheimer's Unit in an ICF

Hall, G. R., Kirschling, M., & Todd, S. (1986). *Geriatric Nursing, 7*(3), 132–136.

Study Problem/Purpose

The purpose of this study was to test the progressively lowered stress threshold (PLST) model in a dedicated Alzheimer's unit.

Hall (1986) reported developing an 18-bed special care Alzheimer's unit in which the PLST model of care was used. The unit controlled for fatigue by keeping activity periods short, providing rest periods twice daily, and limiting caffeine. Changes in unit routines were minimal. Careful attention was paid to reducing noise levels and group sizes and limiting residents' exposure to misleading stimuli, such as television. Residents ate in small groups at tables in the bedrooms. Staff and family were trained to provide positive communications and avoid testing residents' knowledge. Nursing staff performed physical assessments and urine cultures when unrelenting dysfunctional behavior occurred. The responses of 11 residents, 2 men and 9 women, were studied over a 9-month period. They had a mean Global Deterioration Scale (GDS) score of 5.27 at the outset of the study. (The GDS was developed by Reisberg et al., 1982, to assess the stages of cognitive decline. A score of 1 indicates normal cognitive ability, and a score of 7 indicates severe decline.)

Findings

Results included stabilization of residents' weights, although no dietary supplements were used, and gradual decline in residents' ability to perform all activities of daily living except eating. Dramatic increases were found in eating abilities during the first 6 months of the study. However, these reverted in the last 3 months. Night wakening was virtually eliminated, and there were increases in socialization among residents. Use of mood-controlling medications was significantly reduced over the course of the study. Wandering and assaultive behaviors were rare in the facility, but they occurred with even less frequency on the special care unit.

Implications

This study showed that the PLST model of care for persons with cognitive deficits can significantly improve the quality of these persons' lives. In addition, the structure provided helps eliminate catastrophic behaviors and the need for psychoactive medications. Study of environmental manipulation to promote quality of life for demented individuals will lead to important nursing interventions for persons with dementia.

Brief descriptions of other probable irreversible dementias follow. Many of the symptoms are similar to those of AD, with variations as delineated. It should be kept in mind that persons who suffer from dementia are individuals and that the disease presentation is as heterogeneous as the population it affects.

Vascular Dementia

Vascular dementia is a dementia that results from vascular diseases that cause multiple small or large cerebral infarcts. The onset is generally acute, and, unlike AD, the stages are clear-cut or stepwise, with obvious decline associated with each infarct. The client may have a history of transient ischemic attacks, hypertension, strokes, diabetes mellitus, vasculitis, and cardiac arrhythmias. A family history of stroke or cardiovascular disease is common (Read & Jarvik, 1984).

The person with vascular dementia may have more language difficulties than the person with AD, as well as **focal neurological signs** and symptoms, such as speech difficulty or weakness or paralysis of one limb. Emotional lability, depression, and crying spells are frequently observed. Other deficits may include dysarthria (difficulty with speech due to motor deficits), hemineglect (denial of one side of the body), movement disorders, and a subtle paresis (partial paralysis) (see the accompanying display on DSM-IV diagnostic criteria). The course of the disease is fluctuating and intermittent. Delirium may occur with each infarct, clearing with time, with no return to preinfarct cognitive functioning. Some persons with vascular dementia may benefit from anticoagulation therapy and treatment of underlying disease, especially hypertension, which is the most important risk factor.

Pick's Disease (Lobar Atrophy)

Pick's disease is a rare form of presenile dementia that affects women more often than men and most frequently occurs in middle adult life. Cerebral atrophy, particularly of the frontal and temporal lobes, characterizes this degenerative disease. In the atrophied areas, Pick's bodies—swollen, abnormal, and balloon-like neurons—are seen. The ventricles are also enlarged (Adams & Victor, 1985).

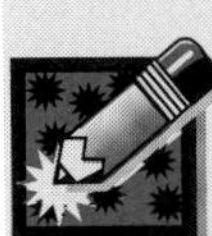

DSM-IV DIAGNOSTIC CRITERIA FOR VASCULAR DEMENTIA

A. The development of multiple cognitive deficits manifested by both
- (1) memory impairment (impaired ability to learn new information or to recall previously learned information)
- (2) one (or more) of the following cognitive disturbances:
  - (a) aphasia (language disturbance)
  - (b) apraxia (impaired ability to carry out motor activities despite intact motor function)
  - (c) agnosia (failure to recognize or identify objects despite intact sensory function)
  - (d) disturbance in executive functioning (i.e., planning, organizing, sequencing, abstracting)

B. The cognitive deficits in Criteria A1 and A2 each cause significant impairment in social or occupational functioning and represent a significant decline from a previous level of functioning.

C. Focal neurological signs and symptoms (e.g., exaggeration of deep tendon reflexes, extensor plantar response, pseudobulbar palsy, gait abnormalities, weakness of an extremity) or laboratory evidence indicative of cerebrovascular disease (e.g., multiple infarctions involving cortex and underlying white matter) that are judged to be etiologically related to the disturbance.

D. The deficits do not occur exclusively during the course of a delirium.

From American Psychiatric Association. (1994). *Diagnostic and statistical manual of mental disorders, fourth edition.* (p. 146). Washington, DC: Author.

The symptoms of Pick's disease may be similar to those of AD, but focal signs are more common and may involve frontal, temporal, or parietal lobes. Unlike AD, behavioral and personality changes precede memory deficits. Dysphasia occurs early in the disease, progressing to muteness. Agnosia (loss of comprehension of sensations with intact sensory sphere) and apraxia (inability to perform purposeful movement) commonly occur if the parietal lobe is involved. Disturbances in gait occur late in the course of the disease, which can last from 2 to 10 years. The etiology of Pick's disease is unknown, but genetic factors are suspected.

Huntington's Disease

Huntington's disease (HD) is characterized by intellectual deterioration, and advanced HD results in impairment of memory, intelligence, and verbal fluency. In the early stages, deficits in learning ability are apparent but verbal fluency is only mildly impaired. Intelligence is within the normal range. Memory is more impaired in recognition than in recall tasks. Impairment in long-term memory is also present. Impairments are also seen in visuospatial capacity, along with personal orientation in space. The classic presentation is general **chorea** (well-coordinated jerky movements), with the intensity of the chorea correlating with the severity of the cognitive deficits. Mild **choreiform** movements are present in the earlier stages, but their severity increases as the disease progresses. The absence of rapid eye movements is the most striking of oculomotor disturbances. HD is genetically transmitted, and genetic counseling of carriers is imperative.

Creutzfeldt-Jakob Disease

Creutzfeldt-Jakob disease is a rare form of presenile dementia. It is a progressive, fatal disease of the CNS that usually begins in late life, after age 50. The disease has been observed in younger persons, however. CJD evolves rapidly, with death occurring within 2 years, although the course of the disease may be longer.

CJD is characterized by loss of neurons in all lobes and the cerebellum, along with a proliferation of hypertrophied **astrocytes.** The brain takes on a sponge-like appearance, which is termed ***status spongiosus*** (Adams & Victor, 1985).

Mental deterioration begins early in CJD and presents as memory loss, behavioral abnormalities, and higher cortical dysfunction (aphasia, apraxia, and agnosia). Myoclonus (shocklike contractions of muscle) develops early in the course of the disease. Sensory stimuli such as loud noises, flashing lights, or movement or touch can produce myoclonus. Visual disturbances, headache, vertigo, and dizziness are common.

The disease progresses rapidly; changes can be noted on a daily basis. With progression of the illness, the person becomes bedridden, mute, and unable to move voluntarily. **Decerebrate** or **decorticate** posturing and rigidity are common in the later stages (Brown et al., 1979), and the person eventually lapses into a coma.

CJD is thought to be caused by a specific virus that is highly resistant to destruction (Roos et al., 1973). The source of the pathogen are blood, CSF, and CNS tissue (Tateishi, 1985). The nurse should follow the Centers for Disease Control and Prevention universal precautions when caring for a person with CJD to prevent exposure to blood, CSF, tissues, or urine. A family history of CJD has been observed in about 10 percent of cases (Wells, 1985a).

Acquired Immunodeficiency Syndrome

AIDS is one of the most serious health problems confronting society today. The human immunodeficiency virus (HIV) is the infecting organism. More than 100,000 persons have died from the disease, and it is estimated that more than 1 million people are infected with HIV. It is among the five leading causes of death for women ages 25 to 44 and is the third leading cause of death for men in that age group (Chu et al., 1990; Osborn, 1990). About 10 percent of persons with AIDS are over age 50.

AIDS transmission is caused by homosexual or heterosexual contact, sharing of needles, or blood transfusion. AIDS dementia complex is frequently misdiagnosed as AD. AIDS dementia complex is a subcortical dementia in which the HIV virus begins to infect the CNS but overt signs of dementia are not observed. Before clinical symptoms occur, cerebral atrophy may be seen on the CT scan. Early symptoms include gradual cognitive impairment, forgetfulness, difficulty with concentration, flat affect, poor insight, and indifference. These symptoms may lead to functional disabilities. Balance problems and leg weakness may occur. Behavioral changes vary and are unresponsive to antidepressant medications. There may be verbal and motor slowing, as well as gait ataxia and hyperreflexia. Later symptoms frequently include a spontaneous tremor or myoclonus, paraparesis, urinary and fecal incontinence, and mutism (Scharnhorst, 1992).

It is estimated that 40 to 70 percent of AIDS clients will develop a discernible neurological syndrome during the course of their illness. In about 10 percent of all HIV-positive persons, the presenting symptom is neurological impairment (Detwiler, 1989). Because the disease is spread through body fluids, psychiatric nurses caring for persons infected with the HIV must use universal precautions to prevent transmission to themselves.

Korsakoff's Disease (Alcohol Amnestic Disorder)

Dementia caused by chronic alcoholism is called **Korsakoff's disease**. In Korsakoff's disease, recent memory is impaired. The person fails to learn and remember new information but can retrieve and use previously acquired knowledge. The person is frequently able to learn and perform complex motor skills but is unable to recall the context in which they were learned (Tariot & Weingartner, 1986). People with Korsakoff's disease frequently lack motivation or initiative and appear apathetic. CNS functions other than memory are usually normal (Sagar & Sullivan, 1988).

Parkinson's Disease and Diffuse Lewy Body Disease

Approximately 20 to 30 percent of patients with **Parkinson's disease** (PD) show clinical evidence of dementia (Sagar & Sullivan, 1988). Like AD, cognitive changes frequently start as mild, insignificant memory lapses. Over time, several intellectual functions become impaired and performance of activities of daily living declines. Unfortunately, some of the drugs used to treat PD can cause confusion, delusions, or hallucinations.

Not all PD clients develop dementia. Old age seems to be a risk factor; older PD clients are significantly more likely than younger ones to develop dementia. It has been theorized that people with PD dementia actually suffer from AD as well. However, studies of the pathology in the brains of persons with PD have shown degenerative changes different from those seen in AD. These changes include loss of a small number of neurons in the brain stem. The remaining cells in the brain stem contain unique deposits, called **Lewy bodies**. The brains of some persons with PD dementia contain neurofibrillary tangles and neuritic plaques identical to those in the brains of AD patients. However, many others contain widespread Lewy bodies. Some researchers now speak of "diffuse Lewy body disease," a previously unrecognized form of dementia.

Many clients with diffuse Lewy body disease present as PD clients who later become demented, whereas others initially thought to have AD later develop the motor difficulties characteristic of PD. Similarly, a few AD clients have been found to develop motor defects very similar to those characterizing PD (Jarvik et al., 1991; Leverenz & Sumi, 1986; McKeith et al., 1992; Morris et al., 1989).

Symptoms of Lewy body dementia include fluctuating cognitive impairment, psychotic features including visual and auditory hallucinations, and paranoid delusions. In addition, the person may present with depressive symptoms, a history of falling, and unexplained losses of consciousness.

Other Cognitive Disorders

Amnestic Disorder Due to a General Medical Condition. The main features of amnestic disorders are the inability to remember recent events and its relative uncommon occurrence in children (APA, 1994). The syndrome may be found in childhood, as well as adulthood, however, if the person has experienced head trauma, hypoxia, lead or carbon monoxide poisoning, or herpes simplex encephalitis. It may also be related to alcohol withdrawal or sedative-hypnotic or anxiolytic intoxication in adults.

Personality Change Due to a General Medical Condition. This syndrome is characterized by a persistent personality disturbance, either a lifelong disturbance or a disturbance that represents a change or exaggeration of a previously characteristic trait, due to a specific organic factor (APA, 1994). Clinical features include emotional instability, aggressive outbursts, impaired social judgment, apathy, and sometimes suspiciousness and paranoid ideation. Common causes include tumors, head trauma, and cerebrovascular disease.

THE NURSE'S ROLE

It is imperative that the psychiatric nurse understand the common physiological and psychosocial changes that occur with normal growth and development and aging. The nurse who understands normal growth processes can deliver holistic care that empowers the client and family and allows for maximum physical and psychosocial functioning. The psychiatric nurse must recognize the importance of support from the family, significant others, the school, and the community and include these resources in all stages of the nursing process. There exists a stereotype, termed "ageism" by Butler (1982), that asserts that all old persons are senile, decrepit, isolated, lonely, and useless. Nothing could be further from the truth. Not all elderly are isolated and lacking family involvement (Shanas, 1979). The psychiatric nurse should recognize the valuable resource available to society in the form of our older population.

As we age, we become more susceptible to chronic diseases. It is estimated that all persons over age 65 suffer from at least one chronic disease, and people in middle age may be beginning to develop chronic disease conditions. Table 13–10 lists the most common chronic illnesses in old age. Many persons suffer from more than one chronic condition. Interactions may occur between illnesses and between drug therapies that may have psychosocial repercussions. For example, some medications can cause depression or mental confusion. It is important for the psychiatric nurse to be cognizant of concomitant illnesses and their symptoms, as well as the psychosocial effect of these illnesses.

COLLABORATION

An interdisciplinary team is important to the design of comprehensive, holistic care for the person with a cognitive disorder. This team consists of nurses; physicians; psychologists; social workers; teachers; and possibly special therapists, such as physical and occupational therapists. The interdisciplinary team develops the plan of inpatient and outpatient care that is the most appropriate for the ill person and his or her family. Community resources such as partial hospitalization, special education, case management, day programs, visiting nurses, and respite are examples. It is important that the psychiatric nurse recognize the importance of caring for the caregiver as well. With a healthy caregiver, positive client outcomes are possible. If the caregiver becomes physically or psychologically ill because of the burdens of caregiving, the consequences can be dire. It is not uncommon for the caregiver of a cognitively impaired person to develop physical illness or even die because of the physical and psychological demands of caregiving. Therefore, it is important that comprehensive community support be marshalled.

TABLE 13–10
Chronic Diseases in Aging

RANK	DISEASE	FREQUENCY IN 65+ (%)
1	Arthritis	55
2	Hypertension	45
3	Hearing impairment	40
4	Heart disease	35
5	Visual impairment	25

MEDICAL DIAGNOSIS AND MANAGEMENT

Data Collection. For any cognitive disorder, the emphasis of data collection is on the underlying general medical or psychiatric condition. A thorough history, a mental status assessment, a medical examination, behavioral observations, a neurological evaluation, neuropsychological testing, and selected laboratory tests are all essential components of the diagnosis and treatment of clients with cognitive disorders.

Symptomatology. There are a limited number of cognitive disorders, but there are innumerable conditions that give rise to them. The same physiological condition can result in several different clinical syndromes, and thus the psychiatric manifestations of a disease depend more on the disease process itself than on etiology. For example, the psychiatric symptoms associated with a brain tumor depend not only on the cellular morphology, but also on the location, size, and extent of tissue involvement and the speed with which the tumor is growing. The clinical expression of symptoms may also be affected by the person's genetic makeup, intelligence, premorbid personality, support network, coping mechanisms, environment, and past experiences.

History. The history probably provides the most important clues to the etiology of a cognitive disorder. The history indicates whether the psychiatric symptoms are acute or chronic, whether they change throughout the day and night, whether there are any recent psychosocial stressors, whether the client's medication or health status has changed recently, and so on. The review of systems, medical history, social history, school history, past psychiatric history, family psychiatric history, and description of current symptoms are essential for making an accurate diagnosis of the underlying etiology of the psychiatric symptoms.

Diagnostic Tests. In the medical examination, the physician looks for any underlying medical disorders that might cause the symptoms associated with the cognitive disorder. The neurological evaluation is not always helpful when the psychiatric symptoms are due to a medical condition. Wells (1985a) noted that the neurological examination is usually normal and remains so until the condition is far advanced.

Neuropsychological Testing. It must be remembered that neuropsychological testing is only a quantitative assessment of several specific behaviors. Cognitive impairment found through neuropsychological testing is no more certain evidence of treatable brain disease than is cognitive impairment demonstrated by mental status assessment. The neuropsychological test may be helpful when a cognitive disorder is suspected but cannot be substantiated on the basis of other diagnostic measures (i.e., history, physical examination, mental status assessment, and laboratory tests). Neuropsychological testing may reveal subtle but undeniable losses that point toward an underlying medical condition. It is also very useful for documenting changes in function over time.

Laboratory and Radiological Testing. Laboratory testing includes a blood chemistry profile (urine and blood cultures if sepsis is suspected), a complete blood count with differential, a Venereal Disease Research Laboratory test, a urinalysis, B_{12}, folate, electrocardiogram, thyroid function tests, and a toxicology screen. A test for Lyme disease may be ordered, because a form of dementia can result from this infection. Further evaluation with a chest x-ray, a CT scan of the brain, magnetic resonance imaging, electroencephalography, and a CSF examination is indicated if the cause has not yet been determined.

Ancillary Diagnostic Procedures. Ancillary diagnostic procedures are essential to the search for the etiology of cognitive disorders. These include neurodiagnostic procedures, such as electroencephalography, average evoked responses, as well as an array of biochemical measures of bodily function. A Continuous Performance Test is used for children being evaluated for ADHD. Wells (1985) noted that it is rare for these tests to point to any particular cerebral disease.

Differential Diagnosis. Differential diagnosis of cognitive disorders from other (i.e., functional) psychiatric diagnoses rests primarily on evidence gathered in the history, physical examination, or laboratory tests of a specific organic factor judged to be etiologically related to the disorder or syndrome. Three types of diagnostic errors may be made related to cognitive disorders: (1) There may be a failure to determine the cause of the psychiatric symptoms when one exists, (2) an underlying general medical condition may be diagnosed when there is none, or (3) a diagnosis of a general medical or psychiatric disorder may be made when, in fact, both are present.

Medical Diagnoses. Diagnosis is based on symptoms, results of physical examination and history, and the most-up-to-date criteria. Diagnostic criteria for delirium, dementia and ADHD are presented in the following boxes.

Summary. The methods of collecting data for the purpose of diagnosing and treating cognitive disorders are very complex and often do not yield definitive results. The progression from history and psychiatric interview to medical examination, observation of behavioral changes, and ancillary diagnostic procedures may or may not lead to an etiological explanation for the psychiatric symptoms. The nurse who cares for patients with mental disorders must learn to function comfortably within a complex framework in which diagnostic uncertainty often exists.

THE NURSING PROCESS

Assessment

The psychiatric interview must contain a description of the client's mental status, with a thorough description of behavior, flow of thought and speech, affect, thought processes/mental content, sensorium and intellectual resources, cognitive status, insight, and judgment. Serial assessment of psychiatric status is necessary for determining fluctuating course and acute changes in mental status. Interviews with family members should be included. In interviews with children and adolescents, it is helpful to include developmental screening.

Nursing Diagnoses

Possible nursing diagnoses for persons with cognitive disorders include the following:

- Altered Thought Processes
- Impaired Verbal Communication
- High Risk for Injury
- High Risk for Violence
- Sensory/Perceptual Alteration
- Altered Growth and Development
- Noncompliance
- Self-Esteem Disturbance
- Sleep Pattern Disturbance
- Impaired Social Interaction
- Altered Family Processes

The etiology of the nursing diagnosis depends on the medical diagnosis. For example, the etiology of Altered Thought Processes in the person with AD would be "probable irreversible brain damage." The etiology of Altered Thought Processes in the person with delirium would be "potentially reversible dementia" or an "acute general medical condition."

Defining characteristics indicate behaviors that need attention. The defining characteristics of Altered Thought Processes related to probable irreversible brain damage include any or all of the following:

- Delusions
- Ideas of reference
- Hallucinations
- Inappropriate social behavior
- Altered sleep patterns
- Inappropriate affect

As discussed earlier, according to Hall's PLST model, losses could include the following for persons with Altered Thought Processes related to an irreversible dementia:

- Cognitive losses
- Affective losses
- Conative losses
- Progressively lowered stress threshold

The defining characteristics of Altered Growth and Development include any or all of the following:

- Impulsivity
- Distractability
- Short attention span
- Restlessness
- Inappropriate social behavior

Planning

Treatment outcomes for cognitive disorders that are potentially treatable differ from disorders that are probably untreatable. In addition, outcome measures that are developmentally appropriate should be used. The psychiatric nurse individualizes care and sets realistic goals.

Outcomes for Potentially Reversible Dementia. The outcomes for a client with a potentially treatable dementia are determined by the client's premorbid personality. The following are possible outcomes:

- Full recovery
- Progression to an irreversible cognitive disorder
- Progression to a functional psychosis
- Death

Although full recovery is common, it is not always swift, and despite effective treatment, delirium may be prolonged, especially in the elderly, with the client manifesting a variety of emotional sequelae before functioning is fully restored. Progression to an irreversible cognitive disorder sometimes occurs, especially in cases in which the etiology cannot be treated effectively. Progression to functional psychosis has been documented, but the incidence is low. Finally, death does occur in some clients experiencing a delirium, but it is presumed that, for the most part, death is due to the disease that caused the delirium and is not a result of the delirium itself.

Outcomes for Probable Irreversible Dementia. Because the condition will probably not improve, it is essential to measure outcomes against cerebral pathology. To evaluate the plan of care, the psychiatric nurse evaluates the client's comfort and safety using the following measures (Hall, 1991):

- The number of hours the client sleeps at night should increase, and episodes of confused night wakening should decrease.
- The client's weight should stabilize or increase without special supplements. Food intake at mealtimes should increase, and caloric expenditure should decrease as pacing and agitation disappear.
- Episodes of combative behavior should be eliminated. Agitated episodes should diminish or be eliminated.
- The client's degree of socialization, including voluntary participation in small-group activities, should increase.
- Functional level may improve briefly as excess disability disappears.
- The need for sedatives and tranquilizers should decrease.
- Once family members understand the care program, their satisfaction with the care plan and empathy with the staff should increase (Hall, 1991).

Implementation

Nursing interventions must be individualized according to the client's needs.

Delirium Management. The following nursing actions are included in delirium management, the goal of which is to provide a safe and therapeutic environment for the client who is experiencing an acute confusional state.*

- Identify the etiologic factors causing the delirium.
- Initiate therapies to reduce or eliminate the factors causing the delirium.
- Monitor the client's neurological status on an ongoing basis.
- Provide unconditional positive regard.
- Verbally acknowledge the client's fears and feelings.
- Provide optimistic but realistic reassurance.
- Allow the client to maintain rituals that limit anxiety.
- Inform the client what is happening and what can be expected to occur in the future.
- Do not make demands for abstract thinking if the client can think only in concrete terms.
- Limit the need for decision making if it is frustrating/confusing to the client.
- Administer medications for anxiety or agitation as needed.
- Encourage visitation by significant others as appropriate.
- Recognize and accept the client's perceptions or interpretation of reality (hallucinations or delusions).
- State your own perceptions in a calm, reassuring, and nonargumentative manner.
- Respond to the theme or tone, rather than the content, of the hallucination or delusion.
- Remove stimuli, when possible, that are misperceived by the client (e.g., a certain picture on the wall or the television).
- Maintain a well-lit environment that reduces sharp contrasts and shadows.
- Assist with the client's needs related to nutrition, elimination, hydration, and personal hygiene.
- Maintain a hazard-free environment.
- Place an identification bracelet on the client.
- Provide the appropriate level of supervision/surveillance to monitor the client and to allow for therapeutic actions as needed.
- Use physical restraints as needed, but judiciously.
- Avoid frustrating the client by quizzing him or her with orientation questions that cannot be answered.
- Orient the client to person, place, and time as needed.
- Provide a consistent physical environment and daily routine.
- Provide caregivers who are familiar to the client.
- Use environmental cues (e.g., signs, pictures, clocks, calendars, color coding) to stimulate memory, reorient, and promote appropriate behavior.
- Provide a low-stimulation environment for the client whose disorientation is increased by overstimulation.
- Encourage the client to use aids that increase sensory input (e.g., eyeglasses, hearing aids, and dentures).
- Approach the client slowly and from the front.
- Address the client by name when initiating an interaction.
- Reorient the client to your identity with each contact.
- Use simple, direct, descriptive statements to communicate.

* Adapted from McCloskey, J. C., & Bulechek, G. M. (1992). *Nursing intervention classifications* (pp. 191–192). St. Louis: C. V. Mosby.

- Prepare the client for changes in usual routine and environment prior to their occurrence.
- Provide new information slowly and in small doses with frequent rest periods.
- Focus interpersonal interactions on what is familiar and meaningful to the client.

Confusion Management. For the patient with Altered Thought Processes related to probable irreversible brain damage, the intervention is confusion management, the goal of which is to provide a modified environment for the client who is experiencing a chronic confusional state. Nursing actions may be individualized according to the needs of the client and include the following*:

- Determine the client's physical, social, and psychological histories prior to confusion.
- Determine the behaviors that may be expected of the client, given his or her level of orientation.
- Identify potential dangers in the environment for the client.
- Place an identification bracelet on the client.
- Provide a consistent physical environment and daily routine.
- Touch the client to convey acceptance.
- Provide unconditional positive regard.
- Provide caregivers who are familiar to the client.
- Use the strategies used by the home caregiver to provide comfort if appropriate.
- Monitor cognitive functioning using an appropriate screening tool.
- Avoid unfamiliar situations when possible.
- Identify the client's usual patterns of behavior for such activities as sleep, medication use, elimination, food intake, and self-care.
- Provide structured rest periods to prevent fatigue and reduce stress.
- Have the client sit in a reclining chair instead of in bed for rest periods as appropriate.
- Avoid frustrating the client by quizzing with orientation questions that cannot be answered.
- Provide a low-stimulation environment for the client whose disorientation is increased by overstimulation.
- Seat the client at a small table in a group of three to five at meals as appropriate.
- Allow the client to eat alone if appropriate.
- Provide finger foods to maintain nutrition in the client who will not sit still to eat.
- Provide the client with general orientation to the season of the year by using holiday decorations.
- Decrease the noise level in the environment by avoiding paging systems and call lights that ring or buzz.
- Select television or radio programs based on the client's interests.
- Arrange one-to-one activities between the client and another client that are geared to the client's cognitive abilities and interests.
- Label photos of people familiar to the client with the names of the people in photos.
- Select artwork for the client's room that features landscapes or scenery (client may misinterpret human or animal figures as real).
- Limit visitors to one or two persons at a time.
- Instruct visitors as to appropriate topics to discuss with the client.
- Limit the number of choices the client has to make.
- Give one simple direction at a time.
- Address the client by name when initiating an interaction.
- Provide positive feedback frequently.
- Provide boundaries, such as red or yellow tape on the floor, when low-stimulus units are not available.
- Place the client's name in large block letters in his or her room and on his or her clothing.
- On signs, use symbols rather than words to help the client locate the room, bathroom, or equipment.
- Instruct the family that it may be impossible for the client to learn new material.
- Do not use physical restraints.
- Monitor the client carefully for physiological causes for increased confusion.
- Use mirrors selectively for clients who are not agitated by them.

* Adapted from McCloskey, J. C., & Bulechek, G. M. (1992). *Nursing intervention classifications* (pp. 179–180). St. Louis: C. V. Mosby.

Limit Setting. Limit setting establishes the parameters of desirable and acceptable behavior. Limit setting involves the following nursing actions*:

- Discuss with the client his or her behavior.
- Identify undesirable behaviors.
- Discuss with the client what is desirable behavior in a given situation or setting.
- Establish reasonable expectations for behavior.
- Establish consequences of occurence/nonoccurrence of desired behaviors.
- Communicate the expectations and consequences to the client in language that is easily understood and nonpunitive.
- Communicate the established behavioral expectations and consequences to other staff involved in the client's care.
- Refrain from arguing or bargaining with the client about the established behavioral expectations and consequences.
- When appropriate, help the client perform desired behaviors.
- Monitor the client for occurrence/nonoccurrence of desired behaviors.
- Modify behavioral expectations and consequences as needed to accommodate changes in the client's situation.
- Initiate the established consequences for the occurrence/nonoccurrence of the desired behaviors.
- Decrease limit setting as the client's behavior approximates the desired behaviors (McCloskey & Bulecheck, 1992).

Pharmacological Management. At times, delirious clients may be so agitated, assaultive, or paranoid that immediate symptomatic control is required, either to prevent these clients from harming themselves and others or to quiet them sufficiently for medical evaluation and treatment. Sometimes a client must be treated symptomatically even before a definite diagnosis can be made. The antipsychotics and benzodiazepines are the drugs most often used to help control clients in these out-of-control situations. There is little evidence that one group is more effective than another in managing delirium. Each class of medication has its advantages

* Adapted from McCloskey J. C., & Bulecheck, G. M. (1992). *Nursing intervention classifications* (p. 330). St. Louis: C. V. Mosby.

and disadvantages. The choice is often made on the basis of the specific effect desired or the specific side effect to be avoided. Many of the same medications are used to manage the behaviors of the person with probable irreversible dementia.

It is imperative that the client's behaviors be monitored before medication is administered to determine possible external causes of the behavior, such as stimuli, time of day, or a certain caregiver. It is also important to monitor behaviors after medication is begun to determine the effect of the medication. In addition, the client should continually be monitored for possible side effects, particularly because he or she is unlikely to be able to voice concerns. The following is an overview of medications used to relieve delirium and dementia. A more in-depth discussion of these medications is provided in Chapter 26.

Of the antipsychotic medications, the new, more potent agents such as haloperidol and thiothixene are the most frequently chosen, because they are very effective without sedation. These drugs can be administered by injection, which is useful in acute psychiatric crisis. Chlorpromazine (Thorazine) may be given orally (PO) to calm the agitated client but it is more sedating than the high-potency antipsychotics. Cardiovascular function should be monitored closely in clients receiving high doses of antipsychotics, but this may be impossible in the severely agitated client. Whether antipsychotics or benzodiazepines are chosen, it is desirable to switch from intravenous (IV) or intramuscularly (IM) to PO administration as soon as the client begins to cooperate with treatment.

Because of the high incidence of extrapyramidal side effects (especially acute dystonic reactions) with antipsychotic agents, particularly in adolescents and young adults, it may be necessary to administer benztropine mesylate (Cogentin) with the antipsychotic agent to treat the extrapyramidal side effects. In older patients, it may not be advisable to add a medication such as Cogentin for two reasons. First, the elderly do not demonstrate dystonic reactions as frequently as young persons do. Second, it may be desirable to avoid the use of potent anticholinergic agents unless they are essential because of side effects.

The benzodiazepines are probably as effective as the antipsychotics in controlling the severe psychiatric manifestations of delirium and dementia, and in many clients they may be the drug of choice. Their effect on cardiovascular and respiratory function is minimal, but they usually are more sedating than the more potent antipsychotic agents. The benzodiazepines are potent anticonvulsants, and this characteristic is desired when working with a person who is delirious from drug or alcohol intoxication or has the potential for seizure activity. In the elderly, it is important to use the shorter-acting (oxazepam or lorazepam) rather than longer-acting (clorazepate or diazepam) benzodiazepine sedatives, because of the extended half-life and the potential for longer-acting agents to accumulate in the aged.

It is important to remember that not all clients with delirium or dementia require psychopharmacological agents for relief or control of their symptoms. On the contrary, because these conditions are manifestations of altered cerebral metabolism and psychopharmacological agents further alter cerebral metabolism, there is a real possibility that these agents will increase, rather than mitigate, confusion or agitation. Pharmacological treatment of the symptoms of delirium and dementia is necessary in the following situations:

- When the symptoms interfere seriously with medical evaluation or treatment
- When client's behavior is dangerous to him- or herself or to others
- When the symptoms cause the client intense personal distress

Specific symptoms targeted for pharmacological treatment include intense anxiety, fearfulness, paranoid delusion, insomnia, hallucinations, irritability, intense anger, restlessness, incessant hyperactivity, assaultiveness, and self-injurious actions. It should be noted that *elderly or debilitated clients should receive one third to one half the initial recommended dosage of antipsychotic or anxiolytic medication,* with the dosage subsequently adjusted upward or downward, depending on the client's response.

In the pharmacological treatment of the symptoms of delirium, the problem is more often the appropriate amount of medication, rather than which drug should be used. Too little will be ineffective; too much may be toxic and may actually worsen the delirium. The client's condition must be assessed repeatedly and interventions initiated to keep the client's condition stable while work toward resolution of the underlying condition progresses.

The use of medication for children with ADHD has been controversial. Psychostimulant medications have been prescribed for nearly 40 years, with various outcomes reported. There are three stimulants currently in use: methylphenidate (Ritalin), dextroamphetamine (Dexadrine), and pemoline (Cylert). All of these medications have been found to have some positive influence on specific target symptoms of ADHD. Although it may seem contradictory to give a hyperactive child psychostimulants, the increase in brain activity precipitated by stimulant use encourages an increase in organized activity.

Of the three drugs, methylphenidate has been the most widely studied and used in the last 10 years. The target behaviors most positively affected by methylphenidate include aimless restlessness, short attention span, and impulsiveness. In several studies, children on methylphenidate have received positive ratings from parents and teachers on behavior checklists (Taylor et al., 1987). It is hypothesized that this behavioral/cognitive improvement may be the result of improved sustained attention, better impulse control, and increased motivation (Weiss, 1991).

Methylphenidate appears to be effective in about 70 percent of children with ADHD, but it is not without side effects (Weiss, 1991), the most common being reduced appetite and difficulty getting to sleep. Some children also report stomachache, headache, and sadness or depression. A slowing or arrest of growth (reduced height and weight) has also been reported, but when children are given drug holidays, a growth rebound is observed. This particular side effect may be dose related, as is seen (more often) with dextroamphetamine. Psychostimulant use may result in small increases in systolic blood pressure and heart rate, but these increases do not appear to be clinically significant. Some children with ADHD treated with stimulant medication appear to be vulnerable to the development of tics associated with Tourette's disorder. It is not clear how stimulant medication might exacerbate or precipitate these tics, however.

Before any medication is prescribed for the treatment of ADHD, a comprehensive diagnosis and evaluation should be performed including elicitation of information from teachers, classroom observation, baseline assessment of target behaviors, and elicitation of a commitment from the youngster's parents and school personnel to collaborate in treatment. Psychostimulants will not cure or eradicate ADHD, which has diverse behavioral, social, and cognitive implications, but when they are used in the right child for the right reasons, they are highly effective in ameliorating target behaviors and providing impetus for change in other areas.

Evaluation

Evaluation of the medical and nursing interventions relies greatly on etiological factors and defining characteristics and should be an ongoing process during intervention.

Case Study: The Client with Alzheimer's Disease (Ann)

The following case study illustrates a useful framework with which to evaluate nursing care of the client with AD. See also Nursing Care Plan 13–1.

Ann is a 77-year-old woman who was admitted to the special care unit of a local nursing facility 2 years ago, with a diagnosis of AD, established 5 years previously. She is in the third stage of AD, moving quickly to the fourth. She had been living in her home with live-in help until her admission, but her mental condition had deteriorated so much that it was unwise to keep her at home. She became increasingly dependent in her activities of daily living (ADLs), began wandering, and experienced night wakening. Her caretaker was unable to cope. It was felt that Ann should be placed in a nursing facility near her younger son's home. Ann also has another daughter and son who live in another state. Ann's only other diagnosis is emphysema with no presenting symptoms and for which she is not treated. Ann takes only a multiple vitamin daily, and PRN medication for constipation.

Ann is dependent in all ADLs. Her son visits infrequently, because Ann no longer recognizes him and it is distressing for him to see her in such cognitive decline. Most of the day, Ann wanders around her room, chattering, and tearing the bedsheets off the beds. She does respond to her name and seems to recognize her frequent caregivers, whom she wants to touch and hug.

Ann's speech is jargon, many words of which are meaningless to others. When focused by the staff, she will follow simple directions, will dance with the staff, and even hum along to old-time songs when the staff are singing to her. Ann hates to be left alone, and she will eat only if she can sit on someone's lap or at least very near the person. She will not nap unless someone lies in bed with her to get her to sleep.

Ann's communication is limited. At times her speech is spontaneous—for example, she'll say "Leave me alone" when someone is doing something she doesn't like, such as combing her hair—and profanity comes easily, illustrating the lowered inhibitions frequently observed in persons with AD. Sometimes she will cry for no apparent reason, but she accepts the comfort offered by the staff. Ann detests bathing or showering, and this is one of the most difficult aspects of her care. The staff are very affectionate with Ann and she seems appreciative of this acceptance.

Ann responds well to touch, which is her main form of communication. Her attention is focused only on certain cues, which include touch, imitation of her chattering, and singing. She listens briefly when her name is called and, when in distress, Ann is able to make appropriate sounds. Her language and reality base have been altered because of her cognitive deficits, but she is able to interpret affection and caring appropriately. According to her family, Ann has never wanted to be alone, and this social response remains intact. She frequently reaches out for caregivers as they pass by her. Her attention span is poor, but hugging, dancing, or singing will maintain her focus for several minutes at a time. She is unable to participate actively in communication unless directed by the staff. Her major strength is her love of human contact, and the warm manner in which she responds to touch.

When developing interventions for Ann, the nurse considered her primary mode of communication. Thus touch and affection are used to get her attention and to comfort her when she is distressed. The staff of the nursing facility have implemented several interventions that flow from Hall's PLST model:

1. The staff always call Ann by name whenever they are communicating with her, and they identify themselves to her. In this way, Ann's attention is focused, even if for only moments, and her social role is preserved.

2. Touch and hugs are used whenever possible, except when Ann is not receptive (when she is angry). Ann is particularly dependent on nonverbal language

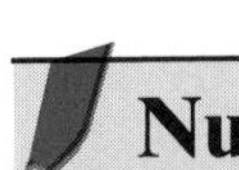

Nursing Care Plan 13–1 The Client with Alzheimer's Disease (Ann)

Nursing Diagnosis: Altered Thought Processes related to destruction of brain tissue

OUTCOME IDENTIFICATION	NURSING ACTIONS	RATIONALES	EVALUATION
1. By [date], the number of hours Ann sleeps at night will increase, and episodes of confused night wakening will decrease.	1a. Identify Ann's usual sleep patterns.	1a. Familiar habits are easy to implement and comforting to client.	*Goal met:* Ann is able to sleep 6 hours throughout night without waking. Documentation: Document number of hours slept and night wakenings.
	1b. Provide structured rest periods.	1b. Periodic rest prevents accumulation of stress and facilitates relaxation.	
	1c. Provide low-stimulation environment.	1c. Low or modified stimulation prevents anxiety and promotes relaxation.	
2. By [date], Ann's weight will stabilize or increase without special supplements.	2a. Identify Ann's usual eating patterns.	2a. Familiarity with foods and rituals optimizes clients' eating abilities.	*Goal met:* Ann maintains or gains weight. Documentation: Document weight and possibly caloric intake if client is undernourished.
	2b. Seat Ann at small table in group of three to five or seat her alone at a table.	2b. Because of clients' inability to process multiple stimuli, eating in small groups or alone reduces stimuli.	
	2c. Provide finger foods.	2c. Client may be unable to sit to eat but will eat finger foods while moving, thus taking in adequate nutrition.	
	2d. Decrease noise levels while Ann is eating.	2d. Noise distracts clients from eating.	
3. By [date], episodes of combative or agitated behavior will be eliminated or diminished.	3a. Determine Ann's physical, social, and psychological histories to find familiar interventions.	3a. Clients find comfort in the familiar and are likely to be more cooperative.	*Goal met:* Episodes of agitation and combative behavior decrease. Documentation: Document episodes of confusion/agitation/combative behavior on log: who, what, when, how, why.
	3b. Determine appropriate behavioral expectations for Ann.	3b. Depending on orientation level, behaviors may or may not be alterable. It is important to set realistic goals.	
	3c. Identify potential changes in Ann's environment.	3c. Because of poor judgment, clients may misinterpret the environment, causing harm or injury	
	3d. Provide consistent routine and environment.	3d. Consistency provides predictability and security for memory-impaired clients.	
	3e. Use touch and unconditional positive regard when interacting with Ann.	3e. Communication, especially nonverbal, determines the tone of interactions.	
	3f. Avoid situations that are unfamiliar to Ann.	3f. The unfamiliar is frightening to memory-impaired clients and can cause catastrophic behaviors.	

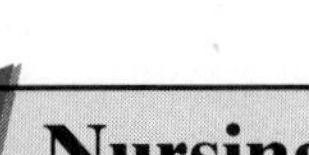

Nursing Care Plan 13–1 The Client with Alzheimer's Disease (Ann) (Continued)

► **Nursing Diagnosis:** Altered Thought Processes related to destruction of brain tissue

OUTCOME IDENTIFICATION	NURSING ACTIONS	RATIONALES	EVALUATION
	3g. Provide structured rest periods.	3g. Rest periods allow clients' stress level to return to baseline.	
	3h. Decrease noise levels and stimulation.	3h. Overstimulation leads to increased confusion and agitation.	
	3i. Monitor causes of increased confusion in Ann.	3i. Agitation and confusion may be caused by fatigue, changes, stimuli, demands, and physiological disorders.	
4. By [date], Ann's socialization will increase.	4a. Determine Ann's previous history of socialization.	4a. Clients are more likely to participate in familiar activities.	*Goal met:* Ann's socializing increases. Documentation: Document participation in activities and episodes of socialization.
	4b. Select activities (using TV or radio carefully) for Ann based on her interests.	4b. Client may not be able to tolerate the stimulation of the TV or radio.	
	4c. Select one-to-one activities as appropriate.	4c. Because of clients' diminished ability to tolerate stimuli, one-to-one and small-group activities are best.	
	4d. Label familiar pictures and objects.	4d. This practice assists caregivers and visitors in identifying important items, events, and people in client's life and provides opportunity for socialization through reminiscence.	
5. By [date], Ann's functional level may improve briefly as excess disability disappears.	5a. Determine Ann's functional history prior to confusion.	5a. It is unrealistic to expect clients to function differently from previous optimal level.	*Goal met:* Ann's functional ability improves. Documentation: Observe ability to perform self-care and document actions that facilitate functioning.
	5b. Provide consistency in all daily activities.	5b. Consistency reduces feeling of insecurity and fear, and enables clients to concentrate on task at hand.	
	5c. Decrease multiple competing stimuli in Ann's environment.	5c. Competing stimuli precipitate frustration and inability to accomplish tasks.	
	5d. Limit the number of choices Ann has to make.	5d. Clients can concentrate on only one or two choices at a time. Breaking down tasks into steps helps simplify and promote self-care.	
	5e. Provide positive feedback.	5e. Provides encouragement to clients.	

Nursing Care Plan 13–1 The Client with Alzheimer's Disease (Ann) (Continued)

► **Nursing Diagnosis:** Altered Thought Processes related to destruction of brain tissue

OUTCOME IDENTIFICATION	NURSING ACTIONS	RATIONALES	EVALUATION
	5f. Instruct family and staff that it may be impossible for Ann to learn new tasks.	5f. Because of loss of cerebral cortex function, new material cannot be learned, and it is frustrating to all for clients to try.	
	5g. Refrain from using physical restraints.	5g. Physical restraints inhibit movement and self-care and cause frustration and agitation.	

and is able to participate actively in physical touch and communication.

3. The staff use exaggerated facial expressions and gestures when communicating with Ann. Thus verbal communication is enhanced with nonverbal cues.

4. The staff mimic Ann's jargon to get her attention, and then proceed with the task at hand. Mimicking serves to catch Ann's attention.

5. The staff sing with Ann, and perhaps dance with her too, in order to have an effective calm time together, especially if Ann has been upset. A sense of security and congruity with the environment and caregivers is instilled in Ann when the staff key into the meaning of Ann's nonverbal attempts at communication.

6. Ann is made an active participant in interactions, to facilitate her communication and enhance her sense of security. The staff do not talk about Ann in her presence, in order to preserve her social functioning and dignity.

7. Ann's inappropriate behavior is redirected. If she is angry or hostile, the nurse leaves and returns in 5 minutes or has another caregiver take over. Because of the impairments in Ann's ability to communicate, it is fruitless for the staff to explain or reason with her. Whatever communication abilities Ann possesses at the time are used, and the staff do not expect more than she is capable of doing.

8. Ann is provided assistance in completing her activities of daily living. She is bathed, dressed, and groomed in privacy, one step at a time.

9. Adequate nutrition is provided.

10. Rest periods are provided.

11. Safety is ensured. All toxic materials, such as cleaning fluids, perfumes, and even some plants, are kept out of reach. Ann's walking ability is assessed, and time for rest is allowed if she seems unsteady. Because of diminished perceptions and interpretation of the environment, the furniture is arranged in a way that maximizes safe ambulation. All areas are well lit but without glare.

► CHAPTER SUMMARY

Cognitive disorders can affect persons of many ages and can have many causes. It is imperative that the psychiatric nurse recognize the disease states, symptoms, and diagnostic criteria to provide adequate nursing care.

Suggestions for Clinical Conference

1. List the suggestions a nurse could give the parents of a 9-year-old boy diagnosed with ADHD regarding limit setting in the home.
2. Identify the topics that need to be reviewed in the education of the parents of a 9-year-old child just given his first prescription for methylphenidate.
3. Identify the topics that need to be included in the education of the 9-year-old.
4. List the nursing interventions for a 20-year-old client recently admitted to the hospital for evaluation of grand mal seizures.
5. Discuss the differences and similarities between dementia and delirium in the elderly and specify assessment and intervention strategies for dementia and delirium.
6. Discuss why it is important to distinguish between reversible and irreversible disorders. What nursing implications are different?

References

Adams, M., & Victor, M. (1985). *Principles of neurology*. New York: McGraw-Hill.

American Psychiatric Association. (1980). *Diagnostic and statistical manual of mental disorders* (3rd ed.). Washington, DC: Author.

American Psychiatric Association. (1987). *Diagnostic and statistical manual of mental disorders* (3rd ed., rev.). Washington, DC: Author.

American Psychiatric Association. (1994). *Diagnostic and statistical manual of mental disorders* (4th ed.). Washington, DC: Author.

Andreasen, N., & Black, D. (1991). *Introductory textbook of psychiatry*. Washington, DC: American Psychiatric Press.

August, G. J., & Stewart, M. A. (1983). Familial subtypes of childhood hyperactivity. *Journal of Nervous and Mental Disease, 171,* 362–368.

Berensin, E. (1985). *Delirium in the elderly: Assessment and management* (Wyeth Monograph Series: *Clinical perspectives in aging*). Philadelphia, Wyeth Publications.

Beresin, E. (1986). Delirium. In L. I. Sederer (Ed.), *Inpatient psychiatry: Diagnosis and treatment* (2nd ed., pp. 126–149). Baltimore: Williams & Wilkins.

Beresin, E. V. (1988). Delirium in the elderly. *Journal of Geriatric Psychiatry and Neurology, 1,* 128.

Blass, J. P. (1982). Dementia. *Medical Clinics of North America, 66,* 1145–1160.

Brown, P., Cathala, F., & Sadowksy, D. (1979). Creutzfeldt-Jakob disease in France: Clinical characteristics of 124 consecutive verified cases during the decade 1968–1977. *Annals of Neurology, 6,* 430–437.

Burgess, A. (1990). *Psychiatric nursing in the hospital and the community*. Norwalk, CT: Appleton & Lange.

Butler, R. (1982). *Aging and mental health* (3rd ed.). St. Louis, MO: Mosby.

Carmichael, A. (1990). Physical development and biological influences. In B. Tonge, G. D. Burrows, & J. S. Werry (Eds.), *Handbook of studies in child psychiatry*. Amsterdam: Elsevier.

Chu, S., Buehler, J., & Berkelman, R. (1990). Impact of the human immunodeficiency virus epidemic on mortality in women of childbearing age. *Journal of the American Medical Association, 264,* 225–259.

Conn, D. K. (1991). Delirium and other organic mental disorders. In J. Sadavoy, L. W. Lazarus, & L. F. Jarvik (Eds.), *Comprehensive review of geriatric psychiatry* (pp. 7311–7336). Washington, DC: American Psychiatric Press.

Cummings, E., & Henry, W. E. (1961). *Growing old: The process of disengagement*. New York: Basic Books.

Dawson, P., Kline, K., Wiancko, D., & Wells, D. (1986). Preventing excess disability in patients with Alzheimer's disease. *Geriatric Nursing, 1,* 298–330.

Deary, I. J., & Whalling, L. J. (1988). Recent research on the causes of Alzheimer's disease. *British Medical Journal, 297,* 807–810.

Farlow M., Gracon, S. I., Hershey, L. A., Lewis, K. W., Sandowsky, C. H., & Dolan-Ureno, J. (1992). A controlled trial of Tacrine in Alzheimer's disease. *Journal of the American Medical Association, 268,* 2523–2529.

Ferri, F. F. (1992). Biology, epidemiology, and demographics of aging. In F. F. Ferri & M. D. Fretwell (Eds.), *Practical guide to the care of the geriatric patient* (pp. 1–12). St. Louis, MO: Mosby.

Fine, W. (1978) Postural hypotension. *Practitioner, 20,* 698–701.

Forster, F., & Booker, H. (1988). The epilepsies and convulsive disorders. In A. Baker & R. Joynt (Eds.), *Clinical neurology* (Vol. 3, p. 31). Philadelphia: Harper & Row.

French, L. R., Shuman, L. M., Mortimer, J. A., Hutton, J. T., Boatman, R. A., & Christians, B. (1985). A case-control study of dementia of the Alzheimer's type. *American Journal of Epidemiology, 121,* 414–421.

Greene, V. L., Monahan, D., & Coleman, P. D. (1992). Demographics. In R. J. Ham & P. D. Sloane (Eds.), *Primary care geriatrics* (2nd ed., pp. 3–19). St. Louis, MO: Mosby.

Grossman, H. J. (1973). *Manual on terminology and classification in mental retardation*. Washington, DC: American Association on Mental Deficiency.

Hall, G. R. (1988). *Evaluating a low stimulus nursing home unit for residents with chronic dementing illnesses*. Unpublished master's thesis, University of Iowa, College of Nursing, Iowa City, IA.

Hall, G. R., (1991). Altered thought processes: SDAT. In M. Maas & K. Buckwalter (Eds.), *Nursing diagnoses and interventions in the elderly* (pp. 332–347). Menlo Park, CA: Addison-Wesley.

Hall, G. R., & Buckwalter, K. C. (1987). Progressively lowered stress threshold: A conceptual model for care of adults with Alzheimer's disease. *Archives of Psychiatric Nursing, 1,* 399–406.

Hall, G. R., Kirschling, M., & Todd, S. (1986). Sheltered freedom: An Alzheimer's unit in an ICF. *Geriatric Nursing, 7,* 132–136.

Ham, R. J. (1992). Confusion, dementia, and delirium. In R. J. Ham & P. D. Sloane (Eds.), *Primary care geriatrics* (2nd ed., pp. 259–311). St. Louis, MO: Mosby.

Havinghurst, R. J., & Albrecht, R. (1953). *Older people*. White Plains, NY: Longman.

Heyman, A., Wilkinson, W. E., Stafford, J. A., Helms, M. J., Sigmon, A. H., & Weinberg, T. (1984). Alzheimer's disease: A study of the epidemiological aspects. *Annals of Neurology, 15,* 335–341.

Jarvik, L. F., Lavretsky, E. P., & Matsuyama, S. S. (1991). Cytoskeletal changes underlying dementias: New evidence from Lewy body research. *Alzheimer's Disease and Associated Disorders, 5,* 265–267.

Jenike, A. J. (1989). *Geriatric psychiatry and psychopharmacology: A clinical approach*. St. Louis, MO: Mosby-Year Book.

Katzman, R. (1986). Alzheimer's disease. *New England Journal of Medicine, 4,* 964–972.

Leverenz, J., & Sumi, S. M. (1986). Parkinson's disease in patients with Alzheimer's disease. *Archives of Neurology, 43,* 662–664.

Levine, M. (1989). Attention deficits: The diverse effects of weak control systems in childhood. *Pediatric Annals, 16*(2), 117–131.

Lipowski, Z. J. (1980). *Delirium*. Springfield, IL: Charles C. Thomas.

Liston, E. H. (1982). Delirium in the aged. *Psychiatric Clinics of North America, 5,* 49–56.

Matteson, M. A. (1988). Age-related changes in the neurological system. In M. A. Matteson & E. S. McConnell (Eds.), *Gerontological nursing: Concepts and practice* (pp. 241–263). Philadelphia: W. B. Saunders

McCloskey, J. C., & Bulecheck, G. M. (1992). *Nursing interventions classification (NIC)*. St. Louis, MO: Mosby.

McKeith, I. G., Perry, R. H., Fairbairn, A. F., Jabeen, S., & Perry, E. K. (1992). Operational criteria for senile dementia of Lewy body type (SDLT). *Psychological Medicine, 22,* 911–922.

Medical news & perspectives: Psychiatrists set to approve *DSM-IV*. *Journal of the American Medical Association, 270,* 13–15.

Morris, J. C., Drazner, M., Fulling, K., Grant, E. A., Goldring, J. (1989). Clinical and pathological aspects of Parkinsonism in Alzheimer's disease. *Archives of Neurology, 46,* 651–677.

Mortimer, J. A., French L. R., & Hutton, J. T. (1985). Head injury as a risk factor for Alzheimer's disease. *Neurology, 35,* 264–267.

Mullan, M., Houlden, H., Windelspecht, M., Fidani, L., Lombardi, C., Diaz, P. L., Rossor, M., Crook, R., Hardy, J., & Duff, K. (1992). A locus for familial early-onset Alzheimer's disease on the long arm of chromosome 14, proximal to the alpha 1-antichymotrypsin gene. *Natural Genetics, 2,* 340–342.

Neugarten, B. (1968). *Middle age and aging*. Chicago: University of Chicago Press.

Osborn, J. (1990). AIDS: Policies for coping with disaster. *AIDS Patient Care, 4*(5), 2–7.

Pericak-Vance, M. A., Bebout, J. L., Gaskell, P. C., Yamaoka, L. H., Hung, W. Y., Alberts, M. J., Walker, A. P., Bartlett, R. J., Haynes, C. A., & Welsh, K. A. (1991). Linkage studies in familial Alzheimer disease: Evidence for chromosome 19 linkage. *American Journal of Human Genetics, 48,* 1034–1050.

Portnoi, J. F. (1979). Digitalis delirium in elderly patients. *Journal of Clinical Pharmacology, 19,* 747–750.

Prusiner, S. B. (1984). Some speculations about prions, amyloid, and Alzheimer's disease. *New England Journal of Medicine, 310,* 661–663.

Purdie, F. R., Hareginan, B., & Rosen, P. (1981). Acute organic brain syndrome: A review of 100 cases. *Annals of Emergency Medicine, 10,* 455–461.

Rabins, P., & Folstein, M. F. (1982). Delirium and dementia: Diagnostic criteria and fatality rates. *British Journal of Psychiatry, 140,* 149–153.

Read, S. L., & Jarvik, L. F. (1984). Cerebrovascular disease in the differential diagnosis of dementia. *Psychiatric Annals, 14,* 100–108.

Reisburg, B., Ferris, S. H., DeLeon, M. J., & Crook, T. (1982). The global deterioration scale (GDS): An instrument for the assessment of primary degenerative dementia. *American Journal of Psychiatry, 139,* 1136–1139.

Richeimer, S. H. (1987). Psychological intervention in delirium. *Postgraduate Medicine, 81,* 173–180.

Ronsman, K. M. (1988). Pseudodementia. *Geriatric Nursing, 9,* 50–52.

Roos, R., Gajdusek, C., & Gibbs, C. (1973). The clinical characteristics of transmissible Creutzfeldt-Jakob disease. *Brain, 96,* 1–19.

Sagar, H. F., & Sullivan, E. V. (1988). Patterns of cognitive impairment in dementia. *Recent Advances in Clinical Neurology, 5,* 47–86.

Scharnhorst, S. (1992). AIDS dementia complex in the elderly: Diagnosis and management. *Nurse Practitioner, 17*(8), 37–43.

Schellenberg, G. D., Bird, T. D., Wijsman, E. M., Orr, H. T., Anderson, L., Nemens, E., White, J. A., Bonnycastle, L., Weber, J. L., & Alonso, M. E. (1992). Genetic linkage evidence for a familial Alzheimer's disease locus on chromosome 14. *Science, 258,* 668–671.

Shanas, E. (1979). The family as a social support system in old age. *The Gerontologist, 19,* 169–174.

Small, G. W. (1992). Tacrine for treating Alzheimer's disease. *Journal of the American Medical Association, 268,* 2564–2565.

St. George-Hyslop, P., Haines, J., Rogaev, E., Mortilla, M., Vaula, G., Pericak-Vance, M., Foncin, J. F., Montesi, M., Bruni, A., & Sorbi, S. (1992). Genetic evidence for a novel familial Alzheimer's disease locus on chromosome 14. *Natural Genetics, 2,* 330–334.

Stolley, J. M. (1992). Fall risk for elderly Alzheimer's patients. In K. C. Buckwalter (Ed.), *Geriatric mental health nursing: Current and future challenges* (pp. 94–101). Thorofare, NJ: Slack.

Strittmatter, W. J., Saunders, A. M., Schmechel, D., Pericak-Vance, M., Enghild, J., Salvesen, G. S., & Roses, A. D. (1993). Apolipoprotein e: High-avidity binding to beta-amyloid and increased frequency of type 4 allele in late-onset familial Alzheimer disease. *Proceedings of the National Academy of Science, 90,* 1977–1981.

Tariot, P. N., & Weingartner, H. (1986). A psychobiologic analysis of cognitive failures. *Archives of General Psychiatry, 43,* 1183–1188.

Tateishi, J. (1985). Transmission of Creutzfeldt-Jakob disease from human blood and urine into mice. *Lancet, 2,* 1074.

Taylor, E., Wieselberg, M., Morley, G., et al. (1987). Changes in family functioning and relationships in children who respond to methylphenidate. *Journal of the American Academy of Child and Adolescent Psychiatry, 26,* 728–732.

Terry, R., & Pena, C. (1965). Experimental production of neurofibrillary degeneration. *Journal of Neuropathology and Experimental Neurology, 24,* 200–210.

Van Broeckhoven, C., Backhovens, H., Cruts, M., DeWinter, G., Bruyland, M., Crass, P. L., & Martin, J. J. (1992). Mapping of a gene predisposing to early-onset Alzheimer's disease to chromosome 14q24.3. *Natural Genetics, 2,* 335–339.

Vicoroff, J. I. (1991). Neurological evaluation. In J. Sadavoy, L. W. Lazarus, & L. F. Jarvik (Eds.), *Comprehensive review of geriatric psychiatry* (pp. 197–222). Washington, DC: American Psychiatric Press.

Weiss, G. (1991). Attention deficit hyperactivity disorders. In M. Lewis (Ed.), *Child and adolescent psychiatry: A comprehensive textbook.* Baltimore: Williams & Wilkins.

Wells, C. E. (1985a). Overview of organic mental disorders. In H. I. Kaplan & B. J. Sadock (Eds.), *Comprehensive textbook of psychiatry* (4th ed.). Baltimore: Williams & Wilkins.

Wells, C. E. (1985b). Organic syndromes: Delirium. In H. I. Kaplan & B. J. Sadock (Eds.), *Comprehensive textbook of psychiatry* (4th ed.). Baltimore: Williams & Wilkins.

Wurtman, R. J. (1985). Alzheimer's disease. *Scientific American, 252,* 62–74.

CHAPTER 14

The Client with a Personality Disorder

SYLVIA WHITING, Ph.D., R.N.,C.S.

OUTLINE

CHAPTER OBJECTIVES

Upon completion of this chapter, you will be able to:
1. Provide an inclusive definition of personality disorders, and differentiate between specific disorder clusters and the disorders within each cluster.
2. Discuss theories relative to possible or probable causes underlying the development and symptom manifestation of personality disorders throughout the life span.
3. Discuss epidemiological information concerning personality disorders.
4. Recognize the need for nursing research in the field of personality disorders.

KEY TERMS

Acting out
Attachment theory
Character
Dysphoria
Ego dystonic
Ego syntonic
Evoked potentials
Internalized relationships
Libidinal object constancy
Object relations
Organic disorders
Patterns
Personality
Psyche organizers
Reality principle
Serotonergic system
Splitting
Traits

Personality is reflected by a person's capacity and skill in managing activities of daily living. Individual responses and interactions to internal and external environmental demands are influenced by the constant interplay of genetic, neurobiological, and psychological factors.

Personality is defined as the characteristic and somewhat predictable traits influencing the cognitive, affective, and behavioral **patterns** of human beings. These patterns evolve over time, are conscious or unconscious, and impact adaptation and response to the environment (American Psychiatric Association [APA], 1994). Adaptation is a central core of all personality theories. Individual adaptation may be adaptive or maladaptive. ***Character*** is generated by early life experiences and is represented by learned personality traits that influence behavioral patterns (Hirschfield, 1986).

Hartmann (1958) considered the mastering of reality to be the basis of adaptation, and he related adaptation to productivity, enjoyment of life, and maintenance of homeostasis. Stress is an integral aspect of living; one's capacity to handle it effectively begins at birth and evolves throughout life. Hartmann asserted that the ***reality principle*** and its relationship to adaptive responses was integral to life and that the struggle to adjust to environmental disruption was an effort to maintain stability. He concluded that "every stimulus disrupts equilibrium, but not every stimulus causes conflict" (Hartmann, 1958, p. 38).

Adaptive personality traits function to maintain homeostasis through healthy interactions. Everyone is capable of adapting to stress, but the level of adaptation is influenced by one's personality structure or **traits.** Maladaptive responses influence and often hamper a person's interpersonal relationships and increase the level of internal stress or the various crises that are thus experienced. Flexibility is needed in dealing with environmental pressures, and the narrowness or rigidity in one's range of responses influences the kind of coping mechanisms demonstrated by the person.

Maladaptive behavioral patterns are the hallmark of personality disorders and are manifested by the degree of rigidity or inflexibility that exists in attitudes and behaviors in the person's coping styles. Once a personality trait is established, it is extremely resistant, but not impossible, to change.

Numerous assumptions have been made regarding personality development. The evolution of personality is a complex issue. It challenges nurses working with clients at various stages of life and requires understanding of adaptive and maladaptive responses that clients use to minimize distress and emotional upheaval.

DEFINITIONS OF PERSONALITY DISORDERS

Kernberg (1984) defined personality disorders as a spectrum of maladaptive traits that produce or influence considerable psychological and emotional disturbance and impair relationships. The 1994 *Diagnostic and Statistical Manual of Mental Disorders* (DSM-IV) (APA) described personality disorders as "personality traits [that] are inflexible and maladaptive and cause either significant functional impairment or subjective distress" (p. 630).

Maladaptive responses such as inflexibility and rigidity are pathological and induce intense anxiety, distress, and depression in clients. Also, these same responses cause difficulty in adapting to environmental stressors, and the ability to perform at optimal levels is compromised. Some clients experience lifelong difficulty in adapting to change and crises and in sustaining meaningful relationships.

Clients often deny existing problems and usually lack insight into their maladaptive behaviors. These behaviors are symptoms that usually are **ego syntonic** (i.e., comfortable for the person but usually uncomfortable for others) and thus acceptable because they represent aspects of the clients' personality that have become typical and gratifying for them. Clients with personality disorders differ from other clients who experience anxiety, depression, or other emotional disorders because the latter experience an uncomfortable and unacceptable **ego-dystonic** state that forces them to seek psychotherapeutic assistance. Because personality-disordered clients are usually comfortable with themselves and their behaviors, they do not recognize the need for, nor do they desire, a change in their condition. These clients usually tax the mental and physical resources of those in charge of their care. They often have an uncanny ability to create crisis and uproar. Nurses and other professionals are challenged in developing innovative treatment strategies that meet the needs and demands of these clients.

PREVALENCE OF PERSONALITY DISORDERS

Many reasons exist for a high prevalence of hospitalized clients with a personality disorder. Although personality-disordered clients may not seek therapeutic assistance, there are many reasons why they require treatment or may be hospitalized. They tend to engage in risky behaviors and may attempt suicide, abuse substances, participate in dangerous activities, or have cognitive-perceptual impairments. As discussed later in the section on specific personality disorders and treatment modalities (see also Table 14–5), clients with personality disorders are diagnosed according to three behavioral clusters (Gunderson, 1988):

1. Odd and eccentric (schizoid, paranoid, schizotypal)
2. Dramatic, emotional, and erratic (histrionic, narcissistic, antisocial, borderline)
3. Anxious, fearful, and introverted (avoidant, dependent, obsessive-compulsive, passive-aggressive)

It is possible to find combinations of these conditions in one person. Clients falling diagnostically within these clusters often present the dilemma of where they should be placed when their behavior brings them to the attention of various social agencies. It is not unusual to hear an official question whether the person belongs in jail or in a hospital. Many end up in prison at the end of a crime spree or some lesser injudicious act, and often they are not likely to receive treatment that might restore them to a healthier position in society.

Widiger and Rogers (1989) suggested the need for assessment of personality disorders in all clients because their prevalence in hospital settings is so great. There are few trained clinicians available for accomplishing this task, however. Studies have shown that researchers who use structured interviews have higher rates of diagnosing personality disorders than do those who merely use client charts (Pfohl et al, 1986; Widiger & Frances, 1987).

It is difficult to obtain prevalence data for personality disorders because of what Gunderson (1988) described as "idiosyncratic or outdated diagnostic systems" that make interpretation difficult. He emphasized the need for caution in the categorization of these disorders because of the inadequacy in the current diagnostic system and decried the fact that a weak empirical base exists currently. However, he has made an attempt to describe the disorders and to provide what information is available relative to prevalence data. Table 14–1 provides a summary of Gunderson's (1988) presentation of available information relative to the 11 personality disorders. He estimated that 15 percent of the general population are likely to meet the criteria for one or more of the personality disorders and that the prevalence rate is likely to increase to between 30 and 50 percent of outpatient and inpatient populations.

Personality disorders often coexist with other personality disorders or with disorders such as major depression, bipolar disorder, and dysthymia (Bellodi et al., 1992; Docherty et al., 1986). Reich (1992) stated that most researchers report that patients who qualify as having one personality disorder usually qualify for two or three additional ones as well. He also stated that "all borderlines are not equivalent" (p. 141). The high prevalence of these disorders suggests the need for greater attention to them by nurses not only for treatment but as areas for research.

CAUSATIVE FACTORS: PERSPECTIVES AND THEORIES

As with other psychiatric disorders, there is no clear-cut single cause of personality disorders. There seem to be different etiological bases for the conditions, with a genetic predisposition most likely for some (e.g., schizotypal and paranoid), environmental causes more likely in others (e.g., narcissism, borderline, dependent, and passive-aggressive), and with mixed causes for still others (e.g., antisocial and obsessive-compulsive). Temperament seems to play a significant role in the etiology of some of these conditions in certain clients. The psychodynamic impact of childhood trauma appears to play a role in many personality-disordered cli-

TABLE 14–1
Available Prevalence Data for Personality Disorders

TYPE OF PERSONALITY DISORDER	PREVALENCE
Paranoid	Unknown
Schizotypal	2–6% inferred from familial studies, but symptoms often overlap with other personality disorders, especially borderline. Twin studies indicate genetic origin
Schizoid	Data suggest 2% or more of the general population; occurs more frequently in males than in females
Narcissistic	Unknown, but symptoms are commonly noted in outpatient settings
Antisocial	2–3% lifetime prevalence and 4–7 times more frequent in males than in females; more prevalent in urban than in rural areas; peak prevalence occurs at ages 24–44 years and decreases sharply in the 45 years of age and older group
Borderline	2–4% prevalence within the general population and three times more frequent in females than in males; the most common personality disorder in outpatient and inpatient populations, constituting from 15–25% of all patients. Most disruptive symptoms diminish over time from the 30s and later
Histrionic	Unknown; much more common in females than in males
Avoidant	Rarely used as a primary diagnosis, but behaviors that meet the criteria for this disorder are commonly seen in outpatient and inpatient populations
Dependent	Early estimates by other investigators (Langner & Michael, 1963) suggested 2.5%; noted more commonly in females than in males
Obsessive-compulsive	Between 2–3% of the general population have identifiable symptoms, with approximately 3/4 of these with symptoms severe enough to be diagnosed as a disorder; more common in females than in males, and more prevalent in people with higher education levels or IQs. Unusual in inpatients, but commonly noted in outpatients

Data from Gunderson, J. G. (1988). Personality disorders. In A. M. Nicholi (Ed.), *The new Harvard guide to psychiatry* (pp. 337–357). Cambridge, MA: Belknap Press.

ents, as do psychosocial factors that, when negative, add to the distress of a growing child. Finally, there is a great deal of research and a growing body of evidence that there are neurobiological effects in some of the conditions, as demonstrated by response to certain types of pharmacological agents. The matter of clear-cut causes continues to be controversial because it is likely that there is much overlap and interplay between internal and external factors (Gunderson, 1988). The literature suggests that personality disorders represent complex entities that challenge nurses and all mental health professionals to assess all maladaptive behaviors and develop an array of creative interventions that facilitate adaptive coping patterns in such clients.

PSYCHODYNAMIC THEORIES

Until the 1970s, Sigmund Freud was the most noted psychoanalytical theorist. Many of his followers and many of those who defected as followers in later years also contributed to the early school of thought regarding personality development. Freud (1961) proposed that the personality developed by a progression through psychosexual stages known as oral, anal, and genital (or oedipal).

Other theorists suggested that these progressions were psychosocial in nature—that is, they were driven by forces other than the libidinal drives proposed by Freud. Harry Stack Sullivan, for instance, suggested that the nature of the relationship between mother and child was the crucial factor in a healthy progression of the infant's or child's development. Erik Erikson (1963) proposed a bridge between developmental stages and social functioning or adaptation. He contended that adaptive responses influenced developmental progression.

Other theorists who made significant contributions to developmental theory during this era included Klein, Mahler, Kernberg, and Bowlby. More recently, an increasing amount of attention has been given to areas such as ego psychology, self-psychology, temperament, and genetics.

Melanie Klein. An English psychiatrist, Klein (1977) contributed to the evolution of the **object relations** concept. Her early work focused on the study of personality development as a transformation of primitive object relations. Object relations, defined in simple terms, are **internalized relationships** recollected from early primary caregivers. This relationship is surmised to be the core of the person's existence, "all other human behavior and experiences . . . are relational derivatives" (Greenberg & Mitchell, 1983, p. 404). Early relationships with caregivers are postulated to be the most significant determinants of the person's ability to adapt and reach optimal growth and health. They are also associated with "emotional gratification (and deprivation) . . . and are believed to form the template for all subsequent relationships" (Cashdan, 1988, p. 23).

Margaret Mahler. Mahler's contribution to psychoanalytical theory also centers around her extensive research and study of object relations. Her work with emotionally ill children allowed her to assess normal growth and development that centered on the faulty object relations between the mother and the child during early infancy. She proposed that bonding and early childhood separation (separation-individuation) laid the foundation for growth, adaptation, and all subsequent relationships. Mahler (1952, 1965a, 1965b) delineated the following three major developmental stages:

1. Autistic (birth to several weeks, when the infant is unaware of others)
2. Symbiotic (when the infant is concerned primarily with meeting basic needs but aware of primary caregiver)
3. Separation–individuation (includes several phases centering around autonomy)

She postulated that successful resolution of the final stage facilitates internalization of the primary caregiver and allows the child to maintain an image of the caregiver when absent. She named this process ***libidinal object constancy,*** a process that allows the child to introject positive and negative images that influence future perceptions of experience and resultant attitudes.

Successful accomplishment of this task serves as the foundation for the child's ability to function independently of primary caregivers and form subsequent healthy interpersonal relationships. In contrast, unsuccessful or incomplete resolution of this task of integrating the primary caregiver as a model image places the child at risk for developing adult maladaptive behavioral patterns such as responding in an overly dependent or independent manner. Klein, a contemporary of Mahler's, termed the inability to achieve resolution as *faulty early object relations* and noted that people with this problem eventually develop psychopathology. These early childhood interactions influence the person's capacity to cope with emotional distress, experience pleasure, and care for others.

Otto Kernberg. Kernberg's (1976, 1984) contribution to object relations theory has been noted in numerous publications and papers. He concurred with other object relation theorists and noted that the basis of severe personality disorders was related to inadequate or impaired object relations that are ingrained in the personality. He also emphasized that the basis for understanding psychological adaptability and integrity stems from the child's relationship with primary caregivers.

John Bowlby. Bowlby's (1969, 1981) **attachment theory** also presented the belief that the infant's relationship with early caregivers influences later interactions. He contended that the function of attachment behavior is a process for the protection and development of early ego function. He further stated that by the end of the first year of life the child has internalized cognitive models of himself or herself and others. Early experiences play crucial roles in children's inferences about their value and acceptability. Additionally, Bowlby (1951) surmised that early experiences with primary caregivers provides the basis for appraisals of all future social interactions and situations throughout the life span.

Bowlby viewed attachment behavior as a natural response in periods when certain needs exist. For example, he considered it natural for people to seek closeness during times of illness and did not consider these behaviors to be regressive or maladaptive as other psychoanalysts had proposed. On the other hand, Bowlby proposed that infants who have healthy interactions with primary caregivers are trusting and able to form enduring, mutually satisfying, and close interpersonal relationships with others in adulthood. Those who have unhealthy interactions with primary caregivers are expected to have difficulty in forming relationships and maintaining closeness; they often experience distrust, fears, and intense anxiety.

Understanding ego development or organization is fundamental to the capacity for adapting effectively to internal and external stressors. Evaluating ego function is a major aspect of the nursing process because it provides data that assist in making accurate diagnoses, planning psychotherapeutic interventions, and bringing about therapeutic outcomes. Table 14–2 provides a framework for assessing ego function. This assessment considers the components of interpersonal relationships, affective capabilities, motivation for treatment, capacity for introspection, insight, defensive behavior, and reality testing.

NEUROBIOLOGICAL THEORIES

Arguments and shifts in beliefs about the personality have occurred throughout the centuries. Hippocrates (c. 460–c. 375 B.C.) asserted that the four body humors—blood, yellow and black bile, and phlegm—were the balancing or homeostatic determinants for a person's behavior. Freudian psychoanalytical theory evolved in the 1880s and prevailed until the 1970s as the dominant theory of personality development. Researchers now dispute the theory that personality is caused solely by psychosocial factors, and evidence exists that suggests neurochemicals influence the development of personality. Several studies have demonstrated that personality disorders have biological, psychosocial, and situational origins (see the Research Abstract display on p. 292.)

Neurotransmitters such as serotonin and dopamine have been associated with the impulsivity, aggression, and suicidal gestures manifested in disordered personalities, especially borderline and antisocial types (Mann et al., 1990). Several studies have demonstrated that low serotonin levels correlated with impulsive and aggressive behaviors. In addition, patients with borderline and antisocial personality disorders have been found to have low platelet levels of monoamine oxidase (which metabolizes dopamine), resulting in higher than normal levels of dopamine, an arousal neurotransmitter (Kaplan & Sadock, 1989).

Kendler et al. (1981) investigated the genetic association of schizotypal personality disorder and found a concordance similar to that of schizophrenic clients. Additional biological similarities exist between clients with schizophrenia and schizotypal personality disorder, such as impaired information processing and abnormal eye movement (Holzman et al., 1984; Siever et al., 1990).

Neuroendocrine studies using the dexamethasone suppression test and the thyrotropin-stimulating hormone test used to diagnose depression have recently been applied to personality-disordered clients and have shown abnormalities that suggest a relationship between disordered personality and depressed mood (Garbutt et al., 1983; Soloff et al., 1982). Additional neurobiological evidence includes a higher incidence of abnormal electroencephalogram waveforms in the temporal and frontal lobe regions in clients with borderline personality disorder when compared with control subjects. Other studies have shown that some clients with antisocial and borderline personality disorders have abnormal evoked potentials (Kutcher et al., 1987; Raine & Venables, 1988). However, Gunderson et al. (1979) found no abnormalities on computed tomography scan in 26 clients who met the criteria for borderline personality disorder, and there continues to be inconclusive evidence of a clear relationship between personality disorders and neurobiological findings.

TABLE 14–2
Assessment of Ego Function

	HIGH	MODERATE	LOW
Quality of Interpersonal Relationships			
Affective Capability of the Ego			
Motivation for Treatment			
Capacity for Introspection			
Insight			
Use of Major Defense Mechanisms			
Capacity for Reality Testing			

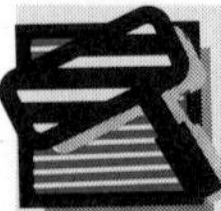

RESEARCH ABSTRACT

Organic Brain Dysfunction and the Borderline Syndrome

Andrulonis, P. A., Glueck, B. C., Stroebel, C. F., Vogel, N. G., Shapiro, A. L., & Aldridge, D. (1981). *Psychiatric Clinics of North America*, *4*, 47–66.

Neurobehavioral Study of Borderline Personality Disorder

van Reekum, R. (1990). Paper presented at the Annual Meeting of the Canadian Psychiatric Association, Toronto.

A 1981 study conducted by Andrulonis et al. examined neurological factors viewed as specific to the development of borderline personality disorder (BPD). The study consisted of retrospective chart review of 91 subjects diagnosed with BPD. The subjects' charts were divided into three categories: (1) a nonorganic group; (2) a minimal brain dysfunction (MBD) group and (3) an organic pathology group (subjects with histories of brain trauma, encephalitis, or epilepsy).

Results demonstrated that MBD or brain pathology occurred in 38% of the subjects. Gender differences were noted: 40% of males compared with 14% of females had attention deficit disorder or learning disabilities, or both, and 52% of males compared with 28% of females had current histories of organic pathology. The researchers concluded that BPD subjects with MBD are predominantly men with an earlier onset of emotional and functional deficits based partially on constitutional deficits.

A 1990 study by van Reekum comparing 48 subjects with BPD with 50 subjects without BPD revealed that the BPD subjects demonstrated a significantly greater prevalence of developmental and acquired brain insults. The author suggested that there may be a correlation between borderline symptoms (impulsivity, cognitive inflexibility, decreased self-monitoring problems, and perseveration) and frontal system dysfunction.

GENETICS

The literature suggests that there are genetic links for certain personality traits such as criminality and other antisocial behavior. Adoption and twin studies suggest a genetic base for antisocial personality (Cadoret et al., 1985). Some twin studies have demonstrated higher incidences of personality disorders among monozygotic twins than dizygotic twins. These findings also suggest a genetic basis for personality disorders (Bouchard et al., 1990; McGuffin & Gottesman, 1984). Other factors are also attributed to criminality, such as alcoholism, family violence, and socioeconomic factors (Le Blanc, 1992).

Goldsmith (1983) has asserted that many adoption and twin studies fall short of providing demonstrable evidence of the link between genetics and personality disorders. He contended that it is difficult to discern the effects of environmental or parental roles and genetics in twin studies. In this regard, Gunderson (1988) stated that "twin and adoptive studies have pointed to a genetic predisposition to this disorder but have also indicated that its development can be modified by good parental care" (p. 347).

Temperament refers to innate, genetically based aspects of personality considered as influential to personality development (Hirschfield, 1986). Thomas and Chess (1977) stressed the impact of temperament as a basis for behavioral disorders and determined that underlying general medical conditions in children that are manifested as personality disorders or behavioral problems increase the likelihood of passivity, hyperactivity, or distractibility. They (1977) also surmised that temperamental differences make themselves apparent within the first few months of life and become much more dramatic in the second 6 months of life.

Thomas and Chess (1977) also associated temperament with a mismatch between the child and the environment. For instance, an anxious child who has an anxious mother is more vulnerable to developing a personality disorder. They attributed this to ineffective parenting styles of parents who are immature and inconsistent. Inadequate parental roles foster family systems that are chaotic and inconsistent. Children from these families often experience intense feelings of anger, abuse, and abandonment.

THE ROLE OF CHILD ABUSE

A number of studies have found a high prevalence of child abuse in the histories of clients with maladaptive behaviors. Clients with borderline personality disorders have a high rate of early childhood traumas. Several studies have demonstrated a significant prevalence of sexual abuse among female clients diagnosed with borderline personality disorders, ranging from 67 percent to 86 percent in the borderline population. In gender-mixed samples, the prevalence of clients reporting histories of physical abuse ranged from 46 to 71 percent (Herman et al., 1989; Shearer et al., 1990; Terr, 1991; Zanarini et al., 1989

Studies of children and adolescents diagnosed with borderline personality disorder provide strong support for the detrimental impact of early childhood traumas on development. Early traumas identified from these studies included chaotic families, abuse in all forms for extended periods, rejection, and attachment issues (Greenman et al., 1986; Herman et al., 1989; Ludolph et al., 1990). Childhood histories of adults who exhibit violent behaviors reveal sexual abuse in their childhood to a large degree (Rubinstein et al., 1993). These findings are consistent with those in other studies of the long-term effects of childhood traumas.

Clients with personality disorders such as borderline and antisocial types exhibit a wide array of maladaptive behaviors such as substance abuse, suicidal gestures, and other self-destructive behaviors. Nursing implications in working with these types of clients require attention to the following:

- Understanding factors associated with personality development
- Recognizing the impact of early childhood traumas on coping styles
- Dealing with intense reactions that occur when working with these clients
- Working with other mental health professionals to develop innovative treatment plans

Assessing personality development entails examining the life span and factors such as early relationships with primary caregivers, the impact of these relationships on ego development, and adaptation and coping styles. Clients with personality disorders are often labeled as difficult because of their need for immediate gratification, their lack of empathy, and the intense affect they use in their frequent outbursts of hostility. They are often noted for **splitting**—a behavior that involves setting up others against each other; it is almost as if they are saying, "Let's you and him fight." It is not uncommon for those with a borderline personality disorder to create splitting among staff members such that the staff become engaged in a serious conflict concerning the appropriate management of the client. Such behaviors often arouse intense negative reactions (countertransference) in nurses and other caregivers.

Understanding the origins of these behaviors can play a key role in minimizing negative reactions toward these clients who are experts in evoking tension in nurses and other professionals. Working with these clients needs to be perceived as a challenge rather than as a burden because it allows nurses to sharpen their skills in patience, self-awareness, creativity, and nonjudgmental approach. Above all, the staff must develop a treatment plan that does not allow for splitting of staff; to accomplish this, they must confer together frequently.

Most personality theories, regardless of their differences, emphasize the significance of primary caregivers in child growth and development. The child must master the initial demands for socialization within the family, where the foundation is laid for the emergence of interpersonal relations with all others. These early interactions mediate the infant's perception of the world (Thomas & Chess, 1977). Understanding key concepts in personality formation such as ego development and organization is crucial for nurses who must assess the meaning of maladaptive behaviors, facilitate adaptive coping behaviors, and evaluate client responses to interventions.

PERSONALITY DISORDERS ACROSS THE LIFE SPAN

The personality is believed to have its origins in the prenatal period. Early childhood experiences and interactions further lay the foundation for the ability to adapt to stress and change and engage in healthy interpersonal relationships. Erikson (1963) stated that the basic component in developing a healthy personality is trust. He described trust as the major issue in personality development because it serves as the basis for expecting that one's needs will be met, that safety will be provided, and that primary caregivers are reliable. His developmental theory describes trust during the first year of life as the foundation for adaptive responses throughout the life span. Freud (1961) divided the personality into three structures: the id, the ego, and the superego. The id is almost totally unconscious and consists of innate drives. It serves the newborn well relative to survival needs with demands for hunger, protection, and warmth and the need for immediate gratification. Characteristics of the id include forces that are unpredictable, spontaneous, creative, uncontrollable, and potentially destructive. Freud contended that the infant does not have the capacity to modulate the drive to gratify instinctual needs.

Freud's oral stage parallels Erikson's stage of trust. During the oral stage, the infant is totally dependent on primary caregivers for survival. It is during this period that the primary caregiver's capacity to nurture and modulate the infant's early emotional, psychological, and neurobiological needs is so important to the infant's survival and emotional development. During the formative years, ego structures (or defense mechanisms) evolve that serve as the basis for modulating affect, dealing with anxiety, mediating thought processes, and activating adaptive responses (see Chapter 2).

Ego Function and Structure. Spitz (1951) proposed that primary caregivers serve as the infant's auxiliary ego, imparting valuable information about the child's world (environment). He also perceived this early parental role as the infant's protective shield by which overwhelming stimuli are minimized.

Ego Mediation of the Id and the Superego. The ego serves as the mediator between the id and the superego in efforts to protect the psyche from intense anxiety and stress. Healthy ego function allows people to adapt to their internal and external environments effectively. The major task of the ego is to maintain homeostasis between internal and external structures. Strong ego function is essential to maturation and to adaptive coping behaviors. Other roles of the ego include channeling mental processes and serving as the core for facilitating adaptive responses in people (Hartmann, 1958).

The superego is totally learned as the child develops in society. It is both conscious and unconscious, but it functions primarily at the unconscious level. Its core components consist of ideals, values, and a moral sense of right and wrong. The child's psychic repertoire of the superego is also influenced by early interactions with primary caregivers, and it evolves throughout childhood and early adolescence. Additionally, the child integrates early identifications through contact with primary caregivers, admired people, teachers, and heroes, and it is in this manner that the foundation for moral standards, values, and ideals is laid. The child's capac-

TABLE 14–3
Comparison of Healthy and Unhealthy Ego Functions

	HEALTHY EGO FUNCTIONING (MATURE)	UNHEALTHY EGO FUNCTIONING (PRIMITIVE)
Defense Mechanisms (conflict resolution)	Repression Sublimation Rationalization Displacement Reaction formation Undoing	Denial Projection Splitting Dissociation Isolation Regression Avoidance Conversion
Modulation of Affect/Impulsivity	Postpones gratification needs Tolerates frustration and stress Maintains gratification through sublimation	Low frustration and stress tolerance Poor impulse control Need for immediate gratification
Self-Esteem (competence)	Mastery of environment Sense of self-worth and confidence	Poor self-esteem Fluctuation in self-worth
Relationship to Others (depth of relationships)	Capacity for object relations Empathic Stable, lasting relationships Capacity to mourn and form new relationships	Places own needs before others Lack of empathy Chaotic relationships Inability to relate to others
Reality Testing	Accurate perceptions and appraisal of inner mental state (insight) Intact ego boundaries Sense of reality	Distorted perceptions Depersonalization Lack of insight into present Fluid ego boundaries Derealization
Cognitive Processes (thinking, learning, judgment)	Tolerates stress Capacity to integrate new experiences Tolerates inconsistency and incongruency in others	Poor tolerance to stress Low capacity to integrate new experiences Rigid, inflexible thinking

ity to integrate these processes will determine the child's ultimate character (Hartmann, 1958).

A person's personality structures represent the degree to which integration of the id, the ego, and the superego has occurred. This integrative process is highly dependent on all the forces that impinge on development. The person's capacity to respond to internal and external stressors throughout life is largely dependent on the degree of integration, and the ability to adapt to stress in healthy ways is crucial in reducing the person's level of distress and maladaptive responses.

If the child perceives the world as loving, accepting, and safe, a healthy ego is likely to evolve. This is a complex process and entails the child's learning how to deal with frustration as well as gratification. Early childhood traumas include conditions such as deprivation, abandonment, abuse, and overindulgence; these conditions hamper the child in developing healthy ego structure. See Table 14–3 for a comparison of healthy and unhealthy ego functions.

INFANCY

Metcalf (1979) has described the concept of **psyche organizers** (an idea originally described by Spitz [1951]) that is concerned with the critical biopsychological periods of development. This is another way of saying that a biopsychological process takes place throughout early development. EEG measurements of these developmental changes are possible. Researchers have determined that it is possible to draw a parallel between EEG development (i.e., brain development) and emotional and psychological development. Research was conducted to obtain EEG data from 80 children who were followed from birth through mid-adolescence. These researchers observed that it is common to find various aberrations in EEGs of normal infants and children and that these variations disappear during early adolescence (Metcalf, 1979). Metcalf (1979) stated that "all experience subsequent to the operation of a new psychic organizer is differently organized than prior to that time in development; it is as if the very reality with which the individual deals is now altered" (p. 64). The particular criterion that must be met to serve as psychic organizer is that of a specific affective behavior. The occurrence of a specific affective behavior (e.g., smiling or, later, stranger anxiety) indicates that a new psychic organizer is present that permits the development to progress. This process leads to a new stage of development, or "psychological organization." The presence of such an affective signal is required to indicate that an intrapsychic change is occurring and that development can proceed to the next level (Metcalf, 1979).

Emde and Robinson (1979) summarized infant research completed in the 1970s by stating that infants are more active than passive and have a preformed organization, rhythmically organized behaviors, and internal states associated with the organization. These authors note a qualitative difference before and after 2 months of age such that classic conditioning is difficult in the early period and not difficult at all after 2 months of age.

Consider, for instance, the erratic sleep patterns of 1-month-old newborns in comparison with those of many 2-month-old infants, who may be sleeping all night as well as demonstrating other pattern regularities.

During the second 6 months of life, the infant definitely prefers and attaches to the maternal figure (Provence, 1979). The infant's awareness and discrimination intensify as an indication of cognitive development and the strengthened maturation of aggressive and libidinal drives. Although self-concept is difficult to measure in infants, nevertheless, there seems to be strong evidence of happy expectation and of satisfaction with self and others in the infant who has been well nurtured. Also, there is evidence of an increasing variety and number of emotional states such as joy, sadness, anxiety, distaste, perplexity, anger, and reproach (Provence, 1979).

When the nurturing caregiver is absent, the child withdraws and may refuse to enter into any relationship. Allnutt (1979) stated that in the absence of an appropriate substitute mother, there is withdrawal of the infant or child and "progressive ego deficits ensue" (p. 376). Thus, the opportunity for trust development is either seriously compromised or diminished altogether.

CHILDHOOD

As the child becomes mobile and realizes that he or she is separate from primary caregivers, a sense of separateness evolves. The child still needs to be reassured by a caregiver's encouraging and applauding steps the child takes toward independence. Healthy families provide this approval and allow the child to wander off in the room with the idea that he or she can return at any time for emotional refueling. Unhealthy families, on the other hand, may be threatened by this newfound sense of freedom and punish the child either by emotional abandonment or other forms of abuse.

The second year is also the period of language acquisition; Miller (1979) stated that it is "the prime example of a rule-directed organization of the ego" (p. 127). Miller referred to other theorists who propose that ego is a *vocal-auditory apparatus,* and it would be difficult to argue that speech and hearing do not strongly influence the way in which one perceives the environment. Furthermore, the thinking aspect of the person is strongly influenced by language. Miller stated that the "concept-matching scheme" and "concept formation" both are parts of a process whereby the ego is enhanced.

Children with early faulty ego development frequently maintain primitive defense mechanisms such as projection, ambivalence, regression, splitting, acting out, and denial. These mechanisms often represent the child's survival tools, and they often persist throughout the life span. These early defense mechanisms are used to ward off bad feelings, depression, anxiety, rage, and intense emotional pain.

Kernberg (1984) has attested that clients use these defense mechanisms to protect the ego from intrapsychic (mental) conflicts by rejecting advice from the unconscious ego. Using primitive defense mechanisms decreases the optimal functioning of the ego structure and further compromises the ability to use adaptive coping behaviors such as crying, talking things out, acknowledging one's own failures or weaknesses, changing the weaknesses or the situation if needed, negotiating, laughing at oneself, and asking forgiveness. The primitive defense mechanisms most often resorted to by clients with borderline personality disorder are splitting and blaming; clients with paranoid personality disorder often resort to projection, and antisocial personalities use repression and denial to a great extent.

Children with faulty ego structures or maladaptive coping patterns often present with behavioral symptoms or conduct disorder. Their histories are frequently dominated by chaotic or dysfunctional family systems. Some psychodynamic theorists suggest a parallel between early childhood traumas and early object losses as common factors in the histories of clients with personality disorders (Freud, 1957; Kernberg, 1984; Masterson, 1976). Many of these losses are attributed to mental illness, substance abuse, and indifference in primary caregivers (Parker, 1984).

It seems appropriate to add the problem of ignorance as another factor in considering causes associated with loss. One of the most important tasks of a lifetime is raising healthy children and yet less attention is given to training in this area than in any other work endeavor. Presently, in the United States the parental role is often given only lip service. Most primary caregivers are female, and these caregivers are underpaid and undervalued. This situation causes concern that the problem of personality disorders rooted in inadequate child care may persist if societal values do not change.

Childen reared in these circumstances usually have poor self-esteem, are distrustful, and have poor social skills. Psychodynamic theorists agree that children with faulty ego function have a developmental arrest that begins in early childhood. The role of psychiatric nurses includes assessing areas of impairment, and the process begins by approaching clients and their significant others in a caring, nonjudgmental manner. This approach facilitates trust building and enhances the potential success of treatment plan outcomes.

Many of these children have disruptive behavior disorders. The DSM-IV (APA, 1994) lists the following diagnoses in this category:

Conduct disorder
  Childhood-onset type
  Adolescent-onset type
Disruptive behavior disorder not otherwise specified

Conduct Disorders

The DSM-IV identifies the essential feature of a conduct disorder as a repetitive and persistent pattern of behavior that violates the basic rights of others or major age-appropriate norms or rules. Certain specific behaviors (at least three) such as lying, truancy, staying out after dark without permission, stealing, vandalism, forced sex, physical cruelty, and use of weapons must have been present during the previous 12 months. The behaviors are grouped according to severity levels of mild, moderate, and severe (APA, 1994). These behaviors are also manifestations of an antisocial personality disorder in clients 18 years of age and older.

Conduct disorder is estimated to affect approximately 9 percent of boys and 2 percent of girls younger than 18 years of age. These children frequently have parents who are substance abusers or who also have antisocial personality disorders (Loeber, 1990).

Causes. The cause of conduct disorders falls into the following categories (Kay & Kay, 1986) (Fig. 14–1):

- Psychological—includes chaotic family dynamics, faulty ego structure (superego) (Keith, 1984), and a lack of parental empathy and affection
- Neurobiological—includes temperament (Cantrell, 1989), alterations in the central nervous system, and genetics (Kay & Kay, 1986)
- Sociological—consists of disturbed parent–child relationships marked by rejection and chaotic interactions (Dadds et al., 1992; Patterson, 1990), lower socioeconomic status, and alcoholism

Interventions and Outcomes. Kay and Kay (1986) have asserted that the prognosis for conduct disorder is poor. Robins (1978) stated that approximately 50 percent of children and adolescents with conduct disorders become adults with an antisocial personality and that the best predictor of antisocial behaviors in adults is that of childhood behaviors.

Conduct-disordered youth are difficult to work with, and they frequently tax the emotional resources of caregivers. They often lack empathy, concern, and anxiety. Their lack of trust and an inability to engage with healthy peers and adults present nurses with many challenges for devising ways to interact with them (Mishne, 1986).

The following are the desired outcomes:

- Establishing rapport
- Completing a comprehensive diagnostic workup (neurobiological, psychological, sociological)
- Understanding the meaning of behaviors and associated thoughts and feelings
- Maintaining a safe, supportive environment
- Improving ego function

Establishing rapport and trust is extremely difficult, but it is crucial if work with these youngsters is to progress. Nurses need to form an alliance with the child and the parents, even though the parent–child relationship is often tenuous. Dysfunctional family dynamics play a crucial role in maladaptive behaviors of children and adolescents (Mishne, 1986), and failure to intervene with parents often results in revictimization of the youngster. Family therapy may be the major treatment modality, or it may be an adjunct to individual therapy with the child.

Adolescents and children may test nurses and other staff by pressing them to break rules or by calling them derogatory names such as "nerd," "stupid," and "geek" in their refusal to comply with demands. Nurses must remain steadfast in rule enforcement and limit setting, and they must maintain their composure and be committed to understanding the meaning of the behaviors and motives. Impaired impulse control underlies **acting-out** behaviors. Children often tend to act rather than to think things out or to allow themselves to feel.

Nurses need to be actively involved in the assessment

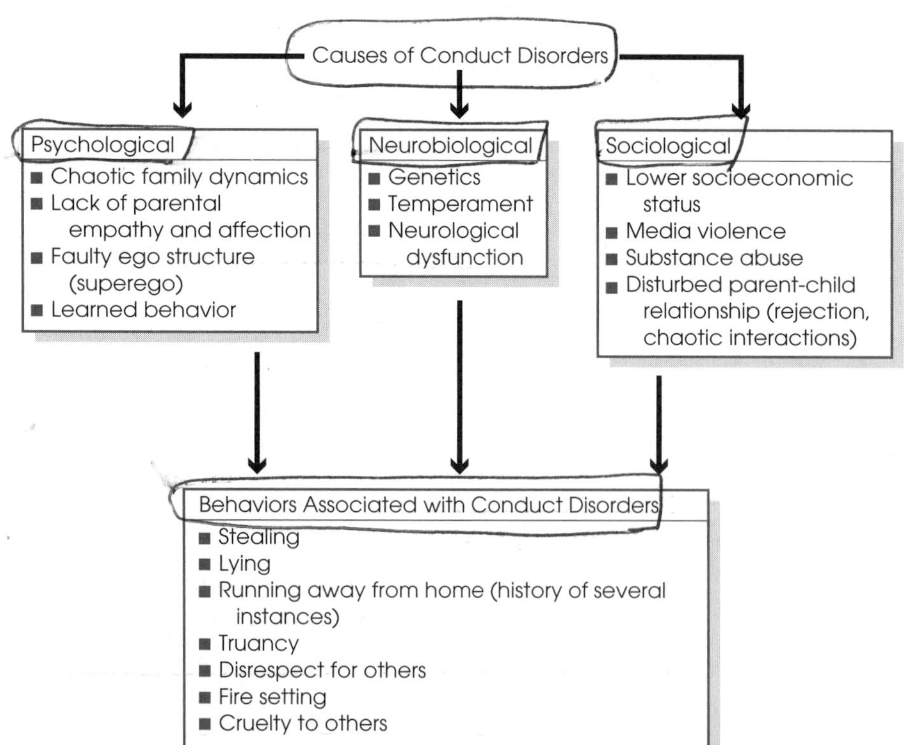

FIGURE 14–1
The interplay of psychological, sociological, and neurobiological factors in conduct disorders, and resulting behaviors (Data from American Psychiatric Association. [1994]. *Diagnostic and statistical manual of mental disorders.* [4th ed.]. Washington, DC: American Psychiatric Association.)

process to determine factors that contribute to the maladaptive behaviors of these children. This process helps in identifying treatment possibilities and determining the possible presence of conditions such as depression, seizure disorder, suicidal attempts, acting-out behaviors, and school problems. The client is likely to feel safe and accepted if the nurse assumes an accepting, nonjudgmental attitude during all interactions. Helping these children and their families appreciate the meaning of their maladaptive behaviors, feelings, and thoughts is crucial to facilitating adaptive responses from the youngster. He or she may ultimately gain insight if a safe and supportive environment is provided. Individual psychotherapy and a therapeutic milieu can foster opportunities for testing and growth as the process of introspection is encouraged and modeled. Group psychotherapy is a helpful intervention modality because it provides an opportunities for peer exchanges to be experienced and for leaders to model healthy behaviors.

Self-esteem is influenced by the experiences that have helped mold the ego. Children who can adapt to changes in their internal and external environments usually feel secure and demonstrate positive self-esteem. In contrast, youngsters with low self-esteem tend to perceive their environments as negative and threatening. Clients with low self-esteem may experience depression and faulty superego function. Building self-esteem is a continuous process and begins with initial contacts in the treatment setting and continues throughout treatment. Acceptance, patience, perseverance, and honest sharing of one's self and time are key ingredients in establishing trust and assisting in the process of improvement in the area of self-esteem in children with disruptive behaviors.

Because it is well known that conduct disorders are multifactorial (Kay & Kay, 1986), the single most crucial need is for a complete diagnostic evaluation. The evaluation should include the neurobiological, psychological, and sociological aspects of the child's history and present condition. Studies to determine the long-term effects of previous interventions such as psychotherapy, biological interventions, and intensive multimodal care should be completed (Kay & Kay, 1986). Juvenile violence remains the major predictor of adult violence (Loeber, 1990), so steps should be taken to assist the child in learning ways to solve problems without resorting to violence. Some important ongoing nursing studies have the intent of creating interventions that are helpful in decreasing violence in youth (Hardin et al., 1993).

Oppositional Defiant Disorder

The primary manifestations of oppositional defiant disorder (APA, 1994) are negative, hostile, and stubborn behaviors, such as

- Difficulty in controlling temper
- Frequent arguing with adults, including parents and teachers
- Frequent refusal to follow rules or to do chores or homework
- Frequently being purposefully annoying to others
- Being easily agitated or upset by others
- Frequent use of profanity

Causes. Weiss (1991) stated that oppositional defiant and conduct disorders co-occur with attention deficit hyperactive disorder (ADHD) in 40 percent or more of hyperactive children. Some investigators claim that these are all variants of the same disorder. Others have given evidence, although at times conflicting, that there is more neglect in conduct-disordered children than in children with oppositional defiant disorder or ADHD.

Finch and Green (1979) observed that children with oppositional defiant disorder develop a passive-aggressive response pattern in which there is chronic rebellion against rules and regulations. The oppositional traits, then, become ingrained and begin to spread to other areas. Finch and Green stated that the child's orientation is primarily anal and that the traits pervade every area of the child's life.

Kalogerakis (1974) reported a number of consistent findings in the families of children with these behaviors, including

- Parental rejection
- Conflict between parents and family chaos
- Punitive discipline
- Inconsistent discipline
- Low self-esteem in primary caregivers
- Defiance in parents
- Permissiveness or aggressiveness

As with other psychological conditions of childhood, medical and neurological examinations are suggested to rule out neurological disorders or other illnesses that may contribute to the behaviors. Psychosocial assessment should attend to the type and quality of parent–child interactions, parental skills in disciplining and rewarding, attachment behaviors, and the child's self-perception.

Because of their passive aggression and poor school performance, these children are often alienated from their peers. Their alienation, coupled with poor self-esteem places these children at risk for depression and self-destructive behaviors such as substance abuse, cult involvement, promiscuity, and suicide. They must be assessed for symptoms of depression and level of risk directed at either themselves or others throughout treatment.

Interventions and Outcomes. Nursing interventions should focus on establishing rapport with the child and parents, teaching parental skills in child management, and promoting positive self-esteem in the child and parents. These children are often searching for reasonable structure or for someone to help them self-regulate their behavior (Marohn, 1992). Realistic limits need to be set and consequences explained in an empathic manner. Therapeutic goals should be established as follows:

1. Establishing trust through a therapeutic relationship

2. Assisting parents to avoid the use of reinforcing behaviors toward the child
3. Helping the child to understand the meaning of self-destructive behaviors and obtaining a "no suicide" pact
4. Finding ways to restore self-esteem
5. Building adaptive coping behaviors in children and their parents

Interventions are most effective when they are begun early to prevent the strengthening of dysfunctional behaviors. The high prevalence rate of child abuse is a major concern to mental health caregivers not only because of its effect on the growing child but also because of the long-term effects on adult behaviors. Nursing interventions include prevention of abuse, assessment of clients for symptoms of abuse, assistance for the child in learning new coping skills, and provision of safety for children in distress.

ADOLESCENCE

Adolescence is characterized as a period of instability in which there are fluctuations of mood, behavior, and ideals. Psychiatric nurses are challenged to differentiate between age-appropriate adaptive and non–age-appropriate maladaptive behaviors. Adolescents demonstrate oppositional defiant and conduct disorders, but now the symptoms may intensify. Other aspects of treatment include assessing attitudes and the level of danger in acting-out behaviors and joining the interdisciplinary team in making a differential diagnosis.

Major stressors for adolescents include authority and control (separation-individuation issues). The younger adolescent is shifting from parents to peers, and the older one may be dealing with intimacy and sexual issues. Positive self-esteem is the core struggle in concert with the search for identity (Kalogerakis, 1992). Erikson (1963) identified the primary task of adolescence as identity and found that firm establishment of identity is dependent on the successful resolution of previous developmental tasks.

Impairments in ego and superego development are considered to be a major cause of maladaptive behavior. Erikson (1963) contended that if the adolescent were unable to attain a healthy identity, the result would be role confusion. Role confusion is another reason for the occurrence of maladaptive behavioral traits. These youngsters are frequently bored and frustrated, and they often experience difficulty dealing with intense feelings such as anxiety, fears, and intimacy (Mishne, 1986; Redl & Wineman, 1951). They also have distorted cognitions (impaired reality testing) and low self-esteem. Other maladaptive behaviors include using primitive defense mechanisms such as acting-out and expressing extreme hostility or aggression toward authority figures. Their ability to solve problems and to control immediate gratification needs (impulsivity) is impaired. Adolescents with personality disorders experience bouts of depression and anxiety and turn to risky tension-reducing activities, including substance abuse, sexual promiscuity, suicidal behaviors and attempts, and various other antisocial acts to help in coping with distress (Egan, 1986).

Assessing the adolescent's level of dangerousness is the same as for adults. Suicidal adolescents present clinicians with a serious emergency situation. Assessing the client's current stressors, the suicide plan, the available means for carrying out the act, and previous personal or family history of suicide and gestures can assist the health care team in making appropriate interventions. The risk of suicide is high—the third leading cause of death in this age group—and the seriousness of the problem is heightened by the impulsivity of youth. Although some adolescents give clear signals, many give none; therefore, if an adolescent is acting differently than is usual for him or her or has escalated acting-out behaviors, it may be a signal that he or she is in serious emotional trouble. If the family has established open communications, it may not be difficult to talk to the adolescent about what is being experienced. On the other hand, if communications of the adolescent and family members are generally closed and they share little together, or if the parents are too busy, a professional may be the only one who can succeed in making contact. As with adults who are suicidal, it is important to determine (1) lethality; (2) intent; (3) maladaptation or emotional instability; (4) association of feelings or behaviors with depression or impulsivity; (5) substance abuse; and (6) presence of depression or psychosis (Kalogerakis, 1992; Shaffer, 1988).

Adolescents with personality disorders can be demanding and disruptive in clinical settings. Many of their behaviors reflect their unconscious need to recreate their own dysfunctional family systems. Their insatiable need to verbally or behaviorally avoid and minimize intense feelings of anxiety or other emotional pain gives rise to great challenges for psychiatric nurses in developing a workable treatment plan for adolescents and their families.

Hospitalization of adolescents for specific personality disorders is indicated when they exhibit destructive behavior toward themselves and others and to property. These may be suicidal acts or threats to self, eating disorders, substance abuse, homicidal acts or threats to others, or destructiveness of property. Failure to respond to treatment, severe depression, psychosis, or severe family dysfunction may lead to inpatient care (Mishne, 1986; Rinsley, 1982).

Inpatient care may include a treatment center other than a hospital because there are fewer reimbursement mechanisms for inpatient care. Therefore, the adolescent may be referred to a residential treatment program or a group home, depending on the seriousness of the condition. Hospital care may be provided only long enough to complete a diagnostic workup. Inpatient care may be brief or long term. Short-term treatment focuses on crisis resolution, and long-term care focuses on the facilitation of behavioral change in the adolescent and his or her family. The overall aim is to minimize acting-out behaviors and to increase ego strengths. Egan (1986) stated that the following purposes are served when the adolescent's ego is strengthened:

- Increased impulse control
- Delayed need gratification
- Improved self-esteem
- Decreased feelings of dysphoria (sadness) and anxiety
- Increased problem-solving skills

Building ego capacity in adolescents and other age groups can be facilitated in therapy, and a variety of therapeutic modalities work successfully, such as individual, group, family, and milieu; activity and educational therapies; behavior modification; and pharmacology. Perhaps the most useful modality for staff nurses is milieu therapy because their function most often is to maintain the client's environment as a safe and therapeutic place. It is important to recognize the significance and particular difficulty inherent in this modality because it most closely simulates a family situation and will most likely elicit the typically difficult behaviors in need of on-the-spot interventions (which families often are unable to make). A detailed discussion of treatment is found in Chapters 21 to 24.

Pharmacological treatment depends on the adolescent's symptoms. For instance, if the youth presents with symptoms of depression, such as dysphoric mood and sleep and appetite disturbances, antidepressants may be prescribed. Symptoms such as aggressive or impulsive behavior may respond to carbamazepine (Tegretol), lithium, or haloperidol (Haldol). Lithium seems to be the drug of choice for treating adolescents or children with aggressive-hostile behaviors because it has fewer adverse effects (Campbell et al., 1984). Psychopharmacological agents are used as an adjunct to behavioral and psychosocial interventions to maximize the treatment. Specific information about psychotropic medications is discussed in Chapter 26

Working with adolescents can be an exhaustive experience. Their endless demands and limit testing tax the patience and fortitude of nurses and the health care team. Nurses and their staff members are probably the most vulnerable of the health care team because they are required to be on the unit with the adolescent throughout the 24-hour period instead of just for an hour or two at a time, as is true for other staff members. Strategies that help maximize resources when working with demanding clients include the following:

- Examining personal reactions to these clients
- Determining the meaning of client behaviors
- Participating in professional and peer supervision activities to sort out feelings and reactions
- Having sufficient time and opportunity to take care of professional needs
- Developing realistic client outcomes

ADULTHOOD

Erikson (1963) divided adulthood into several developmental tasks, including early adulthood (ages 20 to 40 years), middle adulthood (ages 40 to 65 years), and late adulthood (older than 65 years of age). Intimacy and generativity were described by Erikson as the developmental stages for early and middle adulthood.

As previously mentioned, healthy adult behavior depends on mastering early childhood and adolescent tasks and the development of an ego that masters reality and relationships successfully. Capacity for maturation, optimal level of function, and adaptability to life are at their apex (Erikson, 1963). Manifestations of the healthy adult ego are having the following:

- Capacity to trust
- Ability to form and maintain healthy relationships
- Sense of identity that is firmly established and effective
- Capacity to value themselves and others (healthy self-esteem and empathy)
- Capacity for coping and feeling modulation (affect) during change and stressful periods (flexible open system)
- Capacity to balance work and leisure activities

Intimacy refers to one's ability to form and sustain meaningful relationships. It also entails a sense of mutuality or sense of sharing and receiving love from another person. Adulthood is a continuous process, and it encompasses life-long experiences that include work and meaningful relationships such as marriage and family involvements. Other life stressors include losses such as divorce, serious illnesses, financial troubles, relationship breakups, death, and the "empty nest" experience.

Generativity includes more than having a family and raising children. It also is applicable to childless adults who contribute in their own ways to maintaining the next generation. This can be facilitated through a great variety of activities in which the person feels fulfilled and creative and is generous toward others.

Resolving crises and dealing with changes are integral aspects of adulthood. One's ability to use adaptive coping behaviors is influenced by the person's emotional repertoire, the experience and perception of stressors, and available support systems. Adaptive coping methods allow people to reduce, modify, or eliminate their stress. Adults can usually be expected to demonstrate resilience in the face of crisis if internal and external resources are available.

Clients with personality disorders often perceive crises or change as overwhelming. Their lack of internal and external resources compromises their ability to use adaptive coping methods to reduce or eliminate intense feelings. A lack of healthy ego functions interferes with one's ability to perceive stress accurately or realistically, to minimize his or her anxiety effectively, and to establish and maintain healthy relationships. The capacity for intimacy is lacking. Erikson (1963) described self-absorption as the antithesis of intimacy. These clients often experience feelings of emptiness and loneliness in spite of their numerous efforts to form relationships. They may also be extremely demanding of the relationships that they do have, and this is representative of the unmanageable anxiety that they may have but fail to acknowledge because many or most remain in an ego-syntonic state most of the time. Distress usually results from the inability to cope and deal with emptiness, low self-esteem, and intense but unacknowledged emotional pain. Clients experiencing these feelings are at risk for using other maladaptive behaviors such as substance abuse, suicide attempts, and destructive relationships and behaviors. The more florid acting-out and socially disturbing behaviors of earlier years tend to drop out or decrease in intensity as the person grows older (Gunderson, 1988).

LATE ADULTHOOD

Personality disorders are postulated to endure throughout the life span. Clients with these disorders continue to be influenced by internal and external stimuli. Older adults are challenged to use their previous life experience to cope with biological and neurological changes associated with the aging process. Erikson (1963) described the eighth stage of development as old age, with the primary development task of integrity. In some instances, however, despair rather than integrity is the outcome because the person does not perceive himself or herself to have any or many positive experiences for which to be proud; in effect, the task of generativity was not accomplished and possibly neither were other earlier tasks.

As mentioned earlier, the antisocial behaviors that may have been present in earlier years have generally become less of a problem as time passes; however, some of the disorders may intensify (e.g., the suspiciousness of the paranoid personality or the seclusiveness of the schizoid personality) because there are often accentuations in personalities of older persons. This occurs because new ego operations do not develop, and the person exaggerates defense mechanisms already present to cope with increased stress in association with loss, retirement, illness, and other circumstances of later life (Berezin et al., 1988).

Older adults who have never developed healthy ego functions, as well as those with physical and mental problems, are at risk for experiencing despair (Erikson, 1963). Lacking accomplishment, the person may face what is left of life with hopelessness and even helplessness. He or she may believe that any chance to make anything out of his or her life is gone and that there is no reason to be cheerful or ambitious about anything. Because of the numerous losses in this period, there is a vulnerability to depression, and the rate of suicide among men is high (Berezin et al., 1988). Relative to losses, one elderly person remarked, "All my friends have either gone to Florida or to heaven."

Elderly clients need to have complete physical, neurological, and psychological examinations because there is a complexity in these clients that is not found in younger ones. For instance, the elderly often are placed on large doses and mixtures of medications that add to their problems. These clients also have the tendency to shop around from physician to physician either to obtain a more perfect medication, because they do not trust their physician, or they may be confused about what is best. Furthermore, they have a tendency to be unreliable relative to their dosages and may forget to take any at one time, take too many at another time, or borrow and share with others at other times. It usually takes less of a particular medication to bring about the desired effects, but the various circumstances of abuse or misuse may create new and worse problems than those for which the client originally sought medical assistance.

Elderly persons often become clients; however, the effects of deinstitutionalization have reversed the prevalence of inpatient hospitalizations (Berezin et al., 1988), and the elderly who were once the predominant inpatient group in state and county hospitals often cannot receive mental health services for economic and various other reasons. Nevertheless, even though the number of inpatient admissions has decreased, there are still many elderly clients within the mental health service system. They may appear either in clinics, long-term care facilities (mainly devoted to physical problems but also responsive in some instances to the emotional problems), or home health situations. These clients require scrupulous attention and care because of the multiplicity of needs and drug interactions that may seriously affect them. Cultural and age-appropriate behaviors must be assessed in addition to all the physical problems that are likely to be present. Individualized care plans must be established. This is emphasized because there is a tendency for young people to perceive the elderly as all alike, and this is far from the truth. There are very wide variations in behavior and personality just as there are in the physical status of the clients.

There is a need for research to determine age-specific needs of clients with personality disorders. These efforts may be useful in minimizing feelings of helplessness, worthlessness, and hopelessness in the elderly and also in the nurses who work with them as more appropriate and helpful interventions are established.

Table 14–4 presents a summary of the various manifestations of maladaptive coping behaviors across the life span.

SPECIFIC PERSONALITY DISORDERS AND TREATMENT MODALITIES

Table 14–5 summarizes the three clusters of personality disorders, as defined by Gunderson (1988).

CLUSTER I

The first cluster of personality disorders comprises those in which clients are considered withdrawn, odd, or eccentric. These disorders include paranoid, schizoid, and schizotypal personality disorders.

Paranoid Personality Disorder

Kraeplin first coined the term *paranoia,* and he defined it as systemized delusions devoid of global deterioration. People with pervasive distrust and suspiciousness

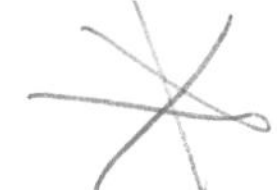

TABLE 14–4

Manifestations of Maladaptive Coping Behaviors Across the Life Span

	MALADAPTIVE BEHAVIOR	POSSIBLE CAUSE
Infancy	Withdrawal, refusal to enter into relationship	Absence of nurturing caregiver
Childhood	Projection, ambivalence, regression, splitting, acting out, denial	Faulty ego development
Adolescence	Boredom, frustration, difficulty dealing with intense feelings, distorted cognitions (impaired reality testing), low self-esteem, acting out, expressing extreme hostility toward authority figures, impaired ability to solve problems, impaired impulsivity control, risky tension-reducing activities (e.g., substance abuse, sexual promiscuity, and suicidal behaviors)	Impairments in ego and superego development, role confusion
Early and Middle Adulthood	Feelings of emptiness, loneliness, and distress; extremely demanding of relationships; low self-esteem; intense but unacknowledged emotional pain; substance abuse; suicide attempts; destructive relationships and behaviors	Lack of healthy ego functions
Late Adulthood	Intensification of earlier behaviors, suicide, feelings of despair, hopelessness, and helplessness	Nondevelopment of new ego operations, exaggeration of existing defense mechanisms to cope with increased stress associated with loss, retirement, or illness

of others such that their motives are interpreted as malevolent are more likely to develop this disorder, and it is the basis for the DSM-IV criteria for paranoid personality disorder. The following characteristics are defined in the DSM-IV (APA, 1994, pp. 637–638):

- Suspects, without sufficient basis, that others are exploiting, harming, or deceiving him or her

TABLE 14–5
Personality Disorders Organized by Cluster

	TYPE OF DISORDER	DESCRIPTION
Cluster I	Paranoid Schizoid Schizotypal	Client is withdrawn and engages in odd or eccentric behavior
Cluster II	Antisocial Borderline Histrionic Narcissistic	Client seeks attention and engages in erratic behavior
Cluster III	Avoidant Dependent Obsessive-compulsive Passive-aggressive	Client seeks to avoid or minimize the experience of anxiety

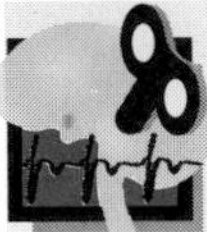

KEY INTERVENTIONS

The Client with Paranoid Personality Disorder

- Establish rapport
- Minimize potential for aggressive behavior
- Support adaptive behaviors

- Is preoccupied with unjustified doubts about the loyalty or trustworthiness of friends or associates
- Is reluctant to confide in others because of unwarranted fear that the information will be used maliciously against him or her
- Reads hidden demeaning or threatening meanings into benign remarks or events
- Persistently bears grudges, i.e., is unforgiving of insults, injuries, or slights
- Perceives attacks on his or her character or reputation that are not apparent to others and is quick to react angrily or to counterattack
- Has recurrent suspicions, without justification, regarding fidelity of spouse or sexual partner

Interventions (see Key Interventions display) are planned to draw the client into a nurse–client relationship, in which a measure of trust can be established. However, all personality disorders are ingrained, fixed patterns of behavior that are extremely resistant to change. Nurses must be scrupulous in keeping their word because the client will "look for chinks in the armor" of any professional who attempts to become involved in a therapeutic relationship. The pattern of suspiciousness was established a long time before any professional relationship; and because the client has not had sufficient reason to trust others, there is no guarantee it will happen in this instance.

These clients rarely seek treatment because of these personality traits. They are distant and guarded, and it is difficult to establish rapport with them because they consistently perceive people as untrustworthy. They are hypersensitive to criticism, and they have impaired interpersonal and work relationships. They have generally not been successful in establishing intimacy.

Clinical Example: The Client with Paranoid Personality Disorder (Mr. Jones)

Mr. Jones came into the psychiatric triage unit with his wife of 6 months. He stated that he is seeking help because his wife is threatening to leave him because of his intense jealousy and constant accusations of infidelity. She reported that he calls her job constantly trying to find out who she is talking to. Her boss has threatened to fire her if he calls again. He denied having a basis for his accusations, but he admitted that when someone calls their home and has the wrong number, he believes it is for his wife. Two weeks ago, he lost his fourth job within a 10-

month period. He admitted that his jealousy has increased during this period. When questioned about the basis of his jealousy, he became argumentative and defensive, stating he doesn't know why his wife feels there is something wrong with him.

Clients with paranoid personality disorder often feel the need to be on guard all the time in an effort to deal with perceived threats or attacks from others. (This characteristic is referred to as *hypervigilance*.) Their moods are irritable and agitated, and they are distant. These behaviors make it difficult for nurses to establish a trusting relationship. Interventions that are helpful in these situations include approaching the client in a calm, empathetic manner, avoiding overzealousness. These suspicious clients may interpret all behavior as threatening and react in an aggressive manner. Nurses need to assess verbal and nonverbal behaviors for cues that suggest increased agitation and aggression. Signs of impending aggression include pacing, speaking loudly, glaring, and clenching of the fists and jaw. These clients are not good candidates for intensive or intrusive therapy, especially group therapy, because these approaches may intensify suspiciousness and increase the risk of escalating aggressive thoughts and behaviors. Some of these clients show a slight response to low-dose neuroleptics, benzodiazepines, and antidepressants for symptoms of agitation, anxiety, or depression.

Schizotypal and Schizoid Personality Disorders

Clients with schizotypal personality disorders have pervasive patterns of impaired interpersonal relationships and a reduced capacity for close relationships (APA, 1994). They are also poor candidates for treatment and are at risk for developing schizophrenia. Clients with schizotypal personality disorder usually have positive neurobiological and genetic markers similar to those found in schizophrenia. Gunderson (1988) stated that there may be greater differences between schizoid and schizotypal personality disorders than has been previously supposed. Isolation, limited peer relationships, social anxiety, school underachievement, hypersensitivity, peculiarities in thought and language, and bizarre fantasies all are characteristics often found in schizotypal personalities as early as childhood or adolescence (APA, 1994). Gunderson (1988) suggested that there may be a need for further delineation between these types if these similarities are borne out.

Clients with schizoid or schizotypal disorders may have positive family backgrounds of schizophrenia (Fish, 1986). Some of these children are at risk for developing schizophrenia in adolescence or later life, but there is dispute about how many actually do. Gunderson (1988) stated that schizotypal patients rarely need institutional care, and schizoid personalities rarely seek treatment because of their interpersonal detachment. Table 14–6 compares the symptoms as they have been identified in the past (APA, 1994); it remains to be seen whether new studies will bring about revisions in the diagnostic criteria.

One can readily see that there are great similarities in the descriptions of the two conditions outlined earlier. Basically, the differences seem to be in degree more than in substance, with the schizotypal-type client more likely to be disabled, more likely to have a genetic predisposition, and demonstrating more ongoing disability than does the schizoid type (Gunderson, 1988). Further differentiation seems to be in the fact that while the schizotypal client fears social interactions, the schizoid client is basically disinterested in them.

Interventions and Outcomes. Working with schizotypal and schizoid clients requires that nurses understand the need for establishing rapport and that the clients are not going to engage in rewarding, positive affective exchanges. Feedback will be limited, but in addition to rapport, the nurse will need to work at establishing a reality base and the development of adaptive behaviors. Specific interventions to achieve these outcomes are listed in the display in the upper left corner of the next page.

TABLE 14–6
Comparison of Symptoms: Schizoid and Schizotypal Disorders

SCHIZOID DISORDER	SCHIZOTYPAL DISORDER
► Neither desires nor enjoys close relationships, including being part of a family	► Ideas of reference (excluding delusions of reference)
► Almost always chooses solitary activities	► Odd beliefs or magical thinking that influences behavior and is inconsistent with subcultural norms (e.g., superstitiousness, belief in clairvoyance, telepathy, or "sixth sense"; in children and adolescents, bizarre fantasies or preoccupations)
► Has little, if any, interest in having sexual experiences with another person	► Unusual perceptual experiences, including bodily illusions
► Takes pleasure in few, if any, activities	► Odd thinking and speech (e.g., vague, circumstantial, metaphorical, overelaborate, or stereotyped)
► Lacks close friends or confidants other than first-degree relatives	► Suspiciousness or paranoid ideation
► Appears indifferent to the praise or criticism of others	► Inappropriate or constricted affect
► Shows emotional coldness, detachment, or flattened affectivity	► Behavior or appearance that is odd, eccentric, or peculiar
	► Lack of close friends or condfidants other than first-degree relatives
	► Excessive social anxiety that does not diminish with familiarity and tends to be associated with paranoid fears rather than negative judgments about self

Adapted from American Psychiatric Association. [1994]. *Diagnostic and statistical manual of mental disorders, fourth edition* (pp. 641, 645). Washington, DC: American Psychiatric Association.

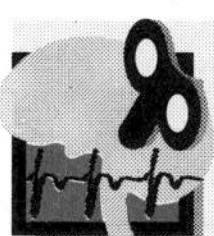

KEY INTERVENTIONS

The Client with Schizoid or Schizotypal Disorder

- Approach client in a calm manner
- Maintain comfortable distance based on client's verbal and nonverbal communication
- Administer psychotropics, and observe client's responses
- Engage supportive groups to provide feedback on client behaviors
- Provide for structured social interactions

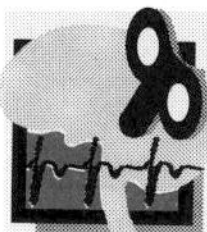

KEY INTERVENTI

The Client with Antisocial Personality Disorder

- Provide role model of positive and healthy interpersonal interactions
- Minimize the success of maladaptive behaviors
- Maintain a firm and structured teamwork approach
- Increase client's self-esteem through socially approved behaviors

CLUSTER II

The second cluster of personality disorders consists of those in which clients seek attention and engage in erratic behaviors. These disorders include antisocial, borderline, histrionic, and narcissistic personalities.

Antisocial Personality Disorder

The oldest known personality disorder is that of antisocial personality disorder (Blashfield & McElroy, 1987). Throughout history it has been given several names, including *moral insanity* by Prichard in 1830, *constitutional psychopathic insanity* by Koch in the nineteenth century, and *sociopathy* in the twentieth century. Regardless of the label, antisocial personality has referred to socially deviant persons who were societal outcasts because they refused to conform to social norms. Gunderson (1988) stated that although these people appear to be enviably free from worry, the essential "flatness and barrenness" from within becomes apparent when their activities fail to provide the desired long-term satisfactions. Typical characteristics include the following (Brooner, et al., 1993; Gunderson, 1988):

- Failure to learn from experience
- Regular engagement in impulsive and risky activity
- Lack of guilt demonstrated toward repetitive misbehavior
- Exploitation of others
- Chronic disregard for rights of others
- Lack of fidelity, loyalty, and honesty

Onset should be documented by antisocial behaviors prior to the age of 15 years and by failure to demonstrate a positive work role after the age of 18 years (APA, 1994).

Specific interventions aimed at achieving positive outcomes are as noted in the display in the upper right corner of this page.

Antisocial clients tend to participate in high-risk behaviors involving substance abuse. The rate of intravenous drug use is estimated to range from 35 to 54 percent in this population (Khantzian & Treece, 1985; Rounsaville et al., 1982). These clients present several treatment problems in that treatment successes are low and there is increased risk for human immunodeficiency viral infection (Brooner et al., 1993). Complete medical and psychiatric workups are needed to assess the behavioral style and resulting illnesses. Other necessary preventive measures include education regarding high-risk behavior and the facilitation of more adaptive coping skills.

Other treatment concerns center around the clients' ability to charm and manipulate because these usually quite intelligent people possess excellent verbal and nonverbal skills. An inexperienced nurse may unwittingly fall into the trap that involves flattery and favors. The nurse, lacking sophistication in this treatment arena, may be swayed to accept the seemingly rational arguments which the client so skillfully presents. When a nurse fails to respond with firm and consistent limits to maladaptive behavior, the behavior is reinforced and greater problems are created.

Mental health professionals are often hesitant, resistant, and pessimistic about treating antisocial clients for a number of reasons because their characteristics include the following (APA, 1994):

- A lack of conformity to social norms and lawful activity by repetitive illegal activity
- A lack of honesty as evidenced in lying, adoption of aliases, and conning others for personal gain
- A lack of planning as seen in impulsive behavior
- A history of fights and assults manifesting irritability and aggression
- A disregard for safety of self or others
- A failure to be consistent in work or financial obligation
- A lack of remorse, evidenced by indifference and rationalization of mistreatment of others

Although these clients have long been considered to be poor candidates for treatment, recent studies have given some hope for success in developing insight. The studies have demonstrated that structure in confined settings, along with peer pressure and confrontations, are essential aspects of treatment (Frosch, 1983; Mc-

Cord, 1982). Professional nurses must learn to approach these clients in a sensitive and nonjudgmental manner to facilitate trust and rapport because they fear and mistrust intimacy and closeness. Their self-destructive and criminal behaviors allow them to maintain distance in relationships.

Borderline Personality Disorder

The next area within this cluster, and one which is frequently encountered inside and outside of hospital settings, is borderline personality disorder. Gunderson (1988) stated that of all the personality disorders, this one is the most varied and unstable. Once thought to be associated with schizophrenia, the condition is now more closely aligned with affective disturbances. In many ways it shares commonalities with several other personality disorders.

Borderline personality has been consistently associated with other illnesses. Deutsch (1942) described the "as if" character; Grinker et al. (1968) called it *borderline schizophrenia*; and Kernberg (1975) described it as a continuum of pathology and associated with severity of symptoms at corresponding levels of development.

Neurobiological studies of these clients have demonstrated abnormal EEGs, and psychopharmacological trials have demonstrated positive results using anticonvulsants and antidepressants for target symptoms of impulsivity or dyscontrol and **dysphoria** (Cowdry et al., 1988).

A wide spectrum of behaviors or symptoms is associated with this disorder, ranging from intense anxiety to psychosis. Numerous factors have been associated with the development of borderline personality such as attachment problems, early childhood traumas or abuse (emotional, physical, or sexual), genetic predisposition, and neurobiological causes (already discussed).

Borderline disorder refers to people who have poorly integrated and fragile ego structures. Their dysfunction manifests itself in the lack of a sense of self-identity, the use of primitive defense mechanisms, and impairment in reality testing. They tend to regress during stressful times and often resort to splitting, denial, and projection. Gunderson (1988) stated that the essential feature of the disorder is fear of and intolerance for aloneness, and clients frequently report intense and excessive feelings of loneliness, emptiness, and rage. Their rage is often translated into self-abusive behaviors such as hitting walls; head-banging; skin scratching and tearing; and suicide attempts, gestures, or threats. Relationships are often unstable and are manifested by devaluation, manipulation, dependency, and self-denial. They may, at times, have psychotic-like perceptual distortions, become dissociative, or experience paranoid episodes (Gunderson, 1988). The DSM-IV (APA, 1994) lists the following behaviors:

- Attempts to avoid abandonment, either real or imagined, that are frantic
- Alternating extremes of idealization and devaluation leading to relationship instability
- Poor and unstable self-image and sense of self
- Self-damaging impulsivity in at least two areas, such as spending, sexual behavior, substance abuse, reckless drinking, binge eating
- Gestures, threats, self-mutilation, or actual suicidal behavior that is recurrent
- Marked mood reactivity, lasting a few hours to days
- Chronic feelings of emptiness
- Anger that is inappropriately intense, uncontrolled, and frequent
- Stress-related paranoid thinking or severe dissociative symptoms that are transient

As with some of the other personality disorders, clients with borderline disorders are particularly difficult to manage and may tax the emotional and physical resources of even the most experienced nurse. This occurs because of the intense demands of dependency or neediness (immense emotional demands), poor insight into their behaviors, and intense fears of abandonment. These behaviors often trigger countertransference responses in nurses and other health care professionals. No other group of clients has a greater ability to create chaos and stress within the system than this one.

Because of their dependency needs, these clients often seek therapeutic assistance in their frequently occurring crises. Their crises may be represented by some stressor (there may be a new crisis every day, and strangely, the one from the previous day may not even be mentioned in the encounter). These clients are prone to abuse of the telephone—they will call for help at any time, especially at night. Crises are most often precipitated by abandonment or separation issues, particularly those that arise in relationships.

Chronic feelings of dysphoria, emptiness, and boredom increase the risk of depression. The prevalence of depression among clients with borderline personality ranges from 23 to 87 percent, with the average at 30 to 40 percent (Shea et al., 1992).

Nursing interventions must center around assessing the meaning of crises, identifying present stressors and coping behaviors, and minimizing self-destructive behaviors. A preferable method of intervention is a careful consideration of the developmental experience of the individual. The need for psychopharmacological intervention must also be considered as treatment for the affective components that frequently accompany this condition. The client is assisted to identify the reasons for the present hospitalization or outpatient experience; the coping methods used in the present situation and the alternative behaviors that might work better; and past coping methods and their outcomes. In addition, these clients are likely to resort to the use of substances and to attempt suicide, so it is important to assess and discuss these issues as unproductive coping methods in therapeutic encounters. The following is a typical example of maladaptive coping behaviors used by a client with borderline personality disorder.

Clinical Example: The Client with Borderline Personality Disorder (Louise)

Louise is a 30-year-old school teacher who has three older brothers. She has a history of broken relationships, having been engaged twice previously, and now she has another broken relationship after 5 months of serious dating and consideration of marriage. Louise has never been married but says she is looking for the perfect man, "like my Granddad." She relates the breakup to her boyfriend's complaints that she was smothering him and that he could not handle her need to control his every move. She admits that these problems were the basis of her previous relationship problems. Her history also shows that she drinks three to four cans of beer at night and that she consumes more during periods of stress. She says that she doesn't drink to get drunk, "just to feel relaxed." She also has a history of several suicidal gestures and had expressed suicidal thoughts just prior to this hospitalization that prompted her eldest brother to take her to the emergency department. She had told her brother, "I might just as well check out since John doesn't seem to want me anymore." None of her suicide attempts have ever been serious enough to cause permanent injury or to be taken seriously by family members, and she has never been hospitalized before; instead, she was treated through crisis intervention. Louise does not appear to be significantly depressed, but she seems to want to latch onto one or two nurses who have become her favorites, and she shows a good bit of disdain toward the others, whom she sees as not catering sufficiently to her needs. When asked about her family relationships, she replies, "None of them ever wanted me; I was an afterthought."

Inpatient treatment typically focuses on crisis stabilization. The challenges in working with these clients has already been described, but it must be stressed that the ego development of these clients is insecure and that they need a great deal of structure, gentle confrontation, and limit-setting similar to that used with the antisocial client (see the Nursing Care Plan display).

Kernberg (1984) defined **splitting** as the dichotomous manner in which clients perceive the world, that is, all good or all bad. These clients have difficulty seeing both positive and negative qualities in one situation or person at a given time. This defect may be the result of early developmental arrests associated with a lack of opportunity or ability to have integrated these qualities from positive and helpful experiences with primary caregivers.

An example of splitting can be seen when the client perceives the nurses as either good or bad, and this depends on some arbitrary and unrealistic perception retained by the client at a given time. Good nurses are seen as those who allow the client to break the unit rules or who rescue (overprotect) the client. Bad nurses are seen as those who are consistent in limit setting or who react negatively to clients. When good and bad nurses argue over what the client needs, intense feelings toward the client emerge along with chaos on the unit. This scenario represents a re-creation of the client's family of origin. Splitting is unconscious and needs to be assessed as a maladaptive coping behavior.

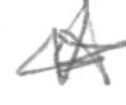

Nursing interventions for these clients are l low.

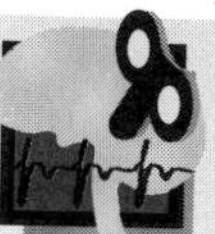

KEY INTERVENTIONS

The Client with Borderline Personality Disorder

- Form a nurse–client alliance based on clearly stated, realistic expectations
- Assist in reduction of self-destructive behavior and intent
- Acknowledge problematic behaviors
- Assist client to develop adaptive coping patterns
- Encourage verbalization of feelings about self

Johnson and Silver (1988) stressed that the treatment of borderline clients is a stressful experience potentially full of conflict between clients and staff. They suggest that these clients probably evoke more intense staff reactions than other clients. Some methods for minimizing conflict and promoting growth in clients are suggested as follows:

- Identify and state the treatment, although not necessarily the goals, from the outset
- Use staff development meetings to discuss conflicts and problem-solving methods
- Seek and use professional staff supervision
- Help create an environment for the honest expression of feelings regarding unit conflicts

Clients with borderline personality disorder generally have difficulty with boundaries, and they may become intrusive into the life and activities of another if permitted to get past appropriate limits. Gutheil and Gabbard (1993) defined boundaries as "parameters of a relationship." The nurse must remain firm from the outset if there is to be some later assurance that there will be no intrusions. Furthermore, the client needs help in understanding the nature of the problem, the expectations of the nurse (and others in the borderline's life), and responsibilities for changing old behavioral patterns surrounding this issue. These boundary problems exist because of the clients' lack of ego integration, and their frail self-identity (or fluid ego boundaries) contributes to difficulty in recognizing where they begin and others end.

Another area of difficulty for clients is placing the blame for their own behavior and its outcomes on others and to avoid any consideration of their own role in continuing the problems in their lives. It is important for them to learn to take responsibility and to recognize that

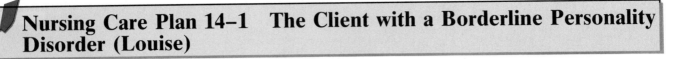

Nursing Care Plan 14–1 The Client with a Borderline Personality Disorder (Louise)

OUTCOME IDENTIFICATION	NURSING ACTIONS	RATIONALES	EVALUATION
Nursing Diagnosis: Impaired Social Interaction related to personal inadequacy as evidenced by behaviors that cause anger in others, low self-esteem, or poor social skills			
1. Form nurse–client relationship.	1a. Approach client in accepting manner.	1a. A nonjudgmental approach is a necessary prerequisite for relationship development. It paves the way for the client to lay aside hesitancy to be open in sharing thoughts and feelings.	*Goal met:* Client is able to interact appropriately with staff and peers. Acting-out behaviors decrease. Client receptive to limit setting and is less demanding. Client actively participates.
	1b. Use active listening.	1b. Active listening demonstrates to the client that he or she is being heard because the nurse repeats the client's statements or pays very close attention.	
2. By [date], client will recognize that this behavior affects relationships.	2. Develop and maintain realistic/consistent limit setting.	2. Clients who are needy, dependent, testy, or manipulative have weak or poorly defined boundaries and benefit best in a therapeutic setting that maintains clear and understandable boundaries.	
3. By [date], client will be able to control impulses to meet immediate gratification needs.	3a. Confront maladaptive responses.	3a. Gentle confrontation offers the client an opportunity to clarify appropriate expectation and establish a stronger sense of boundaries.	
	3b. Actively involve client in treatment.	3b. Clients who are involved in their treatment program are assisted in establishing greater independence of thought and decision making that will ultimately help them become more independent in their overall functioning.	
Nursing Diagnosis: Impaired Social Interactions related to anxiety as evidenced by dependent behaviors			
1. By [date], client will verbalize needs directly.	1. Develop environment that fosters trust.	1. Trust is best established when others are honest, consistent, reliable, and dependable.	*Goal met:* Client asks for assistance. Client adheres to treatment goals. Client is able to make simple decisions.
2. By [date], client will assume responsibility for problem solving.	2a. Maintain consistent limit setting.	2a. Limit setting is essential for clients whose anxiety prevents them from setting their own limits and establishing their own appropriate boundaries.	

Nursing Care Plan 14–1 The Client with a Borderline Personality Disorder (Louise) (Continued)

OUTCOME IDENTIFICATION	NURSING ACTIONS	RATIONALES	EVALUATION
	2b. Offer alternatives/options to present stressors.	2b. Alternatives and options allow clients to decide and choose what makes them comfortable thus promoting growth toward a more independent level of functioning.	
	2c. Encourage client to assess behaviors.	2c. Personal assessment of own behaviors by clients aids them in the cognitive activity required for looking at self and changing.	

► **Nursing Diagnosis:** High Risk for Self-directed Violence related to suicidal gesture as evidenced by history of suicide attempts

OUTCOME IDENTIFICATION	NURSING ACTIONS	RATIONALES	EVALUATION
1. By [date], client will verbalize the absence of suicidal ideations or plan.	1a. Assess level of dangerousness.	1a. Using a suicide risk assessment tool assists in determining the kind of action toward the client that maintains safety.	*Goal met:* Client denies suicidal ideations. Client agrees not to harm self and identifies other options of coping. Client exhibits gradual mood changes and superficial expression of feelings.
	1b. Provide safe environment, e.g., remove potential or actual dangerous objects from environment.	1b. Clients are often impulsive and may use suicidal behavior to gain the attention they need. Safety is a major concern in a psychiatric setting.	
	1c. Discuss "no suicide" verbal contract.	1c. No-suicide contracts have proved to be quite effective in eliciting client's cooperation and in assuring the client that someone else is concerned enough to provide boundaries such as contracts. Many clients do not really want to die but see no other way to get their needs met or to control their environment. Contracts help place control in the client's hands.	
2. By [date], client will discuss options to deal with present stressors.	2a. Encourage examination of available options to cope with present stressors.	2a. An inpatient experience is an excellent place and opportunity for testing evaluation and learning more effective alternative behaviors.	
	2b. Observe for sudden changes in mood.	2b. Mood changes *may* reflect a decision to carry out a suicidal threat if underlying depression is present. The nurse can also use the mood shift to determine behavioral patterns in clients.	

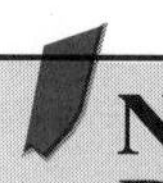

Nursing Care Plan 14–1 The Client with a Borderline Personality Disorder (Louise) (Continued)

OUTCOME IDENTIFICATION	NURSING ACTIONS	RATIONALES	EVALUATION
	2c. Encourage expression of feelings.	2c. The expression of feelings is important for helping clients to get in touch with themselves, something that they are not typically accustomed to doing.	
Nursing Diagnosis: Ineffective Individual Coping as evidenced by fear of abandonment			
1. By [date], client will develop an awareness of the meaning of present behaviors.	1a. Facilitate understanding of client's behaviors.	1a. Cognitive information aids clarity about behaviors that interfere with productive relationships.	*Goal met:* Client returns to previous level of function. Client develops adequate coping skills. Client displays decreased anxiety.
	1b. Assist in problem solving.	1b. Assisted problem solving helps promote greater future independence.	
	1c. Confront maladaptive behaviors.	1c. Fair and consistent confrontation by a trusted model assists in the establishment of needed boundaries.	
Nursing Diagnosis: Self Esteem Disturbance			
1. By [date], client verbalizes feelings of self worth.	1a. Encourage identification of 1 or 2 positive attributes.	1a. This activity promotes cognitive functioning that serves as a foundation for promotion of improved self-esteem based on factual information.	*Goal met:* Client verbalizes at least one positive quality. Client presents self in positive manner (e.g., groomed).
	1b. Provide positive age-appropriate realistic experiences.	1b. This activity provides here-and-now experience that promotes future healthy behavior.	
	1c. Provide constructive feedback regarding accomplishments.	1c. Praise and honest feedback from a trusted model enhance formation of a healthier self-concept.	
2. By [date], client interacts with others assertively.	2. Reinforce adaptive behaviors.	2. Reinforcement in the form of praise and acknowledgment help enhance positive self-esteem.	

it is not "bad" to fail. Clients with borderline disorder often believe that they are bad because they have often received this kind of message about themselves throughout their life. In addition, they have often been sexually abused and often have a great sense of guilt, believing that they were responsible for what occurred to them. Additionally, they may have been held responsible either by the victimizer or even by their mothers.

Because of the circumstances of their entire lives, clients with borderline disorder often believe they are bad, worthless, hopeless, and helpless. These beliefs lead to dysphoria and sometimes to a desire to die. Also, because they feel so alone and often abandoned, they believe that they are of no consequence and have no place in the world. They may feel the need to test these beliefs by threatening suicide to find out if there is anyone who does care enough to rescue them. Therefore, the nurse or other caregivers involved with the client may feel caught in a bind because there is a need to rescue on the one hand and a need not to be manipulated on the other. When a trust relationship has been formed, the nurse can reassure the client that he or she will be there (although not necessarily physically present) and that there is confidence that the client will make a wise decision. The nurse needs to promise to check in later at a specified time to assure the client that he or she is valued and to discuss the issue with problem solving in mind when there is no immediate crisis. When the nurse and client talk the next time, the client will probably have moved on to something else and will seem to have already put the issue in the past. It is almost as if a crisis lasts until the client has been told he or she is significant and then works through it alone so that by the next contact, the issues are changed and the client has a whole new set of concerns. There actually seems to be an incredible amount of personal strength that the client never acknowledges and, in fact, this is true because the client has usually lived through some difficult periods. This particular behavior is reminiscent of la belle indifference, a behavior related to secondary gain in conversion reactions except that, in this instance, it is related to emotional upheaval rather than to physical symptoms.

As stated earlier, these clients often manifest poor impulse control, and it is seen most often in suicidal behavior or self-mutilation. These acts may be carried out as spur-of-the-moment impulses; however, as noted earlier, it also is not unusual for the client to make telephone calls to see if someone will respond. The nurse can make more accurate predictions and determine interventions if there is an accurate assessment of past behaviors already at hand. If the client is in denial or is ashamed about these past events, there may be some 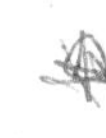 attempt not to share the information. The nurse needs to check the skin of the hands, arm, and face to observe for any scars and record the client's report about the occurrence of self-mutilation or to see if there are old wrist or neck scars as indicators of suicide attempts. Freeman and Gunderson (1989) suggested that these destructive behaviors are germane to maladaptive responses in borderline clients.

Favazza and Rosenthal (1993, p. 134) defined self-mutilation as a "deliberate alteration or destruction of body tissue" without the intent of killing oneself. Self-mutilation is associated with a myriad of conditions encompassing psychosocial, neurobiological, and cultural components (Coccaro et al., 1990; Favazza, 1989). Acts considered to be self-mutilating include plucking eyebrows completely; eye enucleation; castration; head banging; and skin burning, cutting, or carving. Vincent van Gogh provides an example of this behavior in cutting off his ear during an episode of mental derangement.

Favazza and Rosenthal (1990) categorized self-mutilation as three types: major, stereotypical, and superficial or moderate. Major self-mutilation can appear in a wide variety of disorders encompassing psychosis, substance abuse (acute intoxication), and schizoid personality disorder. Clients at risk include those who are religiously or sexually preoccupied. Some of these acts may be responses to command hallucinations. Clients who self-mutilate tend to be calm after the act, suggesting that the act temporarily relieves unconscious emotional pain or conflict. Sterotypical self-mutilation is the most common type. The highest rates are found in autistic children and clients who are mentally retarded. Other clients who may exhibit these behaviors include those with schizophrenia, drug-induced psychosis, brief reactive psychosis, and obsessive-compulsive disorder (Robertson et al., 1989). Typical behaviors include head banging, self-induced seizures, and episodic vomiting. Superficial or moderate self-mutilation is also a common behavior. Favazza and Conterio (1988) estimated that its prevalence ranges from 400 to 1400 in 100,000 annually. Besides its occurrence in the borderline client, it is also found in other personality disorders, eating disorders, multiple personalities, and psychoses. Favazza (1989) suggested that this act is a morbid attempt to temporarily release emotional distress, interrupt depersonalization, and alleviate feelings of alienation and loneliness (see Chapter 15 for more details).

Linehan (1987) stressed the role of the therapist in helping clients gain insight into the meaning of their behaviors, teaching them adaptive coping skills, and continuously assessing their level of dangerousness. Consistent limit setting allows nurses to provide external controls for these clients.

Nurses need to take advantage of any hospital experience that these clients have because it might be the only access that a professional has to a continuous opportunity for interacting and intervening when maladaptive behaviors occur. It can be a time when the client makes tremendous strides if optimal use is made of the time and experience. Hospital stays in the 1990s are not extended stays, and good use needs to be made of extremely limited time.

Other specifically effective treatment methods include cognitive and behavioral psychotherapies. The focus of these therapies include targeting the maladaptive behaviors, feelings, and perceptions associated with interpersonal relationships (Shea et al., 1992). These interventions can teach clients how to modulate their feelings and rage episodes and minimize their feelings of helplessness and sensitivity to criticism. Supportive and group therapies can facilitate development of adaptive social skills associated with learning about how their behaviors affect others (see the Research Abstract display below; also see Chapters 21 and 23).

There has been limited success in the use of psychotropic medications in clients with borderline personality disorder. Antimanic agents (carbamazepine and lithium) and neuroleptics are used to control impulsivity (Cowdry & Gardner, 1988; Links et al., 1990). Other clients have responded favorably to antidepressants such as the tricyclics. A number of studies have demonstrated increased effectiveness of combined psychotherapy and psychopharmacological treatment (Kendall & Lipman, 1991). Shea et al. (1992) have suggested that the response to antidepressant medications is better when the personality-disordered client has an overlying depression. Several researchers postulate that depression found in these clients is not biologically based (Akiskal, 1983; Black et al., 1988).

Stone (1990) considered medications to be helpful in managing aggressiveness, impulsivity, and psychoses. However, he stated that clients with borderline personality disorder are often noncompliant and unreliable about taking psychotropics. If clients can be assisted to see the importance of these drugs in alleviating these problems, their compliance might be increased.

Because the clients with borderline personality disorder have experienced circumstances that affect them seriously, they are likely to have low self-esteem. Un-

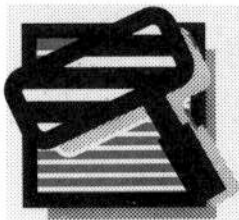

RESEARCH ABSTRACT

Group Therapy for People with Borderline Personality Disorder: Interventions Associated with Positive Outcomes

Nehls, N. (1992). *Issues in Mental Health Nursing, 13*(3), 255–269.

This qualitative study focused on the verification of intended treatment techniques because there had been limited information available about group approaches for borderline personality disorder (BPD).

The clients were located in a community mental health setting and were diagnosed as having BPD. The sample consisted of therapist interventions that were examined using The Hill Counselor Verbal Response Category System-R (HCVRCS-R), a content analytical approach designed to classify counselor responses into nine mutually exclusive categories. These interventions consisted of encouragement/approval/reassurance, reflection/restatement, self-disclosure, confrontation, interpretation, providing information, information seeking, direct guidance/advice, and unclassifiable. Instrument face and content validity were determined to be adequate. Interrater reliability was superior to earlier studies in which Cohen's kappa was .85. Reliability for three videotaped sessions yielded kappa .79, .86, and .85.

Overall, the verbal responses most used during eight sessions were as follows: providing information (55%) information seeking (22%), and reflection/restatement (10%). This indicates that the therapists provided a considerable degree of structure in their sessions. The degree of structure was computed to determine the degree to which "a counselor's messages potentially structure subsequent client responses" (Nehls, 1992, p. 263); it was believed that high-structure responses increase the likelihood that the topic of conversation will remain focused.

Outcomes of the study indicated that success with clients was associated with two interventions: providing and seeking information, and these evolved around methods of coping with loneliness, self-destructive impulses, interpersonal relationships, issues about housing, employment, and problems with the health care system. The women were provided with alternative ways of understanding the issues and empowered with information and strength to manage many problems. The data suggest that for seriously ill people with BPD, an important component of effective group treatment is the meaningful exchange of information. A second implication of the study was that it would have been unrealistic to expect dramatic change in the content or process of interchanges. The data revealed no significant differences across sessions in the quantity or type of therapist response. This finding was contrary to theory that presumed that group process variables change over time. There was, however, no emphasis on the need for change because the group's organizing framework was assisting clients to identify their own goals.

The conclusions in the study were that (1) care of people with BPD is one of psychiatric nursing's major challenges, and (2) caregiving processes that recognize the unique needs and interests of BPD subgroups need to be developed and evaluated.

der extreme stress they are likely to relive early traumatic episodes or posttraumatic stress disorder (PTSD). The symptoms of PTSD include recurrent nightmares, hypervigilance, flashbacks, or intense anger (see Chapter 10). Suggestions have already been made regarding the approach to these clients that will have an impact on the problem of self-esteem.

Histrionic Personality Disorder

Early psychoanalytic literature coined the term *hysteria*, now known as *histrionic personality disorder*. Manifestations of this disorder included exaggerated labile emotions, sexualization of relationships, and dramatic emotional states. The behaviors range from higher ego function (attention-seeking and sociability) behaviors to lower ego function (promiscuity, impulsivity, and psychosis) (Reich, 1949).

Histrionic personality is now considered to be represented by attention-seeking behaviors in which clients exhibit the following behaviors (APA, 1994):

- Discomfort in situations where he or she is not the center of attention
- Inappropriate sexually seductive behavior with others
- Rapidly shifting and shallow emotional expressions
- Use of physical appearance to gain attention on a consistent basis
- Excessively impressionistic style of speech that lacks detail
- Self-dramatization, theatrics, or exaggerated emotional expressions
- Suggestibility
- The attitude that relationships are more intimate than they are

This disorder is most often diagnosed in women. Their interpersonal relationships are superficial, flighty, and their melodramatic expressions are flamboyant, apparently designed to gratify early unmet dependency needs that they anticipate will be met through their therapists. Their ego functioning is disorganized, and they tend to fantasize and idealize their relationships with their therapist; that is, they secretly love them, and they consider themselves special to their therapists (Freeman & Gunderson, 1989). Their major defense mechanisms include repression and dissociation.

Other maladaptive behaviors may include temper tantrums, manipulation, and endless demands. They also tend to evoke intense emotional reactions in nurses, such as anger and a sense of inadequacy. Treatment is similar to that of some other personality disorders and focuses on consistency, understanding, managing countertransference issues, and providing an environment that minimizes maladaptive coping patterns.

In addition to the trust and rapport-building activities and identifying the client's particular maladaptive behaviors, it is also necessary to gain understanding about their infantile fantasies (feelings). As these tasks are accomplished, the client can be helped to develop more adaptive coping skills and to find alternatives to destructive behaviors. The client needs encouragement and assistance in the development and recognition of increased self-worth that leads to new behaviors. The nurse who is skillful in helping the client accomplish these outcomes also needs to recognize how extremely sensitive these clients are to rejection and to experiencing depressive moods and episodes. A detailed discussion of treatment strategies is found in the section on borderline personality disorder.

Psychopharmacological approaches center on depression, anxiety, and psychosis. See Chapter 26 for a further discussion of antidepressants, anxiolytics, and neuroleptics.

Narcissistic Personality Disorder

Narcissus was a young man in Greek mythology who fell in love with his own image reflected in a pool. The term *narcissism* is associated with self-love and self-absorption. Psychoanalytical theory proposes that narcissism is a necessary part of the early developmental stages. Freud described these personality types as having no tension between ego and superego and with no preponderance of erotic needs but mainly interested in self-preservation. They are independent, not easily intimidated, and quite aggressive. They prefer loving to being loved and enjoy being champions for others (Freud, 1957). Freud described three types of narcissism, namely *erotic-obsessional* (superego restriction of libidinal life), *erotic-narcissistic* (unity of opposites so that there is considerable amount of aggressiveness and activity), and *narcissistic-obsessional* (capacity for vigorous action and strengthening of the ego against the superego). Rothstein (1991) summarized earlier theoretical works of Kernberg and Kohut, stating that some narcissistic personalities adapt well vocationally but generally seek help for problems relating to difficulties in intimate relations with others; others suffer in their object relations and seek treatment because they experience neurotic symptoms, sexual difficulties, and chronic feelings of emptiness. The third group functions on a borderline level with nonspecific manifestations of ego weakness.

Children whose parents are aloof, aggressive, rejecting, and emotionally cold are at risk for developmental arrest at the early narcissistic stage because the person is prevented from achieving a sense of self-worth and value. They tend to seek approval and recognition throughout life and experience emptiness, low self-esteem, self-absorption, and somatic symptoms (Kohut, 1971, 1977).

The DSM-IV (APA, 1994, p. 661) states that five or more of the following common characteristics must be present to diagnose this disorder:

- Has a grandiose sense of self-importance (e.g., exaggerates achievements and talents, expects to be recognized as superior without commensurate achievements)
- Is preoccupied with fantasies of unlimited success, power, brilliance, beauty, or ideal love
- Believes that he or she is "special" and unique and can only be understood by, or should associate with, other special or high-status people (or institutions)
- Requires excessive admiration
- Has a sense of entitlement, i.e., unreasonable expectations

of especially favorable treatment or automatic compliance with his or her expectations
- Is interpersonally exploitative, i.e., takes advantage of others to achieve his or her own ends
- Lacks empathy: is unwilling to recognize or identify with the feelings and needs of others
- Is often envious of others or believes that others are envious of him or her
- Shows arrogant, haughty behaviors or attitudes

Because of their self-centeredness, inability to be empathic, greediness, parasitism, and coldness, clients with this disorder experience relationship problems. However, their grandiose façade covers feelings of low self-esteem, insecurity, and inadequacy.

As with other personality disorders, nursing interventions first require that the nurse be aware of his or her own reactions around clients who evoke a great deal of tension in their demands for attention. Kohut (1971) contended that the establishment of therapeutic alliances is important for increasing self-esteem. The nature of narcissism is such that these clients are preoccupied with themselves and need assistance in understanding and valuing events that occur outside their internal environment. To do this, they must first begin to view themselves from a different perspective, and this demands therapeutic intervention requiring much time and effort. Other nursing interventions are the same as those listed in the section on borderline personality disorders.

Inpatient hospitalization is usually precipitated by depression and mood swings that often follow failure or rejection. The primary focus of hospitalization is treatment of these target symptoms, and attention to the underlying cause may be neglected because it would require a longer period to provide such treatment. Clients may avoid group therapy because they are challenged to balance their desire for a special client–therapist relationship and their fear of confrontation by the group members (Freeman & Gunderson, 1989). It may be necessary to provide a period of individual psychotherapy either before or concomitant with a lengthier period of group therapy to achieve the greatest benefit. Individual psychotherapy is often the treatment of choice and allows clients an opportunity to introject or incorporate the adaptive aspects of the therapist (Meissner, 1988) and to avoid the regressive use of primitive defenses such as rage, splitting, and projection.

CLUSTER III

The third cluster of personality disorders comprises conditions in which the prominent symptoms are anxiety and fear. Behaviors in these disorders center around avoiding or minimizing the experience of anxiety. Disorders in this cluster include avoidant, dependent, obsessive-compulsive, and passive-aggressive personalities.

Avoidant Personality Disorder

Major manifestations of avoidant personality disorder are avoidance of activity based on fears of criticism, disapproval, or rejection; unwillingness to be involved without guarantees of acceptance; restraint within intimate relationships becasue of insecurity; preoccupation with criticism and rejection; interpersonal inhibition based on a sense of inadequacy; a view of self as unappealing, inept, and inferior; and a reluctance to engage in new activity because of its potential risk of embarrassment (APA, 1994). Seclusiveness differs from that seen in schizoid personality disorder by the capacity and desire to form meaningful relationships. Fears of rejection coupled with self-doubt interfere with the ability to risk entry into a relationship; these clients are constantly assessing their interactions for signs of devaluation and deception. Even positive social events are avoided so that clients often have no one to whom they relate. They tend to "make mountains out of mole hills" and often attend to negative responses in their environments. They are easily hurt by criticism.

These conditions of distrust make it imperative, then, that nursing interventions facilitate the establishment of trust through the formation of reliable, dependable nurse–client alliances. This helps minimize anxiety sufficiently to permit the exploration of old behaviors and to consider ways to change and feel better. Specific attention needs to be given to relaxing, because mistrust causes hypervigilance, and to developing other relationships in which trust can be expected. The inpatient unit is an ideal place for helping this process, and the nurse is urged to take advantage of every opportunity to promote trust because hospital stays are now so brief. It is also important to recognize the need for outpatient continuation of therapy; appropriate referrals are needed to continue what has already begun in the inpatient setting.

Dependent Personality Disorder

The hallmark of dependent personality disorder is the pervasive pattern of dependency and submissiveness. These clients rely on others exclusively for their support. They rarely make their own decisions, and they place tremendous demands on others for reassurance and advice. They attach and cling tenaciously to anyone who will take care of them, tell them what to do, or make their decisions for them. They are fearful of many things and become the willing shadow of anyone who will take care of them. Their behavior is often childlike in their hesitation to stand on their own as responsible adults.

Dependency is a normal process in nurse–client interactions but must always be redirected as long as the client has the ability to do for himself or herself. These clients require constant redirection when they ask for advice or assistance in doing the things they are able to do. For instance, the client may ask the nurse to make a telephone call and request information that he or she can obtain, or there may be requests for advice that most others would not ask for. The following is an example of an intervention that may occur with a dependent client.

CLIENT: Oh, I'm so upset about getting a job. I have to go to work, and I don't know where to go.

NURSE: You don't know where to go?

CLIENT: No. What do you think I should do?

NURSE: What kinds of things have you thought about doing?

CLIENT: I can't think of anything. I need help with this.

NURSE: What kind of help do you need with this?

CLIENT: Someone to pick out some places for me.

NURSE: What things have you already considered?

CLIENT: I haven't considered anything. I'm waiting for someone to help me.

NURSE: You haven't looked into any possible solutions?

CLIENT: No.

NURSE: Perhaps you would like to get the phone book and look up some possible job placement centers and the newspaper and we can get together this afternoon to talk about some options you have considered.

In this example, the nurse has not given advice but has offered some ways to begin the process of helping the client to begin thinking independently. The nurse has provided support and a broad suggestion about possible job sources along with the offer to listen to problem-solving activities later in the afternoon. Thus, the nurse supports and empowers the client in the beginning steps of a decision-making process. Later it will become possible to promote even more responsibility taking by the client so that there would be no need for suggestions of using the telephone book or newspaper. In this instance, the nurse may say, instead, "Tell me what you think are some of the places where you can find job offerings."

Nurses who need to sustain dependent interactions with clients fail to promote autonomy and growth in their clients and need to examine the meaning of their own dependent needs. Nurses may also err by responding to dependent behaviors by becoming hostile and negative in their responses. These countertransference responses suggest the need for supervision where opportunity is given for exploring and evaluating one's own behaviors.

In all therapeutic endeavors, the most apparent need is the reduction of anxiety, and in nearly all instances there is a concomitant need for increasing self-esteem. This is no less true for dependency. It requires a skillful balancing act to give enough but not too much in the process of helping clients grow into a more adaptive lifestyle. The nurse–client relationship may be the only place where this is given an opportunity to begin. Nurses are urged to consider the dependent-independent-interdependent need structure of themselves and their clients (Whiting, 1994).

Psychotherapeutic intervention may take place through individual therapy that fosters the development of insight and behavioral change. The techniques may be interpersonal, behavioral, analytical, or cognitive. Other appropriate therapy modalities include group therapy, family therapy, and assertiveness training.

Obsessive-Compulsive Personality Disorder

Obsessive-compulsive personality disorder is characterized by a pervasive rigidity and preoccupation with control and power and an exaggerated fear of losing control. These clients tend to be out of touch with their feelings and to intellectualize (Liebowitz et al., 1986). Their emotional expression is extremely constricted, and they give little of anything, either emotionally or materially. They may be described as perfectionists, and these behaviors interfere with interpersonal relationships. These tendencies also interfere with task completion because their overly strict standards cannot be met. Preoccupation with details causes them to lose sight of primary goals (APA, 1994).

The same needs for anxiety reduction and increased self-esteem exist in these clients as with others previously described. Understanding and decreasing maladaptive behaviors are the goals, and they depend on specific manifestations of the disorder. In addition to the nurse–client relationship, psychoanalytical, behavioral, or cognitive therapy may be helpful. Clomipramine (Anafranil) has been shown to effectively reduce symptoms commonly seen in these clients and has offered hope in treatment. This also implies a biological origin for this disorder, and it signals the need for biological research into the other personality disorders. Much of this research is currently ongoing. Chapter 10 offers more specific therapeutic approaches from which these clients may benefit.

THE NURSE'S ROLE

THE GENERALIST NURSE

The generalist nurse will most likely encounter personality-disordered clients in the acute inpatient or community mental health setting. These clients, especially those with borderline or antisocial personality disorders, often look for ways to "penetrate the nurse's boundaries"—they seem to possess an uncanny ability to sense where the nurse is most vulnerable. It is helpful for the nurse to examine personal responses with the following questions:

- What feelings do I have about the client?
- How often do I find myself in conflict with other team members regarding this client?

- What are the client behaviors that trigger the most emotion in me?
- What emotional response do I have when I find myself assigned to this client?

The generalist nurse may need to role-play responses in a supervisory setting or talk about the feelings engendered by such clients. He or she needs to recognize when there is need for a nurse with advanced skills and make proper referral to a nurse clinical specialist as well as to seek supervision from the nurse in advanced practice. The personality-disordered client is particularly difficult to manage and needs the services of a nurse therapist to assist in changing pathological and destructive behavioral patterns. The generalist nurse can provide the helpful collaborative support for change that occurs through therapy.

The care of personality-disordered clients is difficult and often frustrating because they demonstrate behaviors that challenge even the experts. Interventions must be specific to the behaviors, which can vary widely from client to client and even from one time to another for a particular client. Overall, however, one may categorize some of the behaviors of personality-disordered clients according to the behaviors that typify some of the DSM-IV diagnostic groups. Table 14–7 outlines the diagnoses and some typical behaviors within those groups and suggests interventions for the behaviors. It is generally these typical behaviors that have prevented these clients from establishing or maintaining meaningful relationships throughout their lifetimes, and the nurse must take every advantage of the short periods that are available for providing honest confrontation within a milieu that is open and trusting.

THE ADVANCED-PRACTICE NURSE

In addition to treating personality-disordered clients in acute care or community mental health settings, the nurse in an advanced-practice role may encounter these clients in a variety of other clinical settings. Many opportunities exist for providing care either directly or indirectly, in liaison roles, in independent practice, and through supervision and consultation.

Because the predominant etiologic theory for borderline personality disorder is that of separation–individuation, a developmental framework is useful for understanding and guiding treatment. It is also a helpful framework for working with antisocial or other personality-disordered types who seem stuck at the level of "I want what I want when I want it." The nurse in advanced practice will encounter many clients with self-centered, dramatic, seductive, ambivalent, hostile, isolated, dependent, or independent behaviors that challenge the nurse's ability to respond without losing professional control and demeanor.

There are many risks involved in the direct care of clients who use the treatment as a relationship, often to replace relationships they have damaged or destroyed elsewhere. Many clients seek a relationship that is nurturing and expect undivided attention from the therapist they claim as their own. For example, the dependent client may want a "mother," the seductive client a lover, and the narcissistic client an admirer. In contrast, the paranoid client may be mistrusting, the avoidant client afraid, and the obsessive-compulsive client too controlling. The therapist needs to be extremely careful in responding to these demands. Each of the behaviors

TABLE 14–7
Typical Behaviors of Clients with Personality Disorders According to DSM-IV Diagnostic Groups and Suggested Interventions

DIAGNOSES	TYPICAL BEHAVIORS	SUGGESTED INTERVENTIONS
Avoidant Obsessive-compulsive Paranoid Passive-aggressive Schizoid Schizotypal	Anger Dysfunctional independence Isolation Mistrust and suspicion Withdrawal	1. Offer self on a regular basis without intrusion 2. Acknowledge observed behaviors with client 3. Be particularly attentive to commitments that help develop trust 4. Work at drawing client into interactions that promote enjoyment on a 1:1 basis and then on a group level 5. Involve client in establishing at least one relationship and in working toward increasing the number of social involvements
Borderline Dependent Histrionic Narcissistic (sometimes)	Attention-seeking Dependence Neediness	1. Assess the type and frequency of demands for attention 2. Establish a trusting relationship that allows confrontation of dependent or needy behavior, and assist client in acknowledging the behavior 3. Set specific goals and methods for achieving greater independence 4. Provide reinforcement of independent functioning
Antisocial Narcissistic (sometimes)	Aggression Dishonesty Entitlement Manipulation Risk-taking	1. Provide and maintain a team-developed set of rules that are strictly followed 2. Remind client of expectations before the temptation sets in to deviate 3. Develop an atmosphere of trust in which sincere confrontation is possible 4. Provide pleasurable activities that serve as a substitute for the previous deviant activities no longer permitted 5. Recognize that many of these clients have operated dishonestly for a long time and have a pattern of behavior that is difficult to change

challenges the ingenuity of the nurse in trust building and countering certain behaviors toward the establishment of trust.

The nurse in advanced practice is warned to be alert to the skillful maneuvers of seduction and neediness by maintaining constant and clear boundaries. The client feels safe and will honor the boundaries that help keep him or her in control. Also, the nurse in advanced practice needs to recognize that many clients with personality disorders are not suited to brief encounters or therapy. There must be a willingness to commit to a long period and process of building new behavioral patterns. This process is tedious and requires great patience, commitment, and personal strength.

The Nursing Process

Assessment

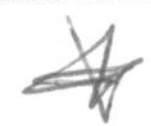

Evaluating ego function is a major aspect of the nursing process because it provides data that assist in making accurate diagnoses, planning psychotherapeutic interventions, and bringing about therapeutic outcomes. This assessment considers the components of interpersonal relationships, affective capabilities, motivation for treatment, capacity for introspection, insight, defensive behavior, and reality testing.

Assessing personality development entails examining the life span and factors such as early relationships with primary caregivers, their impact on ego development, and adaptation and coping styles. Understanding key concepts in personality formation such as ego development and organization is crucial for nurses who must assess the meaning of maladaptive behaviors, facilitate adaptive coping behaviors, and evaluate client responses to interventions.

The role of psychiatric nurses includes assessing areas of impairment, and the process begins by approaching clients and their significant others in a caring and nonjudgmental manner. This approach facilitates trust building and enhances the potential success of treatment plan outcomes. Interventions are planned to encourage the client into a nurse–client relationship in which a measure of trust can be established. However, it is important to remember that all personality disorders are ingrained, fixed patterns of behavior that are extremely resistant to change.

Nursing Diagnoses

Once the assessment is completed, the nurse analyzes the data to arrive at the nursing diagnoses. Personality-disordered clients are difficult to treat, so to determine what is preventing the client from making adequate adjustment and engaging successfully in relationships, it is necessary to identify the specific behaviors that hamper success. It is typical to find, in all personality-disordered clients, a pattern of immaturity, narcissism, inflexibility, and hostility, either overt or covert. Examples of nursing diagnoses include the following:

- Self-Esteem Disturbance
- Altered Thought Processes
- Social Interaction
- Powerlessness
- Ineffective Individual Coping
- Defensive Coping

Planning

Goal setting and outcome criteria enable the nurse to schedule activities that are helpful to the client and to evaluate outcomes. Goals (long term) and outcome criteria (short term) are measurable. Examples of three goals and outcome criteria as related to the diagnoses listed earlier are as follows:

Goal 1. Client will report at least one satisfying relationship in 3 weeks.

Outcome Criteria

1. Client will list at least five positive personal characteristics by the next interaction on [date].
2. Client will describe the type of person with whom she or he would like to be friends with within the next several meetings.
3. Client will identify the things in self that she or he believes are hindering development of relationships within the next three meetings.
4. Client will identify within the next week at least three behaviors that she or he is interested in changing by time of discharge.
5. Client will demonstrate definite effort toward establishing contact with the person who was identified as a desirable friend within 3 weeks.

Goal 2. Client will demonstrate more appropriate cognitive functioning by the time of discharge (or the end of the contract with the nurse).

Outcome Criteria

1. Client will listen to alternative ideas and beliefs as offered by group members (or nurse).
2. Client will accept confrontation of group members (or nurse) within 1 week.
3. Client will verbalize alternatives for faulty thoughts or ideas when challenged by group members (or nurse) within 2 weeks.
4. Client will begin to challenge faulty thinking of other group members within 3 weeks.

Goal 3. Client will demonstrate improved interactions with peers on the unit.

Outcome Criteria

1. Client will become acquainted with peers through attendance at daily group meetings for the next 4 weeks.
2. Client will recognize behaviors in self that group

members identify as detrimental to relationships within 2 weeks.

3. Client will respond to in-group critiques by acknowledging what she or he needs to work on within 2 1/2 weeks.

4. Client will verbalize the behaviors in self that create interpersonal problems within 3 weeks.

5. Client will demonstrate less interest in self and more interest in others within 4 weeks.

Refer again to the Nursing Care Plan display for an example of a care plan for a client with borderline personality disorder.

Interventions

Interventions are planned and carried out in accordance with the steps identified in the section on outcome criteria. All formal and informal interactions are considerate of the goals and outcome criteria. The nurse is aided by remaining cognizant of the specific needs of the client throughout every contact. This means that each contact is goal centered and client centered and aimed at taking advantage of every available moment. This is especially important in these times when treatment contact is short and every contact is significant. Interventions for the above goals may include interactions such as the following:

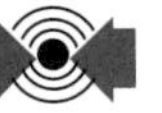

NURSE: Hi, Louise. I see that you have spent only 10 minutes applying your make-up today.

LOUISE: Yes, I remembered what the group said last time, and I didn't want them to jump on me again today.

NURSE: You didn't want them to "jump" on you again today?

LOUISE: No way.

NURSE: Louise, I'm aware that you used to spend 2 hours plus numerous remakes on your make-up each day. What changed?

LOUISE: I think I'm beginning to see that I was spending too much time on that and keeping others away from me by my self-centeredness.

The nurse–client interaction indicates the effectiveness of group intervention coupled with nurse interventions. These occur both internally and externally as the client begins to think and then act out the new behaviors. Nehls (1992) decried the lack of information about group approaches for borderline personality disorder (see the Research Abstract display on group therapy [p. 310] and Chapter 23).

Evaluation

When nursing diagnoses are directly related to goals and outcome criteria that in turn are directly related to the interventions, there is greater likelihood that the client will make obvious progress toward a goal. Personality-disordered clients are, however, likely to regress and need frequent, sometimes constant, reinforcement. It may take years to fully accomplish the original goals, but the client will be able to hear and respond to criticism or confrontation that has been applied skillfully and with sincere care. Personality-disordered clients are capable of identifying the nurse's "weak spots" and often appear to be working to defeat the nurse's attempts to help. Unless the nurse is extremely secure, there may be a tendency to give up in despair of ever helping. The nurse must be willing to persevere, even when success seems elusive.

Evaluations are completed at the times designated in the goals and outcome criteria. The nurse and client experience satisfaction as these are met. The sense of partnership exists when the client can truly acknowledge feeling better or having success in one of the areas that was such a struggle in the beginning. It may be the first time the client has ever experienced any success at anything significant, so it needs to be acknowledged as an accomplishment for the client.

► CHAPTER SUMMARY

Personality development is a complex process that is influenced by innate neurobiological and psychosocial factors. Numerous theories abound about the influence of early caregivers on the developing personality. Maladaptation appears in many forms, and it is imperative that all nurses have an understanding about adaptive and maladaptive forms of relating, both in themselves and in their clients. Therapeutic nurse–client relationships can be effective in developing trust and providing an opportunity for intervening in maladaptive patterns of behavior.

Personality disorders represent a continuum of maladaptive coping patterns and are currently organized into three clusters that center on central characteristics. Overall, the personality disorders are characterized by inflexible and compulsive responses that are specific to the conditions involved. Within these behavioral clusters are generalized distress, rejection issues, restricted expression, insecure attachment, conduct problems, intimacy problems, social impairment, and cognitive distortion (Livesley et al., 1992).

Nurses are challenged to use the nursing process to assess the client experience of chronic distress, fragmented ego functioning, and impaired social skills. Personality-disordered clients often experience an overlay of other psychiatric problems and may present with a complexity of problems. These clients present a challenge to nurses as they offer themselves in distributing a significant amount of powerful and potentially toxic medications and place themselves in situations taut with frustration, tension, manipulation, rejection, and disparagement. Their clients often lack insight and motivation to change, and it takes great energy and interest to sustain involvement with clients who are as maladaptive as those with a personality disorder.

Nurses need to maintain their sense of adequacy and

self-esteem by recognizing these behaviors as representative of client illness and not aimed at personal destruction of the nurse. When the nurse is able to grasp this concept, it becomes easier to be nonjudgmental and caring enough to minimize the overwhelming distress that these clients encounter. Mastery of feeling and response in the nurse can set the stage for the modeling of adaptive behavior so needed by their personality-disordered clients. Nurses are in the unique position of being able to provide what may be the only health-promoting experience of personality-disordered clients in both inpatient and outpatient settings and to the clients across the life span.

Suggestions for Clinical Conference

1. Role-play countertransference reactions such as malice, hate, and anger, and examine feelings and thoughts generated during the exercise.
2. Discuss adaptive and maladaptive behaviors using the nursing process.
3. Analyze developmental issues associated with a client's present behaviors.
4. Compare major concepts of personality theories, and apply them to several case histories.

References

Akiskal, H. S. (1983). Dysthymic disorder: Psychopathology of proposed clinical depressive subtypes. *American Journal of Psychiatry, 140,* 11–20.

Allnutt, B. L. (1979). The motherless child. In J. D. Nospitz (Ed.), *Basic handbook of child psychiatry* (pp. 373–378). New York: Basic Books.

American Psychiatric Association. (1994). *Diagnostic and statistical manual of mental disorders* (4th ed.). Washington, DC: Author.

Bellodi, L., Battaglia, M. A., Gasparini, M., Scherillo, P., & Brancato, V. (1992). The nature of depression in borderline depressed patients. *Comprehensive Psychiatry, 33*(2), 128–133.

Berezin, M. A., Liptzin, B., & Salzman, C. (1988). The elderly person. In A. Nicholi (Ed.), *The new Harvard guide to psychiatry* (pp. 665–680). Cambridge, MA: Belknap Press.

Black, D. W., Bell, S., Hulbert, J., & Nasrallah, A. (1988). The importance of Axis II in patients with major depression: A controlled study. *Journal of Affective Disorders, 14,* 115–122.

Blashfield, R. C., & McElroy, R. A. (1987). The 1985 journal literature on the personality disorders (Review). *Comprehensive Psychiatry, 28*(6), 536–546.

Bouchard, T. J. Jr., Lykken, D. T., McGue, M., Segal, N. L., & Tellegan A. (1990). Sources of human psychological differences: The Minnesota study of twins reared apart. *Science, 25,* 223.

Bowlby, J. (1951). *Maternal care and mental health.* Monograph Series, No. 2. Geneva: World Health Organization.

Bowlby, J. (1969). *Attachment and loss.* Vol. 1: Attachment. New York: Basic Books.

Bowlby, J. (1981). *Attachment and loss.* Vol. 3: Loss: Sadness and depression. Hamondsworth, England: Penguin.

Brooner, R. F., Greenfield, L., Schmidt, C. W., & Bigelow, G. E. (1993). Antisocial personality disorder and HIV infection among intravenous drug abusers. *American Journal of Psychiatry, 150*(1), 53–58.

Cadoret, R. J., O'Gorman, T. W., Troughton, E., & Heywood, E. (1985). Alcoholism and antisocial personality: Interrelationships, genetics, and environmental factors. *Archives of General Psychiatry, 42,* 161–167.

Campbell, M., Small, A. M., Green, W. H., Jennings, S. J., Perry, R., Bennett, W. G., & Anderson, L. (1984). Behavioral efficacy of haloperidol and lithium carbonate: A comparison in hospitalized aggressive children with conduct disorder. *Archives of General Psychiatry, 41,* 650–656.

Cantrell, D. P. (1989). Disruptive behavior disorders. In H. I. Kaplan & B. J. Sadock (Eds.). *Comprehensive textbook of psychiatry/V* (Vol. 2, 5th ed., pp. 1821–1828). Baltimore: Williams & Wilkins.

Cashdan, S. (1988). *Object relations therapy.* New York: W. W. Norton.

Coccaro, E. F., Astilk, J. L., Herbert, J. E., et al. (1990). Psychopharmacologic studies in patients with personality disorders: Review and perspective. *Journal of Personality Disorders, 4.*

Cowdry, R. W., & Gardner, D. L. (1988). Pharmacotherapy of borderline personality disorder: Alprazolam, carbamazepine, trifluoperazine, and tranylcypromine. *Archives of General Psychiatry, 45,* 802–803.

Cowdry, R. W., Pickar, D., & Davies, R. (1985–1986). Symptoms and EEG findings in the borderline syndrome. *International Psychiatry in Medicine, 15*(3), 201–211.

Dadds, M. R., et al. (1992). Childhood depression and conduct disorder: II. An analysis of family interaction patterns in the home. *Journal of Abnormal Psychology, 101*(3), 503–513.

Deutsch, H. (1942). Some forms of emotional disturbances and their relationship to schizophrenia. *Psychoanalysis, 11,* 301–321.

Docherty, J., Fiester, S., & Shea, T. (1986). Syndrome diagnosis and personality disorder. In R. Hales & A. Frances (Eds.), *Psychiatry update: American Psychiatric Association annual review,* vol. 5 (pp. 315–355). Washington, DC: American Psychiatric Press.

Egan, J. (1986). Etiology and treatment of borderline personality disorder in adolescents. *Hospital and Community Psychiatry, 37*(6), 613–618.

Emde, R. N., & Robinson, J. (1979). The first two months: Recent research in developmental psychobiology and the changing view of the newborn. In J. D. Nospitz (Ed.), *Basic handbook of child psychiatry* (pp. 72–105). New York: Basic Books.

Erikson, E. (1963). *Childhood and society* (2nd ed.). New York: W. W. Norton.

Favazza, A., & Conterio, K. (1988). The plight of chronic self-mutilators. *Community Mental Health Journal, 24,* 22–30.

Favazza, A. (1989). Normal and deviant self-mutilation. *Transcultural Psychiatric Research Review, 26,* 113–126.

Favazza, A., & Rosenthal, R. J. (1990). Varieties of pathological self-mutilation. *Behavioral Neurology, 3,* 77–85.

Favazza, A., & Rosenthal, R. J. (1993). Diagnostic issues in self-mutilation. *Hospital and Community Psychiatry, 44*(2), 134–140.

Finch, S. M., & Green, J. M. (1979). Personality disorders. In J. D. Nospitz (Ed.), *Basic handbook of child psychiatry* (pp. 235–248). New York: Basic Books.

Fish, B. (1986). Antecedents of acute schizophrenia break. *Journal of American Academy of Child Psychiatry, 25,* 595–600.

Freeman, P. S., & Gunderson, J. G. (1989). Treatment of personality disorders. *Psychiatric Annals, 19*(3), 147–153.

Freud, S. (1957). On narcissism: An introduction. In J. Strachey (Ed. and Trans.). The standard edition of the complete psychological works of Sigmund Freud (Vol. 19, pp. 69–102). London: Hogarth Press. (Original work published 1923)

Freud, S. (1991). Some character types met within psychoanalytic work. In M. F. R. Kets de Vries & S. Perzow (Eds.), *Handbook of character studies: Psychoanalytic explorations* (pp. 27–54). Madison, CT: International Universities Press.

Frosch, J. (1983). The psychosocial treatment of personality disorders. In J. Frosch (Ed.), *Current perspectives on personality disorders.* Washington, DC: American Psychiatric Press.

Garbutt, J. C., Loosen, P. T., Tipermas, A., & Prange, A. J. Jr. (1983). The TRH test in patients with borderline personality disorder. *Psychiatric Research, 9,* 107–113.

Goldsmith, H. H. (1983). Genetic influences on personality from infancy to adulthood. *Childhood Development, 54*(2), 331–355.
Greenberg, J. R., & Mitchell, S. A. (1983). *Object relations in psychoanalytic theory*. New York: Basic Books.
Grinker, R., Werber, B., & Drye, R. (1968). *The borderline syndrome*. New York: Basic Books.
Gunderson, J. G. (1979). The relatedness of borderline and schizophrenic disorders. *Schizophrenia Bulletin, 5*(1), 17–22.
Gunderson, J. G. (1988). Personality disorders. In A. M. Nicholi (Ed.), *The new Harvard guide to psychiatry* (pp. 337–357). Cambridge, MA: Harvard Press.
Gutheil, T. G., & Gabbard, G. O. (1993). The concept of boundaries in clinical practice: Theoretical and risk-management dimensions. *American Journal of Psychiatry, 150*(2), 188–196.
Hardin, S. B., Pesut, D., Head, K., Mitchell, J., & Stewart, J. (1993). *Intervention to decrease violence in adolescents by enhancing coping, self-efficacy, and support*. Paper presented at the 15th Southeastern Conference of Clinical Specialists for Psychiatric–Mental Health Nursing, Charleston, September 4.
Hartmann, H. (1958). *Ego psychology and problem of adaptation* (D. Rapaport, Trans.). New York: International Universities Press.
Herman, J. L., Perry, J. C., & van der Kolk, B. A. (1989). Childhood traumas in borderline personality. *American Journal of Psychiatry, 146*(4), 490–495.
Hirschfield, R. M. A. (1986). Personality disorders. In A. J. Frances & R. E. Hales (Eds.), *American Psychiatric Association annual review* (Vol. 5, pp. 233–239). Washington, DC: American Psychiatric Press.
Holzman, P. S., et al. (1984). Pursuit of eye movement dysfunction in schizophrenia: Family evidence for specificity. *Archives of General Psychiatry, 41,* 136–139.
Johnson, M., & Silver, S. (1988). Conflicts in the inpatient treatment of the borderline patient. *Archives of Psychiatric Nursing, 2*(5), 312–318.
Kalogerakis, M. G. (1974). The sources of individual violence. In S. Feinstein & P. Giovacchini (Eds.), *Adolescent Psychiatry* (Vol. 3, pp. 323–339).
Kalogerakis, M. G. (1992). Emergency evaluation of adolescents. *Hospital and Community Psychiatry, 43*(6), 617–621.
Kaplan, H. I., & Sadock, B. J. (1989). *Comprehensive textbook of psychiatry* (5th ed.). Baltimore: Williams & Wilkins.
Kay, R. L., & Kay, J. (1986). Adolescent conduct disorders. In A. J. Frances & R. E. Hales (Eds.), *Psychiatry update: American Psychiatric Association annual review* (Vol. 5, pp. 480–496). Washington, DC: American Psychiatric Press.
Keith, C. (1984). Individual psychotherapy and psychoanalysis with the aggressive adolescent: A historical review. In C. Keith (Ed.), *The aggressive adolescent: Clinical perspectives*. New York: Free Press.
Kendall, P. C., & Lipman, A. J. (1991). Psychological and pharmacological therapy: Methods and modes of comparative outcome research. *Journal of Consulting and Clinical Psychology, 39,* 78–87.
Kendler, K. S., Greenberg, A. M., & Strauss, J. J. (1981). An independent analysis of the Copenhagen sample of the Danish adoption study of schizophrenia: II. The relationship between schizotypal personality disorder and schizophrenia. *Archives of General Psychiatry, 38,* 982–984.
Kernberg, O. (1975). *Borderline conditions and pathological narcissism*. New York: Jason Aronson.
Kernberg, O. (1976). *Object relations theory and clinical psychoanalysis*. New York: Jason Aronson.
Kernberg. O. (1984). *Severe personality disorders*. New Haven: Yale University Press.
Khantzian, E. J., & Treece, C. (1985). DSM III psychiatric diagnosis of narcotic addicts. *Archives of General Psychiatry, 42,* 1067–1071.
Klein, M. (1977). Some theoretical conclusions regarding the emotional life of the infant. In M. Klein (Ed.), *Envy and gratitude and other works: 1946–1963* (Vol. 4, pp. 1946–1963). New York: Delacorte Press.
Kohut, H. (1971). *The analysis of self.* New York: International Universities Press.
Kohut, H. (1977). *The restoration of self.* New York: International Universities Press.
Kutcher, S. P., Blackwood, D. H., St. Clair, D., Gaskell, D. F., & Muir, W. J. (1987). Auditory P300 in borderline personality disorder and schizophrenia. *Archives of General Psychiatry, 44,* 645–650.
Le Blanc, M. (1992). Family dynamics, adolescent delinquency, and adult criminality. *Psychiatry, 55,* 336–353.
Liebowitz, M. R., Stone, M., & Trukat, I. D. (1986). Treatment of personality disorders. In A. J. Frances and R. E. Hales (Eds.), *Psychiatry update: American Psychiatric Association annual review* (Vol. 5, pp. 356–393). Washington, DC: American Psychiatry Association Press.
Linehan, M. M. (1987). Dialectical behavioral therapy: A cognitive behavioral approach to parasuicide. *Journal of Personality Disorder, 1,* 328–333.
Links, P. S., et al. (1990). Lithium therapy for borderline patients: Preliminary findings. *Journal of Personality Disorders, 4,* 173–181.
Livesley, W. J., Jackson, D. N., & Schroeder, M. L. (1992). Factorial structure of traits delineating personality disorders in clinical and general population samples. *Journal of Abnormal Psychology, 101*(3), 432–440.
Loeber R. (1990). Development and risk factors of juvenile antisocial behavior and delinquency. *Clinical Psychology Review, 10,* 1–42.
Loeber, R., & Strouthamer-Loeber, M. (1987). The prediction of delinquency. In H. C. Quay (Ed.), *Handbook of juvenile delinquency*. New York: Wiley.
Ludolph, P. S., Westen, D., Misle, B., Jackson, A., Wixom, J., & Wiss, F. C. (1990). The borderline diagnosis in adolescents: Symptoms and developmental history. *American Journal of Psychiatry, 147*(4), 470–476.
Mahler, M. (1952). On child psychosis and schizophrenia: Autistic and symbiotic psychosis. *Psychoanalytic Study of the Child, 7,* 206–305.
Mahler, M. (1965a). On early infantile psychosis: The symbiotic and autistic syndromes. *Journal of the Academy of Child Psychiatry, 4,* 554–568.
Mahler, M. (1965b). On the significance of the normal separation-individuation phase: With reference to research in symbiotic child psychosis. In M. Schur (Ed.), *Drives, affects, behaviors* (Vol. 2, pp. 161–169). New York: International Universities Press.
Mann, J. J., Arango, V., & Underwood, M. D. (1990). Serotonin and suicidal behavior. In P. M. Whitaker-Azmitta & S. J. Peroutka (Eds.), *The neuropharmacology of serotonin* (pp. 476–485). New York: New York Academy of Sciences.
Marohn, R. C. (1992). Management of the assaultive adolescent. *Hospital and Community Psychiatry, 43*(6), 622–624.
Masterson, J. F. (1976). *Psychotherapy of the borderline adult*. New York: Brunner/Mazel.
McCord, W. M. (1982). *The psychopathic and milieu therapy*. New York: Academic Press.
McGuffin, P., & Gottesman, I. I. (1984). Genetic influences on normal and abnormal development. In M. Rutter & L. Hersov (Eds.), *Child psychiatry: Modern approaches* (2nd ed.). London: Blackwell.
Meissner, W. W. (1988). The psychotherapies: Individual, family, and group. In A. Nicholi (Ed.), *The new Harvard guide to psychiatry* (pp. 449–480). Cambridge, MA: Belknap Press.
Meissner, W. W. (1990). Treatment of specific disorders: Paranoid personality. In American Psychiatric Association (Ed.), *Treatment of psychiatric disorders: A task force segment of the American Psychiatric Association*. Washington, DC: American Psychiatric Press.
Metcalf, D. R. (1979). Organizers of the psyche and EEG development: Birth through adolescence. In J. D. Nospitz (Ed.), *Basic handbook of child psychiatry* (pp. 63–71). New York: Basic Books.
Miller, R. (1979). Development from one to two years: Language acquisition. In J. D. Nospitz (Ed.), *Basic handbook of child psychiatry* (pp. 127–144). New York: Basic Books.
Mishne, J. M. (1986). *Clinical work with adolescents*. New York: Free Press.
Nagy, J., & Szatmari, P. L. (1986). A chart review of schizotypal personality disorders in children. *Journal of Autism and Developmental Disorders, 16,* 351–167.
Nehls, N. (1992). Group therapy for people with borderline personality disorder: Interventions associated with positive outcomes. *Issues in Mental Health Nursing, 13*(3), 255–269.
Parker, G. (1984). The measurement of pathogenic parental style and its relevance to psychiatric disorder. *Social Psychiatry, 19,* 75–81.

Patterson, G. R. (1990). *Depression and aggression in family interaction*. Hillsdale, NJ: Erlbaum.

Perry, P. C., et al. (1990). Treatment of specific disorders: Dependent personality disorders. In *American Psychiatric Association, Treatment of psychiatric disorders: A task force report of the American Psychiatric Association*. Washington, DC: American Psychiatric Press.

Pfohl, B., et al. (1986). DSM-III personality disorders: Diagnostic overlap and internal consistency of individual DSM-III criteria. *Comprehensive Psychiatry, 27*, 21–34.

Provence, S. (1979). Development from six to twelve months. In J. D. Nospitz (Ed.), *Basic handbook of child psychiatry* (pp. 113–117). New York: Basic Books.

Raine, A., & Venables, P. H. (1988). Enhanced p3 evoked potentials and longer p3 recovery times in psychopaths. *Psychophysiology, 25*, 30–38.

Redl, F., & Wineman, D. (1951). *Children who hate*. Glencoe, IL: Free Press.

Reich, J. (1992). Measurement of DSM-III and DSM-III-R borderline personality disorder. In J. F. Clarkin, E. Marziali, & H. Munroe-Blum (Eds.), *Borderline personality disorder* (pp. 116–148). New York: Guilford Press.

Reich, W. (1949). *Character analysis*. New York: Noonday Press.

Rinsley, D. B. (1982). *Borderline and other self-disorders*. New York: Jason Aronson.

Robins, L. N. (1978). Sturdy childhood predictions of adult antisocial behavior: Replications from longitudinal studies. *Psychosomatic Medicine, 8*, 611–622.

Rothstein, A. (1991). An exploration of the diagnostic term narcissistic person. In M. F. R. Kets de Vries & S. Perzow (Eds.), *Handbook of character studies: Psychoanalytic explorations* (p. 303–318). Madison, CT: International Universities Press.

Rounsaville, B. J., Weissman, M. M., Kleber, H., & Wilber, C. (1982). Heterogeneity of psychiatric diagnoses in the treatment of opiate addicts. *Archives of General Psychiatry, 39*, 161–166.

Rubinstein, M., Yeager, C. A., Goodstein, C., & Lewis, D. O. (1993). Sexually assaultive male juveniles: A follow-up study. *American Journal of Psychiatry, 150*(2), 262–265.

Sandler, J. (1991). Character traits and object relationships. In M. F. R. Kets de Vries & S. Perzow (Eds.), *Handbook of character studies: Psychoanalytic explorations* (pp. 191–203). Madison, CT: International Universities Press.

Searles H. F. (1984). Transference: Responses in borderline patients. *Psychiatry, 47*, 37–49.

Shaffer, D. (1988). The epidemiology of teen suicide: An examination of risk factors. *Journal of Clinical Psychiatry, 49*(Suppl), 36–41.

Shea, M. T., Widiger, T., & Klein, M. H. (1992). Comorbidity of personality disorders and depression: Implications for treatment. *Journal of Consulting and Clinical Psychology, 60*(6), 857–868.

Shearer, S. L., Peters, C. P., Quaytman, M. S., & Ogden, R. L. (1990). Frequency and correlates of childhood sexual and physical abuse histories in adult female borderline inpatients. *American Journal of Psychiatry, 147*(2), 214–216.

Siever, W., Keefe, R., Bernstein, D. P., Coccaro, E. F., Klar, H. M., Zemishlany, Z., Peterson, A. E., Davidson, M., Mahon, T., Horvath, T., et al. (1990). Eye tracking impairment in clinically identified patients with schizotypal personality disorder. *American Journal of Psychiatry, 147*(6), 740–745.

Soloff, P. H., George, A., & Nathan, R. S. (1982). The dexamethasone suppression test in patients with borderline personality disorder. *American Journal of Psychiatry, 139*, 1621–1623.

Spitz, R. A. (1951). The psychogenic diseases in infancy. *Psychoanalytic Study of the Child, 6*, 255–275.

Stone, M. H. (1990). Treatment of borderline patients: A pragmatic approach. *Psychiatric Clinics of North America, 13*(3), 265–285.

Terr, L. C. (1991). Childhood trauma: An outline and overview. *American Journal of Psychiatry, 14*, 10–20.

Thomas, A., & Chess, S. (1977). *Temperament and development*. New York: Brunner/Mazel.

Weiss, G. (1991). Attention deficit hyperactivity disorder. In M. Lewis (Ed.), *Child and adolescent psychiatry: A comprehensive textbook* (pp. 544–561). Baltimore: Williams & Wilkins.

Whiting, S. A. (1994). A Delphi study of the defining characteristics of interdependence and dysfunctional independence. *Issues in Mental Health Nursing 13*(1), 37–47.

Widiger, T., & Frances, A. (1987). Interviews and inventories for the measurement of personality disorders. *Clinical Psychology Review, 7*, 49–75.

Widiger, T., & Rogers, J. H. (1989). Prevalence and comorbidity of personality disorders. *Psychiatric Annals, 19*(3), 132–136.

Zanarini, M. C., Gunderson, J. G., & Frankenbury, F. R. (1989). Axis I phenomenology of borderline personality disorder. *Comprehensive Psychiatry, 30*, 149–156.

CHAPTER

The Client with a Dissociative Disorder

CATHERINE PAWLICKI, M.S.N., R.N.,C.S.

OUTLINE

CHAPTER OBJECTIVES

Upon completion of this chapter, you will be able to:

1. Define dissociation.
2. Discuss the influence of the nature of the stressor on the identified dissociative disorder.
3. Identify the psychiatric nurse's role and function in the treatment of the client with a dissociative disorder.
4. Assess a client for the presence of dissociation.
5. Intervene with a dissociating client to promote continuity of the self.
6. Identify expected client outcomes for continuity of the self based on developmental level.

KEY TERMS

Alter
Depersonalization disorder
Dissociation
Dissociative amnesia
Dissociative disorder
Dissociative fugue
Dissociative identity disorder
Personality
Secondary gain
Switching
Trauma

One of the most rapidly expanding areas of psychiatric practice is **trauma** and one of its sequelae, dissociation. All aspects of the concept of dissociation are being researched, including the neurobiology of dissociation. Dissociation as a mental mechanism was identified in the 19th century when Janet (Counts, 1990) considered its relationship to hypnosis and Freud (Sanders, 1986) identified the concept of repression as a defense mechanism. Putnam (1985, p. 66) recently defined **dissociation** as

> *a complex psychophysiological process, with psychodynamic triggers, that produces an alteration in the person's consciousness. During this process, thoughts, feelings and experiences are not integrated into the individual's awareness or memory in the normal way.*

Ludwig (1983) defined dissociation as a defense mechanism that holds great survival value for people experiencing trauma, allowing (1) automatization of behavior, (2) resolution of irreconcilable conflicts, (3) isolation of the traumatic experience, (4) discharge of feelings, and (5) escape from reality.

According to Sullivan, dissociation is an anxiety-reducing mechanism that functions by restricting awareness. If circumstances require a child to adapt by using dissociation excessively, the child becomes limited in his or her ability to make meaningful connections between an event and his or her thoughts and feelings about the event (Sullivan, 1953). Using Sullivan's theory, Peplau (1952) operationally defined dissociation. Her definition is presented in Table 15–1.

Continual exposure to overwhelming experiences in the absence of an external comforter can lead to life events being managed by varying degrees of dissociation. Dissociative phenomena exist along a continuum

TABLE 15–1
Operational Definition of Dissociation

1. In early life, certain thoughts, feelings, and/or actions of the client are disapproved by significant other persons.
2. Significant people's standards are incorporated as the client's own.
3. Later in life, the client experiences one of the disapproved thoughts, feelings, or actions.
4. Anxiety increases to a severe level.
5. The feelings are barred from awareness.
6. Anxiety decreases.
7. Dissociated content continues to appear in disguised form in the client's thoughts, feelings, and actions.

Adapted from Peplau, H. (1952). *Interpersonal relations in nursing.* © Springer Publishing Company, Inc., New York 10012; used by permission.

from minor to normative to pathological forms (Putnam, 1984). Minor forms of dissociation can be inconspicuous everyday occurrences of "spacing out," for example, while driving a car or sitting in class. Midpoint on the continuum would be reported out-of-body, near-death experiences, wherein the clients have an experience of viewing their body from a vantage point above or to the side of their body. Clients with out-of-body experiences report various perceptual experiences. The more pathological forms of dissociation are amnesia, fugue, and identity disorder, and they are related to traumatic, intense anxiety antecedents (see Fig. 15–1).

The core conflict in the person experiencing trauma is the wish to deny the horrible experience, while simultaneously wishing to proclaim it to everybody (Herman, 1991). The traumatic experience is usually prolonged and engenders in the victim a deep sense of being helpless to control his or her own survival. The repertoire of coping mechanisms available depends on the age of the victim during the traumatic event and determines the extent to which dissociation serves as the primary or persistent defense mechanism. Research has demonstrated a significant relationship between early childhood traumas, especially sexual abuse, and chronic dissociation.

The degree of self-ownership that is present in a dissociative experience is a gauge of the normal or pathological nature of the process (Allen, 1993). In the normal or minor process of dissociation, the sense of self or of the affect and thought belonging to the self is never lost. In pathological dissociation, the sense of self is disconnected from the experience. Affect or thought is disowned (psychogenic fugue and amnesia) or attributed to another self, or "not me" (dissociative identity disorder). Repeated use of dissociation leads to its indiscriminate use in response to a variety of stressors.

Dissociation does help a person survive and escape an overwhelming reality such as child abuse. It provides relief and time for the person to gather resources to cope with the trauma. When trauma persists, as is usually the case in child abuse, the use of dissociation persists and greatly influences personality development. Estimates of the incidence of child abuse have increased dramatically in the last decade. Ninety percent of clients with dissociative identity disorder have been identified as having been abused as children (Ross, 1992). Until further quantitative research becomes available that links **dissociative disorder** to the major public health problem of child abuse, the psychiatric nurse will be the frontline case finder of these clients. Therefore, the psy-

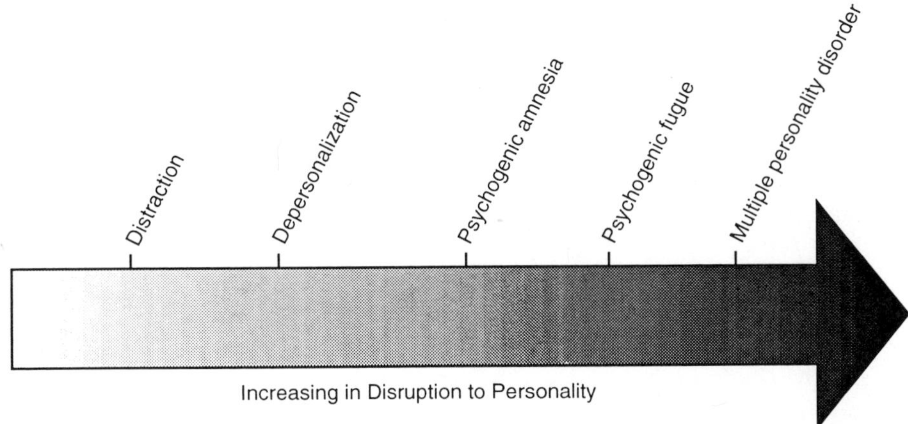

FIGURE 15–1
Dissociative disorder continuum.

chiatric nurse needs to have a firm grasp of dissociative disorders.

CAUSATIVE FACTORS: PERSPECTIVES AND THEORIES

INTERPERSONAL THEORY AND PERSONALITY DEVELOPMENT

A significant part of **personality** development is the lifelong process of assimilating experiences (thoughts, feelings, and actions) and using the assimilated product (understanding) to observe the self and make judgments of present-day interpersonal interactions.

In Sullivan's theory of personality development, Interpersonal Theory, the personality is conceptualized as a *self-system* that consists of three mutually interacting aspects: *good-me, bad-me,* and *not-me*. The development of each aspect is based on significant interpersonal experiences and the intensity of anxiety caused by each experience. According to Sullivan (1953), the self-system, or personality, develops around attempts to modulate anxiety internally in the context of an interaction with a significant other.

Good-me

This good-me aspect of the self-system consists of experiences from infancy on that are soothing and indicative of approval and acceptance by a significant other. Good-me is the part of self that is available to conscious awareness and comfortably revealed to others throughout life. The following example illustrates the good-me dynamic.

A toddler is playing and runs away from her mother into the next room. In a minute, the toddler reappears and races and puts her head into her mother's lap. Laughing, the mother picks up her daughter and hugs her. The daughter smiles, and when she is put down, runs away again.

In this interaction, the toddler is experimenting with separation. The crucial issue is the degree of control over separation that she and her mother can tolerate without either one becoming overwhelmingly anxious.

Bad-me

Experiences that elicit disapproval from significant others and result in a high degree of anxiety for a person constitute that part of the self-system known as bad-me. This aspect of the personality is available to a person's conscious awareness, but defense mechanisms (e.g., splitting or sublimation) are used in an effort to control the internal anxiety experience. The following is an example of the bad-me dynamic (see Chapter 2).

A 5-year-old girl wants the toy her 3-year-old brother is playing with. The brother won't give it to her, so the 5 year old slaps the toy out of his hand. The little boy cries loudly, and their mother comes over, picks her son up, and tries to comfort him. The mother asks the little girl why she did that, and the little girl states she wanted the toy. The mother sternly tells the daughter "That was not nice," and says she shouldn't do it again.

In this incident, the girl tried to meet her need through aggression directed toward her younger brother. As the mother comforted her brother, the little girl became more anxious, because not only did she not get her need met, she also received no comfort. As she assimilates this experience, her bad-me will come to involve the notion that attempting to get her needs met through aggression will cause her more anxiety.

Not-me

Experiences that are intensely overwhelming and elicit little or no soothing from a significant other are relegated to the not-me. This aspect of the self is kept in the unconscious; that is, it is dissociated. Even though this part of the self-system is dissociated, it continues to exert powerful influences on the rest of the person's development, interpersonal world, and behavior (see the Research Abstract display on p. 324). Maturation involves discovering and bringing to conscious awareness this aspect of the self and assimilating it with other known experiences of the self. The mature person expe-

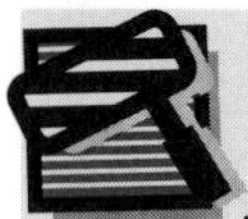

RESEARCH ABSTRACT

Child Maltreatment, Attachment, and the Self System: Emergence of an Internal State Lexicon in Toddlers at High Social Risk

Beeghly, M., & Cicchetti, D. (1994). *Development and Psychopathology*, *6*, 5–30.

Beeghly and Cicchetti examined how the quality of children's attachment relationships with their caregiver affected the children's self-system, including their ability to talk about their feelings. Because the ability to talk about internal states of the self is an age-appropriate development of later toddlerhood (2 1/2 to 3 years), the subjects of this study were 40 toddlers with a history of maltreatment and their biological mothers. The comparison group consisted of 20 toddlers and their mothers. The subjects in the comparison group were verified as having no history of abuse or neglect. Data from this study indicated that maltreatment has a significant negative effect on children's development of language about their internal state. Language is essential to the organization of self/other interactions, and with the negative effect of maltreatment, the toddlers are likely to experience further, more complex disruptions in the development of their personality.

riences the self as whole and continuous. The not-me dynamic is demonstrated in the following example:

A little girl is repeatedly sexually abused by her father. Each time he is done abusing her, he tells her he did it for her own good, but that she must never tell because her mother may die. The little girl never tells and believes she is now responsible for keeping her mother alive. Somehow, she must learn to live with the overwhelming experience of being abused without seeking comfort from significant others.

This little girl will dissociate the abuse experience as well as her feelings and needs associated with it in order to survive the ordeal psychologically and physically. As an adult, she will be vulnerable to self-mutilation and dissociation any time she becomes angry. Her personality development will be seriously compromised because her experiences and feelings are so overwhelming she cannot assimilate them or make emotional and conceptual connections about her self. She will adapt through dissociation, disowning this aspect of her self-system but continuously being affected by it.

NEUROBIOLOGICAL FACTORS

The limbic system is responsible for processing traumatic memories, and the hippocampus is responsible for storing and categorizing such information.

Many years of research with nonhuman primates have indicated that early and prolonged detachment from the significant caretaker directly affects the development of the limbic system (Van der Kolk & Saporta, 1991). Because the limbic system is where memories are processed, early trauma experiences will remain unassimilated to the degree the stress of detachment affected the limbic system. This could account for the hyperarousal caused by stimuli similar to the original trauma that then precipitates dissociation.

Significant early traumatic experiences and the lack of attachment have also been demonstrated to have long-term effects on neurotransmitters, specifically serotonin (see Fig. 9–1). Serotonin is considered to be the neurotransmitter most directly related to regulation of affect (Brown et al., 1982). There is reason to expect that research will demonstrate a positive relationship between dissociation and serotonin levels.

Clients with a dissociative disorder often present with a multitude of somatic complaints. Thus the nurse must thoroughly assess the client's physical status as the first intervention. Simultaneously, the nurse will want to keep in mind that if the client has a history of very early trauma, the somatic complaint may be representative of a memory laid down along primitive neurological pathways that is being stimulated by something in the current environment (Van der Kolk & Saporta, 1991). The client often experiences the nurse's attention to his or her physical complaints and the nurse's education about "body memories" to be helpful and soothing.

Any sudden onset of symptoms of dissociative disorder should first be evaluated for a possible medical etiology (see Table 15–2). Prolonged sleep deprivation, excessive caffeine ingestion, or electrolyte imbalance can present with symptoms of amnesia, depersonalization, or identity disturbance (Good, 1989; Stein & Unde, 1989). Clients with head injury or brain lesions can present with symptoms of dissociation. Clients arriving in the emergency room after overdosing on street drugs also present with dissociative symptoms (Kaplan & Sadock, 1991).

In the nineteenth century, Charcot and others attributed dissociative processes to various forms of epilepsy involving the temporal lobe. Research that continues in this area today presents supporting evidence of temporal lobe involvement in dissociation.

Research on stress and trauma has also demonstrated altered limbic system function in response to chronic stress, with concurrent suppression of hippocampal activity. It is possible that the stress hormones released (cortisol and adrenaline) precipitate dissociative episodes directly, or through influence on the limbic system and hippocampal processes. Dissociation may be precipitated by physiological or emotional changes, and the nurse must thoroughly assess the client in all domains to gain understanding of contributing factors.

TABLE 15–2
Medical and Other Psychiatric Diagnoses with Symptoms Similar to Those of Dissociative Disorders

DISSOCIATIVE DISORDER	SIGNS AND SYMPTOMS	MEDICAL OR OTHER PSYCHIATRIC DIAGNOSIS	SIGNS AND SYMPTOMS
Depersonalization disorder	Parts of body feel unreal Client has sensation of body change Client is aware of perceptual distortions	Accompanies numerous other psychiatric disorders: electrolyte disturbance, seizure disorder	
		Ganser's syndrome (seen in men with severe personality disorder)	Hard to differentiate
		Factitious Disorder: client fabricates symptoms	Has factitious quality—symptoms are worse when client is aware of being observed
		Toxic disorders	Blood chemistry is abnormal
		Neoplasms	Magnetic resonance imaging, computed tomography, and position emission tomography are abnormal
Dissociative amnesia	Begins abruptly Client is aware of memory loss and is alert before and after Depression is usually associated Physical assessment is normal	Transient global amnesia Postconcussion amnesia	Client is upset about amnesia Memory loss is generalized Amnesia *gradually* subsides Central nervous system examination is abnormal
Dissociative fugue	Client travels away from home and takes on a new identity May be associated with alcohol ingestion Evidence of secondary gain is clear	Cognitive disorder	Temporal lobe epilepsy Wandering does not result in socially adaptive behavior
Dissociative identity disorder	Changes in behavior are dramatic or sudden Client experiences either co-consciousness of or amnesia for alters Physical assessment is usually normal	Cognitive disorder	Central nervous system examination is abnormal Intoxication Street drugs are used

THE ROLE OF FAMILY DYNAMICS

The role of family dynamics in the dissociative process is highly potent for the child experiencing trauma such as physical or sexual abuse.

Personality development in the child is fostered by the family and is initially concentrated in the mother–child interaction. Healthy interactions between the mother and child protect and soothe the child when he or she is confronted by anxiety-provoking experiences. Healthy caretaking by the whole family facilitates the child's developing into an adult family member who is able to protect and sooth the self. This ability is manifested in appropriate affect regulation and a continuous experience of the self.

Behaviors such as sucking, crying, clinging, and smiling are evolutionarily adapted to elicit caretaking from the mother (Bowlby, 1969). When the mother responds calmly and reciprocally to the infant, attachment behavior is facilitated. Once young children learn that behavior can elicit comfort and security from the mother figure, they can start to develop a whole range of behaviors that enable them to attach to others and comfort themselves.

The perception of a secure base in the mother generalizes to the family as a whole. The members of a healthy, dynamic family protect and soothe each other through the maintenance of permeable but stable boundaries, defined and fulfilled roles and functions for each family member, resilience in the face of danger, and the ability to communicate across generations and family roles.

In an incestuous family, little if any, protection or soothing occurs. The members of the family experiencing incest are usually closed not only to each other but also to the outside world. Often the father is a controlling figure who dominates through physical force. He may present himself as a quiet family man, good provider, and churchgoer, but often he is actually quite introverted and preoccupied with sex. His relationship with the wife is conflicted. She often is weak or absent (detached) and physically or emotionally disabled. The child experiencing sexual abuse usually has no one to turn to for help (Blake-White & Kline, 1985). The child is living an experience that is violent and overwhelming. The experience and fear drive the child to a desperate search for attachments. When there is no protective figure to attach to, the need is so great that he or she will attach to the abuser. This attachment manifests itself in a phenomenon known as "internalization of the abuser." The child searches for a means to "join" a significant other on an unconscious level. In order to join or to be attached to the other, part of the child's self will mirror and eventually even mold to the abuser's self. This "attachment" is a survival defense for the child's internal self. In dissociative identity disorder, one **alter**, or personality fragment, is usually rageful, sadistic, and potentially homicidal.

A child may react to his or her incestuous family by defensively detaching the abandoning parent. The defensive detachment is usually manifested in a dissociative disorder. Dissociation or detachment protects the child from crying for help and finding no parent there (Barach, 1991). Thus, in a healthy family, the child is able to develop a wide range of soothing behaviors because of effective and protective family response, whereas in an abusive family, the only soothing the child is able to take into adulthood is a well-developed dissociative disorder. Any relationship that signals danger will elicit attachment behavior that is alternated with behavior that maintains distance (e.g., self-mutilation or dissociation).

Incestuous families often deny they have problems. Excessive use of denial by a family is fertile ground for physical and sexual abuse. There is usually always a rationale for abusive behavior, such as claims that it is "deserved," "unintentional," or "forgivable." A child attempting to cope through dissociation and surrounded by a family in denial struggles in treatment with the issue of what is real and what is not real. He or she may go through life excessively seeking validation or engaging in retraumatizing behavior in an effort to make the trauma real and develop some mastery over it.

Family dynamics around the abused child leave him or her with a rigid perception of interpersonal roles. That is, the child perceives all people to fall into one of the following roles: abuser, victim, rescuer, or neglectful or powerless bystander (Herman, 1991).

The nurse interacting with the dissociating client will be placed in one of these roles as the client re-creates the family experience. The nurse needs to observe the role pattern developing and assist the client in describing his or her perception of their interactions. Nursing interventions such as limit setting or confrontation will cause the client to perceive the nurse as an abuser. The client's threats or acts of self-destructive behavior can initiate the dynamic whereby the nurse perceives and experiences himself or herself as a victim or powerless bystander.

As each of these re-created family patterns is enacted, the nurse assists the client to identify his or her present need and to think about how to get it met. The goal is to foster a secure base for the client in the various treatment relationships so that security will eventually be internalized.

Clinical Example

Lucy, a 30-year-old client experiencing episodes of dissociation, visits with the psychiatric nurse at the mental health clinic every 2 weeks. Lucy was severely sexually and physically abused by her father and a neighbor until she was 18 years old and left home. Since that time, she has experienced severe alcohol and drug abuse, self-mutilation, and dissociation. Lucy reports that whenever she was upset at home, her mother would tell her to "put on a happy face."

Lucy has been meeting with the nurse for 3 months, having stated that she wanted to "feel better." Early in treatment, Lucy would start a session stating everything was going "pretty good." However, she would come in the following session with scratches on her arms and say she didn't remember what she had said in the preceding session. After this pattern developed, the nurse pointed out to Lucy that she would come in and say everything was okay but end up mutilating herself a short time later. Lucy and the nurse worked on what the pattern might mean. Eventually, Lucy was able to tell the nurse that she came in determined to talk about her anger but started worrying the nurse couldn't handle hearing about it. Her wish for the nurse to know her anger and her simultaneous fear of the consequences if that should happen resulted in dissociation and self-mutilation. Lucy was afraid of being angry in front of the nurse and believed the nurse "couldn't handle it"—the powerless bystander role. Lucy used the "happy face" her mother had wanted and engaged in dissociation to detach and manage the internal conflict and in self-mutilation to punish and soothe herself.

DISSOCIATIVE DISORDERS ACROSS THE LIFE SPAN

CHILDHOOD

Dissociation is an early primitive defense mechanism available to children until they mature and gain greater psychological capacity to accommodate ambiguity and tolerate conflict—Putnam (1991) labeled this a "normative dissociation." It is normally manifested in fantasy play and other imaginary activities. It is common for children to have elaborate, imaginary companions, and the phenomenon should not be considered pathological unless it is carried into adolescence. Normative dissociation usually peaks at 10 years of age if the child has not experienced a traumatic event and has had supportive and empathetic parenting.

Empathetic parenting allows the child to develop the cognitive and emotional schemata with which to understand ambiguous and conflicting thoughts and feelings. The child is provided comfort and protection while experimenting in the world and can verbalize his or her experience to the parent with a sense of safety.

A child with a dissociative disorder is most likely to have a history of early sexual or physical abuse and has not been able to develop attachment because of the absence of empathetic parenting.

Children with a dissociative disorder are often difficult to differentiate from children with attention deficit disorder. There is increasing evidence that abuse itself can cause hyperactivity (Van der Kolk, 1987). The abrupt changes in behavior and short attention and memory spans seen in hyperactive children are similar to episodes of dissociation. Traumatized boys are more hyperactive and aggressive than traumatized girls (Peterson, 1991). Sadly, children with pathological dissociation will be labeled as liars when they accurately state that they cannot remember homework, behavior, etc. Often, these children suffer self-hatred and appear anxious and depressed. The following are additional symptoms of childhood dissociative disorder (Peterson, 1991):

- Apparent confusion about very basic things
- Odd changes in physical skills
- An imaginary companion the child claims is real
- Inappropriate sexual behavior
- Reference to the self in the third person
- Self-mutilation

ADOLESCENCE

At its best, adolescence is a turbulent time for the individual. Affect and behavior become more erratic than they were in childhood, and the search for identity necessitates some fantasy thinking. Fantasy provides the healthy adolescent an opportunity to redefine his or her power and role in relation to significant others (Hogarth, 1991). It can be normal for adolescents under temporary, severe stress to regress and cope through depersonalization.

Symptoms of pathological dissociation in adolescence can be consistent with the diagnosis of conduct disorder. More defense mechanisms are available to the adolescent, and the dissociative process, the struggle to keep the not-me out of awareness, will be confused with the adolescent's search for identity and intimacy. The adolescent with dissociate identity disorder and an extreme identity problem is likely to be the most pliable to the demands of peer groups and will have alters to meet each demand.

In an effort to counteract a not-me personification of powerlessness, the adolescent may become more aggressive and act out sexually. Denial, along with dissociation, will present in an adolescent who not only does not recall trauma but rejects any suggestion that he or she is the least bit troubled.

Having never experienced parental soothing and attachment, the adolescent who is dissociative will attempt to provide soothing for himself or herself through drug abuse and sexual promiscuity and to meet attachment needs through gang membership. Management of affect, especially sadness, is accomplished by self-mutilation in the form of excessive tattoos or ear piercing.

THE ROLE OF THE NURSE WORKING WITH CHILDREN AND ADOLESCENTS

When working with the child or adolescent with a dissociative disorder, the nurse's first goal is to ensure the client's safety. The protection and soothing that were unavailable in the client's early development must be present in the nurse–client relationship and therapeutic environment. The nurse should accept the experiences of alters in children and adolescents with dissociative identity disorder. Excessive **switching** between alters is usually the result of an environmental or interpersonal trigger similar to past trauma. Reassurance by the nurse, who is in the here and now, is therapeutic. Structure in the nurse–client relationship and physical milieu helps the client experience his or her self in a continuous manner. In addition the continuity of the client's self may be facilitated by the use of clearly defined limits and consequences for inappropriate behavior. Emphasis should be on talking or writing about feelings, rather than acting on them. Children can be encouraged to keep art journals.

The nurse in advanced practice may have success in using a group therapy process for adolescents. An expressive group process will help the adolescent normalize some feelings as well as provide a consistent and healthy peer group experience.

Promotion of clients self-soothing is a major goal for the psychiatric nurse. The child client will need concrete direction in this area. Does he or she have a soothing stuffed toy or a favorite story? something or someone to turn to when frightened? The adolescent can be assisted to use sports or imagery that involves relaxation as a means of soothing.

ADULTHOOD

The healthy adult continues the development of the three aspects of his or her self-system that originated in childhood, with the not-me aspect continually being uncovered and brought into conscious awareness. However, even in healthy adults, the experience of a traumatic event, such as a flood, earthquake, or car crash, may result in dissociation. Dissociation of the experience is adaptive in the sense that it gives the person time to gather his or her defense mechanism resources. This gathering of resources will help the person assimilate the experience without being psychologically overwhelmed. The dissociative process paces the assimilation of the experience into consciousness and modulates the anxiety. For example, after a natural disaster such as a hurricane or earthquake, it is not uncommon for people to not remember the event or to be found wandering, unsure of where they live. It is quite common after a car crash to not remember what happened during the hours immediately after the crash.

As with any other age group, it is important to differentiate between a general medical condition and a psychological etiology for a dissociative process in an adult. In amnesia with an underlying medical condition, such as severe electrolyte imbalance or head injury, general information is lost before personal information. Thus, elderly clients may wander away from home and, when found, be able to state their name but not have a sense of their general location or how long they have been wandering. Clients with psychological amnesia, on the other hand, have no sense of who they are, who their family members are, or what their occupation is.

The psychiatric nurse can make major contributions to the diagnostic process. The nurse observes patterns of apparent dissociation in terms of particular time of day and the presence or absence of possible environmental factors. The nurse correlates these observations with the objective physiological data. The nurse psychotherapist in the community will use his or her extensive knowledge of physiology as well as interviewing skills to identify trauma in the assessment of a client presenting with "lost time" or a sense of "not being myself."

The adult with a dissociative disorder frequently goes undiagnosed or is misdiagnosed (Kluft, 1991). Several factors account for this unfortunate phenomenon. First, the person, having grown up in a chaotic family, may not know that losing time is an abnormal experience. Unless the behavior becomes disruptive, he or she may go through life with a dissociative disorder. Second, some adults may be in the mental health system for years being treated for depression, and the dissociation becomes evident only after a triggering event such as puberty or pregnancy. Adults with dissociative identity disorder have usually developed skill at keeping secret all the alters and their activities. Often, the dissociative disorders of adult survivors of incest will come to the fore when one of their children reaches the age at which they were victimized. Adult men with undiagnosed dissociative disorders end up incarcerated in prison because of aggressive behaviors such as assaults on men or women, serial killing, or drug-related activities. The problem for these men is poor affect regulation, which results in episodes of rage or attempts at intimacy that only re-create the abuse they experienced as children.

SPECIFIC DISSOCIATIVE DISORDERS

DEPERSONALIZATION DISORDER

Depersonalization disorder is a rapid-onset, persistent dissociative process in which the client's experience of the self or perception of the reality of the self or environment is changed. The client is able to observe the process as it occurs and verbalize discomfort (APA, 1994).

Etiology. The client is overwhelmed by feelings during a current event that is similar to a traumatic event in the past (APA, 1994).

Clinical Example

Ted, a 20-year-old hospitalized male, has just had a visit from his family, with whom he has not lived for 5 years. His mother, a recovering drug abuser, would violently beat Ted and then tell him to "forget everything" before he went to school. His greatest concern before the family visit was that he would "just hold it together." After his family left, Ted was observed sitting rigidly in a chair. He reported feeling like the floor was sinking and the walls were falling out. The episode lasted 2 to 3 minutes.

DISSOCIATIVE AMNESIA

Dissociative amnesia is a dissociative process that results in a sudden identity disturbance due to the client's inability to recall significant personal information. Underlying general medical conditions have been ruled out as a possible cause (APA, 1994). A person may experience **secondary gain,** or psychogenic amnesia could be a means of gaining media attention or escaping from financial responsibility.

Etiology. The origin of dissociative amnesia is usually a traumatic event that is psychosocial in nature, for example, the sudden loss of a significant other or impulsive behavior that is unacceptable (APA, 1994).

Clinical Example

Louise was admitted to the psychiatric unit after her daughter found her sitting on her porch. Louise did not recognize her daughter or know her own name or the name of the town she lived in. Louise was given a thorough medical evaluation, and no general medical cause was found for her amnesia. Louise had no history of psychiatric treatment. Louise's daughter told the nurse that her mother had discovered her husband was having an affair and had been planning to divorce him, but he was killed in a car wreck 10 days ago. Louise had told her daughter the day before the accident that she was so angry with her husband that she wished he was dead.

DISSOCIATIVE FUGUE

Dissociative fugue is a dissociative process that results in an identity and memory disturbance manifested by sudden travel away from the home or work environment in conjunction with the development of a new identity. The travel may be for brief or extended periods, and the new identity is usually in contrast to the old (e.g., from somber to jovial) (APA, 1994).

Etiology. The origin of dissociative fugue is usually a traumatic event that is psychosocial in nature (APA, 1994).

Clinical Example

Bob was a 54-year-old insurance salesman with a wife and three teenage children. One day he didn't come home from work, and all efforts to locate him proved unsuccessful. Before his disappearance, Bob had sought a promotion but was passed over for a much younger employee. Bob had always worked 7 days a week. He had been proud of the fact that his wife never had to work outside the home. After hearing he had been rejected for the promotion, Bob got in his car to drive home, but he ended up going to the Northwest coast where he lived alone, worked as a bartender, and gambled on the side. He called himself Rex and felt vague about his past, but he calmed himself by saying, "Life is for having fun and spending money."

DISSOCIATIVE IDENTITY DISORDER

Dissociative identity disorder is a severe dissociative disorder characterized by multiple amnestic episodes and alternating separate and distinct identities (Kluft, 1991). The following are the signs and symptoms of dissociative identity disorder:

- Unremembered behaviors
- The discovery of items in client's possession that the client cannot account for
- Loss of time
- Behavior characteristics that represent distinctly different ages
- Changes in appearance and dress
- Use of different voices

Etiology. An antecedent to dissociative identity disorder is overwhelming sadistic trauma early in life. The trauma is usually severe sexual abuse that overwhelms the child's nondissociative defenses. Subsequently, the abuse experience is dissociated and aspects of the experience (memory of it and affect related to it) later appear in the form of various personalities.

TREATMENT MODALITIES

PSYCHOPHARMACOTHERAPY OF DISSOCIATIVE DISORDERS

There is no particular drug or combination of drugs that is specific to the treatment of a client with a dissociative disorder. Psychopharmacotherapy is usually targeted at relieving some of the intense symptoms and persistent depression that these clients often present (Barken et al., 1986). See Chapter 26 for more information on psychopharmacology.

Anxiety that is persistent and peaks prior to a dissociative episode is a symptom common to all types of dissociation. Thus anxiolytics such as clonazepam (Klonopin) and lorazepam (Ativan) given PRN and in maintenance doses are helpful in stabilizing the client as he or she works to develop nondissociative coping mechanisms.

Depression is also a common presenting symptom of clients with dissociative disorder and may be what first brings them into the mental health system. No particular class of antidepressant is more effective than another; each needs to be evaluated on an individual basis. Monoamine oxidase inhibitors should be cautiously prescribed to clients with dissociative identity disorder, because one of the alters may deliberately violate the food restrictions.

Anger and severe internal disequilibrium will accompany dissociation in varying degrees. Neuroleptics can be a useful adjunct to treatment to assist the client in periods of dyscontrol or rapid dissociation. Haloperidol (Haldol) and chlorpromazine (Thorazine) can be effective. It should be noted that the alters of the client with dissociative identity disorder may have varying degrees of responsiveness to neuroleptics. This is not manipulation but a basic difference in psychological responsiveness.

The nurse's role in psychopharmacotherapy is to educate the client about the medication, including the purpose of the medication, the dosage schedule, and possible side effects. The nurse should assess the client for medication compliance, which can be disrupted by dissociative episodes. An emphasis on client responsibility, especially with clients with dissociative identity disorders, is paramount for medication and safety.

CLIENT GROUNDING TECHNIQUES

Grounding, as a concept, is meant to convey the notion of "not going away," that is, dissociating. The following techniques help clients concentrate on the here and now and move toward verbalizing what is occurring in their internal world. The nurse should teach the client these techniques.

Safe Place. Finding a safe place is a concept very familiar to survivors of abuse. The dissociative person should be encouraged to find a reasonable place in the environment where he or she can go and guarantee the nurse and himself or herself safety and freedom from destructive impulses. A typical place could be a particular chair or room.

Ice in Hands. Ice helps the client focus on a physical sensation that is not harmful. When the warning signs of dissociation are present, the nurse may encourage the client to hold an ice cube securely in each hand until he or she can report feeling calmer.

Wrapping Self in Blanket. A person who is dissociating may start to feel not real or feel that he or she is going to "come apart." Wrapping a blanket around himself or herself like a long cloak helps set the external boundaries and promote a sense of protection.

Counting Forward or Backward. Counting forward or backward is a technique used mostly by clients with dissociative identity disorder. Counting is a form of hypnosis that can be used to let an alter that is overwhelmed go in and another come forward with behavior appropriate to the situation.

CLIENT EDUCATION

Providing clients with skills to cope with their dissociative disorder is an important function of the psychiatric nurse. Essential skills are relapse prevention and journaling.

Relapse Prevention. Relapse prevention is an important skill drawn from work with chemically dependent persons. The client is taught to recognize contributing factors (triggers) to dissociation. The client and nurse then develop a concrete plan to interrupt the stimulation of a dissociative episode. The plan could include activities such as listening to music, staying with people, or engaging in a task. The plan is then shared with the family and other health care professionals involved in the client's treatment to enlist support in implementing the plan whenever it is needed.

Journaling. Writing in a journal helps the client achieve several outcomes: feelings are put into words, a sense of continuity of the self is developed in the journal, and the impact of triggers is diminished.

If the client has not journaled before, he or she should start with a 5-minute daily exercise. The client should be encouraged to pick an event that occurred during the day and write down his or her thoughts and feelings about it. The client should share the journal with the nurse on a regular basis. Journal work should be an essential part of each client's day. The structure can vary according to the client's threshold of dissociation and phase of treatment. Children and adolescents can be encouraged to keep an art journal, rather than a written one.

THE NURSE'S ROLE

THE GENERALIST'S ROLE

The psychiatric nurse is pivotal in the care of the client vulnerable to or diagnosed with dissociative disorder. The generalist in psychiatric nursing will be on the frontline of identifying the undiagnosed dissociative disorder. The nurse's other important role is to help the client develop healthier living skills and achieve basic symptom management, including appropriate use of medications.

THE ROLE OF THE ADVANCED-PRACTICE NURSE

The advanced-practice psychiatric nurse may often engage the client in a psychotherapy/case management process. Psychotherapy is the arena in which the client may retrieve memories in a controlled manner to consider their impact on his or her life. The nurse needs to assess clients' safety continually, and use short hospital stays if necessary, to help clients retrieve their capacity to feel safe.

THE NURSING PROCESS

Assessment

Early case finding is an important function of the nurse working with children. Recognition that a child is being abused or is experiencing early school failure can help to interrupt progression toward a much more problematic dissociative disorder in adulthood.

Psychosocial assessment involves collecting both subjective and objective data. The client may not always be able to report sexual or emotional trauma because the event is dissociated. The nurse watches for signs of abuse: startle reaction, erratic sleep, fear at night, refusal to sleep on the bed, or unexplained fear of objects or other people. Because some clients are not aware they dissociate, the nurse also observes for a pattern of not remembering events and a pattern of unexplained behaviors. Clients with an overt history of self-harm or accident proneness should be assessed for dissociation (Torem, 1989).

More than any other psychiatric disorder, dissociation is assessed basically through observation and a period of repeated interaction with the client. Because dissociation is episodic and not continual, many clients learn to adjust to their dissociation experience. Psychological tests do not always reveal dissociation.

Nursing Diagnosis

Possible nursing diagnoses include

- Alteration in Self-Concept
- Ineffective Coping: escape through dissociation
- Severe Anxiety related to acute stressor

Planning

The client and psychiatric nurse should mutually identify the desired outcomes of their working together. The outcome that is most likely to be achieved is the one the client values. In most cases, clients with dissociative disorders need environmental and interpersonal safety to be established first. A core part of trauma is the person feeling helpless and vulnerable (Speigel, 1986). The process of working to identify desired outcomes is empowering.

Outcomes should be very short-term in nature, so that clients are able to appreciate their progress. Planning, whether in a community or hospital setting, should be reviewed frequently.

Implementation and Evaluation

As the client works with the nurse to implement a plan of care, the client should experience a form of support that has been missing in his or her life. Regardless of setting, intervention should be flexible but emphasize consistency and predictability.

If the nurse is working with a client with dissociative identity disorder, several interventions need to be identified to correspond to the different developmental levels of the alters (Anderson & Ross, 1988).

The client should be encouraged to write in his or her journal about the effectiveness of the care plan as often as possible. Evaluation should be a mutual affair and based on as much behavioral data as possible.

Text continued on page 335

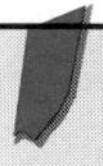

Nursing Care Plan 15–1 The Client with Dissociative Identity Disorder (Penny)

OUTCOME IDENTIFICATION	NURSING ACTIONS	RATIONALE	EVALUATIONS
Nursing Diagnosis: Altered Self-Concept as evidenced by dissociative phenomena.			
1. By [date], Penny will identify at least two warning signs of impending dissociation.	1. Teach Penny to write in journal everyday, especially after a dissociative episode.	1. Keeping a journal is a method of documenting events and feelings that are otherwise difficult to retrieve because of dissociation.	*Goal met:* Penny discovers that her handwriting changes dramatically around 11:00 each evening. Penny has started to list six warning signs by reviewing the past 48 hours of her journal.
	1b. Review Penny's journal with her.	1b. Working with the client on the journal enhances the value of the journal.	
	1c. Have Penny make a list of possible warning signs of dissociation.	1c. The first step in mastering dissociation is achieving conscious awareness of warning signs.	
Nursing Diagnosis: High Risk for Violence: Directed at others, as evidenced by presence of alter (Sue) with homicidal rage.			
1. By [date], Penny will express a sense of responsibility for Sue's behavior.	1. Emphasize to Penny that she is responsible for all parts of herself.	1. Teaches client that the "personalities" are all part of him or her and under his or her control (Braun, 1986).	*Goal met:* Penny makes an effort to communicate verbally with staff about Sue's rage. Chart requested restraints because "didn't want to hurt innocent people" when feeling angry.
	2. Empathize with the original purpose of the rage—to provide protection from sadistic abuse.	2. All defense mechanisms serve a purpose. Behavior cannot be changed without understanding the original motivation for it.	
Nursing Diagnosis: Dysfunctional Attachment Patterns as evidenced by continued wish for idealized parents and lack of integrated sense of self.			
1. By [date], Penny will identify one strategy for managing the feeling of abandonment.	1. Help Penny identify the dysfunctional coping strategy she presently uses when she is feeling abandoned.	1. Expectations of others and behaviors when needs are not met must be brought to client's awareness before they can be changed.	*Goal met:* Penny makes plans to offer "Lily" (the 5-year-old alter) extra time in her room near shift change.
	2. Encourage Penny to develop a coping plan for potential times of feeling abandoned.	2. Anticipation of an event promotes observance of behavior and sense of control over impact of the event.	

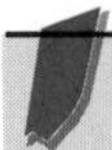

Standard of Care for the Client with a Dissociative Disorder

Nursing Diagnosis: Alteration in Continuity of Self

Client Outcome: By [date], client will demonstrate or verbalize increased continuity in one or all parameters of the self: identity, memory, experience.

Defining Characteristics:

Loss of time
Disorientation to person
Intrusive memories
Object in client's possession for which origin is unknown
History of early severe sexual abuse or neglect
Recent interpersonal/environmental trauma
History of multiple diagnoses
Age-inappropriate behaviors
Hyperarousal
Change in appearance and dress
Change in voice
Mute
Migraine headache
Self-mutilation
History of alcohol and drug abuse
History of eating disorder
Difficulty in trusting
Affect dysregulation

NURSING DOMAIN	CLIENT OUTCOME	NURSING INTERVENTIONS
Psychotherapeutic interventions	1. Client states what personality is interacting with nursing staff.	1a. Collaborate with client in mapping out the alters and the purpose and function of each.
		1b. Instruct client that he or she is responsible for letting staff know which alter is out.
		1c. Identify with client which alters are caretakers (internal self-helpers) and can be elicited in stressful situations.
		1d. Before the client goes off the unit, have him or her contract to have only an appropriate alter out when off the unit.
		1e. Emphasize that all alters are responsible for care and behavior of body.
		1f. Respond to client as a whole person.
		1g. Encourage host personality to engage all alters in writing in a journal.
	2. Client relates memories of self-system to present peer relationship patterns.	2a. Educate client about dysfunctional attachment/trust patterns from past abuse.
		2b. Initiate *brief* contact frequently with client during first 72 hours of hospitalization.
		2c. Problem-solve with client regarding how client may feel safe in presence of another client or nurse who reminds client of trauma.
	3. Client maintains progressively longer experience of here-and-now reality.	3a. Teach client basic structure of journal: Work 5 to 10 minutes daily Choose one event of day Write about thoughts and feelings related to event
		3b. Review journal work with client on regular basis.
		3c. Review nursing care plan and sleep patterns with client on a regular basis.
		3d. Assess client for what, if any, grounding techniques he or she currently uses.

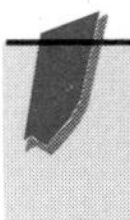

Standard of Care for the Client with a Dissociative Disorder (Continued)

NURSING DOMAIN	CLIENT OUTCOME	NURSING INTERVENTIONS
		3e. Support client in use of following client-appropriate grounding techniques: Going to safe place Holding ice in hands Placing feet on floor and grasping chair Wrapping self in blanket Staying out of room Blowing his or her nose Listening to tapes that provide pleasant memories Washing face Counting forward or backward Requesting quiet room Requesting PRN medication Requesting restraints
Therapeutic milieu	1. Client identifies triggers in environment that lead to dissociation.	1a. Educate client about concept of trigger. 1b. If client rapidly switches, start flow sheet to identify pattern of triggers. 1c. Provide client with feedback about when dissociation was observed.
	2. Client participates in promotion of a safe milieu.	2a. Explore with client how client meets his or her need to feel safe. 2b. Educate client about the need to not allow own behavior to become alarming to other clients (abuse is unacceptable). 2c. Develop plan with client to contain violent or self-destructive alters when and if they come out. 2d. Encourage client to have child alters come out only in privacy of his or her room. 2e. Support client in stating when another client's behavior seems similar to past abuse.
Activities of daily living	1. Client maintains a structured day.	1a. Assess client's ability to make up a daily schedule. 1b. Support client in keeping appointments by providing positive feedback. 1c. Provide client with unit-restricted schedule if he or she is being kept on the unit. 1d. Actively support client in adhering to unit-restricted schedule. 1e. Document any dissatisfaction client expresses with schedule. 1f. Assist client in structuring time for alters to come out appropriately.
	2. Client participates in development of safe nighttime environment.	2a. Help client identify his or her patterns of sleep and wakefulness. 2b. Problem-solve periods of wakefulness. 2c. Encourage identification and use of specific self-soothing techniques as a part of bedtime preparation.

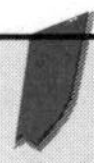

Standard of Care for the Client with a Dissociative Disorder (Continued)

NURSING DOMAIN	CLIENT OUTCOME	NURSING INTERVENTIONS
Health teaching	1. Client verbalizes purpose, side effects, and dose of medication.	1a. Provide client with appropriate information about medications. 1b. Explain value of consistent medication dosage. 1c. Encourage client to identify which alters, if any, are resistant to medication. 1d. Problem-solve resistance to use of medication.
	2. Client verbalizes understanding of nursing care plan development and implementation.	2a. Explore understanding of nursing care plan development and implementation. 2b. Identify with client the value of participating in development of care plan. 2c. With client, practice identifying problem goal and intervention.
	3. Client demonstrates use of journal as tool to facilitate continuity of experience.	3a. Assess client's experience with journal writing: how often: ____ technique: ____ tools: ____ 3b. Teach client journal structure and value of using journal consistently. 3c. Review client's journal writing with him or her. 3d. Encourage journal writing as substitute for acting out and as method to self-soothe.
	4. Client demonstrates use of safe place.	4a. Assess client's history of using safe place: where: ____ when: ____ how long: ____ 4b. Teach client value of still using safe place as adult. 4c. Encourage client to identify safe place on the unit. 4d. When client appears overstimulated, remind him or her of safe place. 4e. If client harms self or others in safe place, repeat b and c. 4f. Encourage client to use safe place for alters via imagery.
Somatic therapies	1. Client adheres to prescribed medication regimen.	1a. Encourage client's input regarding most effective time structure of doses. 1b. Assist client in encouraging resistant alters to help take care of the body. 1c. Teach client to use PRN medication on a preventive basis using warning signs.

Standard of Care for the Client with a Dissociative Disorder (Continued)

NURSING DOMAIN	CLIENT OUTCOME	NURSING INTERVENTIONS
	2. Client uses self-soothing techniques for grounding.	2a. Assess client's current repertoire of self-soothing techniques. 2b. Encourage attendance at group activities promoting body awareness. 2c. Assist client in use of grounding techniques listed under Psychotherapeutic Interventions.
Discharge planning	1. Client develops relapse prevention plan for triggers that lead to dissociation.	1a. Review relapse prevention plan with client. 1b. Practice prevention plan with client. 1c. Help client identify people with whom client will share plan after discharge.

Case Study and Nursing Care Plan

The following case study illustrates the application of the nursing process to the client with a dissociative disorder.

Case Study: The Client with Dissociative Identity Disorder (Penny)

Penny is a 35-year-old woman who suffered sadistic sexual abuse by both of her parents and their friends from infancy through 15 years of age. She is admitted to the hospital in a dissociated state, claiming that she is Mary and doesn't understand how she got to the unit, except that Penny must have tried to commit suicide again. A nursing assessment elicits a description of five alter personalities ranging in age from 6 months (the children) to 35 (Mary). Each of the personalities is described as manifesting a particular affect. The "host" personality is Mary. Lily is 5 years old and looking for a "mommy and daddy." Sue is 16 years old and is the protector; she wishes to kill people when they don't do as she says. Penny is 12 and feels all the pain. Mary states she tries to keep Penny from hearing things that are "going on outside."

Nursing Care Plan 15–1 (p. 331) identifies the desired outcomes for this case study, the nursing actions needed to achieve these outcomes, and the rationales for these actions.

STANDARD OF CARE

The accompanying Standard of Care (p. 332) for clients with a dissociative disorder provides the nurse with a menu of client outcomes and nursing interventions within the six domains of nursing: psychotherapeutic intervention, therapeutic milieu, health teaching, activities of daily living, somatic therapies, and discharge planning.

► CHAPTER SUMMARY

Dissociative disorders are usually the result of trauma. Clients with underlying general medical conditions can present with symptoms of dissociative disorder, and a general medical condition should be ruled out in a thorough evaluation.

The severity of the dissociative disorder is determined by the severity and nature of the trauma, the age at which the trauma was experienced, the neurobiological predisposition of the victim, and the presence or absence of a soothing caretaker.

Dissociative disorders are treated with psychopharmacology, psychotherapy, and client education.

The nurse's role in the care of the client with a dissociative disorder is that of casefinder, consultant, and coach in affect regulation. The nurse helps the client observe the pattern of dissociation and develop coping strategies to interrupt or minimize the process.

Suggestions for Clinical Conference

1. Briefly describe the trauma a client has experienced and identify one factor that has helped him or her survive.
2. Discuss myths you have heard about people with dissociative disorders.
3. Review medications that clients with dissociative disorders in the clinical setting are receiving.

References

Allen, J. (1993). *Dissociative processes: A working model for clinician and patient.* Unpublished manuscript.

American Psychiatric Association. (1994). *Diagnostic and statistical manual of mental disorders* (4th ed.). Washington, DC: Author.

Anderson, G., & Ross, C. (1988). Strategies for working with a patient who has multiple personality disorder. *Archives of Psychiatric Nursing, 2*, 236–243.

Barach, P. (1991). Multiple personality disorder as attachment disorder. *Dissociation, 4*, 117–123.

Barkin, R., Braun, B., & Kluft, R. (1986). The dilemma of drug therapy for multiple personality disorder. In B. Braun (Ed.), *Treatment of multiple personality disorder* (pp. 109–132). Washington, DC: American Psychiatric Press.

Blake-White, J., & Kline, C. (1985). Treating the dissociative process in adult victims of childhood incest. *Social Casework: The Journal of Contemporary Social Work, 66*, 394–402.

Bowlby, J. (1969). *Attachment and loss: Vol. 1. Attachment.* New York: Basic Books.

Braun, B. (Ed.). (1986). *Treatment of multiple personality disorder.* Washington, DC: American Psychiatric Press.

Brown, G. L., Ebert, M. E., Goyer, P. F., Jimerson, D. C., Klein, W. J., Bunney, W. E., & Goodwin, F. K. (1982). Aggression, suicide, and serotonin: Relationships to CSF amine metabolites. *American Journal of Psychiatry, 139*, 741–746.

Counts, R. (1990). The concept of dissociation. *Journal of the American Academy of Psychoanalysis, 18*, 460–479.

Good, M. (1989). Substance induced dissociative disorders and psychiatric nosology. *Journal of Clinical Psychopharmacology, 9*, 88–93.

Herman, J. (1991). *Trauma and recovery.* New York: Basic Books.

Hogarth, C. (1991). *Adolescent psychiatric nursing.* St. Louis: Mosby–Yearbook.

Kaplan, H., & Sadock, B. (1991). Dissociative disorders. In *Synopsis of psychiatry.* (pp. 428–437). Baltimore: Williams & Wilkins.

Kluft, R. (1991). Multiple personality disorder. *American Psychiatric Press Review of Psychiatry, 10*, 161–188.

Ludwig, A. (1983). The psychobiology functions of dissociation. *American Journal of Clinical Hypnosis, 26*, 93–99.

Peplau, H. (1952). *Interpersonal relations in nursing.* New York: G. F. Putnam and Sons.

Peterson, G. (1991). Childhood dissociation. *Dissociation, 4*, 152–166.

Putnam, F. (1985). Dissociation as a response to extreme trauma. In R. Kluft (Ed.), *Childhood antecedents of multiple personality* (pp. 66–97). Washington, DC: American Psychiatric Press.

Putnam, F. (1991). Recent research on multiple personality disorders. *Psychiatric Clinics of North America, 14*(3), 489–502.

Ross, C. (1992). Epidemiology of multiple personality disorder and dissociation. *Psychiatric Clinics of North America, 14*, 503–517.

Sanders, S. (1986). A brief history of dissociation. *American Journal of Clinical Hypnosis, 29*, 83–91.

Spiegel, D. (1986). Dissociating damage. *American Journal of Clinical Hypnosis, 29*, 123–131.

Sullivan, H. (1953). *The interpersonal theory of psychiatry.* New York: G. F. Putnam and Sons.

Stein, M., & Uhde, T. (1989). Depersonalization disorder. Effects of caffeine and response to pharmacotherapy. *Biological Psychiatry, 26*, 315–320.

Torem, M. (1989). Recognition and management of dissociation regressions. *Hypnosis, 16*, 197–217.

Van der Kolk, B. (1987). *Psychological trauma.* Washington, DC: American Psychiatric Press.

Van der Kolk, B., & Saporta, J. (1991). The biological response to psychic trauma: Mechanisms and treatment of intrusion and numbing. *Anxiety Research, 4*, 199–212.

CHAPTER 16

The Client at Risk for Suicide

DEBORAH ANTAI-OTONG, M.S., R.N.,C.S.

OUTLINE

CHAPTER OBJECTIVES

Upon completion of this chapter, you will be able to:
1. Analyze the meaning of high-risk suicidal behaviors.
2. Identify clients at risk for suicide.
3. Develop a nursing care plan for suicidal clients across the life span.
4. Integrate various self-destructive theories.
5. Assess clients for self-destructive behaviors.

KEY TERMS

Hopelessness
Impulsivity
Lethality
Psychological autopsy
Self-destructive
Self-mutilation
Suicidal ideation
Suicide

One of the most demanding and perplexing challenges in psychiatric nursing is the prevention of **suicide**, the intentional taking of one's own life. Suicide is a significant public health problem, ranking as the eighth leading cause of death in the United States (Weed, 1985) and accounting for approximately 25,000 deaths annually. The frequency of suicide in the United States has remained constant since 1950 (National Center for Health Statistics, 1991). These data are conservative because not all suicides are recorded. A large percentage of clients who kill themselves have experienced profound psychological disturbances.

Suicide crosses all boundaries, affecting all age, socioeconomic, and religious groups. Illnesses such as depression, alcoholism, and schizophrenia increase the risk of suicide (Beck et al., 1990; Roy et al., 1984). Fifteen percent of clients with major depression eventually kill themselves (Bulik et al., 1990). Other risk factors include male gender, family history of suicide, social isolation, and aging. Developmental and biological factors also place people at risk for suicide (Table 16–1).

The incidence of adolescent and elderly suicide is increasing, and this presents mental health professionals with challenges to develop innovative strategies of identifying persons at risk. Advances in neurobiology have identified biological markers, such as decreased serotonin levels in depressed clients, that place those clients at risk for suicide and other **self-destructive** behaviors.

TABLE 16–1
Clinical Factors of High Suicide Risk

PSYCHOLOGICAL
Hopelessness Helplessness Depression Cognitive impairment
BEHAVIORAL
History of suicide attempts Poor impulse control Alcoholism Substance abuse
SOCIOCULTURAL
Family history of suicide or attempts Previous attempts Recent significant loss Poor support systems Chaotic or disorganized family systems
NEUROBIOLOGICAL
Neurochemical dysregulation Genetic Hormonal imbalances (e.g., as detected by dexamethasone suppression and thyroid-stimulating hormone tests) Physical illness (e.g., HIV positive, terminal, debilitating)
MAJOR DEMOGRAPHIC
Unmarried (separated, divorced, widowed) Male older than 65 years of age White Protestant Mental illness (e.g., depression, schizophrenia) Alcoholism or substance abuse

HIV, human immunodeficiency virus.

It is a common fallacy that people who threaten to kill themselves are not likely to commit suicide. The opposite is true, and an estimated 80 percent of clients who kill themselves have made previous threats or attempts to do so (Beskow, 1979). The mistaken premise that suicidal threats or gestures are mere manipulative behaviors often generates negative reactions toward suicidal clients and impedes objective decision making. Increased awareness and knowledge about suicide are crucial to evaluating clients at risk for self-destructive behaviors such as suicide. There is no absolute predictor of suicide, and it remains an enigma.

The focus of this chapter is to analyze biological and psychosocial concepts that increase the risk of suicide or other self-destructive behaviors. Psychiatric nurses play a crucial role in assessing, preventing, and evaluating self-destructive behaviors in clients using maladaptive coping patterns.

DEFINITIONS

Suicide. The term *suicide* stems from the Latin word *sui*, "of oneself," and *-cida* from *caedere*, "to kill." Shneidman (1985) described suicide as "the conscious act of self-induced annihilation" (p. 203), and he emphasized the importance of psychosocial stressors and the inability to resolve intolerable pain by stopping "consciousness." **Suicidal ideations** are thoughts of injury or demise of self but not necessarily a plan, intent, or means. A suicidal threat is verbalization of imminent self-destructive action that, if carried out, has a high probability of leading to death (Shneidman, 1985). The following is an example of these terms:

> The child who states, "I want to kill myself" (ideation)
> The adolescent who states, "I am going to hang myself" (threat)

Suicidal ideations or threats must always be taken seriously, especially when they are expressed by children.

Self-Destructive Behaviors. ***Self-destructive*** refers to behavior that tends to harm or destroy the self. Roy (1985) classified self-destructive behaviors as direct or indirect. *Direct pattern of self-destruction* refers to those behaviors that directly affect the client's physical and mental well-being, such as suicide, anorexia, alcohol and substance abuse, and self-mutilation. Indirect patterns of self-destructive behavior include high-risk behaviors that may cause harm, such as promiscuity, prostitution, abusive relationships, dangerous sports, and compulsive gambling.

Self-destructive behaviors occur on a continuum, the most severe of which is suicide. Other actions include self-mutilation behaviors such as hair pulling, nail biting, burning, picking at wounds, and hacking or cutting. Winchel and Stanley (1992) defined **self-mutilation** behaviors as those that cause deliberate harm to one's body. Injuries sustained by these behaviors frequently cause tissue damage or scarring. High-risk groups for self-mutilation are clients who are mentally retarded or those with psychosis or personality disorders (such as the borderline type).

Self-mutilation is frequently described as experiences of depersonalization or dissociative states. These acts of self-induced pain stimulate the opiate system in the brain, producing endorphins. Many clients state that they do not feel pain when they injure themselves (van der Kolk, 1988) (see the section on borderline personality disorder in Chapter 14 for more information on self-mutilation).

CAUSATIVE FACTORS: PERSPECTIVES AND THEORIES

Early perceptions of suicide still affect current beliefs, assumptions, and practices. Most mental health professionals do not consider suicide to be a rational act. The perception of suicide is generally based on religious, cultural, and social factors that have prevailed for centuries. Suicide is considered a taboo by many societies and religions, and it is frequently labeled a sin.

PSYCHODYNAMIC THEORIES

Early psychodynamic theorists described suicide as an escape from intolerable life stressors—an act of valor, insanity, and seductiveness. The act symbolized aggression directed at a loved one or society. Freud's (1961) classic psychoanalytical theory of suicide described suicidal clients as ambivalent, integrating concepts of love and hate in the decision to kill themselves. He surmised that guilt generated by self-destructive impulses toward object relations (early caregivers) motivated clients to suicide. Suicide was perceived as a kind of self-murder and was accepted as internalized aggression.

Karl Menninger's (1938, 1947) contribution to the understanding of suicide was based on Freud's earlier concepts. He postulated that suicide is anger turned inward, and in his classic contributions, *Man Against Himself* and *The Human Mind,* Menninger (1947) linked depression and suicide and described it as an "ever-present spectra" (p. 122). Depressed clients are always at risk for suicide. Additionally, he delineated the following three components of hostility in suicide:

1. The wish to kill
2. The wish to be killed
3. The wish to die

In other words, he perceived suicide as an integration of anger, malice, remorse, retaliation, and despair that were too great to be resolved realistically and that the act is a "flight from reality" or "submission to punishment." This premise proposes that suicide is a symptom of mental illness and the murder of self by self (Menninger, 1947).

SOCIOLOGICAL THEORIES

Emile Durkheim's (1951) classic work, *Suicide,* focused on the sociological aspects of suicide. His writings centered on deaths by suicide, and he analyzed patterns of death from health statistics. He contended that several sociological theories involving the integration and regulation of society contributed to suicide. He defined four types of suicides as follows:

1. Egoistic suicide—the person no longer finds acceptance or is insufficiently integrated into a social group and lacks close, meaningful relationships (higher rates of suicides among singles, socially isolated people)
2. Altruistic suicide—the person is too integrated into society, or the suicidal behavior is a response to a cultural expectation (i.e., cult members who may be willing to kill themselves as part of a group suicide or hara-kari)
3. Anomic suicide—society is insufficiently regulated; there is social instability (i.e., lack of norms or values)
4. Fatalistic suicide—society is too regulated (i.e., group suicide regulated by rigidity and control or suicide pact)

PSYCHOCULTURAL THEORIES

Hendin's 1987 study of youth suicide examined a broad spectrum of cultural and psychosocial aspects of suicide. The subjects of his study were youths from Scandinavian countries, Harlem, the white middle class, and colleges. He explored the relationship of successful suicides and social influences. His findings showed that for the first 70 years in the twentieth century, the suicide rates among New York urban African Americans, aged 15 to 30 years, were consistently higher than rates among Caucasians of the same age group. These findings were consistent with other metropolitan areas across the country (Stack, 1982). High suicide rates among African American youths were related to histories of marked childhood violence and rage (Hendin, 1969, 1971). Overt cultural rejection among young African Americans often reinforced feelings of rage, worthlessness, and powerlessness, which their families cultivated, resulting in distorted self-images. Self-image—personal meaning of life and death—for youths is determined by cultural and subcultural social structures (Hendin, 1971, 1987).

Cultural norms impact the rate of suicide. Societies that value the elderly foster a sense of identity and importance for this age group. Older adults are valued as models for youth. Cultures that place more significance on youth create societies that alienate the elderly. Elderly people are more likely to feel alienated because they lack clear definition of their role and significance. Feelings of alienation, devaluation, loss of identity, and low self-esteem contribute to suicide in the elderly.

Socioeconomic, ethnic, and cultural factors also influence suicide rates. Cultural causes that buffer people from suicide (Gibbs, 1988; Shaffer, 1988) include

Negative perceptions of suicide
Strong social support systems
Networking generated by families who experience discrimination or extreme stress

Conversely, cultures that condone substance abuse, neglect, social isolation, and violence increase the risk of suicide (Gibbs, 1988).

Suicide is a paramount concern of Native American tribes. Suicide rates among this population have increased drastically during the past 10 years. The rates of suicide among the Navajo tribes reflect the national average, approximately 12 in 100,000. In contrast, the Apache tribes have suicide rates as high as 43 in 100,000 (Berlin, 1987). This rate varies among tribes and is related to decreased ties with traditional Native American practices. Tribes that practice traditional rituals are usually stable and promote a sense of belonging and support among members. In contrast, tribes in turmoil that do not support their members have higher rates of substance abuse, feelings of alienation and neglect, alcoholism, and emotional or physical abuse. These factors increase the risk of suicide among adolescents and young adults in Native Americans and other populations (Berman & Jobes, 1991; Wyche et al., 1990).

There are inconsistent research findings about the role of psychocultural influences on the prevalence of suicide. Some of these studies have been criticized for biased sampling that shows a significant number of suicides among the poor (Adams, 1985).

NEUROBIOLOGICAL THEORIES

Recent advances in neurobiology suggest a relationship between suicide and altered neurological factors, such as abnormal neuroendocrine and neurochemical function of the brain. For example, there may be an association between major depression and dysregulation of the hypothalamic-pituitary-adrenal axis. Studies have been done using the dexamethasone suppression test, which is performed to determine the body's response to additional steroid administration. In normal health, the dexamethasone would suppress adrenocortical production of cortisol; however, in major depression, the neuroendocrine challenge shows high production of urinary free cortisol and nonsuppression of plasma cortisol. This has been found in suicidal clients, suggesting that cortisol secretion is poorly regulated by the hypothalamic-pituitary process (Meltzer & Nash, 1988).

Perhaps most significantly, the serotonergic system is believed to play a pivotal role, because serotonin modulates mood and modifies feelings of fearfulness, despondency, and depression (Vogt, 1982). Major depression is manifested by a constellation of neurovegetative behaviors, such as altered mood, abnormal sleep patterns, diminished libido, abnormal eating patterns, and altered cognitive function. These same behaviors are directly affected by abnormalities in the production and metabolism of serotonin and other neurotransmitters such as dopamine and norepinephrine (see Chapter 9). Abnormally low levels and activity of 5-hydroxyindoleacetic acid, a major metabolite of serotonin, have been found in the spinal fluid of depressed suicidal clients (Meltzer, 1990; Meltzer & Lowry, 1987), indicating low brain serotonin production. Furthermore, recent studies demonstrated decreased 24-hour urinary output of dopamine metabolites, homovanillic acid, and dihydroxyphenylacetic acid, suggesting that decreased dopaminergic neurotransmission may play a role in suicidal behavior in depression (Roy, 1993; Roy et al., 1992).

Aggression and self-injurious behaviors have also been linked to decreased serotonergic levels in clients diagnosed with borderline personality and obsessive-compulsive disorders (Coccaro et al., 1989; Goodman et al., 1989). Serotonin reuptake inhibitors have consequently been effective in the treatment of self-injurious behaviors and depression. Additionally, self-injurious behaviors, such as nail-biting and hair-pulling symptoms, have been relieved by fluoxetine (Prozac) and clomipramine (Anafranil) (Primeau & Fontaine, 1987).

Genetic factors have also been linked with the prevalence of major depression and suicidal behavior. Twin and adoption studies suggest that genetic traits play a significant role in the cause of depression and vulnerability to maladaptive coping patterns (Kendler, 1992; Kendler et al., 1993; McGuffin et al., 1991). Despite these findings, the exact role of genetic traits remains controversial. Other environmental factors, such as psychosocial stressor, culture, and modeling, probably also influence depression and suicidal behaviors (Adams, 1985).

The cause of suicide is complex and encompasses neurobiological, psychosocial, and genetic factors that affect one's response to stress. Identifying high-risk populations and behaviors can help nurses explore the client's wish to die and develop interventions that help clients cope with intolerable emotional pain. Exploring the causes of mental illness and suicidal behavior is a continuous responsibility involving the behavioral assessment of psychosocial, cultural, and neurobiological aspects of human beings.

PSYCHOSOCIAL FACTORS

Suicide is a response to a crisis, and it is an effort to cope with intolerable psychosocial and neurobiological stressors generated by life experiences. Developmental crises generate enormous stress for the person who is challenged to master the next life phase. People with close family ties are less likely to commit suicide than are those with distant ties. Meaningful interpersonal relationships can buffer people from experiencing stress as intolerable and decrease the deleterious effects of crisis.

The two developmental stages in which suicide peaks are adolescence and older adulthood. Social problems such as chaotic family systems, divorce, violence, and child abuse increase the likelihood of adolescent suicide. Furthermore, family conflict manifested by rejection, abuse, and ineffective communication patterns are common among adolescents who commit suicide.

Elderly clients who experience significant losses, such as their health, spouse, and financial security, experience enormous psychological and physical stress. Stable, close interpersonal relationships help this age group cope more effectively.

STRESS FACTORS

Living can be thought of as a continuum of stress and adaptation. Perceptions of stress are influenced by the frequency of stressful life events and their severity and the person's ability to mobilize internal and external resources to handle them. Stress plays a major role in adaptation, and an inability to resolve stress results in crisis. Crisis often generates disorganization and feelings of helplessness and **hopelessness.** Reorganization and crisis resolution are determined by ego integrity or are a function of the person's ability to mobilize psychosocial and biological resources (Caplan, 1961). Suicide becomes a viable option in the face of poor ego function and a lack of resources to cope with stress (see Chapter 7).

OTHER RISK FACTORS

Additional risk factors associated with suicide are depression, schizophrenia, previous attempts, lack of psychosocial resources, alcoholism and substance abuse, and major health problems (psychiatric or physical).

Clinical Example: Mr. Jones

Mr. Jones is a 46-year-old man who recently had a massive heart attack. His business is failing, and his wife of 20 years has decided that she does not want to be married to an "invalid." He has few social supports. He is referred for acute psychiatric hospitalization. His mood is sad, and he expresses feelings of hopelessness about his situation and thoughts of dying. He reports a poor appetite, concentration difficulties, and extreme fatigue since the heart attack.

What places Mr. Jones at risk for suicide? He is depressed; he has feelings of hopelessness, a major physical health problem, and is facing an impending divorce; and he is preoccupied with dying.

Understanding the risk factors for suicide provides a basis for understanding nursing interventions and prevention. Predicting suicide remains a mystery, but certain behaviors and circumstances increase its risk. The nursing assessment is a vital part of identifying populations at risk for suicide. The client needs a comprehensive physical and psychosocial assessment to determine reasons for treatment, level of danger, present and past coping patterns, and current support systems.

Depression

Persons with depression or other mental disorders have 3 to 12 times greater risk for suicide compared with other populations. Clients who commit suicide usually have major depression, but not all depressed clients commit suicide. Clients with depression often feel hopeless, worthless, inadequate, and guilty. These clients have already given up and feel they do not deserve happiness. Suicide may be an act of desperation for clients or a way out of immense psychological pain. Preoccupation with suicide reflects the client's perception that current conditions are hopeless. Hopelessness is a fundamental suicide predictor. People who feel hopeless are more likely to kill themselves because they believe that suicide is the only viable option to managing "insoluble problems" (Beck et al., 1985, 1990). Psychotic depression increases the risk of suicide. Symptoms of this disorder include delusions, excessive worrying and guilt, and hallucinations.

Schizophrenia

Fifteen percent of clients with schizophrenia commit suicide. These data parallel those of suicide in clients who experience depression and alcoholism. Young men recently diagnosed with schizophrenia have the highest suicide rates, especially during the first 4 years after the diagnosis is made (Prasad-Ashoka, 1986; Waltzer, 1984). Psychosis is often manifested by command auditory hallucinations, that is, voices telling the client to commit suicide. The nature of psychosis increases **impulsivity** and impairs judgment and cognitive function. These behaviors increase the likelihood of suicide.

Previous Attempts

A previous suicide attempt is often the best predictor of death by suicide (Shaffer et al., 1988). Suicide attempts usually occur 8 to 10 times more often than successful suicide. Most people who commit suicide have made previous attempts. The severity of suicide attempts is a continuum, and the severity of attempts evolves over time until the attempts end with a completed suicide (Garland & Zigler, 1993) (Fig. 16–1).

Past suicide attempts must be explored along with the reasons for their failure. This information is invaluable because it helps the nurse understand about the client's impulsivity, seriousness of intent, and coping behaviors. Nurses can explore the meaning of past suicide attempts by asking clients the following questions:

- How many suicide attempts have you made?
- How have you tried to kill yourself? (actual behavior) Did you want to die? When was the last time?
- What are your feelings about the unsuccessful attempt(s)? (provides clues about the client's attitude regarding the attempt)
- What were the circumstances of each? (e.g., What types of stressors [changes] were you experiencing at the time?)
- Did you plan the attempt, or did you do it on the spur of the moment? (impulsivity)

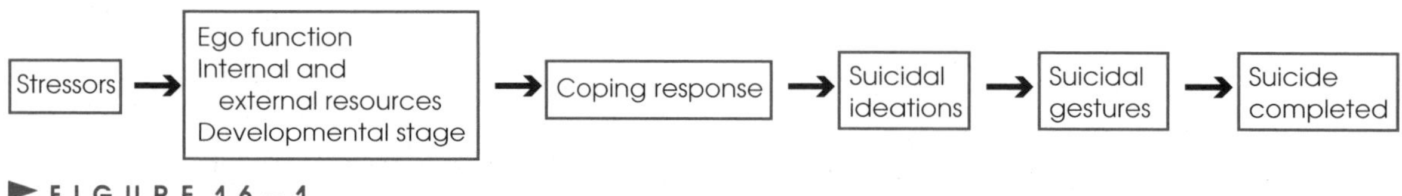

FIGURE 16–1
Suicide continuum.

- Were you drinking or abusing substances at the time or shortly before the attempt?
- What type of treatment did you receive after the attempt?

Questions about past suicide attempts serve as the basis for developing nursing interventions to prevent present or future suicides. Assessing the meaning of present and past coping patterns needs to include verbal and nonverbal cues. An example is the client who admits making attempts in the past and her expression reflects remorse about the impact it has had on family members. Another client may show no affective response when discussing past attempts. The client who exhibits remorse or feelings is more likely to be concerned about the impact of future attempts on the family's well-being. Conversely, the client who displays little affect or emotion is less likely to consider the effect of suicide on others. Each client provides information about coping patterns, substance abuse, and interpersonal relationships. Clients with histories of poor impulse control, such as those with personality disorders, psychosis, and alcoholism, are at risk for suicide.

Lack of Psychosocial Resources

Psychological support is crucial to crisis resolution. Clients who are recently divorced, widowed, or socially isolated are at far greater risk for suicide than those who have strong family ties of interpersonal relationships. Support systems provide emotional renewal and validation of self-worth. Depressed clients may willfully distort their experiences and isolate themselves from loved ones to resolve their perception of being a burden or remorseful of their present illness.

Suicide generally occurs within chaotic and stressful environments or relationships (Helig & Klugman, 1970). Suicidal threats and attempts are forms of communication with families and may represent an attempt to express feelings of stress or despair that the client has difficulty verbalizing. Incidences such as the adolescent who overdoses after failing a class and the man who drives his car off a bridge the day his divorce is final are examples of communicating stress and feelings of helplessness. Clients who commit suicide often generate feelings of helplessness, negative reactions, and anxiety in the nurse. These feelings often stem from the belief that nurses are supposed to save lives, and when clients commit suicide, the inability to save them often triggers anger and guilt (see Controversy display).

Approaching the client in a calm, nonjudgmental manner is the basis of a therapeutic alliance. Effective communication is fundamental to helping the client understand his or her behavior. Assessing suicide risk involves recognizing risk factors and understanding the effect of psychosocial stressors on biological processes and cognitive functioning. Several considerations can assist in evaluating suicide risk. They include the following:

- Determining whether the client has a suicidal plan—the client may express thoughts of dying, such as "I want to kill myself" or "I wish I could go to sleep and not wake up." Most clients who kill themselves have planned their demise. Suicidal plans need to be taken seriously because this indicates that thorough planning and working through have already taken place. A suicide note suggests that the client is resolved to kill himself or herself and the ambivalence of wanting to live and die has been worked through. Assessing for suicidal plans includes asking, "Are you having thoughts of killing yourself?" There is a myth that asking clients about suicide "plants" ideas. Contrary to this belief, clients often welcome the opportunity to discuss their feelings about suicide. Nurses need to make sure that they are speaking the same language as the client, because he or she may not know what the word suicide means. An example is the client who is asked, "Are you have thoughts of hurting yourself?" Her responses may be "no." Actually, she is having thoughts not of hurting herself but of killing herself.

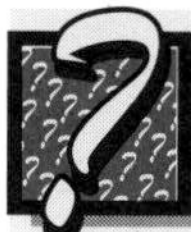

CONTROVERSY: ASSISTED SUICIDE

Suicide generates intense reactions in nurses and other health care professionals: Successful suicides often generate feelings of helplessness, anger, and failure. The notion of mercy killings or assisted suicide is not new. In recent years family members have killed their loved ones with painful or terminal illnesses. In a society intolerant of pain and suffering, suicide by various means has become a viable solution. Unfortunately, this solution has replaced seeking support from family members or professionals who facilitate adaptive resolution of a seemingly helpless situation. It is no wonder that the clinicians who advocate physician-assisted suicide have become a solution to various medical and mental illnesses. As nurses, we have to explore the meaning of suicide and our reactions to it. Do people have the right to seek out the Jack Kevorkians and other mercy killers to resolve stressful life events, or should they stick to traditional means of crisis resolution?

- Determining the dangerousness of the suicide attempt—it is essential to assess the level of **lethality.** The term *lethality* refers to the potential degree of injury caused by suicidal gestures or attempts. Direct questions need to be asked about the suicide to assess the suicidal potential. Degrees of lethality range from high risk (e.g., shooting, hanging, stabbing, or using carbon monoxide) to low risk (e.g., overdosing on 15 acetaminophen tablets). The client's perception of the incident determines the seriousness of the attempt, except in instances when the attempt is minimized.

When the client is assessed to have a definite suicidal plan, the next question involves assessing its lethality. Shneidman (1985) defined ***lethality*** as the probability of the person killing himself or herself in the immediate future. He ranked lethality into four levels: (1) high; (2) medium; (3) low; and (4) absent. The second concern is providing safety and preventing suicide. This is generally done by offering the client referral for acute inpatient psychiatric treatment to provide crisis intervention and further evaluation of suicide potential and the treatment of underlying mental illness.

Preoccupation with suicide or dying is a symptom of distress and ineffective coping reactions. Suicidal thoughts and plans must be thoroughly assessed to determine their duration and how they have been responded to in the past. Acute suicidal ideation is more likely to generate greater concern than are chronic threats. This does not mean that chronic suicidal thoughts are less serious than acute ones, but the client who admits having thoughts of dying for 10 years that he or she has not acted on for whatever reason is indicating some degree of impulse control. This information needs to be documented, and the client needs to be assessed for level of dangerousness at the present time and asked about specific circumstances that would make him or her act on the thoughts.

Suicidal clients are usually ambivalent about dying. That is, a part of them usually wants to die and another part wants to live. The part that wants to live usually communicates despair and pain through verbal and nonverbal cues. These cues must be taken seriously, and their meaning must be thoroughly assessed. The client who has a specific plan, the means, and the intent is at serious risk for suicide. Questions such as, "What has stopped you from acting on these thoughts or plans in the past?" elicits information about the imminence of suicide. Some clients may respond by saying "I don't want to hurt my family" or "I know this is a silly idea." Inquiring about ways they have handled similar thoughts is useful in assessing impulse control and coping patterns.

Alcoholism and Substance Abuse

The risk of suicide increases when alcohol or substance misuse occurs during a crisis, stressful life events, or major losses, and it is likely to occur within 6 weeks of these events. Major losses account for about one third of suicides among clients with alcoholism. Intoxication impairs cognitive function and lowers inhibitions that impair cognitive ability, judgment, decision making, and reality testing. There has been a dramatic increase in the number of adolescents who kill themselves under the influence of alcohol and drugs. Adolescents using violent means tend to kill themselves when intoxicated. An alarming number of clients with schizophrenia also abuse alcohol, further increasing the risk of suicide (Drake et al., 1990). Alcoholism accounts for 15 percent of suicides (Brent et al., 1987; Rich et al., 1988). Nursing implications from these findings indicate the need to assess the client's present and past substance abuse history.

Major Health Problems

Major health problems also generate feelings of hopelessness, helplessness, and despair. These factors play a major role in depression. Chronic illnesses such renal failure, chronic pain, and chronic lung disease interfere with the client's livelihood and quality of life. Clients with chronic and debilitating illnesses need to be assessed for depression and suicide potential.

SUMMARY

Suicide is a significant health care problem because it impacts all societies, communities, families, and people. Nurses are in key positions to identify clients at risk. Risk factors include psychosocial, biological, and developmental components. Recognizing these factors and their impact on human behavior and adaptation is a critical aspect of prevention.

SUICIDE ACROSS THE LIFE SPAN

Suicide crosses all boundaries of the life span. Understanding coping patterns throughout the life span helps the nurse recognize the significance of prevention and health promotion. Table 16–2 summarizes the prevalence and causative factors of suicide across the life span.

CHILDHOOD

Child and adolescent suicide has perplexed poets, composers, artists, and authors for centuries (e.g., Shakespeare's *Romeo and Juliet*). Early descriptions of suicidal children were noted in several nineteenth century foreign journals. The authors postulated that the risk of suicide increased with age and that suicide was more likely to occur in urban than in rural communities. Other commonalities among suicidal children included the death of a significant family member, parent–child strife, and the school's role in providing discipline (Zilboorg, 1937). Freud (1961) asserted that childhood suicides were influenced by parent–child turmoil and incest.

Family factors generally play a major role in childhood suicide. Children and adolescents who commit

TABLE 16–2 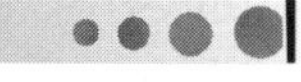

Prevalance and Causative Factors of Suicide Across the Life Span

	PREVALENCE	CAUSATIVE FACTORS
Childhood	Unknown (some accidents may be suicide); predicted to increase 13% for ages 10–14 years by 2000	Affective disorder (depression), family and developmental factors
Adolescence	6–13% have attempted suicide; predicted to increase 94% for ages 15–19 years by 2000	Affective disorders, conduct and antisocial disorders, substance abuse, family disorganization
Early and Middle Adulthood	15% of those with major depression commit suicide; 15% of those with schizophrenia commit suicide; 80% of those who commit suicide have made previous attempts; 15% of alcoholics commit suicide	Depression, schizophrenia, previous attempts, lack of psychosocial resources, alcoholism and substance abuse, major psychiatric and physical health problems
Older Adulthood	17% have attempted suicide	Loss, feelings of isolation, poor physical health status
Total Population	12% have attempted suicide	Mental illness, alcoholism

Data from National Center for Health Statistics. (1991). *Vital Statistics of the United States: Vol. 2. Mortality—part A.* Washington, DC: U.S. Government Printing Office.

suicide typically live in homes of family chaos due to substance misuse with fears of abandonment and inconsistent discipline styles. Negative parent–child relationships generate low self-esteem that arises from anger and rejection. Low self-esteem has been observed in abused, depressed, and suicidal children. These children tend to blame themselves and feel responsible for family problems (Maltsberger, 1986; Shneidman, 1975).

Major predictors of childhood emotional distress and suicide (Shafii et al., 1985) include

- Affective disorder (depression)
- Family factors (chaos, abuse, divorce, or death)
- Developmental factors (including early major losses)

The National Center for Health Statistics (1986) predicts that by the year 2000, childhood suicide will increase 13 percent for children 10 to 14 years of age and 94 percent for those aged 15 to 19 years. Children as young as 2 or 3 years of age have been found to exhibit suicidal behaviors, such as attempting to jump from high places, verbalization of wishes to kill oneself, and attempting to hang oneself or inject poison (Rosenthal & Rosenthal, 1984).

Suicidal behavior is the most common psychiatric emergency in children and adolescents. It is the third leading cause of death in this age group. Demographic findings show that girls contemplate suicide three times as often as boys, but boys kill themselves four times more frequently than do girls (Berman & Jones, 1991; Eisenberg, 1984).

Suicidal ideation is far more serious when expressed by children than when expressed by adults because of the former's immature ego and cognitive function. Ego function is affected by relationships with primary caregivers, previous life experiences, present stressors, and affect modulation. Immature ego function interferes with the capacity to cope with stress, modulate feelings, and feel good about oneself. Depression affects cognitive function and interferes with the way the child thinks of himself or herself and situations. Depression has been positively correlated with suicide as a major risk factor (Pfeffer et al., 1984). When adaptive mechanisms fail to allay the child's emotional pain and distress, the risk of acting on suicidal ideations heightens. Children have a distorted and inadequate sense of time and death. Their limited capacity for abstract thinking interferes with believing the finality and absoluteness of death. The concept of death is beyond their comprehension (Pfeffer, 1986).

Furthermore, children do not grasp a full understanding of death by suicide. They have a difficult time expressing emotional pain and problems, and suicide is often perceived as the solution to immense distress. Although some children report feelings of sadness and hopelessness, others have difficulty verbalizing their thoughts, feelings, and ideas and they may act on them. Children are capable of planning and carrying out suicide, and their behavior provides invaluable cues about their intent. Predominant behaviors and characteristics among suicidal children include aggression, preoccupation with death, social isolation, depression, and antisocial symptoms (Pfeffer, 1985).

Many childhood accidents may have been suicides. Pfeffer (1986) asserted two reasons that children commit suicide accidentally: (1) they misjudge the impact of the suicidal act (e.g., the placement of a gun or the number of pills); and (2) they miscalculate the time required for others to save them. They often use deadly methods such as shooting, hanging, and ingesting poisons. It is difficult to determine if a child's death is accidental or intentional because of social embarrassment, remorse, and cultural and socioeconomic reasons (Pfeffer, 1985, 1986).

The Nursing Process

Children exhibiting suicidal behaviors are experiencing serious distress and emotional pain. Early detection and prevention of childhood suicide are crucial to helping depressed or mentally disturbed children and families. The following clinical example provides a useful framework in which to examine the nursing process.

Clinical Example: The Child at Risk for Suicide (Lillie)

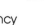

Lillie is a 10-year-old child brought to the emergency department by her mother, who reports that Lillie

TABLE 16–3
Assessing the Suicidal Child: Major Concepts

Understand developmental factors and suicidal behaviors in children
Examine feelings regarding death and suicide
Explore meaning of ideations, thoughts, and attempts
Assess imminence of suicide risk (lethality)
Obtain "no suicide" contract from the child
Actively involve the family
Encourage the child to talk about suicidal feelings and thoughts

Adapted from Pfeffer, C. R. (1986). Basic principles of assessing childhood suicidal risk. In *The suicidal child* (p. 178). New York: Guilford Press.

expressed feeling of wanting to die and join her best friend. Lillie has become increasingly despondent over the past 2 weeks since the death of her friend, who died from complications of cystic fibrosis.

Assessment

Childhood suicidal behaviors often represent a family problem. Assessing the child's role within the family context is important to evaluating the meaning of suicidal behavior. Factors such as motivation and current stressors play key roles in the child's ability to cope. Motivations of childhood suicidal threats include manipulation, revenge, escape from distress, desire to join a dead friend, or response to auditory hallucination. (Table 16–3 presents guidelines for assessing the suicidal child.)

In the clinical example, Lillie was depressed about the death of her friend. Additionally, her mother reported a recent separation from Lillie's father and a current custody dispute. Shortly after her father moved out the home, Lillie's grades began to drop, her appetite decreased, and she spent more time with her best friend until the friend's death. The nurse interviewed the child and mother separately and together to assess the parent–child interaction. Major family stressors identified involved the several losses, mainly the death of a close friend, family disorganization generated by an impending divorce, and Lillie's fears of losing her parents.

Pfeffer (1986) asserted that suicidal children often have fantasies and wishes to be cared for by kind and devoted people, and these fantasies can be fulfilled during the initial family–child assessment. The child becomes the center of attention during this process, acquires a sense of hopefulness, and renews the wish to live and work out problems rather than to commit suicide.

Nursing Diagnosis

- High Risk for Violence: Self-Directed
- Ineffective Individual Coping

Planning

Nursing Care Plan 16–1 identifies the desired outcomes for the nursing diagnoses listed earlier and delineates the nursing actions needed to achieve these outcomes, along with the rationales for these actions.

Families should never be blamed for the client's suicidal behavior. Nurses need to provide emotional support to families coping with crisis and form therapeutic relationships to protect the child. Crisis intervention is a useful strategy to teach parents and the child to identify and enhance their strengths, teach effective coping skills, reinforce family cohesiveness, and increase the family's ability to handle stress (Langley & Kaplan, 1968). Each situation must be assessed to determine interventions that ensure the child's safety and effective resolution of crisis situations.

Implementation

Major nursing interventions include the following:

- Establishing rapport with the child and parents
- Ensuring the child's safety
- Assessing the parent–child relationship
- Assessing the family system
- Teaching the family about legal rights regarding treatment

Crisis intervention with the child and parents reestablishes effective communication and expression of feelings and thoughts about the family crisis. It also helps the nurse identify family stressors, strengths, resources, and vulnerabilities. Involving the family in the initial assessment infers the seriousness of the situation and an understanding that the child's behavior reveals family problems. Additionally, the nurse is able to assess the family's understanding and willingness to make rapid changes to ensure the child's safety.

Encouraging the child to talk about suicidal behavior during the initial assessment emphasizes the significance of this behavior. Verbalization of feelings may be difficult for some children, and other means of communication, such as play and art therapy, can be useful in assessing the child's behavior.

Evaluation

In the clinical example, Lillie stated that she wanted to live and that she would not kill herself. Her mother reassured her that she would not leave her and she loved and wanted her. They were given biweekly parent–child (family therapy) followup appointments, and Lillie was discharged from the emergency department. Her mother was encouraged to observe the child for behavioral changes that suggested despondency, suicidal ideations, and social isolation. She was also instructed to call the nurse or family therapist in case of emergency. The child agreed to report any recurrent suicidal ideations to her mother or other family members (see the Nursing Care Plan display).

ADOLESCENCE

There is growing concern about the increasing suicidal rate among adolescents. This apprehension is legitimate, because in 1988, 2059 adolescents between 15 and 19 years of age committed suicide (National Center for

Nursing Care Plan 16–1 The Child at Risk for Suicide (Lillie)

OUTCOME IDENTIFICATION	NURSING ACTIONS	RATIONALES	EVALUATION
Nursing Diagnosis: High Risk for Violence: Self-Directed			
1. By [date], Lillie will verbalize the absence of suicidal ideations or plans.	1a. Assess the level of danger.	1a. All suicidal threats, plans, or ideations must be explored to determine if the child is at risk of harming or killing herself.	*Goal met:* Lillie ► denies suicidal ideations. ► does not harm self. ► is able to identify options. ► shows gradual mood changes. ► is able to express superficial feelings.
	1b. Provide a safe environment. Remove potential or actual dangerous objects from the environment.	1b. A safe environment provides structure and the controls needed to reduce impulses to harm or kill oneself.	
	1c. Establish an agreement with the child to inform the staff/nurse of suicidal ideations or aggressive behavior.	1c. This agreement provides an agreement and understanding between the child and the nurse and stresses the seriousness of the child's suicidal ideations.	
2. By [date], Lillie will discuss options to deal with present stressors.	2a. Encourage examination of available options to cope with present stressors.	2a. Exploring options and resources enhances coping skills.	
	2b. Observe for sudden changes in mood.	2b. Sudden mood changes, especially decreased depression, may signal the increased energy needed to act on suicidal ideations or plans.	
	2c. Encourage expression of feelings.	2c. Expression of feelings decreases internalization of emotional distress and mechanism to process meaning of present stressors/crisis.	
	2d. Encourage participation in therapeutic group activities with peers.	2d. Enhances social interactions and facilitates the grief process.	
	2e. Teach the child to identify symptoms of sadness, preoccupation with death, and suicide.	2e. Encourages expression and understanding of feelings.	
Nursing Diagnosis: Ineffective Individual Coping			
1. By [date], Lillie will develop an awareness of the meaning of present behaviors.	1a. Facilitate an understanding of Lillie's present behaviors.	1a. Understanding the meaning of maladaptive behaviors enhances adaptive coping responses and provides an opportunity for growth and mobilization of adaptive coping behaviors.	*Goal met:* Lillie ► returns to previous level of functioning. ► develops adequate coping skills. ► displays less anxiety.
	1b. Assist in problem solving.	1b. Crisis situations often overtax coping and problem-solving skills. This action affords an opportunity to enhance coping and problem solving.	

Nursing Care Plan 16–1 The Child at Risk for Suicide (Lillie) (Continued)

OUTCOME IDENTIFICATION	NURSING ACTIONS	RATIONALES	EVALUATION
	1c. Confront maladaptive behaviors.	1c. Confronting maladaptive behaviors allows the client to understand the meaning of them and develop adaptive coping responses.	
2. By [date], Lillie's family will understand and use available community resources.	2. Provide the family with information about local resource groups for suicide prevention.	2. Group participation can provide an environment that enables the client to express feelings and thoughts.	

Health Statistics, 1991). Garland and Zigler (1993) surmised that there was a profound increase in suicides among adolescents. The suicide rate in this age group increased more than 200 percent compared with an increase of 17 percent in the general population from 1968 to 1991. Adolescent males tend to use more violent means, such as shooting and hanging, than do females.

Approximately 6 to 13 percent of youngsters have attempted to kill themselves at least once in their lifetime. Most adolescents who attempt suicide do not seek or receive psychiatric treatment. Suicidal ideations are quite prevalent among adolescents, but only 10 percent have specific plans (Meehan et al., 1992; Smith & Crawford, 1986).

Risk Factors. Adolescence is a time of intense emotional and biological changes. Puberty increases vulnerability to stress and impaired self-concept as the youth searches for identity within society. Ineffective coping patterns, poor self-esteem, and inadequate support systems increase the risk of maladaptive responses to stress. Suicidal behavior is a symptom of maladaptive coping skills.

Principal precipitants of adolescent suicide include a history of mental illness (in the child as well as family members), previous attempts, ineffective coping skills, family disorganization, and substance abuse. Most adolescents who commit suicide have at least one mental disorder. Major mental illnesses include affective (mood) disorder, conduct or antisocial disorder, and substance abuse. They tend to perform poorly academically and experience family conflict and legal problems (Rhode et al., 1991).

Depressed adolescents, like depressed adults, usually experience impaired cognitive function and coping skills. They also tend to view themselves and the world as negative or hopeless. Ineffective interpersonal and problem-solving skills further compromise their ability to express emotional pain and worries effectively.

Gibbs (1988) stressed the significance of sociocultural factors in assessing depression in adolescents. She noted that African American youths from lower socioeconomic families are more likely to communicate depression and suicidal feelings with verbal abuse, hostility, and acting out in school and with their peers and society. Furthermore, Gibbs associated these expressions with underlying feelings of isolation, pessimism, and discouragement generated by enormous life stressors.

Family disorganization also increases the risk of mental illness and suicide in adolescents. Numerous studies support the notion that family competence affects coping behaviors in its members. Mental illness and substance abuse affect the parent's ability to provide stable, nurturing environments. Changing times, a mobile society, and a lack of extended families increase stress in the youth (Downey & Coyne, 1990).

Healthy families provide emotional and physical support for the adolescent during a turbulent period of rapid biological and emotional changes. A lack of this support, coupled with inadequate structure and limit setting, increases stress in the adolescent. Furthermore, poor parent–child relationships heighten the risk of maladaptive behaviors, such as substance abuse and suicidal and other self-destructive acts, to soothe emotional turmoil and pain (Pattison, 1984).

Additionally, peer groups are also significant to adolescents. They serve functions similar to those of families, providing a sense of belonging, validation, acceptance, and comradery. Interpersonal communication and sharing serve as psychosocial buffers and enable youths to effectively cope with crisis situations.

Treatment Modalities. Treating youths at risk for suicidal behaviors requires an interdisciplinary approach to ensure safety, reduce acute suicidal behaviors, decrease risk factors, and reduce vulnerability to future suicidal behavior (Pfeffer, 1986). This process must start as soon as possible and include making dynamic efforts to assess the client's mental and physical status.

The youth with a history of previous suicidal attempts must be protected and probably hospitalized to evaluate the risk for harm. The cause of suicidal behavior is complex and comprises psychosocial, cultural, and neurobiological factors. Treatment strategies are usually multimodal, consisting of psychodynamic, psychopharmacological, cognitive, behavioral, and family therapy. An emphasis on building hope and establishing healthy family interaction is vital to all treatment approaches. Assessing family interaction, strengths, manner of discipline, roles, and nurturing patterns provides information that can improve communication between the youth and his or her parents (Pfeffer, 1986) (see Chapter 22 for an in-depth discussion of family therapy).

Adolescence is a time of great emotional and biological stress. It is also a time for growth and health that allows the youth to move into adulthood using adaptive coping skills. The youth who attempts or completes suicide has immense emotional pain and is unable to cope with the turbulence of adolescence. Nurses play a major role in helping troubled adolescents and their families by identifying high-risk behaviors and working with these clients to build adaptive coping behaviors that protect the youth and promote health.

ADULTHOOD

Adults face numerous stressful life events. How is it that some people can handle tremendous pressures and stress, whereas others resort to suicide or other maladaptive responses to reduce stress? The answer to this question has been discussed in the first part of this chapter, which focuses on several issues, such as theories of suicide and causative factors, that affect young and middle-aged adults.

OLDER ADULTHOOD

Elderly clients have the highest rate of completed suicide, and they account for approximately 17 percent of suicides in this country (McIntosh, 1985). The highest rate of suicide is in depressed older, widowed or divorced, medically or mentally ill Caucasian men. Many of these clients had visited a physician within 6 months of their suicide (Miller, 1978; Murphy, 1975a, 1975b, 1983). Elderly clients make fewer attempts than do younger clients, but they have a higher rate of completed suicides because they tend to use more lethal means.

Risk Factors. What factors contribute to suicidal behavior in the elderly? Several factors, in addition to those shown in Figure 16–2, have been found to be consistent predictors of suicidal behaviors in the elderly, including loss, aging stereotypes, feelings of isolation, and poor physical health.

Loss. The first factor is loss. Elderly clients face numerous losses that consist of health, financial and social status, and the death or deteriorating health of a loved one. Inadequate or ineffective coping skills also increase the risk of depression and maladaptive responses to loss. Depression is a major predictor of suicide among the elderly, and assessing it is critical to prevention and the development of effective treatment.

Aging Stereotypes. Myths and stereotypes about the aging process may interfere with assessing depression in the elderly. Nurses can dispel these misconceptions by working with the mental health team to assess age-related symptoms and those associated with depression. Contrary to popular belief, dementia is not a nor-

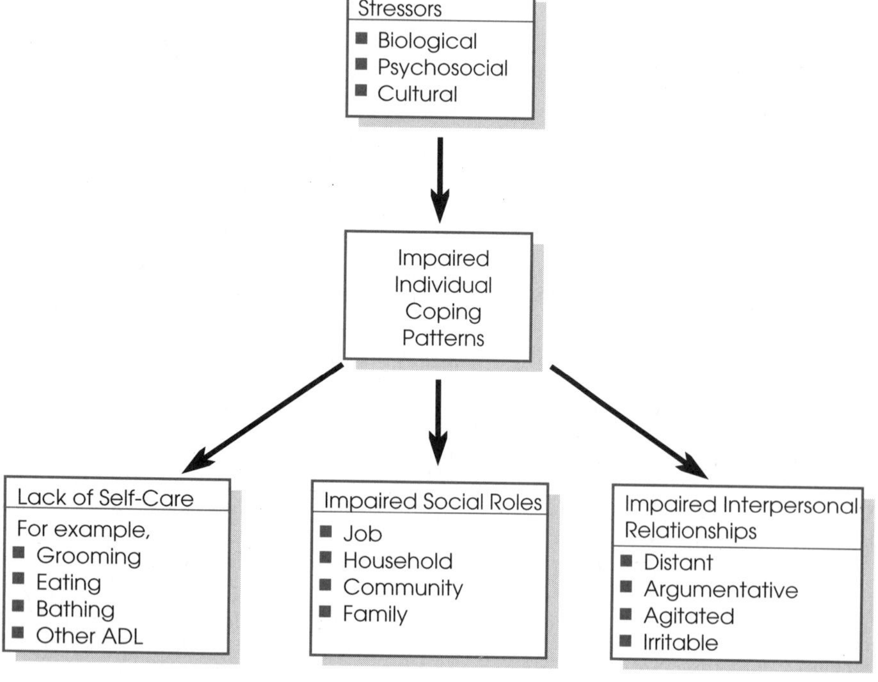

FIGURE 16–2
Factors that may put the elderly at high risk for suicidal behaviors. (Data from Miller, L. [1979]. *Toward classification of aging behaviors. Gerontologist, 19,* 283–290.)

mal aging process, and clients who present with cognitive impairment (such as memory loss and acute mood changes) need to be assessed for depression. Depression in the elderly is significant because of its relationship to suicidal behavior (Antai-Otong, 1990, 1993), and ignoring suicidal behaviors in the elderly can be deadly. Elderly clients perceive this unresponsiveness as indifference and rejection, which reinforces their sense of worthlessness and hopelessness (Osgood, 1985).

Feelings of Isolation. The third factor is social ties and a sense of belonging. Elderly clients with strong family ties and a sense of integrity are less likely to become depressed or suicidal than those who are socially isolated. Roskow (1967) believed that many elderly clients feel alienated from society because their social roles are devalued.

Poor Physical Health. The final factor is physical status. Physical illness places tremendous stress on the elderly, threatening their quality of life, comfort, and sense of well-being. These stressors compromise coping mechanisms, self-esteem, and interpersonal relationships and generate feelings of despair (Cohen & Lazarus, 1979). Coping with physical illness is influenced by the client's personality and coping style and whether mental illness and alcoholism are present.

The elderly client with physical illnesses needs to be assessed for depression because he or she is at risk for suicide. Involving families or significant others in the client's care is helpful. Major treatment goals include helping clients express their feelings and mobilizing psychosocial resources (Horton-Deutsch et al., 1992).

Suicidal behaviors of the elderly, as in other age groups, must be assessed early, and measures to prevent it are major nursing goals. Establishing therapeutic relationships is critical to this process because nurses can identify client resources and develop effective treatment that increase self-esteem and adaptive coping skills.

THE NURSE'S ROLE

THE GENERALIST NURSE

Suicidal clients challenge nurses to develop innovative strategies that facilitate adaptive coping skills and reduce the risk of suicide. The role of the generalist nurse includes identifying clients at risk for suicide, assessing coping behaviors, and intervening to minimize the risk of suicide among all age groups in various clinical settings. Additionally, the generalist nurse collaborates with clients, families, and other mental health professionals to develop a comprehensive plan of care that reduces the risk factors of suicide. Major strategies include crisis intervention, case management, psychoeducation, administration of psychotropics, and monitoring of client response.

THE ADVANCED-PRACTICE NURSE

Nurses in the advanced-practice role must respond to complex needs of clients in distress, and the suicidal client is a particular challenge in this regard. The complexity of suicidal behaviors suggests a need to understand the factors that increase the risk for self-destructive behaviors, such as biochemical aspects of mental illness, developmental issues, and family dynamics. Major interventions include prescriptive authority, case management, individual and family psychotherapy, and working with other disciplines to develop a comprehensive plan of care.

The Nursing Process

Suicidal clients often generate feelings of uneasiness, anger, and helplessness in the nurse. These feelings usually stem from conflicts associated with personal values and ethical and professional considerations. Nursing is a helping profession, and life is valued—suicide is the antithesis of this premise. Suicidal clients challenge nurses to use sensitive and caring approaches to manage profound emotional pain and suffering. Regardless of the number of suicide attempts, each one depicts the client's inability to cope effectively. Some nurses may even have difficulty relating to suicidal clients because they perceive their problems as self-imposed. Nurses must explore their own perceptions and attitudes about suicide and death.

Assessment

Suicidal clients can be effectively managed by an interdisciplinary approach, and nurses are crucial to this process. Initially, there must be an evaluation of the level of suicide risk or danger. Evaluation is a continuous process that requires accurate and prompt documentation of the client's behavior and response to treatment.

The therapeutic relationship is the basis of the assessment process. Encouraging clients to discuss suicidal ideations and plans allays their anxiety and disputes the notion that asking about suicide "puts thoughts into the client's head." Suicidal clients are frightened about their impulses and wishes to kill themselves. Suicidal thoughts must be assessed in all clients as part of the mental status examination. Questions such as, "Are you having thoughts of killing yourself?" or "Have you attempted to kill yourself in the past?" are parts of this assessment. Most suicidal clients feel relieved about the opportunity to discuss these feelings. Most clients who eventually kill themselves have communicated clues about their intent. Exploring suicidal intent communicates that the cry for help has been assessed and relief is achievable.

Once the client has been assessed to be a suicide risk, the decision to hospitalize is considered. Criteria for hospitalization is based on several factors

- The nature of the suicide attempt (e.g., gunshot, hanging, carbon monoxide)
- The client's expression of a plan and the means to carry out the plan
- History of previous attempts or impulsivity
- Lack of a social support system

Clients presenting with suicidal ideations realize that they are in trouble. Hospitalization is a viable option to further protect the client from suicide and evaluate psychosocial and biological stressors. This process can begin with discussing treatment options with the client and the family. If the client is unwilling to voluntarily enter the hospital and this is clearly indicated, an involuntary admission may be initiated by the psychiatrist. Laws governing this process vary, and nurses must familiarize themselves with their state's statutes for emergency detention and involuntary admissions (see Chapter 5 for an in-depth discussion of this process).

The first priority when caring for the suicidal client is managing the client with the least restrictive treatment to ensure his or her safety. This can be accomplished by the following (Hanke, 1984):

- Placing the client in a room free of sharp or dangerous items that can be used to harm oneself or others, such as glass, razors, knives, and metal
- Checking the client's personal belongings and clothing for medication or potential weapons
- Making sure that the client is not left alone
- Placing the client in a hospital gown or pajamas

Even when safety measures are instituted by hospitalization, the risk for suicide exists throughout treatment. A small number of clients may commit suicide on psychiatric units, especially during the first week of hospitalization. Preventing suicide begins with recognizing high-risk behaviors, minimizing the risk, and developing effective treatment plans that ensure safety and effective coping behaviors. Times of high risk within the hospital routine include weekends and holidays, visiting hours (if the client has no visitors), change of shifts, or mealtime or when there is rotation of staff or unit chaos (Copas & Robin, 1982; Hankoff, 1980).

When clients are determined to commit suicide, the greatest efforts do not stop them. These clients tend to wait and watch for opportunities when there is chaos or minimal staff on the unit or when they leave on pass or by elopement (without medical advice or approval). High-risk clients need to be observed continuously and assessed for change in mood, behaviors, or ideations. A sudden change in mood from a depressed to elated or energetic mood increases the risk of suicide because of improved cognitive function and ability to carry out a plan.

Clinical Example: The Client at Risk for Suicide (Mr. Leonard)

Mr. Leonard is a 45-year-old man who has reported having thoughts of killing himself after his 13-year-old son recently died of bone cancer. He is despondent and expresses guilt because he was unable to spare his son from intense pain and suffering. He has a history of chronic back pain and associates this pain with his son's suffering. His mood is depressed, and he cries often during the assessment. He denies having made suicide attempts in the past or actively abusing alcohol or drugs. He has thoughts of shooting himself. When questioned about the reasons for not acting on these thoughts in the past, he replied that his son would not have approved of it.

Nursing Diagnosis

- High Risk for Violence: Self-Directed, suicidal ideations with a plan
- Ineffective Individual Coping
- Dysfunctional Grieving

Mr. Leonard is in tremendous emotional pain, and his suicidal thoughts and plans place him at high risk for lethality. He is currently on one-to-one suicide precaution, which means that a staff person is constantly with him until his condition improves (i.e., he no longer expresses suicidal ideations or plans). Suicidal clients need to be encouraged to express their feelings and thoughts about their problems and suicide. This helps them sort out the reality of their situation and incorporate adaptive coping patterns through crisis intervention. Mr. Leonard openly discussed his pain and feelings of despair about losing his son. His sense of helplessness in not being able to save his son mirrored his intense emotional suffering. Conveying care and instilling hope are major aspects of prevention.

Planning

The following are the desired outcomes identified for Mr. Leonard:

- Expresses feelings and thoughts of suicide rather than acts on them
- Identifies reasons for wanting to die
- Develops adaptive coping skills
- Develops hope regarding the future
- Develops adequate support systems

Nursing Care Plan 16–2 delineates the nursing actions needed to achieve some of these outcomes and the rationales for these actions.

Implementation

The primary intervention of working with the suicidal client is prevention.

Evaluation

Mr. Leonard was discharged after a brief hospitalization. He was assessed for suicidal tendencies during hospitalization and at the time of discharge. He was not suicidal after the first day, and he began to openly express his pain and sadness. He decided that suicide was not the solution to his present stressors. At discharge he was referred to a day hospital program for several weeks. He was able to use group treatment to resolve his grief and develop effective coping skills. No medica-

Nursing Care Plan 16–2 The Adult at Risk for Suicide (Mr. Leonard)

Nursing Diagnosis: High Risk for Violence: Self-directed, suicidal ideations with a plan

OUTCOME IDENTIFICATION	NURSING ACTIONS	RATIONALES	EVALUATION
1. By [date], client will verbalize the absence of suicidal ideations or plans.	1a. Assess the level of danger.	1a. This enables the nurse to identify interventions to reduce suicidal risk.	*Goal met:* Mr. Leonard ► denies suicidal ideations. ► does not harm self. ► is able to identify options. ► shows gradual mood changes and is able to express superficial feelings
	1b. Provide a safe environment. Remove potential or actual dangerous objects from the environment.	1b. Removing objects reduces access to lethal weapons and lessens the risk of suicide.	
	1c. Discuss a "no suicide" verbal contract.	1c. Encouraging the client to agree to a "no suicide contract" helps him or her understand the seriousness of the situation and verbalize feelings regarding suicide.	
2. By [date], client will discuss options to deal with present stressors.	2a. Encourage the examination of available options to cope with present stressors.	2a. Increasing the client's options decreases the lone option of suicide; it also enhances the client's coping skills.	
	2b. Observe for sudden changes in mood.	2b. Sudden mood changes (decreased depression) signal increased energy and ability to carry out a suicide plan.	
	2c. Encourage the expression of feelings.	2c. Expression of feelings reduces tension and frustration and is an important aspect of the nurse–client relationship.	

Nursing Diagnosis: Ineffective Individual Coping

OUTCOME IDENTIFICATION	NURSING ACTIONS	RATIONALES	EVALUATION
1. By [date], client will develop an awareness of the meaning of present behaviors.	1a. Facilitate an understanding of the client's present behaviors.	1a. Understanding the meaning of maladaptive behaviors enhances adaptive coping responses and provides an opportunity for growth and mobilization of adaptive coping behaviors.	*Goal met:* Mr. Leonard ► returns to previous level of functioning. ► develops adequate coping skills. ► displays less anxiety.
	1b. Assist the client in problem solving.	1b. Crisis situations often overtax coping and problem-solving skills. This action affords an opportunity to enhance coping and problem-solving skills.	
	1c. Confront maladaptive behaviors.	1c. Confronting maladaptive behaviors allows the client to understand the meaning of them and develop adaptive coping responses.	

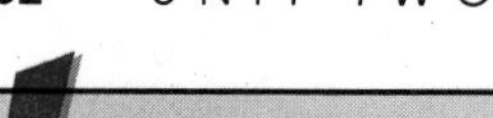

Nursing Care Plan 16–2 The Adult at Risk for Suicide (Mr. Leonard) (Continued)

Nursing Diagnosis: Dysfunctional Grieving

OUTCOME IDENTIFICATION	NURSING ACTIONS	RATIONALES	EVALUATION
1. By [date], client will realistically accept loss.	1a. Form a meaningful nurse–client relationship.	1a/1b. This relationship provides emotional support and enables the nurse to assess the significance of the loss.	*Goal met:* Mr. Leonard ► forms a meaningful relationship with the nurse. ► expresses feelings regarding the death of his son and how life has been without him. ► begins working through the grief process and works through his guilt. ► reestablishes a relationship with family members.
	1b. Assess the meaning of the loss to the client.		
	1c. Determine stage of grief.	1c. This helps the nurse to assess the client's needs and conveys empathy.	
2. By [date], client will actively participate in the grief process.	2a. Provide a calm, accepting, and empathic environment.	2a. This alleviates anxiety and promotes trust.	
	2b. Encourage expression of feelings regarding loss.	2b. This facilitates understanding the meaning and acceptance of the loss.	
	2c. Educate the client and family about the grief process.	2c. This facilitates understanding of and participation in the grief process.	
3. By [date], client will participate in activities that promote social interaction.	3. Encourage participation in social activities.	3. This decreases social isolation and facilitates the establishment of new and meaningful relationships.	

tion was prescribed at the time of discharge to the day hospital program.

This clinical example demonstrates how crisis intervention can be used to help a suicidal client. All situations do not end this way, and the client sometimes completes a suicide. Completed suicides can be devastating to nurses and families. How can these situations be dealt with?

WHEN A CLIENT COMMITS SUICIDE

In spite of heroic efforts to save clients, some of them manage to kill themselves. The suicidal client is not the only victim when this occurs. Family members and friends have to deal with the emotional aftermath of completed suicides. General staff reactions include, "what did I miss?" or "I should have been able to prevent this suicide." Feelings of guilt, helplessness, inadequacy, and anger are common staff reactions when a client commits suicide. Similar reactions emerge in the relative or friend survivors of suicide. Many of them openly attack the nurses and other staff, projecting their own sense of guilt, helplessness, and anger about losing a loved one. Nurses can work through these feelings and form an interdisciplinary approach with a psychological autopsy.

Litman et al. (1963) defined **psychological autopsy** as a mechanism to evaluate whether a death was suicidal or accidental. Components of the psychological autopsy include

- Interviewing the family or significant others who were familiar with the client
- Reviewing the client's behavior prior to death
- Discussing the client's medical and psychiatric history
- Identifying the client's significant family history
- Determining the presence or absence of substance or alcohol abuse

This process facilitates interaction among the staff and provides opportunities for the expression of feelings and thoughts about the suicide. Team members can work though the crisis of suicide while grasping the reality that the client had made the decision to follow through with the act.

Interviewing significant others provides the staff with pertinent information about family interactions, lifestyle, personal attributes, and coping patterns. The family may be hesitant to discuss these issues with the staff because of guilt and remorse generated by the suicide. Families can be referred to age-appropriate community support groups for survivors.

NURSING RESEARCH

The emergence of behavior-based approaches to understanding the psychosocial and neurobiological aspects of suicidal and other self-destructive behaviors prompts psychiatric–mental health nurses to explore these major concepts. Nurses can examine and identify factors that increase the risk for or vulnerability to suicide as part of data collection from clients, families, and medical records (see the Research Abstract display). Collaborating with other disciplines is a critical aspect of research because it integrates the expertise of a team approach to assessing, intervening in, and evaluating self-destructive behaviors across the life span. Other studies involve investigating the effects of psychotropics on behavior. Major nursing roles in drug trials include prescribing specific agents, administering research drugs, observing clients for desired and adverse responses, and participating in structured interviews and treatment planning.

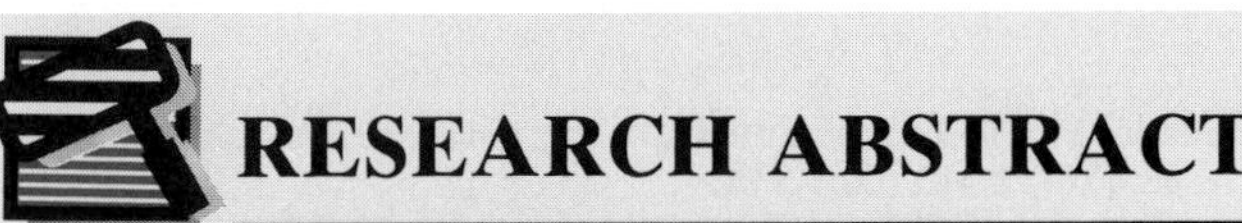

RESEARCH ABSTRACT

Suicidal Behaviors in Adult Psychiatric Outpatients: I. Description and Prevalence

Asnis, G. M., Friedman, T. A., Sanderson, W. C., Kaplan, M. L., van Praag, H. M., & Harkavy-Friedman, J. M. *American Journal of Psychiatry, 150*(1), 108–112.

Study Purpose

Evaluate the prevalence of suicidal behaviors among clients with a spectrum of psychiatric illnesses in a large general psychiatric outpatient population.

Methods

Six hundred fifty-one outpatient subjects participated in the study between 1987 and 1989. Each participant was interviewed and given a self-rating survey package with the Harkavy-Asnis Suicide Survey and the Hopkins Symptom Checklist-90.

Results

Fifty-five percent of the participants had a history of suicidal ideation, and 25 percent reported at least one suicide attempt. Major methods of suicide included overdosing, jumping, and wrist cutting. These behaviors were found among clients with major psychiatric disorders, particularly those with major depression and other mood disorders. These findings suggest that suicidal behaviors commonly exist among most outpatients seeking treatment.

Nursing Implications

Clients seeking psychiatric treatment must be thoroughly assessed for suicidal risk.

►CHAPTER SUMMARY

Suicide is a significant health problem that affects approximately 12 percent of people in the United States. Adolescents and the elderly are the age groups most likely to commit suicide. Additionally, clients with histories of mental illness and alcoholism are more likely to attempt suicide.

The complexity of suicide suggests that nurses must identify clients at risk and collaborate with other mental health professionals to develop effective interventions to prevent suicide. This process involves recognizing the relevance of psychosocial, neurobiological, and cultural components of human responses. Prevention is crucial to alleviating stress and a sense of crisis. Through therapeutic relationships, nurses provide immediate emotional support, mobilize resources, and promote a sense of hope in otherwise overwhelming situations.

Suggestions for Clinical Conference

1. Interview a suicidal client and family in the presence of a registered nurse or other personnel, and present the data to peers. Discuss the feelings generated by an interview regarding suicidal behaviors.
2. Present a case history of a client with self-destructive behaviors.
3. Role-play as suicidal client with a peer, and discuss the interactions and feelings generated.
4. Present a case history of a suicidal client using the life span approach.
5. Discuss the complex entities associated with suicidal behavior, including psychosocial, cultural, and neurobiological aspects.

References

Adams, K. S. (1985). Attempted suicide. *Psychiatric Clinics of North America, 8*(2), 183–201.

Antai-Otong, D. (1990). Suicide risk? *Geriatric Nursing, 11*(5), 228–230.

Antai-Otong, D. (1993). Cognitive and affective assessment of the geriatric patient. *MEDSURG Nursing, 2*(1), 70–74.

Beck, A. T., Brown, G., Berchick, R. J., Stewart, B. L., & Steer, R. A. (1990). Relationship between hopelessness and ultimate suicide: A replication with psychiatric outpatients. *American Journal of Psychiatry, 147*(2), 190–195.

Beck, A. T., Steer, R. A., Kovacs, M., & Garrison, B. (1985). Hopelessness and eventual suicide: A 10-year prospective study of patients hospitalized with suicidal ideation. *American Journal of Psychiatry, 142*, 559–563.

Berlin, I. N. (1987). Suicide among American Indian adolescents: An overview. *Suicide and Life-Threatening Behaviors, 17*(3), 218–232.

Berman, A. L., & Jones, D. A. (1991). *Adolescent suicide: Assessment and intervention.* Washington, DC: American Psychological Association.

Beskow, J. (1979). Suicide and mental disorders in Swedish men. *Acta Psychiatrica Scandinavica Supplement, 277*, 1–138.

Brent, D. A., Perper, J. A., & Allman, C. J. (1987). Alcohol, firearms, and suicide among youth: Temporal trends in Allegheny County, Pennsylvania, 1960 to 1983. *Journal of the American Medical Association, 257*, 3369–3372.

Bulik, C. M., Carpenter, L. I, Kupfer, D. J., & Frank, E. (1990). Features associated with suicide attempts in recurrent major depression. *Journal of Affective Disorders, 18*, 29–37.

Caplan, G. (1961). *An approach to community mental health.* New York: Grune & Stratton.

Coccaro, E. F., Siever, L. J., Klar, H. M., Maurer, G., Cochrane, K., Cooper, T. B., Mohs, R. C., & Davis, K. L. (1989). Serotonergic studies in patients with affective and personality disorders: Correlates with suicidal and impulsive aggressive behavior. *Archives of General Psychiatry, 46*(7), 587–599.

Cohen, F., & Lazarus, R. (1979). Coping with stresses of illness. In G. Stone, F. Cohen, & N. Adler (Eds.), *Health and psychology: A handbook* (pp. 217–255). San Francisco: Jossey-Bass.

Copas, J., & Robin, A. (1982). Suicide in psychiatric patients. *British Journal of Psychiatry, 141*, 503–511.

Downey, G., & Coyne, J. C. (1990). Children of depressed parents: An integrative review. *Psychological Bulletin, 108*, 50–76.

Drake, R. E., Osher, F. C., Noordsy, D. L., Hurlbut, S. C., Teague, G. B., & Beaudett, M. S. (1990). Diagnosis of alcohol use disorders in schizophrenia. *Schizophrenia Bulletin, 16*, 57–68.

Durkheim, E. (1951). *Suicide* (2nd ed.) (J. A. Spaulding & G. Simpson, Trans.). New York: Free Press (Original work published 1897)

Eisenberg, L. (1984). The epidemiology of suicide in adolescents. *Pediatric Annals, 13*, 47–54.

Freud, S. (1961). Economic problems of masochism. In J. Strachey (Ed. and Trans.), *The standard edition of the complete psychological works of Sigmund Freud* (Vol. 19, pp. 159–170). London: Hogarth Press. (Original work published 1923)

Garland, A. F., & Zigler, E. (1993). Adolescent suicide prevention. *American Psychologist, 48*(2), 169–182.

Gibbs, J. T. (1988). Conceptual, methodological, and sociological issues in black youth suicide: Implications for assessment and early intervention. *Suicide and Life-Threatening Behavior, 18*(1), 73–89.

Goodman, W. K., Price, L. H., & Charney, D. S. (1989). Fluoxamine in obsessive-compulsive disorder. *Psychiatric Annals, 19*(2), 92–96.

Hanke, N. (1984). *Handbook of emergency psychiatry.* Boston: Collamore Press.

Hankoff, L. (1980). Suicidal behavior in the institutional setting. *Journal of Psychiatric Treatment and Evaluation, 2*, 19–24.

Helig, S. M., & Klugman, D. J. (1970). The social worker in suicide centers. In H. J. Parad (Ed.), *Crisis intervention: Selected readings* (5th ed., pp. 274–283). New York: Family Service Association of America.

Hendin, H. (1969). Black suicide. *Archives of General Psychiatry, 21*(4), 407–422.

Hendin, H. (1971). *Black suicide.* New York: Harper & Row.

Hendin, H. (1987). Youth suicide: A psychosocial perspective. *Suicide and Life-Threatening Behavior, 17*(2), 151–165.

Horton-Deutsch, S. L., Clark, D. C., & Farran, C. J. (1992). Chronic dyspnea and suicide in elderly men. *Hospital and Community Psychiatry, 43*(12), 1198–1203.

Kendler, K. S. (1992). A population-based twin study of major depression in women: The impact of varying definitions of illness. *Archives of General Psychiatry, 49*(9), 257–266.

Kendler, K. S., Kessler, R. C., Neale, M. C., Heath, A. C., & Eaves, L. J. (1993). The prediction of major depression in women: Toward an integrated etiologic model. *American Journal of Psychiatry, 150*(8), 1139–1148.

Langley, D., & Kaplan, D. (1968). *Treatment of families in crisis.* New York: Grune & Stratton.

Litman, R. E., Curphey, T., Shneidman, E. S., Farberow, N. L., & Tabachnick, N. (1963). Investigation of equivocal suicides. *Journal of the American Medical Association, 184*, 924–929.

Maltsberger, J. T. (1986). *Suicide risk.* New York: New York University Press.

McGuffin, P., Katz, R., & Rutherford, J. (1991). Nature, nurture and depression: A twin study. *Psychological Medicine, 21*(2), 329–335.

McIntosh, J. L. (1985). Suicide among the elderly: Levels and trends. *American Journal of Orthopsychiatry, 55*(2), 288–293.

Meehan, P. J., Lamb, J. A., Saltzman, L. E., & O'Carroll, P. W. (1992). Attempted suicide among young adults: Progress toward a meaningful estimate of prevalence. *American Journal of Psychiatry, 149*(1), 41–44.

Menninger, K. A. (1938). *Man against himself.* New York: Harcourt, Brace.

Menninger, K. A. (1947). *The human mind.* New York: Alfred A. Knopf.

Meltzer, H. Y. (1990). Role of serotonin in depression. *Annals of the New York Academy of Sciences, 600*, 486–499.

Meltzer, H. Y., & Lowry, M. T. (1987). The serotonin hypothesis of depression. In H. Y. Meltzer (Ed.), *Psychopharmacology: The third generation of progress* (pp. 513–526). New York: Raven Press.

Meltzer, H. Y., & Nash, J. F. (1988). Serotonin and mood: Neuroendocrine aspects. In D. Granten & D. Pfaff (Eds.), *Current trends in neuroendocrinology* (Vol. 8, pp. 183–210). Heidelberg: Springer-Verlag.

Miller, L. (1978). Geriatric suicide: The Arizona study. *Gerontologist, 18*(5), 488–495.

Miller, L. (1979). Toward classification of aging behaviors. *Gerontologist, 19*(3), 283–290.

Murphy, G. E. (1975a). The physician's responsibility for suicide: I. An error of commission. *Annals of Internal Medicine, 82*, 301–304.

Murphy, G. E. (1975b). The physician's responsibility for suicide: II. Errors of omission. *Annals of Internal Medicine, 82*, 305–309.

Murphy, G. (1983). On suicide prediction and prevention. *Archives of General Psychiatry, 40*(3), 343–344.

National Center for Health Statistics. (1986). Births, marriages, divorces, and deaths for January 1986 (provisional data). *Monthly Vital Statistics Report, 35*, 1–12.

National Center for Health Statistics. (1991). *Vital statistics of the United States: Vol. 2. Mortality—part A* [for the years 1966–1988]. Washington, DC: U.S. Government Printing Office.

Osgood, N. J. (1985). *Suicide in the elderly.* Rockville, MD: Aspen.

Pattison, E. M. (1984). Types of alcoholism reflective of character disorders. In R. Zales (Ed.), *Character pathology: Theory and treatment* (pp. 362–378). New York: American College of Psychiatry, Brunner/Mazel.

Pfeffer, C. R. (1985). Self-destructive behavior in children and adolescents. *Psychiatric Clinics of North America, 8*(2), 215–226.

Pfeffer, C. R. (1986). *The suicidal child.* New York: Guilford Press.

Pfeffer, C. R., Zuckerman, S., Plutchik, R., & Mizruchi, M. S. (1984). Suicidal behavior in normal school children: A comparison with child psychiatric inpatients. *Journal of the American Academy of Child Psychiatry, 23*(4), 416–423.

Prasad-Ashoka, J. (1986). Attempted suicide in hospitalised schizophrenics. *Acta Psychiatrica Scandinavica, 74*(1), 41–42.

Primeau, F., & Fontaine, R. (1987). Obsessive disorder with self-mutilation: A subgroup responsive to pharmacotherapy. *Canadian Journal of Psychiatry, 32*(8), 699–701.

Rhode, P., Lewinsohn, P., & Seeley, J. R. (1991). Comorbidity of unipolar depression: Comorbidity with other mental disorders in adolescents and children. *Journal of Abnormal Psychology, 100*(2), 214–222.

Rich, C. L., Fowler, R. C., Fogarty, L. A., & Young, D. (1988). San Diego Suicide Study: III. Relationships between diagnoses and stressors. *Archives of General Psychiatry, 45*(6), 589–592.

Rosenthal, P. A., & Rosenthal, S. (1984). Suicidal behavior by preschool children. *American Journal of Psychiatry, 141*(4), 520–525.

Roskow, I. (1967). *Social integration of the aged.* New York: Free Press.

Roy, A. (1985). Suicide and psychiatric patients. *Psychiatric Clinics of North America, 8*(2), 181, 227–241.

Roy, A. (1993). Genetic and biologic risk factors for suicide in depressive disorders. *Psychiatric Quarterly, 64*(4), 345–358.

Roy, A., Karoum, F., & Pollack, S. (1992). Marked reductions in indexes of dopamine metabolism among patients with depression who attempt suicide. *Archives of General Psychiatry, 49*(6), 447–450.

Roy, A., Mazonson, A. & Picar, P. (1984). Attempted suicide in chronic schizophrenia. *British Journal of Psychiatry, 144,* 303–306.

Shaffer, D. (1988). The epidemiology of teen suicide: An examination of risk factors. *Journal of Clinical Psychiatry, 49*(Suppl.), 36–41.

Shaffer, D., Garland, A., Gould, M., Fisher, P., & Trautman, P. (1988). Preventing teenage suicide: A critical review. *Journal of the American Academy of Child and Adolescent Psychiatry, 27*(6), 675–687.

Shafii, M., Carrigan, S. Whittinghill, J. R., & Derrick, A. (1985). Psychological autopsy of completed suicide in children and adolescents. *American Journal of Psychiatry, 142*(2), 1061–1064.

Shneidman, E. S. (1975). Psychiatric emergencies: Suicide. In A. M. Freedman, H. Kaplan, & B. J. Sadock (Eds.), *Comprehensive textbook of psychiatry* (Vol. 2, pp. 1774–1785). Baltimore: Williams & Wilkins.

Shneidman, E. S. (1985). *Definition of suicide.* New York: Wiley.

Smith, K., & Crawford, S. (1986). Suicidal behavior among "normal" high school students. *Suicide and Life-Threatening Behavior, 16*(3), 313–325.

Stack, S. (1982). Suicide in Detroit: Changes and continuities. *Suicide and Life-Threatening Behavior, 12*(2), 67–83.

van der Kolk, B. A. (1988). The biological response to psychic pain. In F. M. Ochberg (Ed.), *Posttraumatic therapy and victims of violence* (pp. 25–38). New York: Brunner/Mazel.

Vogt, M. (1982). Some functional aspects of central serotonergic neurons. In N. N. Osbow (Ed.), *Biology of serotonergic neurotransmission* (pp. 299–316). Chichester, England: John Wiley & Sons.

Waltzer, H. (1984). Suicide risk in the young schizophrenic. *General Hospital Psychiatry, 6*(3), 219–225.

Weed, J. A. (1985). Suicide in the United States: 1958–1982. In C. A. Taube & S. A. Barrett (Eds.), *Mental health in the United States: 1985* (pp. 135–155). Rockville, MD: National Institute of Mental Health.

Winchel, R. M., & Stanley, M. (1992). Self-injurious behavior: A review of behavior and biology of self-mutilation. *American Journal of Psychiatry, 148*(3), 306–317.

Wyche, K., Obolensky, N., & Glood, E. (1990). American Indian, black American, Hispanic American youth. In M. J. Rotheram-Borus, J. Bradley, & N. Obolensky (Eds.), *Planning to live: Evaluating and treating teens in community settings* (pp. 355–389). Tulsa: University of Oklahoma Press.

Zilboorg, G. (1937). Consideration on suicide, with particular reference to that of the young. *American Journal of Orthopsychiatry, 7,* 15–31.

CHAPTER 17

The Client with Addictive Behaviors

ARDYCE A. PLUMLEE, M.N., R.N., C.A.R.N.

OUTLINE

CHAPTER OBJECTIVES

Upon completion of this chapter, you will be able to:

1. Describe six models for explaining chemical dependency.
2. Identify the signs, symptoms, and behaviors of substance abuse.
3. Identify expected effects, toxic effects, and withdrawal effects of alcohol and other depressants, stimulants, narcotics, cannabis, and hallucinogens.
4. Use the nursing process to plan care for clients across the life span who abuse chemicals or are dependent on them.
5. Discuss changes that occur in the family as a result of chemical abuse.
6. Explain the processes of addiction and recovery.
7. List the components of effective treatment for substance abuse.
8. Identify current use of psychopharmacological agents to treat chemical dependency and discuss the effects.
9. Identify referral sources for persons and family members affected by substance abuse.

KEY TERMS

Addiction
Al-Anon
Alcoholics Anonymous
Alcohol withdrawal delirium
Amotivation syndrome
Blackouts
Cachectic
Co-dependency
Delirium tremens
Drug
Dysfunction
Ego competency
Enabling
Fetal alcohol effects
Fetal alcohol syndrome
Initiation phase
Maintenance phase
Mind-altering substance
Nar-Anon
Narcotics Anonymous
Neurotransmitter
Recovery
Relapse
Shame
Status epilepticus
Substance abuse
Substance dependence
Tolerance
Withdrawal

DEFINITIONS OF MIND-ALTERING SUBSTANCES AND ADDICTION

A **drug** is a substance that by its chemical nature alters the structure or function of the living organism. A **mind-altering substance** is any chemical substance that alters mood, perception, or consciousness and is misused to the apparent injury of the person or society (U.S. Drug Enforcement Agency). **Addiction** is a dysfunctional pattern of human response that is characterized by one or more of the following: (1) some loss of self-control capability, (2) episodic or continuous maladaptive behavior or abuse of some substance, and (3) development of dependence patterns of a physical or psychological nature (American Nurses' Association [ANA], 1987).

MIND-ALTERING SUBSTANCES AND THE BRAIN

Clients who use mind-altering substances report that they use these drugs to achieve a feeling of well-being or euphoria. They seek "enhanced" insight, and heightened or exhilarated experiences, believing that these chemicals enhance brain function. This is contrary to brain research. One brain researcher, Michael Gazzaniga, has stated that each child is born with the optimum structure and function of the brain to cope with and enjoy life and that brain function cannot be enhanced. He declared that all studies to date have shown that environmental influences can only maintain this optimum function or affect the brain in a negative way (Gazzaniga, 1985).

What, then, is the appropriate use of mind-altering substances? Many prescribed medications are targeted for the brain; however, they all have side effects in addition to the effects for which they are prescribed. For any medication to be approved for use in treating disease, it must be subjected to extensive controlled trials to determine whether its benefits outweigh the risks of taking it. This, ideally, is the determinant for acceptable use of mind-altering substances. When it has been determined by carefully controlled research that the benefits of the drug outweigh the risks, then that drug is approved and appropriate for prescribed use. In practice, however, use of prescribed medications may not follow the ideal.

The target organ for abused substances is the brain. For the drug to achieve its effect, it must alter the brain's function in some way. Because natural chemicals are produced in controlled and minute amounts and appear in the right place in the right amount at the right time, this system must be altered to produce a change in perception and experience. The brain has its own protective system, the blood–brain barrier, which keeps certain substances from reaching the neurons. The only way for a compound to invade this center of thought, emotion, and control is to fool it. This is exactly what mind-altering substances do, and if a substance can invade the brain, it can penetrate and affect all other organs in the body (Inaba & Cohen, 1989). Substances must be lipid soluble to diffuse across the cell membranes and into the lipid-rich brain material. Mind-altering substances (psychoactive drugs) inhibit, stimulate, or distort the release of **neurotransmitters** or stimulate or inhibit the actions of the neurotransmitters once they are released (Fig. 17–1). This alters the neurotransmitter messages in the brain, disrupting the user's ability to think and reason. Because the brain controls all other systems, use of psychoactive substances alters these other systems also. A minuscule quantity of some of these drugs can have a profound effect on neurotransmitters. Many brain neurotransmitters may be affected by drugs or alcohol; however, the ones most implicated in addiction are dopamine, serotonin, and norepinephrine.

People can take drugs into their body through (1) their digestive system, by eating or drinking; (2) their lungs, by smoking; (3) their veins, by intravenous (IV), intramuscular, or subcutaneous injection; (4) their skin, by contact; and (5) the mucosa of the nasal passages, by snorting. The chemical travels in the bloodstream to reach the central nervous system (CNS). The magnitude of a drug's effect is determined by the quantity and nature of the drug taken, route and speed of absorption, and how the drug is metabolized in the body.

PREVALENCE OF SUBSTANCE ABUSE

Few persons have been unaffected by drug and alcohol use in the world today. According to a survey conducted by the U.S. Department of Health and Human Services, about 43 percent of U.S. adults (about 76 million people) have been exposed to alcoholism in their own family (National Council on Alcoholism and Drug Dependence [NCADD], 1991). Nurses encounter substance-abusing clients in all health care settings, although the clients' substance abuse may not be recognized and diagnosed. People who abuse substances come from all socioeconomic groups and may appear little different from people who do not use mind-altering substances. In 1988, the National Household Survey on Drug Abuse found that 105.8 million Americans were current drinkers of alcohol. Among young adults, 90 percent had tried alcohol, 65 percent during the month surveyed. Approximately 12 million Americans were alcoholics, and 11.5 to 15.7 percent of the population will become alcoholic during their lifetime. Men were five times more likely than women to be diagnosed with **substance abuse** or **dependence,** although the incidence is rising in women. The actual number may be hidden because of the lifestyle of many women, e.g., housewives drinking alone in their homes (National Institute on Drug Abuse [NIDA], 1989).

That same survey found that 37 percent of the American population age 12 or older had tried illicit drugs at least once in their lifetime. Five and a half percent of the U.S. population were projected to have a problem with drug abuse during their lifetime, with twice as many males as females involved. After alcoholism and depression, drug abuse was the third most common psychiatric diagnosis of men, with minimal difference between races or educational levels (NIDA, 1989).

Substance abuse has a major impact on a person's health and precipitates a variety of health problems. As many as 45 percent of medical/surgical inpatients and 20 percent of outpatients have substance abuse as a primary problem (Lewis, 1989). Fetal alcohol effects are the first or second leading cause of mental retardation, depending on the survey. Alcohol-related problems cause 100,000 excess deaths per year, 50 percent of fatal auto accidents, 68 percent of drownings, 54 percent of fires, and 48 percent of serious falls (NCADD, 1991).

Approximately 40 percent of the psychiatric population has an alcohol or drug problem. Fifty percent of children referred to child guidance clinics have an alcoholic parent (Lewis, 1989). It is readily apparent that clients using mind-altering substances are seen frequently in the health care setting. Nurses are in a position to identify these clients and play a significant role in helping them receive treatment and recover.

CAUSES OF ADDICTION: PERSPECTIVES AND THEORIES

In contrast to other abused drugs, on which research is in a less advanced stage, there has been extensive research on the use of alcohol. Therefore most of the data presented in this section pertain to alcohol use. Six models of addiction are explained: psychodynamic models, the disease model, the behavioral model, the biochemical model, the family systems model, and the biopsychosocial model.

PSYCHODYNAMIC MODEL

There are several psychodynamic theories of addiction. The client may be seen as fixated at the oral stage. Ingestion of substances may be seen a response to this fixation. Treatment and recovery consist of psychotherapy to remove the fixation. The client may also be seen to have excessive dependency needs. The addiction is an attempt to meet these needs, and treatment is psychotherapy for the excessive dependency needs. Neither of these theories is currently widely accepted.

DISEASE MODEL

The disease model of addiction conceptualizes addiction as a chronic, progressive, relapsing, incurable, and potentially fatal disease. The client has inherited a predisposition to addiction, and use of the substance triggers the disease under favorable environmental circumstances. "The susceptible user quickly experiences a compulsion to use, a loss of control, and will continue the use despite negative physical, emotional, or life consequences" (Inaba & Cohen, 1989, p. 218). The disease model of addiction is widely accepted by substance abuse treatment providers and by many persons who describe themselves as "recovering." Because clients are considered to have a disease, they are not to blame for their condition, but they *are* responsible for their recovery. **Recovery** consists of abstinence first and then physical, emotional, and spiritual healing. Recovery is thought to continue over the life span, and complete recovery is not considered possible; hence the term *recovering*.

BEHAVIORAL MODEL

The behavioral–social learning model conceptualizes addiction as developing and progressing according to the laws of learning theory. According to this model, the first phase of addiction is the **initiation phase**, when the person learns to drink or use drugs. If use is positively reinforced, or if negative reinforcement occurs in the form of relief from pain, the person will continue

HOW DRUGS AND ALCOHOL ALTER BRAIN MESSAGES

Drugs can enter the body in various ways: through the digestive system by eating or drinking, through the lungs by smoking, directly by injection, through the skin by contact, or through the nasal mucosa by snorting. In all cases the target organ is the brain. Since the brain controls all other body sytems, use of psychoactive substances influences these systems as well.

Drugs work by inhibiting, stimulating, or distorting the release or action of neurotransmitters in the brain, as detailed below. Many brain neurotransmitters are affected by drugs or alcohol, but the ones most implicated in addiction are dopamine, serotonin, norepinephrine, and acetylcholine.

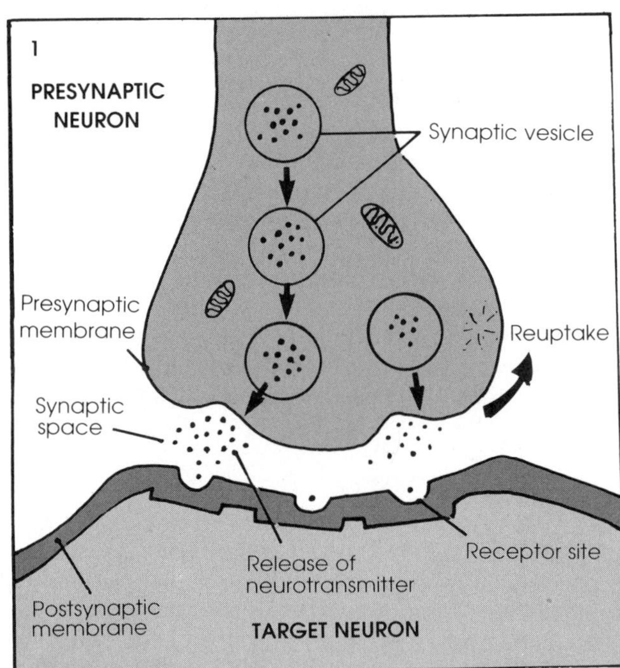

1. Normal Neurotransmitter Action

Neurons (nerve cells) manufacture neurotransmitters and store them in vesicles. When a neuron is stimulated, the vesicles migrate to the presynaptic cell membrane and release the neurotransmitter into the synaptic cleft in controlled amounts as needed. The neurotransmitter diffuses across the synaptic cleft to the postsynaptic membrane of the adjacent or target neuron, where it is taken up by receptor sites. Neurotransmitter action is ended by reuptake into the presynaptic cell or through breakdown by enzymes. *(See also Figure 2-4, Anatomy of a Synapse.)*

2. Some Drugs Stimulate Neurotransmitter Production

Cocaine, amphetamines, and other stimulants greatly increase the production of the excitatory neurotransmitters dopamine, serotonin, norepinephrine, and acetylcholine and the rate of their release into the synaptic cleft. This excessively stimulates the postsynaptic cell membrane and ultimately causes hyperstimulation of the central nervous system. The physiological effects include heightened energy, increased tolerance to pain, and improved intellectual performance. Initially, tolerance to the drug develops, with larger amounts needed to create the desired effects. Then, over time, the chronic demand placed on receptor sites by an overabundance of neurotransmitters results in supersensitivity of the postsynaptic membrane, which can stimulate the creation of additional receptor sites. A subsequent drop in the neurotransmitter level will result in an artificial shortage and understimulation, causing craving for the drug or withdrawal symptoms.

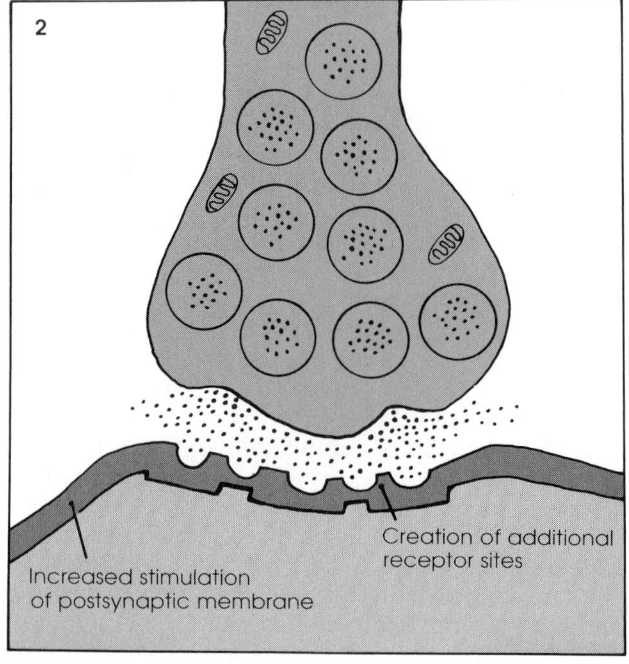

FIGURE 17–1
The effects of mind-altering substances on neurotransmitters. (Illustration concept: Gail Kongable, M.S.N., C.N.R.N., C.C.R.N., Department of Neurosurgery, University of Virginia Health Sciences Center. Illustration by Marie T. Dauenheimer.)

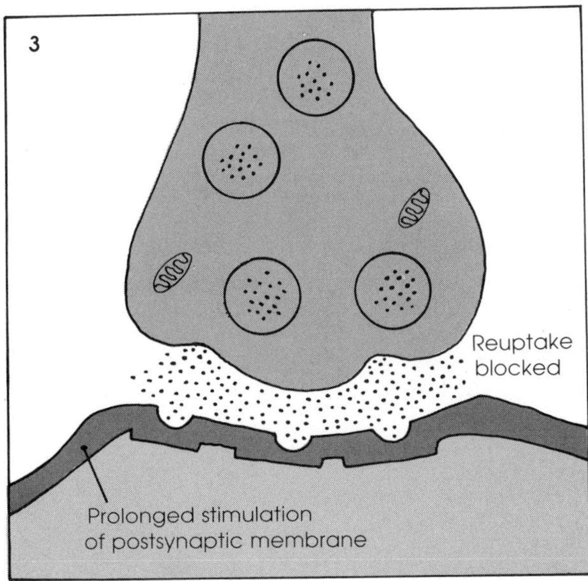

3. Some Drugs Block Neurotransmitter Reuptake

When neurotransmitters are released into the synaptic cleft, excess amounts normally "recycle" into the presynaptic neuron in a process called *reuptake*. Some drugs block reuptake, increasing the supply of neurotransmitters in the synaptic cleft. This lengthens stimulation of the postsynaptic cell membrane, and prolongs stimulation of the central nervous system. Cocaine, for example, blocks reuptake of serotonin and dopamine, allowing a greater than normal amount of these excitatory neurotransmitters to reach the target neurons. The ultimate effect is the euphoric feeling associated with this drug. Alcohol, barbiturates, and benzodiazepines, on the other hand, block reuptake of the modulating neurotransmitter gamma-aminobutyric acid (GABA) and enhance GABA binding to the receptor sites in the target neurons. The characteristic calming or sedative effects of alcohol, barbiturates, and benzodiazepines result from the "hypermodulation" due to the greater-than-normal availability of GABA. *(See Figure 10-1, GABA Pathways and Receptors.)*

4. Chronic Drug Use Slows the Rate of Neurotransmitter Production and Release

With chronic use of a drug, the neurotransmitters cannot be produced and released into the synaptic cleft at a rate fast enough to keep up with the new demand. Because of this artificial shortage of the neurotransmitters, the receptor sites are now understimulated. Withdrawal symptoms occur, and the person experiences a craving for the desired physiological effects that can be satisfied only by larger amounts of the drug (tolerance).

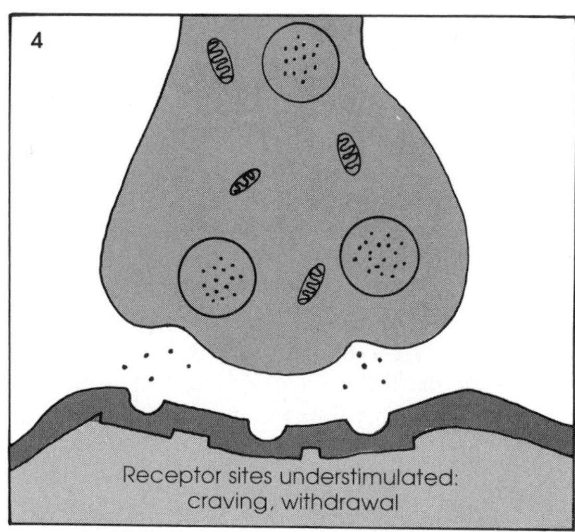

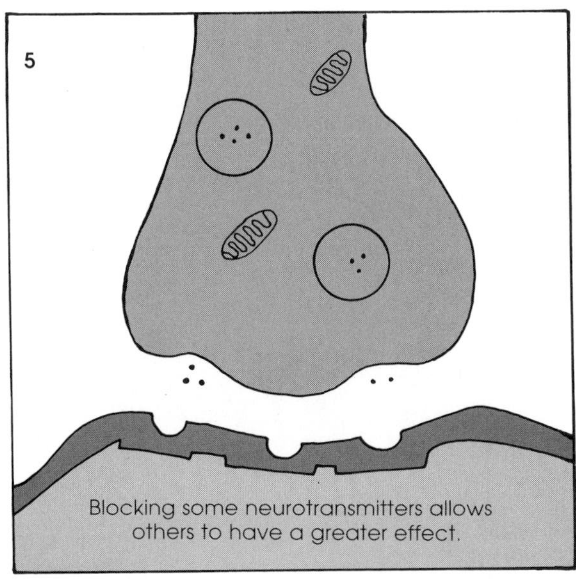

5
Blocking some neurotransmitters allows others to have a greater effect.

5. Some Drugs Reduce or Block Neurotransmitter Production

Hallucinogenic drugs such as LSD and PCP greatly reduce the supply of serotonin and GABA in the synaptic cleft. The reduction in the amounts of these neurotransmitters permits excessive activity of dopamine and acetylcholine, wtih resultant hallucinations, delusions, and paranoia.

using the substance. The second phase is the **maintenance phase**, in which use is sustained by the development of tolerance and the desire to avoid experiencing painful withdrawal symptoms. Use is also maintained by the desire to block the pain and guilt from the accumulation of many negative consequences from the use. Recovery results from choosing to cope differently and learning to do so. Relapse is prevented by identifying one's triggers and developing new methods of coping.

BIOCHEMICAL MODEL

The biochemical, or CNS deficiency, model integrates knowledge gained by research on addiction (Inaba & Cohen, 1989). It acknowledges that the beginning of addiction may be explained in different ways. The end result, however, is change in the neurotransmitters of the brain. No matter how the deficiency or disruption of brain neurons occurs, "whether it's heredity, overuse of the drug, or environmental factors, it's the brain chemistry that's disrupted, and most often that disruption causes a deficiency of certain transmitters" (Inaba & Cohen, 1989, p. 221). Once they have developed, all addictions share a common brain change, that of deficiencies in certain neurotransmitters. The end result is that once they begin using the substance, users are unable to predict how much of the substance they will use or how long they will use it.

People are born with different degrees of sensitivity to mind-altering substances. As a person experiments with substances, sensitivity is enhanced. The higher the inherited sensitivity, the greater the chance of habitual use and the greater the chance that use will progress to addiction. If the person uses a substance heavily or on a long-term basis, the level of inherited sensitivity determines how long it may take for addiction to occur. For the highly sensitive person, it may only take 2 months; for someone else, it may take 3 to 4 years, depending on the substance and the person's age. When the former

TABLE 17–1
Risk Factors for Alcohol and Other Drug Abuse (AODA) by Category

BIOLOGICAL
► Family history of AODA (there appears to be a genetic basis to the relative risk of at least some kinds of alcohol and other drug dependency)
► Past history of AODA
► Relative sensitivity to the effects of the drug
PSYCHOLOGICAL
► School failure
► Rebelliousness and alienation
► Early antisocial behavior
► Early, heavy use of alcohol and other drug, associated with continuing use
► Need for immediate gratification
► Lack of empathy
► Easy and frequent lying
► Insensitivity to punishment
FAMILY
► Family history of AODA
► Family history of antisocial behavior
► Inadequate parental direction and discipline
PEER
► AODA by best friends and other peers
► Choice of friends who use drugs
► Choice of peers over adults
► Older siblings who are involved with alcohol and drugs
COMMUNITY/CULTURAL
► High level of mobility
► High levels of crime and delinquency
► High population density
► Community disorganization
► Poverty and deprivation

From U.S. Office for Substance Abuse Prevention. (1992). *Nurse training course: Alcohol and other drug abuse prevention.* Rockville, MD: National Training System, U.S. Public Health Service.

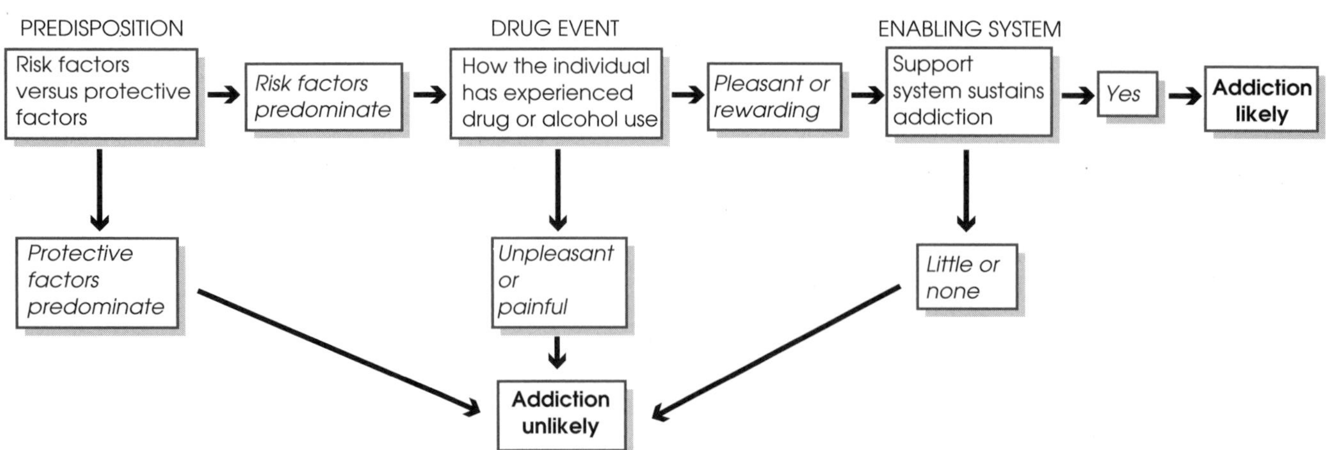

FIGURE 17–2
The biopsychosocial model of addiction. (Adapted from the U.S. Office for Substance Abuse Prevention. [1992]. *Nurse training course: Alcohol and other drug abuse prevention.* Rockville, MD: National Training System, U.S. Public Health Service.)

TABLE 17–2
Risk Factors for Alcohol and Other Drug Abuse by Life Span

CHILDHOOD

- Fetal exposure to alcohol and other drugs (AOD)
- Parents who are substance abusers
- Physical, sexual, or psychological abuse
- Economic disadvantage
- Delinquency
- Mental health problems such as depression and suicidal ideation
- Disability

ADOLESCENCE

- AOD use by parents
- Low self-esteem
- Depression
- Psychological distress
- Poor relationship with parents
- Low sense of social responsibility
- Lack of religious commitment
- Low academic performance and motivation
- Peer use of AOD
- Participation in deviant, aggressive behavior

YOUNG ADULTHOOD

- Exposure to drug users in social and work environments
- Marital and work instability
- Unemployment
- Divorce
- Psychological or psychiatric difficulties

MIDDLE ADULTHOOD

- Bereavement, especially as a result of loss of spouse or significant other
- Adverse work conditions or unemployment
- Changes in health status or appearance
- Socioeconomic stressors
- Environmental changes or relocation
- Divorce, separation, or remarriage
- Difficulties with children or changes in child-rearing responsibilities

ELDERLY

- Retirement or role status change
- Loss of loved ones
- Changes in health status and mobility
- Increased sensitivity to effects of alcohol and other drugs
- Housing relocations
- Affective changes (e.g., anxiety and depression)
- History of previous misuse or abuse of AOD
- Solitude or social contexts that foster use of AOD
- Negative self-concept

From U.S. Office for Substance Abuse Prevention. (1992). *Nurse training course: Alcohol and other drug abuse prevention.* Rockville, MD: National Training System, U.S. Public Health Service.

user abstains from use, his or her enhanced sensitivity to the chemicals does not subside. Therefore, upon relapse and return to use, addiction is acquired much more quickly than it originally occurred (Inaba & Cohen, 1989).

FAMILY SYSTEMS MODEL

The family systems model explains addiction as serving to maintain homeostasis in the family (Kaufman, 1985; Stanton & Todd, 1982; Steinglass, 1981). Stanton and Todd (1982) hypothesized that a young adult becomes addicted to preserve the parent's marriage. Steinglass (1981) compared alcoholic and nonalcoholic family response patterns and found that drinking served a stabilizing function for the family. Cermak (1990) concluded that many children growing up in severely dysfunctional homes suffer from posttraumatic stress disorder. A number of authors have hypothesized that addictions develop as a sequel to abuse and neglect within a dysfunctional family in which the child has difficulty developing a healthy sense of self (Black, 1981; Brown, 1988; Cermak, 1990). This family **dysfunction** can result from a number of sources, including drug or alcohol abuse, mental illness, physical illness, or neglect or violence by the adult caretakers. Recovery involves treatment for the family system, either family therapy or therapy with the recovering person to resolve pain and dysfunction from childhood neglect or abuse (see Chapter 22).

TABLE 17–3
Protective/Resiliency Factors That Help Immunize a Child to the Risks of Addiction

- A relationship with a caring adult role model
- An opportunity to contribute and be seen as a resource
- Effectiveness in work, play, and relationships
- Healthy expectations and positive outlook
- Self-esteem and internal locus of control
- Self-discipline
- Problem-solving/critical thinking skills
- Sense of humor

From U.S. Office for Substance Abuse Prevention. (1992). *Nurse training course: Alcohol and other drug abuse prevention.* Rockville, MD: National Training System, U.S. Public Health Service.

BIOPSYCHOSOCIAL MODEL

The biopsychosocial model of addiction includes all factors of etiology (U.S. Office of Substance Abuse Prevention, 1992). It is believed that addiction develops as a result of a complex interplay of many factors (Fig. 17–2). Many risk factors (Tables 17–1 and 17–2) interact with protective factors (Table 17–3) to develop a predisposition toward abuse of drugs or alcohol. This predisposition, along with the quality of the experience of the person when drugs or alcohol is first used and whether the person's support system enables continued use, determines whether addiction develops and is maintained. **Enabling** is any behavior that promotes continued substance abuse by the addicted person and protects the affected person from the consequences of the abuse (Bakdash, 1978). Treatment consists of altering the predisposition by reducing risk factors or strengthening protective factors and changing the support system to stop the enabling. Substance abuse is prevented by changing any one of the major elements of the model. Predisposition may be changed by strengthening resiliency factors or removing risk factors. The first experience of use of the substance can be changed by delaying

TABLE 17 – 4

Drugs with Addictive Characteristics, by Category

DRUGS	PRESCRIPTION BRANDS OR STREET NAMES	PSYCHOLOGICAL DEPENDENCE	PHYSICAL DEPENDENCE	TOLERANCE	POSSIBLE EFFECTS	OVERDOSE EFFECTS	WITHDRAWAL SYNDROME
Stimulants					Increased alertness, excitation, euphoria, dilated pupils, increased pulse rate and blood pressure, insomnia, loss of appetite, increased energy, increased sexual stimulation	Agitation, increase in body temperature, hallucinations, convulsions, possible death, arrhythmias, respiratory collapse	
Amphetamines	Benzedrine, dexedrine uppers, speed, bennies, dexies, ice, crank	High	Possible	Yes			Apathy, long periods of sleep, irritability, depression, disorientation, paranoia
Cocaine	Snow, coke, crack, rock, blow, lady	High	High	Yes			
Nicotine	Tobacco products	High	High	Yes			
Caffeine	Coffee, tea, cola, chocolate	Moderate	Moderate	Yes			Headache, nausea and vomiting
Depressants					Slurred speech, disorientation, drunken behavior, decreased inhibition, sedation, increased sociability, decreased tension and anxiety	Shallow respiration, cold and clammy skin, dilated pupils, weak and rapid pulse, coma, possible death	Anxiety, insomnia, tremors, delirium, convulsions, possible death
Barbiturates	Phenobarbital, Seconal, Tuinal	High	High	Yes			
Sedative-hypnotics	Quaalude, Soper, Ludes	High	High	Yes			
Tranquilizers	Librium, Valium, Equanil, Miltown	Moderate	Moderate	Yes			
Alcohol	Beer, wine, spirits	High	High	Yes			
Narcotics					Euphoria, drowsiness, respiratory depression, constricted pupils, nausea	Slow and shallow breathing, clammy skin, convulsions, coma, possible death	Watery eyes, runny nose, yawning, loss of appetite, irritability, tremors, panic, chills and sweating, cramps, nausea, vital sign changes
Opium	Paragoric (O)	High	High	Yes			
Morphine	(M), Hard Stuff	High	High	Yes			
Codeine	School Boy	Moderate	Moderate	Yes			
Heroin	H, Horse, Smack, Junk, Mexican Brown, Porcelain, China White	High	High	Yes			
Fentanyl	Tar	High	High	Yes			
Methadone		Moderate	Moderate	Yes			
Hallucinogenics					Illusions and hallucinations, poor perception of time and distance, heightened awareness of reality	Longer, more intense "trip" episodes, psychosis, possible death, distortions in body image, impulsive violence	
Mescaline	Peyote	Possible	No	Yes			
LSD	Acid, Lucy in the sky with diamonds	Possible	No	Yes			
PCP	Peace Pill, Angel Dust, Hog	Possible	No	Yes			
STP, MDA							
Psilocybin (mushrooms)	Magic mushrooms	Possible	No	Yes			
Inhalants					Disorientation, slurred speech, dizziness, nausea, poor muscular control	Unconsciousness, coma, liver, kidney, and brain damage, possible death from asphyxiation	Restlessness, anxiety, irritability
Gasoline	Trash drugs	Moderate	No	Yes			
Toluene acetone	Rush	Moderate	No	Yes			
Cleaning fluids		Moderate	No	Yes			
Airplane cement		Moderate	No	Yes			
Amyl nitrate	Poppers	Moderate	No	Yes			
Cannabis							
Marijuana, hashish, THC	Pot, grass, joint, reefer, weed	Yes	Yes	Yes	Sense of well-being, relaxation, altered perceptions, euphoria	Flashbacks, bronchitis, personality changes	Craving, general anxiety, restlessness, insomnia

Note. LSD = lysergic acid diethylamide, PCP = phencyclidine, STP = 2,5, dimethoxy, 4, methyl amphetamine, MDA = methylene-dioxy-phenyl-iso-propanolamine, THC = tetrahydrocannabinol.
From U.S. Office for Substance Abuse Prevention. (1992). *Nurse training course: Alcohol and other drug abuse prevention.* Rockville, MD: National Training System, U.S. Public Health Service.

first contact with substance through early education or community restriction of use. Enabling can be reduced by family education or therapy.

TYPES OF ADDICTIVE DRUGS

There are several groups of drugs that have qualities that are addictive. These include CNS depressants, CNS stimulants, opiates (i.e., narcotics, most of which are used for pain medication), hallucinogens, inhalants, and cannabis (Table 17–4). Although at one time it was thought that each group of drugs affects the brain in a different manner, new research is identifying a common pathway in the brain for addictive substances. All abused drugs seem to influence the "pleasure center" in the brain at various points along the neural pathway.

CENTRAL NERVOUS SYSTEM DEPRESSANTS

CNS depressants depress the CNS's functioning to induce sedation and drowsiness and can produce coma and, ultimately, death. This group includes alcohol, sedatives-hypnotics, and anxiolytics. The sedative-hypnotics can be divided into several groups: barbiturates, barbituratelike drugs, benzodiazepines, and some miscellaneous drugs. Opiate drugs also depress the CNS, but they are discussed in a separate section because of their unique qualities.

Alcohol

Alcohol has the longest history of use and is the most widely used and abused drug. It is absorbed quickly from the stomach and the small intestine and metabolized by the liver at a fixed rate, about one drink (1 oz.) an hour. Alcohol is both fat and water soluble and is distributed throughout the body. In its concentrated form it is toxic to nerve cells; in the diluted form of alcoholic beverages, it irritates nerve cells. Thus, long after the drinker eliminates the alcohol from his body, a hangover of irritated nerve cells remains. See Table 17–5 for a description of blood alcohol levels.

Frequently, clients are treated for a physical problem resulting from the alcohol use, but the alcohol abuse is neither identified nor treated. Chronic alcohol use affects all body systems and predisposes a person to many diseases. Chronic liver disease, gastrointestinal ulcers, esophageal varices, pancreatic disease, cardiac disease, peripheral neuropathy, increased risk for cancer, nephropathy, and increased respiratory infection are all associated with heavy alcohol use. Recent research on the relationship between alcohol use and acquired immune deficiency syndrome (AIDS) indicates that alcohol depresses immune function and lowers resistance to the disease (National Institute on Alcohol Abuse and Alcoholism [NIAAA], 1992). In addition, alcohol use is related to increased sexual risk-taking, also increasing the opportunity for AIDS infection.

Tolerance to alcohol use develops rapidly. **Withdrawal** from alcohol causes nerve cell excitation, leading to hyperarousal in the form of anxiety, irritability, insomnia, loss of appetite, tachycardia, and tremulousness. In the majority of persons, this state is mildly resolved; however, in others, it may be precipitous and severe. **Alcohol withdrawal delirium (Delirium tremens**, or DTs) is the most serious form of alcohol withdrawal. About one fifth of clients experiencing DTs died in past years; currently there is about a 1 to 2 percent mortality (Kinney & Leaton, 1987). The delirium consists of hallucinations, confusion, and disorientation. The tremens includes all the symptoms of severe stimulation of the autonomic nervous system: elevated vital signs, tremulousness and agitation, and the same symptoms of early withdrawal, only worse. It is important for the nurse to carefully monitor alcohol withdrawal and identify potentially serious withdrawal symptoms, because they are best prevented. Usually a benzodiazepine such as chlordiazepoxide (Librium) or diazepam (Valium) is given in decreasing doses to facilitate safe withdrawal from alcohol.

TABLE 17–5
Blood Alcohol Levels

20–99 mg%	Impaired coordination with euphoria
100 mg%	Legal drunkenness in most states
100–199 mg%	Ataxia, decreased mentation, poor judgment, labile mood
200–299 mg%	Marked ataxia and slurred speech, poor judgment, labile mood, nausea and vomiting
300–399 mg%	Stage I anesthesia, memory lapse, labile mood
400+ mg%	Respiratory failure, coma, death

Note. These figures are approximations, and effects depend on the amount of tolerance the person has acquired.
From Schuckit, M. A. (1989). *Drug and alcohol abuse: A clinical guide to diagnosis and treatment* (3rd ed.). New York: Plenum.

Sedative-Hypnotics and Anxiolytics

These groups of CNS depressants include drugs which are frequently prescribed for medical reasons, most commonly, the benzodiazepines. Barbiturates and a similar group of drugs are now rarely prescribed, but they continue to be used illegally. The sedative-hypnotics and anxiolytics are usually taken orally and have varying addictive potential. The shorter acting drugs have rapid blood level peaks and are the most highly addicting. Death can result from overdose of CNS depressants used alone (except benzodiazepines) and from the use of one type of CNS depressant with another (including alcohol). Intoxication is similar to that of alcohol. Withdrawal from these drugs can be extremely serious. When the severe CNS depressant effects of the drugs are removed, the resultant hyperactivity may result in fatal **status epilepticus**.

NARCOTICS

Narcotics are the most effective drugs available for the relief of pain. Pain messages in the brain are communicated via the neurotransmitter called *substance P*. The endorphins, a group of neurotransmitters, normally assist the body to reduce pain. Narcotics attach to the endorphin receptors and can block the pain by blocking release of substance P. They are derived from the opium poppy and include opium, morphine, heroin, and codeine. Synthetic narcotics that are similar to the naturally occurring opiates in their chemical structure and effects are hydromorphone (Dilaudid), meperidine (Demerol), methadone (Dolophine), fentanyl (Duragesic), propoxyphene (Darvon), oxycodone (Percodan), pentazocine (Talwin), and diphenoxylate (Lomotil).

All narcotics relieve pain to a varied extent, and all depress parts of the CNS. Use of these substances results in euphoria, drowsiness, relief from pain, respiratory depression, constipation, nausea, and constricted (pinpoint) pupils, the last being used as diagnostic for the presence of narcotics. Coma or death from overdose occurs from severe respiratory depression. This respiratory depression can be reversed, however, with the administration of a narcotic antagonist. Within seconds of injection, the narcotic antagonist, such as naloxone (Narcan) or nalorphine, replaces the narcotic on the neuroreceptors and immediately reverses the effects. This puts the client in a state of acute withdrawal that must be monitored carefully. Withdrawal from these drugs is not life threatening, but it is extremely distressful to the client and is therefore avoided at all costs. The client experiences flulike symptoms, extreme nausea and diarrhea, panic, and chills.

STIMULANTS

CNS stimulant drugs range from very potent ones, such as cocaine, to mild ones, such as caffeine. Stimulant drugs activate the sympathetic branch of the autonomic nervous system, forcing the release of adrenergic neurotransmitters such as dopamine, norepinephrine, and serotonin in the brain. The powerful release of neurotransmitters, along with their rapid depletion, results in intense craving for more. This craving may be present for months or years after use of cocaine. The stimulants are the most highly addictive drugs known. They suppress the appetite and users are likely **cachectic**. Toxic effects reflect the extreme stimulation of the sympathetic nervous system: vital signs are elevated, and excessive anxiety or psychosis may accompany the euphoria. Generally, there are no physical symptoms of withdrawal, but some persons may appear profoundly depressed.

HALLUCINOGENS

Hallucinogens mimic psychosis, altering the person's sensory perception; the effects on neurotransmitters are not known. The emotional makeup of the user and the mood at the time the drug is used seem to influence the perceptions of the user. A person may experience a "bad trip" sometimes and a "high" other times. The hallucinogens include lysergic acid diethylamide (LSD), other similar chemicals, and the mushrooms: psilocybin and mescaline. Phencyclidine (PCP), an animal tranquilizer, has become one of the more widely abused drugs in Western culture. It suppresses the function of the cortex, so that control of behavior and judgment is performed by the more primitive brain centers, resulting in sometimes violent behavior while peripheral nerves are anesthetized.

CANNABIS

A group of substances that are widely abused are those derived from cannabis plants. The effects of smoking marijuana range from the very mild to moderate, because of variations in the concentration of the major active ingredient (tetrahydrocannabinol) in marijuana. The drug has some stimulant and some depressant properties, as well as some hallucinogenic properties at high dose. A possible mechanism of action is the stimulation of dopamine production. Andreasson et al. (1987) found that schizophrenia occurred in 6 percent of marijuana users, in contrast to 1 percent of the general population. Because it is thought that people with schizophrenia have excess dopamine in their brains, it is possible that heavy use of marijuana could precipitate the disease in those so predisposed (see Chapter 12). Long-term use may result in **amotivation syndrome**, memory difficulties, susceptibility to upper respiratory infections, and possible birth defects of children.

INHALANTS

The fumes from some gaseous substances are inhaled for their effects. These substances are organic solvents found in paints, glues, volatile nitrites, and nitrous oxide (also known as "laughing gas" and used as an anesthetic). An altered mental state is achieved partially by the effects of these chemicals on the brain and partially by the anoxia that results from inhalation. These substances can cause serious and permanent system damage, such as exploded or frozen lung tissue or brain damage.

DESIGNER DRUGS

The term *designer drug* originates in the practice of altering the chemical structures of drugs to evade legal prosecution. A drug is designed to create the same effect of a banned substance, but with a changed chemical structure that is no longer illegal. There have been some disastrous results from this practice. One drug, a synthetic meperidine derivative, called China White, was found to destroy cells in the substantia nigra portion of users' brains, precipitating irreversible Parkinson's disease. Another designer drug is ecstacy (also called ADAM), a synthetic, psychoactive drug with hallucinogenic and amphetaminelike properties. Both China White and ecstacy were classified as illegal once they were found to cause severe problems in users.

DRUG INTERACTIONS AND CROSS-TOLERANCE

Polydrug use, or the abuse of two or more drugs, is more common than the use of one substance alone. Users will often substitute another drug when the drug of choice is not available, usually staying within the category of choice. Some users inject a combination of drugs with "opposite effects" (e.g., heroin and cocaine), anticipating an enhanced experience, but they may experience an unpredictable result: death. Several prominent entertainers have died from this combination. Rarely do combinations of drugs cause the sum of the effects of the drugs; rather, the drugs react synergistically. The result often is multiplication or exponential increase in effects, possibly leading to death. A frequent cause of drug death is the use of a sedative-hypnotic in combination with alcohol.

One effect commonly observed in the hospital setting is the cross-tolerance of one drug with another. A heavy user of one drug will exhibit tolerance to another. For example, the heavy alcohol user will require larger amounts of medication to relieve pain. This may be problematic because of the slower development of tolerance to respiratory depression.

SUBSTANCE ABUSE ACROSS THE LIFE SPAN

CHANGES IN ADDICTED FAMILIES

When an adult family member becomes addicted, he or she will gradually fail to fulfill family responsibilities. Others assume these responsibilities, with the family either changing to include the chemical dependency or excluding the addicted member. Because of the insidiousness of the onset of the disorder, many families deny the existence of the addiction and seek to rationalize or explain the deviant family member's behavior. Black (1981) described the resulting dysfunctional family roles as *don't talk, don't trust, and don't feel.*

Effects of Addiction in the Family on Children in the Family. Children who grow up in severely dysfunctional homes experience alterations in their basic sense of self. Neglected children have had their trust in their parents violated by their parents' inability or unwillingness to provide for their needs. Children who have been physically or sexually abused experience fear and pain from caretaking adults. Children are totally dependent on adult caretakers for survival, and acknowledgment of their parents' incompetence is often unthinkable, because of overwhelming anxiety about abandonment. Subsequently, the children view the situation as occurring because of their own defectiveness or badness. In addition, family abuse or neglect is characteristically denied within and outside the family. The result of this denial is that the children do not discuss or validate their painful feelings with significant others. This scenario is experienced as an overwhelming sense of **shame**. The children learn to hide the internal sense of badness, defectiveness, and shame from themselves and others and develop a false, external self.

Wegscheider-Cruse (1981) identified five roles assumed by children growing up in a severely dysfunctional family: the enabler, the hero, the scapegoat, the lost child, and the mascot. The *enabler* will try to alleviate consequences resulting from the behavior of others. The *hero* assists the family to maintain self-esteem by shining for all to see. The *scapegoat* is an acting-out child to whom the family can point as the cause of the family's pain. The *lost child* is quiet and unobtrusive, often going unnoticed and avoiding upsetting anyone. The *mascot* diverts the family's attention from the problems at hand by being cute or funny. Some famous comedians were mascots in their alcoholic families during childhood. All children from dysfunctional homes experience life as excessively stressful and painful, even though many function at or above the level of others in society (see Chapter 22).

Co-Dependency. One behavior resulting from dysfunctional families is **co-dependency**. There is no agreed-on definition of the term among health care providers; however, the pain experienced as co-dependency is becoming more and more recognized. Originally the term was used to describe the spouse of an alcoholic who becomes more and more focused on the alcoholic, trying to control the alcoholic's behavior and drinking and the consequences on the family. Wegscheider-Cruse (1981) defined co-dependency as a condition characterized by preoccupation and extreme dependency (emotionally, socially, and sometimes physically) on a person or object. Eventually, the co-dependent's excessive dependency on the object or person becomes a pathological condition that affects all of the co-dependent's other relationships. Beattie (1987) described a co-dependent person as one who has let another person's behavior affect him or her and who is obsessed with controlling that person's behavior (see Table 17–6 for a description of co-dependent behaviors). Black defined co-dependency as a set of beliefs that results in hurtful behaviors and emanates from a basis of shame that is most often the result of having been raised in a rigidly hurtful, painful family (C. Black, personal communication, 1992). An example is an adult woman who, because of her mother's alcoholism, assumed adult responsibilities in her home as a child. She believed that she was at fault for her mother's drinking and experienced herself as "not enough." In adulthood, she had three failed marriages, had difficulty making decisions, and felt that "I don't know who I am." Two of her husbands were abusive, and the other was absent; all are alcoholics. Such persons have chronic low self-esteem, excessive difficulty maintaining relationships, and difficulty expressing feelings and seek others' counsel for personal choices. Black characterized co-dependent persons as having difficulty living with themselves, protecting themselves, identifying themselves

TABLE 17–6
Characteristics of Co-Dependent People

EXTERNAL FOCUS
▸ Have inordinate need to control self, others, and outside events ▸ Have chronic low self-esteem because of difficulties controlling life
CHRONIC CARETAKING
▸ Care for others at expense of self
DIFFICULTIES WITH INTERPERSONAL RELATIONSHIPS
Boundary Difficulties ▸ Let others infringe on their boundaries ▸ May infringe on others' boundaries ▸ May not know appropriate boundaries **Intimacy Dysfunction** ▸ Have excessive dependency needs ▸ Fear abandonment ▸ Fear engulfment (being controlled by others) ▸ Have difficulty trusting others
ATTRACTION TO PERSONS WITH INTERPERSONAL PROBLEMS
▸ Such problems seem normal to co-dependent ▸ May bond to first available person ▸ May tolerate abusive situations
COMMUNICATION DIFFICULTIES
▸ Use denial excessively ▸ Use projection ▸ Punish self-disclosers in family
ARRAY OF BEHAVIOR AND AFFECTS
▸ Anxiety ▸ Depression ▸ Personality disorders ▸ Compulsive behaviors or addictions ▸ Constriction of emotions ▸ Hypervigilance ▸ Stress-related medical illnesses

Data are from Beattie, M. (1987). *Codependent no more.* New York: Harper & Row; Cermak, T. (1990). *Evaluating and treating adult children of alcoholics* (Vols. 1 and 2). Minneapolis: Johnson Institute; Scheitlin, K. (1990). Identifying and helping children of alcoholics. *Nurse Practitioner, 15*(2), 34–47.

TABLE 17–7
Comparison of Co-Dependent Versus Caring People

CODEPENDENT	CARING
Have low self-esteem and are self-critical and perfectionistic	Are sure of own identity and able to accept and learn from mistakes
Act out of guilt and fear, especially toward authority figures	Act out of freedom and choice
Seek approval, need to be liked, want rewards and acknowledgment; try to meet others' expectations	Are self-confident and truly altruistic, not needing recognition; Want to meet Higher Power's expectations and make self-expectations congruent with those of Higher Power
Are extremely loyal, even when loyalty is not merited	Are able to confront others and say no when appropriate
Are intimidated by angry people and personal criticism	Are able to listen to others' anger and criticism and use it constructively
Are attracted to dysfunctional people and feel the need to care for them	Form primary relationships with healthy, caring people
Avoid conflict; may appear superficially sweet, but underneath feel angry and resentful	Use conflict for growth and creativity; even enjoy appropriate confrontations
Feel guilty when acting assertively	Are naturally assertive
Deny, or do not remember, childhood traumas and the feelings associated with them; lose ability to express current feelings	Recall both the joys and difficulties of childhood; can look back on them with appropriate emotion
Afraid of rejection or abandonment; tend to stay in jobs or relationships that are harmful	Are able to terminate jobs and relationships with hopeful attitude toward future
Have difficulty with intimate relationships and are unable to trust others	Form deep, mutually trusting relationships in which emotions can be freely expressed
Become enmeshed in another person's needs and emotions, living other person's life as own	Are able to empathize and care for another without losing own identity
Base behavior on shame	Base actions on a solid sense of self-worth
Cannot accept limitations; take on role of Higher Power	Accept human finitude and limitations

From John, S. (1991). Codependency versus caring. *Journal of Christian Nursing, 8*(2), 22.

and sharing that identity with others, taking care of themselves, becoming interdependent with others, and being moderate. Black considered shame to be the basis for co-dependency and, underlying it, the fear of being abandoned. The experience of feeling abandonment is a result of the child's boundaries of the self being distorted or undefined at the time in life when identity and self worth should be being developed. See Table 17–7 for a comparison of co-dependency versus caring behaviors.

PREGNANCY

More than five million (9 percent) of the nearly 60 million women of childbearing age (ages 15–44) have used an illicit drug in the past month, and three of every five women of childbearing age currently drink alcoholic beverages (NIDA, 1989). These chemicals cross the placenta and enter the bloodstream of the unborn child, causing a variety of detrimental effects on the baby. The most profound effects are produced when the drugs are used in the first 8 weeks of pregnancy, when the mother may be unaware of her pregnancy, resulting in gross structural changes in or death of the embryo. After the eighth week of pregnancy, drug use is more frequently associated with growth retardation, prematurity, and neurological damage. Drug use near the time of delivery may precipitate labor and can be hazardous. The most consistent sequelae from use of any drug or alcohol during pregnancy are intrauterine growth retardation and smaller than normal head and chest measurements. In addition, sexual promiscuity may develop or the client may have sexual encounters with IV drug users, thus exposing the fetus to AIDS and other sexually transmitted diseases.

Common effects of alcohol are interference with the delivery of maternal nutrients to the fetus and impairment of oxygen supply. Alcohol may impair fertility and cause obstetrical complications, spontaneous abortion, stillbirth, and premature delivery. Marijuana affects fertility in both males and females and has been associated with increased numbers of spontaneous abortions and stillbirths. Women who use cocaine and crack may become obsessed with the use of these drugs and disregard their effects on themselves and the child. The user may become cachectic because of appetite suppression, radically impairing nutrition to the fetus. Because of cocaine's strong vasoconstrictive properties, the fetus's life support system may be damaged, resulting in a high rate of spontaneous abortion, early onset of labor, and complications such as abruptio placentae (premature detachment of the placenta). Women using narcotics have many medical problems. Low self-esteem, depression, and histories of child neglect and abuse are common in narcotics users. Narcotics use has been implicated in altered neural development and pregnancy complications. From 10 to 15 percent of pregnant women who use narcotics develop toxemia that may lead to eclampsia (Cook et al., 1990).

Experience has shown that most expectant mothers desire a healthy baby and, given adequate information, will make changes in their lifestyle to ensure their child an excellent opportunity for health. The nurse should bear in mind that if a woman continues to use mind-altering substances while pregnant, she probably is unable to decrease use or remain abstinent without help. Assessment for substance use and abuse and referral for treatment are critical for the prevention of further damage to the child. Treatment facilities for pregnant women have not always been available; therefore, it is important for the nurse to acquire a knowledge of treatment facilities in the community. Cessation of use, even late in pregnancy, decreases risk of damage and offers the hope that parenting will become more competent. However, drug withdrawal during pregnancy is risky and requires special monitoring.

TABLE 17–8
Manifestations of Fetal Alcohol Syndrome

- Prenatal and postnatal growth retardation—infant is abnormally small in weight, length, and/or head circumference for age.
- Central nervous system disorders—infant shows signs of abnormal brain functioning, delays in behavioral development, and/or intellectual impairment.
- At least two of the following abnormal craniofacial features—small head, small eyes or short eye openings, poorly developed philtrum (the groove above the upper lip), thin upper lip, short nose, or flattened midfacial area.

Data from Cook, P. S., Peterson, R. C., & Moore, D. T. (1990). *Alcohol, tobacco and other drugs may harm the unborn.* Rockville, MD: U.S. Department of Health and Human Services.

FETAL AND INFANT DEVELOPMENT

The infant born to parents using mind-altering substances is in double jeopardy, being exposed both to the damaging effects of drugs in utero and to impaired parenting. Fetal exposure to alcohol or drugs may cause suffering from a variety of aftereffects, ranging from severely altered growth and development to subtle neurological changes not evidenced until the child is school age. Fetal exposure to alcohol most consistently presents as intrauterine growth retardation. Manifestation of this may be a mild condition called **fetal alcohol effects** (FAE), or a severe condition called **fetal alcohol syndrome** (FAS) (see Table 17–8). Alcohol and its metabolites have been shown to be directly toxic and may result in physical abnormalities or mental retardation for which alcohol is the most common cause in the United States. The cognitive functioning of children with FAS with the most severe CNS involvement does not improve, even with remedial instruction (Cook et al., 1990).

A newborn whose mother has been using marijuana may exhibit increased tremulousness, altered visual response patterns to a light stimulus, and withdrawallike crying. In a large study in Boston, Cook et al. (1990) found that marijuana use correlated with a syndrome similar to FAS.

Cocaine use during pregnancy is most consistently associated with increased risk among newborns for intrauterine growth retardation (Cook et al., 1990). Infants tend to be jittery, to cry shrilly, and to startle at the slightest stimulation. They may demonstrate abnormal sleep patterns, poor feeding responses, tremors, and hypertonia; these behaviors make them difficult to console, adding to the difficulties in bonding between mother and infant.

Narcotic use during pregnancy results in intrauterine growth retardation in the newborn. About 80 percent of babies born to heroin-addicted mothers have such serious medical problems as hyaline membrane disease, brain hemorrhage, and respiratory distress syndrome (Cook et al., 1990). Newborns of mothers addicted to narcotics may have dramatic withdrawal symptoms after birth. They demonstrate CNS irritability that may last from 1 to 3 months and are difficult to console (Cook et al., 1990).

CHILDHOOD IN A HOME IN WHICH SUBSTANCE ABUSE EXISTS

Studies of children whose parents use mind-altering substances have largely been conducted with children of alcoholics (Kumpfer, 1987). Children of alcoholic mothers may demonstrate developmental problems such as hyperactivity, distractibility, short attention spans, language difficulties, and delayed maturation even when measured intelligence scores are within the normal range (Cook et al., 1990). These children do not catch up to normal children in physical growth and have decreased attention spans and delayed reaction times. It is difficult to separate the effects of having been subjected to toxic drugs during fetal development and the alterations in family functioning that occur when one or both parents are using drugs or alcohol. In two studies, more children of alcoholics than children from families without alcoholism were found to have difficulties such as repeating grades, failing to graduate from high school, and requiring referrals to school psychologists (Miller & Jang, 1977; Knop et al., 1985). Behavioral problems found more frequently among children of alcoholics than among children from nonalcoholic families are lying, stealing, fighting, truancy, and school behavior problems (West & Prinz, 1987). They are often diagnosed with a conduct disorder and are at greater risk for low self-esteem and depression and especially for substance abuse themselves (Anderson & Quast, 1983; Schuckit & Chiles, 1978).

In spite of many reports of behavioral and adjustment problems in these children, there are also reports that the majority of them function quite well. Werner (1989) described characteristics that were protective for children of alcoholics: the ability to obtain positive attention from other people, adequate communication skills, average intelligence, a caring attitude, a desire to achieve, and a belief in self-help. O'Sullivan (1991) found that children having a mentor developed resiliency against the affects of alcoholism in the family. Wolin et al. (1980) found that if family rituals, such as mealtimes or celebrations such as birthdays and holidays, were not disrupted by the parent's alcoholism, children's risk for later development of alcoholism was greatly diminished. Tweed and Ryff (1991) found that adult children of alcoholics exhibited many indications of wellness.

ADOLESCENCE

Following a period of epidemic drug and alcohol use, increases in adolescent suicide, and increasing crime rates, new statistics that demonstrate reduced rates of drug and alcohol use by teens are hopeful. Compared with high school seniors in 1979, increased numbers of youth now appear to view chemical use as a danger. Nevertheless, alcohol is involved in 45 to 60 percent of all accidents and at least 40 percent of suicides and homicides among teens (Robinson & Greene, 1988). Accidents, suicides, and homicides account for 80 percent of all adolescent deaths, with the rate rising for 15–24 year olds.

Adolescence is the most frequent time for initiation into alcohol or drug use. Among teens who try use of either alcohol or drugs, 1 in 10 will develop an addiction. One study found that nearly four fifths of the population of an inpatient treatment facility had begun using chemicals before the age of 18 (Kashani et al., 1987).

Adolescents may try drugs or alcohol to experience pleasurable feelings, to cope, to "have a good time," to feel a part of their peer group, or to take their mind off their problems. Significant use of drugs or alcohol by an adolescent halts normal emotional maturation and intensifies acting-out behavior. Tendencies toward impulsiveness, destructiveness, mistrustful behavior, irresponsibility, and general immaturity are demonstrated (Hartford & Grant, 1987). Severe acting-out behavior usually occurs in the areas of (1) more substance abuse, (2) sexual promiscuity, or (3) criminal behavior. Thus the chemical use becomes a vicious cycle.

An adolescent's drug or alcohol use may progress to addiction much faster than an adult's drug or alcohol use. Whereas an adult male may take 15 to 20 years to become addicted to alcohol, an adolescent may become addicted within 2 years. Cocaine addiction develops within a period of months. Changes in development, personality, and emotional and behavioral responses can be dramatic. Development of good judgment, tolerance of frustration, and problem-solving skills are impaired; school performance drops rapidly; and values may change radically because of cocaine use. A formerly responsible young person may begin associating with school dropouts or people with criminal behaviors. As usage increases, the adolescent may hide his or her use and lie when asked about it. The adolescent may feel alone and isolated. Suicide risk is increased.

Treatment for the adolescent is comprehensive and involves the entire family in an attempt to return the teen to normal growth and development. Prevention of drug and alcohol use in the first place is of prime importance. The most successful programs include parents, the schools, and community organizations in a coordinated approach. Reduction of initiation of use was found to occur when students were assisted in raising their self-esteem and taught interpersonal skills and social skills in refusing pressure from peers (DuPont, 1987).

ADULTHOOD

Evidence of addiction is most likely to appear during middle adulthood. Most people who are going to initiate chemical use during their lifetime will have done so by this time, and those who began using chemicals in their teen or pre-teen years will likely evidence the consequences of abusive use by the time they are adults. A number of factors determine when a person has crossed the line into abusive use or dependence. The substance used, the amount used, and the frequency and pattern of use are primary determinants. In addition, the user may accelerate use at a time of stress and at that time encounter difficulties with the substance.

Jellinek (1952) described four phases in the development of alcoholism. These phases fit into the disease model of alcoholism. Phase 1, the *prealcoholic phase*, is characterized by occasional relief drinking and an increase in alcohol tolerance. Phase 2, the *prodromal phase*, begins with the onset of blackouts, an early symptom, and then sneaking drinks and feeling guilty. During a **blackout**, a person appears to be functioning normally but remembers nothing of these periods when sober. Phase 3, the *crucial phase*, begins with the onset of loss of control and describes a progressive deterioration in relationships, responsibilities, and emotional stability. Phase 4, the *chronic phase*, begins with the onset of prolonged intoxications and includes the physical and mental deterioration many think of as chronic alcoholism. Jellinek studied males in the latter stages of alcoholism, however, so that all persons do not fit into this pattern. On the basis of later studies, Jellinek defined a number of other types of alcoholics, including those whose abusive drinking is periodic.

Some authors have attempted to derive phases in development of addiction to other substances, but they have been less well accepted. Many patterns occur in the use and abuse of mind-altering substances in the adult population. Routine screening for alcohol or drug use is imperative because, as can be seen from Jellinek's phases of alcoholism, some of the symptoms that are commonly perceived as indicating alcoholism do not occur until the late or chronic phase. This progression can be interrupted, and alcoholism and drug addiction can be treated.

LATE ADULTHOOD

It has long been thought that alcoholism and other drug abuse diminish greatly by old age. Recent reports, however, have disputed this claim. In one study of elderly people seeking health care, 18 percent of the women and 56 percent of the men had a substance abuse problem (Krach, 1990; Gomberg, 1982). A complex set of interacting factors place some elderly at high risk for use of these drugs. The elderly experience many stressors, such as major losses and role changes and possibly reduced resources to deal with them.

In addition, because of physiological changes, the elderly become more sensitive to drugs or alcohol. Sometimes as small amount as one drink a day can cause large changes in function. Prescription drugs either alone or in interaction with other prescription drugs, over-the-counter medication, or alcohol can greatly alter an elderly person's physiological, cognitive, or emotional function.

Several patterns of substance abuse may be seen in the elderly. First, there are those who have abused alcohol or drugs for many years and continue to do so and are usually in a debilitated state of health. Second, there are those who began using drugs or alcohol abusively late in life as a result of grief or the emptiness of finding themselves alone. Third, there are those who used drugs and alcohol safely in younger years but that find the same rate of use is now toxic because of aging.

Many family members and nurses regard substance abuse in the elderly as harmless and something they can still enjoy. They do not realize the many detrimental effects that accrue to the person. Quality of life for the elderly may improve dramatically with abstinence. When appropriately confronted with the reality that many physical and cognitive problems are caused by use of chemical substances, many elderly people are willing and able to quit and enjoy an enhanced quality of life.

SUBSTANCE ABUSE AND PSYCHIATRIC DISORDERS

EGO COMPETENCY AND SUBSTANCE ABUSE

Alcoholism or drug abuse and psychiatric disorders appear to be related in a number of ways. First, addiction and a psychiatric disorder can originate independently. Second, drugs could cause the psychiatric disorder. Third, people with psychiatric disorders are more likely to indulge in chemical use. In addition, withdrawal from chemicals can produce a syndrome that can mimic a psychiatric disorder (NIAAA, 1991).

Use of mind-altering drugs interferes with the functioning of the ego, causing competency to decrease from previous levels; this may masquerade as the onset of a mental illness. Conversely, when a person has a mental illness, altered **ego competency** in the form of impaired thinking, impaired impulse control, and poor judgment may result in the decision to use mind-altering drugs. Drug use may further impair ego competency, leading to addiction in a vicious circle (see the Research Abstract display below). In addition, some clients may use a mind-altering substance in an attempt to medicate or relieve the symptoms of a preexisting psychiatric disorder.

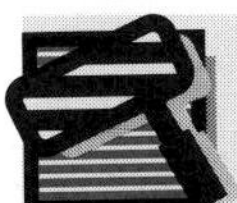

RESEARCH ABSTRACT

Psychopathology as an Antecedent to, and as a "Consequence" of, Substance Use in Adolescence

Friedman, A. S., Utada, A. T., Glickman, N. W., & Morrissey, M. R. (1987). *Journal of Drug Education, 17,* 233–244.

Friedman et al. examined the relationship between psychopathology and substance use in 232 9th, 10th, and 11th graders. They found that psychopathology (as assessed by the Brief Symptom Inventory) predicted substance use 17 months later and that earlier substance use predicted later psychopathology. Data indicated an additive or cumulative interaction effect, in which having psychiatric symptoms (psychopathology) contributed to the tendency to use drugs, and using drugs added to the tendency to have psychiatric symptoms. Among the nine types of psychiatric symptoms measured, obsessive–compulsive symptoms, hostility, paranoid ideation, and depression were more predictive of later increase in substance use than were other types of psychiatric symptoms (e.g., somatization); phobic anxiety was not predictive in any way.

Estimates vary widely, but there is strong evidence that substance abuse and psychiatric disorders frequently occur in the same person (NIAAA, 1991). Drug use may precipitate a psychiatric disorder in a person so predisposed. Use of CNS depressants or withdrawal from stimulants precipitates at least temporary depression, whereas use of stimulants or withdrawal from CNS depressants may precipitate anxiety (Brown & Schuckit, 1988; Ross et al., 1988). Use of drugs or alcohol may precipitate a manic episode in persons with bipolar disorder. Stimulant intoxication or overdose or intoxication from marijuana may precipitate a psychotic disorder. A number of disorders occur more frequently in alcoholics than in the general population, but this relationship is poorly understood. Compared with nonalcoholics, alcoholics are 21 times more likely to also have a diagnosis of antisocial personality disorder, the behaviors of which may disappear with treatment for the alcoholism (Helzer & Pryzbeck, 1988). Vaccani (1989) stated that alcoholism and borderline personality often occur simultaneously in the same person. "They both manifest similar pathologic ego-defense mechanisms and they frequently occur together making differential diagnoses difficult" (p. 113). Other disorders that occur more frequently in alcoholics are bulimia, depression, and anxiety.

An addictive personality has never been found, but most substance abusers sooner or later develop a particular group of personality characteristics, seen also in those with antisocial personality disorder, that result from the chronic chemical use. These characteristics are altered coping skills, passivity and dependency, low frustration tolerance, impulsivity, and a tendency to manipulate others.

EGO DEFENSE MECHANISM

Denial is a core component of the disease of chemical dependency; as the disease develops, so develops the denial system. It protects the person against the consequences of the disease, but it also locks him or her into a pattern of self-destruction. To facilitate the denial, these people use *rationalization*. They will find a plausible explanation for everything that occurs. They separate the problems from the use of the substances by externalizing and using the defense mechanism of *projection* to explain what they experience. They project their own feelings and problems on the people around them, blaming everyone but themselves.

RECOVERY AND TREATMENT

Recovery, a long process that involves learning to live and cope without chemicals, begins, but does not end, with abstinence. True recovery means recovering from being a "dry drunk," that is, having the distorted thinking and values that resulted from the substance use. It also means picking up emotional and personality development where it left off. Emotions must be felt and dealt with, and relationships with others must be reestablished. In some cases, vocational training will be needed to aid the person in becoming a productive member of society.

Most people will need some kind of treatment to recover from substance abuse. The treatment setting may be inpatient or outpatient, depending on economics or the severity of illness. Indications for inpatient treatment are risk for severe withdrawal symptoms and the lack of job or family support system. A working person can attend outpatient treatment during the evenings, with the length of treatment varying from one to four evenings a week for a set period of time. Unfortunately, many facilities are available for the treatment of the client with insurance coverage or adequate finances, but few such facilities exist for poor or unemployed clients. As a result, those without private resources face long waiting lines before treatment may begin. These clients may have the essential motivation at the time of enrollment for treatment, but they may have lost this motivation by the time the bed materializes.

Successful treatment settings are structured so that strong cohesiveness with others develops in the recovering person. The person can then begin to cope through depending on relationships with other people, rather than on chemicals. One important task of treatment is identification of the *triggers* that set in motion the person's desire for the chemical. **Relapse** is known to be a part of the disease; therefore, the recovering person needs to prepare for the eventuality that he or she will become tempted to indulge again and must develop a strategy to maintain sobriety when these triggers occur. Before the client is discharged from the inpatient setting, support groups need to be identified in the community to which the client will return. In addition, some persons will require psychotherapy for underlying psychiatric disorders or pain from childhood trauma (Young, 1990). Generally, only supportive counseling is used for the first year or two, to give the brain time to recover from the chemical use before intensive psychotherapy is begun.

The most common models of treatment consist of the following components:

1. Intense and ongoing education about the disease of alcoholism or drug addiction to break the abuser's denial
2. Initiation of the Twelve Steps of **Alcoholics Anonymous** (AA) (see Table 17–9)
3. Required reading from literature from AA and **Narcotics Anonymous** (NA)
4. Attendance at the meetings of these groups
5. Skill building to maintain abstinence

AA and NA support groups are sources of social support and structure for the healing process. Early in recovery, the person may attend groups daily or even more frequently. Clients participate in meditative readings and share their stories, that is, the unfortunate experiences and consequences they suffered as a result of chemical use. This sharing facilitates emotional support and a sense of oneness and commonality. Each member

TABLE 17–9
The Twelve Steps of AA

1. Admitted we were powerless over alcohol—that our lives had become unmanageable.
2. Came to believe that a Power greater than ourselves could restore us to sanity.
3. Made a decision to turn our will and our lives over to the care of God *as we understood Him.*
4. Made a searching and fearless moral inventory of ourselves.
5. Admitted to God, to ourselves, and to another human being the exact nature of our wrongs.
6. Were entirely ready to have God remove all these defects of character.
7. Humbly asked Him to remove our shortcomings.
8. Made a list of all persons we had harmed, and became willing to make amends to them all.
9. Made direct amends to such people wherever possible, except when to do so would injure them or others.
10. Continued to take personal inventory and, when we were wrong, promptly admitted it.
11. Sought through prayer and meditation to improve our conscious contact with God *as we understood Him*, praying only for knowledge of His will for us and the power to carry that out.
12. Having had a spiritual awakening as the result of these steps, we tried to carry this message to alcoholics, and to practice these principles in all our affairs.

chooses a *sponsor*, a person more experienced at sobriety, from whom he or she will receive individual support. The programs operate around the Twelve Steps, which the client works on one at a time, with the sponsor's supervision. Members of these groups claim that emotional and spiritual healing is possible through the program; however, there are persons who recover from chemical dependency without the use of these groups.

The psychiatric client who abuses drugs or alcohol produces special challenges. Treatment for the dual-diagnosis client needs to be directed at both the psychiatric disorder and the substance abuse problem. If only one of the disorders is addressed, the outcome frequently is failure. The psychiatric client, who already has difficulty coping with life, needs additional support to function independently without drugs or alcohol. In addition, the message against the use of *any* medications that many substance abuse treatment facilities give results in the client's refusing to take medication for the psychiatric disorder. Nurses who care for these clients need knowledge of both psychiatric and substance abuse disorders.

THE NURSE'S ROLE

THE GENERALIST'S ROLE

The nurse may work with the substance abuser at any level of care and in a number of roles (Fig. 17–3). The generalist nurse uses knowledge of basic addictions theory in carrying out the nursing process with all clients. Self-awareness and skill in self-assessment assist the nurse to apply this knowledge therapeutically. The skills needed are basic therapeutic communications skills and health teaching skills. Nursing plays a key role in the identification and assessment of substance abuse and referral for any client in any setting. In addition, nurses who work in the community and in pediatric settings participate in primary prevention (Tables 17–10 and 17–11).

THE ROLE OF THE ADVANCED-PRACTICE NURSE

Addictions specialist nurses have advanced theoretical knowledge and clinical skills and may work in a variety of settings in a variety of capacities both to assist with identification and treatment of substance abuser and to prevent abuse. Some may provide comprehensive holistic assessment, serve as a primary therapist for clients, or implement treatment with a variety of clients. Others may serve as a consultant and liaison or perform program development and evaluation. Other roles of the addictions specialist nurse are supervisor, administrator, consultant, researcher, and educator.

THE NURSING PROCESS

Table 17–12 lists the standards of addictions nursing practice.

Assessment

How to Take a Substance Abuse History. Assessment of the client who is using mind-altering substances is sometimes a difficult process because of the pervasiveness of the client's denial. In addition to the client's resistance, there are nurse-centered variables, such as the nurse's own attitudes, that may hinder the process. For example, a nurse from an alcoholic family, reminded of unresolved angers and pain may judge the client harshly, making the developing of a therapeutic relationship difficult. It is imperative for nurses to be aware of their own attitudes toward clients' use of mind-altering substances and to accept clients as people in need of help. The process of self-searching may uncover the pain inflicted earlier on one by a substance abuser, but it is possible to set aside this pain and give caring and humane nursing care when one is motivated to do so. This may even be a time for seeking a therapist to assist in one's own recovery or healing process, enabling one to become an even more knowledgeable and helpful nurse.

The drug and alcohol history is a natural part of the health history. Because chemical abuse interferes with all spheres of life, all aspects of the person's life must be assessed. Identification of problematic use of mind-altering substances often hinges on identifying the consequences of use of these substances.

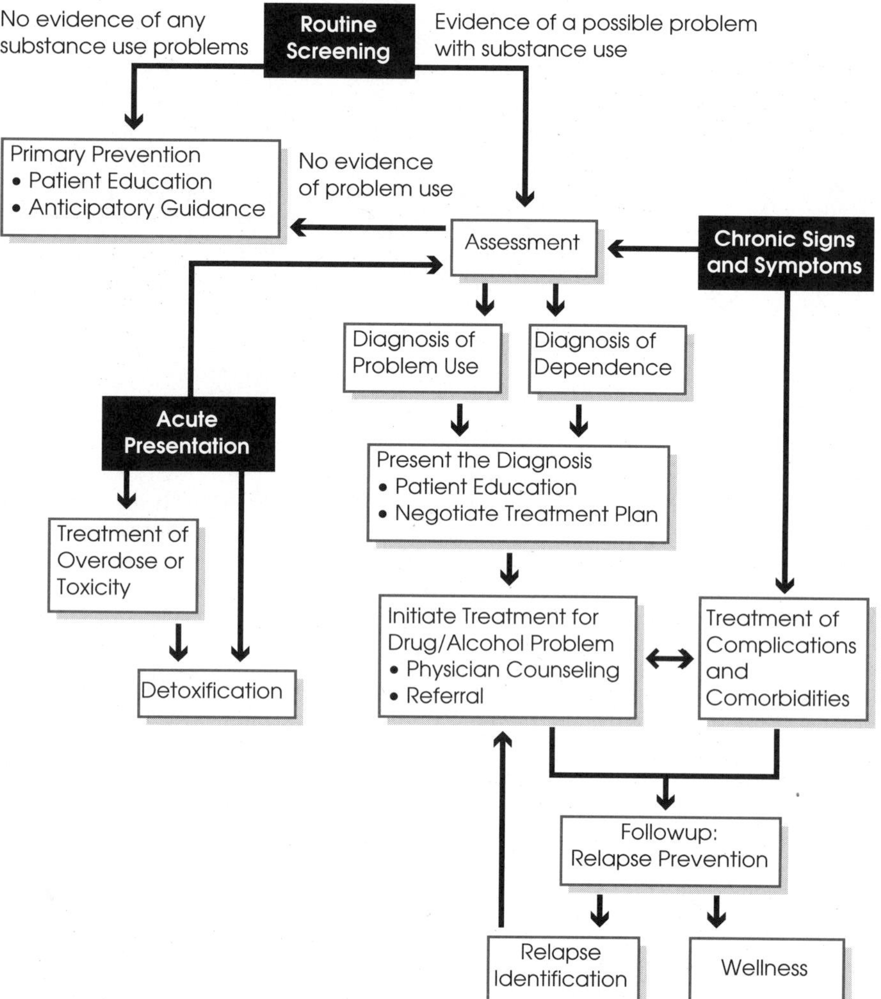

FIGURE 17–3
Assessing and treating the client with a substance abuse problem. (Courtesy of Project ADEPT, Brown University, ANA/NNSA 10/1/92.)

Assessment of drug and alcohol use includes the use of all drugs. Assessment begins with use of the least threatening drugs, such as caffeine and tobacco, and then proceeds to alcohol and prescription and non-prescription drugs, and lastly street drugs. People who are abusing drugs or alcohol *will* underestimate the quantity and frequency of use. Therefore, questions must be asked in such a way as to provide as accurate an assessment as possible. When beginning to assess for abuse of a substance, the nurse asks the following questions in order:

1. Whether the substance is used at all,
2. When the substance was last used,
3. How much of the substance was used on that occasion,
4. How often the person uses the amount used on the last occasion,
5. Whether that is the amount usually taken.

Continued followup questions are asked to clarify use and frequency. It is *very important* to determine the risks of possible withdrawal from a substance and when withdrawal might occur.

Screening Tests. When the nurse ascertains from the initial assessment that the individual does use a substance, it is important to follow up and screen for problem use. The CAGE questionnaire is short and easy to

TABLE 17–10
Characteristics of an Effective Prevention Program

1. Is comprehensive, addressing multiple systems (youth, families, school, clients, community organizations, and media) and using multiple strategies (e.g., providing accurate information, developing life skills, creating positive alternatives, training influential people, changing community policies and norms).
2. Involves the whole community in prevention efforts.
3. Addresses everyone, not just those identified as at high risk.
4. Is part of a broader, generic effort to promote health and reduce or eliminate risk.
5. Offers interventions across the life span and programs of duration (not just one-shot programs).
6. Is integrated into family, school, work, and community life.
7. Builds a supportive environment that enhances protective/resiliency factors.
8. Is culturally sensitive and specific.

From U.S. Office for Substance Abuse Prevention. (1992). *Nurse training course: Alcohol and other drug abuse prevention.* Rockville, MD: National Training System, U.S. Public Health Service.

TABLE 17–11
Characteristics of a Health Promotion Program

1. Focuses on maintenance/enhancement of existing levels of health.
2. Usually targets individuals or groups who are not currently ill or addicted.
3. Involves programs, community activities, and services to assist people to achieve positive change and reduce risk.
4. Uses approaches that provide people with resources to confront stressful life conditions constructively.
   a. Disseminates information on
      The effects of alcohol/drugs
      Prevention services and availability
      Treatment services and availability
      Prevention approaches and strategies
      Information about healthy lifestyle
   b. Develops life coping skills, including
      Decision-making skills
      Communication techniques
      Goal-setting skills
      Values clarification skills
      Problem-solving techniques
      Self-responsibility/self-care
      Responsible attitude toward alcohol/drugs
      Stress management/relaxation techniques
   c. Provides alternative activities that will
      Contribute to use of and growth in personal skills
      Create more positive self-image
      Develop satisfaction and self-esteem
      Develop respect for self and others
      Create opportunity for positive interactions with others
      Provide identification with appropriate role models
      Alleviate boredom, unrest, and apathy

From U.S. Office for Substance Abuse Prevention. (1992). *Nurse training course: Alcohol and other drug abuse prevention.* Rockville, MD: National Training System, U.S. Public Health Service.

TABLE 17–12
Standards of Addictions Nursing Practice

Standard I. Theory: Nurse uses appropriate knowledge from nursing theory and related disciplines in practice of addictions nursing.

Standard II. Data Collection: Data collection is continuous and systematic and is communicated effectively to treatment team throughout each phase of nursing process.

Standard III. Diagnosis: Nurse uses nursing diagnoses congruent with accepted nursing and interprofessional classification systems of addictions and associated physiological and psychological disorders to express conclusions supported by data obtained through nursing process.

Standard IV. Planning: Nurse establishes plan of care for client that is based on nursing diagnoses, addresses specific goals, defines expected outcomes, and delineates nursing actions unique to client's needs.

Standard V. Intervention: Nurse implements actions independently and/or in collaboration with peers, members of other disciplines, and clients in prevention, intervention, and rehabilitation phases of care of clients with health problems related to patterns of abuse and addiction.

Standard VA. Intervention: Therapeutic Alliance—Nurse uses "therapeutic self" to establish relationship with clients and to structure nursing interventions to help clients develop the awareness, coping skills, and behavior changes that promote health.

Standard VB. Intervention: Education—Nurse educates clients and communities to help them prevent and/or correct actual or potential health problems related to patterns of abuse and addiction.

Standard VC. Intervention: Self-Help Groups—Nurse uses knowledge and philosophy of self-help groups to assist clients in learning new ways to address stress, maintain self-control or sobriety, and integrate healthy coping behaviors into their lifestyle.

Standard VD. Intervention: Pharmacological Therapies—Nurse applies knowledge of pharmacological principles in nursing process.

Standard VE. Intervention: Therapeutic Environment—Nurse provides, structures, and maintains therapeutic environment in collaboration with individual, family, and other professionals.

Standard VF. Intervention: Counseling—Nurse uses therapeutic communication in interactions with client to address issues related to patterns of abuse and addiction.

Standard VI. Evaluation: Nurse evaluates client's responses and revises nursing diagnoses, interventions, and treatment plan accordingly.

Standard VII. Ethical Care: Nurse's decisions and activities on behalf of clients are in keeping with personal and professional codes of ethics and in accord with legal statutes.

Standard VIII. Quality Assurance: Nurse participates in peer review and other staff evaluation and quality assurance processes to ensure that clients with abuse and addiction problems receive quality care.

Standard IX. Continuing Education: Nurse assumes responsibility for his or her continuing education and professional development and contributes to professional growth of others who work with or are learning about persons with abuse and addiction problems.

Standard X. Interdisciplinary Collaboration: Nurse collaborates with interdisciplinary treatment team and consults with other health care providers in assessing, planning, implementing, and evaluating programs and other activities related to addictions nursing.

Standard XI. Use of Community Health Systems: Nurse participates with other members of community in assessing, planning, implementing, and evaluating community health services that attend to primary, secondary, and tertiary prevention of addictions.

Standard XII. Research: Nurse contributes to nursing care of clients with addictions and to addictions area of practice through innovations in theory and practice and participation in research, and communicates these contributions.

Reprinted with permission. *Standards of addictions nursing practice with selected diagnoses and criteria.* © 1993, American Nurses Association, Washington, DC.

TABLE 17–13
CAGE Screening Tool for Alcohol or Drug Abuse

1. Have you ever tried to **c**ut down your use (of a substance)?
2. Have others ever **a**nnoyed you by complaining about your use (of the substance)?
3. Have you ever felt **g**uilty by your use (of the substance)?
4. Have you ever used (the substance) in the morning to avoid feeling nervous? (**e**yeopener)

Note. One positive response is suspicious for a drug or alcohol problem. Two positive responses are diagnostic.

From Ewing, J. A. (1984). Detecting alcoholism: The CAGE questionnaire. *Journal of the American Medical Association, 252*(14), 1905–1907. Copyright 1984, American Medical Association.

use, having only four questions (Table 17–13). Other screening tests are the Michigan Alcohol Screening Test (MAST) and the Trauma Scale (Tables 17–14 and 17–15). Meyer (1992) found that two thirds of the trauma clients admitted to an emergency department had a history of substance abuse.

After assessing the substance-abusing client, the nurse will find a variety of nursing diagnoses encompassing the entire sphere of nursing care. The American Nurses Association (1987) has identified the most frequently encountered diagnoses and categorized them according to the four dimensions of practice: biological, psychosocial, cognitive, and spiritual (discussed below).

Nursing Diagnoses

Mind-altering chemicals affect the client physically, emotionally, socially, cognitively, spiritually, and behaviorally, causing many chronic problems:

Biological
- Sensory–Perceptual Alteration
- Potential for Injury
- Self-Care Deficit
- Sexual Dysfunction
- Potential for Infection
- Sleep Pattern Disturbance
- Alterations in Nutrition: less than body requirements
- Alteration in Comfort: pain
- Altered Growth and Development: biological

Psychosocial
- Impaired Communications
- Ineffective Individual Coping
- Alteration in Self-Concept
- Anxiety
- Fear
- Social Isolation
- Dysfunctional Family Process
- Altered Parenting
- Altered Growth and Development: Psychosocial
- Potential for Violence

Cognitive
- Knowledge Deficit
- Alteration in Thought Process
- Noncompliance

TABLE 17–14
Brief Michigan Alcoholism Screening Test (MAST)

POINTS		
(2)	*1.	Do you feel you are a normal drinker?
(2)	*2.	Do friends or relatives think you are a normal drinker?
(5)	3.	Have you ever attended a meeting of Alcoholics Anonymous?
(2)	4.	Have you ever lost friends or girlfriends/boyfriends because of drinking?
(2)	5.	Have you ever gotten into trouble at work because of drinking?
(2)	6.	Have you ever neglected your obligations, your family, or your work for 2 or more days in a row because you were drinking?
(2)	7.	Have you ever had delirium tremens (DTs) or severe shaking, heard voices, or seen things that weren't there after heavy drinking?
(5)	8.	Have you ever gone to anyone for help about your drinking?
(5)	9.	Have you ever been in a hospital because of drinking?
(2)	10.	Have you ever been arrested for drunk driving or driving after drinking?

Note. Negative responses to questions marked by asterisk are alcoholic responses.

Scoring is as follows: 3 points or less = nonalcoholic, 4 points = suggestive of alcoholism, 5 or more points = alcoholism.

From the *American Journal of Psychiatry, 129*, 342–345, 1972. Copyright 1972, the American Psychiatric Association. Reprinted by permission.

Spiritual
- Spiritual Distress
- Powerlessness
- Hopelessness
- Grief

In the fourth edition of the *Diagnostic and Statistical Manual of Mental Disorders* (DSM-IV; American Psychiatric Association, 1994), there are two categories of substance abuse disorders: psychoactive substance dependence and psychoactive substance abuse (see DSM-IV Criteria displays on p. 377).

TABLE 17–15
Trauma Scale

Since your 18th birthday:
1. Have you had any fractures or dislocations to your bones or joints?
2. Have you been injured in a road traffic accident?
3. Have you injured your head?
4. Have you been injured in an assault or fight (excluding injuries during sports)?
5. Have you been injured after drinking?

Note. Two or more positive answers are suggestive for alcoholism or drug dependence.

Reproduced with permission from Skinner, H. A., Hoth, S., Schuller, R., Rey, J., & Israel, Y. (1984). Identification of alcohol abuse using laboratory tests and a history of trauma. *Annals of Internal Medicine, 101*, 847–851.

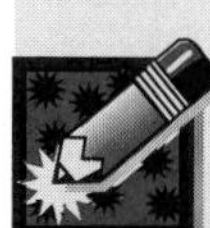

DSM-IV CRITERIA FOR SUBSTANCE DEPENDENCE

A maladaptive pattern of substance use leading to clinically significant impairment or distress, as manifested by three (or more) of the following, occurring at any time in the same 12-month period:

(1) tolerance, as defined by either of the following:
  (a) a need for markedly increased amounts of the substance to achieve intoxication or desired effect
  (b) markedly diminished effect with continued use of the same amount of the substance
(2) withdrawal, as manifested by either of the following:
  (a) the characteristic withdrawal syndrome for the substance (refer to Criteria A and B of the criteria sets for Withdrawal from the specific substances)
  (b) the same (or a closely related) substance is taken to relieve or avoid withdrawal symptoms
(3) the substance is often taken in larger amounts or over a longer period than was intended
(4) there is a persistent desire or unsuccessful efforts to cut down or control substance use
(5) a great deal of time is spent in activities necessary to obtain the substance (e.g., visiting multiple doctors or driving long distances), use the substance (e.g., chain-smoking), or recover from its effects
(6) important social, occupational, or recreational activities are given up or reduced because of substance use
(7) the substance use is continued despite knowledge of having a persistent or recurrent physical or psychological problem that is likely to have been caused or exacerbated by the substance (e.g., current cocaine use despite recognition of cocaine-induced depression, or continued drinking despite recognition that an ulcer was made worse by alcohol consumption)

From American Psychiatric Association. (1994). *Diagnostic and statistical manual of mental disorders, fourth edition* (p. 181). Washington, DC: Author.

DSM-IV CRITERIA FOR SUBSTANCE ABUSE

A. A maladaptive pattern of substance use leading to clinically significant impairment or distress, as manifested by one (or more) of the following, occurring within a 12-month period:

(1) recurrent substance use resulting in a failure to fulfill major role obligations at work, school, or home (e.g., repeated absences or poor work performance related to substance use; substance-related absences, suspensions, or expulsions from school; neglect of children or household)
(2) recurrent substance use in situations in which it is physically hazardous (e.g., driving an automobile or operating a machine when impaired by substance use)
(3) recurrent substance-related legal problems (e.g., arrests for substance-related disorderly conduct)
(4) continued substance use despite having persistent or recurrent social or interpersonal problems caused or exacerbated by the effects of the substance (e.g., arguments with spouse about consequences of intoxication, physical fights)

B. The symptoms have never met the criteria for Substance Dependence for this class of substance.

From American Psychiatric Association. (1994). *Diagnostic and statistical manual of mental disorders, fourth edition* (pp. 182–183). Washington, DC: Author.

Planning

There are four main goals of nursing care for clients using mind-altering substances:

1. To provide safe and humane care
2. To help clients recognize their use and abuse of substances
3. To develop a relationship that provides clients with safe and caring support
4. To know where and how to refer clients and their families

The following case study and Nursing Care Plan 17–1 illustrate how a nurse would approach caring for a client with addictive behaviors.

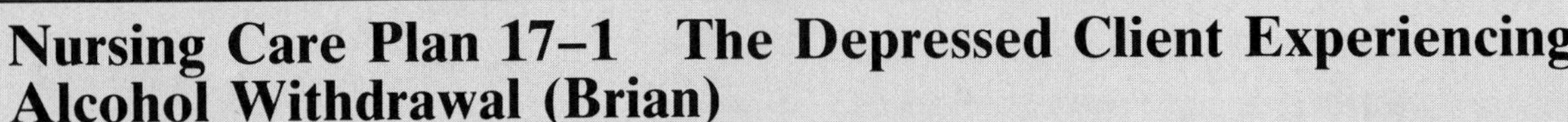

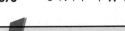

Nursing Care Plan 17–1 The Depressed Client Experiencing Alcohol Withdrawal (Brian)

OUTCOME IDENTIFICATION	NURSING ACTIONS	RATIONALES	EVALUATION
► Nursing Diagnosis: Sensory–Perceptual Alterations related to withdrawal from multiple psychoactive substances			
1. By [date], Brian will maintain vital signs within normal limits.	1. Collect data about Brian's drug and alcohol use in history.	1. Client's current state, history of use, and course of previous detoxifications are important to indicate time, type, and severity of withdrawal.	*Goal met:* Brian's vital signs stay below the midnight elevation previously recorded.
2. By [date], Brian will have maintained orientation throughout detoxification.	2. Assess Brian for stage of withdrawal, orientation, presence of hallucinations, speech pattern, and need for continuing safety measures.	2. Orientation is a key measure to determine the severity of withdrawal. In addition, a disoriented client is at increased risk for injury. Hallucinations and speech patterns provide additional clues to the severity and stage of withdrawal.	When asked, Brian is able to state the current time, the fact that he is in the hospital, and his current feelings. Brian detoxifies without incident.
3. By [date], Brian will detoxify from alcohol with minimum psychological and physiological effects.	3a. Monitor Brian's vital signs frequently, observing his reactions to medications.	3a. Medications must be closely monitored to determine whether the dosage is correct. More may be needed to counteract severe withdrawal; if withdrawal is light, the client may be overmedicated. Vital signs are good indicators of the course of withdrawal.	
	3b. Provide a safe, calm environment for Brian, with a reduced amount of stimuli.	3b. Because of possible perceptual distortion, the client must be protected. The environment must be quiet and calm to avoid overstimulating an already irritated central nervous system.	
	3c. Promote restful sleep without chemicals.	3c. Sleep is disturbed in withdrawal. Client needs assistance to sleep without using more chemicals.	
► Nursing Diagnosis: Ineffective Individual Coping related to use of denial in acknowledging the addiction process			
1. By [date], Brian will acknowledge that he has a problem controlling use of alcohol.	1a. Develop a therapeutic relationship with Brian.	1a. The addicted client has difficulty trusting others. It is important to develop a trusting relationship.	*Goals partially met:* Brian acknowledges that lately he had been drinking too much, but he still attributes this to his depression.
	1b. Use a supportive approach while Brian is detoxifying. Avoid confronting Brian at this time.	1b. The client is physically ill during detoxification. He or she needs comfort and support during this time.	Brian becomes tearful and sad when discussing his recent behavior of staying in bed and not going to work.

Nursing Care Plan 17–1 The Depressed Client Experiencing Alcohol Withdrawal (Brian) (Continued)

OUTCOME IDENTIFICATION	NURSING ACTIONS	RATIONALES	EVALUATION
	1c. After detoxification, when feeding back data about Brian's behavior and physical condition, state in objective terms.	1c. The addicted client manipulates people and is suspicious of overly solicitous behavior. Honesty, genuineness, and a matter-of-fact approach attain his or her trust.	Brian acknowledges that his recent heavy drinking did not help his depression and in fact may have worsened it. Brian continues to deny that he could not control his use of alcohol once he began drinking.
	1d. Use a genuine, matter-of-fact, nonjudgmental approach when interacting with Brian. Focus interactions on the present circumstances and facts, rather than past behavior.	1d. The client withdrawing from chemicals usually experiences overwhelming guilt. Current information is easier to tolerate than past information.	
	1e. Avoid use of labeling terms such as "alcoholic" or "addict."	1e. Labeling terms alienate the client and hinder cooperation.	
2. By [date], Brian will describe and own his feelings associated with his addictive behavior.	2a. Be persistent in obtaining responses from Brian. Never discuss his alibis, excuses, rationalizations, or other inaccurate or vague explanations of the problems with him.	2a. The client's denial is deeply entrenched. It will be difficult for him or her to "hear" information that is contrary to his or her usual perceptions.	
	2b. Reflect back Brian's feeling tone.	2b. This begins the client's process of learning about him- or herself. In addition, it may diffuse hostility the client shows to deflect focus away from the substance abuse.	
3. By [date], Brian will identify specific ways his life has become unmanageable because of his use of alcohol.	3a. Teach Brian about disease states associated with addictions, support and self-help groups' philosophies, positive communications skills, and new coping skills.	3a. The client needs this information to begin to understand and cope with addictive disease. These are coping skills the client needs in order to recover from addiction and lead a satisfying lifestyle.	
	3b. If Brian continues to deny, do not push, but approach him at a later time.	3b. Additional pushing when the client obviously is not interested will only alienate him or her. At a later time, the client may be in a more receptive mood.	

Case Study: The Depressed Client Undergoing Alcohol Withdrawal (Brian)

Brian, 46 years old, was admitted to the psychiatric unit at 4:00 A.M. for severe depression and suicide ideation. His wife sought help after she found him in the garage with a gun to his head. At the time of admission, his breath smelled of alcohol and his speech was slurred. When he was asked how much he had drunk, he replied, "I've had a couple of beers." Blood alcohol level was found to be .185. Vital signs at admission were as follows: blood pressure, 150/90, temperature, 98.7, pulse, 75, and respirations, 15.

Brian was a new car salesman and was normally one of the top salesmen for the agency. In the past

2 months, his sales had been dropping off and he had failed to report to work for the past 2 weeks, lying in bed and appearing to be sleeping. At the time of admission, he was unshaven and declared that he hadn't slept in weeks. His movements were slowed, his head bowed, and his gait slumped and slow. He averted his eyes and answered questions in grunts and monosyllables; his wife provided most of the assessment information. She stated that they had three children, all grown except one still in college, and she could give no reason why he had become so depressed. She considered their marriage to be happy and spoke of the many good times they had. When asked whether Brian used substances, she said the he smoked two packs of cigarettes per day and "liked his beer." She acknowledged that he had several beers an evening and on weekends sometimes drank until he was drunk.

The first night after admission, Brian had his call light on frequently. He complained of difficulty sleeping and "shakiness." At midnight, his vital signs were blood pressure, 180/100, temperature, 100.1, pulse, 90, and respirations, 20. He asked and received medication for sleep and slept for several hours. It was decided that he was withdrawing from alcohol, and he was therefore transferred to the dual-diagnosis treatment unit, where a protocol for alcohol withdrawal was established.

After Brian had passed the acute phase of alcohol withdrawal, he was assigned to participate in the treatment program. This consisted of treatment for both alcoholism and depression. Brian acknowledged that he was depressed but denied that he had a problem with alcohol. He maintained that the reason he drank was because he was depressed. "As soon as I get over this depression, I won't drink so much. I can take it or leave it."

Brian's difficulties with sleep did not improve after alcohol withdrawal. He complained of severe nightmares and difficulty initiating and maintaining sleep. He was placed on an antidepressant medication, but he still asked for sleeping medication each night. When he was told he could no longer receive medication for sleep, he became irate.

TABLE 17–16
Management of Delirium (Unawareness of the Environment) in Alcohol or Drug Withdrawal

1. Keep room adequately lit—it is important that there be a window to prevent misperceptions such as illusions and hallucinations.
2. Avoid low voice conversations with others within the client's hearing.
3. Elevate the head of the bed. Being flat in bed increases the chances of hallucinations occurring.
4. If possible, have people and objects familiar to the client at hand.
5. Provide properly functioning eyeglasses and hearing aids if needed.
6. Provide information for orientation.
7. It is helpful to have the same personnel caring for the person if possible.
8. Use restraints **only** as a last resort.
9. Use one-on-one observation.
10. Inform the client frequently of his or her condition and progress.
11. Do not awaken the client during the night if at all possible.
12. Use kind firmness when client is agitated.
13. Reassure client that he or she is safe and you are there to help.

Courtesy of N. Thompson, Department of Nursing, University of Kansas Medical Center, Kansas City, Kansas.

Implementation

Acute Care. An intoxicated client needs careful monitoring that implements all the precautions used with any client with altered consciousness (see Table 17–16 for an explanation of the management of delirium in alcohol or drug withdrawal). Head trauma may cause restlessness or violence. Identification of the quantity of substance used, time of last use of the substance, and time span of use is vital to facilitation of safe drug or alcohol withdrawal. It is important to monitor the client's vital signs and mental and neurological status. It is also important to obtain a urine sample at the time of admission to the emergency department, because some chemicals are eliminated rapidly. If there is no order for the screen, the sample can be frozen until the order has been made.

Alcohol and drugs alter the absorption and metabolism of certain vitamins and minerals. Thiamine deficiency can become so severe that the brain damage of Wernicke-Korsakoff syndrome or thiamine dementia occurs. Symptoms are ophthalmoplegia, sixth-nerve palsy, nystagmus, ptosis, ataxia, confusion, and coma. When a client is comatose from alcohol intoxication, the nurse should never infuse glucose until thiamine is given, because brain damage may be induced. Thiamine is necessary to metabolize the glucose; without thiamine, the glucose will damage the cells (see Chapter 13).

Special Consideration for Medications. There are two special considerations for the management of pain in the person abusing substances. It has been shown that the best protection against addiction is timely and adequate pain relief (McCaffery, 1991). However, cross-tolerance between the narcotic pain medication and the abused substance may require such a high dose for the relief of pain that respiration is depressed. Moreover, the pain medication may trigger a craving for the drug, causing relapse in the abstinent client. It is important for the nurse to recognize this threat, discuss it with the client, and plan nursing care to assist the client in maintaining abstinence. For severe pain, narcotic pain relievers may be given, with additional support provided by the nurse or the client's own support system. For less severe pain, nonnarcotic pain relievers can be given.

Nearly all antianxiety and sleep medications are addictive, and because cross-tolerance is a probability, the likelihood of their effectiveness in providing relief for the substance-abusing client is limited. Frequently, addicted clients who are unable to obtain the drug of choice persist in seeking any addictive drug. It is thus preferable to refrain from giving these drugs to actively abusing clients. The recovering client will usually request that these drugs not be given to him or her because of their triggering effect. In the event that antianxiety or hypnotic drugs are prescribed, it is important for the nurse to discuss these difficulties with the physician. For invasive procedures, they may be given anyway, or another drug, such as an antihistamine, may be given. The problems with sleep and anxiety are particularly vexing for the client who is withdrawing from mind-altering substances, frequently causing severe difficulty in either initiating or maintaining normal sleep patterns. Because most of the abused drugs alter the normal stages of sleep, especially REM sleep, withdrawal may induce intense and bizarre nightmares. It is important for the nurse to teach the client that sleep disorders are typical and to assist him or her to sleep without medication. Measures that promote healthy sleep are

- Exercise during the daytime hours
- Relaxation during the evening
- Regularity of meal and awakening times
- Exposure to sunlight

A cool, quiet, darkened room provides the best setting for sleep. Staying awake during the daytime and restricting caffeine intake assist nighttime sleep. When sleep fails to come, the nurse may provide warm milk or a back rub. If the client is still unable to sleep, allowing him or her to engage in quiet activity may allow for sleep later in the night.

Dealing with Denial. Many times, health professionals inadvertently enable a client's denial by allowing his or her view of the world to stand. The client must at least question whether he or she has a problem in order to obtain help. The client protects the denial system in several ways: by maintaining that something is not so; by downplaying the significance of the problem; by blaming others (projection); by providing excuses; by intellectualizing the problem, that is, talking and thinking about it in academic or theoretical terms; by diverting attention away from the subject; or by becoming hostile to stop the nurse from confronting the substance abuse.

There are several means for overcoming a client's denial: First, the confrontation of denial should take place within a trusting relationship in an atmosphere of caring. The nurse must communicate in a nonjudgmental, objective, and accepting manner. Second, the nurse should be patient and persistent, not expecting the client to acknowledge his or her chemical dependency right away. Third, the nurse must reject the client's use of the above-listed defense mechanisms; alibis or rationalizations, for example, cannot be accepted. Fourth, the nurse needs to establish the connection between drinking or other drug use and repeated harmful consequences. Fifth, inconsistencies in statements and behavior need to be pointed out. Finally, the nurse should back up the diagnostic conclusion with evidence (*Dealing with Denial*, 1975).

The first task for the nurse is to increase his or her own comfort level and be courageous enough to be a role model for colleagues. Because the client needs much emotional support during the withdrawal period, it is not an appropriate time to confront him or her about the chemical use. After withdrawal, however, it is important to work toward assisting the client to become aware of the difficulties he or she is experiencing as a result of substance abuse. Use a warm, gentle approach and gently explain to the client the consequences he or she has suffered as a result of the use of drugs. Do not make excuses for the client regarding his or her inadequacies. Maintaining silence about the chemical use will continue denial; therefore, it is important to talk with the client about this.

The nurse uses a businesslike and matter-of-fact approach when working with a chemically dependent person, focusing on the present and not the past. After supporting data are obtained, feedback is stated in objective terms and is given privately, out of earshot of others. Labeling terms such as "alcoholic," "addict," or "drunk" are not to be used. The nurse asks open-ended, specific, factual questions that are difficult to answer with evasions or vague generalities, reflecting back the client's feeling tone. After a hostile response, the nurse reflects back the stated or implied feelings. Tactfully, but insistently, the nurse probes for details, never taking responses at face value or accepting vague or general answers. Sidestepping the issue or diversionary tactics such as changing the subject should not be allowed. The nurse must simply stick to the task, focusing exclusively on areas that need to be covered by the interview. The client's alibis, excuses, rationalizations, or other inaccurate explanations of the problems should never be discussed. It is common for the drug or alcohol abuser to blame chemical use on the consequences of use, rather than vice versa.

It can be discouraging for the nurse to work to try to get the client to face the chemical dependency while the client persists in denying it. The effects of the nurse's efforts may not be evident initially and the nurse's efforts may need reinforcing by others at a later time. If the client hears the same information from different sources, perhaps eventually it will provoke a response. Therefore, the nurse who does not succeed in getting the client to hear that he or she has a problem should not push. The nurse may be successful the next time; if not, others may succeed.

Health Teaching. Teaching is a pivotal part of the nursing care of any client who is using and abusing substances. Typically, the client needs to be made aware of the effects the substance has on him or her and of the addictive disease process. The nurse must plan care to teach and assist the client with methods of coping with-

TABLE 17–17
Teaching the Addicted Client

1. Repeat information frequently. Remember that the client will have at least some temporary cognitive alterations as a result of the chemical abuse.
2. Reinforce learning with auditory and visual aids.
3. Use the philosophy of the support groups in the teaching process.
4. Present information in a nonthreatening, nonjudgmental learning environment.
5. Present factual information about the addiction, recovery, and relapse process.
6. Present concepts from the simple to the complex.
7. Develop learning material that includes the client in the process.
8. Support any positive response to learning made by the client.
9. Find individualized motivations to support the client in using adaptive behaviors in place of the addictive behaviors.
10. Provide frequent opportunity for the client to provide questions or comments or to apply the information to him- or herself.

From American Nurses' Association and National Nurses' Society on Addictions. (1988). *Standards of addictions nursing practice with selected diagnoses and criteria.* Kansas City, MO: American Nurses' Association.

out chemicals, such as discussing concerns with others, developing problem-solving skills, delaying gratification, learning relaxation techniques, and developing interpersonal skills. Many clients have no knowledge of what constitutes a healthy lifestyle and need to be taught about nutrition, proper exercise, and rest. It is common for substance-abusing clients to lack a repertoire of healthy recreational activities. There is a whole range of skills that the nurse may help the recovering client obtain (Table 17–17).

Other Interventions. Because clients who use chemicals have a chronically low self-esteem, interventions that raise self-esteem are important. The nurse assists clients to identify their feelings, validate these feelings with clients, and give clients emotional support without discounting their perception and reality. Encourage clients to share their feelings with other clients, so that they realize they are not alone in their pain. This experience has profound positive effects on clients' self-esteem and hence recovery. Because the impact of chemical use may involve a wide range of systems, nursing care may range from physical care to growth-producing interventions that assist the client in lifestyle change. If any previous coping skills existed, they were replaced by the chemical use and now must be built or reclaimed. Personal interests and values that were set aside must be reexamined and reclaimed, or new ones developed.

The nurse can also serve as a liaison among the various disciplines in assisting the client to find help. Because the break in denial is usually for a short time only, any willingness by the client to seek treatment must be acted on promptly. The nurse assists the client by contacting the appropriate colleague and helping to initiate the referral, whether it is to a social worker, a psychiatrist, the psychiatric liaison nurse, the chemical dependency nurse, the community health nurse, or the discharge planning person. It is important for the nurse to suggest that the client attend AA or NA groups and "work the program" to grow emotionally and spiritually. Many clients claim renewed zest for life from the camaraderie, support, and growth they find in these groups.

Psychopharmacology. A number of medications may be prescribed to assist the client to maintain abstinence from the chemical. Disulfiram (Antabuse), which blocks alcohol metabolism and makes the client severely ill when alcohol is ingested, is given to discourage its use. Clients must be taught to never ingest alcohol when taking Antabuse and that occasionally the result is fatal. Naltrexone, a narcotic antagonist, has been experimentally given to block craving for a number of agents, including alcohol (Swift, 1992). Methadone, a long-acting narcotic that can be given orally once a day, has been a controversial treatment for narcotic addicts. Desipramine/imipramine, fluoxetine, bromocriptine, and amantadine are frequently used to help cocaine abusers maintain abstinence.

Nutrition. A client who has been chronically using mind-altering chemicals usually exhibits alterations in nutrition. Some clients, especially those using cocaine, are cachectic. Multivitamins with large doses of thiamine are given routinely to persons who are addicted. Balanced diets are provided to replenish the depleted nutrition.

Assisting and Supporting the Family. There is a great need for understanding and emotional support in the family of the substance abuser, especially if there are children. Conversely, if children exhibit symptoms indicative of abuse or neglect, caretaking adults need to be assessed for use of mind-altering substances. Any child who displays any chronic symptoms of being hungry, angry, lonely, or tired should be assessed further. If there are any signs of sexual or physical abuse, the nurse should talk to the child privately, ensuring the child that what he or she says will *not* be reported to his or her parents. If the child reports abuse, the nurse tells the child that he or she will let persons know who can provide protection and explains that he or she is legally required to do so. The nurse praises the child for being brave enough to share what has occurred. If there is suspicion of physical or sexual abuse, the nurse sees that the child is protected and reports this to authorities.

If there is suspicion of spouse abuse, the nurse talks to the spouse alone, offering help and emotional support. The spouse is encouraged to discuss her concerns. Because she alone knows most accurately the extent of her danger, and she is an adult, it is important to listen to her and respect and follow her wishes as to the course of action. Even if help is refused at that time, be sure she has emergency numbers and procedures available should she desire help at a later time.

Family members need to be educated about alcoholism and drug addiction. They need a listening ear to hear their pain and anger. Usually, family members are grateful to receive literature that explains chemical dependency and to find there are resources in the community such as **Al-Anon** and **Nar-Anon**, which are support groups for family members and friends of people who abuse alcohol or drugs. Al-Anon and Nar-Anon also have a Twelve Step approach and encourage their members to share their experiences with each other and to work on growth and healing within themselves. Some family members will deny the loved one's chemical dependency and will continue to play out a co-dependent role, inadvertently enabling the chemical dependency.

Evaluation

The following are the major criteria for evaluation of the nursing care of the client who is using mind-altering substances:

1. The client safely undergoes detoxification and withdrawal.
2. The client realizes that the use of the substance is detrimental to him or her. This is a major criterion, and the likelihood that it will be accomplished in one short-term hospital stay is dim; therefore, a small increment toward this end can be used for evaluation.
3. The client connects use of the substances to the problems he or she encounters. An appropriate evaluation criterion would be a single, concrete, realistic step toward making this connection.
4. The client and the family agree to continued care toward recovery from substance abuse.

An outcome criterion should be stated in terms of the client's or family's response to a nursing measure. In addition, there are many outcome criteria that reflect the appropriate nursing diagnoses for a particular client.

RESOURCES AND REFERRAL SOURCES

All nurses need to know a repertoire of referral and other resources for the chemically dependent client. Included in the repertoire should be a certified addictions nurse, professionals from other disciplines with expertise in the care of the substance abuser, and professionals with expertise in evaluating and/or treating the substance-abusing client. The nurse needs to identify and keep a list of such professionals so that he or she may make referrals as needed. These professionals will assist the nurse to find the name of one or more treatment facilities to which clients may be referred.

The nurse also needs to have a collection of literature available to distribute to clients who use mind-altering substances and members of their families. An excellent source of literature is the National Council on Alcohol and Drug Dependency (NCADD). This organization offers a wide variety of services including evaluation of a client; referral; and community classes for professionals, clients, and clients' family members.

It is always appropriate for the nurse to refer a client or a family member to a support group when indicated. Of course, receptivity to this kind of intervention first must be assessed. AA, NA, Al-Anon, Adult Children of Alcoholics, and Codependents Anonymous groups are often listed in the telephone directory. If the desired group is not listed, often a telephone number or address may be obtained by calling the AA number. AA has informational literature available for distribution to clients.

Usually, each state has a center where listings of resource professionals, treatment centers, and support groups and literature on drug and alcohol abuse may be obtained. In addition, there are sources of information at the federal level. The National Clearinghouse for Alcohol and Drug Information is one such source: Information Services, P.O. Box 2345, Rockville, MD 20852. There is also a drug abuse information and treatment referral line: 1-800-662-HELP. By using these resources, the generalist nurse may access a variety of information sources for whatever information is needed in the care of a client.

►CHAPTER SUMMARY

The use of mind-altering substances is prevalent in today's society. The financial, personal, and family costs of this use and abuse are staggering. People who abuse substances are heavily represented in the population seeking health care. It is imperative that the nurse identify and provide safe care for substance-abusing clients. In addition, the nurse needs to be skilled in giving appropriate care to facilitate these clients' recovery.

The etiology of substance abuse is not entirely understood. It is generally accepted that substance abuse arises from a complex set of factors, including genetic predisposition, learned behavior, response to past stress from a dysfunctional family, and current stressors. A key model for understanding substance abuse is the disease model, which is used extensively in treatment settings. This model conceptualizes substance abuse as a disease that arises once substance abuse is initiated. It follows the course of a chronic disease, with describable symptoms and an inclination toward relapse.

A number of substances may be a source of addictive behavior: Alcohol is the most frequently used; other CNS depressants, narcotics, CNS stimulants, hallucinogens, cannabis, and inhalants are also used. These substances may be ingested, smoked, snorted, or injected. They cause a variety of physiological, emotional, cognitive, spiritual, behavioral, and social changes. People of all ages are affected in some manner or another.

Denial, projection, and rationalization are ego defense mechanisms that substance abusers use to protect themselves from the consequences of abuse. The defense mechanisms make assessment and care for the user problematic, because the user does not acknowledge the excessive use, the problems or consequences of the excessive use, or the relationship between the two. The nurse is challenged to identify the user and to plan and intervene.

Twenty-six nursing diagnoses have been identified as common in the care of substance abusers. Care for the substance abuser requires knowledge and practice of the principles of safety for the intoxicated or withdrawing client. Knowledge of key medications is important because of the special considerations for the addicted or recovering person. Skill is needed in developing a therapeutic relationship and in assisting the client to acknowledge that there is a problem. In addition, it is important to communicate with the client in a way that does not enable continued use of the substance. Communication must focus on breaking the denial. Any time a client or family member is at all receptive, it is important to refer him or her to an appropriate resource.

Suggestions for Clinical Conference

1. Call you local AA and request that a recovering person attend a clinical conference. Ask that person to describe how he or she became addicted and how he or she came to recover.
2. Discuss your attitudes about substance abuse and where these attitudes might have originated. Discuss how current attitudes might influence nursing care on a psychiatric unit; on an adult medical unit; and on a pediatric unit, if the parent were the addicted person.
3. Describe the behaviors of addicted persons you have encountered. What would be the difficulties in confronting clients who demonstrated these same behaviors?
4. Obtain names of persons and facilities in the community with expertise in dealing with the substance-abusing client. Find out from these persons and facilities how their expertise can assist the practicing nurse.
5. Attend an open AA meeting as a clinical group. Discuss what happened. What feelings did you experience?

References

Alcoholics Anonymous World Services. *Alcoholics Anonymous* (3rd ed.). (1976). New York City: Author.

American Nurses' Association, Drug and Alcohol Nursing Association, and National Nurses Society on Addictions. (1987). *The care of clients with addictions: Dimensions of nursing practice.* Kansas City, MO: American Nurses' Association.

American Nurses' Association and National Nurses Society on Addictions. (1988). *Standards of addictions nursing practice with selected diagnoses and criteria.* Kansas City MO: American Nurses Association.

American Psychiatric Association. (1994). *Diagnostic and statistical manual of mental disorders* (4th ed.). Washington, DC: Author.

Anderson, E., & Quast, W. (1983). Young children in alcoholic families: A mental health needs-assessment and an intervention/prevention strategy. *Journal of Primary Prevention, 3,* 174–187.

Andreasson, S., Allebeck, P., Engstrom, A., & Rydberg, U. (1987). Cannabis and schizophrenia. A longitudinal study of Swedish conscripts. *Lancet, 2,* 1483–1486.

Bakdash, D. (1978). Essentials the nurse should know about chemical dependency. *Journal of Psychiatric Nursing and Mental Health Services, 16*(10), 33–37.

Beattie, M. (1987). *Codependent no more.* New York: Harper & Row.

Black, C. (1981). *It will never happen to me.* Denver, CO: MAC Printing and Publications Division.

Brown, S. (1988). *Treating adult children of alcoholics: A developmental perspective.* New York: John Wiley & Sons.

Brown, S. A., & Schuckit, M. A. (1988). Changes in depression among abstinent alcoholics. *Journal of Studies on Alcohol, 49,* 412–417.

Cermak, T. (1990). *Evaluating and treating adult children of alcoholics* (Vols. 1 and 2). Minneapolis, MN: Johnson Institute.

Cook, P. S., Petersen, R. C., & Moore, D. T. (1990). *Alcohol, tobacco, and other drugs may harm the unborn.* Rockville, MD: U.S. Department of Health and Human Services.

Dealing with denial. (1975). Center City, MN: Hazelden Educational Materials.

DuPont, R. L. (1987). Prevention of adolescent chemical dependency. *Pediatric Clinics of North America, 34,* 495–505.

Gazzaniga, M. (1985). *The social brain.* New York: Basic Books.

Gomberg, E. (1982). Alcohol use and alcohol problems among the elderly. In *National Institute on Alcohol Abuse and Alcoholism, Special Population Issues* (pp. 263–290). Washington, DC: U.S. Government Printing Office.

Hartford, T., & Grant, B. (1987). Psychosocial factors in adolescent drinking contexts. *Journal of Studies on Alcohol, 48,* 551–557.

Helzer, J. E., & Pryzbeck, T. R. (1988). The co-occurrence of alcoholism with other psychiatric disorders in the general population and its impact on treatment. *Journal of Studies on Alcohol, 49,* 219–224.

Inaba, D. S., & Cohen, W. E. (1989). *Uppers, downers, all arounders.* Ashland, OR: Cinemed.

Jack, L. (Ed.). (1989). *Nursing care planning with the addicted client* (Vols. 1 and 2). Skokie, IL: National Nurses Society on Addictions and Midwest Education Association.

Jellinek, E. M. (1952). Phases of alcohol addiction. *Quarterly Journal of the Studies on Alcohol, 13,* 672.

John, S. (1991). Codependency versus caring. *Journal of Christian Nursing, 8*(2), 22.

Kashani, J. H., Solomon, N. A., Dugan, K., & Joy, F. (1987). Differences between early and late onset of substance abuse: An inpatient experience. *Southern Medical Journal, 80,* 554–557.

Kaufman, G. (1985). *Shame: The power of caring.* Cambridge, MA: Schenkman Books.

Kinney, J., & Leaton, G. (1987). *Loosening the grip.* St. Louis, MO: Times Mirror/Mosby College.

Knop, J., Teasdale, T. W., Schulsinger, F., & Goodwin, D. W. (1985). A prospective study of young men at high risk for alcoholism: School behavior and achievement. *Journal of Studies on Alcohol, 46,* 273–278.

Krach, P. (1990). Discovering the secret: Nursing assessment of elderly alcoholics in the home. *Journal of Gerontological Nursing, 16*(11), 32–38.

Kumpfer, K. L. (1987). Special populations: Etiology and prevention of vulnerability to chemical dependency in children of substance abusers. In *Youth at High Risk for Substance Abuse* (DHHS Pub. No. (ADM) 90-1537, pp. 1–72). Rockville, MD: U.S. Department of Health and Human Services.

Lewis, D. C. (1989). *Project ADEPT: Curriculum for primary care physician training.* Providence, RI: Brown University.

McCaffery, M. (1991). Opioid use: Pain control versus addiction. *Perspectives on Addictions Nursing, 2*(1), 4–6.

Meyer, C. (1992). Trauma patient? Look for substance abuse. *American Journal of Nursing, 92*(8), 12.

Miller, D., & Jang, M. (1977). Children of alcoholics: A 20-year longitudinal study. *Social Work Research and Abstracts, 13,* 23–29.

National Institute on Alcohol Abuse and Alcoholism. (1991). *Alcoholism and co-occurring disorders.* (Alcohol Alert No. 14, PH302). Rockville, MD: U.S. Department of Health and Human Services.

National Institute on Alcohol Abuse and Alcoholism. (1992). *Alcohol and kids.* (Alcohol Alert No. 15, PH311) Rockville, MD: U.S. Department of Health and Human Services.

National Institute on Drug Abuse. (1989). Highlights of the 1988 National Household Survey on Drug Abuse: National Institute on Drug Abuse. In *NIDA capsules* (pp. 1–4). Rockville, MD: Author.

National Council on Alcoholism and Drug Dependence. (1991). *The Alcoholism Report*, *20*(3), 3.

O'Sullivan, C. M. (1991). The relationship between childhood mentors and resiliency in adult children of alcoholics. *Family Dynamics Addiction Quarterly*, *1*(4), 46–59.

Robinson, D. P., & Greene, J. W. (1988). The adolescent alcohol and drug problem: A practical approach. *Pediatric Nursing*, *14*, 305–310.

Ross, H. E., Glaser, F. B., & Germanson, T. (1988). The prevalence of psychiatric disorders in patients with alcohol and other drug problems. *Archives of General Psychiatry*, *45*, 1023–1031.

Scheitlin, K. (1990). Identifying and helping children of alcoholics. *Nurse Practitioner*, *15*(2), 34–47.

Schuckit, M. A. (1989). *Drug and alcohol abuse: A clinical guide to diagnosis and treatment* (3rd ed.). New York: Plenum Medical Book Company.

Schuckit, M. A., & Chiles, J. A. (1978). Family history as a diagnostic aid in two samples of adolescents. *Journal of Nervous and Mental Disease*, *166*, 165–176.

Stanton, M. D., & Todd, T. C. (1982). *The family therapy of drug abuse and addiction*. New York: Guilford Press.

Steinglass, P. (1981). The impact of alcoholism on the family. *Journal of Studies on Alcohol*, *42*, 288–303.

Swift, R. M. (1992, November). *Effect of naltrexone on ethanol intoxication in non-alcoholic humans*. Paper presented at the National Conference for the Association for Medical Education and Research in Substance Abuse, Washington, DC.

Tweed, S. H., & Ryff, C. D. (1991). Adult children of alcoholics: Profiles of wellness amidst distress. *Journal of Studies on Alcohol*, *52*, 133–41.

U.S. Drug Enforcement Administration. (Undated). *Controlled substances: Use, abuse, and effects*. Washington, DC: U.S. Department of Justice.

U.S. Office for Substance Abuse Protection. (1992). Nurse Training course: *Alcohol and other drug abuse prevention*. Rockville, MD: National Training System, U.S. Public Health Service.

Vaccani, J. M. (1989). Borderline personality and alcohol abuse. *Archives of Psychiatric Nursing*, *3*, 113–119.

Wegscheider-Cruse, S. (1981). *Another chance*. Pompano Beach, FL: Health Communications.

Werner, E. E. (1989). High risk children in young adulthood: A longitudinal study from birth to 32 years. *American Journal of Orthopsychiatry*, *59*, 72–81.

West, M. O., & Prinz, R. J. (1987). Parental alcoholism and childhood psychopathology. *Psychological Bulletin*, *102*, 204–218.

Wolin, S. J., Bennett, L. A., Noonan, D. L., & Teitelbaum, M. A. (1980). Disrupted family rituals: A factor in the intergenerational transmission of alcoholism. *Journal of Studies on Alcohol*, *41*, 199–214.

Young, E. B. (1990). The role of incest issues in relapse. *Journal of Psychoactive Drugs*, *22*, 249–258.

CHAPTER 18

The Client with an Eating Disorder

HOLLY BERCHIN, M.S.N., R.N.,C.S.
HOPE TITLEBAUM QUALLO, M.S., R.N.,C.S.

OUTLINE

CHAPTER OBJECTIVES

Upon completion of this chapter, you will be able to:

1. Discuss the similarities and differences among the various eating disorders.
2. Identify possible causative factors of eating disorders.
3. Discuss the neurobiological implications associated with eating disorders.
4. Identify special populations at risk for eating disorders and their unique needs.
5. Discuss specific modalities used in the treatment of eating disorders.
6. Plan nursing care specific for the treatment of a client with an eating disorder.

KEY TERMS

Alexithymia
Anorexia nervosa
Binge
Body image disturbance
Bulimia
Eating disorder
Fear of fatness
Purge

Eating disorders have become increasingly prevalent in American society. They are characterized by an extreme disturbance in eating-related behaviors. Most people with eating disorders are greatly ambivalent about seeking treatment. Anorectic clients tend to be socially insecure and somewhat isolated. They lack spontaneity and can be extremely rigid in their thinking; they are perfectionistic and, consequently, may be highly successful in their work or academically. Usually there is an element of depression that accompanies anorexia, and there may be a tendency toward obsessive-compulsive disorder. Outwardly, anorectic clients may appear pleasant and compliant, but a will of steel underlies this facade. After all, their emaciation is a special achievement that few can match. Anorexia is the method to maintain "control" over life.

Clients with bulimia are more likely to acknowledge the need for help. Usually they are more aware of their own emotional distress. Bulimic clients may also experience a concurrent affective disorder. They have difficulty with impulsivity, including shoplifting, suicidal behavior, and substance abuse. They can be very histrionic. Usually, they are more socially skilled in relationships than their anorexic counterparts. Although anorexia nervosa and bulimia nervosa are classified as separate disorders by the Diagnostic and Statistical Manual of Mental Disorders (DSM-IV) (American Psychiatric Association [APA], 1994), they can exist concurrently.

DEFINITIONS AND CRITERIA

ANOREXIA NERVOSA

Anorexia nervosa can be defined as self-induced starvation resulting from **fear of fatness** rather than from true loss of appetite. The word *anorexia* is derived from Greek and is translated as "loss of appetite due to nerves," but the term is a misnomer. Persons with anorexia continue to feel hunger but persist in denying themselves food. Hilde Bruch (1966), a pediatrician who later became a psychoanalyst, described one of the central features of this disorder as "the relentless pursuit of thinness." Other features include amenorrhea, an intense fear of gaining weight or becoming fat, and a distorted body image.

Although anorexia has been described in the medical literature for hundreds of years, it was not until the 1960s that the disorder was considered a treatable psychiatric condition. Clients with this disorder usually are not seen in the treatment setting until the weight loss or failure to gain expected weight is marked. The DSM-IV (APA, 1994), in considering the patient's age and height, uses less than 85% of expected weight as the guide (see the display on diagnostic criteria for anorexia nervosa). With profound weight loss, a variety of metabolic changes are seen, as well as hypothermia, hypotension, bradycardia, edema, and lanugo (neonatal-like) body hair.

Anorexia occurs 8 to 12 times more frequently in females than in males. Prevalence rates for adolescent girls range from 0.3 percent to 1 percent, or from 1 in

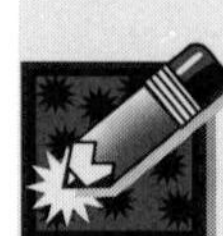

DSM-IV DIAGNOSTIC CRITERIA FOR ANOREXIA NERVOSA

A. Refusal to maintain body weight at or above a minimally normal weight for age and height (e.g., weight loss leading to maintenance of body weight less than 85% of that expected; or failure to make expected weight gain during period of growth, leading to body weight less than 85% of that expected).

B. Intense fear of gaining weight or becoming fat, even though underweight.

C. Disturbance in the way in which one's body weight or shape is experienced, undue influence of body weight or shape on self-evaluation, or denial of the seriousness of the current low body weight.

D. In postmenarchal females, amenorrhea, i.e., the absence of at least three consecutive menstrual cycles, (A woman is considered to have amenorrhea if her periods occur only following hormone, e.g., estrogen, administration.)

From American Psychiatric Association. (1994). *Diagnostic and statistical manual of mental disorders, fourth edition*. Washington, DC: Author.

800 to as many as 1 in 100 females, according to studies of samples of different populations. Amenorrhea usually follows weight loss, but it is not unusual for this symptom to appear before noticeable weight loss has occurred. In premenarchal anorexia, termed *early onset anorexia,* there may be no weight loss, but there is failure to gain during this active growth phase. In this younger population (8 to 14 years of age) comprising 10 percent of anorectic clients, pubertal growth and development are delayed.

The course of anorexia varies: it most often consists of a single episode with return to normal weight, but it may be episodic or unremitting until it leads to death. Reportedly mortality rates of this disorder range from 5 percent to 18 percent. Outcome studies indicate that one third of anorectic clients will successfully recover, one third will repeatedly relapse (Butler, in Scott, 1988).

There are biological mechanisms and genetic factors related to anorexia. Twin studies have shown a higher concordance rate among monozygotic twins than dizygotic twins. Anorexia is more common among sisters and mothers with the disorder than among the general population. The literature also reports a higher than expected frequency of major depression and bipolar disorder among first-degree biological relatives of anorectic clients (Brownell & Foreyt, 1986). There is an established disturbance in the hypothalamic-anterior pituitary-gonadal axis (Garfinkel & Garner, 1982).

BULIMIA NERVOSA

The term ***bulimia*** is translated as "ravenous appetite" and refers to a syndrome of episodes of binge eating, followed by self-induced vomiting, or **purge** behavior, accompanied by an excessive preoccupation with weight and body shape. There is a feeling of a lack of control over eating behavior when bingeing, and the measures to prevent weight gain include use of laxatives, cathartics, and diuretics; periods of strict dieting or fasting; and strenuous exercise. Some bulimic clients discover and abuse syrup of ipecac, a high-risk behavior because of the drug's cardiotoxicity.

DSM-IV (APA, 1994) defines a **binge** as "eating in a discrete period of time an amount of food that is definitely larger than most individuals would eat under similar circumstances" (see the display on diagnostic criteria for bulimia nervosa). Typical binge food is sweet and high in calories. It is consumed rapidly with little chewing and often in secret.

Bulimic clients may be of normal weight, overweight, or underweight. Clients with this disorder characteristically have a thin body with swollen cheeks due to enlarged salivary glands and exhibit signs of fluid retention. The skin tends to be dry with cuts and abrasions, particularly over the knuckles, owing to the repeated trauma of putting the fingers down the throat to induce vomiting (Russell's sign). The repeated vomiting causes erosion of the dental enamel, and any of the purging mechanisms may lead to dehydration and electrolyte imbalance, particularly of potassium. More rarely, serious complications may include cardiac arrhythmias, esophageal tears, gastric ruptures, and even sudden death.

Bulimia nervosa usually begins in adolescence or early adulthood, and the disorder can follow a chronic and intermittent course over many years. Parents of clients with this disorder are frequently obsese, and there is a higher rate of major depression in first-degree relatives than expected. Bulimic clients themselves commonly have a depressive disorder and may concurrently abuse psychoactive substances, most frequently alcohol, sedatives, amphetamines, or cocaine. Johnson et al. (1984) described a psychological profile of these clients as impulsive, anxious, depressed, self-critical, intolerant of frustration, and troubled by feelings of helplessness, inadequacy, and an exaggerated sense of guilt.

DSM-IV DIAGNOSTIC CRITERIA FOR BULIMIA NERVOSA

A. Recurrent episodes of binge eating. An episode of binge eating is characterized by both of the following:

1. Eating, in a discrete period of time (e.g., within any 2-hour period), an amount of food that is definitely larger than most people would eat during a similar period of time and under similar circumstances
2. A sense of lack of control over eating during the episode (e.g., a feeling that one cannot stop eating or control what or how much one is eating)

B. Recurrent inappropriate compensatory behavior in order to prevent weight gain, such as self-induced vomiting; misuse of laxatives, diuretics, enemas, or other medications; fasting; or excessive exercise.

C. The binge eating and inappropriate compensatory behaviors both occur, on average, at least twice a week for 3 months.

D. Self-evaluation is unduly influenced by body shape and weight.

E. The disturbance does not occur exclusively during episodes of Anorexia Nervosa.

From American Psychiatric Association. (1994). *Diagnostic and statistical manual of mental disorders, fourth edition.* Washington, DC: Author.

BINGE EATING DISORDER

Binge eating disorder (BED) is a disorder newly described in the DSM-IV (APA, 1994) (see the display on research criteria for binge eating disorder). Clients with BED experience recurrent binge eating but do not regularly engage in the purging behaviors or compulsive exercise that bulimic clients use to avoid weight gain. Spitzer et al. (1993) studied 2802 subjects drawn from client and nonclient community samples. More than one half of the total sample (1785 subjects) were participants in weight control programs, and 20 percent of these met the criteria for BED. In both the weight control and community samples, BED was associated with a lifetime history of fluctuating weight and severe obesity. The female-to-male ratio in the Spitzer et al. study was 3:2. In an earlier study, Spitzer et al. (1992) found a 71 percent frequency of BED in a sample of subjects from Overeaters Anonymous, an organization that addresses two central features of BED: episodic eating and loss of control.

Characteristics of the BED population include impairment in work and social functioning; preoccupation with weight and shape; general psychopathology; significant time and energy devoted to dieting; and a history of depression, alcohol, or drug abuse and treatment for emotional problems (Spitzer et al., 1993).

OBESITY

Obesity is recognized as a serious health problem but is not classified by itself as an eating disorder, at least in the DSM-IV (APA, 1994). Many medical diseases and complications are associated with obesity, including hypertension, gallbladder disease, diabetes, trauma to weight-bearing joints, and increased risk of cardiovascular disease, especially when there is an excess accumulation of fat in the abdominal region.

Obesity is defined as a condition in which a person's weight is 20 percent greater than the ideal weight as determined by standard height-weight tables (Logue, 1991). Freemouw and Damer (1992) defined obesity as "a biological condition that is the product of a complex interaction between heredity, metabolism, and eating–exercise behaviors" (p. 2). Prevalence statistics indicate that obesity is found more commonly in women than in men and that the condition increases with age up to 60 years, when it begins to decrease. In the United States, obesity is more prevalent in lower socioeconomic groups, although it is found in all groups and cultures. Studies of the eating behavior of adults who are obese have shown no clear or consistent differences from those of people who are of normal weight. Obesity is common in children and is estimated to range from 15 percent to 25 percent of children in the United States (Lucas, 1991). Most of these children were obese infants, and 60 percent of them will become obese adults.

Bray (1978) reported that 10 percent to 50 percent of the population of the United States is obese; 90 percent of these are mildly obese or 20 percent to 40 percent

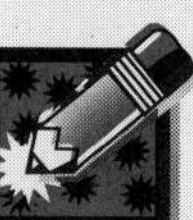

DSM-IV RESEARCH CRITERIA FOR BINGE EATING DISORDER

A. Recurrent episodes of binge eating. An episode is characterized by both of the following:
1. Eating, in a discrete period of time (e.g., within any 2-hour period), an amount of food that is definitely larger than most people would eat during a similar period of time under similar circumstances.
2. A sense of lack of control during the episode (e.g., a feeling that one cannot stop eating or control what or how much one is eating).

B. The binge-eating episodes are associated with three (or more) of the following:
1. Eating much more rapidly than normal.
2. Eating until feeling uncomfortably full.
3. Eating large amounts of food when not feeling physically hungry.
4. Eating alone because of being embarrassed by how much one is eating.
5. Feeling disgusted with oneself, depressed, or feeling very guilty after overeating.

C. Marked distress regarding binge eating is present.

D. The binge eating occurs, on average, at least 2 days a week for 6 months.

Note: The method of determining frequency differs from that used for bulimia nervosa; future research should address whether the preferred method of setting a frequency threshold is counting the number of days on which binges occur or counting the numbers of episodes of binge eating.

E. The binge eating is not associated with the regular use of inappropriate compensatory behaviors (e.g., purging, fasting, excessive exercise) and does not occur exclusively during the course of anorexia nervosa or bulimia nervosa.

From American Psychiatric Association. (1994). *Diagnostic and statistical manual of mental disorders, fourth edition.* Washington, DC: Author.

overweight. Nine percent of the obese population is described as moderately (41 percent to 100 percent overweight) or severely obese (more than 100 percent overweight). Although it has not been established that obesity is genetically determined, it is certainly strongly influenced by genetic factors. Forty percent of children with one obese parent become obese, whereas 70 percent of those with two obese parents are similarly affected.

In spite of the widespread popularity of weight loss programs, most studies from the 1970s have shown that significant weight loss is rare and losses that do occur are not well maintained. More promising results have been shown recently with the use of a combination of maintenance medications.

Although obesity is not considered an eating disorder in the psychiatric nomenclature, it is considered a risk factor for anorexia nervosa and bulimia nervosa. With the new category of BED, people with simple obesity must be differentiated from those with the more complex features of that disorder.

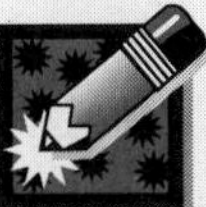

DSM-IV DIAGNOSTIC CRITERIA FOR PICA

A. Persistent eating of nonnutritive substances for a period of at least 1 month.

B. The eating of nonnutritive substances is inappropriate to the developmental level.

C. The eating behavior is not part of a culturally sanctioned practice.

D. If the eating behavior occurs exclusively during the course of another mental disorder (e.g., Mental Retardation, Pervasive Developmental Disorder, Schizophrenia), it is sufficiently severe to warrant independent clinical attention.

From American Psychiatric Association. (1994). *Diagnostic and statistical manual of mental disorders, fourth edition*. Washington, DC: Author.

PICA

Pica refers to the persistent eating of a nonnutritive substance. The name is derived from the Latin word for magpie, a bird known to eat a variety of objects. Infants with this disorder may eat hair, cloth, plaster, paint, or string, and older children may eat sand, leaves, insects, pebbles, or animal droppings. Almost all children occasionally ingest such substances, and the behavior is not considered abnormal in children 18 months of age and younger. Pica is common in children as old as 6 years of age, with greater occurrence in several mentally retarded or psychotic children. Pregnant women may also exhibit pica.

Pica is believed to result from iron and zinc deficiencies or to be related to lack of stimulation and adult supervision. Medical complications include lead poisoning from the ingestion of paint or paint-soaked plaster. *Toxoplasma* or *Toxocara* infections may result from the ingestion of feces or dirt. Hairball tumors may cause intestinal obstruction.

The DSM-IV (APA, 1994) includes only two diagnostic criteria for pica, as listed in the accompanying display.

RUMINATION DISORDER

Rumination disorder is a rare phenomenon, seen equally in male and female infants. It usually appears between 3 months and 1 year of age but may show up later in children who are mentally retarded or in adolescents. This disorder can be serious, with a reported 25 percent mortality rate from malnutrition. Even when children with this disorder survive, the failure to gain expected weight and malnutrition may lead to general developmental delays and severe impairment.

This disorder is marked by repeated regurgitation of food, with resultant weight loss or failure to gain expected weight (see the display on diagnostic criteria for rumination disorder of infancy). It develops following a period of normal functioning. There is no accompanying

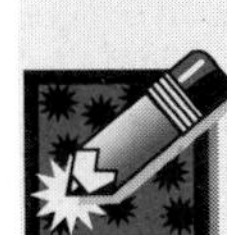

DSM-IV DIAGNOSTIC CRITERIA FOR RUMINATION DISORDER

A. Repeated regurgitation and rechewing of food for a period of at least 1 month following a period of normal functioning.

B. The behavior is not due to an associated gastrointestinal or other general medical condition (e.g., esophageal reflux).

C. The behavior does not occur exclusively during the course of Anorexia Nervosa or Bulimia Nervosa. If the symptoms occur exclusively during the course of Mental Retardation or a Pervasive Developmental Disorder, they are sufficiently severe to warrant independent clinical attention.

From American Psychiatric Association. (1994). *Diagnostic and statistical manual of mental disorders, fourth edition*. Washington, DC: Author.

self-disgust, nausea, vomiting, or other associated gastrointestinal disorder. Ruminating infants typically regurgitate milk and partially digested food either spontaneously or after inserting their fingers into their mouth. They may chew and reswallow the regurgitated food, or they may vomit the food. The characteristic posture is described as straining and arching the back with the head held back.

Even though the infant seems to be satisfied, as evidenced by sucking movements and sounds, the parent or caretaker may avoid the infant. This avoidance behavior occurs either because of frustration or discouragement with failure to gain or because of the noxious odor of the regurgitated food. Thus there is a danger of disrupted bonding or understimulation. An additional feature is that the infant is often irritable and hungry between episodes of regurgitation. There are no known predisposing factors.

Rumination disorder must be differentiated from other disorders that cause regurgitation, such as pyloric stenosis and infections of the gastrointestinal system. When the disorder occurs in adolescence, the behavior appears involuntary and may be related to a disturbance of esophageal motility. Some of these affected adolescents have a history of self-induced vomiting and a fear of becoming fat. They are able to achieve vomiting more and more easily over time, and then the disorder resembles rumination of infancy.

COMORBIDITY ISSUES

Multiple diagnoses in the same person are commonly identified in psychiatry yet are just now in the 1990s receiving deserved attention. "When disorders are observed to co-occur at a rate that differs from that expected by chance, this finding is of theoretical and practical importance: it may imply shared etiological factors, and it may affect response to treatment" (Taylor et al., 1993, p. 147).

AFFECTIVE DISORDERS

Hsu (1990) reported that about 20 percent of anorectic clients and 40 percent of bulimics meet the criteria for major depression. There is much debate in the literature concerning whether eating disorders are variants of an affective illness (Garner & Garfinkel, 1985). This hypothesis is supported by family studies that demonstrate an increase in the prevalence of affective illness in the first-degree and second-degree biological relatives of clients with an eating disorder. In addition, activation of the hypothalamic-pituitary-adrenal axis that occurs in the eating disorders is a biological finding in affective disorders (Hsu, 1990). Hsu believed, however, that the link between affective illness and eating disorders is not as clear or significant as the growing evidence that persons with affective illness are more vulnerable to the development of an eating disorder once they start a diet.

Garner and Garfinkel (1985, p. 26) recommended a careful assessment of "the nature of the depressive experience" to discriminate a primary affective disorder from a reactive or more psychological depression. The patient with more anaclitic depression is characterized as highly dependent with a strong need for attachment, impulsive, and helpless. (*Anaclitic depression* refers to an acute reaction of lethargy and apparent despondency in infants abruptly separated from their mothers or deprived of mothering.) Clients with more introjective depression present with more obsessive symptoms and perfectionism. (*Introjective depression* refers to an unconscious process of directing unacceptable hatred or aggression toward the self, as a defense against the hatred or rage toward another person.) A complicating assessment factor is that symptoms of disturbance of appetite, fatigue, gastrointestinal distress, and impaired concentration are diagnostic in depression and eating disorders. The comorbidity of depression is correlated with a poorer prognosis of the eating disorder and thus requires ongoing assessment, evaluation, and treatment.

OBSESSIVE-COMPULSIVE DISORDER

Obsessive-compulsive traits are observed and documented in the eating disordered population, particularly related to the obsessive drive toward thinness at all costs and the compulsive nature of the binge-purge or food-restricting behaviors. As in obsessive-compulsive disorders, the binge-purge cycle appears to be strongly linked with anxiety (Brownell & Foreyt, 1986). Eating elicits the anxiety (or morbid fear of weight gain), and purging reduces the anxiety. Binge eaters who do not vomit or purge, sometimes referred to as compulsive eaters, also experience a drive to eat accompanied by anxiety reduction as they "fill the emptiness." This is in contrast to bulimics, whose anxiety level rises with the sensation of fullness.

The obsessive nature of the preoccupation with food, weight, and body shape is thought to be more a result of starvation than a primary cause. The ego-syntonic nature (compatible with the conscious self-concept) of the obsessive-compulsive traits in clients with eating disorders differentiates it from true obsessive-compulsive disorder in which the thoughts and rituals are experienced as ego-dystonic or ego-alien (Brownell & Foreyt, 1986). (*Ego-dystonic* refers to thoughts, impulses, or wishes that are unacceptable or repugnant to the ego or self.)

SUBSTANCE ABUSE

Hsu (1990) reported that alcohol and substance abuse occurs in about one third of all bulimic clients. The Toronto group (Toner et al., 1986), using a Diagnostic Interview Schedule, found significant differences in substance use disorders between bulimic-anorectic clients (42.9 percent) and restrictive-anorectic clients

(23.1 percent). Taylor et al. (1993) studied 52 female attendees at an alcohol clinic and confirmed earlier studies that clinical eating disorders and disturbed eating habits and attitudes are more prevalent in women receiving treatment for alcohol problems than in a comparable community sample. The association between substance abuse and eating disorders in many clients may represent one aspects of a borderline personality organization with a variety of impulse-dominated behaviors. An alternative hypothesis is that use of alcohol and other substances may be a coping response to the isolation and dysphoria commonly associated with eating disorders. In the study by Taylor et al. (1993), an improvement in one problem led to deterioration in the other, supporting the impulse control explanation. More research is clearly indicated, but again the data reinforce the importance of careful and thorough assessment.

BORDERLINE PERSONALITY DISORDER

When a client has an eating disorder coexistent with a diagnosed borderline personality disorder, "the eating disorder is secondary to a more serious problem of understructured internal resources" (Garner & Garfinkel, 1985, p. 31). These clients present with labile affect, diffuse boundaries, and a dependence on external sources for tension regulation and self-management. They use primitive defenses such as splitting, denial, and projective identification. Bingeing may be experienced as depersonalization and purging as a form of masochism, like self-injury, as an attempt to ward off self-fragmentation. Garner and Garfinkel (1985) suggested that eating disorder symptoms in this population usually remit only after the client experiences the holding environment of the treatment setting.

Three hundred inpatient female medical records between 1978 and 1990 were studied by Koepp et al. (1993), who found that 23 percent had eating disorders and 11 percent had a concomitant borderline personality disorder, according to DSM-IV criteria (APA, 1994). These are clients with serious psychopathology who test nurses' patience and skills and usually require long-term treatment. (See Chapter 14 for an in-depth discussion of personality disorders.)

SEXUAL ABUSE

Clinicians have observed that many clients with eating disorder behaviors and diagnosed disorders also report histories of sexual abuse. Studies have shown that from 30 percent to 50 percent of adult women with eating disorders also report unwanted sexual experiences as children or adults. The literature is just beginning to explore this link, and the cause-and-effect relationship remains unclear.

Waller (1992) concluded in his study that the nature of the abuse is more relevant than the presence of such history. The women in Waller's study binged more frequently if they reported unwanted sexual experience that occurred at an early age or that member. Purging behaviors, particul be repeating the experience of gagg concomitant wish or need to "throw u nated material associated with forced oral pe Individual or group therapy with other abuse surviv can be helpful to clients in understanding and overcoming the eating disorder symptoms that may be related to past sexual abuse.

When abuse is severe and prolonged, other disorders such as posttraumatic stress disorder, dissociative disorders, or even dissociative identity disorder may coexist with the eating disorder. The following statements were written in a journal by a depressed bulimic young woman with diagnosed dissociative identity disorder:

> *Every day I feel hungry and it's real hard to fight that feeling every day and sometimes I break and give in and that's just one more failure. I just feel worse when that happens. I'm not doing very good at this. . . . Maybe I should consider ipecac. . . . It seems like all the fun has gone out of life. . . . I can't even eat just to enjoy it. . . . It feels like I'm trapped.*

CAUSES OF EATING DISORDERS: PERSPECTIVES AND THEORIES

There are three different theories about the cause of eating disorders. They are derived from biological, psychodynamic, and psychosocial perspectives.

BIOLOGICAL FACTORS

There are a number of possible explanations concerning the biological factors associated with eating disorders. One theory proposes that the amenorrhea resulting from the nutritional deprivation and extreme exercise disrupts the functioning of the hypothalamus, which then results in loss of appetite (Palmer, 1990). A second explanation involves an excess secretion of cortisol in anorectic clients. This excess cortisol may act on the hypothalamus, causing a decrease in the response to hunger. "Excess secretion of cortisol may also cause depression, resulting in decreased appetite and weight loss" (Palmer, 1990, p. 12).

There may be genetic factors associated with the etiology of eating disorders. In their study of 34 twin pairs, Holland et al. (1984) found a significant occurrence of anorexia in monozygotic twins but a much smaller occurrence in dizygotic twins. It has also been observed that certain personality traits are usually present in anorectic clients. Strober (1991) suggested that "an essential core of anorexia nervosa lies in genotypic personality structures that predispose the individual to rigid and perseverative avoidance behaviors with marked obsessional, anxious-depressive coloring" (p. 11). In summary, it is clear that the role, if any, of specific genetic factors in the etiology of eating disorders is a question yet to be resolved.

Neurobiological Factors

The most common eating disorder is bulimia nervosa in women who maintain normal weight. These women exhibit symptoms usually found in women with anorexia nervosa, such as disturbed appetite, abnormal body image, depression, and neuroendocrine changes that precipitate menstrual irregularities. However, as these women are of normal weight, the changes cannot be attributed to weight loss.

Kaye and Weltzin (1991a) have contributed significant information to the neurochemical pathophysiology of the eating disorders. They suggest that bingeing and purging may have reinforcing properties. Stress and tension may be reduced by binge eating because neurochemical levels fluctuate with food intake, and this may cause a reduction in anxiety. Vomiting may also serve the same purpose. In addition, bulimic women could have abnormalities of the serotonin neurotransmitter system that predispose them to disturbances in appetite or mood, or both.

The pathophysiology of the relationship between disturbances in mood, feeding, weight, and neuroendocrine function is unknown; however, Kaye and Weltzin (1991a) have suggested a hypothesis about the connection. Each of the above systems is regulated by the same monoamine neurotransmitters: serotonin and norepinephrine. "It is possible that a disturbance of the neurochemical integrity within one behavior or neuroendocrine system could spread, through disruptions of monoamine functional activity, into other systems dependent on monoamine activity" (p. 22).

Kaye and Weltzin (1991a) suggested that a number of central nervous system neurotransmitter systems may have a specific role in the regulation of feeding. Neurotransmitters such as norepinephrine, serotonin, and opioids regulate the size of meals as well as the selection of carbohydrates and protein in animals. Theoretically, the abnormalities found in the neurotransmitters of bulimic clients may contribute to a specific disturbance in feeding behaviors.

The fact that antidepressants are helpful in the treatment of bulimia further supports the possibility that bulimic clients experience alterations in norepinephrine and serotonin regulation (Kaye & Weltzin, 1991a). Some antidepressants appear to have a specific antibulimic effect, as the result of their administration is a decrease in binge eating and vomiting behaviors. Antidepressants decrease binge eating but do not affect the consumption of normal-sized meals. In addition, these antibulimic properties occur independent of the presence of depression (Kaye & Weltzin, 1991a).

In anorexia nervosa, there are complex disturbances in the reproductive biochemistry. Because amenorrhea is a central feature of the disorder, great importance has been assigned to the hypothalamic-pituitary-gonadal axis (Weiner, 1989). During recovery from anorexia, a person may regain lost weight but may not ovulate or menstruate for years. Weiner (1989) discussed extremely delicate changes that occur with anorexia such as in the hormones related to thyroid function. In addition, there are changes in estradiol levels and metabolism, including changes in luteinizing hormone and follicle-stimulating hormone levels.

Brain serotonin activity and its contribution to satiety has been studied extensively by Kaye and Weltzin (1991b). "Theoretically, bingeing behavior is consistent with reduced serotinin function, whereas anorexia nervosa is consistent with increased serotonin activity" (p. 41). Low serotonin levels in the brain may also contribute to pathological manifestations such as dysphoria, lack of impulse control, and obsessive behavior.

Disturbances of serotonin have been found in acutely ill anorectic clients. Tryptophan, an essential amino acid, is the precursor of serotonin. Therefore, serotonin disturbances could be the result of the anorectic client's dietary abnormalities (Kaye & Weltzin, 1991b). Because disturbances in serotonin regulation are also present in bulimic clients, it is highly possible that the dietary abnormalities of both groups contribute to these changes.

According to Kaye and Weltzin (1991b), it is possible—given that tryptophan is the precursor of serotonin—that dietary abnormalities produce a disturbance in the regulation of serotonin leading to a disruption that may continue even after a healthy weight has been attained by the client with anorexia.

PSYCHODYNAMIC FACTORS

Bruch, the renowned theorist in the study of eating disorders mentioned earlier, believed that anorexia and bulimia were related to "underlying deficits in the individual's sense of self-identity and autonomy" (1982, p. 1532). She was the first to formally suggest that there was an actual disturbance of body image in anorexia nervosa. Bruch (1962) stated that "what is pathognomonic of anorexia nervosa is not the severity of the malnutrition per se . . . but rather the distortion of body image associated with it: the absence of concern about emaciation, even when advanced" (p. 187). She believed that the extreme denial of the emaciation was an expression of a delusional disturbance in body image.

Body image disturbance is an essential characteristic of anorexia. Although it is related to a more generalized misperception of internal states, such as hunger and emotions, it specifically involves the anorectic client's inability to identify his or her appearance as abnormal. This misperception can be extremely dangerous because it can become almost delusional as the anorectic client defends an emaciated body shape.

In the psychoanalytical framework, eating disorders are viewed as a form of neurosis representing a regression to the oral stage of development. Just as Freud connected oral drives and sexual drives, Bruch (1973) expounded on this connection when she addressed the anorectic client's abhorrence to his or her own sexuality.

Within the framework of object relations theory, the understanding of eating disorders can be broadened.

Winnicott (1965) focused on the interaction between the mothering one, or the object, and the infant by exploring how they accomplish the tasks of attachment and separation. The concept of the transitional object (Winnicott, 1975) is an integral part of the mother–infant relationship. As the infant begins to separate from the mother, he or she uses a transitional object such as a blanket or teddy bear to facilitate the illusion of good mothering (Winnicott, 1965). The key function of the transitional object is to act as a calming agent. The soothing abilities of the transitional object are illustrated by the child's reaching for it at times of stress or when the mother is unavailable. In this situation, the transitional object replaces the mother until she herself returns. Just as a transitional object can represent good-enough mothering, it may also reflect not-good-enough mothering (Winnicott, 1975). The latter may be more applicable when dealing with clients who are experiencing eating disorders. "Since eating patterns, like transitional objects, are created by the individual and soothe one during times of stress, it is probable that eating patterns reflect the infant–mother pattern of relating" (Jacobson, 1988, p. 111).

Humphrey and Stern (1988) stated the following about object relations theory and its impact on the family system:

> *Whereas in anorexia nervosa the child's developing self is enfeebled by negative responses to separation coupled with more positive responses to dependent and regressive behavior, in bulimic families there is a paucity of positive responses to any behavior. Instead, the child's separate self is criticized, ignored, or enlisted in meeting the parents' needs* (p. 343).

PSYCHOSOCIAL FACTORS

Familial Factors

The genesis of eating disorders may be viewed from a family systems theory framework. Ideally, the family is to provide a child with the nurturance and opportunities needed to develop as an individual. This is done through parental guidance and promotion of the autonomy needed in adult life. However, the family interactions of the anorectic or bulimic child discourage the development of independence and autonomy. This results in a self-perception of powerlessness and helplessness on the part of the child.

Minuchin (1978) has identified characteristics often present in the families of children with eating disorders as enmeshment, overprotectiveness, rigidity, and lack of conflict resolution, based on extensive studies of the interactions of the child and the family. He has spoken at length about the concept of *enmeshment,* which is "an extreme form of proximity and intensity in family interactions" (p. 30). This extreme closeness results in a lack of definite boundaries between the parent and child roles, which become blurred. In the enmeshed family, "the individual gets lost in the system" (p. 30).

Overprotectiveness manifests itself in an unusually high degree of concern for each family member's welfare. "In such families, the parents' overprotectiveness retards the children's development of autonomy, competence, and interests or activities outside the safety of the family" (Minuchin, 1978, p. 31).

Finally, Minuchin (1978) addressed the *rigidity* within these families, which refers to their inflexible nature and their desire to maintain the status quo. The *lack of conflict resolution* refers to the family's inability to negotiate any type of compromise or any kind of solution to an identified problem. Family conflicts are usually polarized into a "win or lose" situation, with no one wanting to be on the losing end (see Chapter 22).

Sociocultural Factors

Until recently, research regarding the cause of eating disorders has focused on the previously discussed areas. Yet it is obvious that we live in a diet-conscious society in which thinness is viewed as attractive and healthy. Advertisements promote weight loss and exercise. It seems that dieting has become necessary to achieve our culture's image of thinness. The phenomenon of eating disorders has been described mainly in Western culture, where there is an extreme idealization of thinness.

In addition, there is tremendous pressure on women today to achieve in separate arenas simultaneously. They must be successful, independent, and competitive professionally while competently maintaining their traditional role as wife, mother, and homemaker. The stressors inherent in this situation may be overwhelming to those women who may be predisposed to eating disorders.

None of the previously discussed theories can explain the current increase in the incidence of eating disorders or why it mostly affects middle-class and upper-class Caucasian women. Researchers are beginning to examine possible sociocultural factors that predispose young women to problems related to dieting and food consumption. Steiner-Adair (1986) is exploring the possibility of repressive cultural forces that may be present at this time, concluding that "it may be that certain sociocultural influences make anorexia, bulimia, and anorexic-like behavior a seemingly adaptive response to the development demands of growing up female in certain populations at this time in history" (p. 93).

The conceptualization of eating disorders as a failure to separate and individuate is being challenged by theorists such as Gilligan (1982), who suggested that the female personality develops through attachment to others and interdependent relationships. This is in contrast with boys, for whom their masculine identity is confirmed through separation and autonomy (Erikson, 1968).

Theorists such as Gilligan (1982) and Chodorow (1978) are working toward a model of female development that presents the identity process as one of self-differentiation within the context of relationships. Developmental theory for females may need to shift from the male-based model that emphasizes detachment to one that emphasizes individuation within the context of relationships. According to Chodorow (1978), "in any given society, feminine personality comes to define itself in relation and connection to other people more than masculine personality does" (p. 187).

Intimacy and Marital Issues

Issues of disturbance in sexuality and intimacy have been associated with the eating disorders, but Garner and Garfinkel (1985) suggested that problems with sexuality may reflect more basic issues with autonomy and self-regulation. Persons who restrict food intake appear to have decreased libido and be less interested in sex, whereas those who binge or binge and purge seem to have more frequent sexual activity and interest. The latter is sometimes interpreted as part of the larger issue of impulse control, but it may also be due to age differences. Anorexia has been interpreted psychologically as a fear of sexuality or an attempt to delay or prevent sexual development and menses. Thus, instead of making age-appropriate explorations with boys or having intimate conversations about boys, the adolescent anorectic is preoccupied with weight loss, diet, and exercise. The bulimic woman may be sexually active or even promiscuous, but often sex is more of a compulsive or impulsive behavior and less an expression of intimacy.

The eating-disordered person with obesity also experiences a fear of intimacy and may use food as a substitute. Food is more dependable and does not evoke issues of trust and vulnerability that emerge in relationships, including marriage. Most eating-disordered clients experience shame and disgust with their bodies, whether they are obese, of normal weight, or very thin. These feelings obviously interfere with any enjoyment or pleasure in physical touching or joining. Related behaviors include hiding or not showing their bodies to partners or spouses and projecting feelings of disgust when looked at or touched. Some obese women have reported much anxiety when dieting in the context of becoming more attractive and thus sexually appealing. It would appear that the eating disorder syndrome may provide comfort, safety, and anxiety reduction when the client is presented with the fears and conflicts of intimacy.

Populations at Risk

Certain populations with associated weight expectations or specific weight criteria for participation have been shown to create a higher risk of the development of eating disorders. Generally, athletes have more problems than do control groups, and the risk increases with sports such as wrestling and gymnastics that are characterized by specific weight requirements or appearance expectations.

Women are at higher risk than men because of the cultural desire for thinness, with the resulting dietary restraint being more prevalent among young women than their male peers (Brownell & Foreyt, 1986). The already existing societal pressure for thinness is exacerbated in professions such as fashion modeling and dancing. Any environment that emphasizes slimness and competitiveness appears to be associated with an increase in the incidence of eating disorders and suggests that for some people, dieting may lead directly to the onset of an eating disorder (Hsu, 1990).

EATING DISORDERS ACROSS THE LIFE SPAN

Through the continued study of clients with eating disorders, various presentations have emerged. A major area of research has started to focus on the increasing prevalence of eating disorders in children and adolescents. These groups present unique circumstances that must be taken into account. Theories of growth and development must be used when dealing with a person experiencing an eating disorder who is not an adult. See Table 18–1 for an overview of when specific eating disorders occur in relation to the life stage.

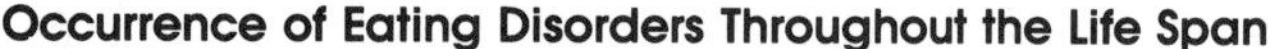

TABLE 18–1

Occurrence of Eating Disorders Throughout the Life Span

	ANOREXIA	BULIMIA	OBESITY	RUMINATION DISORDER	PICA	BINGE EATING DISORDER
Infant (Birth–1 yr)				✓		
Toddler (2–5 yr)					✓	
Early School Age (6–9 yr)			✓			
Late School Age (10–12 yr)	✓		✓			
Adolescence (13–18 yr)	✓	✓	✓			✓
Adulthood (18 yr +)	✓	✓	✓			✓

EARLY CHILDHOOD

The young child with an eating disorder is one who is in a prepubertal stage of development and is considered to be preadolescent—classic DSM-IV criteria may not be applicable. However, DSM-IV now addresses feeding disorders that occur in childhood before the age of 6 years (see the display on diagnostic criteria for feeding disorder of infancy or early childhood). For instance, a child does not have to lose the percentage of weight appropriate for an adult with an eating disorder. Prepubertal children have a lower percentage of body fat. A child who is thin at the start of the weight loss process may reach an unhealthy state quickly. In addition, children tend to eliminate fluids, including water, as well as food. It is helpful to continually plot out the child's progression on the growth chart, accounting for both height and weight. This important tool quickly shows developmentally inappropriate positions on the chart that need specific attention. In addition, both boys and girls present with childhood anorexia, whereas bulimia is not as prevalent in childhood. Symptoms of depression are also usually present and need to be addressed.

Within the psychotherapeutic process, developmental theory continues to be of great importance. Younger children are still very involved in the family and may react strongly to changes within the household and stressful family events. A major component of treatment should be family therapy. Individual therapy for the child may also prove helpful.

DSM-IV DIAGNOSTIC CRITERIA FOR FEEDING DISORDER OF INFANCY OR EARLY CHILDHOOD

A. Feeding disturbance as manifested by persistent failure to eat adequately with significant failure to gain weight or significant loss of weight over at least 1 month.

B. The disturbance is not due to an associated gastrointestinal or other general medical condition (e.g., esophageal reflux).

C. The disturbance is not better accounted for by another mental disorder (e.g., Rumination Disorder) or by lack of available food.

D. The onset is before age 6 years.

From American Psychiatric Association. (1994). *Diagnostic and statistical manual of mental disorders, fourth edition.* Washington, DC: Author.

ADOLESCENCE

The clinical picture presented by the adolescent also needs to be considered within a developmental framework. Central to the eating disorder are those issues relative to puberty, such as increased independence from the family and increased autonomy in problem solving; peer pressures, including sexuality; and initiation into the process of major life choices.

The issue of sexuality is noteworthy because anorectic clients tend to have difficulty with interpersonal intimacy and closeness. Both anorectic and bulimic groups may reveal a history of childhood sexual trauma, which would have implications for future sexual relationships. The adolescent with an eating disorder can benefit from multimodal therapy including individual, family, and group work.

ADULTHOOD: SPECIAL POPULATIONS

The Adult Male

Eating disorders typically present in the male with the same core psychopathological features as in the female; however, there are some unique features. According to Anderson (1984), males tend to be less focused on their exact weight and more intent on attaining the idealized masculine shape of large shoulders and narrow waist and hips. What they fail to appreciate is the role of testosterone in this idealized male shape and that testosterone production decreases in proportion to weight loss. It is estimated that males constitute approximately 10 percent of the population presenting with eating disorders (Anderson, 1984). Males usually share a history of involvement with sports such as wrestling prior to the development of the eating disorder. In addition, males tend to exhibit more sexual anxiety related to issues of homosexuality and bisexuality.

The Client with Diabetes

The prevalence of eating disorders among the diabetic population is unknown, yet the lethality possible in this combination cannot be overemphasized. Food is an integral component of the diabetic regimen. According to Krakoff (1991), diabetes may predispose one to the development of an eating disorder, because a person can attempt to control weight by manipulation of an insulin dosage. Many diabetic women equate insulin usage with weight gain and therefore reduce their insulin dosage to decrease their weight. This method results in glycosuria and the life-threatening consequence of diabetic ketoacidosis (DKA). An eating disorder should be suspected in a diabetic female who presents with a history of multiple incidents of DKA and unexplainable difficulties in the regulation of blood glucose levels. This situation becomes even more complex in an adolescent who is confronting developmental issues in addition to those related to the chronic nature of diabetes. The health care professional may want to monitor the results of the glycosylated hemoglobin tests. This blood test monitors the diabetic client's glucose levels over the past 3 months. The normal values for this test range from 4 percent to 8 percent, so a result between 12 percent and 20 percent would indicate uncontrolled blood glucose levels. In other words, if a diabetic client claims to have had normal blood glucose levels at home, a glycosylated hemoglobin test will validate or invalidate this claim. Most important, appropriate control of the diabetes must be the first goal of treatment.

TREATMENT MODALITIES FOR EATING DISORDERS

THE MULTIDISCIPLINARY TEAM APPROACH TO TREATMENT

The care of the person with an eating disorder is complex and multifaceted. The optimal form of treatment is via the team approach. This method helps diffuse the heavy burden of dealing with these clients and their families. The ability to share the responsibilities with others helps each professional maintain perspective because working with these clients is quite challenging. Essential members of the team include a family physician or pediatrician, a psychotherapist from one of the designated mental health professions, a dietitian, a consulting psychologist to administer standardized tests, and a consulting psychiatrist to assess the need for psychotropic medication. During inpatient hospitalization, the nursing staff plays an integral role in the care also (see the section on the nurse's role later in this chapter).

Clients receiving treatment for an eating disorder can be extremely manipulative and may try to "split" the professionals on the team. It is essential that team members communicate and firmly abide by the boundaries of their particular role; otherwise, the goals of treatment may be sabotaged. A major function of the team is to provide support, clarification, and feedback to the mental health professional acting in the role of primary therapist. Team conferences need to be held frequently and regularly to optimally aid the client and family being treated.

PSYCHOTHERAPY

The use of psychotherapy in treatment may take more than one form—many clients benefit from a combination. For instance, a 15-year-old anorectic client may find both individual and family work necessary for recovery. A 30-year-old bulimic client may need both individual and marital therapy. Many clients with eating disorders, especially bulimia, seem to benefit from group work. The primary goal of any therapeutic relationship is the establishment of trust. The issue of confidentiality should be addressed early in therapy. However, any indication of an issue involving self-harm (or sexual trauma in the case of a child) needs to be addressed with family members. This should be explicitly shared with the identified client, and the family, if appropriate.

Individual Therapy

A primary goal of individual therapy is to strengthen the person's self-esteem and autonomy. Assertiveness training can be helpful in the accomplishment of this goal. Clients with an eating disorder must learn how to recognize their own emotions and other internal states such as hunger. As they become more aware of their feelings and their unique right to have them, they may increase awareness of themselves as distinct entities. This may encourage a sense of self-responsibility. Clients must learn to see that efforts to please everyone are futile and ego-dystonic, or incongruent, to the building of a healthy personality. They must see that their extreme compliance to the wishes of others has deprived them of the right to make their own decisions. They must acknowledge their own right to get angry.

Family Therapy

All the issues discussed earlier also need to be addressed within family therapy if the identified client lives with his or her parents. However, the family usually defines the problem in the context of eating behaviors and weight. They believe that if the client would give up these behaviors, then any remaining problems would be solved. This misconception will need further clarification as the family will need insight into the working of the family as a system. They need to see how the person with the eating disorder has contributed to the functioning of the family system. Some family members become extremely angry and upset when the therapist suggests that everyone needs to work on changes, not just the person with the eating disorder. Conflicts and disagreements need to be openly acknowledged and compromises worked out. This open acknowledgment of conflict and problems can be threatening to these families, because the image of perfection may be extremely important to them.

Marital Therapy

Sometimes within the context of individual or family therapy, the need for marital therapy will be uncovered. This may occur with an adult client attempting to deal with relationship issues in his or her own marriage, or this may occur within family work when it becomes clear that the marital dyad is experiencing difficulties. Leadership, power, autonomy, and decision-making issues may need further exploration within the privacy of marital sessions.

Group Therapy

Group work can be an effective tool in the treatment of clients with an eating disorder. Bulimic clients especially seem to benefit from the support of a group. Anorectic clients may have difficulty with the group setting because it may be too threatening to speak so openly about relevant issues. The anorectic client is usually less skilled socially than the bulimic client and may fear the intimacy created by the group situation. The group leader must be aware of the potential for competition in the group. For instance, the anorectic members may begin to compete with each other in weight loss to see who can be the thinnest. These groups need the supervision of a trained professional who is knowledgeable in group dynamics and can anticipate potential problems before the therapeutic process is sabotaged.

PHARMACOTHERAPY

Many different drugs have been used in the treatment of eating disorders, including antipsychotic agents (e.g., chlorpromazine), anxiolytic agents (e.g., benzodiazepines), appetite stimulants (e.g., cyproheptadine), opiate antagonists (e.g., naloxone and naltrexone), and lithium carbonate. There has been limited success with these pharmacologic agents.

Depression occurs in many clients experiencing an eating disorder, although it may present differently in anorectic clients than it does in those with bulimia. Restrictive anorectic clients usually manifest a more introjective type of depression characterized by feelings of hopelessness and worthlessness. Antidepressant medication may not be indicated in this type of clinical situation. There may be some lessening of depressive symptoms once a healthier nutritional state has been reached. **Alexithymia,** or an inability to recognize internal emotional state, needs to be explored in psychotherapy. Often, the depression remains even after a healthy weight has been established. In addition, the characteristic obsessive-compulsive tendencies seen in the restrictive anorectic clients may be reduced with the use of clomipramine (Anafranil).

On the other hand, a more classic picture of major depression usually presents in bulimic clients and those anorectic clients who use purging behaviors. These clients tend to respond more favorably to antidepressant medication. The tricyclic antidepressants have been administered most frequently, although there has been some use of the monoamine oxidase inhibitors. Common side effects of the tricyclics include tachycardia, dry mouth, urinary retention, blurred vision, and orthostatic hypotension. Cardiac status must be assessed prior to the initiation of a tricyclic antidepressant because these drugs interfere with the conductivity of the heart.

Fluoxetine (Prozac) has been shown to reduce the obsessive-compulsive behavior, anxiety, and depression seen in classic anorexia (Kaye et al., 1991). In addition, a large 13-center study (Fluoxetine Bulimia Nervosa Collaborative Study Group, 1992) explored the use of fluoxetine with bulimic clients and showed marked improvement in depressive symptoms, carbohydrate craving, and other pathologic eating behaviors. It is believed that fluoxetine, a serotonin uptake inhibitor, decreases the desire for carbohydrates, thereby decreasing the incidence of binge eating and purging behaviors. However, much research is still needed in this area, and careful study concerning the use of fluoxetine in anorexia and bulimia is continuing.

Another area of research may occur in the future concerning the use of sertraline hydrochloride (Zoloft) in the treatment of eating disorders. Currently, this drug is being used in the treatment of depression, and it may also prove useful in the treatment of anorexia and bulimia. Its mechanism of action is similar to fluoxetine in that it also inhibits the uptake of serotonin (see Chapter 26).

MEDICAL CONSIDERATIONS

Ideally, an outpatient regimen is the method of choice when treating a person with an eating disorder. After the initial evaluations with the eating disorders team, the client may carry on with usual daily activities. Concurrently, he or she meets regularly with the therapist, dietitian, family physician, and psychiatrist as needed. In this way, progress is monitored closely, and any indication of need for hospitalization will be noted quickly and acted on accordingly. Seriously ill or emaciated clients may need to be hospitalized when seen for the first assessment on an outpatient basis. This may be done on an involuntary basis to prevent death. Anorectic clients are especially upset at the need for hospitalization because they may be in a state of profound denial. Most bulimic clients acknowledge the pathological aspects of their eating behaviors but may still resist an inpatient stay.

Indications for Stabilization by Hospitalization

According to Anderson (1983), the four most frequent indications for an inpatient stay consist of (1) extremely low body weight; (2) severe metabolic abnormalities resulting from vomiting, laxative, or diuretic abuse; (3) suicidal ideation; and (4) failure in outpatient treatment.

Physical Manifestations

Anorectic clients will present themselves as "fine," although that is a far cry from reality. There is often a history of lethargy or frenetic energy, or both. Owing to impaired gastric emptying, constipation, bloating, and abdominal pain are frequent. There may be cardiovascular symptoms such as bradycardia, orthostatic hypotension, mitral valve prolapse, and electrocardiographic (ECG) abnormalities. Endocrine abnormalities include amenorrhea, osteoporosis, hypothermia, elevated growth hormone levels, and changes in thyroid function. During fluid restriction there may be changes such as an increased blood urea nitrogen (BUN) level, decreased glomerular filtration rate, renal calculi, and edema. Dermatological abnormalities include hair loss, dry skin, and development of lanugo hair. Metabolic changes include trace mineral deficiencies (e.g., zinc), osteopenia, and increased plasma cholesterol and triglyceride levels. The anorectic client may show signs of anemia, leukopenia, and thrombocytopenia.

Bulimic clients also present a complex clinical picture. They report gastrointestinal symptoms such as constipation, bloating, abdominal pain, and nausea owing to delayed gastric emptying. Chronic laxative abuse can result in the loss of normal peristalsis, and recurrent vomiting of stomach acid can result in esophagitis. Forceful vomiting can cause tears in the esophagus (Mallory-Weiss syndrome) and possible gastrointestinal bleeding—esophageal rupture is a life-threatening situation. Chronic vomiting causes salivary and parotid gland enlargement. The cardiac system is affected in bulimia. Symptoms include dehydration, orthostatic hypotension, arrhythmias due to electrolyte imbalance (e.g., potassium), bradycardia, myocardial changes related to ipecac poisoning, and possible congestive heart failure. Endocrine changes include irregular menses. Pulmonary complications usually take the form of aspiration pneumonia secondary to vomiting. Fluid and electrolyte imbalance is extremely serious and results in dehydration, hypokalemia, hypochloremia, metabolic acidosis and alkalosis, hypophosphatemia, hyponatremia, and hypocalcemia. Vomiting induced with the use of a finger produces calluses and abrasions on the fingers and knuckles. The teeth are eroded by stomach acid, and there may be increased dental caries. An elevated BUN level is usually noted owing to fluid restriction and loss. Another renal symptom includes a reduced glomerular filtration rate. There may be polydipsia and polyuria.

Medical Management

The medical management of the client with an eating disorder is vitally important. Along with the history, laboratory examination should augment the physical examination. Laboratory tests include determination of the following:

- Complete blood count
- Renal function
- Thyroid function
- Electrolytes
- Blood glucose
- Trace minerals
- Cholesterol and triglycerides
- Liver enzymes
- Muscle enzymes

Urinalysis may be used to detect the use of laxatives or diuretics. An ECG may also be helpful.

The main goal of a medical admission is the stabilization of physical crisis. Correction of the anorectic client's body weight is of supreme importance. Liquid supplements or tube feedings may be employed along with intravenous fluids. Extreme care is needed to prevent fluid overload that may result in congestive heart failure.

In the bulimic client, the focus may be on the interruption of the binge-purge cycle and the associated abuse of laxatives, diuretics, and ipecac. The abrupt cessation of laxatives results in constipation, whereas the discontinuation of diuretics may result in reflex edema. The constipation may be handled through the use of roughage intake, exercise, and hydration. The normalization of fluid balance should occur on its own.

Nutritional Management

During hospitalization, the dietitian plays a major role in the rehabilitation process. Using a nonjudgmental approach enables the dietitian to provide support and establish rapport. The dietitian supplies nutritional education, helps the client explore extreme misperceptions and use of food, and recommends realistic goals to the client and the treatment team. The dietitian attempts to reestablish regular eating patterns with the client. Many dietitians are using the body mass index as a measure of nutritional status (Table 18–2):

$$\text{Body mass index} = \text{Weight (kg)} \div \text{Height}^2\text{ (m)}$$

This method is replacing the charts based on ranges of ideal body weight.

The Inpatient Stay

Overall, weight restoration is a central goal during the hospitalization of the anorectic client. A behavioral management program may be employed using both positive and negative reinforcements, and this may influence the rate at which the anorectic client progresses. Lenient behavioral plans may be as effective as the strict programs because they enlist the client's cooperation and increase the sense of control and autonomy. A drawback of the strict behavioral regimen is that conflict may develop between the client and the staff over "control" of the client. This may be a reproduction of the power struggle already occurring at home for the adolescent client who is rebelling against his or her parents. The behavioral plan must be carefully delineated by the involved professionals and clearly understood by everyone involved. Even then, misunderstandings between the client and the staff occur over the parameters of the plan. Clear limits need to be established with the client.

The length of hospital stay may vary depending on factors such as physical acuity, resolution of emotional crises, and financial status. Some clients may require multiple hospitalizations for their eating disorder, as this illness can take a course of chronicity.

TABLE 18–2
How to Calculate Ideal Weight Using the Body Mass Index

Body mass index (BMI) is a measure of relative body weight, where the weight in kilograms (2.2 lb) is divided by the square of the height in meters (39.37 inches). For example,

$$\frac{\text{Weight (kg)}}{\text{Height}^2\text{ (m)}} = \frac{35\text{ kg}}{(1.54\text{ m})^2} = \frac{35\text{ kg}}{2.37\text{ m}} = 14.76\text{ (BMI)}$$

This is an example of an anorectic woman who is approximately 5′½″ tall and weighs 77 lb. A desirable BMI is in the range of 19–23. As can be seen, her BMI is far lower than would be expected for a healthy woman.

From Bray, G. A. (1978). Definition, measurement, and classifications of the syndromes of obesity. *International Journal of Obesity, 2,* 99–112.

THE NURSE'S ROLE

THE GENERALIST NURSE

The treatment of a person with an eating disorder can be quite challenging for all the professionals involved, and considerable knowledge, skill, and energy are required. The staff nurse plays an integral role as a member of the treatment team on an inpatient unit. In this role, the responsibility for care is shared with the other staff nurses. The members of the eating disorders team need to meet with the nursing staff on a regular basis to delineate the goals and objectives of treatment and to facilitate clear communication among the professionals involved. Ideally, a primary nurse assumes responsibility for the care plan.

Primary nurses have an important role to play because they enforce the therapeutic milieu of the unit. They must be empathetic and supportive but clearly able to define boundaries and set appropriate limits with these clients. There is commonly manipulation and "splitting" done by this type of client, and staff nurses need to be aware of these dynamics as they occur; otherwise, the goals of the treatment may be critically undermined as the health professionals are set up to "take sides." Most primary nurses are invaluable in their ability to establish trust within the therapeutic relationship. Their conversations and exchanges with the eating-disordered client may serve to strengthen and augment the relationship between the client and the primary psychotherapist.

THE ADVANCED-PRACTICE NURSE

The advanced-practice nurse, or clinical specialist (CS), may participate in a variety of roles. The CS may participate as part of the specialized eating disorders team as a primary psychotherapist. In this role, the CS is responsible for individual, family, marital, or group therapy. The CS with advanced skills and knowledge of eating disorders may coordinate the eating disorders team in the role of program director. The CS may act as a consultant to other professionals concerning treatment issues. The CS in private practice may see a client with an eating disorder in short-term or long-term outpatient therapy. Finally, the CS may be an active participant in a research project concerning a particular aspect of eating disorders. In general, the role of the nurse in the treatment of clients with eating disorders is governed by the practitioner's level of education and experience with the treatment of this special population.

THE NURSING PROCESS

Clients with eating disorders present with complex psychopathology, physical symptoms, and maladaptive eating and coping behaviors. The nursing process is used to develop an individualized, comprehensive, continuous plan of care.

Assessment

Assessing the client with an eating disorder is a multifaceted process that must include a biological history of the client and a comprehensive psychosocial history of both the client and the family.

The client's medical condition must be assessed to determine the extent of nutritional deprivation and potential complications. A complete physical examination includes laboratory tests and cardiac evaluation. The following case study provides a useful framework in which the nursing process can be examined.

Case Study: The Client with Anorexia Nervosa (Sara)

Sara Smith, a 15-year-old, was seen with her mother for an initial family interview in an eating disorders program for children and adolescents. This first meeting was conducted on an outpatient basis. Mrs. Smith expressed concern about her daughter's physical status. Sara is 5′4″ tall and weighs 80 lb. She has lost 40 lb from her original weight of 120 lb over the last 8 months, and she has experienced amenorrhea for the last 4 months. Sara admitted to eating very little food, consisting mostly of raw green vegetables. She drinks only water and diet soda on a restricted basis. She admitted to using vomiting only when her mother forced her to eat. She denied any use of diuretics, laxatives, or ipecac, although she did complain of constipation. Sara has exercised every day for 2 hours but can no longer do this because she is too exhausted. Lanugo hair was evident on both her forearms, and her lips were dry and cracked. Sara wore layers of clothing and complained of constantly being cold. She kept her coat on throughout the interview. Her affect was flat, and she said little. She maintained minimal eye contact on interview. She was tearful at times. Answers given by Sara were slow and laborious in coming.

Family history revealed that Mr. and Mrs. Smith had divorced when Sara was 3 years old. She has two older sisters. Mrs. Smith stated that Mr. Smith had been physically abusive of her and their girls. She also questioned the possibility of sexual abuse of Sara by her father. Sara has always denied this. The family history was positive for depressive disorder on the paternal side. Sara admitted to long-standing insomnia, decreased concentration, and suicidal ideation. Sara continues to attend high school, where she maintains a 4.0 grade point average. Sara used to be active in school clubs, cheerleading, and dance. However, she has withdrawn from all extracurricular activities and stays home isolated in her room. She rarely spends time with friends.

Because of the findings revealed by the interview, Sara was hospitalized immediately in a children's hospital on an adolescent medical unit. Her primary care physician was a pediatrician who consulted the eating disorders team, including the team's child psychiatrist. A complete physical examination was done and appropriate laboratory tests were ordered. These showed severe metabolic acidosis, hypophosphatemia, elevated cholesterol and low serum zinc levels, and anemia. She was bradycardic in the range of 45 to 49 beats per minute. An ECG was done, and Sara was placed on strict bed rest with a cardiorespiratory monitor. She was started on intravenous fluids, and a nasogastric tube was placed for feedings. The team dietitian met with Sara and began to work on food-related issues. A CS on the team was designated as primary therapist. The team psychiatrist recommended a trial dose of fluoxetine. A behavioral plan was instituted. A full psychological profile was later conducted by the team psychologist. The primary nurse worked closely with the eating disorders team and constructed a plan of care for Sara (see the Nursing Care Plan display).

Psychosocial assessment begins with establishing a trusting relationship with the client and family members. Major components of the psychosocial assessment include identifying the client's reasons for seeking treatment, present and past history of impaired eating and coping patterns, family involvement, and the impact of family members on the client's well-being. A complete family assessment is a critical part of assessing clients with eating disorders. Assessing family interactions, personal boundaries, coping patterns, and management of stress are major aspects of this process (see Chapter 22).

Other aspects of the assessment process include the mental status examination, identification of present and past psychiatric treatment, identification of resources, assessing the client's level of danger to self or others, identification of individual and family strengths, and assessment of current stressors.

Nursing Diagnoses

Major nursing diagnoses for eating disorder clients include

- Alterations in Nutrition: Less Than Body Requirements related to self-starvation
- Constipation related to erratic eating patterns
- Decreased Cardiac Output related to inadequate caloric and fluid intake
- Ineffective Individual Coping related to feelings of lack of control, fears of growing up, and symptomatic response to family stress
- Ineffective Family Coping: Disabling related to impaired interactions and ineffective management of stress

Planning

Planning for and implementing a plan of care for clients with eating disorders is a detailed process that requires a multidisciplinary, comprehensive, and continuous approach. The health care team often includes an internist, the nursing staff, a dietitian, a child psychiatrist, and a psychiatric clinical specialist. Expected outcomes include an increase in oral intake, appropriate weight gain, and alleviation of the physical manifestations of food deprivation. Expected psychosocial outcomes include an increase in the client's expression of feelings, recognition by the client of unrealistic self-expectations, the use of viable coping behaviors to deal with negative self-perceptions, and improved communication patterns within the family.

Intervention

Medical interventions depend on the extent of nutritional alterations and include measures that restore fluid and caloric intake while monitoring for medical complications, such as cardiac arrhythmias. Furthermore, close monitoring of laboratory studies, cardiac status, intake and output, and vital signs enables the health care team to assess responses to treatment.

Psychosocial interventions include behavioral-cognitive and assertiveness techniques and family psychoeducation. Behavioral-cognitive techniques increase self-awareness, including realization of low self-esteem and maladaptive coping patterns. Assertiveness techniques encourage self-expression, improve interpersonal skills, and increase self-esteem. Family psychoeducation facilitates improved communication patterns and increases knowledge of underlying family dynamics in anorexia nervosa.

Because treatment for the client with an eating disorder is long term, the family will need to continue treatment on an outpatient basis.

Evaluation

The evaluation of client and family response to treatment is continuous and based on outcome identification.

DIRECTIONS FOR FURTHER RESEARCH

The care of clients with eating disorders is extremely complex. At times, it can be frustrating because much is still unknown about these illnesses. Some information is still speculative. More formal research is needed because the study of disturbed eating patterns is relatively recent. The following are required:

- Continued development of sophisticated measurement tools
- Longitudinal study of the different eating-disordered populations
- Longitudinal study of the long-term effects of eating disorders on health status
- Continued study of at-risk populations and identification of causative factors
- Exploration of the impact of different stages in the life span
- Continued study in the neurobiological area and other physiological implications of an eating disorder

Nurses and clients with eating disorders have a major commonality: both groups consist mainly of females. As nursing advances in the development of theory, perhaps nurses will play a significant role in further research in the area of eating disorders.

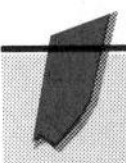

Nursing Care Plan 18–1 The Client with an Eating Disorder (Sara)

OUTCOME IDENTIFICATION	NURSING ACTIONS	RATIONALES	EVALUATION
Nursing Diagnosis: Altered Nutrition: Less than Body Requirements related to self-starvation			
1. By [date], Sara will verbalize increased understanding of appropriate nutritional needs.	1. Discuss fundamentals of healthy nutrition, i.e., basic four food groups and or food pyramid.	1. Increased understanding of basic nutritional requirements may encourage more appropriate food intake.	*Goals met:* Sara expresses understanding of need to eat more and increases food intake. Sara has fewer complaints of bloating and gas, and there is no sign of cardiac overload. Improvement is noted in phosphorus and carbon dioxide levels. Sara's weight has increased.
2. By [date], Sara will increase oral intake.	2a. Provide small frequent feedings.	2a. Small, frequent feedings limit stress on the gastrointestinal and cardiac systems.	
	2b. Monitor intake and output.	2b. Appropriate intake and output will ensure meeting of caloric requirements.	
3. By [date], Sara will show appropriate weight gain as specified by team dietitian.	3a. Monitor weight gain.	3a. Weight gain will validate appropriately met metabolic needs.	
	3b. Monitor results of laboratory studies.	3b. Laboratory studies will indicate improvement in metabolism.	
4. By [date], Sara will cooperate with tube feeding regimen.	4. Educate client and family concerning rationale for tube feedings.	4. Client may be unable to meet caloric needs by oral intake. Tube feedings provide a caloric supplement.	
Nursing Diagnosis: Constipation related to erratic eating patterns			
1. By [date], Sara will have more frequent bowel movements.	1a. Provide small, frequent feedings.	1a. Small, frequent feedings will improve intake and limit stress on the gastrointestinal system.	*Goal met:* Sara exhibits more normal bowel habits.
	1b. Monitor bowel function.	1b. Regular assessment will indicate whether or not there is improvement in bowel function.	
Nursing Diagnosis: Decreased Cardiac Output related to inadequate caloric and fluid intake			
1. By [date], Sara will experience alleviation of bradycardia and increased normalization of pulse.	1a. Provide small, frequent feedings.	1a. Small, frequent feedings limit stress on the cardiovascular system.	*Goal met:* Sara shows improvement in cardiac status and increased metabolism. Laboratory results are improved. No sign of respiratory or cardiac distress.
	1b. Monitor vital signs. 1c. Use cardiorespiratory monitor.	1b–c. Regular vital sign readings and use of monitor will help with assessment of pulse and cardiac status.	
2. By [date], Sara will avoid congestive heart failure during the refeeding process.	2a. Monitor serum electrolytes, urine specific gravity, and blood urea nitrogen.	2a. Regular assessment of laboratory studies will indicate improvement in cardiovascular system.	

Nursing Care Plan 18–1 The Client with an Eating Disorder (Sara) (Continued)

OUTCOME IDENTIFICATION	NURSING ACTIONS	RATIONALES	EVALUATION
	2b. Offer small amounts of fluid.	2b. Small amounts of fluid will prevent cardiac overload.	
	2c. Measure intake and output.	2c. Appropriate intake and output will ensure meeting of caloric requirements.	

Nursing Diagnosis: Ineffective Individual Coping related to feelings of lack of control, fears of growing up, and symptomatic response to family stress

OUTCOME IDENTIFICATION	NURSING ACTIONS	RATIONALES	EVALUATION
1. By [date], Sara will explore and identify feelings associated with perception of self.	1a. Encourage expression of feelings. 1b. Explore misperceptions between perceived and actual self.	1. These actions will contribute to increased self-awareness and realization of low self-esteem.	*Goals met:* Sara ► Begins to express feelings, both positive and negative ► Begins to use assertiveness techniques in discussions with her mother ► Expresses awareness of her own unrealistic expectations of self ► Begins to go to activity room on her own accord ► Is able to verbally share her positive traits.
2. By [date], Sara will use viable options for coping with negative feelings and self-perceptions.	2a. Explore use of assertiveness techniques.	2a. Use of assertiveness technique enables client to express herself.	
	2b. Encourage realistic expectations of self.	2b. Encourages examination of perfectionism.	
3. By [date], Sara will actively participate in social activities.	3. Encourage participation in unit activities.	3. Anorectic clients tend to be socially isolated and have limited interpersonal skills.	
4. By [date], Sara will verbalize a more positive perception of self.	4. Encourage positive verbalization about self.	4. Anorectic clients tend to have extremely low self-esteem.	

Nursing Diagnosis: Ineffective Family Coping: Disabling related to impaired interactions and ineffective management of stress

OUTCOME IDENTIFICATION	NURSING ACTIONS	RATIONALES	EVALUATION
1. By [date], Sara will improve patterns of family communication as family increases knowledge of underlying dynamics in anorexia nervosa.	1a. Develop a trusting relationship with family.	1a. Trust is the basis for therapeutic relationships.	*Goals met:* Sara and her family ► Freely voice worries and concerns. ► Begin to express perceptions and needs more clearly ► Begin to implement more effective methods of conflict resolution. ► Begin to examine with therapist what changes in communication patterns need to occur ► Agree to long-term plan of care
	1b. Assess patterns of family communication.	1b. Lack of healthy family communication contributes to anorexia.	
	1c. Assist family in the identification of inherent patterns of communication.	1c. Family may not be aware of ineffective patterns of communication, i.e., may need to learn more appropriate methods of conflict resolution.	
	1d. Encourage expression of thoughts and feelings.	1d. Family may not encourage expression of conflicts or differences.	
	1e. Share information on the process of anorexia nervosa with the family.	1e. Increased knowledge will increase awareness of need to examine family communication patterns.	
2. By [date], Sara's family will be in agreement with extended therapeutic plan of care.	2. Assist family in the development of a long-term plan of care.	2. Family will need to continue treatment on an outpatient basis as treatment is long term.	

▶ CHAPTER SUMMARY

The client with an eating disorder can present with complex symptoms and clinical findings. There are similarities between the different eating disorders, but there are also distinctly unique features. Theories concerning possible causality encompass the neurobiological, psychological, and psychosocial perspectives. Treatment of the eating-disordered client is optimally managed by a multidisciplinary team whose members focus on the medical, nursing, psychological, and nutritional needs of the client. A great deal of research is needed to better understand the complexities of the eating-disordered client.

Suggestions for Clinical Conferences

1. Discuss the similarities and differences of the individual eating disorders.
2. Discuss how nursing care of the anorectic client may differ from that of the bulimic client.
3. Discuss the need to be supportive, yet objective, while caring for the client with an eating disorder, in view of the manipulative quality inherent in the disorder.
4. Explore the possibility that cultural expectations support the continuation of eating disorders.

References

American Psychiatric Association. (1987). *Diagnostic and statistical manual of mental disorders, 3rd edition, revised.* Washington, DC: Author.

American Psychiatric Association. (1994). *Diagnostic and statistical manual of mental disorders* (4th ed.). Washington, DC: Author.

Anderson, A. (1983). Anorexia nervosa and bulimia: Diagnosis and comprehensive treatment. *Comprehensive Therapy, 9,* 9–17.

Anderson, A. (1984). Anorexia nervosa and bulimia in adolescent males. *Pediatric Annals, 13,* 901–907.

Bray, G. A. (1978). Definition, measurement, and classifications of the syndromes of obesity. *International Journal of Obesity, 2,* 99–112.

Brownell, K. D., & Foreyt, J. P. (1986). *Handbook of eating disorders: Physiology, psychology, and treatment of obesity, anorexia, and bulimia.* New York: Basic Books.

Bruch, H. (1962). Perceptual and conceptual disturbances in anorexia nervosa. *Psychosomatic Medicine, 24,* 187–194.

Bruch, H. (1966). Anorexia nervosa and its differential diagnosis. *Journal of Nervous and Mental Disease, 141*(3), 555–566.

Bruch, H. (1973). *Eating disorders: Obesity, anorexia and the person within.* New York: Basic Books.

Bruch, H. (1982). Anorexia nervosa: Therapy and theory. *American Journal of Psychiatry, 139,* 1531–1538.

Chodorow, N. (1978). *The reproduction of mothering.* Berkeley: University of California Press.

Erikson, E. (1968). *Identity, youth and crisis.* New York: W. W. Norton.

Fluoxetine Bulimia Nervosa Collaborative Study Group. (1992). Fluoxetine in the treatment of bulimia nervosa. *Archives of General Psychiatry, 49,* 139–147.

Freemouw, W., & Damer, D. (1992). Obesity. In P. H. Wilson (Ed.), *Principles and practice of relapse prevention.* New York: Guilford Press.

Garfinkel, P. E., & Garner, D. M. (1982). *Anorexia nervosa: A multidimensional perspective.* New York: Brunner/Mazel.

Garner, D. M., & Garfinkel, P. E. (1985). *Handbook of psychotherapy for anorexia nervosa and bulimia.* New York: Guilford Press.

Gilligan, C. (1982). *In a different voice.* Cambridge, MA: Harvard University Press.

Holland, A., Hale, A., & Murray R. (1984). Anorexia nervosa: A study of 34 twin pairs. *British Journal of Psychiatry, 145,* 414–419.

Hsu, L. K. G. (1990). *Eating disorders.* New York: Guilford Press.

Humphrey, H., & Stern, S. (1988). Object relations and the family system in bulimia: A theoretical integration. *Journal of Marital and Family Therapy, 14*(3), 337–350.

Jacobson, J. (1988). Speculations on the role of transitional objects in eating disorders. *Archives of Psychiatric Nursing, 2,* 110–114.

Johnson, C., Lewis, C., & Hagman, J. (1984). The syndrome of bulimia: Review and synthesis. *Psychiatric Clinics of North America, 7,* 247–273.

Kaye, W., & Weltzin, T. (1991a). Neurochemistry of bulimia nervosa. *Journal of Clinical Psychiatry, 52,* 21–28.

Kaye, W., & Weltzin, T. (1991b). Serotonin activity in anorexia and bulimia nervosa: Relationship to the modulation of feeding and mood. *Journal of Clinical Psychiatry, 52,* 41–48.

Kaye, W., Weltzin, T., Hsu, L., & Bulik, C. (1991). An open trial of fluoxetine in patients with anorexia nervosa. *Journal of Clinical Psychiatry, 52,* 464–471.

Koepp, W., Schildbach, S., Schmager, C., & Rohner, R. (1993). Borderline diagnosis and substance abuse in female patients with eating disorders. *International Journal of Eating Disorders, 14*(1), 107–110.

Krakoff, D. (1991). Eating disorders as a special problem for persons with insulin-dependent diabetes mellitus. *Nursing Clinics of North America, 26,* 707–713.

Logue, A. W. (1991). *The psychology of eating and drinking.* Salt Lake City: W. H. Freeman.

Lucas, A. L. (1991). Eating disorders. In M. Lewis (Ed.), *Child and adolescent psychiatry: A comprehensive textbook.* Baltimore: Williams & Wilkins.

Minuchin, S., Rosman, B., & Baker, L. (1978). *Psychosomatic families: Anorexia nervosa in context.* Cambridge, MA: Harvard University Press.

Palmer, T. (1990). Anorexia nervosa, bulimia nervosa: Causal theories and treatment. *Nurse Practitioner, 15,* 12–21.

Steiner-Adair, C. (1986). The body politic: Normal female adolescent development of eating disorders. *Journal of The American Academy of Psychoanalysis, 14,* 95–114.

Strober, M. (1991). Family-genetics studies of eating disorders. *Journal of Clinical Psychiatry, 52,* 9–12.

Taylor, A. V., Peveler, R. E., Hibbert, G. A., & Fairburn, C. G. (1993). Eating disorders among women receiving treatment for an alcohol problem. *International Journal of Eating Disorders, 14*(2), 147–151.

Toner, B. B., Garfinkel, P. E., & Barner, D. M. (1986). Long-term follow-up of anorexia nervosa. *Psychosomatic Medicine, 48,* 520–529.

Waller, G. (1992). Sexual abuse and bulimic symptoms in eating disorders: Do family interaction and self-esteem explain the links? *International Journal of Eating Disorders, 12*(3), 235–240.

Weiner, H. (1989). Psychoendocrinology of anorexia nervosa. *Psychiatric Clinics of North America, 12,* 187–205.

Winnicott, D. (1965). *Ego integration in child development: The maturational processes and the facilitating environment.* New York: International University.

Winnicott, D. (1975). *Transitional objects and transitional phenomena: Through pediatrics to psychoanalysis.* New York: Basic Books.

CHAPTER

19

Physical and Sexual Abuse

CHRISTINE GRANT, Ph.D., R.N.

OUTLINE

CHAPTER OBJECTIVES

Upon completion of this chapter, you will be able to:

1. Discuss the types of abuse directed at children and adults.
2. Identify the causative factors contributing to individual risk for violence or violent behaviors.
3. Identify the effects of abuse throughout the life span.
4. Recognize and discuss the nurse's role in interacting with child protective services and legal resources.
5. Apply the nursing process to victims and perpetrators of violence.

KEY TERMS

Abuse
Battering
Incest
Pedophile

Violence is an inescapable reality in today's society. The statistics on children who are hurt each year in the United States are incomprehensible. The incidences of elder and spouse **abuse** are disturbing. Human beings inflict an unbelievable array of unspeakable acts on each other. Perhaps overwhelmed by the magnitude of the problem, we become numb to the staggering crime rate.

Despite the fact that violence is commonplace in our lives, the concepts of violence and abuse are complex. At the same time that, as persons, we recognize the public images of child abuse, spouse abuse, and elder abuse, as professionals we must realize that these concepts do not share a theoretical perspective or common vocabulary. Nurses, physicians, sociologists, psychologists, lawyers, and social service practitioners all have their own conceptualizations of violence and abuse. These competing theories create controversy and urgency. The consequences of abuse require that as nurses we educate ourselves about the joint enterprise to which we must contribute to intervene on behalf of victims and victimizers.

The nurse will encounter abuse victims and perpetrators in all settings. *The Diagnostic and Statistical Manual of Mental Disorders,* fourth edition (DSM-IV) (American Psychiatric Association [APA] 1994), includes a section on categorization of severe mistreatment (Table 19–1). Knowledge of the incidence, dynamics, and causative factors of abuse is essential. In addition, at each juncture, nurses will be asked to examine their own feelings regarding abuse. Sadness, rage, anger, and frustration are just a few of the emotional consequences of working with abuse victims. Introspection and processing of her or his own feelings regarding caring for victims and perpetrators are important exercises for the nurse. The reader is referred to Chapters 20 and 21 for discussions of therapeutic relationships with these clients. This chapter focuses the reader on the realities of violence within a family context and on the nursing process throughout the life span with victims and victimizers.

TABLE 19–1
Problems Related to Abuse or Neglect as Defined in the DSM-IV

- The focus of clinical attention is harsh abuse of one person by another (e.g., physical and sexual abuse or child neglect).
- Specify whether the client is a victim or a perpetrator.
- The following categories apply:
  1. Physical Abuse of Child
  2. Sexual Abuse of Child
  3. Neglect of Child
  4. Physical Abuse of Adult (e.g., spouse battering, elder abuse)
  5. Sexual Abuse of Adult

Adapted from American Psychiatric Association. (1994). *Diagnostic and statistical manual of mental disorders, fourth edition.* Washington, DC: Author.

DEFINITIONS AND INCIDENCE OF ABUSE

INCEST

Incest, familiar to most as a form of sexual abuse, is actually a legal term that is defined by each state's civil and criminal laws. Although many of these laws are fashioned from federal legislation, the nurse should be aware of the definition(s) of the state in which he or she practices. For example, in Pennsylvania, the State Code defines incest as sexual intercourse with a blood relative or a relative by adoption, including whole or half relations. Incest is illegal in all states, but the behaviors that are considered incestuous may vary from state to state. Incest encompasses a wide variety of sexual behaviors and has enormous effects on the victims.

Researchers have reported that 1 in every 4 women (Russell, 1984a) and 1 in every 6 men (Finkelhor et al., 1990) will have experienced some form of childhood sexual abuse during their childhood years (Finkelhor & Hotaling, 1984). However, because of the hidden nature of the act, it is virtually impossible to determine the true incidence of sexual abuse. Professionals estimate that there is a major problem of underreporting and that if 15 percent of women and 5 percent of men say they were sexually abused (low estimates according to survey research), then there would be 300,000 to 400,000 new child victims per year. These numbers are two or three times higher than the current reported statistics (Finkelhor et al., 1990), indicating a serious problem of underreporting to authorities.

CHILD ABUSE

Child abuse takes many forms in the United States. This chapter focuses on serious physical injury, neglect, sexual abuse, and serious mental injury.

Serious Physical Injury

Serious physical injury creates a condition in the child wherein physical functioning is either permanently or

TABLE 19–2
Forms of Child Physical Abuse

- Skin and soft tissue injury (i.e., bruises, hematomas, and abrasions)
- Internal injuries
- Dislocations and fractures
- Loss of teeth due to shaking, slapping, punching, kicking, striking, and hitting
- Throwing of child or throwing of objects against child
- Branding or loop or restraint marks made by belt buckles, handprints, electric cords, ropes, or ligatures
- Hair loss due to pulling the child by the hair
- Burns due to spills, immersions, flames, and branding
- Wounds due to gunshots, knives, razors, or other sharp objects

temporarily impaired. The harm causes severe pain to the child and may be accompanied by a pattern of separate, unexplained injuries (see Table 19–2 for forms of child physical abuse). Dr. C. Henry Kempe of the University of Colorado Medical School is credited with creating the term *battered child syndrome*, which refers to a diagnosis of physical abuse of a child made through radiological techniques that detect old bone fractures. Dr. Kempe's work brought into public awareness the seriousness of the problem of the battered child and initiated a nationwide campaign to have each state mandate that physicians report cases of child abuse. The physical abuse of a child is any nonaccidental injury inflicted by the child's caretaker. Physical abuse can be a single episode or repeated events.

Neglect

Neglect is defined by individual state law, but on a practical basis it is difficult to discern. Neglect is distinguished by the failure to provide for the child's basic needs for subsistence, including food, housing, clothing, education, medical care, and emotional care (see Table 19–3 for types of neglect and behaviors indicating neglect). The Child Welfare League of America (1973) described child neglect as not providing the child with the love, care, guidance, and protection needed for healthy growth and development. The definition of child neglect is nebulous because of the fact that the consequences of neglect lie on a continuum. The situations of neglect cannot be circumscribed, and there are many variations on the term "healthy growth and development." At its most extreme, neglect can result in death, especially in very young children.

Serious Mental Injury

Serious mental injury is a psychological condition caused by the acts or omissions of a perpetrator who renders a child chronically and severely anxious, depressed, withdrawn, or psychotic (Ludwig & Kornberg, 1992). The true incidence of mental abuse is impossible to measure, because mental abuse leaves no clear indicator and typically occurs within the context of the home environment. The Study of National Incidence and Prevalence of Child Abuse and Neglect (1988) concluded that emotional abuse occurs in three to four children per thousand and may affect as many as 4 percent of the children in the United States. Emotional abuse and neglect take many forms, but they may begin early in the child's life, when the parent(s) fail to interact with the infant. Lack of stimulation can lead to emotional deprivation, which can have enormous consequences for the child (Owen & Coant, 1992). Emotional neglect and abuse have also been defined as a passive lack of nurturing and differ from other types of abuse and neglect in that the child's psyche is violated.

Garbarino (1989) described five areas of the process of emotional abuse as follows:

1. Rejecting—failing to acknowledge the child's worth and importance
2. Isolating—separating a child from friends to prevent the child from learning through social relationships
3. Terrorizing—using verbal abuse to frighten the child and to create fears
4. Ignoring—failing to provide the child with stimulation
5. Corrupting—forcing a child to engage in antisocial behavior (e.g., purchasing of drugs, shoplifting, and stealing)

Emotional injury, or maltreatment, can also include bizarre forms of punishment, such as locking a child in a dark closet or tying the child to a chair or stair rail. Emotional injury or abuse may be exhibited in forms

TABLE 19–3
Types of Neglect and the Behaviors Indicating Neglect

TYPE OF NEGLECT	BEHAVIOR INDICATING NEGLECT
Failure to protect	Ingestion of poison, accidents (including falls, electric shocks, and burns), and disregard for child's safety. Lack of appropriate supervision.
Physical neglect	Failure to provide food, clothing, and shelter. Failure to provide adequate heating, diet, and hygiene. Indicators include diaper dermatitis, lice, odors, scabies, and dirty appearance. Additional indicators are inappropriate clothing for the season, lack of adequate bedding, and a living environment infested with insects or rodents. Other signs include failure to immunize, poor dental hygiene, malnutrition, and failure to provide child with hearing or seeing aids.
Medical neglect	Failure to provide for the medical needs of the child, including failure to seek timely intervention or failure to comply with prescribed medical treatment. Indicators include repeated urgent health care visits, delayed diagnosis, physical incapacity, and avoidable complications.
Emotional neglect and nonorganic failure to thrive	Failure to provide nurturing and psychological support. Indicators include delayed growth and development, depression, poor school performance, acute psychiatric manifestations (withdrawal, phobias, hyperactivity, and acting out), and difficulties with relationships (inability to trust, attention-seeking behaviors, or suspiciousness).

TABLE 19–4
Types of Sexual Abuse Behaviors

- Penile penetration of the anus and/or vagina
- Insertion of object into the anus and/or vagina (e.g., fingers)
- Fellatio and cunnilingus
- Masturbation of the victim
- Masturbation of self in front of the victim
- Manipulation of the genitals (e.g., touching, caressing)
- Exposure of the perpetrator's genitals to the victim
- Exposure of pornography to the victim (e.g., sexually explicit magazines, books, videos, or computer graphics)

such as facial tics, racing movements, and eccentric reactions to adult authority.

SEXUAL ABUSE

Sexual abuse, a form of child abuse, is differentiated from incest in that sexual abuse of children can involve a wide variety of perpetrators, not just blood relatives. Sexual abuse is often defined as sexual contact with a person 5 or more years older than the child victim, whether by force or consent. The sexual contact includes a wide variety of sexual behaviors, such as touching and exposing of the child's sexual parts for the sexual gratification of the perpetrator, sexual intercourse, oral and anal penetration, rape, the prostitution of children, and the use of children in pornography. The sexual contact can also be observed contact (i.e., exposing the genitals to the child or having the child view sexually explicit activity) (Table 19–4 lists types of sexual abuse behaviors). Some adults who sexually abuse children are attracted to them sexually. The term for such a person is ***pedophile.*** The fourth edition of the DSM-IV (APA, 1994) defines pedophilia under the paraphilias category of the sexual and gender identity disorders (see the display on the DSM-IV diagnostic criteria for pedophilia).

Child abuse recognition and reporting has increased dramatically since the creation of the Society for the Prevention of Cruelty to Children in New York City in 1874, in response to the plight of one little girl, Mary Ellen Wilson:

Case Study: Mary Ellen Wilson

Mary Ellen Wilson was abandoned as an infant and was taken in and raised by Mary McCormack Connolly. In the winter of 1873, Etta Wheeler, a missionary from St. Luke's Methodist Church in New York City, became aware that Mary Ellen was being beaten, starved, and imprisoned by her stepparents. Mrs. Wheeler contacted the police, who declined to get involved with the case, even though Mary Ellen was being beaten daily with a whip and locked in a dark, unventilated room. Mrs. Wheeler then approached the president of the Society for the Prevention of Cruelty to Animals and enlisted his aid. The child's court testimony read as follows:

My name is Mary Ellen. I don't know how old I am. My mother and father are both dead. I have had no shoes or stockings in this winter. I have never been allowed to go out of the rooms except in the night time . . . my bed at night is only a piece of carpet on the floor underneath a window. Mamma has been in the habit of whipping and beating me almost every day with a rawhide-twisted whip. The whip always left black and blue marks on my body. The cut on my head was made by a pair of scissors in mamma's hand. I have never been kissed by mamma. Whenever she went out she locked me in the bedrooms. I do not want to go back to live with mamma because she beats me so (Lazoritz, 1990, p. 143).

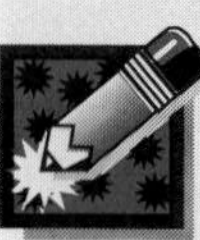

DSM-IV DIAGNOSTIC CRITERIA FOR PEDOPHILIA

302.2 Pedophilia

A. Over a period of at least 6 months, recurrent, intense sexually arousing fantasies, sexual urges, or behaviors involving sexual activity with a prepubescent child or children (generally age 13 years or younger).

B. The fantasies, sexual urges, or behaviors cause clinically significant distress or impairment in social, occupational, or other important areas of functioning.

C. The person is at least 16 years and at least 5 years older than the child or children in Criterion A.

Note: Do not include an individual in late adolescence involved in an ongoing sexual relationship with a 12- or 13-year-old.

Specify if:
Sexually attracted to males.
Sexually attracted to females.
Sexually attracted to both.

Specify if:
Limited to incest.

Specify type:
Exclusive type (attracted only to children)
Nonexclusive type.

Used with permission from American Psychiatric Association (1994). *Diagnostic and statistical manual of mental disorders, fourth edition.* Washington, DC: Author.

Between 1976 and 1987, reports of suspected child abuse and neglect in the United States rose from an estimated 669,000 to 2,163,000, an average increase of more than 10% per year (Finkelhor, 1993). Although incidence figures are impossible to substantiate, authorities believe that a large number of child abuse incidents are still not reported each year. Aggressive reporting of child maltreatment is crucial, and, as mandated reporters, all nurses are responsible for contributing to the identification of serious child abuse.

In 1974, the Child Abuse Prevention and Treatment Act was signed into law. All states have enacted statutes requiring that maltreatment of children be reported. Nurses are responsible for reporting suspected child maltreatment as mandated by these state reporting laws. All the states and U.S. territories have laws and statutes requiring the reporting of child abuse and neglect to designated agencies or officials. Nurses who care for children and their families are in key positions to identify possible incidents of child abuse and neglect. Each state's reporting laws specify how to report, to whom, when, and the contents of the report. Most states have legal provisions to protect nurse reporters from civil lawsuits and criminal prosecution resulting from the reporting made in "good faith." Failure to report abuse by a designated mandated reporter, such as a nurse, can result in criminal penalties. All nurses are urged to obtain copies of their state's reporting laws.

ABUSE OF OLDER ADULTS

The term *elder abuse* is not well defined, because the definitions used by both legal and social service agencies are ambiguous and contradictory. Steinmetz and Straus (1974) incorporated the phenomenon of elder abuse under their general definition of family violence: "the intentional use of physical force on another person" (p. 4). A broader definition of the abuse of older adults would include not only physical abuse but also verbal abuse; emotional and psychological abuse in the form of threats and insults; medical abuse, which would include the refusal to offer medication or needed medical treatment; and neglect (Block & Sinnott, 1979; Fulmer & O'Malley, 1987; Phillips, 1983; Steinmetz, 1988). Pillemer (1993) and Steinmetz (1993) both argue that abuse of the older adult in the United States is related to the stress, frustration, and feelings of burden experienced by the caregivers of the dependent elderly. They conclude that because of the demands placed on the caregiver, the older adult is at risk for abusive and neglectful treatment. Estimates for the prevalence of abuse of the older adult vary considerably. Pillemer and Finkelhor (1988) interviewed by telephone a random sample of individuals age 65 or older in Boston and found that the abusive family member was often dependent on the elder and in nearly 60% of the cases was a spouse.

BATTERED WOMEN

One in 10 American women is abused by an intimate partner (Sampselle, 1992). Estimates of physical abuse of women in the United States range from 1.8 to 4 million yearly incidents (Hotaling et al., 1988; Straus et al., 1980). **Battering** of women is the foremost cause of injury to women, and researchers have reported that 40 to 60 percent of battered women are abused during pregnancy (Fagan et al., 1983; Walker, 1984). The battered woman is exposed to repeated trauma as a result of physical, sexual, and/or psychological assault inflicted on her by an intimate partner. Research reveals that these women are often sexually abused or raped in addition to experiencing the physical and psychological battering. Brendtro and Bowker (1989) and Campbell (1989) found that at least 45 percent of all battered women are also being sexually assaulted.

Walker (1979) delineated the psychological effects of battering on women and coined the term *battered woman syndrome*. The syndrome is a group of transient psychological symptoms that are observed in a particular recognizable pattern in women and is a subcategory of post-traumatic stress disorder (see Chapter 10 for more information on post-traumatic stress disorder).

BATTERED MEN

Little is known about the battered male. Dutton (1988) and Stets and Straus (1990) concluded that men underreport their own assaults. Data are not available on the number of men who are assaulted by their female partners. Some studies suggest that because men do not sustain serious injury or chronic severe assaults, they feel that police reports are not warranted. In addition, it may be difficult for men to admit that they cannot handle their women partners (Kaufman-Kantor & Straus, 1990). Men may also tolerate a certain level of violence from their spouse or partner as a result of traditional cultural norms.

Nurses need to be aware of the reality that men can be victims of battering. The man who has been assaulted by his partner cannot be ignored or dismissed.

CAUSES OF ABUSE: PERSPECTIVES AND THEORIES

Psychological and sociological factors are important to consider in attempting to understand family and interpersonal violence. Psychologists emphasize individual characteristics and personalities as the roots of the aggression. Certain personalities, such as the suspicious, paranoid, and sadistic types, have been associated with a proclivity to abuse.

PSYCHOANALYTICAL THEORY

Psychoanalytical theory proposes that the basic instinct of aggression is expressed or suppressed as a result of a wide variety of internal and external factors. The tenet of psychoanalytical thought is that because some basic need (or needs) of the person is not met, the person instinctively responds in a violent manner. This instinctivist theory proposes that aggression is an innate drive and that humans are fundamentally motivated by aggression (for an in-depth discussion of aggression, see Ardrey, 1966, and Lorenz, 1966).

NEUROPHYSIOLOGICAL THEORY

Neurophysiological theory concludes that violence is the result of many environmental and physical factors (Moyer, 1976). Laboratory studies indicate that animals' aggression is caused by stimuli and is not simply spontaneous.

The biological theory related to aggression suggests that the limbic system and the neurotransmitters play a role in the development of violent behavior. Within the limbic system's influence is the mediation of the aggressive sexual and emotional responses (deGroot & Chusid, 1988). Interference with the processes of information through brain lesions, substance use, head injury, malnutrition, and medical conditions such as epilepsy may contribute to the expression of aggression (Harper-Jacques & Reimer, 1992). The limbic system influences memory storage, information interpreting and processing, and the autonomic functions of the nervous system.

Additionally, research has suggested that exposure to trauma can evoke persistent biological abnormalities (Friedman, 1993). Post-traumatic stress disorder, often diagnosed in victims of sexual and physical trauma, has been associated with a hyperadrenergic state, hypofunctioning of the hypothalamic-pituitary-adrenocortical system, and dysregulation of the endogenous opioid system (Friedman, 1993). Physiological changes include sympathetic hyperarousal, excessive startle reflex, abnormalities in sleep physiology, and traumatic nightmares. Post-traumatic stress disorder is often viewed as a disorder of arousal (Everly & Benson, 1989), which has direct implications for nursing interventions. Successful planning for the victim and the perpetrator must include reducing the pathognomonic arousal through a variety of behavioral interventions such as cognitive restructuring and relaxation techniques.

SOCIAL LEARNING THEORY

Social learning theory has also provided explanations for aggression and violence. Bandura (1973) postulated that aggression is stimulated and can be learned through modeling, observation, or direct experience. The models for aggression are found within families, the mass media, and society at large.

SOCIOLOGICAL THEORIES

Sociological theories of violence address cultural attitudes toward aggression, societal structures that permit aggression, and social frustration and fragmentation. Violence as a cultural attitude is reflected in the glorification of violent behavior in movies and television. Our society reflects a permissive attitude toward violence in our willingness to accept aggression as part of daily living.

The sociologist Gelles (1983; Straus & Gelles, 1990) has stated that the problem of domestic violence is simply a reflection of our violent society. From survey research, Gelles has concluded that violence in the family is committed equally by men and women and is an overall response to stress. The stress is a result of social and economic inequities that families experience. On the other hand, sociologists emphasize the violent nature of American society and our tolerance of the violence. Our society accepts certain levels of violence, and the social ethos in America is such that we are conditioned to strike out at those who trouble or frustrate us (Ziegler & Hall, 1989).

PSYCHOSOCIAL FACTORS

The psychosocial factors or characteristics of abusive families have also been identified. Psychologists (Starr, 1988; Wolfe, 1987) have identified a set of risk factors or correlates for child abuse that includes the following:

- Isolation from family and friends
- High ratio of negative to positive interactions with various family members
- High level of expressed anger and impulsivity
- Inappropriate expectations of the child
- Relatively high rates of both actual and perceived stress

Irrespective of the theoretical account of child abuse, there are certain factors that are consistently mentioned in the literature. Impulse control, anger control, conditioned emotional arousal, weak personality development, and emotion-focused coping are examples of the factors cited in the child abuse literature (Widom, 1989; Wolfe, 1985). In addition, the family unit has changed considerably over the last century, with the result that children no longer live with extended family members. Many parents thus do not have adult support in the raising of their children, and the family is isolated. If there is abuse in the family, the family may respond by becoming even more isolated.

Yet families' increased isolation is only one factor and in itself does not explain the abuse of children. In the 1970s, the popular belief was that abusive parents had personality disorders that predisposed them to aggressive impulses and acting out. However, that view discounts social and cultural factors. Violence against children is better seen as an interaction of various factors, including psychological, sociological, cultural, situational, and societal influences.

GENERAL SYSTEMS THEORY

The psychological perspective looks for causes of violence within the individual, whereas the sociological view looks at the structure of the family. Straus et al. (1980) claimed that the family is society's most violent social institution. Straus (1973) presented the following eight propositions to illustrate how general systems theory relates to family violence:

1. Violence between family members has many causes and roots. Normative structures, personality traits, frustrations, and conflicts are only some.
2. More family violence occurs than is reported.
3. Most family violence is either denied or ignored.
4. Stereotyped family violence imagery is learned in early childhood from parents, siblings, and other children.
5. Family violence stereotypes are continually reaffirmed for adults and children through ordinary social interactions and the mass media.
6. Violent acts by violent persons may generate positive feedback—that is, these acts may produce desired results.
7. Use of violence, when contrary to family norms, creates additional conflicts over ordinary violence. The conflict now becomes the *use of violence*, not the behavior that elicited that response in the first place.
8. Persons who are labeled violent may be encouraged to play out a violent role, either to live up to others' expectations of them as violent or to fulfill their own concept of themselves as violent or dangerous.

THE FEMINIST PERSPECTIVE

Abuse of partners has been discussed from several theoretical vantage points, all of which vary considerably. The feminist perspective holds that wife abuse is the result of attitudes in our patriarchal society that support the inequality of women (Dobash & Dobash, 1992). Some literature suggests that battered women are masochistic (Shainess, 1984) or think they deserve the abuse because of some personality defect (Snell et al., 1964). Other literature has focused on the psychological nature of the interactions between the partners and emphasizes the dyadic patterns in the relationships (for a discussion of dyads, see Chapter 22). O'Leary (1988) and Rosenbaum and Maiuro (1990) described the relationships as being characterized by physical aggression and abuse.

Feminists (Ferree, 1990; Goldner et al., 1990; Schechter, 1982) refer to domestic violence as *wife battering* and assert that it is a means of keeping women in a subordinate position. Feminist theory goes on to explain that although only some men batter, all men benefit from the atmosphere of intimidation that it creates.

THE SOCIAL PSYCHOLOGIST PERSPECTIVE

Social psychologists focus on the social learning that contributes to violence. They note that batterers and, less often, the women who are battered, come from violent families. When people grow up in a family context of violence, they learn that violence is a legitimate form of communication. Families socialize their children into violence, creating an intergenerational transfer of violent behavior.

ROLE OF STRESS

The theoretical perspectives on the causes and correlates of abuse are many and varied. Some models focus on the individual etiological model, but an erroneous implication of this model is that one should be able to identify a potentially abusive person. Research has shown that it is not useful to have lists of characteristics of potential abusers, because people do not fall into neat categories. Therefore, some researchers use interactive theories, which combine several mutually affective forces (Zigler & Hall, 1989). Basic to these theories are social stresses, including families' interactions with society and the resulting pressures on the families. The role of stress, particularly in the area of child abuse, has been repeatedly emphasized. Garbarino (1983) and Gaudin and Pollane (1983) are only two examples of researchers who have noted that stressed parents are socially isolated, seldom have close ties with extended family or community, and are economically deprived. These families are presumed to have greater stresses than other families and, because of their greater disconnectedness from the community, are more likely to abuse. Other studies have revealed that there are high levels of child abuse in military families, connecting this fact to the transience associated with military life (James et al., 1984), and in families whose members' lives are complicated by new babies and expensive health problems, prematurity, or the departure of one parent from the workforce (Zigler & Hall, 1989). The psychosocial approach to abusive families has also identified a high level of life stress as a correlate to abuse. Life changes, physical illnesses, poor emotional health, and weak kinship associations all may be predisposing factors for the maltreatment of a child or other family member.

ROLE OF COPING AND ADAPTATION

Determining the predisposition for violence involves looking beyond pathology to maladaptive characteristics (Table 19–5). Role disturbance, power imbalance, and marital dissatisfaction all are correlates of abuse. Failure to cope with or adapt to stress leads to low frustration tolerance, which in turn can exacerbate a situation to a crisis level. The solution to the perceived crisis is violence and aggression. Families with members who engage in maltreatment tend to exhibit a pattern of coping characterized by a low level of social exchange, low responsiveness to positive behavior, and high responsiveness to negative behavior. These families cope ineffectively and demonstrate inconsistent punishment and discipline (Garbarino, 1984).

Alcohol abuse and substance abuse also play a role in abuse in the family. Maladaptive coping in the form of substance abuse can interfere with a person's ability to parent.

Lack of parenting skills, difficulties with intimacy, and generalized poor interpersonal skills may result in a proclivity for maltreating behaviors. Yet none of these

TABLE 19–5
Effects of Abuse on the Family

IMMEDIATE EFFECTS
Yelling, screaming, verbal outbursts
Erratic discipline
Corporal punishment
Isolation of members
Unrealistic expectations
Disengagement or enmeshment
Role disruption
Power struggles
LONG-TERM EFFECTS
Psychopathology/mental disturbances
Separation or divorce
Running away
Court intervention
Social service involvement
Disturbances in school and work
Health problems
Drug or alcohol abuse
Intrafamilial homicide

characteristics has direct causation. There is no single cause of violence, and violence occurs in all socioeconomic, religious, and ethnic groups.

Child abuse, for example, is an exceedingly complex problem. To characterize the problem as stemming from one underlying cause, no matter what the theoretical viewpoint, would be an oversimplification. Child abuse in the 1990s is the result of complicated interplay of several factors: poor parenting skills, social isolation, poverty, substance abuse, or a combination of these things. Family members' methods of coping and their ability to adapt to stress is but one influence in the development, escalation, or intervention of violence.

ABUSE ACROSS THE LIFE SPAN

IMMEDIATE EFFECTS OF CHILD ABUSE

The immediate effects of child abuse on the victim and the family are enormous. Regardless of the type of abuse a child sustains, research suggests that maltreated children demonstrate the following effects at varying levels of severity: disruptions in relationships, behavioral symptomatology, and developmental deficits (see Aber et al., 1989, for a review).

Disruptions in relationships can be observed in children through their interactions with their primary caregivers. Abused and neglected children may have difficulties in exploring and coping with the demands of new relationships and may demonstrate distortions in their relationships with their caregivers. These distortions include a tendency to be passive with the abusing parent rather than either difficult or compliant. Some abused children may exhibit excessive dependency, wariness, and an inability to form interpersonal relationships.

Critical to an understanding of the effects of abuse on the child and adolescent is an appreciation of the components of the abuse. The nature of the act; the relationship of the perpetrator to the child; the response of other caregivers to the abuse; the frequency of the abuse; the duration and the severity of the abuse; and child-specific factors such as gender, coping and adaptation ability, and developmental level must be taken into account.

Children who are abused and neglected present with a wide variety of immediate effects. The nurse needs to consider the various defense mechanisms children may use to cope with the reality of the abuse. Like adults, children need to protect themselves from the emotional pain of the abuse. Common defense mechanisms used by children include denial, regression, projection, dissociation, and repression. Nurses also need to be aware of the immediate effects seen in children who are abused and neglected, some of which are delineated in Table 19–6. The nurse is cautioned, however, to remember that many of the effects will also present in the long term in the child.

Although the immediate effects of childhood victimization are varied, an overriding effect is the erosion of trust. Without the ability to trust, a child cannot develop healthy relationships or meet the daily challenges of life. Children who are abused also have a confused sense of self. The loss of self-esteem, directly related to the abuse, creates a child who is filled with self-doubt, self-blame, and self-hatred. The nurse may recognize the immediate effects of child abuse through the child's expression of shame, embarrassment, guilt, and a sense of being different from other children.

TABLE 19–6
Immediate Effects of Abuse on the Child and Adolescent

BEHAVIORAL

- Acting out
- Aggression
- Hyperactivity
- Self-destructive acts
- Antisocial and delinquent behaviors (e.g., cruelty to animals, fire setting, or fecal smearing)
- Sexual acting out (promiscuity, prostitution, or sexualization)
- Withdrawal and avoidance
- Somatic complaints and psychosomatic symptomatology

EMOTIONAL

- Depression
- Anxiety
- Anger
- Fears and phobias
- Psychotic processes
- Self-deprecating thoughts

COGNITIVE

- Distractibility
- Inability to concentrate
- Memory impairment
- Poor judgment

INTERPERSONAL

- Poor peer relationships
- Conflictual family relationships
- Disrespect and disregard for authority

CONTROVERSY

What is the false memory syndrome?

Current debate has focused on the long-submerged memories of childhood sexual abuse that resurface to consciousness after years or decades of repression. The number of adults who claim to retrieve repressed memories of childhood sexual abuse has increased dramatically, and divergent professional opinions have emerged. One response by professionals has been to believe the victims, even after decades of amnesia, because of the nature of traumatic memories. On the opposite side, professionals claim that memories are fabricated by overzealous therapists who "invent" rather than discover sexual abuse histories.

One response to this controversy has been the formation of the False Memory Syndrome Foundation, a private organization, in 1992 in Philadelphia, Pennsylvania. This group's purpose and function are to understand the proliferation of the false memory syndrome (a term the group coined), to prevent the exacerbation of the syndrome, and to assist the victims, both primary and secondary, who are harmed by the syndrome. The debate among professionals will no doubt continue for years as each side argues the malleability of memories and the psychological processes of the unconscious mind.

The effect of child abuse on the family can be disruptive and reflective of the child's adaptation. Family members may respond to the disclosure of abuse with disbelief, denial, anger, hostility, and feelings of revenge (see the Controversy display above).

IMMEDIATE EFFECTS OF BATTERING

Women's responses to repeated acts of violence within an intimate partner relationship have been described in the nursing literature in great depth. Campbell's (1989) research on battered women delineated the responses into physical, psychological, and behavioral areas. Battering of men by female intimate partners can produce the same immediate physical and psychological symptoms.

The immediate, overt physical effects of battering include bruises, swellings, lacerations, fractures, hematomas, blackened eyes, abdominal injuries (especially during pregnancy), burns, and open wounds. Yet the victim may explain all of these physical effects as the result of something other than battering. Women are often embarrassed, humiliated, and fearful to disclose that they are being abused by an intimate partner. They may feel the need to protect the batterer by excusing his behavior or may cover for the batterer in an attempt to be viewed favorably by either the batterer or others. Battered women may develop sleep problems, eating problems, and physiological reactivity to the abuse. These women report pain, headaches, and panic reactions.

The immediate psychological effects of battering on women include depression, low self-esteem, anxiety, and stress response. These effects are directly related to the destructiveness, unpredictability, and uncontrolled nature of the violence. The attacks—verbal, physical, and sexual—typically occur without warning or can be in response to some minor infraction that the batterer uses as an excuse to assault the woman. The battered woman realizes that she cannot reason with her attacker and is helpless in her attempts to resist the attacks. It is during these acute battering incidents that the woman feels psychologically trapped (Walker, 1989).

The behavioral responses of the battered woman are a direct result of the abuse. For example, many women learn that to respond to the violence with physical fighting serves only to escalate the man's violence toward them. Battered women are often isolated from supportive resources and outside intervention and thus remain in the relationship because they do not have adequate resources to leave. Battered women endure abuse to protect their children, to protect other relatives, and in some instances, to protect what is familiar to them. The women often assume responsibility for the marriage and believe that to end the relationship indicates personal failure. One of the extreme behavioral responses to battering is the realistic fear of homicide. Battered women who kill their abusive partners are responding out of fear: these women believe that killing is the only way for them to stay alive. Only 12 percent of the homicides in the United States are committed by women, most of whom killed a violent partner (Browne & Williams, 1989).

As mentioned earlier, many women who have experienced battering in an intimate relationship develop a recognized pattern of psychological symptoms called *battered woman syndrome* (Walker, 1993). These symptoms are usually transient but are observed in a recognizable pattern in women who have been physically, sexually, or seriously psychologically abused by their partner. Components of battered woman syndrome are consistent with post-traumatic stress disorder. For example, it is usual for battered women to experience flashbacks to the battering incidents, and when the intrusive memories are too overwhelming, it is not uncommon for battered women to dissociate from the memories. Battered women experience avoidance of thoughts about the abuse, depression, and anxiety-based symptoms.

IMMEDIATE EFFECTS OF ABUSE OF OLDER ADULTS

The older adult who is a victim of abuse and neglect may present with physical injuries, often unexplained, such as fractures, bruises, abrasions, and hematomas. He or she may appear dehydrated, untidy, malnourished, and in some cases, oversedated. The elderly victim may be in need of hearing, vision, and walking appliances, indicating that his or her physical needs are not being met. The psychological effects present in the elderly victim are commonly withdrawal, passivity, hopelessness, and nonresponsiveness. The older adult may resist talking about the injuries, especially if the person believes he or she is dependent on the perpetrator for his or her livelihood. The abused older adult is often embarrassed, humiliated, and defensive.

CONTROVERSY

Are abused children more likely than nonabused children to become abusers?

Research has not confirmed the popular notion that abuse in childhood creates circumstances for the victim to become a victimizer. Most persons with histories of abuse do not grow up to abuse their own or anyone else's children. The intergenerational transmission of violence must not be blindly accepted; rather, the nurse must carefully examine the history of abuse as one risk factor for becoming abusive. Researchers claiming to have found support for the intergenerational hypothesis have not used comparison subjects and prospective, longitudinal designs in their studies.

For further reading, see Kaufman, J., & Zigler, E. (1989). The intergenerational transmission of child abuse. In D. Cicchetti & V. Carlson (Eds.), Child maltreatment: Theory and research on the causes and consequences of child abuse and neglect *(pp. 129–150). Cambridge, England: Cambridge University Press.*

LONG-TERM EFFECTS OF ABUSE

In Children. The long-term consequences of child abuse are complex and insidious. The human cost of the mistreatment of children is staggering. Children who are abused inherit a litany of psychological effects, poor interpersonal relationships, cognitive and developmental deficits, and low self-esteem. In the long term, many of these children present with behavior problems and psychopathology, some of which last a lifetime.

Children who are physically abused, neglected, or sexually victimized grow up with fundamental deficiencies in trust, autonomy, and initiative (Herman, 1992). The challenges of adulthood, such as achieving independence and forming intimate relationships, are compromised. The child has a reduced ability to care for himself or herself, to trust others, and to create a satisfying life. Without intervention, these children grow up haunted by the fear of abandonment or exploitation (Herman, 1992). In response to these fears, it is not unusual for the adult to seek out powerful authority figures who appear to be special caretakers. The adult survivor of abuse has difficulty in protecting himself or herself in the context of intimate relationships and may experience intense, unstable relationships. The adult survivor is at risk of repeated victimization later in life (Herman, 1992).

Another risk for victims, although not the majority of victims, is to become perpetrators of violence themselves. There is much argument concerning "the cycle of violence" or the intergenerational transmission of violence (see the Controversy display on this page). Clearly, there are victims who become perpetrators, but most survivors neither abuse nor neglect their children. Many adults who were victimized are terribly fearful of hurting their own children and go to great lengths to avoid the possibility. The experience of abuse in childhood leaves a legacy of disequilibrium that at any juncture can manifest itself in the form of symptomatic effects or psychiatric disorder.

Battering. The consequences of violence against intimate partners are enormous. The physical injuries women experience can be severe and long-lasting. The psychological effects can include passivity, lack of self-esteem, inability to deal with anger, and failure to nurture the self (Walker, 1993). The woman may remain socially isolated, be financially unstable, and engage in self-blame. Battering creates feelings of terror, constant anxiety, apprehension, and lingering self-doubt about the ability to cope. Other long-term effects from the battering, which includes marital rape, include sexual dysfunction, confusion regarding intimacy, negative feelings toward men, and fear of men.

Women who have been battered are changed forever. Their experiences can be integrated through therapy, and the nurse needs to be aware of four areas of assessment over the long term (Mackey, 1992):

- Social support disturbances
- Sexual dysfunction
- Affective disturbances
- Post-traumatic stress disorder

Table 19–5 summarizes the general immediate and long-term effects of abuse on the family.

In Older Adults. The long-term physiological and psychological effects of elder abuse are similar to the immediate effects of abuse and include permanent injuries, such as fractures, dehydration or electrolyte imbalance, and possible death. Feelings of helplessness, hopelessness, and persistent despondency and depression often evolve over time. Elder abuse also increases the risk of suicide, particularly when coupled with depression. As previously mentioned, the elderly client may be dependent on his or her abuser and reluctant to discuss circumstances surrounding injuries.

TREATMENT MODALITIES

INTERVENTIONS FOR FAMILIES AND PARENTS

Parents who abuse their children may present with issues of chronic low self-esteem, depression, dependency, immaturity, impulsiveness, suspiciousness, and lack of empathy. Environmental stresses include financial problems, intergenerational family myths (i.e., parents usually raise their children the way they were brought up), or difficulties with family structures (i.e., single-parent families, large families, or blended families). The stresses can contribute to serious family dysfunction, resulting in child maltreatment. The nursing interventions are to teach or improve stress management, to foster positive parent–child interactions, and to help parents manage their conflicts. The collaboration of different service providers may be needed. However, nurses need to be aware that the involvement of too many professionals or services may frustrate a family and engender feelings of powerlessness.

INTENSIVE HOME-BASED SERVICES

Intensive home-based (family preservation) services are becoming increasingly popular. This provides short-term, intensive interventions aimed at preventing the removal of the children from the home. Short-term concrete behavioral objectives for the family are jointly contracted with the professional.

INDIVIDUAL THERAPY

Individual therapy ranges from insight-oriented psychotherapy to behavioral treatment. The specific type of therapy used with a family is determined by the family's or victim's current situation, ability to verbalize feelings, and willingness to effect change. The following are some of the issues discussed in individual therapy:

- Past history of abuse
- Attitudes toward violence
- Meaning ascribed to events
- Anger/impulse control
- Sexuality and intimacy
- Stress
- Substance abuse

Therapy for abusing parents focuses on the parents' ability to protect their child and meet the child's developmental needs. See Chapter 21 for further description of individual therapy.

COUPLES THERAPY

Couples therapy can be beneficial when parents realize that their anger toward and frustration with each other are being redirected onto the children. Couples can be taught direct styles of communication that encourage expression of their feelings, listening techniques, and effective verbalizations.

In families in which incest is occurring, the focus of couples therapy is on the effect of the incest on the dyad. Issues in therapy include the couple's capacity for intimacy, sexual relations in the relationship, communication, respect, and an examination of roles and responsibilities.

FAMILY THERAPY

Family therapy can also be a productive intervention if the family members are verbal, the children are old enough to participate, and the level of anger in the family is controlled. The goal of intervention is to prevent further maltreatment. The following are examples of family therapy objectives:

- Confrontation of the abuse
- Identification of the patterns of abuse
- Setting of short- and long-term goals for the family in relation to the abuse
- Discussion of family rules and roles

Issues discussed with abusive families include the following:

- Impulse control
- Judgment errors
- Conflicts with authority
- Manipulative behaviors
- The tendency to act out rather than talk
- Blurred boundaries
- Role dysfunction
- Imbalance of power
- Communication skills
- Trust and intimacy

See Chapter 22 for further discussion of family and couples therapy.

GROUP THERAPY

Group therapy interventions provide unique opportunities for family members to work on issues of trust, differentiation, and responsibility. Group therapy enhances interpersonal communication and provides safe opportunities for social relationships. Groups reduce isolation by bringing parents together and improve self-esteem by introducing parents to other families who are struggling. Groups help parents learn to trust and receive and give support. During the group process, members confront their use of denial, projection, and rationalization defenses.

Group therapy is often the treatment of choice for child sexual offenders. It may also be the treatment of choice for adult survivors of childhood sexual abuse. Chapter 23 provides more information on group therapy.

PSYCHIATRIC HOSPITALIZATION AND PHARMACOLOGICAL INTERVENTIONS

Psychiatric assessment should be considered when clients are chronically depressed or express affective or thought disorders (see Chapter 9). Advanced-practice nurses may be involved in providing individual, group, couples, or family treatment. A referral to a psychiatrist may be necessary if medication or inpatient hospitalization is indicated.

SUBSTANCE ABUSE THERAPY

Substance abuse therapy provides medical treatment, addictions treatment, and support services for nonabusers. Most communities have services for drug and alcohol abusers, including

- Detoxification programs
- Inpatient hospital programs
- Outpatient programs
- Health Services
- Parent education classes
- Employment training or retraining
- Self-help or support groups (e.g., Parents Anonymous; see Chapter 23 for discussions of types of self-help groups)
- Educational support (i.e., graduate equivalent degree [GED] courses)
- Legal referrals and resources

TREATMENT FOR CHILDREN

Art Therapy. *Art therapy* allows children to express their feelings and conflicts. Art therapy is helpful as both a diagnostic and therapeutic tool.

Group Therapy. *Group therapy* allows abused children to regain their status as children. The group provides peer interactions and age-appropriate tasks. Victims are validated for their feelings and reinforced that they are not at fault. Groups for sexually abused children can help correct the distortions in the parent–child relationship. Groups should be a safe place for children to talk and play out their feelings. The group leaders are role models and help the children learn to relate to peers who have also been abused.

Individual Therapy. *Individual therapy* is suggested for children who can verbalize their feelings and needs. Therapy is directed toward their fears, conflicts, and the disclosure of the trauma associated with the abuse. Therapy helps the child process the abuse.

Play Therapy. *Play therapy* is indicated for children too young to have the capacity for introspection and verbalization (toddlers to 6 year olds). Play therapy allows the children to demonstrate their feelings through their actions. The abusive behaviors are observed in their play.

Special Education Programs. *Special education programs* for the physically, developmentally, or emotionally disabled children should be considered by the nurse when these children present with maltreatment.

Therapeutic Day Schools. *Therapeutic day schools* are also available for maltreated children. These programs provide a safe environment in which children can develop the ability to trust. The consistent routines with professionals allow children to test their feelings and actions, such as anger and fear, in an accepting environment.

Other Services. Other services for children include early childhood intervention programs, supportive services such as community or church groups, and, when indicated, out-of-home placement.

THE NURSE'S ROLE

LEGAL AND ETHICAL ISSUES

Violence is clearly a significant health problem in the United States. Nurses are in a key position to prevent and identify abuse and intervene on behalf of both victims and offenders. Nurses need to remain alert to women's and children's increased risk of abuse. Nurses have a mandate to question the health care system's management of victims and victimizers and to explore alternative ways in which the needs of these special populations can be met.

Questions and statements that can encourage discussion include the following:

- What behaviors should be defined as violent?
- What behaviors, including aggressive communication, should be defined as morally intolerable?
- Are certain personality traits associated with violence?
- Should abused children be placed in foster care?
- Does corporal punishment constitute maltreatment of children?
- Is abuse of children not recognized and/or underreported by professionals because many fear the consequences of recognition?
- Do children have rights?
- Is abuse the woman's problem, and must she accept responsibility to leave the relationship?
- Can violent offenders be rehabilitated?
- Can nurses' attitudes toward violence impede the progress of victims?

THE NURSE'S ROLE IN THE LEGAL SYSTEM

Nurses have a mandated responsibility to report suspected child abuse and neglect (see earlier discussion in the section on definitions and incidence of abuse). To report suspected abuse or neglect, nurses should follow the procedures specified by their employer.

Clients' right to confidentiality is typically waived in regard to child abuse reporting. All professionals are required to report their suspicions, even if the information comes from the client. The majority of states have laws protecting the mandated professional from civil lawsuits or criminal prosecution as a result of reporting child abuse in good faith. Many states have penalties for failure to report. Each nurse needs to become familiar with his or her state laws regarding reporting, because reporting procedures vary from state to state (see Table 19–7).

TABLE 19–7
Child Abuse: How the Nurse Fits into the Reporting and Intervention Process

STEPS 1 THROUGH 3: THE NURSE'S ROLE

1. The nurse suspects reportable child abuse. A case conference is convened as indicated.
2. Reports are made to the state authority (child protective services or law enforcement) by telephone or in person.
3. A written report may be required. The content should include the following:
   a. Demographics of the child and the family
   b. Nature and content of injuries, in detail
   c. Caretaker information

STEPS 4 THROUGH 7: THE STATE'S ROLE

4. The state agency initiates an investigation. High-risk assessments require response within 24 to 48 hours.
5. Family assessment takes place.
6. Case management ensues. If abuse is indicated, the child protective service workers may initiate any or all of the following:
   a. Treatment
   b. Referrals
   c. Court intervention
7. Closure of case is implemented.

Policies and protocols for reporting are well established. Typically, the following are specified:

- Roles and responsibilities of the professional nurse
- Definition of abuse and neglect
- Type and specificity of information needed
- Intervention styles
- Description of necessary documentation
- Legal rights of the nurse
- Coordination and collaboration procedures

Nurses can play a major role in the child protection system and judicial system. They are instrumental in identifying and reporting suspected child abuse (see Chapter 5).

GENERALIST'S ROLE

The generalist nurse is integral to the mental health team that intervenes on the behalf of victims and their families. The generalist nurse has the skill and expertise to provide interventions at all junctures for the client. The nurse in the psychiatric setting implements the nursing process to assist the client to explore feelings related to the abuse. The nurse acts as advocate while helping the client negotiate the many systems (such as health care and child protective services; schools; the workplace; community agencies; grassroot service organizations [food banks, day care centers, shelters, self-help or support groups]; fraternal organizations; ethnic, cultural, and religious organizations; and social and recreational groups) that may affect the client. The generalist nurse assesses the client's functional health status and mental status and establishes the goals of the nurse–client relationship. The generalist nurse works in collaboration and coordination with all health professionals.

Nurses are in a key position to assess, understand, and evaluate a victim's emotional responses following traumatic experiences. The nurse has the skill to develop and implement the one-to-one therapeutic relationship that is so important for the client's optimal functioning.

ADVANCED-PRACTICE NURSE'S ROLE

Advanced-practice nurses conduct evaluations of children and families, provide treatment for victims and perpetrators, and provide clinical consultation to other professionals. They provide testimony in court, either as expert or as fact witnesses. The expert nurse witness offers an opinion about the particular case. The opinion is based on the nurse's education, training, and experience and is in a substantive area (e.g., battering or sexual abuse). The expert nurse is asked to explain the basis for his or her opinion. Expert testimony involves offering factual material about the case and the methodology used to analyze the information.

THE NURSING PROCESS

The family who is experiencing violence requires careful assessment and intervention. Because child maltreatment and adult violence are the result of multiple interacting factors, the nurse's intervention needs to address as many issues as possible.

Assessment

The initial assessment of the family includes a careful history of all members. In obtaining the history, the nurse needs to pay close attention to the following factors:

1. Family structure and function
2. Sex role socialization and role strain
3. Social functioning of each member
4. Ability for each member to fulfill task performance
5. Coping style of each member
6. Resources available to the family in home and community
7. Daily stresses experienced by family
8. Expression of frustration and anger
9. Beliefs about aggression and violence
10. Health status of family

Each factor needs to be explored in depth with the family members. The psychiatric nurse needs to develop a style of interviewing that is comfortable but adaptive to each individual family. Table 19–8 presents guidelines for assessing patterns of physical abuse of a child.

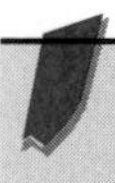

Nursing Care Plan 19–1 The Child Experiencing Sexual Abuse (Kerrie)

► **Nursing Diagnosis:** Fear

► Kerrie, age 5, reveals to her mother that she doesn't like being licked. On questioning, Kerrie reveals that when she visits her father on weekends, he crawls into her bed, lifts up her nightgown, and engages in cunnilingus. Kerrie's mother contacts the local counseling center and is referred to a nurse specialist.

OUTCOME IDENTIFICATION	NURSING ACTIONS	RATIONALES	EVALUATION
1. By [date], Kerrie will engage in discussions/therapeutic play sessions about sexual abuse.	1a. Assess post-traumatic stress response.	1a. Specific behavioral affective and cognitive responses correlate with post-traumatic stress disorder (see text).	*Goals met:* Kerrie participates in therapeutic plan.
	1b. Reassure Kerrie that she is not to blame.	1b. Children do not understand the concept of consent and the motives of the offender.	Kerrie verbalizes that she is not responsible for abuse.
	1c. Encourage Kerrie to express feeling about abuse through play, the use of puppets or dolls for reenactment, stories or role play, or artwork.	1c. Developmentally appropriate interventions facilitate children's expression of trauma and associated memories.	Kerrie experiences a full range of emotions through self-expression. Kerrie expresses appropriate physical boundaries within relationships.
	1d. Record Kerrie's disclosure and clarify with mother the child's use and meaning of unfamiliar words (e.g., "pee pee" may mean vagina to the child).	1d. Contributions by family members can provide corrective information and an accurate understanding of the events. Family participation can assist the child's recovery.	Family provides empathy to Kerrie and reinforces responsibility of abuser. Kerrie perceives parental figures as protective and available.
2. By [date], Kerrie will express feelings of fear, guilt, and anger.	2a. Provide nurturant behaviors.	2a. Enhances trust and models positive behaviors for parents.	Family is receptive to educational and supportive approaches.
	2b. Guide mother to offer love and support to Kerrie.	2b. Fears of blame and retaliation can emerge in the child without continuous parental support.	
3. By [date], Kerrie's mother will develop a plan to assist in Kerrie's recovery.	3. Identify Kerrie's coping skills and assess her educational needs.	3. The parent and child require an accurate understanding of abuse dynamics.	

► TABLE 19–8
Guidelines for Assessing Physical Abuse of a Child

- History of injury given by caretaker does not match injury observed
- Delay in seeking treatment for the child
- Past history of unexplained injuries
- Concealment of injuries by parents
- Recurrent injuries
- Failure to gain appropriate weight

Nursing Diagnosis

The following are possible nursing diagnoses that may be applied to families and individuals who have experienced violence. The list is not comprehensive, but may serve as a reminder.

- Anxiety
- Coping, Ineffective Family: compromised
- Coping, Ineffective Family: disabling
- Coping, Ineffective Individual

Nursing Care Plan 19–2 The Older Adult Experiencing Physical Abuse (Mattie)

► **Nursing Diagnosis:** Hopelessness, related to being a victim of violence (battering)

► Mattie, a frail 84-year-old woman, was referred to the psychiatric nursing consultation service after she appeared in the emergency department with signs of being overmedicated and unexplained bruises on her back. Mattie was accompanied by her 53-year-old son, who stated to the pyschiatric nurse, "You don't know what I've been through. She's always wetting herself. I can't do it all!"

OUTCOME IDENTIFICATION	NURSING ACTIONS	RATIONALES	EVALUATION
1. By [date], Mattie will recognize the abusive behavior she has experienced.	1a. Assure Mattie of confidentiality.	1a. Assurance is essential for the client to feel comfortable opening up because denial is a common defense mechanism when one is abused by a loved one.	*Goal met:* Mattie verbalizes knowledge of abusive behaviors.
	1b. Respect Mattie's right to make her own decisions.	1b. Allowing the client to make her own decisions will restore a sense of self and feelings of being in control.	
	1c. Interview Mattie alone to ensure she does not experience pressure by abuser.	1c. The client may not feel safe in the presence of her son, especially to disclose abusive events that are painful to recall, humiliating, and embarrassing. The client may feel disloyal to her son and, because of the perceived disruption she is creating in the family, she may feel pressure to recant.	
2. By [date], Mattie will express feelings of fear, anxiety, and helplessness related to the abuse.	2a. Spend time with Mattie to promote expression of feelings.	2a. Abusive experiences by her son may be perceived by the client as a loss of an important relationship; therefore, the client will need to re-establish trust through her relationship with the nurse to feel comfortable in revealing her feelings.	Mattie verbalizes acceptance of her feelings about the abuse as valid.
	2b. Be nonjudgmental and be aware of personal feelings.	2b. A nonjudgmental approach is critical, because the client may be reluctant to disclose her feelings if she senses blame by the nurse. Issues of abuse may evoke ambivalent, confusing feelings in the nurse and may interfere with the therapeutic relationship.	
	2c. Accept Mattie's ability to reveal abuse and pace interviews accordingly.	2c. Acknowledgment of the reality of the abuse can be frightening and painful;	

Nursing Care Plan 19–2 The Older Adult Experiencing Physical Abuse (Mattie) (Continued)

OUTCOME IDENTIFICATION	NURSING ACTIONS	RATIONALES	EVALUATION
		therefore, assist clients in the retrieval of memories so as not to overwhelm them. Traumatic memories may be retrieved in fragments, so allow time for processing. When abuse is disclosed, client may feel powerless over the situation and overwhelmed by the disclosure.	
3. By [date], Mattie will not present as a danger to herself (potential for self-injury).	3a. Assess Mattie's potential for suicide and any suicide ideation or plan.	3a. Disclosure and discussion of the abuse may trigger feelings of worthlessness and hopelessness. The client may believe she is a burden to her family and therefore deserves to die.	Mattie expresses anger and hopelessness appropriately.
	3b. Refer Mattie for counseling if she verbalizes suicidal plan.	3b. Referral is necessary to protect the client from herself and any suicidal impulses.	
4. By [date], Mattie will be provided with alternative methods of care.	4a. Investigate need for a complete physical assessment of Mattie.	4a. A client's health status is affected by abuse. Basic needs in terms of hydration, nutrition, and elimination may not be met.	Mattie and family participate in community programs designed for the family and caretakers.
	4b. Enlist assistance from other family members.	4b. Additional assistance will provide stress relief to caregiver.	
	4c. Refer Mattie and her family to day programs, day care centers for the elderly, and respite care.	4c. Alternative programs will relieve stress on family and provide the client with maximum attention to her needs.	

- Denial, Ineffective (especially in the case of the offender, who refuses to acknowledge the abuse)
- Family Processes, Altered
- Fear
- Growth and Development, Altered (as exemplified by the young child who is neglected)
- Hopelessness
- Injury, High Risk for (in the case of a battered woman)
- Parenting, Altered
- Parenting, Altered, High Risk for
- Post-Trauma Response
- Powerlessness
- Rape Trauma Syndrome
- Self-Esteem Disturbance
- Trauma, High Risk for
- Violence, High Risk for: self directed or directed at others

Planning

The nursing care plan for a family or individual who has experienced violence is derived from the nursing diagnoses, which are made on the basis of careful data gathering during assessment. The plan contains the goals and objectives for the care. These goals and objectives are set within realistic time frames and prioritized. For example, the battered woman needs a plan that is mutually derived, one that it specifically sensitive to her desire to end or leave the battering relationship. A short-term goal of separating from her husband would be unrealistic if she had not thought through the consequences of her actions, because leaving the abusive

Nursing Care Plan 19–3 The Child Experiencing Physical Abuse (Charlie)

► **Nursing Diagnosis:** Situational Low Self-Esteem related to physical abuse

► Charlie, an 8-year-old boy, is transferred to the child psychiatry unit after a court-ordered psychiatric evaluation. Charlie has a known history of being abused by his natural mother. A recent attempt to reunite mother and son ended when Charlie reported to the school nurse that his mother was beating him.

OUTCOME IDENTIFICATION	NURSING ACTIONS	RATIONALES	EVALUATION
1. By [date], Charlie will identify feelings of self-worth.	1a. Encourage Charlie to verbalize his thoughts and feelings related to his mother and her abusive actions.	1a. Understanding of the client's perception of abuse and role in the experience is essential to validate the client's feelings.	*Goal met:* Charlie is able to express one positive attribute about himself.
	1b. Offer acceptance to Charlie. Do not use direct confrontation, yet support Charlie in his attempts to verbalize.	1b. Clients need to be viewed as worthwhile persons regardless of their experiences. Positive feedback gives clients the recognition they need to experience success.	
2. By [date], Charlie will express fears related to abuse.	2a. Support Charlie's ventilation of feelings.	2a. Memories of the abuse may evoke distress in Charlie.	Charlie is able to demonstrate trust in his relationship with the nurse by continuing to discuss feelings.
	2b. Create situations to discuss feelings in a safe manner.	2b. Indirect explorations of fears through play, storytelling, and board games can alleviate feelings of anxiety and fear.	
	2c. Anticipate Charlie's stress related to fears and provide problem-solving techniques.	2c. Increased stress interferes with a child's ability to cope. Teaching the child to handle fears will decrease anxiety of relating abuse.	
3. By [date], Charlie will demonstrate improved ability to deal with the effects of physical abuse.	3a. Spend time with Charlie to help him with full expression of a range of feelings.	3a. The child's ability to express feelings is critical to successful healing.	Charlie verbalizes his feelings and thoughts freely and openly.
	3b. Accept all feelings Charlie expresses as valid.	3b. Successful emotional processing of abuse must occur in a wide variety of expressions.	
	3c. Encourage Charlie to explain his feelings.	3c. Clients' distortions and misperceptions need to be corrected.	
	3d. Continually expose Charlie to the realities of his abuse and legal proceedings that may be occurring.	3d. Realization of future outcomes will help clients grieve their losses.	

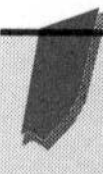

Nursing Care Plan 19–4 The Woman Experiencing Battering (Shelley)

▶ **Nursing Diagnosis:** Fear and Anxiety related to physical threat to self by batterer

▶ Shelley, a 34-year-old mother of four, has been married to Jay for 9 years. Jay, an executive, demands perfection in his job and in his family. Over the past 3 years, since the birth of their fourth child, Jay has become increasingly hostile, belligerent, and abusive. Shelley has repeatedly been to her family physician with vague physical complaints. On New Year's Day, she went to the emergency department for a head injury she claimed occurred when she fell on the ice. In reality, Jay beat her during one of his angry rages. Shelley received 10 stitches above her eye, and examination revealed a mild concussion. Desperate for help, Shelley contacted the Victim Resource Center for counseling with a psychiatric clinical nurse specialist.

OUTCOME IDENTIFICATION	NURSING ACTIONS	RATIONALES	EVALUATION
1. By [date], Shelley will describe the abuse and identify her fears.	1a. Approach Shelley nonjudgmentally. Ensure privacy and confidentiality.	1a. Conveying respect and empathy supports the client's self-worth.	*Goal met:* Shelley reports the extent of her abuse and her need for protection. Shelley is knowledgeable about community resources. Shelley identifies supportive family members and enlists their help.
	1b. Assess level of danger to her by assessing her home situation and available resources. Inquire of Jay's escalating violence.	1b. Enhances the client's awareness of the potential for further injury.	
2. By [date], Shelley will express the need for external resources.	2a. Provide Shelley with information on services available for battered women.	2a. The client's ability to be autonomous and in control is increased through knowledge, education, and outside resources.	
	2b. Explore with Shelley whether she can disclose her situation to trusted family members.	2b. Disclosure of abuse to others facilitates the potential for ending the abuse.	
	2c. Explore Shelley's fears related to contacting resources and informing supportive family members.	2c. The client may be afraid of retaliation by her husband's family and fear that her disclosure of abuse will not be believed. Victims of battering may hold incorrect beliefs about their "causing" the abuse. Allowing Shelley to freely discuss her fears will provide the nurse with the opportunity to provide information and education about the dynamics of battering.	
3. By [date], Shelley will devise a plan to leave the home if needed.	3. Provide local service information, and refer Shelley to a support group if she desires. Allow Shelley to verbalize an escape plan.	3. Information gathering provides client with opportunities for increased self-awareness and facilitates control of self.	Shelley verbalizes a plan of action to ensure the safety of herself and her children.

partner is the most dangerous time for the battered woman.

During the planning stages, the nurse develops the outcome criteria, or anticipated results, by which he or she may determine whether the goals of the nursing care plan were met. The outcome criteria reflect the client's behavior and are extremely individualized.

See Nursing Care Plans 19–1 through 19–4 for examples of how to plan care for a child who is experiencing sexual abuse, an older adult who has been physically abused, a physically abused child, and a battered woman.

Implementation

The implementation phase is the individualized application of the plan of care to the client and the client's unique experience. During the implementation phase, the nurse accepts a variety of roles to help the client achieve his or her goals. The nurse responds to the client as educator, advocate, therapist, and health promoter.

Evaluation

The final phase is the evaluation phase. The nursing care is evaluated in the context of the stated outcome criteria. The evaluation phase is not a discrete entity but rather occurs throughout the nursing process. When the nurse examines the outcome criteria, he or she also examines his or her own behavior and feelings in relation to the client and the care that was offered. The nursing process is an important and significant part of the client's total care, especially when the client has been traumatized by violence.

►CHAPTER SUMMARY

Violence is a significant health problem in the United States. Psychiatric nurses are in a key position to identify, intervene, and treat the victims and perpetrators of violence. It is imperative for psychiatric nurses to have an understanding of the complexities of violence in a family context and to appreciate the cues that signify that violence is occurring and the events that trigger it. Nurses need careful preparation to help families at risk based on the study of life span issues as they relate to abuse. Nurses need to recognize their role in case finding because they are in the forefront of the effort to identify and assess victims. The therapeutic relationship between the psychiatric nurse and the client is a powerful force, and it is within this relationship that victims can learn to trust and change.

Suggestions for Clinical Conference

1. Discuss individual perceptions, attitudes, and beliefs regarding the disciplining of children. Suggested questions include the following:
   a. Should parents be allowed to use corporal punishment on their children?
   b. Should schools be permitted to use corporal punishment on students?
   c. Do parents who abuse their children have a psychopathological disorder?
2. Discuss the following statements:
   a. Men beat women to gain control and power.
   b. A battered woman who stays in the relationship has a personality disorder or defect.
   c. Battered women are masochistic because they stay.
   d. All women who are battered develop battered woman syndrome.
3. The United States is a violent country. Discuss the factors that contribute to the high incidence of violence in the United States, including handguns, drugs, poverty, and racism.
4. The intergenerational-transmission-of-violence theory proposes that a child learns to be violent. What factors contribute to a person's expressing him- or herself through violent means?
5. Blaming the victim is a powerful force in cases of sexual assault, particularly in cases of teenage victims of incest. Discuss this phenomenon.
6. Discuss how you would evaluate a caretaker's stress in regard to caring for an elderly dependent parent. How would you plan to evaluate the elderly client?
7. Discuss how violence may differentially affect various cultures.
   a. Homicide is the leading cause of death in African American men.
   b. Family is all-important in the Hispanic culture.
   c. Divorce is shameful in Asian cultures.

References

Aber, J. L., Allen, J. P., Carlson, V., & Cicchetti, D. (1989). The effects of maltreatment on development during early childhood: Recent studies and their theoretical, clinical and policy implications. In A. Cicchetti & V. Carlson (Eds.), *Child maltreatment: Theory and research on the causes and consequences of child abuse and neglect* (pp. 579–619). Cambridge, England: Cambridge, University Press.

American Psychiatric Association. (1994). *Diagnostic and statistical manual of mental disorders* (4th ed.). Washington, DC: Author.

Ardrey, R. (1966). *The territorial imperative*. New York: Antheneum.

Bandura, A. (1973). *Aggression: A social learning analysis*. Englewood Cliffs, NJ: Prentice-Hall.

Block, M. R., & Sinott, J. D. (1979). *The battered elder syndrome: An exploratory study*. College Park: Division of Human and Community Resources, University of Maryland.

Brendtro, M., & Bowker, H. L. (1989). Battered women: How nurses can help. *Issues in Mental Health Nursing, 10*, 169–180.

Browne, A., & Williams, K. R. (1989). Exploring the effect of resource availability and the likelihood of female-perpetrated homicides. *Law and Society Review, 23*(1), 75–94.

Campbell, J. (1989). Women's response to sexual abuse in intimate relationships. *Health Care for Women International, 8*, 335–347.

Child Welfare League of America. (1973). *Standards for Child Protective Service* (Rev. ed.). New York: Author.

deGroot, J., & Chusid, J. G. (1988). *Correlative neuroanatomy*. East Norwalk, CT: Appleton & Lange.

Dobash, R. P., & Dobash, R. E. (1992). *Women, violence, and social change*. New York: Routledge.

Dutton, D. G. (1988). *The domestic assault of women: Psychological and criminal justice perspectives*. Boston: Allyn & Bacon.

Everly, G. S., & Benson, H. (1989). Disorders of arousal. *International Journal of Psychosomatics*, *36*, 15–22.

Fagan, J., Stewart, D., & Hansen, K. (1983). Violent men or violent husbands: Background factors and situational correlates. In D. Finkelhor, R. Gelles, G. Hotaling, & M. Straus (Eds.), *The dark side of families* (pp. 49–67). Beverly Hills, CA: Sage.

Ferree, M. M. (1990). Beyond separate spheres: Feminism and family research. *Journal of Marriage and the Family*, *52*, 866–884.

Finkelhor, D. (1993). The main problem is still underreporting, not overreporting. In R. J. Gelles & D. R. Loseke (Eds.), *Current controversies on family violence* (pp. 273–287). Newbury Park, CA: Sage.

Finkelhor, D., Hotaling, G., Lewis, I. A., & Smith, C. (1990). Sexual abuse in a national survey on adult men and women: Prevalence, characteristics, and risk factors. *Child Abuse and Neglect*, *14*, 19–28.

Finkelhor, D., & Hotaling, G. (1984). Sexual abuse in the National Incidence Study of Child Abuse and Neglect: An appraisal. *Child Abuse and Neglect*, *8*, 22–23.

Friedman, M. J. (1993). Psychobiological and pharmacological approaches to treatment. In J. P. Wilson & B. Raphael (Eds.), *International handbook of traumatic stress syndromes* (pp. 785–794). New York: Plenum Press.

Fulmer, T., & O'Malley, T. (1987). *Inadequate care of the elderly: A health care perspective on abuse and neglect*. New York: Springer.

Garbarino, J. (1984). What have we learned about child maltreatment? In *Perspectives on child maltreatment in the mid 80's* (DHHS Publication No. OHDS 84-30338). Washington, DC: U.S. Government Printing Office.

Garbarino, J. (1983). What we know about child maltreatment. *Children and Youth Services Review*, *5*, 3–6.

Garbarino, J. (1989). The psychologically battered child. *Pediatric Annals*, *18*, 502.

Gaudin, J. M, & Pollane, L. (1983). Social networks, stress and child abuse. *Children and Youth Services Review*, *5*, 91–102.

Gelles, R. J. (1983). An exchange/social control theory. In D. Finkelhor, R. J. Gelles, G. T. Hotaling, & M. A. Straus (Eds.), *The dark side of families: Current family violence research* (pp. 151–165). Beverly Hills, CA: Sage.

Goldner, V., Penn, P., Sheinberg, M., & Walker, G. (1990). Love and violence: Gender paradoxes in volatile attachments. *Family Process*, *29*, 343–364.

Harper-Jaques, S., & Reimer, M. (1992) Aggressive behavior and the brain: A different perspective for the mental health nurse. *Archives of Psychiatric Nursing*, *6*(5), 312–320.

Herman, J. (1992). *Trauma and recovery*. New York: Basic Books.

Hotaling, G., Finkelhor, D., Kirkpatrick, J., & Straus, M. (Eds.). (1988). *Family abuse and its consequences*. Newbury Park, CA: Sage.

James, J. J., Furukawa, T. P., James, N., & Mangelsdorf, A. D. (1984). Child abuse and neglect reports in the United States Army Central Registry. *Military Medicine*, *149*, 205–206.

Kaufman-Kantor, G., & Straus, M. A. (1990). Response of victims and the police to assaults on wives. In M. A. Straus & R. J. Gelles (Eds.), *Physical violence in American families: Risk factors and adaptations to violence in 8,145 families* (pp. 151–166). New Brunswick, NJ: Transaction.

Lazoritz, S. (1990). Whatever happened to Mary Ellen? *Child Abuse and Neglect*, *14*, 143.

Lorenz, K. (1966). *On aggression*. New York: Harcourt, Brace & World.

Ludwig, S., & Kornberg, A. E. (1992). *Child abuse: A medical reference*. New York: Churchill Livingstone.

Mackey, T. F. (1992). The wake of trauma. In C. M. Sampselle (Ed.), *Violence against women* (pp. 181–204). Washington, DC: Hemisphere.

Moyer, K. E. (1976). *The psychobiology of aggression*. New York: Harper & Row.

O'Leary, K. D. (1988). Physical aggression between spouses: A social learning theory perspective. In V. B. Van Hasselt, R. L. Morrison, A. S. Bellack, & M. Hersen (Eds.), *Handbook of family violence* (pp. 11–55) New York: Plenum.

Owen, M., & Coant, P. (1992). Other forms of neglect. In S. Ludwig & A. E. Kornberg (Eds.), *Child abuse: A medical reference* (pp. 349–356). New York: Churchill Livingstone.

Phillips, L. R. (1983). Abuse and neglect of the frail elder at home: An exploration of theoretical relationships. *Journal of Advanced Nursing*, *8*, 379–392.

Pillemer, K. (1993). The abused offspring are dependent. In R. J. Gelles & D. R. Loseke (Eds.), *Current controversies on family violence* (pp. 237–249). Newbury Park, CA: Sage.

Pillemer, K., & Finkelhor, D. (1988). The prevalence of elder abuse: A random sample survey. *The Gerontologist*, *28*, 51–57.

Rosenbaum, A., & Maiuro, R. (1990). Perpetrators of spouse abuse. In R. T. Ammerman & M. Hersen (Eds.), *Treatment of family violence* (pp. 280–309). New York: Wiley.

Russell, D. (1984a). *Rape in marriage*. New York: Macmillan.

Sampselle, C. (1992). *Violence against women*. New York: Hemisphere.

Schechter, S. (1982). *Women and male violence: The visions and struggles of the battered women's movement*. Boston: South End.

Shainess, N. (1984). *Sweet suffering: Women as victim*. Indianapolis, IN: Bobs-Merrill.

Snell, J., Rosenwald, R., & Robey, A. (1964). The wife-beater's wife: A study of family interaction. *Archives of General Psychiatry*, *11*, 107–112.

Starr, D. H. (1988). Physical abuse of children. In V. B. Van Hasselt, R. L. Morrison, A. S. Bellack, & M. Hersen (Eds.), *Handbook of family violence* (pp. 119–155). New York: Plenum.

Steinmetz, S. (1993). The abused elderly are dependent. In R. J. Gelles & D. R. Loseke (Eds.), *Current controversies on family violence* (pp. 222–236). New Park, CA: Sage.

Steinmetz, S. (1988). *Duty bound: Elder abuse and family care*. Newbury Park, CA: Sage.

Steinmetz, S. K., & Straus, M. A. (1974). *Violence in the family*. New York: Harper & Row.

Stets, J. E., & Straus, M. A. (1990). Gender differences in reporting marital violence and its medical and psychological consequences. In M. A. Straus & R. J. Gelles (Eds.), *Physical violence in American families: Risk factors and adaptations to violence in 8,145 families* (pp. 151–166). New Brunswick, NJ: Transaction.

Straus, M. A. (1973). A general systems theory approach to a theory of violence between family members. *Social Science Information*, *12*, 105–125.

Straus, M. A., & Gelles, R. J. (Eds.). (1990). *Physical violence in American families: Risk factors and adaptations to violence in 8,145 families*. New Brunswick, NJ: Transaction.

Straus, M., Gelles, R. J., & Steinmetz, S. K. (1980). *Behind closed doors: Violence in the American family*. Garden City, NY: Anchor/Doubleday.

U.S. Department of Health and Human Services. (1988). Study findings: Study of national incidence and prevalence of child abuse and neglect. Washington, DC: U.S. Government Printing Office.

Walker, L. (1989). *Terrifying love*. New York: Harper & Row.

Walker, L. (1993). The battered woman syndrome is a psychological consequence of abuse. In R. J. Gelles & D. R. Loseke (Eds.), *Current controversies on family violence* (pp. 133–153). Newbury Park, CA: Sage.

Walker, L. (1984). *The battered woman syndrome*. New York: Springer.

Walker, L. (1979). *The battered woman*. New York: Harper/Colophon.

Widom, C. S. (1989). Does violence beget violence? A critical examination of the literature. *Psychological Bulletin*, *106*, 3–28.

Wolfe, D. A. (1987). Child abuse: Implications for child development and psychopathology. Newbury Park, CA: Sage.

Zigler, E., & Hall, N. (1989). Child abuse in America. In D. Cicchetti & V. Carlson (Eds.), *Child maltreatment: Theory and research on the causes and consequences of child abuse and neglect* (pp. 38–75). Cambridge, England: Cambridge University Press.

CHAPTER 20

The Client with a Sexual Disorder

MARGARET BRACKLEY, Ph.D., R.N.,C.S.

OUTLINE

CHAPTER OBJECTIVES

Upon completion of this chapter, you will be able to:

1. Define sexual health.
2. Explain the various theories of sexual development.
3. Identify two different organizational systems that health care professionals use to define sexual problems.
4. Discuss sexual issues across the life span.
5. Explore the professional nursing roles in relation to sexual themes and issues.

6. Cite clinical examples of and relevant research in sexual health care.
7. Assess the sexual health of a client.
8. Analyze the data obtained in the assessment to determine appropriate diagnoses.
9. Identify outcomes of care for the client.
10. Develop a plan of care for the client.
11. Make a referral to an appropriate health care provider if the client is unable or unwilling to execute necessary interventions.
12. Implement the client's plan of care.
13. Evaluate the plan of care for its effectiveness and revise it if necessary.

KEY TERMS

Gender
Love
Self-awareness
Sexual dysfunction
Sexual health
Sexual orientation
Sexual patterns

All human beings are sexual beings. The World Health Organization (WHO) (1975) has defined sexual health as holistic and inseparable from other aspects of health and well-being. In this chapter, a variety of theories on sexual development and health are presented. Sexual issues and themes that the professional nurse will encounter are explored, and the organizational systems that health care professionals use to classify sexual problems are explained. The roles of the generalist and the advanced practice nurse are then described. To begin at the beginning, however, let's consider a definition of sexual health and nurses' need to be aware of their responses to persons who present with sexual issues and problems.

DEFINITIONS OF SEXUAL HEALTH

According to WHO (1975), **sexual health** is the "integration of the somatic, emotional, intellectual and social aspects of sexual being, in ways that are positively enriching, and that enhance personality, communication and love" (p. 3). The WHO is describing a gestalt, a whole, whereby the sexual self cannot be separated from the rest of the self. A sense of unity within the individual thus reflects sexual health as well as nonsexual health. Sexual health is personal. It is defined by each person within the context of his or her physical, emotional, intellectual, social, cultural, and spiritual environment.

THE NURSE'S ATTITUDE TOWARD SEXUALITY

The field of nursing has traditionally recognized and appreciated humans' holistic nature. However, in spite of a fundamental belief in the importance of the total health of the person, until recently, the nursing profession had neglected the sexual aspects of health care. There are a number of reasons for this neglect. Human sexuality has traditionally been ignored and its importance downplayed in Western health care in general. In addition, the field of nursing emerged during the Victorian era; when one considers the attitudes and values of that era, along with the religious undertones and traditions of nursing, one can readily grasp why nurses neglected the sexual aspects of health.

However, nursing professionals have also traditionally supported knowledge as a method to empower individuals and groups. For example, in the 1920s, Margaret Sanger led the fight to educate women about their bodies and birth control. The American Nurses Association (ANA) has resolved in the 1980s and 1990s to (1) support birth control knowledge and access for men and women, even adolescents, and (2) work to preserve the availability of abortion as an alternative to unwanted pregnancy.

SELF-AWARENESS

Self-awareness and awareness of others are key attributes nurses need to address sexual issues or themes in clients and their families. First, nurses must be aware of their own attitudes, values, and beliefs regarding sexual health. Second, nurses must become aware of their clients' sexual issues. Third, nurses must be aware of how their personal attitudes, values, and beliefs affect their ability to recognize, and their reactions to, clients' sexual issues and themes.

For example, the nurse who is having conflict in intimate relationships over sexual issues may be affected by this conflict in several ways. The nurse may see the conflict in a client's intimate relationship as sexual in nature when it is not or may fail to recognize the sexual themes in a client's conflicts. If the nurse focuses on personal awareness, the nurse questions his or her assumption that the conflict was sexual in nature or seeks consultation to ensure that sexual themes are not overlooked. The nurse who has self-awareness is able to do quality checks on the nursing care he or she delivers. The unaware nurse is unable to do this.

REACTIONS TOWARD OTHERS

A word of caution is appropriate here. Untoward reactions have been observed in nurses faced with sexual issues/themes. Strong reactions may indicate the need for the nurse to seek help to address personal issues that prevent his or her own sexual health. Seeking outside help to work through and resolve sexual issues/themes is strongly encouraged. Both the nurse and his or her clients will benefit from resolution of issues that prevent self-awareness in the nurse.

Throughout history and across cultures, many standards for sexual behavior have been accepted. One current standard for human sexual behavior is that pleasure should be maximized while the coercion of others and giving or receiving of pain is minimized. Thus a wide range of human sexual behavior exists. It is often unsettling and even upsetting to the nurse who has not examined his or her own sexual attitudes, values, and beliefs to be faced with the diversity of sexual behaviors that human beings exhibit from person to person and culture to culture. As in all other types of nursing care, the nurse is expected to be nonjudgmental in delivering sexual health care. Being nonjudgmental does not imply agreement with others' values and beliefs. By definition, the nurse "diagnoses and treats human responses to actual or potential health problems" (ANA, 1980, p. 1) that affect human beings. Caring about the client is another recurrent theme in nursing (Benner & Wrubel, 1989). If the nurse cares about the client, the client's experience is worthy of concern, regardless of how it differs from the nurse's.

HEALTHY SEXUALITY

PHYSIOLOGY OF HUMAN SEX

According to Masters and Johnson (1966), who conducted basic research in the 1950s and 1960s on sexual physiology, there are four stages in the human sexual response. This research team observed more than 700 men and women in approximately 10,000 cycles of sexual arousal and orgasm. On the basis of their observations, they identified the following stages of sexual response: excitement, plateau, orgasm, and resolution. The physiological processes of vasocongestion (increased blood flow to the genital area) and myotonia (muscle contraction throughout the body) occur during sexual activity.

The *excitement* phase begins with arousal. Vasocongestion produces an erection in the male sex organ, the penis, and lubrication in the female sex organ, the vagina. During the excitement phase, the woman's clitoris and breast tissues swell. The inner and outer lips of the vagina swell and flatten out, while the vagina balloons out and the cervix pulls up internally. Both the man and woman may develop a sexual flush that resembles a measles rash on the upper abdomen and chest. Pulse and blood pressure increase in both sexes. The skin of the man's scrotum thickens, the scrotal sac tenses, and the contents of the sac pull up closer to the body. The spermatic cord shortens, elevating the testes.

During the *plateau* phase, the man's penis is completely erect, testes become engorged, and a few drops of fluid appear at the tip of the penis. This fluid may contain live sperm. In the woman, the outer third portion of the vagina swells and thickens. The vagina becomes smaller, the clitoris retracts into the body. Vasocongestion and myotonia continue to build until the resultant tension produces an orgasm.

The *orgasm* phase in the man is characterized by rhythmic contractions. Ejaculate is forced into a bulb at the end of the urethra, and then the urethra bulb and the penis itself contract rhythmically to force semen out. In the woman, the process is similar. Rhythmic contractions of the muscles occur in the man and woman in about 0.8-second intervals. Both the woman and man experience sudden increases in pulse rate, blood pressure, and breathing. Muscles contract throughout the body.

In the *resolution* phase, the body returns to the unaroused state. The processes of vasocongestion and myotonia are reversed. In the woman, breast swelling and sex flush disappear rapidly, and the genital changes that occurred during arousal disappear. Resolution occurs in 15 to 30 minutes, unless the woman did not reach orgasm, in which case resolution can take up to 1 hour. In both the man and woman, pulse rate, blood pressure, and breathing gradually return to normal. In the man, penile erection is lost immediately. A refractory period occurs in which the man is incapable of arousal. The length of the refractory period varies with age and other individual differences. In older men, it may last up to 24 hours, while in some younger men it lasts only a few minutes. A refractory period is not present in women.

Kaplan (1974) suggested an alternative to the Masters and Johnson model based on her work as a sex therapist. This biphasic model was divided into vasocongestion and muscular contractions. Later, a third phase—sexual desire—was added. Because vasocongestion and muscular contraction are controlled by separate parts of the nervous system, the parasympathetic and sympathetic nervous systems, respectively, this approach has merit. In clients with sexual problems, treatment depends on the part of the central nervous system affected. Sexual desire also has a neurophysiological component.

The nervous system and sex hormones are important parts of sexual desire and behavior. The sex hormones testosterone, an androgen secreted by the male testes, and progesterone, an estrogen secreted by the female ovaries, are regulated by the anterior lobe of the pituitary gland and the hypothalamus, located on the lower side of the brain. The hypothalamus, pituitary and gonads, the testes and ovaries work together in sexual functions such as the menstrual cycle, pregnancy, puberty, and sexual behavior (Hyde, 1986).

The human sexual response is complex. Sexual disorders and difficulties can arise from multiple sources. Some of these are discussed in the remainder of this chapter. But first, a word about love.

LOVE

Love is a very human trait that is not mentioned often in nursing textbooks or sex education textbooks. Love is important and therefore must not go unmentioned. Not much research has been conducted on love. Romantic love and sexual activities appear to go together, and yet there is discomfort in talking about the relationship between them. These concepts are elusive. More about the relationship between love and sex is offered in the section on helping people change their sexual behavior.

SEXUAL ORIENTATION

The American Psychiatric Association considers variations in **sexual orientation**, that is, homosexuality and bisexuality, as healthy sexuality. No one knows why a person becomes gay, lesbian, or bisexual. Theories that have posited that nonheterosexual sexual orientations result from disturbed family relationships, labeling of opposite-gender-linked behavior (boys playing with dolls), or an unpleasant sexual experience have not been supported through scientific study. It seems plausible that there is a biological basis for differences; twin studies have tended to support this notion (Holden, 1992). There is a growing body of scientific knowledge that links sexual orientation to the brain (Witelson, 1993). However, some scientists believe it is too simplistic to blame biology alone for sexual orientation. In truth, a complex interaction between sexual development within the context of social and familial milieu and individual temperament and personality traits may influence a person's sexual orientation (Byne & Parsons, 1993).

SEXUALITY: PERSPECTIVES AND THEORIES

It is important to know the different theoretical perspectives on sexuality. No theory can claim to be the real truth. This chapter, while acknowledging the different viewpoints of theorists, focuses on the here-and-now problem of the client, the perception and awareness of both the client and nurse, and the nurse's role in helping the client solve the identified problem. In sexual health care, as in all nursing activity, the nurses's therapeutic use of the self is expected. The therapeutic interaction between nurse and client should never be underestimated. The nurse's concern for and acceptance of the client and the problem can have a profound influence on the health care outcome.

BIOLOGICAL THEORIES OF GENDER DEVELOPMENT

Two types of biological theories have been used to explain human sexuality, one of which has for the past several centuries been referred to as "biology is destiny." The focus of this and similar theories is that a person responds in all aspects of life on the basis of whether a male (XY) or female (XX) chromosome pattern is present in the person. Boys are seen as aggressive, independent, productive, and rational, whereas girls are thought to be nurturing, passive, dependent, and intuitive. A neurochemical explanation for sexual differences is the basis of this theoretical stance. No allowance for culture and learning is included in this theory. Sexual intercourse and reproduction are explained as biochemical responses to external and internal factors.

Another biological explanation of human sexuality is sociobiology, the attempt to explain human behavior by evolutionary concepts (Wilson, 1975). Sexual behavior is seen as patterned social behavior that ensures a large gene pool and numerous offspring; through natural selection, the fittest of the human species survive. Sociobiologists suggest that everything from dancing, which allows the potential spouse to see the physical abilities of his or her mate, to the accumulation of wealth, which offers evidence of the ability to support future children, is rooted in the genetic makeup of the human species. What a culture considers attractive in a mate may be none other than characteristics of healthy people (Symons, 1979).

The criticism of biological theories of sexual behavior is that they espouse biological determinism, while ignoring culture and learning sources of behavior, and assume that the sole function of sex is reproduction, which may not be true today. In addition, biological theories have been criticized for not taking into consideration human innovations such as genetic engineering.

PSYCHOANALYTICAL THEORIES

In his theory of personality development, Sigmund Freud (1962) stated that parts of the personality are unconscious. This theory has become most influential in Western thought. Freud developed an idea of sexual energy or drive that he called *libido*. Libido is the major motivating force behind human behavior, according to Freud. He believed that sexual energy was behind many nonsexual behaviors, such as creativity, aggression in the workplace and elsewhere, and many other human endeavors. Students should review the discussion of the defense mechanism sublimation in their psychiatry textbooks for an explanation of this mechanism in action.

In psychoanalytical theory, the personality is subdivided into three sections: the id, ego, and superego. The *id* is the source of psychic energy; it contains the libido and operates on the pleasure principle. The *ego* helps keep the id's energy under control. It acts in concert with the reality principle. The *superego*, or conscience, operates in response to an ideal principle. For example, if left on its own, the id would seek out pleasure without regard to social mores or consequences of its behavior. The id must have a functioning ego to keep it from doing what is unacceptable to others in public, such as masturbating while riding on the subway. The superego checks both pleasure and reality-oriented behavior by adhering to ideal behavior as taught within the context of a particular culture. For example, a person has been taught that it is wrong to let another person believe a relationship will be ongoing when sexual intercourse is really all that is sought. The id wants intercourse, the ego knows the potential sexual partner wants involvement as well as intercourse, and the superego prevents the ego and id from promising a commitment that is not really felt. As other examples, a person's superego may believe that one must not receive pleasure by giving another person pain or that one should not engage in sexual intercourse before marriage.

Freudian theory has had a profound influence on how Americans in particular view human development and behavior. Even though Freud has fallen into disfavor in recent years, this theory of personality remains the standard against which we hold all others accountable.

In terms of psychosexual development, Freud believed the child passed through developmental stages, each focused on a different erogenous zone. An erogenous zone is a part of the body—such as the lips and mouth, genitals, and anus and rectum—that is a source of pleasure. Sucking and defecating cause pleasure, as does rubbing the genitals. According to Freud, a person could become fixated, or stuck, in a stage if passage through it was blocked. Nailbiting or thumbsucking might be considered evidence of being fixated at the oral stage, for example.

The position of women in psychoanalytical theory has been examined in recent times. Freud espoused that "anatomy is destiny." He saw women as biologically inferior because they lacked penises. Believing themselves inferior, women were thus destined to be passive, masochistic, and narcissistic, Freud said. It is no wonder that feminists object to Freud's viewpoint and resultant therapy for women. Feminists argue that Freud was speaking and acting on his own biased Victorian viewpoint of women, rather than on the basis of scientific evidence (Donovan, 1988).

BEHAVIORAL THEORIES

Learning theories are based on the notion that the frequency with which a behavior is enacted is related to reinforcement or punishment from something or someone within the individual's internal or external environment. Some rewards, like food and sex, are considered primary. That is, they are intrinsically rewarding. If a person is hungry, food decreases the hunger, rewarding the person. Other rewards are conditioned reinforcers. Recall Pavlov's experiments with dogs, in which a bell was rung as food was given. After several times, the dog salivated (indicating its readiness to eat) when the bell was rung even if food was not simultaneously presented.

Sexual behavior is thought to be influenced by learning theory. A person whose first experience with sex-related activities was positive is more likely to increase the frequency of these activities than is a person whose first sex-related experience was not positive. If the first encounter with sex involves punishment, like the pain of rape or the guilt of being caught and severely punished for masturbating, the behavior is less likely to occur later or may occur in an altered form. An example of sex of an altered form is a woman's becoming a prostitute after undergoing prolonged sexual abuse as a child. Perhaps as a child, she received extra spending money for keeping silent about the abuse and now associates sex with money, not love.

Human beings are complicated creatures and, unlike Pavlov's dogs, can find rewards in complex behaviors. For example, consider an Olympic athlete. Training appears to be painful as physical limits are pushed and sports records broken. Injuries have been experienced by most people who seek gold medals. Few rewards are given during training, and some athletes work several jobs to support themselves during training. There is no guarantee that an athlete will be chosen for the Olympic team, and if the athlete is not selected, all the sacrifice of training will go unrewarded. And yet every 4 years, the world community watches as athletes represent their countries. A few win and receive medals while standing on a platform as crowds cheer and their national anthem is played. Is winning the result of endorphin release, the reinforcement of fans, both, or neither?

Punishment and reward must be immediate to shape behavior. If a person does something "bad" and is not caught and punished until time passes or is not punished every time the behavior is enacted, chances are the frequency of the behavior will not decrease. In fact, it may increase. *Behavior modification*, the use of operant conditioning to change behavior, has become popular in educational as well as therapeutic settings. Aversion therapy, or punishing the behavior until it no longer occurs, has also been used in sex therapy.

SOCIAL LEARNING THEORY

Bandura (1969) added the concepts of *imitation* and *identification* to operant conditioning. Many sexual behaviors are thought to occur in this way. For example, children dress up in adult clothing and pretend to be adults in order to develop adult sex roles. Adolescents imitate the dress and mannerisms of rock musicians and film stars to attract boyfriends and girlfriends.

In the dominant American culture, social learning of sexual behaviors is not direct. Sexual activities occur behind closed doors and on the screen in movie theaters. Even in the movies, sexual intercourse is restricted to people over 18 years of age. Consequently, much learning about sex is through indirect example and innuendo, which opens up the possibility of misunderstanding and lack of information.

SELF-ACTUALIZATION THEORIES

Humanistic psychologists, notably Maslow (1970) and Rogers (1951), view humans as growth oriented. Sex is viewed as one of many means of achieving *self-actualization*, one's human potential. Sex is not merely for reproduction, but rather is a means of having fun, giving and receiving pleasure. Impersonal sex, in which another human being is treated as a sex object, is incongruent with the tenets of self-actualization. The goal of being an authentic person cannot be achieved through using another for sexual gratification.

SOCIOLOGICAL THEORIES

The structural–functional theory of families addresses sexual behavior. According to this point of view, sex roles are fixed and oriented toward maintaining the structure of society. The belief is that society regulates sexuality in an effort to preserve order and prevent chaos. Regulation occurs through laws, religious teaching, accepted behaviors of the group, and division of labor.

CAUSES OF SEXUAL DISORDERS

KNOWLEDGE DEFICIT

People's lack of knowledge about sex can give them problems. There has been a great debate in America over the last several decades as to what children should be taught about sex and when and by whom should they be taught it. One segment of the population views sex and reproduction education as a private family matter, while another faction views sex and reproduction as social issues that affects the population as a whole, thereby requiring public education. Some people believe that if adolescents have knowledge of sex and birth control, they will be promiscuous leading to the breakdown of the social fabric of society.

As mentioned earlier, nursing has traditionally supported knowledge as a method to empower individuals and groups. Sex education has become a part of nursing practice, whether the nurse works in a school, birth control clinic, or hospital. Nurses must be knowledgeable about sex and aware of a client's need for information. Getting in the habit of asking clients about sex-related issues or whether they have any questions about sex issues is a good idea. The nurse who cannot or is unwilling to address clients' sex-related questions is obligated to make a referral to a specialized sex educator or therapist.

LACK OF COMMUNICATION

The failure to communicate is often the source of people's sex-related problems. The dominant American culture does not openly discuss sex, and thus it does not encourage people, especially women, to ensure that their sexual needs are met through openly discussing problems with their partners. Several factors contribute to the lack of open discussion of sex. First, communication in general is not stressed as a way to get human needs met. Children are often told they are selfish or self-centered if they directly ask to have their needs met. Second, history has not helped. The Victorian era, in which men and women did not talk about their bodies at all, greatly influenced our thinking. "Nice" girls had no sexual feelings at all, so how could such a girl discuss her sexual needs? These taboos remain for some segments of our society today. Finally, even some cultures in American society that were not influenced by Victorian attitudes discourage talking about sex and sexual needs.

In this age of human immunodeficiency virus (HIV) infection, we have now begun a public campaign to educate sexually active people about the need to use condoms during sexual intercourse. It is difficult to imagine how partners convey the message "Please wear a condom" if communication is lacking. Whether the message is about condoms or the failure to reach orgasm, communication is a fundamental aspect of sex. Nurses are well advised to learn to talk with their clients about the use of clear, direct communication and to role model it themselves.

Messages that use "I" are the most powerful. For example, "I need for you to hold and cuddle me" instead of "all you want is sexual intercourse" lets the sexual partner know what is needed to make intimacy satisfying.

BODY IMAGE DISTURBANCE

A person's body image may be the source of his or her sexual problems. We all have in our minds an ideal body image that has been shaped by our culture. Both male and female Americans have been found to be dissatisfied with some aspects of their bodies.

Spectatoring is when a person observes and judges his or her own sexual performance rather than living the sexual experience (Masters & Johnson, 1970). Body image distortions contribute to this problem. When a person begins to ask "Is my stomach flat enough?", "Is my penis big enough?", or "Are my breasts large enough?" instead of experiencing the sensations of the sex act, he or she is spectatoring. People with disabilities can also suffer from body image problems that affect their sexual function.

PAST EXPERIENCE OF ABUSE

Past experience of abuse can lead to sexual problems. Sexual abuse in childhood, rape both in and out of marriage, and other traumas can have lasting effects on sexuality. Sometimes, the experience of past abuse has been repressed to such a degree that the abuse survivor has no awareness or memory of the abuse. Sexual problems may appear bizarre and unexplainable. For example, a couple, Joe and Ann T., came for therapy because their sexual desire was unequal—Joe wanted more sex than Ann wanted. To solve this problem, Joe would stop by a bar where he could purchase oral sex from young men. He saw no problem with this arrangement. He denied homosexuality or bisexuality. Ann was distressed; she did not consider her husband's behavior normal. After a detailed sexual history, the nurse therapist learned that as a child, Joe had been involved in a sex ring in which older men purchased sex from young, homeless boys. The selling and buying of sex was a common occurrence for Joe. He had not dealt with or even allowed himself to be aware of his victimization. For Joe, bartering sex was just a way to survive.

Nurses must always ask about past sexual abuse (see Chapter 19). Many clients in substance abuse units in hospitals have histories of abuse. It is more difficult to assess the prevalence of history of abuse among clients in general psychiatric wards; however, it is thought to be widespread.

FEAR

Fear is yet another cause of sexual problems. For example, fear of pregnancy or sexually transmitted diseases such as HIV infection can interfere with sexual satisfaction. Although nurses must encourage and explicitly teach clients avoidance of risky sexual practices, giving the idea that sex is dangerous and all aspects of human closeness should be avoided is shortsighted and irresponsible. Sex is a basic human need that involves much more than intercourse. Nonrisky behaviors such as cuddling, necking, petting, and mutual masturbation can be encouraged as alternatives to risky behaviors. To encourage unattainable standards like total abstinence may lead to hopeless, helpless feelings that end in the client's abandoning any effort to control unsafe sex practices.

Fear of intimacy can also cause sexual problems. People with schizoid personality disorder and schizophrenia have the fear of being "swallowed up" if they get too intimate with another person. Unlike what you would expect, some of these people often have sexual relations with many partners (Frost & Chapman, 1987). So you may see people who avoid sex at all costs and those who seek out sexual experiences frequently. The latter group will avoid getting close to others emotionally but can tolerate physical closeness if it is sexual in nature.

WOMEN'S CULTURAL POSITION

Women's position in American dominant culture can interfere with their sexual activity. In a culture in which women are told their proper place is in the home raising children and keeping a husband happy, rebellion is a natural response. Add to this message the message that women are sex objects and the economic reality that women must work, and it is easy to see why women's sex lives may suffer.

Some women directly confront the situation and avoid relationships with men. Some try to treat them as sex objects by seeking out clubs with male strippers and buying sexual magazines about men. Women who try to meet all the demands placed on them by becoming a supermom, a great employee, and a superwife often find themselves too tired to have sexual relations at all. It appears that women in America are in a transition period.

HOMOPHOBIA

Homophobia, the irrational fear of homosexuality, is a common occurrence in American life. Groups as varied as political campaigns, church ruling bodies, and the American Psychiatric Association (APA) have studied homosexuality in our culture. Opinions range from homosexuality is immoral to a normal sexual variation. In 1974, the APA voted that homosexuality is not a mental disorder. In spite of this, gay men and lesbian women are subjected to discrimination, ridicule, and hate campaigns.

AGGRESSION

Aggression can be played out sexually in our culture. Rape is an example of using sex as a weapon in an aggressive act.

NEUROBIOLOGICAL CAUSES

As mentioned earlier, sexual activity is a complex endeavor that involves many factors. The neurobiological aspects of sexuality are affected by age, genetic makeup, disease, use of mood-altering substances, nutrition, and many other variables.

Depression. Underlying depression may lead to fatigue and feelings of unworthiness. Lack of libido from neurochemical sources is probable. Depressed people often report no interest in sexual activity.

Use of Mood-Altering Substances. Use of mood-altering substances changes the neurochemistry of the brain and the rest of the nervous system. Lack of libido, arousal disorders, and impotency in males have been noted with both short- and long-term substance use. Sexual themes and issues often emerge during recovery from addiction. See *Substance-Induced Sexual Dysfunction* for more information.

ROLE OF STRESS AND COPING

Benner and Wrubel (1989) posited that what a person cares about defines what can be stressful for the person. They defined stress as the "disruption of meanings, understandings and smooth functioning so that harm, loss, or challenge is experienced and sorrow, interpretation, or new skill acquisition is required" (Benner & Wrubel, p. 59). For example, when people who define themselves as a breadwinner and provider for their family lose their job, they feel a high degree of stress. Stress has a physiological effect on the body. It changes a person's neurochemistry, and because sex is regulated by neurochemistry, sexual function may be altered. It is easy to see why sexual disorders may begin during periods of stress.

According to Benner and Wrubel (1989), coping is not the "antidote for stress" (p. 62), but rather is what one does when one is experiencing stress. Choices for coping are not unlimited. Each human being lives within a cultural and historical context. The context provides meanings and hence possibilities for stress and coping. In the age of the HIV and acquired immunodeficiency syndrome (AIDS) epidemic, knowledge of unsafe sexual practices may produce stress in an individual who has just had an unsafe sexual encounter. The meanings attached to the experienced stress may lead to coping actions ranging from the fatalistic attitude "Oh well, since I have already been exposed, I might as well do whatever I please because I am probably infected already" to "I had better get tested and hope I am uninfected, but in either case I need to change my behavior." Nurses can enable clients to change their behavior by exploring the meanings attached to stressful experiences and by considering the possibilities for coping. This nurse–client interaction is discussed later in this chapter.

SEXUALITY AND SEXUAL DISORDERS ACROSS THE LIFE SPAN

Sexual themes and issues are present throughout the life span. Nurses should incorporate sexual histories in their assessments. See Table 20–1 for a summary of sexual issues across the life span.

TABLE 20–1

Sexual Issues Across the Life Span

Childhood:	Identification with gender
Adolescence:	Identity development vs. role confusion
Young Adulthood:	Intimate relationship development
Adulthood:	Generativity, guiding children
Middlescence:	Redefinition of identity and roles
Old Age:	Changing physical and mental conditions

CHILDHOOD

Sexuality is a lifelong phenomenon that begins with birth, when the nurse midwife or physician announces, "It's a girl" or "It's a boy." The culture in which the child grows up defines and limits boundaries of sexual behavior. By the time the child reaches 3 years old, he or she proclaims to be a boy or a girl.

The following case study illustrates a potential problem that arises in childhood—sexual gender disorder.

Case Study: Sexual Gender Disorder

Frank was brought to the clinic by his mother at his kindergarten teacher's insistence. Frank, now 5 years old, had insisted that he was a girl for as long as his mother could remember. He often played quiet games with stuffed animals or dolls. He liked to wear nightshirts and long tee-shirts which he pretended were dresses. Frank refused to stand to urinate; he preferred to sit down for this activity. Once his estranged father, who was currently not living at home because of conflicts with Frank's mother about his son's behavior, showed him the "correct" way to urinate. During this demonstration, Frank screamed, fell on the floor, and yelled, "I am a girl and this (pointing to his penis) will fall off soon." Frank's teacher complains that Frank will not line up with the boys, plays alongside the girls, and refuses to enter the boys' restroom.

The nurse would encourage the parents not to respond to Frank in a negative way that could harm his self-esteem. The nurse could work collaboratively with the child psychiatric treatment team to develop a plan for behavioral therapy aimed at helping Frank fit in with his peers. Behaviors such as going to the boys' bathroom would be expected, while the nurse and teacher remain aware that Frank may be taunted and possibly abused by his age peers. His safety and self-esteem are of most importance.

ADOLESCENCE

Erikson (1964) described a theory of ego development that was based on Freud's work. Erikson conceptualized ego development as occurring in eight stages over a life span. Adolescence is characterized as the years from 12 to 20, when a person tackles the task of creating an identity in the midst of confusion. If the goal of identity development is not achieved, unresolved conflicts will result in behavioral disorders.

Case Study: Identity Versus Role Confusion

Eighteen-year-old Ann Marie has aroused the concern of her family, the faculty at the community college she attends and her co-workers at the fast food restaurant at which she works. The source of this concern is her impulsive and sometimes self-destructive behavior. Ann Marie is not doing well in school; she is indecisive about her career goals, as indicated by her changing majors every semester. Co-workers complain that she is late for work and say she appears not to care that she might be fired. Along the same line, Ann Marie's parents worry because their daughter goes out with a different boyfriend every night. There is reason to believe that she is having sex with these various boys. Drinking behavior is suspected.

Ann Marie needs for the nurse to help her set limits on her behavior while improving her sense of self-worth. The college counselor can help with career goal development. Marie needs to be taught in terms she can understand the dangers in her present course: alcohol use which lowers inhibition coupled with a number of sexual contacts can result in sexually transmitted diseases including HIV and unplanned pregnancy.

YOUNG ADULTHOOD

The major task of young adulthood is development of an intimate relationship. Erikson (1964) identified isolation as the outcome of the failure to develop intimacy.

Case Study: Isolation as a Result of Failure to Develop Intimacy

Jay, age 28, avoids social interactions in his work as a computer programmer. He lives with his parents, as he always has done. His older sister worries that he is "not doing what 28 year old men do." She has tried involving Jay in her life by inviting him to parties to meet her friends. He has refused her efforts. Jay fears he will say or do the wrong thing. He becomes anxious and extremely sensitive to questions that family acquaintances ask him about his social life.

Any help the nurse can give that breaks down Jay's isolation is essential. Intimacy is difficult for Jay so that pushing him to do too much too fast will fail. Small steps toward socialization might include getting involved in a computer network, a computer interest group, or anything that moves him toward people at a pace he can tolerate.

ADULTHOOD

The task of adulthood is generativity, that is, guiding children and being constructive and creative in work. Failure results in stagnation and self-indulgence. In recent years, infertility has become a problem of adulthood.

Case Study: Stress of Infertility on a Relationship

George and Annie began seeking treatment for infertility 3 years ago without success. All of their sexual activities have revolved around Annie's fertile periods and attempts to conceive. The stress has resulted in marital problems, and the couple has discussed divorce. During this ordeal, many couples begin to lose feelings of love and closeness and begin to doubt the commitment of marriage.

An infertility support group lead by a nurse with knowledge and experience in this area will help this couple share their experiences with others and learn they are not alone. It is important that a knowledgeable health professional be the group leader because misinformation is a real danger in leaderless support groups or psychotherapy groups lead by someone who does not understand infertility and its treatment.

MIDDLESCENCE

Middlescence is the period around the middle of the life span heralded by hormonal changes in both sexes that lead to gradual decline in reproductive function.

During midlife, both sexes begin to redefine themselves. Because our culture idolizes youthful sexuality, the perception of lost youth may cause anxiety. Most people succeed in making the transition to middlescence in a healthy manner. Some do not. Those who are unwilling to accept this transition may face a crisis situation with a variety of possible outcomes.

Case Study: Anxiety over Lost Youth

On Janis's 50th birthday, she decided to change her life. She went to a spa to tone up her always youthful-looking body. When she returned home, she informed her husband that she had filed for divorce and was leaving him. She refused to discuss her plans with her children, rationalizing that she had devoted her life to them and now it was time to think of herself first. She opened a business in real estate, bought a luxury car, and began to date younger men. Janis bragged to her new friends that she found happiness and would never return to her former life.

The nurse can suggest family therapy; however, Janis may resist. Regardless of what Janis does, the rest of this family needs help to pick up the pieces of their family life. The nurse will want to prevent further dissolution of the family unit if possible. Active listening to Janis's husband and children can help them sort out their feelings and perhaps tell them to Janis.

OLDER ADULTHOOD

Old age is now divided into young old and old old. Sexuality and sexual function vary according to the person's gender and physical and mental conditions. Sexual activity may decline somewhat in old age, but many people remain sexually active into their 80s and 90s. Decline in sexual activity may have more to do with attitudes about aging and the death of a spouse than with dysfunction. Although physical changes do occur that make sex in old age different from sex in other periods of life (women experience less lubrication and elasticity and declining estrogen levels, resulting in thinner vaginal walls; men produce less testosterone, take longer to achieve an erection, and experience a longer refractory period), adjustments can be made for all of these changes so that sexual activity need not stop in old age.

Case Study: Aging and Sexuality

Mary and James, 76 and 80 years of age, respectively, had always had a satisfactory sex life in their marriage. Sexual intercourse has decreased in frequency to twice a month because James has difficulty achieving an erection. Both Mary and James view this as an acceptable change in behavior. Neither one wants to lose the closeness of sexual expression. For this reason, the regularity of cuddling and touching has remained constant. The couple continues to experience sexual satisfaction in their marriage.

It is possible that James' erection problems have a physiological source that can be treated. The nurse can suggest a medical work-up with a urologist if it has not been done recently. Otherwise this couple appears to be satisfied with their sex life so that the nurse can offer assistance if future problems arise. Acknowledging that people in old age still need and have sex is essential to good nursing care for this group.

SPECIFIC SEXUAL DISORDERS AND TREATMENT MODALITIES

Table 20–2 lists the sexual disorders recognized by the American Psychiatric Association (1994) (APA) in the fourth edition of the *Diagnostic and Statistical Manual of Mental Disorders* (DSM-IV). These disorders are described below.

TABLE 20–2
Sexual and Gender Disorders

GENDER IDENTITY DISORDERS
SEXUAL DYSFUNCTIONS
Sexual Arousal Disorders
Sexual Desire Disorders
Orgasmic Disorders
Sexual Pain Disorders
Sexual Dysfunction due to General Medical Condition
Substance-Induced Sexual Dysfunction
PARAPHILIAS

Data from American Psychiatric Association. (1994). *Diagnostic and statistical manual of mental disorders* (4th ed.). Washington, DC: Author.

GENDER IDENTITY DISORDERS

Sexuality is an integral part of a person's life; it is not limited to sexual intercourse. **Gender** identity is inborn and culturally defined. At various times, the average male or female may contemplate what it would be like to be the opposite sex. At times, for example, at Halloween or at a masquerade party, a person of either sex may try on the role of the other sex by putting on gender-identified clothing or adopting gender-typical mannerisms.

Gender identity disorder is not allowing oneself to experience the role of the other; rather, it is a pervasive distress over being a boy or a girl. A child with a gender identity disorder may be preoccupied with the dress and behavior stereotypical of the opposite sex. In addition, the child persists in asserting that he or she will develop the sex organs of the other sex. In adulthood, this condition is referred to as *transsexualism*. The person is persistently (for at least 2 years) preoccupied with getting rid of current primary and secondary sexual characteristics.

Other identity problems are seen in children and adults who cross-dress, that is, wear culturally appropriate dress of the opposite sex. This cross-dressing is not to be confused with wearing clothes of the opposite sex for the purpose of feeling sexual arousal.

SEXUAL DYSFUNCTIONS

Arousal Disorders

Sexual arousal disorders are primary disorders in people who have an inadequate physiological response during the period of sexual arousal. In women, the problem is a persistent or recurrent inability to attain or maintain lubrication and swelling of the vagina during the excitement phase. In men it is a persistent or recurrent inability to attain or maintain an erection. For a diagnosis of sexual arousal disorder in both men and women, no other Axis I diagnosis should be evident. For example, major depression, substance abuse, and sexual dysfunction related to a medical condition (e.g., spinal cord injury) all cause changes in a person's physiological ability for sexual arousal.

Desire Disorders

Disorders in sexual desire are primary problems as identified by the person experiencing them or by the clinician during assessment. The disturbance must cause marked distress or difficulty in interpersonal relationships. Sexual desire may be hypoactive, or there may be an aversion to all sexual activity. Hypoactive desire disorder is marked by low or absent sexual fantasy or activities. The person's age, sex, and life context (culture, relationship, etc.) must be taken into account.

An aversion to sexual activity is a persistent and extreme avoidance of all or almost all genital sexual contact with a partner. The presence of another Axis I diagnosis, such as depression or obsessive–compulsive disorder, must be ruled out before a sexual desire disorder diagnosis is made.

Orgasmic Disorders

Both men and women can suffer from orgasmic disorders. In the DSM-IV, the APA (1994) has made an effort to account for the variations in normal female functioning. The APA assumes that women have more frequent orgasms as they age and become more experienced. The type of stimulation also plays an important role in female sexual response.

An orgasmic disorder is a persistent or recurrent delay in or absence of orgasm following a normal sexual excitement phase. The disorder may be further categorized as generalized (occurs every time) or situational (orgasm may occur with self-stimulation or occurs with only a particular partner).

Premature ejaculation is another type of orgasmic disorder. The condition must be persistent or recurrent, and the situation must be taken into account.

Sexual Pain Disorders

Persistent or recurrent genital pain in men or women before, during, or after intercourse that cannot be explained by other medical or psychiatric conditions is called *dyspareunia*. *Vaginismus* refers to an involuntary spasm of the musculature of the outer two thirds of the vagina that interferes with intercourse. Like other sexual conditions identified in the *DSM–IV*, the sexual pain disorders must be persistent or recurrent to warrant diagnosis and treatment. Both sexual pain disorders must cause a problem for the person individually and interpersonally.

TABLE 20–3
Medical Conditions That Affect Sexual Function

NEUROLOGICAL
Spinal cord injury
Cervical disc problems
Multiple sclerosis
VASCULAR
Atherosclerosis
Sickle cell anemia
ENDOCRINE
Addison's disease
Cushing's syndrome
Hypothyroidism
Diabetes mellitus
SYSTEMIC DISEASE
Liver disease
Renal disease
Pulmonary disease
Arthritis
Cancer
GENITAL DISEASE IN FEMALES
Infections
Cancers
Allergies to spermicide
GENITAL DISEASE IN MALES
Prostatitis
Orchitis
Tumor
Trauma
SURGICAL PROCEDURES

For a detailed discussion of these conditions and nursing interventions, see Fogel & Lauver (1992).

TABLE 20–4
Drugs That Affect Sexual Function

Prescription drugs
Antianxiety agents
Alprazolam (Xanax)
Diazepam (Valium)
Doxepin (Sinequan)
Anticholinergic agents
Homatropine methylbromide (Homapin)
Mepenzolate bromide (Cantil)
Methantheline bromide (Banthine)
Propantheline bromide (Pro-Banthine)
Anticonvulsant agents
Phenytoin (Dilantin)
Antidepressant agents
Most can cause changes
Antipsychotic agents
Most can cause changes
Antiarrhythmic agents
Disopyramide (Norpace)
Antihypertensive agents
Beta blockers
Diuretics
Sympatholytics
Others
Cimetidine (Tagamet)
Sulfasalazine (Azulfidine)
Over-the-counter drugs with anticholinergic properties
Social drugs
Alcohol
Amyl nitrate
Cocaine
Lysergic acid
Marijuana
Heroin
Methadone

Sexual Dysfunction Due to General Medical Condition

A sexual difficulty with evidence of a nonpsychiatric medical condition etiology causes a great deal of distress, disruption of sexual functioning, and interpersonal problems (Fogel & Lauver, 1990; Lubkin, 1986). The sexual dysfunction may result in secondary male erectile disorder, secondary dyspareunia, secondary vaginismus, or another secondary sexual dysfunction. Table 20–3 lists nonpsychiatric medical conditions that affect sexual functioning.

Substance-Induced Sexual Dysfunction

In substance-induced sexual dysfunction, a prescription or recreational drug causes sexual dysfunction (Rogers, 1990). Usually, the substance was ingested within 6 weeks of the sexual problem's appearance. The specific substance should be identified as the etiology of the problem. Table 20–4 lists drugs that are known to affect sexual function.

PARAPHILIA

Paraphilia is an umbrella term for variations in sexual behavior. Hyde's (1984) definition of abnormal sex may be used to give an overall framework to paraphilia. Sex is abnormal when it (1) is uncomfortable for the person doing it, (2) is inefficient in that it causes problems in that person's life (e.g., results in arrest), (3) is viewed by the person's culture as bizarre, and (4) does harm to the person and others.

The *DSM–IV* identifies sexual variations that are problematic to the individual. The problem may be viewed as mild (the person is distressed by the urge but does not act on it), moderate (occasionally the urge is acted on), or severe (the person repeatedly acts on the urge). Table 20–5 presents a list of the paraphilias and their definitions.

THE NURSE'S ROLE

A gestalt theoretical approach may be used to address sexual issues and themes. The advantage of this theory is that it views the body as inseparable from the mind, the basic tenets of gestalt theory are that the power is in the present moment, experience counts most, the therapist—in this case the nurse—is the instrument for change, and therapy is too good to waste on the sick (Polster & Polster, 1973). Because the power is in the present, the nurse can deliver care and comfort to clients in the immediate present. All that is required is the nurse's presence and awareness of a client concern. From this vantage point, nurses can attend to physiological concerns as well as any emotional discomfort the client may experience. The nurse does not have to work only with a diagnosed disease; well people can improve their lot in life, too. Because the nurse is the instrument of change, no other health professional has to be involved if the nurse is capable of intervention.

Any time a nurse and client interface, sexual concerns may be addressed. In dealing with any client, from the client who comes to a teen clinic with a complaint of acne to the client who comes to geriatric clinic for treatment for hypertension, the nurse can take a sex history and open up the topic for the client to express any concern. All the nurse must do is give the client permission to speak about sex. Then the nurse must be willing to listen or must refer to someone who will. In this way, sexual issues and themes can be addressed openly in a way that gives comfort to the client.

The psychiatric–mental health nurse is in a key position to support sexual behavior changes in groups at risk for HIV infection. More effort in developing effective counseling and educational programs is needed. Psychiatric–mental health nurses are uniquely qualified to provide holistic care, counseling, and education to clients at risk of HIV infection. In addition, in an administrative role, the nurse can ensure that groups at risk are targeted for appropriate and effective services. In a scientific role, the nurse can generate and test theories regarding interventions that may be used in clinical settings to support behavior changes in people at risk for HIV infection.

TABLE 20–5
Definitions of Paraphilia

Exhibitionism: exposure of one's genitals to strangers
Fetishism: sexual fixation on an object to which erotic significance is attached
Frotteurism: sexual fantasies involving touching and rubbing against a nonconsenting individual
Pedophilia: sexual fantasies and activities with prepubescent children
Sexual masochism: sexual fantasies comprising being humiliated, beaten or bound, or made to suffer
Sexual sadism: sexual fantasies, behaviors, or acts that generate psychological or physical suffering of another person
Transvestic fetishism: recurrent and intense sexual urges and sexual fantasies involving cross-dressing
Voyeurism: sexual arousal at secretly viewing the nude body
Paraphilia not otherwise specified include the following: *Telephone scatologia:* obscene phone calls *Necrophilia:* sexual fantasies and acts involving corpses *Partialism:* exclusive sexual focus on a part of the body, for example, the feet *Zoophilia:* sexual fantasies and acts with animals *Coprophilia:* feces hold sexual meaning for the individual *Klismaphilia:* sexual fantasies and arousal involving enemas *Urophilia:* urine produces sexual response

Data from American Psychiatric Association. (1994). *Diagnostic and statistical manual of mental disorders* (4th ed.). Washington, DC: Author.

THE GENERALIST'S ROLE

A generalist in psychiatric–mental health nursing is a registered nurse working in a specialized setting. Clients often confide in the generalist information of an intimate nature. The generalist uses the therapeutic relationship to listen and express caring concern to the client. The listening and caring activities of the generalist are vital to the client's healing process.

Sexual themes and problems are addressed by the generalist in the same way he or she addresses other problems—through the nursing process. The nurse must feel comfortable asking about clients' sexual concerns and listening to their problems. After assessment, the nurse develops methods to increase the client's awareness of the problems and potential solutions. Increasing awareness involves education and counseling skills. The generalist is responsible for knowing his or her personal limitations, be they lack of knowledge of sexual issues, discomfort in discussing sexual issues, or lack of skill in. The nurse can overcome limitations in knowledge or skills or differences in values and beliefs by assisting the client through referral or consulting with appropriate professionals.

ROLE OF THE ADVANCED-PRACTICE NURSE

The clinical specialist (CS) is a nurse with a master's degree in psychiatric and mental health nursing who may or may not specialize in sex therapy. Regardless of whether the CS is a sex therapist, he or she can help determine what interventions are indicated for the client with a sexual problem and should be the first resource considered by the generalist.

Advanced practice as outlined in the ANA's *Standards of Psychiatric and Mental Health Clinical Nursing Practice* (1994) requires at least a master's degree in the specialty. The CS functions as a psychotherapist with individuals, families, and groups. The CS who specializes in sex therapy should be recognized by the state in which he or she practices as a clinical specialist. In addition, in-depth training in sex therapy should be evident. The American Association of Sex Educators, Counselors and Therapists has identified qualifications for practice in this area and issues a directory of certified professionals.

THE NURSING PROCESS

Sexual health promotion requires the client's active participation and, ultimately, assumption of responsibility for care. The client must use an organized, systematic process to choose a specific course of action for behavior change. Psychiatric clients may have difficulty with decision making. Being faced with choices for behavior change may create conflict within the person and the family. Feelings of helplessness in the client may encourage unnecessary dependence on the nurse. It is the nurse's job to enable the client to operate free of help as quickly as possible, while ensuring the client's self-care potential.

Enabling sexual change begins with the nurses' assessing the meaning the client attaches to sexual behavior. Educational plans are then developed that help the client identify alternative sexual methods or nonsexual methods of finding meaning. For example, if John, a late adolescent, is engaging in sexual activities in order to satisfy the need for touch, then safe-sex ways of touching must be explored (see Nursing Care Plan 20–1). A wealth of information indicates that simply pointing out the dangers of an activity does not bring about change (Hochhauser & Greensweig, 1992). The nurse must be willing to discuss openly and nonjudgmentally the meaning of John's desire for sexual activity, instead of simply reciting its dangers.

A sexual history includes all aspects of sexuality and therefore is holistic. An overall health assessment, including a thorough physical examination, is basic to good problem identification, because sexuality includes neurological, vascular, muscular, hormonal, psychosocial, and other components. A sexual history should include the context in which the problem emerged and the context in which it currently exists, awareness of both the nurse's and client's underlying anxieties and prejudices, a description of the experience as it is lived by the client, the meaning of the problem from the client's perspective, and the support currently available to the client and the nurse.

Case Study: The Client with Sexual Problems (John)

John, an 18-year-old diagnosed as schizophrenic, confides in Nurse Jones that he has difficulty with his girlfriend, who is also an inpatient. The nurse collects the following data.

Context. John and his girlfriend went on a therapeutic pass last Sunday. He felt no desire to kiss or get close to his girlfriend, even though she indicated to him that she wanted to be close.

Awareness. Although John became anxious whenever his girlfriend got close to him, he was aware that he wanted to please her. Nurse Jones is aware that John's illness sometimes creates problems in closeness. She also remembers that a possible side effect of his antipsychotic medication is decreased sexual desire. In addition, she recognizes that she did not know that John had a girlfriend and is aware that she has mixed feelings about John's expressed desire to become sexually active.

Lived Experience. John expresses his isolation and loneliness. He wants to be, as he says, "a normal guy, get married and have children. But my illness prevents all this." Since his recent diagnosis of mental illness, he has begun to feel hopeless about his future.

Meaning. John believes that a powerful force is manipulating his life in a negative way. He feels hopeless and lost. Reaching out to his girlfriend is like "an anchor in a storm" to him, he says.

Support. Nurse Jones believes she can support John through daily therapeutic one-to-one interactions. John identifies his girlfriend and his mother as two supportive people. There is a schizophrenic support group beginning on the unit that also might help break down some of the isolation John experiences.

Assessment

The North American Nursing Diagnosis Association (NANDA) lists the following diagnoses with human sexuality as the phenomenon of concern:

Sexual Dysfunction. Sexual dysfunction is the person's experience of change in sexual function. The person views this change as unsatisfying, unrewarding, inadequate, or socially inappropriate.

Sexual dysfunction can arise from various etiologies across the spectrum of human sexual response. Numerous examples emerge from individual human response to stress, surgery, value conflicts, body image changes, loss of meaning as well as many other sources. Disruption within the body, the family, or community can create this problem (Sheahan, 1989).

Alteration in Sexual Patterns. Sexual variations or paraphilias come under this category. For the person to achieve sexual arousal and orgasm, stimulation from an unusual object or situation is needed. If this object or

Nursing Care Plan 20-1 The Client with Sexual Problems (John)

► Nursing Diagnosis: Potential Sexual Dysfunction Related to Fear of Closeness

OUTCOME IDENTIFICATION	NURSING ACTION	RATIONALE	EVALUATION
1. By [date], John will state his satisfaction with the amount of closeness he can tolerate with his girlfriend.	1a. Explore with John what he expects out of being close to his girlfriend.	1a. Sex is often used for non-sexual reasons during adolescence (e.g., peer approval).	*Goals met:* John discusses his expectations and fears with nurse and supportive others. John tolerates one-to-one interaction with his girlfriend.
	1b. Support John's efforts to communicate appropriately with others.	1b. Sexual expression and touch are basic forms of human communication.	
	1c. Allow John to express his fear of closeness to others.	1c. Patients with boundary problems often fear closeness.	

► Nursing Diagnosis: Perception of Alteration in Sexual Patterns Related to Misinformation

OUTCOME IDENTIFICATION	NURSING ACTION	RATIONALE	EVALUATION
1. By [date], John will report acceptance of his sexual pattern.	1a. Assess John's perception of the problem.	1a. Misperceptions about sexuality are common.	*Goals met:* John states he did not realize the variations of sexual frequency that people might experience. John states he has decided to not have sexual intercourse with his girlfriend. He says he has decided to wait until he feels ready.
	1b. Assess own beliefs and values about sexuality.	1b. If the nurse is judgmental, meaningful dialogue is impossible.	
	1c. Assess frequency of sexual activity in the past and currently.	1c. John may have no sexual experience or be unable to determine what his pattern is.	
	1d. Explore the meaning of sexual behavior to John.	1d. Patients with cognitive impairment may not know a behavior is inappropriate.	

► Nursing Diagnosis: Knowledge Deficit Related to Age and Lack of Experience

OUTCOME IDENTIFICATION	NURSING ACTION	RATIONALE	EVALUATION
1. By [date], John will demonstrate adequate knowledge of sex.	1. Provide information about sexuality and sexual health.	1. Sex education is not provided by many families or schools. John may have misinformation that has created stress and anxiety.	*Goals met:* John describes basic anatomy and physiology of sex. John states that his medication may change his sexual function. John is willing to explore ways to solve his perceived sexual difficulties. John verbalizes the importance of continuing his medications.
2. By [date], John will demonstrate adequate knowledge of how his illness and his medication affect his sexual activity.	2. Provide information on the effects John's mental illness and the psychotropics he takes may have on his sexuality.	2. Schizophrenia can affect sexual functioning and loss of impulse control. Nearly all psychotropic medications decrease libido and inhibit ejaculation. This effect may be reversed by changing or decreasing medication. It is important to discuss the effects of stopping his medication. Sexual dysfunction is one reason why medications are not taken.	

situation involves the coercion of an unwilling or unaware partner, then enabling change in sexual behavior is needed. Coercive sexual **patterns** are illegal and people who practice them are subject to arrest and punishment. Noncoercive sexual patterns require communication and negotiation between partners (McFarland et al., 1992).

Other NANDA Diagnoses. Other NANDA diagnoses that may apply are Alteration in Family Process, Ineffective Individual Coping, Spiritual Distress, Anxiety, Fear, Pain, Personal Identity Disturbance, Body Image Disturbance, and Knowledge Deficit.

Planning

Working in partnership with the client, family, and interdisciplinary team to enable the client's sexual behavior change involves open communication and cooperation. All parties must be aware of the nature of the problem and how to work toward a satisfactory change. This involvement is not always easy; conflict and discomfort may arise. Encouraging participants' expression of differences in value and beliefs while advocating acceptance of the client's wish to change should be the focus of nursing interactions.

Nursing Care Plan 20–1 identifies the nursing diagnoses and desired outcomes for the case study of John presented earlier and specifies the nursing actions needed to achieve these outcomes and the rationales for these actions.

Implementation

Treatment should be aimed at (1) removal of the cause of the problem, (2) symptom management for problems that cannot be readily treated because their etiology is unknown or effective treatment is unavailable, (3) case management for the client with chronic problems, and (4) family support. Of course, treatment varies with each condition.

Evaluation

The outcome of nursing interventions should be that the client reports satisfactory and socially appropriate sexual functioning within the context of his or her situation. Concern for the sexual partner if there is one is also an expected client outcome (McFarland et al., 1992).

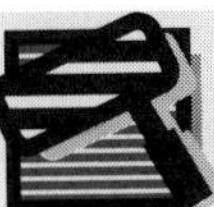

RESEARCH STUDY

Women and HIV Infection: State of the Science

Smeltzer, S. C., & Whipple, B. (1991). *Image: Journal of Nursing Scholarship, 23,* 249–256.

This article summarizes what is known about the human immunodeficiency virus (HIV) and women. Nurses are in a key position to help women assess the behavior that creates risk of infection. Because women were not identified initially with the risk groups for HIV infection, some women are unaware that their sexual practices or intravenous drug use can expose them to the HIV. Women are not diagnosed with acquired immunodeficiency syndrome (AIDS) as often as men are because of the way in which the Centers for Disease Control and Prevention (CDC) has set forth criteria for this disease. Opportunistic infections that are specific to homosexual contact and intravenous drug use are used as criteria. Women develop gynecological problems that are not included on the CDC list. Problems specific to women with HIV, as opposed to men with HIV, include candida infections; sexually transmitted diseases like herpes, syphilis, chancroid, and human papilloma virus; pelvic inflammatory disease; problems caused by the natural immune changes during pregnancy; and perinatal transmission of HIV.

The researchers suggest that nurses need to use empowerment models of intervention to help women improve their communication and negotiation skills. Empowering women to control the transmission of HIV through prevention is the goal of this type of nursing intervention. Women should be encouraged to use barrier methods of protection that they can use themselves, instead of relying on male partners to provide protection. Women are reluctant to make demands on male partners that could result in abandonment, physical abuse, or loss of financial support. Empowerment would help these women change their behaviors to decrease their risk. Educational programs aimed at helping women change risky behaviors must be culturally, religiously, and ethnically sensitive to the groups they are targeting. More research by nurses is needed that addresses the special needs of women in the prevention and treatment of HIV disease.

RESEARCH ON SEXUAL ISSUES RELEVANT TO PSYCHIATRIC NURSING

Nurses are expected to provide sex education and counseling to various groups of clients across the life span. Nurses have often been frustrated by the traditional approach to health education, that is, to tell the client what the risk is and what to change to decrease that risk and then presume that the client will change the behavior to avoid the risk. This model of health education often does not work and creates conflict in the nurse–client relationship when it fails.

In the last decade, the risk of exposure to HIV infection and the resulting morbidity and mortality has led to increased research on behavior change. Some of the findings have implications for the practice of the psychiatric–mental health nurse. Flaskerud and Nyamathi (1989) studied African American and Hispanic American women's knowledge, attitudes, values, and beliefs about AIDS. They found that a higher level of knowledge of AIDS was not related to positive behavior. They also found that whereas negative attitudes in the Hispanic American women led to safer sexual behaviors, these same attitudes in African American women were related to unsafe behaviors. The authors concluded that because of differences among ethnic and cultural groups, health education interventions must assess the effects of attitudes and values on the behavior of the target group.

In a related study, Bevier et al., (1991) sought to determine whether HIV risk behaviors were reduced after counseling and to evaluate the determinants of behavior change in clients enrolled in a sexually transmitted disease clinic. Subjects ($N = 1016$) completed a questionnaire at enrollment and again 6 months after counseling regarding HIV risk behavior. Behaviors before and after counseling were assessed. The major behavior changes were (1) a reduction in the number of clients who were sexually active, (2) a reduction in the number of partners, and (3) an increase in the number of sexual contacts with these fewer partners. Men significantly decreased their number of partners and number of contacts with prostitutes. Women reduced their total number of partners, but they did not decrease their number of contacts with intravenous drug users. The frequency of contact with intravenous drug users increased for both sexes; condom use increased slightly (the women used condoms in 10% of their contacts with intravenous drug users). Bevier et al. concluded that whereas the single counseling session was somewhat effective, intensive counseling of people at high risk is needed, and strategies different from those used with men are needed to help women change their behaviors.

Smeltzer and Whipple (1991) supported the conclusions of Bevier et al. (1991) in a state-of-the-science article on women and HIV infection. These authors summarized the issue of women's being at greater risk for HIV infection through heterosexual transmission. Because women have only recently been targeted as a risk group for HIV infection, significant gaps in knowledge are apparent. HIV disease appears in female-specific symptoms different from the male presentation. Little is known about the manifestations, treatment, or course of this illness in women. Smeltzer and Whipple called for increased attention to women at risk of HIV infection or already infected with the virus (see the Research Study display on p. 441).

► CHAPTER SUMMARY

The person who presents for nursing care and concern is a holistic being. He or she has been sexual from birth. Nurses are in a privileged position of intimacy with the client and family. During the course of generalist and advanced nursing practice, sexual themes and issues are present. The competent nurse asks questions about the client's sexual health, gives permission for the client to discuss problems or concerns of a sexual nature, and seeks appropriate intervention for the client and family. What is an appropriate intervention depends on the nature of the problem. Education, advice, therapeutic intervention, and referral are possible actions the nurse may take in promoting the client's sexual health.

Suggestions for Clinical Conference

1. Discuss ways in which children are taught about sexual identity by their families, culture, schools, and other institutions.
2. Bring to conference and discuss items from the media that stereotype men and women in particular ways.
3. Think of various words (slang, profanity, words from foreign languages) that are used to describe male and female genitalia and sexual activities. Write these words on the board. Keep track of the feelings these words provoke in you. As a group, discuss the emotional effects of the words.
4. Discuss the position of women in American society. How does women's position in society influence both men's and women's ideas about sexuality? Do the same with age or race. How do these ideas affect people's ideas about sexuality?
5. Invite gay, straight, and bisexual men and women to a panel discussion of sexual orientation.
6. Interview someone in recovery from addiction and ask the person to describe how addiction affected his or her sexual identity and behavior.
7. Invite representatives of the National Alliance for Mental Illness to discuss problems and issues in the sexual health of the mentally ill.

References

American Nurses' Association. (1980). *A social policy statement*. Kansas City: Author.

American Nurses Association. (1994). *A statement on psychiatric–mental health clinical nursing practices and standards of psychiatric–mental health clinical practice*. Washington, DC: Author.

American Psychiatric Association. (1994). *Diagnostic and statistical manual of mental disorders* (4th ed.). Washington, DC: Author.

Bandura, A. (1969). *Principles of behavior modification*. New York: Holt, Rinehart & Winston.

Benner, P., & Wrubel, J. (1989). *The primacy of caring: Stress and coping in health and illness*. Menlo Park, CA: Addison-Wesley.

Bevier, P., Ewing, W., Hilderbrandt, D., Castro, K., & Chiasson, M.A. (1991). Effect of counseling on HIV behavior at a New York City sexually transmitted disease clinic. *International Conference on AIDS*, June 16–21, 7(2):458 (Abstract No. WD 4281).

Byne, W., & Parsons, B. (1993). Human sexual orientation: The biological theory reappraised. *Archives of Psychiatry, 50*, 228–239.

Donovan, J. (1988). *Feminist theory*. New York: Continuum.

Erikson, E. (1964). *Childhood and society*. New York: W. W. Norton.

Flaskerud, J. H., and Nyamathi, A. M. (1989). Black and Latina women's AIDS-related knowledge, attitudes, and practices. *Research in Nursing and Health, 12*, 339–346.

Fogel, C. I., & Lauver, D. (1990). *Sexual health promotion*. Philadelphia: W. B. Saunders.

Freud, S. (1962). *Three essays on the theory of sexuality*. New York: Avon.

Frost, L. A., & Chapman, L. J. (1987). Polymorphous sexuality as an indicator of psychosis proneness. *Journal of Abnormal Psychology, 96*, 299–304.

Hyde, J. S. (1986). *Understanding human sexuality* (3rd ed.). New York: McGraw-Hill.

Hochhauser, M., & Greensweig, E. (1992). *Why do people have sex? Implications for AIDS education*. Paper presented at *The Sixth International Conference on AIDS Education*, Washington, DC.

Holden, C. C. (1992). Twin study links genes to homosexuality. *Nature, 255*, 33.

Kaplan, H. S. (1974). *The new sex therapy*. New York: Brunner/Mazel.

Lubkin, I. M. (1986). *Chronic illness: Impact and interventions*. Boston: Jones & Bartlett.

Maslow, A. H. (Ed.). (1970). *Motivation and personality*. (2nd ed.). New York: Harper & Row.

Masters, W. H., & Johnson, V. E. (1966). *Human sexual response*. Boston: Little, Brown.

Masters, W. H., & Johnson, V. E. (1970). *Human sexual inadequacy*. Boston: Little, Brown.

McFarland, G. K., Wasli, E. L., & Gerety, E. K. (1992). *Nursing diagnoses & process in psychiatric mental health nursing* (2nd ed.). Philadelphia: J. B. Lippincott.

Rogers, A. (1990). Drugs and disturbed sexual functioning. In C. I. Fogel & D. Lauver (Eds.), *Sexual health promotion*. Philadelphia: W. B. Saunders.

Rogers, C. R. (1951). *Client-centered therapy: Its current practice, implications, and theory*. Boston: Houghton Mifflin.

Polster, E., & Polster, M. (1973). *Gestalt therapy integrated*. New York: Brunner/Mazel.

Sheahan, S. L. (1989). Identifying female sexual dysfunctions. *The Nurse Practitioner, 14*(2), 25–34.

Smeltzer, S. C. & Whipple, B. (1991). Women and HIV infection. *Image: The Journal of Nursing Scholarship, 23*, 249–256.

Symons, D. (1979). *The evolution of human sexuality*. New York: Oxford University Press.

Wilson, E. O. (1975). *Sociobiology: The new synthesis*. Cambridge, MA: Harvard University Press.

Witelson, S. F. (1993, April). *Sexual orientation: Biologic and psychosocial issues*. Paul C. Weinberg Lectureship presented at University of Texas Health Science Center at San Antonio, San Antonio, Texas.

World Health Organization. (1975). *Education and treatment in human sexuality: The training of health professionals*. (Technical Rep. No. 572). Geneva, Switzerland: Author.

Unit 2 Study Questions

See Appendix I for answers.

CHAPTER 9

1. Which factors are not predictive of greater risk for depression in adolescence?
   a. Parental illness.
   b. Higher socioeconomic status.
   c. Family history of depression.
   d. Emotional abuse.

2. Characteristics of depression common in the elderly include all of the following *except*
   a. Guilt feelings.
   b. Complaints of depressed mood.
   c. Ruminations.
   d. Somatic complaints.

3. Suicide is a serious complication of depressive disorders and is most common in
   a. Childhood.
   b. Adolescence.
   c. Middle adulthood.
   d. Older adulthood.

4. The most common form of treatment for dysthymia is
   a. Electroconvulsive therapy.
   b. Individual insight–oriented psychotherapy.
   c. Family therapy.
   d. Tricyclic antidepressants.

5. Risk factors for a pathological grief reaction include all of the following *except*
   a. Lack of social supports.
   b. Multiple losses.
   c. Chronic physical illness in self.
   d. Dependent relationship with the deceased.

CHAPTER 10

1. M. B. is a 21-year-old woman who presents in the emergency department crying and distraught, complaining that her date raped her. After a complete physical examination and laboratory studies, she is referred to a nurse for further assessment. The nurse can most effectively help this client by
   a. Reassuring her that the man will be prosecuted.
   b. Referring her to a rape crisis center.
   c. Putting her at ease using active listening techniques.
   d. Providing her with a tranquilizer to decrease her anxiety.

2. M. B. begins screaming and stating she feels so ashamed and maybe the rape was her fault. What is an appropriate nursing response?
   a. "I can see this is very upsetting to you."
   b. "Please lower your voice because you are disturbing other sick clients."
   c. Remain quiet, and allow her to ventilate feelings and thoughts.
   d. Offer her a tranquilizer because she is out of control.

3. J. F., a 15-year-old girl, is admitted to the hospital with numerous somatic complaints, including generalized ache, stomach pain, and nausea. Her mother reports that she has had these symptoms for several weeks. J. F. agrees with her and states that she is sick of school and has refused to attend for several days. What information is most pertinent to the treatment in assisting them to make a definite diagnosis?
   a. History of substance abuse.
   b. Social relationships.
   c. History of these symptoms in the past.
   d. Present stressors.

4. H. M. is seen in his home complaining of fears of going outdoors and grocery shopping. Additionally, he is complaining of intense anxiety manifested by tachycardia, shortness of breath, and lightheadedness. What should the nurse do in this situation?
   a. Inquire about his last dose of alprazolam (Xanax).
   b. Call an ambulance or emergency backup.
   c. Check his vital signs.
   d. Encourage him to express his feelings.

5. Manifestations of childhood anxiety disorders include all of the following *except*
   a. Inability to form trusting relationships.
   b. Crying and following in infancy.
   c. Overconcern for the safety of primary caregivers.
   d. Excessive handwashing and counting.

CHAPTER 11

1. M. J., a 45-year-old woman, is in the ambulatory care unit for the third time this week complaining of itching and a skin rash that has not responded to a topical cortisone cream. She is noticeably anxious, tense, and demanding. Which of the following questions reflects an understanding of her situation?
   a. "What recent changes have you experienced over the past 6 months?"
   b. "I noticed that you look pretty anxious. Are you being treated for this condition?"
   c. "When was the last time you had a complete physical?"
   d. "You need to try another medication since this is not helping you."

2. Type A and type B personality coping styles affect one's health status. Manifestations of type A personality include all *except*
   a. Laid back and reposed.
   b. Highly driven.
   c. Hesitancy to take vacations.
   d. Need to be "perfect."

3. Type A personality coping style is associated with an increased risk of
   a. Peptic ulcer disease.
   b. Coronary heart disease.
   c. Asthma.
   d. All of the above.

4. Stress increases the risk of certain physiological disorders. Which of the following does not represent an alteration in the immune system?
   a. Cancer.
   b. Gastroenteritis.
   c. Herpes.
   d. Epstein-Barr virus.

5. Jody, a 6-year-old, has been seen in the pediatric emergency department several times over the past 2 weeks. His breathing is presently not labored or distressed. He is tense and slightly anxious. His asthma had been under control until 2 weeks ago. His interaction with his parents is age-appropriate. His parents report that his asthma medication has been ineffective over the past week and they are very concerned about his health. An appropriate response to the parents is
   a. "What major changes have occurred in the family over the past 2 weeks?"
   b. "Are you having family problems?"
   c. "I am concerned about his health; explain how you have been giving his medication."
   d. "What kind of relationship do you have with your son?"

6. The nurse learns that Jody's grandfather died 3 weeks ago. He was very close to his grandfather. Additionally, he began first grade 2 weeks ago. An important nursing intervention at this time is to
   a. Encourage Jody and his parents to talk about the recent events.
   b. Talk to the parents alone and encourage them to talk to their son when they go home.
   c. Assess the family dynamics and the role of the child's illness in keeping the family together.
   d. Refer the family to the psychiatric clinical specialist for family therapy.

CHAPTER 12

1. Twelve-year-old N. P. is brought into the pediatrician's office by his parents, who express concern about his behavior. Over the past year he has become progressively more agitated and isolative. His grades have dropped from Bs to failing. Additionally, his teacher has expressed concern about his inappropriate smiling. Which of the following *best* describes his symptoms?
   a. Anger toward his parents.
   b. Rebellion associated with adolescence.
   c. Impaired thought processes.
   d. Impaired coping behaviors.

2. What is the best initial response to N. P.'s parents?
   a. "He is just going through a difficult stage."
   b. "This must be a difficult time for you."
   c. "Has he been treated for these symptoms in the past?"
   d. "What major changes has the family had recently?"

3. What is the most accurate description of positive symptoms of schizophrenia?
   a. Paranoia, hallucinations, pressured speech.
   b. Elated mood, delusions of grandeur, tangential speech.
   c. Coherent thoughts, poor eye contact, blunted affect.
   d. Apathy, few relationships, flat affect.

4. The primary teaching goal of interrupting hallucinations is to
   a. Show its relationship to mental illness.
   b. Help the client relate them to stress.
   c. Assist the client in controlling them.
   d. Understand their meaning and relationship to illness.

5. Which is the most effective approach with the suspicious client?
   a. Cautiously extend the hand.
   b. Introduce self and explain the reasons for the visit.
   c. Avoid eye contact, but extend the hand.
   d. Introduce self and extend the hand.

CHAPTER 13

1. N. L., an 8½-year-old boy recently diagnosed with attention deficit disorder, has just begun taking 5 mg of methylphenidate (Ritalin) at 7:30 A.M. and 11:30 A.M. His current weight is 45 lb and his height is 46 in. His mother is concerned that he may experience appetite suppression and weight loss. Which of the following approaches should the nurse take?
   a. Reassure her that her son looks quite healthy and has always had a robust appetite.
   b. Record the youngster's vital signs, including height and weight, on a growth chart, and let the mother know that a record will be maintained at each visit.
   c. Suggest that the mother try to increase this child's food intake in anticipation of his potential weight loss by offering several snacks during the day.
   d. Suggest that the mother contact a registered dietitian and plan all the child's meals and snacks to maximize the benefit of his eating habits.

2. A. S. is an 80-year-old client admitted with a preliminary diagnosis of Alzheimer's disease (AD). She was living alone prior to this hospitalization and developed sudden confusion and anxiety. Why would you question this diagnosis?
   a. AD does not occur after 70 years of age.
   b. Persons with AD cannot live alone.
   c. AD does not develop suddenly.
   d. We never question a medical diagnosis.

3. In obtaining a history of A. S. and reviewing her laboratory reports, you find that she has a urinary tract infection (UTI) and mild renal failure. What could you conclude?
   a. The UTI is insignificant regarding A. S.'s confusion.
   b. The UTI, coupled with mild renal failure, probably caused delirium, and A. S.'s confusion is acute and reversible.
   c. A. S. has poor hygiene habits.
   d. Mild renal failure is insignificant in an 80-year-old woman.

CHAPTER 14

1. H. R. is a 27-year-old woman who is admitted because of a recent overdose of fluoxetine (Prozac). This is her third suicidal attempt in the past year. The nurses show little empathy for her and even though she is on one-to-one observation, she continues to have numerous demands. What term can be used to define the behavior of nurses in this situation?
   a. Transference.
   b. Countertransference.
   c. Projection.
   d. Rescuing.

2. H. R.'s demands continue, and she begins to have rage episodes. The best approach to this client is to
   a. Point out the inappropriateness of her rage behavior.
   b. Explain that the rage behavior will not be tolerated.
   c. Assess the meaning of the behavior.
   d. All of the above.

3. Major manifestations of poor ego function include
   a. Poor self-esteem.
   b. Impaired reality testing.
   c. Distorted cognitions.
   d. All of the above.

4. Clients with personality disorders *differ* from clients in psychiatric settings because they
   a. Experience their symptoms as ego-syntonic.
   b. Are more compliant in treatment.
   c. Seldom exhibit addictive behaviors.
   d. Experience their symptoms as ego-dystonic.

5. Increasing self-esteem in clients is a major nursing goal. What is the *least* effective approach?
   a. Ignoring acting-out behavior.
   b. Setting limits.
   c. Encouraging expression of feelings.
   d. Allowing special privileges.

6. Which statement represents the clearest evidence of *dependent personality disorder*?
   a. "I am having trouble deciding what to wear. I would like your opinion about this sweater."
   b. "I think I'll wear this sweater because it looks good with this skirt. What do you think?"
   c. "I think you should wear younger-looking clothes."
   d. "Tell me if I should wear this sweater."

7. B. J. is a 9-year-old boy who is seen by the school nurse after he gets into a fight with another child. This is the third time he has come in the infirmary with a bloody nose, and he is verbally abusive and hostile as the nurse assesses his injuries. The nurse also remembers seeing B. J. in the principal's office several weeks ago after he was accused of taking another child's lunch. Based on the child's present and past history, what is the best *initial* approach to establishing a therapeutic alliance?
   a. Have a parent–child conference to assess the family system.
   b. Ask B. J. what his reasons are for exhibiting behavioral problems.
   c. Ask B. J. if he would like to talk about his recent fight.
   d. Use a firm approach, and let B. J. know that verbal abuse is not allowed.

8. G. S., a 24-year-old hairdresser, arrives in the emergency department from a nightclub, where she and her boyfriend began an argument that escalated into a physical fight. She is bleeding from a cut over her eye sustained when she fell against a table. She has a strong odor of alcohol on her breath and refuses to cooperate with the nurse who asked her to lie on the examining table. She is very angry and curses loudly about the partner with whom she had fought. The medical resident comes in to examine G.S., and she suddenly becomes very docile. She lies on the table and displays her leg seductively, She tells the resident that she is "through with Jimmy, but I have time for you if you get that nurse out of the room." In the *Diagnostic and Statistical Manual of Mental Disorders, Fourth Edition,* the diagnosis most suited to G. S.'s behavior is
   a. Obsessive-compulsive personality disorder.
   b. Schizotypal personality disorder.
   c. Histrionic personality disorder.
   d. Paranoid personality disorder.

CHAPTER 15

1. R. P. brings 8-year-old T. X. to the clinic for a checkup. T. X. is in R. P.'s care as a foster child, having been removed from his parents because of profound neglect and abuse. As part of a psychosocial assessment to rule out any chronic dissociative pattern of coping on T. X.'s part, the nurse would ask about
   a. The presence of other siblings in the home.
   b. Play patterns with other children.
   c. Odd, contradictory displays of behavior.
   d. Twenty-four-hour nutritional intake.

2. You and other clinic team members diagnose T. X. as having a dissociative disorder. One of the areas you will want to intervene in first is the development of
   a. Better study habits.
   b. Age-appropriate self-soothing skills.
   c. Language skills.
   d. A sense of interpersonal and environmental safety.

3. S. F., a 20-year-old college junior, was seen by her friends wandering in the street. Her friends brought her to the college health clinic where you practice. The friends say that when they asked S. F. what she was doing, she didn't recognize them. S. F. has just finished her final exams for the academic year. One of the first factors you want to assess is
   a. How much coffee and sleep has she had in the past few weeks.
   b. Whether S. F. has a history of sexual trauma.
   c. Whether S. F. has a history of head injury.
   d. What could be the secondary gain from acting "weird."

4. W. T. is admitted to the psychiatric unit with a diagnosis of depersonalization. One of your nursing interventions is to teach W. T. how to use a journal. The expected outcome of this nursing intervention is that
   a. W. T. will develop better writing skills.
   b. W. T. will have a record of his week to show his psychotherapist.
   c. W. T. will not experience depersonalization.
   d. W. T. will develop a greater and continuous sense of self.

5. Medications that may be helpful to W. T. are
   a. Anxiolytics.
   b. Antipsychotics.
   c. Mood-altering agents.
   d. Barbiturates.

CHAPTER 16

1. C. O. is a 21-year-old man who presents with symptoms of weight loss, poor appetite, and difficulty concentrating the past 3 weeks. His girlfriend is expressing concerns about his health because he sleeps all the time and he does not enjoy life anymore. His physical examinations and diagnostic tests are normal. As his nurse, your next questions should be
   a. "Have you had psychiatric treatment in the past?"
   b. "Are you having thoughts of killing yourself?"
   c. "What kind of relationship do you have with your girlfriend?"
   d. "Do you have a family history of suicide?"

2. Based on C. O.'s presenting symptoms, what is the most important implication for nursing?
   a. Assessing his level of dangerousness.
   b. Administering an antidepressant.
   c. Establishing rapport to assess his emotional pain.
   d. Maintaining his nutritional status.

3. The most important suicidal indicator for children and adolescents is
   a. The presence of hallucinations.
   b. Chaotic parent–child relationship.
   c. Poor academic performance.
   d. Disorganized family system.

4. Older adults tend to kill themselves more than adolescents because
   a. Their physical health is more frail.
   b. Their methods are more lethal.
   c. Their mental state is compromised.
   d. Their thinking processes are usually impaired.

5. Suicide is a complex act. Which of the following is the most important indicator for suicide?
   a. Decreased energy in the depressed client.
   b. A sense of hopelessness.
   c. A lack of support systems.
   d. The death of a loved one.

6. The hospitalized depressed client is at a higher risk for suicide at which time?
   a. When symptoms of depression are decreasing.
   b. During the second hospitalization for an overdose.
   c. When symptoms of depression are intense.
   d. When the client is preparing for a weekend pass.

CHAPTER 17

1. K. M., a 52-year-old man, is admitted to your unit for observation with chest pains. On the morning of his second day on the unit, he yells and complains about the noise on the unit. His vital signs are as follows: temperature 38°C; pulse, 90 beats per minute; blood pressure, 160/95

mm Hg; and respirations 20 breaths per minute. You call his physician. What assessment do you need to make next?
a. Neurological assessment.
b. Family history.
c. Alcohol and drug use history.
d. Mental status examination.

2. S. M., a 29-year-old woman with a diagnosis of bipolar disorder, manic phase, and marijuana abuse is admitted to the psychiatric unit. She lived with her parents until 2 years ago when they decided that they couldn't take care of her anymore. She was brought to the hospital by the police when they found her naked by the side of the highway. She indicated that her belongings were under an overpass where she lived. After 10 days, S. M. is no longer psychotic. An important nursing diagnosis for this client at this time is
a. Spiritual Distress related to psychosis.
b. Ineffective Individual Coping related to an inability to care for herself.
c. Noncompliance related to taking off clothes in public.
d. Potential for Violence related to the diagnosis of bipolar disorder.

3. Now that S. M.'s psychosis is stabilized, the focus of her care is to assist her with her substance abuse problem. Which one of the following goals is the next step for her at this time?
a. S. M. will acknowledge that the marijuana use is causing her problems.
b. S. M. will no longer use marijuana.
c. S. M. will attend Alcoholics Anonymous meetings.
d. S. M. will use marijuana safely.

4. E. D., a 19-year-old man, is admitted to the trauma unit after an automobile accident. His blood alcohol level when admitted was .330. On the day before his discharge, he tells you, "I can't wait to get out of this place. I need a drink!" Your *best* response is
a. "Yeah, I'll bet. You have been through a lot!"
b. "You shouldn't be drinking like that. Look where it got you!"
c. "I can understand why you want to get out of here. I would, too."
d. "Getting a drink seems to be important to you. Tell me more about that."

5. S. G., a 39-year-old woman, has been hospitalized for cocaine abuse. As a nurse working on the addiction unit, you have been working with her family. Many codependent behaviors have been identified in family interactions. Which of the following are appropriate outcome criteria for this family?
a. The family members assume responsibility for S. G.
b. S. G.'s parents take her back into their home to "reparent" her.
c. Each family member speaks only for himself or herself.
d. Each family member lets S. G. know how he or she feels.

CHAPTER 18

1. J. S., a 16-year-old girl, has been admitted to a medical unit due to complications from her out-of-control bulimia. She is 5 ft., 4 in. tall and weighs 125 lb. She has a number of binge episodes each week and purges three times per day. When the nurse asks, J. S. admits to irregular "heartbeats" (pulse) at times and menstrual periods. J. S. is tearful throughout the interview and admits to sporadic suicidal thoughts and chronic insomnia. She denies any history of a suicidal gesture. The nurse is assessing J. S.'s current physical status. Which of the following would be most likely seen in a client with bulimia nervosa?
a. Lanugo hair, amenorrhea.
b. Swollen parotid glands, callused knuckles.
c. Hepatomegaly.
d. Hair loss.

2. Restoration of fluid and electrolyte balance is important in the care of the bulimic client. Disturbance of which electrolyte is most often responsible for the bulimic client's irregular pulse?
a. Zinc.
b. Potassium.
c. Magnesium
d. Chloride.

3. In planning J. S.'s comprehensive nursing care *while she is in the hospital*, which nursing diagnosis would assume initial priority?
a. Self-Esteem Disturbance.
b. Altered Nutrition.
c. Fluid Volume Deficit.
d. Impaired Social Interaction.

4. J. S. continues to say that she feels "bloated and fat." Which response by the nurse would be most appropriate?
a. "You look just fine."
b. "You're too thin."
c. "You may perceive yourself as fat, but you are at a healthy weight for your height."
d. "Why would you feel that way?"

5. Family therapy has been ordered while J. S. is in the hospital, with the hope that it will continue once she is discharged. The parents are "not sure" that they need to participate. What would be the most helpful response by the nurse in reference to the parents' ambivalence?

a. "As parents, you need to understand how you helped to cause this."
b. "You can't expect J. S. to handle this by herself."
c. "You need to go because your physician has ordered the therapy."
d. "Participation in family sessions may help everyone understand how family relationships impact J. S.'s eating disorder."

CHAPTER 19

1. Increases in the reporting of child maltreatment and abuse are attributed to
   a. Improved investigations.
   b. Greater awareness of the problem, resulting in a willingness to report.
   c. The frequency of witnessing abuse.
   d. More child protective service workers in hospitals.

2. Nurses working with families at risk for violence can assess family members by
   a. Caring for the infant individually.
   b. Interviewing mothers individually.
   c. Interviewing all members about their contributions to the child's care.
   d. Interviewing extended family members.

3. Of the following categories of young children, which is most at risk for violence?
   a. Emotionally stable children.
   b. Premature and colicky infants.
   c. Highly intelligent children.
   d. Physically and mentally disabled children.

4. A mother of two small children has decided to remain with her husband even though she has experienced 2 years of battering. A desirable response is
   a. "Let's discuss a plan of safety."
   b. "You'll leave when you're ready."
   c. "I think you are at risk. Please reconsider."
   d. "I can't work with you any longer."

5. To effectively plan for the care of an older abused client, the nurse needs to appreciate that the elderly
   a. Have diminished cognitive capacity.
   b. Are often disoriented.
   c. Are prone to reminiscing about past events.
   d. Are often humiliated and defensive when asked about abusive experiences.

CHAPTER 20

1. A. D., age 20, and B. J., age 25, have been dating for several months. B. has been pressuring A. to have sexual intercourse with him. A. has been reluctant to agree to this activity; she has not experienced sexual intercourse before and had planned on waiting for marriage. One cause of A.'s reluctance is her belief about sex outside marriage. From Freud's perspective, the part of this personality that contains this belief is
   a. Ego.
   b. Id.
   c. Superego.
   d. Spiritual.

2. According to Erikson, B. is attempting to
   a. Reproduce.
   b. Resolve aggression issues.
   c. Fulfill his intimacy needs.
   d. Gain respect of his peers.

3. A. and B. have been socialized in a culture where young people engage in sexual activity at the beginning of puberty. In this context, A.'s desire to wait until marriage would be likely to be considered as
   a. Unusual.
   b. Pathological.
   c. A cultural variation.
   d. An individual choice.

4. L. L. is a 40-year-old banker with a drinking problem who recently separated from his wife of 15 years. His typical intake of alcohol is two gin martinis at lunch, two vodka on the rocks before dinner, a bottle of wine with dinner, and a couple of brandies after dinner. Recently, his day has begun with an "eye-opener" of a shot of vodka. L. L. is in for a checkup for stomach pain. He mentions to the nurse that he doesn't feel like himself, his sexual desire has decreased, and he has had one or two episodes of impotence. The nurse attributes L. L.'s problems to
   a. Stress.
   b. Marital discord.
   c. Alcohol intake.
   d. An undiagnosed condition.

5. In an effort to help L. L., the nurse
   a. Enrolls L. L. in a stress management class.
   b. Schedules a meeting with his estranged wife to open lines of communication.
   c. Gives L. L. the meeting times for Alcoholics Anonymous.
   d. Waits for the medical diagnosis before doing anything.

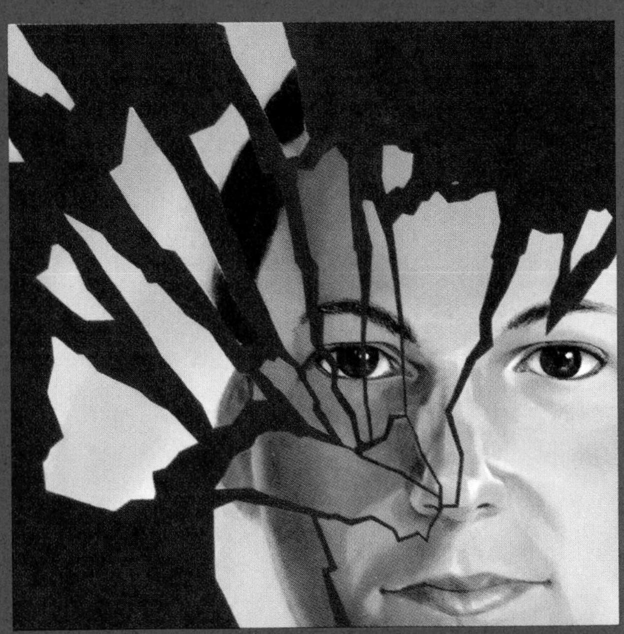

UNIT

3

Therapeutic Interventions

CHAPTER 21

Individual Psychotherapy

DEBORAH ANTAI-OTONG, M.S., R.N.,C.S.

OUTLINE

CHAPTER OBJECTIVES

Upon completion of this chapter, you will be able to:
1. Identify the major theories of individual psychotherapy.
2. Recognize the significance of psychotherapy across the life span.
3. Discuss essential qualities of psychotherapists.
4. Analyze the role of psychotherapy in facilitating adaptive behaviors.
5. Gain awareness of personal reactions to specific clients.

KEY TERMS

Catharsis
Confrontation
Countertransference
Eclecticism
Insight
Play therapy
Psychotherapy
Self-disclosure
Termination
Therapeutic alliance
Transference

Psychotherapy is the global term for the use of professional help to resolve problems, promote personal growth, and reduce maladaptive responses. Achieving an understanding of their feelings and behaviors is a major goal for people who undertake psychotherapy. Psychotherapy is a valuable form of treatment in which the nurse and client engage in an interactional relationship that promotes adaptive changes, encourages insight, and facilitates optimal functioning. Psychotherapy is based on a therapeutic nurse–client relationship that the client uses to understand and change his or her maladaptive behaviors and distorted cognitive processes and to learn how to improve interpersonal relationships. In this chapter, the major concepts of individual psychotherapy and the usefulness of individual psychotherapy in improving communication across the life span are discussed.

HISTORICAL PERSPECTIVES

Psychotherapy has its roots in the early works of Sigmund Freud. His work with Josef Breuer involving the use of hypnosis with a client named Anna O. generated much data that furthered the understanding and treatment of neurosis. Freud's work with Breuer as well as his other clinical experiences with neurotic clients such as Anna are the basis of psychoanalysis. Psychoanalysis is a form of psychodynamic psychotherapy in which the therapist and client explore the client's conscious and unconscious conflicts and coping patterns. The major techniques used in psychoanalysis include free association, transference, and therapeutic alliance.

Psychoanalytical concepts have been integrated into other forms of psychotherapy. Corsini (1984) described psychotherapy as a process that focuses on changing the client's cognitions (thought processes), affect (feelings), and behaviors. Clients' ability and willingness to change help them explore the meaning of their maladaptive behaviors and develop effective coping behaviors. Many clients seek treatment because they want to change.

Hildegarde Peplau (1968), a pioneer in psychiatric nursing, believed that clients with sociopsychological and emotional problems are appropriate candidates for psychotherapy. She described individual psychotherapy as an interpersonal process between a therapist and a client that consists of three phases: orientation, working through, and termination (1968).

Another noted nurse, June Mellow (1967), developed a form of nursing psychotherapy on the basis of her extensive work with a woman experiencing an acute psychotic schizophrenic episode prior to the advent of psychotropics. She used the nurse–client relationship to establish trust, provide safety, and assess and meet the client's psychosocial needs.

THEORIES AND CONCEPTS OF INDIVIDUAL PSYCHOTHERAPY

The success of a helping relationship hinges on the client's ability to form open, trusting relationships. The client brings to psychotherapy an array of present and past experiences that affect his or her perceptions of the nurse and present stressors and his or her motivation to change. The nurse also brings past and present experiences to this relationship, and the meaning the nurse assigns to the client's responses to stressors is influenced by the nurse's theoretical orientation and self-awareness. Many therapists use an eclectic approach to psychotherapy. The term ***eclecticism*** in psychotherapy means the use of two or more theories to meet a client's needs and develop effective treatment (Norcross, 1991). An eclectic approach increases the likelihood that psychotherapy will be successful and provides the client with an assortment of interventions.

Several factors contribute to the lack of development of a therapeutic relationship. Major factors include the

TABLE 21–1
Psychotherapies: Theoretical Approaches

	GOAL	SPECIFIC ILLNESS	DURATION	TECHNIQUES
Psychoanalytical	► Restructure personality	► Oedipal conflict	► 3 to 6 years	► Free association ► Therapeutic alliance ► Transference ► Interpretation ► Exploration of defenses
Supportive	► Support reality testing ► Promote adaptation and restoration of coping skills	► Ego deficits ► Overwhelming stress ► Cognitive impairment	► Days to years	► Ego strengthening ► Reality-based interactions ► Administration of psychotropics
Brief	► Assess nature of defense mechanisms	► Anxiety, impulsivity ► Childhood conflicts	► <12 months	► Interpretation ► Transference ► Exploration of defenses
Interpersonal	► Improve interpersonal skills and communication	► Depression	► 12 to 16 weeks	► Reassurance ► Assessment of meaning of feelings ► Empathy ► Emotional support

client's noncompliance, the client's inability to form trusting relationships, and premature termination (Basch, 1980; Frank & Gunderson, 1990).

There is no single determinant of successful or unsuccessful psychotherapy. The effectiveness of psychotherapy varies. A number of studies dating back to the 1950s confirm the success of psychotherapy in helping clients in distress (e.g., Piper et al., 1991; Stevenson & Meares, 1992; Wolpe, 1958). However, in other studies, little difference in outcome was found between therapy clients and control groups who did not receive treatment (Seeman et al., 1964; Truax, 1963).

Overall, psychotherapy is a facilitative process in which the therapeutic relationship is used to promote the client's health, growth, and development of adaptive coping behaviors. Successful client outcomes depend on accurate assessment of complex client needs and the integration of various psychotherapy concepts into treatment and evaluation.

Table 21–1 lists some individual psychotherapies and their goals, duration, and techniques, along with examples of disorders in which these therapies may be used.

PSYCHOANALYTICAL PSYCHOTHERAPY

Psychoanalytical psychotherapy has its roots in Josef Breuer's early work with a young neurotic woman, Anna O. This woman, who showed alterations in perception during consciousness, was observed under hypnosis to be free of symptoms. Sigmund Freud's later work and collaboration with Breuer on hysteria provided the foundation of the major concepts of psychoanalytical theory. Breuer's and Freud's work became the foundation of their publication, *Studies on Hysteria*.

Freud eventually developed the technique of free association, in which the client says the first thing that comes to mind, without restrictions, in response to something the therapist says. Free association is the heart of psychoanalytical psychotherapy. It provides verbal **catharsis,** the healthy release of ideas that help the client gain insight into conflicts and early developmental turmoil.

The therapist who uses psychoanalytical therapy is called an *analyst*. An analyst is usually a psychiatrist or other mental health professional who has been trained in psychoanalysis. Treatment focuses on creating an environment that promotes regression, interpretation of free associations and dreams, and transference. Ideally, analysts themselves have been through psychoanalysis as part of their training and are able to maintain neutrality. Duration of treatment may range from four to five sessions per week for 3 to 5 years (Karasu, 1989).

Goals

The goals of psychoanalytical psychotherapy include (1) facilitating the resolution of conflict generated by repressed memories of traumatic childhood psychosexual issues to achieve reorganization of the client's personality, (2) settling unconscious discord, and (3) increasing insight. Psychoanalytical psychotherapy is long-term treatment that involves a gradual integration of repressed conflicts into the personality. Kaplan and Sadock (1991) described analysis as a process similar to putting together the pieces of an immense and complicated puzzle.

Treatment Techniques

The following are the major treatment techniques of psychoanalytical psychotherapy:

- Therapeutic alliance
- Interpretation of transference
- Resolution of countertransference
- Free association
- Neutrality

Therapeutic Alliance. The **therapeutic alliance** is the trusting relationship that the therapist and client have established that lets the client feel free to explore interpersonal and intrapersonal conflicts and gain insight into his or her maladaptive behaviors. Purposes of this relationship involve developing trust, and assessing and curing the client's presenting symptoms.

Interpretation of Transference. The hallmark of psychoanalysis, **transference**, is the clients' unconscious displacement onto the therapist of their feelings and attitudes toward significant figures in their childhood. Transference is an integral aspect of psychoanalysis and is a powerful tool that can be used to explore and understand the meaning of clients' unresolved conflicts with their parents or other significant persons in their childhood. Transference is unconscious and may be positive or negative in tone. In positive transference, clients displace their feelings of warmth, esteem, or love for someone else onto the therapist. In negative transference, clients react to the therapist with the hate, anger, or rage they feel toward some other particular person. Regardless of what feelings, thoughts, or attitudes are expressed, they reveal the client's need to resolve infantile conflicts (Piper et al., 1991).

In interpreting the client's transference, the therapist helps the client examine and understand the origins and meaning of the specific transference reactions and their relationship to early childhood experiences. The interpretation of the transference links the "here-and-now" disturbance with the client's "there-and-then" experience (Kernberg, 1984). A client's expression of anger and feelings of rejection after a session is canceled is an example of transference. The therapist's pointing out that the client expressed similar reactions when dealing with feelings of abandonment by a mother who worked all the time is an example of interpretation of transference.

Resolution of Countertransference. Psychotherapy tends to evoke strong reactions in not only the client, but also the therapist. The therapist's emotional reactions to the client are referred to as ***countertransference.***

Like the client's transference, the therapist's countertransference may be positive or negative and may stem from feelings toward early childhood figures.

Freud (1958) suggested that countertransference should be overcome or minimized because it interferes with the therapeutic relationship. In contrast, others suggested that it is a significant part of the therapeutic process (Heimann, 1950). Countertransference, like transference, has unconscious components stemming from unresolved conflicts. Singer (1970) delineated three categories of countertransference as

- An overly kind and concerned reaction
- An overly hostile and angry reaction
- Intensive anxiety

Singer asserted that the therapist's countertransference reactions may occur during sessions or in fantasies or dreams. Resolution of countertransference is crucial to therapists' understanding of themselves and their clients. Professional supervision and psychoanalysis are forums through which therapists can resolve these conflicts.

Free Association. Free association is clients' spontaneous expression of their thoughts, and it is central to psychoanalysis. The goal of free association is to minimize the conscious screening of thoughts or verbal expressions that allow clients to present rational, logical, and relevant explanations of things. Because clients are free to say the first thing that comes to mind, regardless of whether it is appropriate or embarrassing, their unconscious censorship is reduced. This technique facilitates a deeper understanding of maladaptive behaviors and conflicts. Like other psychoanalytical techniques, it brings areas of conflict into the conscious, or the here and now, so that the client can resolve them (English & Finch, 1964).

Neutrality. Neutrality is another psychoanalytical technique that places the therapist in a passive and permissive role. It enables the client to project onto the therapist certain feelings or attitudes from early childhood relationships (Kernberg, 1984). Like other psychoanalytical techniques, it evokes feelings and thoughts that can be explored and understood in terms of the need to develop adaptive coping behaviors.

BRIEF PSYCHOTHERAPIES

Brief, or short-term, psychotherapy stems from Franz Alexander and Thomas French's work in the 1940s with clients suffering psychosomatic illnesses. They found that brief psychotherapy helped their clients resolve emotional problems that affected biological processes.

Brief psychotherapy refers to any treatment in which the number of sessions is limited, usually to 15 or fewer, and clients are helped to relate present stressors to past experiences. It is useful in treating acute distress, but it is not useful in treating severe symptoms that require immediate resolution, such as suicidal ideations. The client with a spastic colon can benefit from brief psychotherapy. This client may present with acute gastrointestinal symptoms, yet the diagnostic workup may be negative. Brief psychotherapy can alleviate acute physical and emotional symptoms and help the client gain insight into past experiences and current stressors. Positive client outcomes are influenced by the client's motivation to understand the meaning of present symptoms and ego function.

Ego is a psychoanalytical term that refers to the part of the personality that mediates and controls basic biological urges by trying to gratify them within socially acceptable domains. The ego represents the "I" part of the psyche. It is mainly conscious and is the part of the psyche most closely connected with reality or the environment. Self-awareness, perception, and adaptive coping behaviors influence ego function. Clients with healthy ego function have high self-esteem, have good impulse control, adapt positively to stress, tolerate frustration, manage anxiety effectively, and form healthy, meaningful interpersonal relationships. In contrast, those with poor ego function have low self-esteem; poor impulse control; low tolerance for stress, anxiety, and frustration; and distorted perceptions of themselves and others. Their inability to form meaningful interpersonal relationships interferes with the formation of a therapeutic relationship.

Goals. The major goals of brief psychotherapy are to assess the client's problems, remove distressful symptoms, support adaptive coping behaviors, develop treatment goals, and promote optimal functioning. Therapeutic interactions evolve through the use of trust, patience, and flexibility (Davanloo, 1978).

Interpersonal Psychotherapy

Interpersonal psychotherapy is one type of short-term psychotherapy. Interpersonal psychotherapy is based on the assumption that a person's mental processes and behaviors stem from his or her relations with others. A person's interpersonal style is the foundation of his or her coping patterns. It is based on early interactions with primary caregivers, evolves over time, and is inherent in the person's interactions with others (Millon, 1969).

Goals. The major goals of interpersonal psychotherapy are to assess maladaptive interactions and teach adaptive coping skills. Providing guidance, facilitating problem solving, and helping the client gain insight into maladaptive behaviors are major interventions. Clients with impaired social skills can benefit from interpersonal psychotherapy.

Stress-Reducing Therapy

Supportive, or stress-reducing, psychotherapy is used to strengthen clients' adaptive behaviors and promote homeostasis (Rogers, 1942). People who are experiencing stress often feel inadequate and isolated. Stress-reducing therapy gives them emotional and biological support with medication during crisis or stress.

Goals. The major treatment goals of supportive therapy are to promote restoration of health, maintain adaptive coping behaviors, strengthen ego function, improve coping behaviors or patterns, enhance problem-solving skills, and mobilize resources and options.

Creating a supportive climate begins with the establishment of a therapeutic nurse–client relationship that initially encourages dependence and later promotes independence. Supportive therapy reduces stress that interferes with optimal functioning. Clients with schizophrenia or dementia can benefit from supportive therapy because it provides an empathetic and encouraging relationship that facilitates reality testing or ego functioning and monitoring of clients' responses to treatment. Ongoing emotional support increases social interaction and promotes growth and independence. Crisis intervention and administration of psychotropics can enhance supportive psychotherapy (Kaplan & Sadock, 1991).

Behavioral Therapy

Behavioral therapy originated in 1920, at which time Watson and Rayner described their renowned case of Little Albert. This experiment involved a child who was fearful of a white mouse and all furry objects. They surmised that conditioning could help the youngster deal with his fears of these objects, but they were unable to test these strategies because the child was discharged from the hospital. Several years later, however, Jones (1924) used Watson and Rayner's strategies to treat children with phobias.

Behavioral therapy is based on the assumption that human behaviors, or responses, are learned and therefore may be unlearned. In addition, adaptive and maladaptive responses are influenced by a stimulus response that is mediated by the nervous system. Wolpe (1958, 1973) asserted that a behavior is a response; the stimulus occurs before the response; and the activation of the afferent nerves is modulated by sensory stimuli. For example, the client who walks into a crowd (stimulus) and panics (response), experiencing dizziness, heart palpitations, and dry mouth (arousal of the sympathetic nervous system), is experiencing a stimulus response that is mediated by the autonomic nervous system.

Clients with anxiety disorders, phobias, and depression can reduce their distress through various behavioral therapies, such as systematic desensitization, flooding, participant modeling, aversion therapy, positive reinforcement, assertiveness and social skills training, and various psychotropics. Table 21–2 describes these behavioral therapy techniques. See Chapters 10 and 26 for specific psychopharmacological interventions.

Cognitive Therapy

The term *cognitive* stems from the Latin word *cogitare*, meaning "to know." Cognitive therapy helps clients recognize their distorted cognitions and maladaptive behaviors. Major strategies include homework assignments, interruption of irrational belief systems, and reduction of feelings generated by distorted cognition(s) (Beck, 1976; Beck et al., 1979).

The benefits of cognitive therapy are illustrated in the following case study, in which the nurse gently questions the client's overgeneralization and negative self-talk.

Case Study: Using Cognitive Therapy Techniques with a Depressed Client (Phil)

Phil, a depressed client, complains that "today has been a terrible day and everything has gone wrong." After questioning Phil, the nurse discovers that only one negative thing has transpired: a co-worker

TABLE 21–2
Behavioral Therapy Techniques

	DEFINITION	TECHNIQUES AND EXAMPLES
Systematic Desensitization	► Client is exposed to stimulus that produces anxiety	► Relaxation training ► Hierarchy construction ► Desensitization of stimulus (Wolpe, 1958, 1973)
Flooding	► Intensive exposure to anxiety-producing stimulus	► Expose to specific phobia, both real and imagined
Participant Modeling	► New behavior is learned through observation	► Behavioral rehearsal
Assertiveness and Social Skills Training	► Client is taught how to behave appropriately and in a confident manner	► Role modeling ► Positive reinforcement ► Desensitization
Aversion Therapy or Conditioned Reflex Therapy	► Association of abstinence responses with behavior that has offensive consequences (exposure to noxious stimulus)	► Administration of Antabuse in client who has alcoholism ► Exposure to specific phobia
Positive Reinforcement	► Reward is given for desired behavior change	► Token economies ► Positive feedback

turned down Phil's invitation to lunch. After questioning by the nurse, Phil was able to identify several positive occurrences, including an outstanding job appraisal. The nurse pointed out a lack of congruency between Phil's negative thoughts and feelings, and events at work. The nurse gave Phil a "homework assignment" of keeping a log or diary of events and thoughts that occurred prior to his feeling "depressed and down." Follow-up sessions allowed the nurse to confront Phil's overgeneralization and negative self-talk and the lack of congruency between his thoughts and feelings and reality.

Johnston (1990) asserted that the capacity to form a collaborative nurse–client relationship and the client's motivation to change determine the success of cognitive therapy. The nurse's ability to establish a working alliance is crucial to the success of cognitive therapy. It enables the nurse to establish a nonthreatening climate that helps the client recognize irrational belief systems that distort reality and thereby generate distress. Cognitive therapy has been helpful in treating clients with anxiety, personality and depressive disorders (Beck, 1979; Beck & Freedman, 1990). Chapter 10 describes the use of cognitive therapy to treat anxiety.

INDIVIDUAL PSYCHOTHERAPY ACROSS THE LIFE SPAN

Numerous studies attest to the effectiveness of psychotherapy at different stages in the life span. Approaches to individual psychotherapy are based on individual needs and vary with clients' developmental stage, cognitive abilities, ego integrity, and motivation for treatment. See Table 21–3 for a summary of effective techniques of individual psychotherapy for clients of different ages.

CHILDHOOD

The practice of child psychotherapy dates back to 1909, when Freud published his work with a 5-year-old phobic boy (1959a, 1959b). Erikson (1959) and Piaget (1969) contributed to the understanding of the normal developmental stages of childhood and adolescence. Later, the child guidance clinic model (Kanner, 1955) specified that while one therapist works with the child, a second therapist works with the parents. Successful outcomes required focusing on maladaptive interactions between the child and the family system. Currently, child psychotherapists lean toward increasing information about adaptive and maladaptive developmental responses, developing adept assessments and effective treatment, and understanding the causes of childhood mental disorders (Vernberg et al., 1992).

Protecting children from profound distress and facilitating their adaptive coping patterns are germane to the mental health of future generations. The prevalence of emotional and behavioral disorders among the young is approximately 12 to 17 percent, or 7.5 to 14 million (Institute of Medicine, 1989; U.S. Congress, Office of Technology Assessment, 1986). These staggering figures challenge psychiatric nurses to identify children and families at risk and to develop primary, secondary, and tertiary prevention strategies to promote health (see Chapter 4 for more information on prevention strategies).

The following are predictors of psychosocial and neurobiological health in children and adolescents (Compas, 1987; Mallinckrodt, 1992):

- The capacity to use various support systems
- A sense of self-worth and competence
- A sense of belonging
- The ability to respond to developmental crises
- Parents' or caregivers' competence

Treatment strategies are determined by the child's developmental stage, the severity of symptoms in the

TABLE 21–3

Individual Psychotherapy Across the Life Span

	EFFECTIVE PSYCHOTHERAPEUTIC TECHNIQUES	NURSING CHALLENGES
Childhood	► Supportive therapy ► Play therapy ► Behavioral modification ► Cognitive therapy	► Client's immature ego function and inability to express feelings ► Motivation for treatment ► Establishment of trust
Adolescence	► All types	► Establishment of working relationship with client
Young and middle adulthood	► All types	► Role transitions ► Developmental stress (marriage, divorce, parenthood) ► Financial concerns ► Careers
Older adulthood	► All types	► Understanding of aging process, role of medications, presenting symptoms, and coping patterns ► Motivation for treatment

child, and the parents' coping skills. Establishment of a therapeutic relationship is the basis of all psychotherapies. A climate that fosters trust, safety, and growth is the major goal of child psychotherapy.

Types of Child Psychotherapy

Child psychotherapy includes supportive, play, behavior modification, and cognitive therapies.

Supportive Psychotherapy. Supportive psychotherapy enables children who are experiencing normal developmental stress to maintain and improve their adaptive coping behaviors.

Play Therapy. **Play therapy** gives children a symbolic way to express their feelings, anxiety, aggressions, and self-doubt. In play therapy, a simple playroom setting is used as a therapeutic tool. The premise behind play therapy is that because their verbal skills are inadequate, children usually communicate better through play than verbally (Axline, 1955).

Playrooms are an essential part of psychotherapy with children. These rooms usually have an array of playthings and toys that allow the child to communicate fantasies and express feelings. The typical playroom contains special drawers or storage space; multigenerational families of dolls of various races; toy soldiers and policemen; dollhouse furnishings; crayons and clay; puppets; sponge-like balls; tools such as play hammers; rubber knives and guns; building blocks; cars, trucks, and airplanes; and cooking and eating utensils (Everstine & Everstine, 1993).

Behavior Modification. Behavior modification teaches the child how to modify maladaptive target behaviors through positive reinforcement or a token reward system. Modeling plays a vital role in behavior modification, and success is contingent upon training the parents to provide positive reinforcement, so that behavior modification occurs at home (Gordon et al., 1979).

Cognitive Therapy. Cognitive therapy enables the impulsive child to correct negative, distorted cognitive processes and improve self-image (Meichenbaum, 1977).

Psychotherapy Issues Particular to Children

The success of any treatment requires active parent–child participation. Parents act as role models, and in some cases as therapists, and reinforce and encourage adaptive coping behaviors. Various forms of psychotherapy are appropriate for all age groups.

The major differences between child psychotherapy and adult psychotherapy relate to specific developmental needs and tasks. There are four major differences between children and adults seeking treatment. First, children have immature ego function and defense mechanisms. Childhood traumas and problems can result in permanent impairment of personality and physical development. Second, children typically do not present for treatment voluntarily. They are usually brought in by their parents, who want them to be "fixed" after the parents have exhausted their coping and problem-solving skills. This challenges the nurse to motivate the children for treatment while attempting to establish trust. Third, children tend to externalize internal conflicts to work through their distress. They have difficulty solving problems and verbalizing their feelings, except through changing things in their environment. Finally, children are inclined to reenact their feelings in new situations and eagerly engage in new experiences (Mishne, 1986). The nurse can use these attributes to engage children in the therapeutic relationship and facilitate adaptive changes.

Because children's problems are complex and their abilities and levels of understanding that differ from those of adults, play therapy, parental behavioral modification programs, and the various psychotherapies must be tailored to meet the unique needs of each child and his or her parents.

ADOLESCENCE

Adolescence is a time of turmoil and transition. Adolescents have to balance feelings generated by their needs for both separation and dependence, cope with underlying poor self-esteem, and determine an identity. Typical adolescent behaviors include poor impulse control, mood swings, and poor frustration tolerance. Erikson (1959) described adolescence as the final stage of childhood and a time during which personal identity is formed. Piaget (1969) defined adolescence as a period in which abstract thinking and intellectual development are achieved. Adolescence is further influenced by cultural, ethnic, neurobiological, and psychosocial factors.

Assessment Foci

The assessment of adolescents, like the assessment of children, is based on age-appropriate behaviors and mastery of developmental tasks. The assessment process is frequently complicated by the turbulence of adolescence, but Kessler (1966) suggested that assessment of the adolescent should address the following:

1. Behaviors appropriate to the child's chronological age
2. Duration, frequency, and number of symptoms
3. Degree of social dysfunction
4. Severity of behavior
5. Adaptive and maladaptive responses (personality traits)
6. Degree of subjective distress

Transference Issues

The transference reactions of children and adolescents differ from those of adults because they still live with their significant early objects or caregivers. As a rule, they do not displace their feelings toward and perceptions of these significant figures onto other objects. Instead, their behavior and attitude usually relate to their parents in the here and now. They perceive the therapist as an extension of their parents. Transference reactions provide therapists with opportunities to explore impaired thought processes and distorted cognitions (Sandler et al., 1980).

Countertransference Issues

Countertransference, like transference, emerges in psychotherapy with adolescents. Adolescence often being a period of turmoil, teenage clients have a natural ability to evoke strong reactions in the therapist because of their need to express feelings generated by neurobiological and psychosocial stressors. Their tendency to express feelings through acting out rather than through words frequently generates stress in the therapist (Giovacchini, 1985). Therapists can use their interpretations of their countertransference to enhance their self-awareness and understanding of the adolescent client's symptoms.

Establishing a Working Relationship with an Adolescent

Successful identification of the adolescent client's needs and development of effective interventions depend on the quality of the nurse–client relationship. The nurse's initial task is to establish alliance with the adolescent and the parents. Initially, adolescents presenting for treatment are likely to be more provocative, more intense, and cruder than adults seeking treatment. They are less trusting and open during early stages of treatment, frequently denying their problems and blaming their parents. Furthermore, the adolescent, through transference, is likely to act out against authority figures, rather than express feelings. Acting out may include self-destructive behaviors such as substance abuse, truancy, promiscuity, or suicide attempts.

Establishing working relationships with adolescents challenges nurses to use patience and draw on their understanding of adaptive and maladaptive developmental tasks. The major desirable client outcomes include enhancement and maintenance of self-esteem; development of adaptive coping skills; and formation of healthy, meaningful relationships.

Factors that interfere with the formation of a therapeutic relationship with an adolescent include cognitive impairment, which may be seen in psychotic or depressive disorders or substance abuse, and a lack of trust in the family of origin. Anticipation of these behaviors is thus crucial to working with this age group.

YOUNG AND MIDDLE ADULTHOOD

The transition from adolescence to adulthood generates tremendous stress. Major adult transitions include establishing a career, entering into marriage or divorce, managing financial problems, parenting, and caring for aging parents. Stressful life events often generate crises or maladaptive coping patterns. Psychotherapy can be used to identify individual strengths and limitations that enable clients to develop adaptive coping patterns and interactions. Psychotherapy provides an atmosphere of trust, acceptance, and opportunity for growth.

Clients seeking treatment have complex needs and experience various forms of distress, such as depression, anxiety, and somatic complaints. Psychotherapy may be used alone or in conjunction with a case management approach to meet complex client needs. The case management approach includes psychotherapy, monitoring client responses to an array of interventions such as medications, other somatic therapies, and psychosocial interventions. The depressed client who has recently had a myocardial infarction and is now taking an antidepressant and participating in psychotherapy can benefit from case management. Initial contact with the client often begins in an acute or ambulatory care setting, such as the emergency department, and continues for an expanded period in the community. Collaboration with various community health professionals such as psychiatrists, cardiologists, and social service workers is important to ensure continuous comprehensive care.

OLDER ADULTHOOD

Older adults represent the fastest growing segment of the American population. They constitute 12 percent of the population, or approximately 25 million people, and it is estimated that by 2050, this figure will more than double (U.S. Bureau of the Census, 1989). These statistics suggest a need for theory development and research regarding the effectiveness of psychotherapy in meeting the needs of the elderly.

Historically, the effectiveness of working with this age group has been debated. Freud (1959) suggested that the elderly were not appropriate for psychoanalysis, but his colleague, Abraham, disputed this notion and suggested that they could benefit from treatment (Fenichel, 1945). In spite of early debate, the number of elderly clients who seek treatment continues to lag behind that of other age groups, and only 4 percent of mental health clinics and 3 percent of private practitioners treat them (U.S. General Accounting Office, 1982; Vandenbos et al., 1981). Various explanations account for these figures, including older adults' hesitancy to confide in younger therapists, older adults' self-reliance, and therapists' hesitancy to work with older people.

Even though the number of elderly clients who seek treatment is less than that of other age groups, this population is at risk. The elderly experience numerous losses, such as the deaths or debilitating illnesses of loved ones and declines in socioeconomic well-being and mental and physical functioning. The high rate of successful suicides among elderly white males suggests that nurses need to identify stressors and formulate effective interventions that support adaptive coping behaviors and relieve physical and mental distress.

Individual psychotherapy is a useful treatment strategy for the elderly. Understandings of the normal aging process, the role of medications, presenting symptoms, coping patterns, and motivation for treatment are major elements of successful individual psychotherapy with this group.

Teri and Logsdon (1992) stated that the following are essential qualities for psychotherapists working with the elderly:

1. An interest in the elderly and a perception of working with the elderly as a challenge, rather than as a hopeless endeavor
2. Specialized training on the aging process
3. A caring attitude toward the elderly
4. Ability to set realistic and individual treatment goals

They described work with the elderly as challenging and rewarding and an opportunity to appreciate the uniqueness and complexity of the human aging process. Psychotherapy with this age group "maximizes the full spectrum of human knowledge," Teri and Logsdon (p. 86) stated, integrating theories and research findings toward the development of effective interventions.

SUMMARY

Individual psychotherapy across the life span challenges nurses to understand and appreciate the uniqueness of each developmental stage. It reveals the full spectrum of human development and people's methods of coping with the daily stress of living. Individual psychotherapy is a treatment modality that uses the nurse–client relationship to facilitate effective coping responses and promote optimal health. It also encourages self-awareness and growth in clients, which are necessary for clients to understand their behaviors and maximize their resourcefulness.

THE NURSE'S ROLE

Individual psychotherapy focuses on changing personality structure and maladaptive behaviors. The outcome of individual psychotherapy is determined by the quality of the therapeutic alliance, the client's perception of presenting symptoms or behaviors, and motivation for change, and neurobiological and psychosocial factors. Certain conditions must exist to facilitate a positive outcome. A key player in the psychotherapy process is the psychotherapist.

THE GENERALIST NURSE

Psychotherapy is limited to nurses who are at least master's prepared and clinically competent to assess and oversee complex client needs. Conducting psychotherapy requires an in-depth understanding of human behavior and various psychosocial, psychiatric, and biological theories and their application to complex client problems. Generalist nurses are educationally and clinically unprepared to conduct psychotherapy. However, they can provide other therapeutic interventions such as crisis intervention or grief counseling to clients and families and support them during stressful periods. These are effective strategies that provide immediate emotional support, mobilize resources and adaptive coping behaviors, and foster problem solving during crisis situations.

THE ADVANCED-PRACTICE NURSE

The American Nurses Association (ANA, 1994) defines the nurse psychotherapist as an advanced-level (master's degree or higher) clinical nurse specialist who is educated and clinically prepared and certified to provide psychotherapy. The nurse psychotherapist independently performs various forms of psychotherapy and is accountable for his or her practice and health care delivery. The ANA (1994) specifies that the nurse psychotherapist is responsible for

1. Structuring a therapeutic nurse–client agreement
2. Collaborating with health professionals to facilitate effective treatment
3. Maintaining and refining his or her professional skills through continuing education and collaboration with other psychotherapists
4. Providing clinical supervision, role modeling for nurses and other mental health students, and offering inservice education
5. Integrating biological concepts into practice through prescriptive authority within state regulations

PHASES OF THE THERAPEUTIC RELATIONSHIP

Psychotherapy is a powerful treatment modality that enables the nurse to form a therapeutic relationship with the client to assess and relieve the client's distress, to change the client's maladaptive coping patterns, and to promote the client's growth and development (ANA, 1994).

What constitutes a therapeutic relationship? Peplau (1968) stated that the therapeutic process consists of three phases: orientation, the working relationship, and termination.

Orientation—The first phase of the therapeutic relationship is the orientation phase. In this phase, the nurse sets the ground rules and decides the format and process of the therapeutic relationship.

The Working Relationship—The second phase is the working relationship. Peplau (1968) stated that the working relationship is based on several premises: First, the client is responsible for the work done in psychotherapy, and the therapist is a facilitator who provides an environment that fosters trust, empathy, and genuine interest in the client's problems and growth. Second, this climate must enable the client to develop adaptive or competent behaviors that encourage growth and problem resolution. Competencies must consist of cognitive and interpersonal components. Finally, interactions must center on problematic situations.

Termination—As adaptive behaviors and growth emerge, the third phase, termination, begins. During the termination phase, clients' accomplishments are reviewed, and their feelings regarding the ending of the relationship are explored.

Psychotherapy is an interactive process that evolves over time between the therapist and the client. Patience and genuine interest are crucial to a successful outcome, because they facilitate verbal and nonverbal communication that promotes a greater understanding of the complex process of client responses.

THE NURSING PROCESS

Assessment and Diagnosis

In the initial stage of psychotherapy, the client's symptoms and present stressors are assessed. Present and past coping patterns are assessed in a manner that conveys a caring and concerned attitude. Clients are often reluctant to discuss their problems with a stranger because of shame, guilt, or distrust. These feelings can be allayed by active listening that helps the nurse identify common themes, both verbal and nonverbal, in the client's presenting symptoms. A common theme among depressed clients is the feeling of being a failure or loser, which suggests a lack of control or feelings of helplessness.

The specific theoretical framework being followed determines how the client is approached, information is elicited, treatment strategies are developed, and responses to interventions are evaluated. In addition, theoretical concepts determine the focus of observation, such as the here and now rather than past events, and the data collection process. Data collection helps in the development of the nursing and medical diagnoses.

Client education is a major component of psychotherapy. During the assessment process, the nurse educates the client about psychotherapy and about the specific roles and expectations of each of them. This discussion addresses boundary issues and the collaborative nature of psychotherapy. The client is encouraged to play an active role in psychotherapy and share responsibility for outcome identification and response to treatment.

Planning

Outcome identification, or goal setting, is a collaborative endeavor between the nurse and client. This involves problem identification and identification of expected outcomes of interventions. Active client participation in this process fosters independence and responsibility in treatment.

Intervention

The specific interventions used are determined by the client's problems of diagnoses, motivation for treatment, cognitive processes, and developmental stage, as well as the time frame for treatment. In addition, the nurse's theoretical perspective influences interventions. For instance, if the client has cognitive distortions that have activated maladaptive responses, a cognitive–behavioral approach may be helpful in facilitating adaptive coping behaviors. This eclectic approach (i.e., both cognitive and behavioral therapies) is more flexible than a simple perspective because it integrates several theories that are based on the client's needs, ability to learn, and developmental stage.

As the nurse–client relationship evolves, several treatment issues may arise. Countertransference, client resistance, client insight, confrontation, self-disclosure by the nurse, and confidentiality are integral aspects of

TABLE 21–4
Therapeutic Issues and Interventions

ISSUE	INTERVENTIONS
Countertransference: interferes with nurse's ability to provide objective client interventions	▸ Recognize personal reactions to specific clients, e.g., anger, hostility, rescuing, or overprotectiveness
Resistance: maintains client's status quo and interferes with working-through process and development of adaptive coping	▸ Assess meaning of resistance to client ▸ Prescribe no change in resistance (paradoxical intent, or asking client to do the opposite of what is wanted)
Insight: basis for client's motivation for therapy and understanding of course of illness and treatment outcome	▸ Provide client and significant others with education regarding illness, treatment outcome, and course/outcome of interventions ▸ Encourage ventilation of feelings and concerns regarding illness/treatment ▸ Clarify client's and family's feelings ▸ Avoid interpreting behaviors too quickly
Self-disclosure: based on nature of nurse–client relationship; excessive use interferes with therapeutic process	▸ Limit information to what you are comfortable with sharing, such as, "Yes, I am married"
Confidentiality: basis of trust, but absolute confidentiality is unrealistic with children and adolescents	▸ Discuss record keeping with client and family ▸ Maintain computerized records ▸ Follow legal and ethical protocols for duty to warn and duty to protect ▸ Discuss specific issues with client and significant others

psychotherapy (see Table 21–4). Countertransference has already been discussed in this chapter.

Resistance. Resistance is a phenomenon that occurs during early treatment, and clients use it to ward off uncomfortable feelings, particularly anxiety, generated by underlying repressed conflicts. Symptoms of resistance include missed appointments, tardiness, and refusal to do homework assignments.

Insight. **Insight** refers to the client's self-awareness and understanding of the meaning and reason for his or her behavior or motives. This term generally means that the client or significant other has knowledge of the illness and is aware of behaviors that contribute to remission or exacerbation of symptoms. An example of a client with insight is the man who comes to the emergency department or nurse's office requesting a refill of lithium because he knows that he will become manic or psychotic and require hospitalization if he stops taking the drug. In contrast, an example of the client with poor insight is the man who stops taking lithium, becomes manic, and requires an involuntary admission. Poor insight in psychotherapy interferes with restoration of health and optimal functioning.

Nurses cannot instill insight into clients, but they can provide therapeutic climates that increase its likelihood. Resisting the temptation to interpret clients' behaviors and letting them understand the link between maladaptive behaviors and persistent distress can be helpful. Insight often overwhelms the client with feelings and ideas that need to be backed up with behavioral changes. If insight does not exist, the client experiences little change (Carkhuff & Berenson, 1967).

Resistance and poor insight often require nursing interventions that facilitate clients' understanding of results of their persistent maladaptive responses.

Confrontation. **Confrontation** is useful in pointing out parts of the client's assessment and treatment process that are contradictory or confusing, and it reduces vagueness and incongruencies in client affect, behavior, or communication. Trust, patience, and empathy are prerequisites to confrontation (Kernberg, 1984). Its effectiveness lies in its potential to help clients develop adaptive coping responses by clarifying the meaning of resistance, distortions, and poor insight.

Self-Disclosure. **Self-disclosure** on the part of the nurse therapist is an important part of the nurse–client relationship. Judith Simon (1988) described self-disclosure as the antithesis of the detachment or neutrality advocated by psychoanalytical theory. She noted that self-disclosure can enhance the therapeutic alliance and the therapist's self-awareness and modeling role, validate reality for the client, and increase the therapist's satisfaction with a case. Some degree of self-disclosure is a natural part of the nurse–client relationship; in the course of therapy, for example, nurses may reveal their marital status, professional specialty, and family situation. A picture of a child or spouse provides information about the nurse's family, and certificates or diplomas indicate the nurse's professional training and formal education. Knowledge of the nurse's education level and clinical expertise is important to most clients seeking psychotherapy, because it informs them of the nurse's competency.

The degree of self-disclosure by the nurse depends on the nature of the nurse–client relationship, the nurse's comfort in sharing personal information with clients, and the appropriateness of clinical situations. Too little self-disclosure reduces the opportunities for reality testing, slowing the development of a trusting relationship and making the client feel less comfortable disclosing pertinent information about him- or herself. On the other hand, too much self-disclosure may blur boundaries between nurse and client. Negative consequences of self-disclosure can be decreased by avoiding discussion of emotionally provocative and very personal subjects.

Confidentiality. Confidentiality and the right to privacy are the basis of all therapeutic relationships, but they are no longer easily achieved. They are affected by several factors, including legal and ethical matters and developmental stage. The complexity of legal and ethical dilemmas associated with confidentiality challenges psychotherapists to create environments of trust and maintain open communication with clients and significant others about information that remains in therapy and that which has to be shared with others when appropriate. The client who comes into therapy threatening to shoot his wife is an example of a situation that affects confidentiality, which cannot be maintained for several reasons. First, the therapist has a legal and ethical duty to warn and protect the client's wife, to notify the police, and to use sound judgment to intervene appropriately (Tarasoff *v* Regents of University of California, 1976). Second, the client must understand that this information will not be kept confidential, especially if he is deemed imminently dangerous.

Clients must feel that information shared with the psychotherapist remains private and confidential. Concerns such as sexual orientation, mental and physical illnesses, and participation in psychotherapy are personal matters. Respecting and appreciating the significance of information divulged by the client are critical to maintaining a trusting relationship. Discussing and maintaining client records are additional aspects of confidentiality.

Even though confidentiality is the basis of trust, it is unrealistic to maintain it with children and adolescents. Parents must be informed when the need for protection, structure, and safety exists, such as acting out, self-destructive behaviors, or threats to harm self or others.

Evaluation

Nurses can evaluate the effectiveness of psychotherapy by comparing client outcomes with their own and the client's expectations. Evaluation is an ongoing process in which objective and subjective data are integrated.

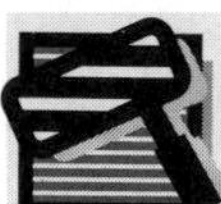

RESEARCH STUDY

An Outcome Study of Psychotherapy for Patients with Borderline Personality Disorder

Stevenson, J., & Meares, R. (1992). *American Journal of Psychiatry, 149,* 358–362.

Study Problem/Purpose

The aim of this study was to evaluate the effectiveness of psychotherapy in an outpatient setting for clients diagnosed with personality disorders.

Method

Thirty clients diagnosed with borderline personality disorder were seen twice weekly for outpatient psychotherapy for 12 months. The outcome criteria used to judge the effectiveness of the therapy were compliance with prescription drug regimen, avoidance of illicit drug use, decrease in episodes of self-destructive behavior, keeping of appointments with medical professionals, fewer absences from work, fewer hospitalizations and inpatient treatments, and decline in severity of personality disorder symptoms as noted on self-report index.

Results

Participants demonstrated significant improvement over a 12-month period. One third of the subjects met the criteria for borderline personality disorder.

Nursing Implications

These findings suggest that clients with borderline personality disorder can benefit from a specific type of psychotherapy.

Termination is an integral aspect of psychotherapy and the evaluation process. It is a painful process for most clients, and they must be encouraged to verbalize their feelings about termination. The ending of psychotherapy is just as crucial as the beginning and working phases. It must begin as soon as possible and can be initiated with a discussion of the duration of treatment. Often terminating practices, including summarizing therapy, reviewing client outcomes, dealing with the client's anxiety and fears associated with the loss of the relationship, and identifying the benefits of treatment, should be performed over a period of several months, if feasible (see the Research Abstract display).

Premature termination occurs when a client leaves intensive psychotherapy before the agreed-upon time frame. Frayn (1992) stated that the following factors increase the likelihood of premature termination:

- Extreme anxiety
- Lack of trust
- Denial or lack of insight
- Negative therapeutic alliance
- Substance abuse
- Personality disorder
- Negative reactions to the therapist
- Poor ego functioning manifested by poor impulse control, low tolerance for frustration, and poor social adaptation

Early identification of these behaviors helps the nurse assess their appropriateness for individual psychotherapy, rather than other treatment modalities.

Premature termination can be a highly stressful experience for therapists, generating anxiety, anger, or sense of powerlessness (Searles, 1986). Frayn (1992) reassured therapists that premature termination does not reflect a failure of treatment outcome. Professional assistance in managing countertransference reactions can help nurses effectively explore intense reactions to clients who terminate treatment prematurely.

The following case study illustrates the nursing process using individual psychotherapy.

Case Study: Individual Psychotherapy for a Client with Borderline Personality Disorder (Mrs. Lively)

Mrs. Lively is admitted with a diagnosis of borderline personality disorder. Her history reveals present and past hospitalization associated with recurrent suicidal ideations and prescription drug abuse. She is demanding and goes into rages with little provocation. The mental health team has recommended individual psychotherapy because she has been disruptive in groups during past hospitalizations.

Theory. Personality disorder: Borderline personality disorder (American Psychiatric Association, 1994). (See Chapter 14 for discussion of borderline personality disorder.) Major psychodynamic issues include intense fear of abandonment and dependency needs, poor ego functioning (poor impulse control, fluid boundaries, poor self-esteem, and distorted cognition), intense affect (rage, anger).

Theoretical Approach. Eclectic (cognitive, interpersonal, and supportive)

Assessment

Data Collection. Mrs. Lively is interviewed by the Psychiatric Clinical Specialist. The client and nurse discuss the therapeutic contract, which specifies the purpose, time, place, and confidentiality of sessions. Issues such as the clients' expectations of treatment, problem identification, and the client's perception of her role in therapy are addressed. During the initial session, Mrs. Lively denies having a problem and states that just because she drinks too much does not mean she is nuts.

Nursing Care Plan 21–1 Individual Psychotherapy for a Client with Borderline Personality Disorder (Mrs. Lively)

Nursing Diagnoses: Ineffective Individual Coping; Self-Esteem Disturbance; High Risk for Violence: Self-Directed

OUTCOME IDENTIFICATION	NURSING ACTIONS	RATIONALES	EVALUATIONS
1. By [date], Mrs. Lively will develop adaptive, long-term coping behaviors.	1. Meet with Mrs. Lively twice per week for 45 minutes.	1. Enables nurse to form intensive and therapeutic relationship with client.	*Goals met:* Mrs. Lively's angry outbursts have decreased from 2–3 times per day to once per day.
2. By [date], Mrs. Lively will identify several positive attributes.	2. Clearly delineate client and nurse roles.	2. Enables client to take responsibility in treatment process.	Mrs. Lively is able to identify one positive attribute.
3. By [date], Mrs. Lively will verbalize feelings rather than acting on them.	3. Discuss Mrs. Lively's progress with mental health team.	3. Provides ongoing feedback about areas of improvement/change.	Mrs. Lively did not try to harm herself during this hospitalization and denied having suicidal ideations on discharge.
	4. Use cognitive, interpersonal, and supportive therapies with Mrs. Lively's agreement.	4. Eclectic approach provides client with diverse treatment to meet complex needs.	

Data collection is an ongoing process. Mrs. Lively has been seen in individual psychotherapy twice a week for several weeks and has continued to deny having problems or difficulty coping with present stressors. Information from the mental health team and her record suggest that Mrs. Lively is noncompliant. Assessment findings are as follows:

- Poor ego functioning manifested by poor impulse control and clinging behaviors
- Self-destructiveness manifested by substance abuse and suicidal ideations
- Impaired ability to form trusting interpersonal relationships
- Noncompliance
- Poor insight
- Anger and rage

Nursing Diagnoses

- Ineffective Coping, Individual
- Self-Esteem Disturbance
- Violence, High Risk for: Self-directed

Planning

A care plan is drawn up to achieve the following desired client outcomes:

- Client develops adaptive, long-term coping behaviors.
- Client identifies several positive attributes.
- Client verbalizes feelings rather than acting on them (see Nursing Care Plan 21–1).

Interventions

Therapeutic Contract. The nurse meets with Mrs. Lively twice per week during this admission at 9:00 A.M. for 45 minutes. The client's and nurse's roles in treatment are clearly delineated.

Collaboration. Mrs. Lively's progress is discussed with her and with the mental health team.

Clinical Supervision. The nurse consults with the clinical supervisor to deal with transference and countertransference issues, enhance clinical skills, and promote personal and professional growth.

Partnership with Client. The nurse and Mrs. Lively agree on an eclectic approach using cognitive, interpersonal, and supportive therapies.

Evaluation

Evaluation is an ongoing process, with feedback on progress toward the outcome criteria in the nursing care plan provided to Mrs. Lively during each session. For example:

- The client's present adaptive coping responses are difficult to assess this early in treatment, but her anger outbursts have decreased from two to three times per day to once per day.
- She is able to identify one positive attribute.
- She is able to recognize reasons for feeling anger.
- She did not try to harm herself during this hospitalization, and she denied having suicidal ideations upon discharge.

Discharge Planning. Mrs. Lively will continue weekly sessions with the nurse psychotherapist.

► CHAPTER SUMMARY

There is no magic way to produce adaptive changes in clients. However, nurses can use individual psychotherapy to explore the meaning of clients' maladaptive responses, collaborate with clients to identify desired outcomes of therapy, and evaluate clients' response to interventions. Although both the nurse and the client are players in this interactive process, the client is ultimately responsible for resolving underlying conflicts and developing adaptive coping behaviors. Psychotherapists facilitate this process through therapeutic relationship, promoting insight, and increasing self-esteem.

Suggestions for Clinical Conference

1. Ask the psychiatric clinical specialist to provide a case history of a psychotherapy client, discussing treatment goals, interventions, and evaluation.
2. Identify the maladaptive behaviors of the client in the case history.
3. Identify the role of the staff nurse and clinical nurse specialist in assisting the client's development of adaptive coping behaviors.
4. Role-play confrontation and self-disclosure with other nursing students.

References

Alexander, F., & French, T. M. (1946). *Psychoanalytic therapy: Principles and applications*. New York: Ronald Press.

American Nurses Association. (1994). *Statement on psychiatric–mental health nursing practice*. Washington, DC: Author.

American Psychiatric Association. (1994). *Diagnostic and statistical manual of mental disorders* (4th ed.). Washington, DC: Author.

Axline, V. M. (1955). Play therapy procedures and results. *American Journal of Orthopsychiatry*, *25*, 618–626.

Basch, M. F. (1980). *Doing psychotherapy*. New York: Basic Books.

Beck, A. T. (1976). *Cognitive therapy and emotional disorders*. New York: International Universities Press.

Beck, A. T., Rush, A. J., Shaw, B. F., & Emory, G. (1979). *Cognitive therapy of depression*. New York: Guilford Press.

Beck, A. T., Brown, G., Berchick, R. J., Stewart, B. L., & Steer, R. A. (1990). Relationship between hopelessness and ultimate suicide: A replication with psychiatric outpatients. *American Journal of Psychiatry*, *147*, 190–195.

Beck, A. T., & Freedman, A. (1990). *Cognitive therapy of personality disorders*. New York: Guilford Press.

Breuer, J., & Freud, S. (1955). *Studies in hysteria*. New York: Basic Books.

Carkhuff, R. R., & Berenson, B. G. (1967). *Beyond counseling and therapy*. New York: Holt, Rinehart & Winston.

Compas, B. E. (1987). Coping with stress during childhood and adolescence. *Psychological Bulletin*, *101*, 393–403.

Corsini, R. J. (1984). *Current psychotherapies* (3rd ed.). Itasca, IL: F. E. Peacock.

Davanloo, H. (1978). *Basic principles and techniques in short-term psychotherapy*. New York: Spectrum.

English, O. S., & Finch, S. T. (1964). *Introduction to psychiatry*. New York: W. W. Norton.

Erikson, E. (1959). *Childhood and society*. New York: W. W. Norton.

Everstine, D. S., & Everstine, L. (1993). *The trauma response*. New York: W. W. Norton.

Fenichel, O. (1945). *The psychoanalytic theory of neurosis*. New York: W. W. Norton.

Frank, A. F., & Gunderson, J. G. (1990). The role of the therapeutic alliance in the treatment of schizophrenia: Relationship to course and outcome. *Archives of General Psychiatry*, *47*, 228–236.

Frayn, D. H. (1992). Assessment factors associated with premature psychotherapy termination. *American Journal of Psychotherapy*, *46*, 250–261.

Freud, S. (1958). The dynamics of transference. In J. Strachey (Ed. and Trans.), *The standard edition of the complete psychological works of Sigmund Freud* (Vol. 12, pp. 97–108). London: Hogarth Press. (Original work published 1910).

Freud, S. (1959a). Analysis of a phobia in a five-year-old boy. In A. Strachey & J. Strachey (Trans.), *Collected papers* (Vol. 3, pp. 149–289). New York: Basic Books.

Freud, S. (1959b). On psychotherapy. In J. Riviere (Trans.), *Collected papers* (Vol. 1, pp. 249–263). New York: Basic Books.

Giovacchini, P. (1985). Introduction: Countertransference responses to adolescents. In S. Feinstein, et al. (Eds.), *Adolescent psychiatry: Vol 12. Development and clinical studies*. (pp. 447–448). Chicago: University of Chicago Press.

Gordon, S. B., Lerner, L. L., & Keefe, E. J. (1979). Responsive parenting: An approach to training parents of problem children. *American Journal of Community Psychology*, *7*, 45–56.

Heimann, P. (1950). On countertransference. *International Journal of Psycho-Analysis*, *31*, 81–84.

Institute of Medicine. (1989). *Research on children and adolescents with mental, behavioral, and developmental disorders*. Washington, DC: U.S. Government Printing Office.

Johnston, N.E. (1990). Cognitive therapy. In A. Baumann, N. E. Johnston, & D. Antai-Otong (Eds.), *Decision-making in psychiatric and psychosocial nursing* (pp. 108–109). Philadelphia: B. C. Decker.

Jones, M. C. (1924). Elimination of children's fears. *Journal of Experimental Psychology*, *7*, 382–390.

Kanner, L. (1955). Child psychiatry (3rd ed.). Springfield, IL: Charles C. Thomas.

Kaplan, H. I., & Sadock, B. J. (1991). *Synopsis of psychiatry* (6th ed.). Baltimore: Williams & Wilkins.

Karasu, T. B. (1989). Psychoanalysis and psychoanalytic psychotherapy. In H. I. Kaplan & B. J. Sadock (Eds.), *Comprehensive textbook of psychiatry* (Vol. 2, 5th ed., pp. 1442–1461). Baltimore, Williams & Wilkins.

Kernberg, O. F. (1984). *Severe personality disorders*. New Haven, CT: Yale University Press.

Kessler, J. (1966). *Psychopathology of childhood*. Englewood Cliffs, NJ: Prentice-Hall.

Mallinckrodt, B. (1992). Childhood emotional bonds with parents, development of adult social competencies, and availability of social support. *Journal of Counseling Psychology*, *39*, 453–461.

Meichenbaum, D. H. (1977). *Cognitive-behavior modification*. New York: Plenum.

Mellow, J. (1967). Evolution of nursing through research. *Psychiatric Opinion*, *4*, 15–21.

Millon, T. (1969). *Modern psychopathology*. Philadelphia: W. B. Saunders.

Mishne, J. M. (1986). *Clinical work with adolescents*. New York: Free Press.

Norcross, J. C. (1991). Prescriptive matching in psychotherapy: An introduction. *Psychotherapy*, *28* (3), 439–443.

Peplau, H. E. (1968). Psychotherapeutic strategies. *Perspectives in Psychiatric Care*, *6*, 264–289.

Piaget, J. (1969). The intellectual development of the adolescent. In G. Caplan, & S. Levovici (Eds.), *Adolescence: Psychosocial perspective* (pp. 22–26). New York: Basic Books.

Piper, W. E., Azim, H. F., Joyce, A. S., & McCallum, M. (1991). Transference interpretation, therapeutic alliance, and outcome in short-term individual psychotherapy. *Archives of General Psychiatry*, *48*, 946–953.

Rogers, C. R. (1942). *Counseling and psychotherapy*. Boston: Houghton Mifflin.

Sandler, J., Kennedy, H., & Tyson, P. L. (1980). *The technique of child psychoanalysis: Discussions with Anna Freud*. Cambridge, MA: Harvard University Press.

Searles, H. F. (1986). *My work with borderline patients*. London: Jason Aronson.

Seeman, J. A., Barry, E., & Ellinwood, C. (1964). Interpersonal assessment of play therapy outcome. *Psychotherapy Theory, Research, and Practice, 1*, 64–66.

Simon, J. (1988). Criteria for therapist self-disclosure. *American Journal of Psychotherapy, 43*, 404–415.

Singer, R. (1970). *Key concepts in psychotherapy*. New York: Basic Books.

Stevenson, J., & Meares, R. (1992). An outcome study of psychotherapy for patients with borderline personality disorder. *American Journal of Psychiatry, 149*, 358–362.

Teri, L., & Logsdon, R. C. (1992). The future of psychotherapy with older adults. *Psychotherapy, 29*, 81–87.

Truax, C. B. (1963). Effective ingredients in psychotherapy: An approach to unraveling the patient-therapist interactions. *Journal of Clinical Psychology, 10*, 256–263.

U. S. Bureau of the Census. (1989). Projections of the population in the United States by age, sex, and race: 1988 to 2080 (Current Population Reports, Series P-25, No. 1057). Washington, DC: U.S. Government Printing Office.

U.S. Congress, Office of Technology Assessment. (1986). *Children's mental health: Problems and services. A background paper* (OTA-BP-H-33). Washington, DC: U.S. Government Printing Office.

U.S. General Accounting Office. (1982). *The elderly remain in need of mental health services* (Document No. HRD-82-112). Washington, DC: U.S. Government Printing Office.

Vandenbos, G. R., Stapp, J., & Kilburg, R. R. (1981). Health service providers in psychotherapy: Results of the 1978 APA human resources survey. *American Psychologist, 36*, 1395–1418.

Vernberg, E. M., Routh, D. K., & Koocher, G. P. (1992). The future of psychotherapy with children: Developmental psychotherapy. *Psychotherapy, 29*, 72–80.

Watson, J. B., & Rayner, R. (1920). Conditioned emotional reactions. *Journal of Experimental Psychology, 3*, 1–4.

Wolpe, J. (1958). *Psychotherapy by reciprocal inhibition*. Stanford, CA: Stanford University Press.

Wolpe, J. (1973). *The practice of behavior therapy* (2nd ed.). New York: Pergamon Press.

CHAPTER

22

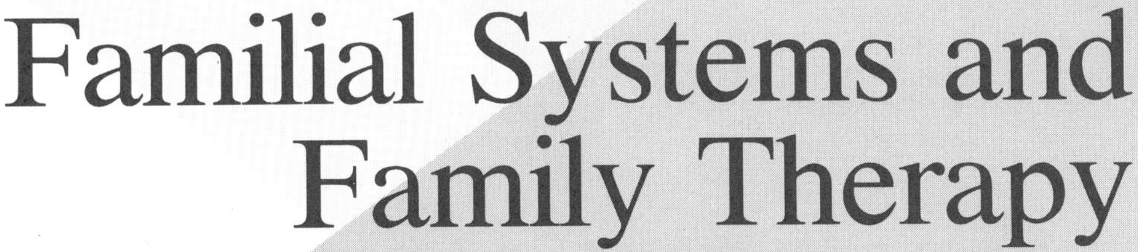

Familial Systems and Family Therapy

DEBORAH ANTAI-OTONG, M.S., R.N.,C.S.

OUTLINE

CHAPTER OBJECTIVES

Upon completion of this chapter, you will be able to:

1. Recognize societal trends and their impact on family structure.
2. Analyze family structures.
3. Integrate major general systems theory into family systems.
4. Recognize maladaptive family communication patterns.
5. Appreciate cultural diversity and coping patterns.
6. Discuss the evolution of families across the life span.
7. Develop a nursing care plan for the family experiencing crisis.

KEY TERMS

Boundaries
Disengagement
Double-bind messages
Dyad
Enmeshment
Family roles
Family structure
Feedback mechanism
Marital schism
Marital skew
Open system
Pseudomutuality
Scapegoating
Subsystems
Triangulation

The American family is transforming, and this transformation parallels immense societal changes. Since the early 1960s, young adults have delayed marriage and have chosen to use effective birth control. The result of this is that fewer children are being born, and parents are older than was typically the case a couple of decades ago. In addition, over the past few decades there has been a surge in the divorce rate and the prevalence of single-parent families has increased. Researchers assert that 60 percent of the children in the United States will live in single-parent homes during their younger years (Hodgkinson, 1989; Zylke, 1991).

Furthermore, family structures have evolved from the traditional couple with 2.4 children to single-parent families, gay and lesbian couples, and single-person households. Traditional couples and families still exist, however, and for many people, the traditional family is the only definition of a "real" family. Nurses are challenged to accept people in various relationships as familial systems.

Regardless of its composition, the family serves numerous purposes within a society. Early family interaction is the basis of lifelong relationships and adaptive processes, such as effective problem solving and communication. In addition, families give their members a sense of identity through cultural transmission, safety, belongings, and social parameters (Minuchin, 1974).

This chapter explores familial interactions and their influence on the development of adaptive and maladaptive behaviors in social contexts. The major concepts of family therapy are discussed, drawing on the work of pioneers such as Salvador Minuchin, Jay Haley, Carl Whitaker, and others. These family therapists' contributions are the foundation of current approaches to family and marital therapy.

CHARACTERISTICS OF FAMILIAL SYSTEMS

Numerous societal changes have made it difficult to define the term *family*. This term stems from the Latin word *familie*, meaning "household or dwelling place." Simply speaking, a family is a dynamic system of people living together who are united by meaningful emotional bonds. The family has two major functions: It ensures survival of the species, and it transmits culture. Families are complex systems. Their ability to integrate biological, psychosocial, and cultural factors and master developmental tasks is determined by family structure and roles (Ackerman, 1958; Baumann & Beckingham, 1990; Satir, 1967).

FAMILY STRUCTURE

Family structure refers to the forms a family takes in adapting and maintaining itself (Minuchin, 1974). The heart of the family structure is the dyad. A **dyad** is a two-person relationship, either an adult–adult relationship or an adult–child relationship. Dyads determine roles, culture, and function. The increased divorce rate and the increase in single male parents and gay couples with children have contributed to a change in the definition of family structure. Thus there is an increased need for nurses to understand family interactions and function and their role in promoting the health of family members.

Table 22–1 lists some types of family structures. The nuclear family and the extended family are two examples. The extended family consists of a nuclear family and three generations living under the same roof (Walsh, 1982). Historically, extended families have been a vital source of care for the young, elderly, and sick. Less traditional family structures, such as stepfamilies, unmarried couples, and single-parent families, have gained acceptance over the past few years.

Overall, the family structure determines how family members interact and carry out their functions in the family. Specifying what constitutes a family is a complex process that is greatly influenced by societal trends and tolerance of diversity.

TABLE 22–1
Definitions of Family Structures

Nuclear family: Parents and children (adopted or conceived)
Blended families, or stepfamilies: Remarried members with children from previous marriage or relationship
Extended (multigenerational) family: At least two generations residing together (e.g., nuclear family and grandparents)
Single-parent family: One-parent family (parent is male or female and is widowed, divorced, or separated or has never married)
Other familial systems: Individuals living together because of common bonds, loyalties, and goals

FAMILY ROLES

Family roles are the behavior patterns or specific behaviors that are expected of persons within the family context. These roles are learned, goal directed, and transmitted within the family. Roles help the family fulfill its functions. In addition, they are the foundation of children's early interactions with primary caregivers, who provide a repertoire of responses to children needs. People's roles and relationships with others in adulthood are built on their early interactions with their primary caregivers (Spiegel, 1957). Industrialization conferred traditional family roles to institutions such as nursing homes and extended care and day care centers.

Women's gender role has evolved from staying at home and raising the children to working to bring a second paycheck into the household. Furthermore, women are permitted to pursue various careers that were traditionally held by men. These social changes have resulted in increased responsibilities for women. For example, by desire or default, they are the primary caregivers of children and housekeepers, as well as employees outside the home. Role overload can affect their emotional closeness with partners. Reductions in quality time, intimacy, and emotional support increase the likelihood of marital and family stress. Family crisis often erupts under these conditions (Alger, 1991).

Epstein and Bishop (1981) divided family roles into two categories: necessary family functions and other family functions.

Necessary Family Functions

Necessary family functions are those family roles that are critical to the health and well-being of the family's members. Epstein and Bishop (1981) identified the following as necessary family functions:

- Allocation of resources (e.g., food, water, shelter, and financial)
- Nurturance and emotional support (e.g., validation, reassurance, and comfort)
- Sexual gratification of the marital partners or couple (e.g., initiating and responding to each other's sexual needs)
- Life skills development (e.g., academia and personal development)
- Maintenance and management of family systems (e.g., negotiating and problem-solving skills, managing finances)

Duvall (1977) conceptualized family function as major family tasks; these tasks are listed in Table 22–2.

Other Family Functions

Epstein and Bishop (1981) defined *other family functions* as roles that are not essential for adaptive functioning but are part of the family developmental process. These functions may be adaptive or maladaptive. Maladaptive functions are related to parental conflict. Healthy families allocate roles, use authority effectively, and are flexible in adapting to role changes. These qualities maintain and promote the health of the family members.

TABLE 22–2
Duvall's Major Family Tasks

MAJOR FAMILY TASK	EXAMPLES
Physical support	Providing basic physical needs, such as safe environment, nutrition, clothing, etc.
Sharing of resources	Providing basic human essentials, including physical, emotional, and psychological needs.
Division of chores	Assigning chores, tasks, and family roles
Social preparation of members	Nurturing and guiding development of acceptable societal behaviors.
Procreation and separation of family members	Bearing and rearing children and participating in nuclear and extended family activities
Maintenance of unity	Using effective communication channels, rules, and appropriate limit setting/structure
Preparing members to enter society	Encouraging participation in various activities, such as school or church activities, and providing safety from harmful external influences
Maintenance of discipline and validation of members	Praising and encouraging members for accomplishments, nurturing self-actualization, and managing family/individual crisis and conflict resolution effectively

THEORETICAL CONSIDERATIONS

HEALTHY FAMILY SYSTEMS

Defining a healthy family system is difficult. Most family theory research has focused on unhealthy family systems. Over the past 30 years, however, research has identified some healthy family patterns and strengths. Family strength has been defined as familial interactions and relationships that foster self-esteem and a positive outlook on life in family members (Otto, 1962).

In systems theory, healthy or functional families are open systems composed of individuals, couples, children, and communities. Cultural factors are an integral aspect of open systems and govern system members' behavior inside and outside the system. In functional families, members' biological, psychosocial, and cultural needs are met. Health is correlated with adaptation to change or crisis generated by developmental stages. The McMaster model of family function (Epstein et al., 1982) is based on systems theory and defines six areas of family function that contribute to healthy outcomes in times of crisis or change:

1. *Problem solving* that provides basic human needs
2. *Communication* that is clear, congruent, and direct

3. *Role allocation* that suits family members' interests and is otherwise appropriate and that allows for role sharing
4. *Affective responsiveness*, wherein emotions are expressed freely, validated, accepted
5. *Affective involvement* in that family members are sensitive to each other's needs
6. *Behavior control*, in the form of flexible rules and feedback mechanisms

Family function evolves throughout the life span. Societal and technological changes continue to shape family norms. Each generation perpetuates the former generation's culture and adaptive processes. Nurses' personal family experiences and perception of the family are critical to their understanding of the role of family dynamics in modeling family members' behavior, enabling members to respond to change, and promoting health.

GENERAL SYSTEMS THEORY

In their classic works, von Bertalanffy (1968) and Miller (1965) surmised that the human organism is part of a system and critical to its maintenance. Systems theory delineates the major components of systems and the hierarchy of subsystems that comprise the whole. A number of theorists have described families as systems that function as interdependent parts or members. Furthermore, families are **subsystems** within larger social systems and within a suprasystem composed of individual members and their biological systems (Bronfenbrenner, 1979; Haley, 1962).

As a dynamic social system, the family provides intimacy for the mates within the family, opportunities for procreation, economic well-being, cultural transmission, education on both verbal and nonverbal communication, and modulation of emotions. Family structure determines the rules, roles, and communication patterns of the family (Napier & Whitaker, 1978).

According to general systems theory, the major components of a system are (1) the interrelatedness of parts, (2) boundaries, (3) tension and stress modulation, (4) equilibrium, and (5) feedback mechanisms. Systems require continuous feedback and resist major changes to ensure maintenance of homeostasis.

Interrelatedness of Parts

Interrelatedness, or wholeness, infers that change in one part affects the entire system.

Boundaries

System identification is determined by its members, social interactions, and boundaries. Boundary delineation is the basis of family function, the rules of the family, and the roles and hierarchy of the members of the family, all of which govern the action and participation of the family members (Minuchin, 1974). In addition, **boundaries** maintain the individuality of the system's members, that is, the separateness between and within subsystems. The family defines the role and hierarchy of its members through boundaries that govern their action and participation in the system. Furthermore, boundaries protect certain aspects of the system members' roles, expectations, and communication patterns. Clearly defining boundaries, serving as the mechanism for transmitting data (energy), and maintaining some degree of freedom for the system are capabilities of functional family systems. Predictable family environments provide safety, security, and growth. Conversely, blurred, rigid, or inconsistent rules and boundaries increase the likelihood of crisis or symptoms in members. Blurred or undefined boundaries include triangulation, disengagement, and enmeshment (Minuchin, 1974). **Triangulation** refers to a three-person or triad emotion interaction. **Disengagement** implies that family boundaries are rigid and impermeable. **Enmeshment** implies overinvolvement or a lack of separateness of family members. Blurred boundaries can be seen in the case of incest. A sexual relationship between a child and a parent is unacceptable and inappropriate because it involves crossing intergenerational boundaries between the adult (parent) and the child. Incest may be acceptable within the family, but society shuns it and considers it unacceptable.

Modulation of Tension and Stress

Tension and stress are inherent in systems because of the diversity among system members, which manifests itself in interactions, actions, and reactions. Regulation of system pressures is vital to sustaining equilibrium. Families that are experiencing tension and stress must respond effectively to reduce the likelihood of maladaptive responses or crisis.

Clinical Example

The Carter family's oldest daughter was physically assaulted by a female gang member after a football game. She returned home emotionally distressed. Her parents called the police to have the gang member arrested. The daughter has had difficulty coping with the situation and was initially emotionally withdrawn and depressed. Her parents became upset because they were unable to help their child. Tension in the family mounted as members became irritable and agitated. The school nurse referred them to family counseling. After several sessions, they began to express feelings about the incident and pull together as a family. The daughter began to interact with family members in the sessions and at home. Tension and stress were lowered, and the family returned to a precrisis level of function.

This clinical example demonstrates several system components. The family members' ability to seek help from each other indicates that the Carter family was an open system. In **open systems**, members are interrelated and are responsive to each other's needs (Miller, 1965; von Bertalanffy, 1968). In addition, open systems nurture self-worth, value, and appreciation of change (Satir, 1967). Mr. and Mrs. Carter exhausted their coping skills, but they recognized the need to help their daughter through a stressful ordeal. Family counseling provided crisis intervention, which represented an exchange of energy or feelings across boundaries and information about the environment or trauma. It mobilized resources, supported adaptive behaviors, and encouraged the formation of new coping skills.

In contrast, *closed systems* limit the exchange of energy and information about the environment. Had the Carters ignored their daughter's feelings and behavior, she may have become seriously disturbed, depressed, or suicidal. Closed systems are chaotic, destructive, and dysfunctional because members have distorted perceptions of themselves and the world (Satir, 1967).

The Carter family was able to restore equilibrium by using internal and external resources. Their coping skills were adequate psychosocial and biological resources and allowed them to manage and reduce family tension and stress.

Equilibrium

A system's *equilibrium* is sustained when sufficient resources are available for the system to manage and reduce tension and stress. Maximizing resources reduces the risk of maladaptive responses and illness and provides buffers to restore and maintain homeostasis.

As living systems, families evolve and change throughout the life cycle. Family evolution is a complex process that involves biological, psychosocial, and developmental components. Living systems are maintained by organization and coherence, which continuously create and sustain life (Maturana & Varela, 1991). Developmental crises such as the birth of a child require families to use adaptive coping processes to facilitate growth and maintain equilibrium in members and the system.

Feedback Mechanisms

Feedback mechanisms permit the exchange of energy and matter across various boundaries. Systems are influenced by and affect their environments. Feedback mechanisms enable systems to modify their structure to encourage growth and change within acceptable parameters. Feedback mechanisms determine whether a system is open or closed. An example of a feedback mechanism in a system is shown in the clinical example involving the Carter family presented later in the chapter.

Summary

People are social beings who continuously interact within social contexts and have experiences that are psychological, biological, and sociocultural in nature. Humans function within social systems or families that have expectations, roles, communication patterns, and rules that maintain equilibrium.

COMMUNICATION OR TRANSACTION THEORY

The word *communication* stems from the Latin word *communicatus*, which means "to impart, participate, or share." Communication is verbal and nonverbal and involves the conveying and receiving of thoughts, feelings, and ideas within a social context. Communication is more than simply sending a message; it includes how the message is "qualified, modified, reinforced, contradicted, and specially framed" (Weakland, 1976, p. 117). Clear communication patterns facilitate healthy interactions and interpersonal relationships. Healthy family interactions arise from clear communication patterns. In contrast, unclear, incongruent, or impaired communication patterns interfere with social interaction and increase the risk of maladaptive responses that lead to unhealthy family interactions.

Incongruent Communication

Incongruent communication occurs when more than one message is sent and the messages contradict each other. Incongruence between what is said and what is meant produces confusion. These messages are usually accompanied by inconsistent smiling, frowning, or tone of voice (Satir, 1967). The mother who slaps her child while saying "I love you" and the husband who, with a smile, tells his wife that he hates her are examples of incongruent communications. Family members often make statements that are contradictory or qualified. Early in the history of family therapy, impaired communication was considered the sole basis for serious mental illnesses, such as schizophrenia, and was related to family chaos and confusion (Haley, 1959). Recent advances in neurobiological research have dispelled this myth and indicate a relationship among neurobiology, genetic, and psychosocial factors as the cause of mental illness. In spite of biological advances, family transactions continue to play a vital role in creating and maintaining system function. Healthy family transactions involve various roles and processes that foster problem solving, negotiating, and effective communication.

The burden of deciphering communication rests on the receiver. Effective communication is vital to healthy family function and is particularly important during infancy and early childhood, because people's perceptions of themselves and the world are based on their early interactions with their primary caregivers. Communicating trust and love during formative years is crucial to developing healthy adult relationships. In addition, family roles, function, and culture are transmitted by verbal and nonverbal communication. Furthermore, impaired communication patterns interfere with problem solving, self-esteem, coping, and negotiation, subsequently increasing stress and tension among members.

Impaired Communication

Impaired communication patterns play major roles in family crisis. A number of theorists have defined impaired communication patterns. They include scapegoating, marital schism, marital skew, double-bind messages, and pseudomutuality.

Scapegoating. **Scapegoating** involves blaming a family member for the actions of another family member. It is a form of displacement whereby more threatening issues may be shunned. An example of scapegoating is the adolescent whose mother yells at him for his tardiness at school when really she is angry at her husband for being out all night. Scapegoating tends to keep the marital dyad from focusing on their problems. In this case, the wife focused on problems with the adolescent to divert attention from marital conflict.

Marital Schism. **Marital schism** occurs when one spouse consistently belittles the other, there is chronic and severe marital discord (Lidz et al., 1965), and one or both parents actively secure a child as an ally in the marital conflict. An example is the father who criticizes his wife in front of the children, seeking an alliance against her. Serious parental conflicts are minimized or discounted by marital schism, but intimacy is compromised, and the parents fail to provide the children's emotional, social, and cultural needs.

Marital Skew. **Marital skew** is when the dominant parent exhibits maladaptive behaviors and the other accepts it without question. For example, a husband feels powerless because his wife is sexually aloof and cold. Dependency and masochism would be the major themes in this marital or couple dyad. Emotional and physical abuse within the dyad are examples of dependency and masochism. Lidz et al. (1965) surmised that these conflicts contribute to distortions, denial, and irrationality in children.

Double-Bind Messages. **Double-bind messages** are transactions that involve a binder and a victim. The victim cannot escape the binding situation and is "caught up in an ongoing system which produces conflicting definitions of the relationship and consequent distress" (Bateson et al., 1962, p. 157). In other words, the conflicting messages cause the person to question relationships with the family. The victim is unable to respond to or get out of the situation. A clinical example is the adolescent who attempts to separate from his family by forming close relationships with his peers. The parents express dismay and use guilt to keep their son from becoming autonomous. Bowing to the pressure, he cancels a date and stays home with his parents. The parents' overprotectiveness and smothering focus on the youth rather than marital conflict. But he perceives unclear communication of affection generated by parents evoking guilt and punishment for seeking autonomy or separation. Double-bind messages are an example of incongruent communication patterns, discussed below.

Pseudomutuality. **Pseudomutuality** is a transaction that implies a sense of relatedness and emotional connectedness but in reality represents a shallow and empty relationship. This term is synonymous to "fitting together as a family at the expense of self differentiation" (Gurman & Rice, 1975, p. 35). A distorted, superficial, or inflated sense of unity tends to prevent intimacy and create distance and turmoil in the family. Deluded family transactions hinder change because they maintain the status quo. The child learns that there is inconsistency between what is real (e.g., her parents are always fighting) and what is said (e.g. "We don't disagree or argue about anything because we have a perfect marriage"). Confusion and chaos are sustained because making changes would force the parents to admit they are denying marital conflict.

Congruent Communication

Congruent communication patterns afford members with clear and consistent boundaries and roles and effective problem-solving skills. Like incongruent communication, congruent communication involves more than one message, but in this case, the messages do not contradict each other. An example is the man who looks at his child and says "I love you" and reaches out and gently caresses her on the head. The verbal and nonverbal messages are congruent because both convey warmth and caring.

At the heart of effective family communication is the communication ability of the marital or couple dyad. Clear, open, direct, and honest communication between the two members of the dyad is crucial to healthy family function. Healthy communication also includes spontaneity, validation, and responsiveness to new input or new ideas (Lewis et al., 1976). Differences and disagreements are perceived as acceptable rather than threatening to the health of the system. Problem solving, negotiating, and conflict resolution are skills passed on by healthy couples. Healthy, stable dyads provide family members with psychosocial and biological support that fosters autonomy and self-esteem. These behaviors are critical to the family's ability to manage crisis and maintain health.

CULTURAL CONSIDERATIONS

Culture provides people with a repertoire of values, beliefs, traditions, and perceptions of themselves and the world. The characteristics of culture are that it is (a) learned or conveyed through generations, (b) adaptive and evolving, and (c) composed of unique components and patterns (Mead, 1955; Young, 1944). Understanding ethnicity is pertinent for professionals working with families, because ethnicity determines cultural norms and values associated with family function, problem solving, and methods of caretaking. Moreover, ethnicity and cultural factors also affect nurses' therapeutic approaches to care (Boyd-Franklin, 1989; McGoldrick et al., 1982). Culture links intergenerational values, beliefs, and rituals. Intergenerational "connectedness" also generates a sense of belonging, comfort, and self-validation within family systems. Because family development is influenced by cultural factors as well as psychosocial and biological ones, nurses' understanding of individuals and families can be strengthened by appreciating cultural needs and uniqueness.

CULTURAL INFLUENCES ON FAMILY ROLES

Family roles are usually determined by cultural factors that are related to access to community systems. For example, being able to provide for the basic needs of family members has a profound effect on a person's self-concept and place within the family and society.

To cite one segment of the population, the African American man's provider role recurrently depends on his access to community systems or the work force. Those who access these systems are viewed the same as other ethnic groups. They have financially enabling factors—social, economical, and emotional resources—that help them provide for themselves and their families. The quality of the *provider role* affects decision-making and child-rearing practices and the quality of the marital relationship. However, barriers that reduce access to community systems such as education and financial equity often inhibit African Americans and other ethnic groups from filling the role of family provider (McAdoo, 1993).

ASSESSING THE ROLE OF CULTURE IN FAMILY FUNCTIONING

The American population is a diverse population made of a number of subcultures. Assessing families' cultural needs involves approaching them with the awareness that each family has unique needs. Stereotypical perceptions of families can interfere with objective data collection and formulation of interventions. Assessment of the influence of culture on adaptation and health is complex and must take into account such things as dietary restrictions, health practices, management of stress, and roles (Boyd-Franklin, 1989; Morris, 1990).

Knowledge of cultural diversity is crucial to understanding the experience of clients and family needs. It also promotes self-awareness and appreciation of and sensitivity to differences in people. Nurses need to anticipate that there will be differences among clients from foreign countries and from different regions of the United States. See Chapter 3 for a detailed discussion of cultural issues.

THE EVOLUTION OF FAMILIES ACROSS THE LIFE SPAN

FAMILY DEVELOPMENT

The concept of family cycle refers to the evolution of family systems. This process is influenced by functional and dysfunctional coping styles that affect the provision of basic needs, interactional patterns, and procreation. Historical patterns, maintenance of behaviors, and survival describe the evolution of a family in terms of a three-generation concept that unites older and younger generations.

Persons, like families, evolve over time. Families depict persons in stages across the life span. Developmental stages are marked by enormous energy and potential for growth and change, as Erikson (1963) noted in his description of normal (adaptive) developmental stages and abnormal (maladaptive) responses of growth and development. Duvall (1977) identified the stages of the family cycle and their role in creating and maintaining culture and meeting members' individual needs (see Table 22–2). Her work provides a classic explanation of expected family developmental tasks. Like Erikson, she asserted that each stage is predictable and parallels individual and family development. Other family therapists have described families in terms of changing family cycles. These stages are based on family patterns that parallel societal shifts (e.g., decreased birth rates and increased elderly population) and are referred to as (1) the individual; (2) the couple; (3) families with children (expansion and consolidation stages; (4) families with adolescent children; (5) middle-aged couples (contraction and partnership stages); and (6) older couples (disappearance stage) (Carter & McGoldrick, 1988; Howells, 1975). Mastery of each stage affects subsequent stages of adaptation and is modulated by internal and external demands placed on the system, which maintains continuity and growth.

THE INDIVIDUAL

Securing a place in society, sexual gratification, and a sense of intimacy are major developmental issues for young adults. The adult enters relationships at various developmental stages, seeking to separate from his or her family of origin and form a sense of identity. Identity often integrates professional goals and sexuality. Biological, psychosocial, and cultural factors, as well as ego function, are crucial to the success of this developmental task. The effort to prove that one is capable of independent living and proficient decision making produces stress. Mastering intimacy depends on successful resolution of previous developmental crises. Whether one received trust, love, and acceptance from one's primary caregivers is at the heart of whether one can achieve intimacy later (Erikson, 1963).

Self-assuredness and the ability to form meaningful relationships enable young adults to take responsibility for their general well-being. Joining the workforce, finding an apartment, and buying a new car promote a sense of accomplishment and strengthen self-esteem and independence. Managing daily household chores and negotiating boundaries with family of origin facilitate separateness and individuation in extended families. These transitions are the foundation of intimate relationships. Intimate relationships can meet psychosocial, cultural, and physical needs (Thomas, 1992).

THE COUPLE (DATING/COURTSHIP AND EARLY MARRIAGE STAGES)

Two people may be brought together by complementary needs and a sense of completeness, commitment, belonging, and sharing. Creation of a viable union involves negotiating one's relationship with one's family of origin. Separation issues play a key role in this success. Successful mastery of intimacy is vital to successful intimate interpersonal relationships. Delineation of roles and boundaries, negotiation of differences, and acceptance of each other's limitations and strengths are key transactions during courtship. Later, negotiation of differences and conflicts is undertaken and continue during early marriage (Skynner, 1976).

Satir (1988) noted that people in successful relationships

1. Believe that people are human (e.g., imperfect),
2. Understand and know themselves (e.g., have a sense of identity and are capable of self-differentiation),
3. Are responsible for their behavior and able to stand on their own feet (e.g., are independent and have clear boundaries).

Marriage is usually the culmination of these relationships; however, couples may choose to remain unmarried. Commitment to the new family challenges the couple to develop a sense of self-worth, risk taking, and potential for growth (Satir, 1988). Many cultures perceive marriage as a bond and commitment between two people. Both partners bring a repertoire of biological, psychosocial, and cultural qualities that affects their perception of themselves and the world and their ability to manage stress and maintain meaningful relationships. Individual and couple strengths are linked to the management of conflicts and adaptation to change across the life span (Thomas, 1992).

When two people fall in love and decide to marry, there is the hope that life will be happier. Love between two people is generally considered to be one of the most rewarding human experiences (Erikson, 1968). Self-worth is often tied to the quality of the relationship. People with high self-esteem are inclined to need less validation from their partners than do those with low self-esteem. People with low self-esteem are more likely to depend on their partners for fulfillment of emotional needs, a sense of self-worth, and survival. Satir (1988) claimed that couples have three parts: "you, me, and us" (p. 145). The development of each is crucial to a healthy marriage or meaningful relationship. These terms imply self-differentiation, which fosters healthy adult relationships.

As the relationship evolves, the couple learns how to relate to each other and appreciate their similarities and differences. These qualities are pertinent to the formation of meaningful relationships. Trust promotes autonomy and effective problem solving. Healthy couples have a clear sense of identity, independence, and intimacy. The developmental tasks of early marriage are (1) formation of particular dyad boundaries, (2) initiation of relationships with in-laws, (3) formation of a satisfactory sexual relationship, (4) planning for children, and (5) formalizing of careers (Thomas, 1992).

BLENDED OR STEPFAMILIES

America's divorce rate has risen over the past two decades and has played a part in the increased prevalence of blended families, or stepfamilies. Major conflicts in stepfamilies arise from members' attempts to adjust to different roles and rules and their sense of family loyalty. The person who marries someone with children from a previous marriage has the monumental task of adjusting to a ready-made family. The problems are compounded when both persons have children. Children often feel loyal to their natural parents and perceive the new marriage as betrayal (Whiteside, 1983).

The major tasks of the blended family are listed in Table 22–3 (Kuhn et al., 1993). Time is a key aspect in the resolution of stepfamily issues.

THE FAMILY WITH CHILDREN (EXPANSION AND CONSOLIDATION STAGES)

The Family with Young Children

Pregnancy and the birth experience precipitate major developmental changes. Anticipation of the new arrival places tremendous stress on the couple and the children already in the family. Major stressors include the couple's uncertainty of their competency as parents, the need to provide adequate caretaking, and the need for stable employment. The birth of and bonding with a child are major developmental tasks for the new parents. Appreciation of parental roles and support for

TABLE 22–3
Major Tasks of Stepfamilies

- To mourn loss or resolve issues from previous relationship or marriage
- To establish new family traditions and rituals
- To develop a stable relationship with spouse or partner (give enough time to restructure roles and functions)
- To form new relationships

From Whiteside, M. (1983). Families of remarriage: The weaving of many life cycle threads. In H. A. Liddle (Ed.), *The family life cycle: Implications for therapy* (pp. 100–110). Rockville, MD: Aspen.

each other buffer couples against feelings of inadequacy and promote healthy interactions and growth.

Recent changes in men's gender roles place them in active parental roles. Men are discovering the emotional and biological rewards of forming intimate relationships with their children. Fathers who willingly accept their role functions in the process of child rearing gain self-esteem and fulfillment (Pruett, 1993). The arrival of a child has a profound effect on the marital and family relationships. The couple move from nurturing each other to caring for a human being totally dependent on them for fulfillment of biological and psychosocial needs (Skinner, 1981). As the child becomes mobile and more independent, the healthy couple encourages and validates the child's autonomy. The toddler's newfound independence promotes self-esteem and separateness. The emergence of identity begins as the child realizes that boundaries exist between him- or herself and parents. Parents' tolerance of autonomy is critical to the child's mastery of this developmental stage. Resolution of attachment or bonding aids the child in moving from relationships with parents to society (Bowlby, 1969).

The child's progression through various developmental stages coincides with the family cycle. Adaptation and mastery of developmental milestones maintain homeostasis. The phase of consolidation centers on managing stress generated by problems of adolescence, independence in children, and conflicts between parents and siblings. Conflicts create tension and stress within the family system. Change fosters growth, spontaneity, and health.

The Family with Adolescent Children

Each developmental phase places enormous stress on families. Adolescence is one of the most stressful times in the family cycle. The adolescent tests the issues of control and autonomy with family renegotiation. As the adolescent's cognitive abilities mature, a search for identity begins, and the youth starts to integrate and evaluate his or her relationships with peers and to question parental authority. Developmentally, adolescence generates tension and intensifies family turmoil. Functional parents support, reinforce, and favor the adolescent's autonomy, self-direction, and independence. Increased family involvement in decision making increases internal motivation and positive self-esteem. Flexible family boundaries empower adolescents with some form of freedom in moving back and forth across them (Eccles et al., 1993).

The family's successful mastery of transitions is determined by its repertoire of biological, psychosocial, and cultural resources. Developmental stages challenge parents to provide safe, caring, and open systems that promote trust, autonomy, initiative, industry, and identity (Erikson, 1963). Chapters 7 and 14 present detailed descriptions of developmental tasks.

Functional and Dysfunctional Families

Table 22–4 lists the characteristics of functional and dysfunctional familial systems. Functional, or healthy, families adapt to changes effectively, promoting developmental transitions. Boundaries remain well defined yet flexible, and adequate feedback mechanisms are in place to sustain the open system.

In dysfunctional families, boundaries are rigid or blurred. The marital dyad is the heart of family health or dysfunction. When parents fail to adapt to their children's changing developmental needs, the risk of maladaption increases (Atwood & Stolorow, 1984). Biological and psychosocial factors, such as mental illness, impaired nutrition, and coping skills, play key roles in maladaptation. Distant alliances with extended families or exhausted social networks compromise access to larger social systems, increasing the risk of crisis (Saulnier & Rowland, 1985).

An example of maladaptive coping behaviors is the case of a mother who has not separated from her family of origin and who subsequently has difficulty tolerating autonomy and independence in her children because they represent extensions of her family. When her children attempt to separate, the mother experiences enormous anxiety. Normal childhood behaviors (e.g., auton-

TABLE 22–4
Characteristics of Functional Versus Dysfunctional Familial Systems

COMPONENTS	FUNCTIONAL FAMILIES	DYSFUNCTIONAL FAMILIES
Family structure	Provides for members' basic needs (i.e., biological, psychosocial, and cultural) Clear role delineation	Neglects members' basic needs Irrational and confused role delineation
Differentiation (the degree of individuality and togetherness)	Parents well differentiated Loyalty to nuclear family and separation from family of origin	Parents undifferentiated (fusion, enmeshment, and lack of autonomy) Lack of separation from family of origin
Communication patterns	Spontaneous, congruent, clear, direct, honest	Distorted, superficial, vague, exaggerated, contradictory Incongruent communication (scapegoating, marital skew, double-bind messages)
Boundaries (rules defining and maintaining individuality between subsystems)	Clearly delineated between members and subsystems Flexible and adaptable to change	Blurred or rigid Fail to adapt to change and tension
Emotional/affective responsiveness	Genuine warmth and affection expressed between subsystems (i.e., parent–parent, parent–child, sibling–sibling)	Distance, hostility, coldness, aloofness, and superficial relationships

omy and independence) are perceived as threatening and unacceptable. To minimize this discomfort, the mother may punish children by emotional withdrawal and abandonment or by physical abuse or neglect (Mahler, 1968; Masterson, 1988).

Chaos and turmoil are common in dysfunctional families, increasing the risk of maladaptive responses throughout the life span. The intensity of maladaptation or symptoms, such as inadequate or impaired communication or conflict resolution skills, is influenced by the couple's ability to solve problems, manage stress, and cope with life span transitions. Biological and psychosocial factors also play key roles in the couple's ability to manage family tension. Biological factors include depression in a parent or poverty, which contributes to a parent's inability to provide for his or her family's basic physical needs. The significance of a parent's failing to meet his or her family's biological needs is seen in the example of a father who is severely depressed and therefore is unable to work and provide for his family. He is emotionally inaccessible to his wife and children. His wife feels neglected and angry, and she triangles one of the children into the parental dyad to diffuse her feelings. The children in this family are likely to feel fearful and uncertain about their well-being. Symptoms of maladaptation may take the form of poor academic performance, depression, delayed growth and development, and substance abuse. Dysfunctional family patterns worsen with the family's increasing inability to reduce tension and mobilize internal and external resources. Family crisis usually results.

THE MIDDLE-AGED COUPLE (CONTRACTION AND FINAL PARTNERSHIP STAGES)

The major developmental tasks of middle adulthood include creating and guiding the next generation. As the last child leaves home, the couple is once again alone and their relationship is highlighted. Reduced involvement with their children and the need for new interests surface. Couples who have renewed their relationships throughout the years see this developmental transition as an opportunity to spend time together, solidifying the intimacy of their relationship.

Physiological changes such as mood swings and fluctuation in weight related to menopause may affect a woman's perception of herself and her relationship with her spouse (Lederer, 1984). Watching their waists and hair lines change, men are increasingly concerned about their body image and experience reduced self-esteem. Alterations in body image caused by the aging process challenge couples to reassess their assets and strengths. Aging is an inevitable process to which most people eventually reconcile themselves over time. The healthy couple recognize they cannot stay young forever, and they accept the biological changes occurring in each other. A sense of contributing to society and satisfaction with overall accomplishment are important psychosocial factors affecting this transition. Positive self-esteem is crucial to a successful mastery of this developmental task. Transmission of generational traditions and cultural values to grandchildren is another rewarding experience for the middle-aged couple.

Failure to master previous developmental tasks increases the risk of maladaptive responses to the aging process. The evidence of growing older may threaten the couple's self-esteem, limiting their ability to recognize lifelong strengths and assets. A negative self-image further compromises their ability to move through the life span realistically. Grandchildren may remind them that they are growing old, rather than engaging them in contributing to the next generation. Longstanding maladaptive coping responses, such as substance abuse, self-destructive behaviors, and ineffective coping skills, further increase the likelihood of depression or suicide.

Some middle-aged couples are now experiencing the dilemma of caring for aging parents and also coping with adult children who have returned home. These stressors often compromise the couple's financial stability and newly found freedom.

THE OLDER COUPLE (DISAPPEARANCE STAGE)

Older couples are faced with the task of retirement. Retirement presents couples with the opportunity to explore lifestyles other than that of the worker. Couples fortunate enough to own their businesses or have careers that are not affected by forced retirement have the option of continuing their job or developing other hobbies and fun endeavors. Healthy couples often have little difficulty coping with aging and retirement. Active involvement with grandchildren and great-grandchildren and other family members is important.

Aging confronts couples with significant losses. Possible losses during this developmental stage include loss of one's spouse, independence, income, and health. The death of the couple means that the original family has disappeared, but the couple lives on through other family systems (Howells, 1975). Perpetuation of families is maintained through the legacy of families who have died.

SUMMARY OF FAMILY EVOLUTION

Families evolve over time. They are established when individuals enter relationships and end with the death of a spouse or the couple. Milestones include marriage, the births of children, children's graduations, children's marriages, and the arrival of grandchildren. Transitional stages challenge families to adapt to and manage stress generated by necessary changes within and outside the system that involve biological, psychosocial, and cultural factors. Functional, or healthy, families resolve crises effectively and grow and mature over time. Members of these systems tend to develop adaptive coping behaviors. Conversely, dysfunctional families are more likely to impede change by using maladaptive coping

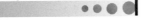

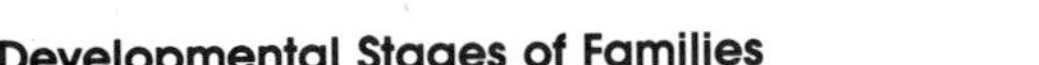

Developmental Stages of Families

STAGE	TASKS
Individual	Identity and separation
Dating/courting	Intimacy
Early marriage	Separation from family of origin
Expansion	Parenting
Consolidation	Conflict resolution and adaptation to parent–child conflict
Contraction	Last child has left home
Final partnership	Renewal of couple relationship, care of aging parents, adaptation to changes in body image
Disappearance	Adjustment to retirement and losses, focus on new generation

responses in managing stress. Family members from these systems often develop maladaptive coping behaviors. See Table 22–5 for a summary of the developmental stages of families.

THE NURSE'S ROLE

When should families seek family or couple's therapy? The psychiatric nurse can answer this question by exploring and assessing the meaning of client symptoms and how they maintain dysfunctional family interactions. Families seeking treatment for a symptomatic child or adolescent need immediate help to deal with maladaptive coping responses. Because of the complexity of a dysfunctional family system, the psychiatric nurse must develop innovative assessment skills and interventions. Recognition that families are *not* the sole cause of mental illness is vitally important. Vulnerable individuals are placed at risk for responding in maladaptive ways not only by how they communicate with their family system, but also by the combination of genetic, biological, and psychosocial factors.

ROLE OF THE ADVANCED-PRACTICE NURSE

Family and marital therapies are forms of psychotherapy that require a minimum of a master's degree in the behavioral or social sciences, nursing, or medicine. Professional supervision and ongoing training are crucial aspects of a career working with families and couples in crisis.

The psychiatric clinical nurse specialist has a master's degree with special training in psychotherapy. The behavioral, biological, and social sciences serve as the basis for assessment, identification of client outcomes, and development of interventions to address maladaptive familial interactions and impaired communication patterns. The nurse often plays an active role in therapy sessions; otherwise, family turmoil escalates and minimizes the nurse's effectiveness (Whitaker, 1976). Most nurses use an array of theories, or an eclectic approach, and tailor them to meet complex needs of each family.

CO-THERAPY

Family interactions and processes are multifaceted and can be emotionally exhausting. They require that the nurse be actively engaged in the family system as well as an observer of interactions. Co-therapy, in which one therapist actively interacts with the system while the other observes verbal and nonverbal family–therapist interactions, is an effective strategy. It provides a parental subsystem and role model for functional interactions. In addition, co-therapists provide each other professional and emotional support to deal with the anxiety and perplexities of therapy. Co-therapy can be extremely useful in the assessment of the active therapist's verbal and nonverbal transactions with family (Olds, 1977).

The disadvantages of co-therapy are that it is a complex process, time consuming, and is expensive, and the coordination of the two therapists' schedules is difficult. There is no consensus on the usefulness of co-therapy, but it is wise to terminate a co-therapy relationship when an impasse exists. This reduces the effectiveness of co-therapy and compromises the treatment process (Olds, 1977). Proponents of co-therapy assert that it provides a major source of support (Whitaker, 1965), while critics contend that it is unnecessary because therapists should be able to handle families alone (Berne, 1966; Kuehn & Crinella, 1969).

Nurses should consider the feasibility and usefulness of co-therapy, because it can be very helpful with severely dysfunctional families. Co-therapy can also be a rewarding and fulfilling experience between two therapists.

MARITAL THERAPY AND FAMILY THERAPY

Marital therapy and family therapy are useful, specialized interventions that focus on maladaptive interactions within the family system. Couples and families usually seek therapy when they are unable to resolve stress using their usual coping skills.

Marital Therapy. *Marital therapy* is a therapeutic approach that alters the marital or couple dyad. Major goals are to help couples understand maladaptive interactions and modify how they satisfy mutual needs (Gurman & Rice, 1975). Recent studies suggest that couples in which one spouse is depressed can affect family function. Marital therapy and antidepressants are effective in alleviating depression and improving role task performance (Keitner & Miller, 1990).

Family Therapy. *Family therapy* is also a specialized intervention that is used to treat clients within a social context, rather than alone. The advantage of this approach over individual psychotherapy is its effectiveness in changing a system and the behaviors of its individual members. In essence, family therapy provides a realistic perspective of a client's world, because input from various members decreases distortions or hearsay information. In addition, interactions with family members facilitate an in-depth assessment of family structure and development of healthy family outcomes (Bandler & Grindler, 1975; Grindler & Bandler, 1976).

Families often present for therapy with what has been called the *identified client*. The client's symptoms are the focus and serve as the reasons for seeking treatment. Interventions are defined by theoretical frameworks that target maladaptive behaviors. The maladaptive behaviors of one member, such as an adolescent's abuse of alcohol, are seen as representing a family problem. Framo (1982) noted that the most effective way to promote health in children is to help the parents. Symptomatic children mirror the quality of the parental subsystem.

STRUCTURAL FAMILY THERAPY

One approach the psychiatric clinical specialist may take in treating families in crisis is Minuchin's (1974) structural family therapy. Structural family therapy involves systems and various subsystems. This approach is based on the premise that certain family structures or arrangements affect transactional and communication patterns. Family transactions are the bases of rules that organize the way members relate to each other while modulating behavior. The family's adaptability to change within and outside the system affects homeostasis.

The major concepts of structural family therapy are boundary, alignment, and power. Identified clients or members cannot relinquish or change family dynamics without modification of family structure or function. Impaired family transactions maintain symptoms in the identified client. Therapy aims to modify impaired family transactions.

Structural therapy focuses on the here and now, rather than on the past. Assessment data are obtained from inspection of family transactions and interpersonal processes. Successful outcomes are based on alleviation or reduction of symptoms and feedback from family members.

THE NURSING PROCESS

The major concepts of structural family therapy are demonstrated in the following case study.

Case Study: The Family Experiencing Crisis (Jerry, Judy, and Amie Carter)

Jerry and Judy present with their 15-year-old daughter, Amie, reporting that her grades have fallen over the past semester and she has had a weight gain of 15 pounds. She is rebellious and frequently argues with her mother. The psychiatric clinical specialist gets the referral from the school counselor, who reports that Amie has become increasingly despondent and is sleeping in class.

Assessment

Parental conflict and divorce often affect children's well-being. The risk of maladaptive responses in adolescents increases with family turmoil, which is a severe stressor for children and adolescents and interferes with competent parenting and marital performance. Bringing children into the marital conflict further compromises the parent–child relationship (Amato, 1986; Amato & Keith, 1991).

The following are the major treatment goals of structural family therapy:

- Reduce tension
- Facilitate effective communication
- Clarify family rules and roles
- Improve problem-solving skills
- Delineate clear boundaries between family members

Ultimately, family structures should be changed, in that maladaptive transactions are altered into adaptive ones.

The nurse begins to establish a therapeutic alliance by joining the family and positioning him- or herself as the leader to accommodate transactional patterns. *Joining* allows the nurse to orchestrate and relate to the family system. *Accommodation* entails adjusting to facilitate the joining process. This does not mean that maladaptive interactions are condoned, but rather asserts appreciation of the family function and structure. In essence, the nurse therapist becomes a part of the family structure and thus part of the status quo, which enables family themes and areas of support and strength to be assessed (Minuchin, 1974).

Assessment involves exploring areas in the family structure that are unable to maintain function. The nurse observes the client's behavior and maladaptive responses other than the presenting symptoms. This can be seen in the man who feels inadequate (presenting symptom) but avoids closeness (behavior) with his wife because of fear of rejection. Data gathered during assessment provide the basis of therapeutic interventions and outcomes. Pertinent data include the interactions of parent–child subsystems and of the couple. *Family mapping* is an assessment tool that may be used to illustrate here-and-now interactions between members of the systems and its subsystems (Minuchin, 1974). Table 22–6 summarizes the components of family assessment.

Nurses need to collect as much information about the child's presenting symptoms as possible, including recent stressors and changes. Observing the interactions

TABLE 22–6
Components of Family Assessment in Structural Family Therapy

	ROLE OF THE THERAPIST
1. Establishment of therapeutic alliance.	Is active participant and directs own behavior toward communication and influencing of specific family transactions
2. Major aspects of assessment	Helps family understand interactional patterns. Assesses family patterns: ► communication ► decision making ► boundaries ► coping behaviors/patterns ► developmental stage of couple/parents
3. Major tasks (outcome identification)	Develops rational social context that encourages changes in social interactional patterns around issues associated with identified problems. Participates actively with family members in therapy
4. Interventions	Facilitates transactions Discourages family interaction by promoting interactions between self and members Escalates stress, which encourages members to adapt or restructure interactions Assigns family tasks (during session and homework) Uses symptoms to restructure (e.g., exaggerating, minimizing focus, relabeling) Clarifies meaning of behavior or symptoms Supports family system Provides psychoeducation Empowers members
5. Evaluation	Bases evaluation on family outcomes, feedback from members, and observation

of the couple and of parent–child subsystems during the initial interview provides vital information about the family structure and function. Family members need to speak for themselves and avoid speaking for other members. Data are generally collected within sessions in which the family's assessment of its transactions and its members' attempts to maintain status quo positions are observed (Minuchin, 1974).

In the case involving Jerry, Judy, and Amie, Amie was the identified client, and her major symptoms were failing grades, changed eating patterns, and social isolation. The problem lay not just in her rebelliousness and arguments with her mother, but in how these symptoms maintained the couple dyad or subsystems. In cases such as this, the child should not be approached immediately, because this reinforces the family label of the sick role. However, if the child is scapegoated, the nurse needs to align with him or her to minimize this process.

Several areas were identified during the assessment of Amie's family:

- Arguments were increasing between Jerry and Judy over Jerry's long work hours.
- Jerry spent most of his free time with Amie rather than with Judy.
- Judy expressed anger and resentment toward Amie.
- Judy frequently criticized Amie's weight gain.

Nursing Diagnoses

The major *nursing diagnoses* for the Amie case study were as follows:

- Ineffective Family Coping related to inability to express feelings directly to get needs met
- Disturbance in Self-Concept related to feelings of inadequacy and lack of trust (couple)
- Disturbance in Self-Concept related to parental criticism
- Potential for Self-Harm, suicide (adolescent)

Planning

Therapeutic interventions are based on problem identification and strategies that will reduce or alleviate symptoms in the identified client. Restructuring interventions such as joining and accommodation modify impaired transactions. "Joining" and "accommodation" refer to the therapist's entering and conforming to a family system with the goal of initiating a therapeutic relationship. This relationship is used to identify maladaptive transactional or communication patterns and help family members form adaptive ones (Minuchin, 1974).

The following client outcomes were identified for Amie's family:

- Amie's family develops adaptive and coping skills to manage stress.
- Boundaries between marital and parent–child subsystems are clearly defined and maintained.
- Amie avoids engaging implicitly or explicitly in her parents' conflict.
- Subsystems clarify and communicate their feelings and thoughts appropriately.
- Amie identifies positive assets and develops adaptive coping skills.
- Amie expresses feelings, rather than acting on them.

Nursing Care Plan 22–1 identifies the nursing actions needed to achieve these outcomes, along with the rationales for these actions.

Implementation

Alternative transactions are explored when the nurse enters alliances with family subsystems and develops a therapeutic contract. Therapeutic techniques preserve family members' self-identity and support mutuality, or the sense of belonging. The major techniques of structural family therapy are as follows:

- Dissuade present members from talking about or for each other in session.
- Encourage the family to discuss its strengths and competencies.
- Support the scapegoated or identified client.
- Maintain age-appropriate behaviors associated with independence.

The nurse psychotherapist interacts with family members. This process begins with discussing options to disengage from maladaptive transactional patterns and pointing out adaptive ones. New scenarios are created by asking the adolescent to talk to a parent and vice

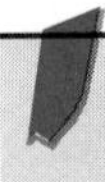

Nursing Care Plan 22–1 The Family Experiencing Crisis (Jerry, Judy, and Amie)

OUTCOME IDENTIFICATION	NURSING ACTIONS	RATIONALES	EVALUATION
► **Nursing Diagnosis:** Ineffective Family Coping			
1. By [date], Amie's family will develop adaptive coping skills to manage present crisis.	1a. Establish rapport and assess reasons why Amie's family is seeking treatment at this time.	1a. Alliance is developed and basis and duration of crisis are determined.	*Goal met:* Alliance and therapeutic contract are established.
	1b. Assess transactional patterns and coping behaviors of Amie's family.	1b. Jerry begins to focus on present marital problems.	Jerry focuses primarily on concerns for Amie's behavior. Jerry answers most questions; Judy is silent.
	1c. Direct questions to Jerry and Judy.	1c. Communication patterns improve in the marital dyad.	
► **Nursing Diagnosis:** Altered Family Processes Related to Situational Stressors			
1. By [date], Amie's family will share their feelings appropriately.	1a. Encourage Amie's family to express their feelings and thoughts regarding present stressors.	1a. Amie is able to express anger appropriately toward her mother.	*Goal met:* Amie expresses anger towards Judy. Judy remains silent while Jerry inquires about meaning of Amie's anger.
	1b. Encourage Judy and Jerry to express their feelings.	1b. Judy is able to express her anger to Jerry, specifying her reasons, and Jerry is able to share his feelings about family and marital stress.	Judy angrily tells Jerry that he is never home and that she is lonely most of the time.
2. By [date], Amie's family will recognize their family roles.	2. Assess what Judy and Jerry want from their relationship.	2. Attention turns to dyad conflict.	Jerry states he was not aware of Judy's anger and that it was being taken out on Amie.
► **Nursing Diagnosis:** Self Esteem Disturbance Related to Present Crisis			
1. By [date], Amie's family members will identify positive assets and qualities.	1. Encourage Amie, Judy, and Jerry to talk about positive qualities and assets.	1. Family can identify their strengths.	*Goal met:* Amie, Jerry, and Judy identify positive attributes qualities.
► **Nursing Diagnosis:** High Risk for Violence: Self-Directed (Adolescent)			
1. By [date], Amie will express feelings, rather than acting on them.	1. Observe Amie for signs and symptoms of depression.	1. Adolescents are at risk for acting out.	*Goal met:* Amie verbalizes feelings and denies suicidal ideations. She interacts more with family/friends. Communication between Jerry and Judy and Amie and her parents improves. The family's coping skills improve.

versa, rather than talking through the therapist. This is an experiential (emotions are generated by specific interactions between members and the nurse) process that centers on the family's presenting symptoms. Joining and accommodation can prompt modification in transactional patterns.

Evaluation

As family members change, their transactions also change. The degree of family restructure is assessed throughout treatment. Client outcomes and the family's and nurse's perceptions regarding adaptive coping behaviors are the basis of evaluation. Structural family therapy involves meeting with the child and couple for 6 months. Response to family therapy depends on reasons for seeking treatment, insight, economic factors, and severity of symptoms.

Termination begins during the initial stage of therapy and involves assessing problem areas, identifying outcomes, establishing interventions, and evaluating outcomes. In the last session, the nurse helps the family members discuss their roles in attaining treatment goals, supporting and accepting each other, and recognizing the strengths that will help them maintain family structure during a crisis.

RESEARCH ON FAMILIAL SYSTEMS

Familial systems mediate clients' responses across the life span. Research is needed at all levels of the nursing process. Assessment of family function can be obtained by researching the effectiveness of family therapy. Research on the effectiveness of the psychiatric clinical nurse specialist as a psychotherapist is sparse. There is a national health care trend toward the use of advanced nurse practitioners as primary caregivers. Primary prevention of high-risk groups is a prime focus of health care reforms. High-risk families include those with a mentally ill parent and those in which substance abuse or poverty is present.

Methods that increase the understanding of the relationships between developmental stages and various roles and patterns in different ethnic and cultural groups are crucial to identifying high-risk groups and promoting primary prevention. Interdisciplinary research can also assist nurses and other mental health professionals in developing qualitative and quantitative methods of examining the roles of fathers in various populations (McAdoo, 1993).

Nurses have always been a major force in health care delivery. Families enter the health care system through numerous portals. The child with hemophilia, the pregnant woman with acquired immune deficiency syndrome, and the middle-aged couple dealing with a parent with Alzheimer's disease all bring familial roles into the health care arena. Nurses can collaborate with families and other health professionals to explore factors that affect family function. Psychoeducation, crisis intervention, supportive therapy, and psychopharmacology are a few areas in which nurses can evaluate family involvement (see the accompanying Research Study display).

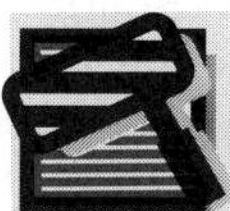

RESEARCH STUDY

Perceptions of Familial Caregivers of Elder Adults

Sayles-Cross, S. (1993). *Image: Journal of Nursing Scholarship*, *25*, 88–92.

Study Problem/Purpose

The aim of this study was to identify the perceptions of 139 familial caregivers of older adults to answer the question, Is there a significant relationship among appraisal, social distance, and the cost of caring for an elder family member?

Method

The study was guided by three research questions: (1) What is the relationship between social distance and the expense of caring for an older family member? (2) What is the association between primary or secondary appraisal and the expense of caring for an older family member? and (3) Which factor (family distance or primary or secondary appraisal) best predicts cost of caring?

A comparative survey was sent to 139 caregivers. The self-report questionnaires consisted of the Age Social Distance Scale, the What's At Stake Scale, the Emotions Scale, and the Cost of Care Index.

Findings

Social distance and the caregiver's degree of understanding and sympathy significantly influenced caregivers' appraisals of the cost of caring for older family members. These results suggest that increased social distance correlates with increased anger and disgust in familial members caring for older family members.

Nursing Implications

Families at risk can benefit from measures that foster self-care and primary prevention. Major nursing interventions include providing psychoeducation, enhancing support systems, and making appropriate community referrals.

►CHAPTER SUMMARY

Families are important aspects of the health care system, and the nurse's daily interactions with them submits the need to understand how they function and manage stress. Recognizing the influence of family roles on maintenance and promotion of clients' adaptive and maladaptive behaviors is vital to outcome identification.

Family and marital therapies are invaluable approaches to managing clients' crises and maintaining health. Through family therapy, family members learn effective communication patterns, grow, express feelings, and clarify boundaries. Boundaries are a barometer of family function. Understanding systems theory helps nurses assess clients as a whole rather than a part.

Research is needed to identify the effectiveness of nursing interventions and assess the impact of factors such as cultural diversity, the changing roles of fathers and mothers across the life span, and age-specific factors on the family system. The effectiveness of various family therapy techniques needs to be explored by psychiatric clinical specialists. Staff nurses also play a major role in biological and psychosocial therapies, such as psychopharmacology and psychoeducation. Identifying client and family needs and developing individualized teaching plans promote formation of adaptive coping behaviors in families experiencing crisis.

Suggestions for Clinical Conference

1. Present and discuss a case history of a family in crisis.
2. Role-play functional and dysfunctional family systems.
3. Identify current societal trends that influence mental health and family structure.
4. Role-play congruent and incongruent communication.
5. Invite a clinical specialist to discuss aspects of working with families experiencing crisis.
6. Develop and present a family psychoeducational program that addresses psychopharmacology or stress management.

References

Ackerman, N. W. (1958). *The psychodynamics of family life*. New York: Basic Books.

Alger, I. (1991). Marital therapy with dual-career couples. *Psychiatric Annals*, 21, 455–458.

Amato, P. R. (1986). Marital conflict, the parent–child relationship, and child self-esteem. *Family Relations, 35,* 103–110.

Amato, P. R., & Keith, B. (1991). Marital conflict, the parental–child relationship, and child self esteem. *Family Relations*, 35, 103–110.

Atwood, G. E., & Stolorow, R. D. (1984). *Structures of subjectivity: Explorations in psychoanalytic phenomenology*. Hillsdale, NJ: Analytic Press.

Bandler, R., & Grindler, J. (1975). *The structure of magic*. Palo Alto, CA: Science and Behavior Books.

Bateson, G., Jackson, D. D., Haley, J., & Weakland, J. H. (1962). A note on double bind. *Family Process*, *2*, 154–161.

Baumann, A., & Beckingham, A. C. (1990). Blended families. In A. Baumann, N. E. Johnston, & D. Antai-Otong (eds.), *Decision-making in psychiatric and psychosocial nursing* (pp. 166–167). Philadelphia: B. C. Decker.

Borne, E. (1966). *Principles of group treatment*. New York: Grove.

Bowlby, J. (1969). *Attachment and loss* (Vol. 1). New York: Basic Books.

Boyd-Franklin, N. (1989). *Black families in therapy: A multisystems approach*. New York: Guilford Press.

Bronfenbrenner, U. (1979). *The ecology of human development*. Cambridge, MA: Harvard University Press.

Carter, B., & McGoldrick, M. (1988). *The changing family cycle*. New York: Gardner Press.

Duvall, E. (1977). *Family development* (3rd ed.). Philadelphia: J. B. Lippincott.

Eccles, J. S., Midgely, C., Wigfield, A., Buchanan, C. M., Reuman, D., Flanagan, C., & MacIver, D. (1993). Development during adolescence. *American Psychologist*, *48*, 90–101.

Epstein, N. B., & Bishop, D. S. (1981). Problem centered systems therapy of the family. *Marital and Family Therapy*, *7*, 23–31.

Epstein, N. B., Bishop, D. S., & Baldwin, L. W. (1982). McMaster model of family functioning: A view of the normal family. In E. Walsh (Ed.), *Normal family processes* (pp. 115–141). New York: Guilford Press.

Erikson, E. H. (1963). *Childhood and society* (2nd ed.). New York: W. W. Norton.

Erikson, E. H. (1968). *Identity: Youth and crisis*. New York: W. W. Norton.

Framo, J. L. (1982). *Explorations in family and marital therapy: Selected papers of James L. Framo*. New York: Springer.

Grindler, J., & Bandler, R. (1976). *The structure of magic II*. Palo Alto, CA: Science and Behavior Books.

Gurman, A. S., & Rice, D. G. (1975). *Couples in conflict*. New York: Jason Aronson.

Haley, J. (1959). Family of the schizophrenia client: A model system. *Journal of Nervous and Mental Disorders*, *129*, 357–374.

Haley, J. (1962). Whitaker family therapy. *Family Process*, *1*, 69–100.

Hodgkinson, H. L. (1989). *The same client: The demographics of education and service delivery systems*. Washington, DC: Institute for Educational Leadership.

Howells, J. G. (1975). *Principles of family psychotherapy*. New York: Brunner/Mazel.

Keitner, G. I., & Miller, W. (1990). Family functioning and major depression: An overview. *American Journal of Psychiatry*, *147*, 1128–1137.

Kuehn, J., & Crinella, F. M. (1969). Sensitivity training: Interpersonal "overkill" and other problems. *American Journal of Psychiatry*, *126*, 841–845.

Kuhn, D. R., Morhardt, D. J., & Monbrad-Framburg, G. (1993). Late-life marriages, older stepfamilies, and Alzheimer's disease. *Families in Society: The Journal of Contemporary Human Services*, *74*, 154–162.

Lederer, W. J. (1984). *Creating a good relationship*. New York: W. W. Norton.

Lewis, J. M., Beavers, R. W., Gassett, J. T., & Phillips, V. A. (1976). *No single thread: Psychological health in family systems*. New York: Brunner/Mazel.

Lidz, T., Fleck, S., & Cornelison, A. (1965). *Schizophrenia and the family*. New York: International Universities Press.

Mahler, M. (1968). *On human symbiosis and the vicissitudes of individuation: Vol. I. Infantile psychosis*. New York: International Universities Press.

Masterson, J. F. (1988). *The search for the real self*. New York: Free Press.

Maturana, H. R., & Varela, F. J. (1991). *The tree of knowledge* (2nd ed.). Boston: New Science Library.

McAdoo, J. L. (1993). The roles of African-American fathers: The ecological perspective. *Families in Society: The Journal of Contemporary Human Services*, *74*, 28–35.

McGoldrick, M., Pearce, M., & Giordano, J. (1982). *Ethnicity and family therapy*. New York: Guilford Press.

Mead, M. (1955). *Cultural patterns and technical change*. New York: New American Library Mentor Books.

Miller, J. G. (1965). Living systems: Basic concepts, structures, and process: Cross-level hypothesis. *Behavioral Sciences*, *10*, 193–237, 337–411.

Minuchin, S. (1974). *Families and family therapy*. Cambridge, MA: Harvard University Press.

Morris, T. M. (1990). Culturally sensitive model of psychosomatic illness in children: Family assessment devices used with Hawaiian-American and Japanese-American families. *Family Process*, *29*, 105–116.

Napier, A. Y., & Whitaker, C. (1978). *The family crucible*. New York: Harper & Row.

Olds, V. (1977). Use of co-therapist in family therapy. In J. Buckly, J. J. McCarthy, E. Norman, & M. A. Quaranta (Eds.), *New directions in family therapy* (pp. 132–137). Oceanside, NY: DABOR Science Publications.

Otto, H. A. (1962). What is a strong family? *Marriage and Family Living*, *24*, 77–81.

Pruett, K. D. (1993). The paternal presence. *Families in Society: The Journal of Contemporary Human Services*, *74*, 46–50.

Satir, V. (1967). *Conjoint family therapy*. Palo Alto, CA: Science and Behavior Books.

Satir, V. (1988). *The new peoplemaking*. Mountain View, CA: Science and Behavior Books.

Saulnier, K. M., & Rowland, C. (1985). Missing links: An empirical investigation of network variables in high-risk females. *Family Relations*, *34*, 557–560.

Skynner, A. C. R. (1976). *Systems of family and marital psychotherapy*. New York: Brunner/Mazel.

Spiegel, J. P. (1957). The resolution of role conflict within the family. Psychiatry, *20*, 1–16.

Thomas, M. B. (1992). *An introduction to marriage and family therapy*. New York: Merritt.

von Bertalanffy, L. (1968). *General systems theory: Foundations, development, applications* (rev. ed.). New York: George Braziller.

Walsh, F. (1982). *Normal family process*. New York: Guilford Press.

Weakland, J. (1976). Communication theory and clinical change. In P. J. Guerin (Ed.), *Family therapy* (pp. 111–128). New York: Gardner Press.

Whitaker, C. (1965). *Acting out: Theoretical and clinical aspects*. New York: Little.

Whitaker, C. (1976). The hindrance of theory in clinical work. In P. J. Guerin (Ed.), *Family therapy* (pp. 154–164). New York: Gardner Press.

Whiteside, M. (1983). Families of remarriage: The weaving of many life-cycle threads. In H. A. Liddle (Ed.), *The family life-cycle: Implications for therapy* (pp. 100–110). Rockville, MD: Aspen Systems.

Young, K. (1944). *Social psychology* (2nd ed.). New York: F. S. Crofts.

Zylke, J. W. (1991). Care for working parents' children grows as a challenge for the nation. *Journal of the American Medical Association*, *266*, 3255–3257.

CHAPTER

Group Psychotherapy

MARTHA BUFFUM, D.N.Sc., R.N.,C.S.
ERIKA MADRID, D.N.Sc., R.N.,C.S.

OUTLINE

CHAPTER OBJECTIVES

Upon completion of this chapter, you will be able to:

1. Define group therapy.
2. Explain the contributions of Pratt, Metzl, Adler, Moreno, and Slavson to group therapy.
3. Describe the purpose and practices of marathon groups.
4. Discuss Yalom's therapeutic factors.
5. Describe the different theoretical models of group therapy.
6. Identify the function of the psychiatric–mental health nurse in the role of group leader, therapist, and co-therapist.
7. Explain the differences between process and content.

8. Identify the types of psychosocial groups that adults use to cope with life stressors.
9. Describe issues that are the focus of groups for specific populations, such as children, adolescents, and the elderly.
10. Discuss current trends in research or group therapy.
11. Identify types of groups on an assigned psychiatric unit.
12. Discuss with clients appropriate groups for specific problems.
13. Prepare a list of self-help groups in the community.
14. Describe the psychiatric–mental health nurses' involvement on an assigned psychiatric unit and in the community.
15. List outcome measures for evaluating the effectiveness of groups.

KEY TERMS

Activity
ANA Standards of Psychiatric and Mental Health Nursing Practice
Behavioral/cognitive model
Communication/systems model
Content
Encounter groups
Existential/gestalt model
Group leadership
Group process model
Group therapy
Insight-oriented or process-oriented group
Interpersonal model
Marathon groups
Process
Psychodrama
Psychodynamic model
Psychoeducation groups
Role playing
Task groups
T-groups
Therapeutic factors

A group is two or more people who are together for a purpose or a common reason (Crenshaw, 1989). Therapy is a treatment used for its beneficial effects. In mental health, **group therapy** is a modality of treatment for more than one person that provides therapeutic outcomes for each individual. This chapter discusses the history of group therapy and its evolution in the psychiatric–mental health arena, the theoretical foundations on which group therapy is based, the specific role of the psychiatric nurse in group therapy and the application of the nursing process to group therapy, types of groups relevant to particular people and needs, and current trends in research on group therapy.

HISTORICAL PERSPECTIVES

There is disagreement about the exact origins of group therapy (Dreikurs, 1959; Mullan & Rosenbaum, 1967). Although therapeutic group interaction may have occurred throughout the world, such as in Greek drama, medieval plays, and Franz Mesmer's hypnotic institute, no documentation acknowledged the beneficial effects or therapeutic intentions of such interactions. Modern group therapy has been documented as beginning in 1905 with Joseph Hersey Pratt, a Boston internist (Mullan & Rosenbaum, 1967). See Table 23–1 for a summary of researchers' contributions.

TUBERCULOSIS AND THE HOME SANATORIUM (EARLY 1900s)

Pratt worked with tuberculosis clients who were living at home. He recognized the social as well as physical elements of the disease, noting that the clients felt discouraged about their plight. His treatment regimen involved weekly meetings of a small class of 15 to 20 clients. All of the members of the class had tuberculosis, were poor, and were from varied racial and religious backgrounds. Selection for the class depended on a client's and his or her family's willingness to follow strict guidelines regarding the need for open air, no work, a particular diet, rest, and hygiene. All levels of illness were included. The class meetings continued over 1 year.

Pratt lectured at each class about the care and treatment of tuberculosis. He had each client keep a record book in which he or she documented the details of his or her life, including daily temperature, diet, and rest periods. Pratt noted the camaraderie that developed. The clients did not talk about their symptoms. They were supportive and encouraging, as was Pratt. Symptom improvement was more encouraging than in the tuberculosis sanatoriums.

When Pratt's experiment was repeated by physicians in the sanatoriums, the exact results were not reproduced. Although Pratt had not written about his own influence on the clients, it appeared evident that his strong personality had an important impact on them. Furthermore, part of Pratt's treatment regimen included nurse visits to clients' homes. These additional acts of caring and reinforcement of education most likely contributed to clients' feelings about themselves, their illness, and their membership in the class. Pratt's (1906) philosophy was that his clients improved because a large amount of care was given to a small number of clients. His work continued, evolving in the area of emotional re-education on the basis of the philosophy that group therapy has a beneficial effect because of the interpersonal dynamics involved and group members' influence on each other.

TABLE 23–1
Selected Researchers' Contributions to the Early History of Group Psychotherapy

RESEARCHER	TIME PERIOD	FOCUS OF GROUP WORK	DESCRIPTION OF GROUP	TREATMENT	CONTRIBUTIONS
Pratt	1900s	Tuberculosis (TB) and the home sanatorium	15–20 poor clients representing a variety of racial and religious backgrounds	Education on care and treatment of TB. Each client kept a record of temperature, diet, rest, etc. Nurse visited clients' homes.	Noted camaraderie, support, and encouragement among clients. Symptom improvement was greater than in sanatorium.
Metzl	1920s	Treatment for alcoholism	Clients had individual counseling, acknowledged their alcoholism, and were of same socioeconomic background.	Group members used power of suggestion that sobriety was possible. Members promised not to drink for 1 week.	Pioneered systematic approach to group treatment of psychiatric clients and made distinction between individual and group counseling.
Moreno	1930s	Psychodrama	Clients were actors and audience, therapist was director, and staff served as auxiliary egos.	Client acted role emphasizing problem, and rest of group provided sounding board of public opinion.	Coined terms *group psychotherapy* and *group therapy*. Established connection between group therapy and psychiatry.

ALCOHOL TREATMENT (1920s)

Dr. Julius Metzl, a police physician in Vienna, developed a method of group counseling for alcoholics. Metzl's groups involved persons who had had individual counseling, who acknowledged their alcoholism, who were accepted into the group by fellow members, and who were from the same socioeconomic level. Some of the principles he used were later adopted by Alcoholics Anonymous. His work was published in an obscure journal on alcoholism in 1927 and later by a colleague, Rudolf Dreikurs, in 1928 in a psychiatric journal. At that time, alcoholics were considered psychiatric patients. Metzl's work pioneered a systematic approach to the group treatment of psychiatric patients (Dreikurs, 1959).

Metzl's work also pioneered the distinction between individual and group or collective counseling (Dreikurs, 1959). With alcoholic clients, group methods appeared to be more successful than individual counseling. In individual counseling, limited time was allowed per person, and only one counselor had the opportunity to affect the client. The counselor's intellectual ability was assumed to be a powerful force against one individual's reasoning. In contrast, group or collective counseling afforded the group the benefit of any one individual's confrontation by the counselor or any group member. The group approach offered a forum in which the achievement of sobriety could be displayed, the belief that one could accomplish what another did was generated, and members were convinced that successful sobriety was possible. The power of suggestion, then, was a force that each member could bring to the group, and each member was influential. In the alcoholic groups, all members were expected to participate, and all members voluntarily promised after their first session not to drink for 1 week.

COLLECTIVE COUNSELING AND GROUP PSYCHOTHERAPY (1920s AND 1930s)

The term *collective counseling* was established in Vienna by Adler and his co-workers in 1921 at the Counseling Center for Parents and Children (Dreikurs, 1959). Psychiatric thinking in the Adlerian sense included the group as a natural setting. That is, the whole family was in treatment when a child was emotionally disturbed.

PSYCHODRAMA (1930s)

Jacob Moreno claimed that he used group therapy in Vienna as early as 1910, and in 1932 he presented his findings to the American Psychiatric Association. This presentation may have established the connection between group therapy or group psychotherapy and psychiatry.

Moreno came to the United States in 1925, and he is credited with coining the terms *group psychotherapy* and *group therapy*. Moreno's specific method of therapy was known as **psychodrama**—the exploration of the truth through dramatic means. The five instruments used in the group setting included the following:

1. The stage, which gave the client the opportunity of expression
2. The subject or client, who enacted a role emphasizing a past or present problem
3. The director, who was the therapist and producer of the drama
4. The staff of therapeutic aides (auxiliary egos), who were responsive to the producer and acted as real or imagined persons in the client's life

5. The rest of the group, who acted as an audience and sounding board of public opinion (Moreno, 1946). For further discussion of psychodrama, see "Psychodrama and Role-Playing Techniques."

Moreno's contributions also included the publishing of the first journal devoted to group therapy, *Impromptu*. For 18 years, he edited *Sociometry*, which he founded in 1937. In 1944, he turned this journal over to the American Sociological Association, which devoted it to social psychology. In 1947, Moreno founded the publication *Sociatry*, the name of which he later changed to *Group Psychotherapy*.

Other individuals were applying group methods to specific populations during the 1930s. Samuel Slavson, originally an engineer, began an **activity** group therapy at the Jewish Board of Guardians. This type of therapy combined group work, education, and psychological analysis. He emphasized the use of the group setting for the acting out of impulses, conflicts, and behavior patterns. Primarily, the activity group therapy was for children from 8 to 15 years. He practiced this therapy for 9 years, presenting it in 1943 and calling it *situational therapy* (Mullan & Rosenbaum, 1967). This was the forerunner of children's group play therapy.

INFLUENCE OF COMMUNICATION BEFORE WORLD WAR II

In contrast to the United States, many physicians in Europe in the early 1900s did not present or publish their experiences with groups. Freud was interested in the group mind and the influence of the group on the individual, but he did not work with groups. The field of psychiatry was new and busy defining itself. Thus internists' work in the area of group therapy methods went unnoticed by psychiatrists. To the Adlerian psychologists, use of group methods with families was part of individual counseling and went undocumented. According to Dreikurs (1959), German, Austrian, Russian, and Danish psychotherapists had been using group methods before 1930. All public forms of group therapy ceased during the period of fascism in Austria between 1927 and 1934 (Dreikurs, 1959). Furthermore, the lives and work of Metzl and other pioneers in group therapy became obscured by the Holocaust.

AFTER WORLD WAR II (1940s–1960s)

There was much growth in the use of group therapy at the end of World War II, because there was a shortage of trained personnel and many clients needed treatment. New methods that required briefer treatment periods were explored. Group therapies now included support, education, inspiration, emotional expression, and reconstruction.

Differences in approach existed in each type of therapy. The purpose of the group and the role of the therapist varied, depending on the therapist's theoretical stance. Styles ranged from didactic to nondirective. Effectiveness was based on outcomes such as enhanced self-concept, better interpersonal relationships, diminished symptoms, support for new communication and behaviors, problem solving, and better understanding of one's personality. Although group therapy was simultaneously used extensively in Great Britain, it seemed to develop in the United States with little influence from the British, as reflected in the American literature (Mullan & Rosenbaum, 1967).

According to Ruitenbeek (1969), most group therapy was conventional, and little variety was seen in this modality until the 1950s. That is, groups would convene once a week for 1 or 1 1/2 hours, and the 8 to 10 members would interact as they exchanged problems and interpretations. Generally, the therapist was passive, offering some guidance and interpretations.

Therapy groups began to be observed for research in the 1950s (Whitaker & Lieberman, 1969). These included psychiatric patients at the Veterans Administration Hospital in Chicago and the Department of Psychiatry at the University of Chicago. Different therapeutic approaches and styles were observed in short-term groups of hospitalized veterans who suffered from acute states of anxiety or severe character pathology.

Interest in the group method extended beyond therapy and problem-oriented work during the 1950s. An understanding of group dynamics was an objective of the training of group therapists. The **T-group**, or basic skills training group, was specifically designed for the experience of being in a group, understanding the group process, studying leadership style, and examining group functions for efficient problem solving. The first T-groups met in Bethel, Maine, in 1948 and 1949 (Goldberg, 1970). Feedback and training for leadership in human relations were part of the education of the participants, who included business persons, community workers, and members of the Armed Forces (Bradford et al., 1964). The groups were so successful in training and educating therapists in group dynamics and interpersonal communication that the National Training Laboratories was established in 1950 within the National Education Association (Yalom, 1985). T-groups led to a desire for intensity of interpersonal interactions, which led to therapy groups for the general population in the form of encounter groups and marathons.

According to Fromm (1957), humans exist in a social context and need to feel related to fellow humans. Furthermore, he asserted that people have a strong need to know themselves and other humans. This philosophy was the basis of the approach in the innovative groups of the 1950s and 1960s that were developed in a sensitivity-group movement that occurred throughout the United States. **Encounter groups,** which were intensive T-groups, and marathon groups provided a type of therapy to the interested population at large. For example, the Esalen Institute in California, founded on Perls's (1969) gestalt psychology, devoted itself to group training and group workshops wherein the marathon group was practiced.

Marathon groups took place in a safe, secluded, private setting. A selected group of 10 to 14 participants stayed together for 2, 3, or up to 4 days. The workshop would extend nonstop through the first 24 hours or longer. The participants used many methods of communication, including nonverbal, dramatic, creative, touch, verbal, and activity techniques. Honesty, intimacy, a feeling of connectedness to others, and authentic communication were the objectives. The group setting gave the participants the opportunity to express genuine feelings openly without fear of social conventions. Some marathons were specialized for couples, business executives, group psychotherapists, or researchers (Bach, 1966).

With a few exceptions, most marathon groups selected persons without a psychiatric diagnosis, persons who wanted to grow, change their relationships, alter their communication or behavior patterns, and learn about themselves. Mintz (1967) described a sequence of phases experienced by members of the marathon group. At the beginning of the group, members demonstrated their usual defense systems. During the second phase, members fluctuated between hostility and dependency. In the third phase, they expressed deep appreciation for one another and a desire for further contact. According to Mintz, more research was needed to determine the beneficial long-term effects of marathon groups. For unknown reasons, however, marathon groups lost their popularity in the 1980s.

The power of group suggestion is strong. The Synanon community, originally a residential treatment program designed for persons addicted to drugs, opened to growth movement individuals who believed in group process. All aspects of life were managed communally, with decisions made by group process. Members learned genuine assertion of expression and recognition that the group's power was greater than that of any individual.

FAR EAST WAR EXPERIENCES (1970s TO PRESENT)

Postwar traumas have emerged in men who had been prisoners of war during World War II, the Korean War, and the Vietnam War. *Post-traumatic stress disorder* became an ever more frequently used term in the 1980s, when veterans began revealing the devastation of their lives due to the reliving of trauma and the extreme difficulty they have had adjusting to civilian life. Several Veterans Administration (now called Department of Veterans Affairs) hospitals have attended to veterans' needs through group therapy and group psychoeducational methods (Koller et al., 1992; Perconte, 1988).

THERAPEUTIC FACTORS OF GROUP THERAPY

All therapy groups are designed to benefit the members. **Insight-oriented or process-oriented** therapy groups are for individuals with high levels of cognitive functioning. Yalom (1985) proposed 11 **therapeutic factors** of insight-oriented or process-oriented group therapy, which are presented in Table 23–2. They can also be applied to education, activity, and task groups, which may be more beneficial for people with cognitive impairments. However, because no two individuals view one event in the same manner, these therapeutic factors may not be of equal value to all participants of all groups. Each person has unique needs, wants, and life experiences. The therapeutic benefits of group participation vary with participants' perceptions, levels of functioning, degree of experience with groups, insights into problems, durations of psychological treatment, and relationships with others in the group. According to Yalom (1985), any group experience offers potential benefit or harm or may be important or meaningless.

TABLE 23–2
Yalom's Therapeutic Factors for Group Therapy

Imparting of information. Information is presented through lecture or teaching aids, or information is shared among members.

Instillation of hope. The therapist and group have the attitude that the client will get better and that the treatment modality is beneficial.

Universality. Problems, thoughts, feelings are shared by other group members—no one is alone or isolated with one's own issues.

Altruism. Each group member gives to another within the group; this process is therapeutic and increases the giver's self-esteem.

Corrective recapitulation of the primary family group member. The members' responses are influenced by past family experiences. Members gain insight into their behavior when they learn that their reactions to others are similar to their reactions to their own family members.

Development of socializing techniques. By accepting feedback about their interpersonal communication and behavior, members become more socially skillful in relationships.

Imitative behavior. Growth is demonstrated when the client identifies with other members, imitating the healthy aspects of other members of the group.

Interpersonal learning. Interpersonal learning results from feedback from others and insight into oneself. This learning is transferrable to other situations, enabling clients to assert themselves, trust others, test reality, give to others, and expect caring from others.

Group cohesiveness. There is a feeling of connectedness among group members. Cohesiveness is demonstrated when positive as well as negative feedback can be given in an atmosphere of acceptance, without group disintegration.

Catharsis. Clients express their deeply felt emotions.

Existential factors. Clients realize that loneliness, death, and the meaning of existence are issues for all men and women; that there is a limit to how much control humans have over these issues; and that there is universal learning about human existence.

Data from Yalom, I. (1985). *The theory and practice of group psychotherapy* (3rd ed.). New York: Basic Books.

ADVANTAGES AND DISADVANTAGES OF GROUP THERAPY

The advantages of group therapy are based on the purpose of the group and the motivation of the participants. For example, a psychoeducational group for families with a member who has Alzheimer's disease offers information to a large number of people simultaneously.

The use of staff is cost-effective. Likewise, an inspiration group such as Alcoholics Anonymous is most effective in large numbers. Usually the members of such groups are motivated to learn, to participate, and to help others in the process of helping themselves.

Group therapies offer people a chance to help each other, to feel less alone in the world, to learn about themselves and other people, to practice new behaviors, to practice problem-solving skills, to improve communication, and to foster better relationships. Self-esteem is enhanced as a result of feeling important and worthwhile in an atmosphere of mutual helping. Persons in group therapy can feel strengthened and hopeful from the process of sharing, from feeling accepted and supported, and through helping others.

A major disadvantage is that a participant's individual needs may not be addressed to his or her satisfaction. Attention to individual problems is not the focus of group therapy, as it is in individual therapy. Persons who need more attention from the therapist may feel frustrated with feedback only from peers. Also, each person's problems may not get addressed in every session. A person may get overlooked for many sessions in a group environment. Talkative members may monopolize the group meetings, and shy persons may not know how to interject their concerns. A person's needs may be incongruent with those of other group members, so there may not be "goodness of fit" for every member in the group. The therapist's style and skills need to blend with the purpose of the group, the experiences and needs of the members, and the personalities of the individuals.

Not all individuals profit from group therapy. That is, persons undergoing an acute psychotic episode, an acute manic phase of bipolar illness, or confusion related to dementia are examples of persons who could probably not participate productively in an insight-oriented group. Moreover, during these acute phases of illness, these persons would be disruptive to a group session focused on verbal expression. For these individuals, exercise or task-centered groups are more useful, helping them discharge energy and focus attention on physical activities.

Psychotic clients can participate in some groups once their thoughts are slowed, verbalizations are mostly coherent, and perceptual distortions are diminished. Usually, regulation on antipsychotic medication facilitates such improvement.

Little has been written specifically about the effect of psychotropic medication on clients' abilities to participate in group therapy. According to Sandison (1959), less dream and fantasy material is presented at group meetings when clients are influenced by psychotropic medications. However, some clinicians report that medication interferes with expression of feelings because of sedation. On the other hand, more people are accessible to treatment because medication allows them to be present in the group for the entire session. Furthermore, the group method offers an opportunity to conduct medication teaching. The challenging issue is timing—the client should not be undersedated or oversedated if he or she is to gain any benefit from the group.

GROUP THERAPY AND PSYCHIATRY

Moreno (1946) first brought group therapy to the attention of psychiatrists. Today, most psychotherapists are trained in group therapy. The American Group Psychotherapy Association is the organization within psychology that is dedicated exclusively to group therapy. Members of this organization include psychologists, psychiatrists, nurses, social workers, and other mental health professionals.

THEORETICAL FOUNDATIONS

Theoretical frameworks that are the foundations for group therapy practice are derived from the behavioral sciences of psychology, social psychology, and sociology. These sciences seek to understand both individual and group behavior, the two often being quite different. Individuals have been observed to act differently when they are part of a group. Different motivations for their behavior are at work, making it necessary to apply different explanatory theories.

Group theory, in general, focuses not only on the treatment of people in groups but also on the properties of groups themselves (Marram, 1978). *Group behavior theories* describe and predict the behavior of members of groups as a function of being in a group. *Group therapy theories* prescribe interventions that effect positive change in the group members.

Psychoanalytical theory and group dynamics theory were the main models of group therapy practice 50 years ago, when group therapy began. Currently, there are several group therapy theoretical models (Dies, 1992). The six main theoretical models are the psychodynamic/psychoanalytical model, the interpersonal/interactional model, the communication/systems model, the group process/analysis model, the existential/gestalt model, and the behavioral/cognitive model.

PSYCHODYNAMIC/PSYCHOANALYTICAL MODEL

The **psychodynamic model** of group therapy has its origins in Freud's psychoanalytical theory of human behavior and shares some of the same basic assumptions as Freudian theory (Rutan, 1992). Psychoanalytical theory assumes the existence of the id (pleasure principle), the superego (internalized parent or conscience), and the ego (reality principle that mediates between the id and the superego) as the psychological determinants of human behavior (Breuer & Freud, 1957). In the psychodynamic model of group therapy, the problems of the members of a group are viewed as similar to the problems a person would present in individual therapy. That is, the problems of the people in the group are conceptualized to center on unconscious conflicts and basic love–hate instincts (constructive versus destructive forces).

One main principle of Freudian theory that is applied to group therapy is the existence of unconscious motives, referred to in groups as *latent content*. This implies that the group as a collective body has unconscious fears and desires, as if the group as a whole had a psyche of its own (Rutan, 1992). These unconscious conflicts have meaning to all the members, but they are not fully aware of them. Frequently, the group experiences simultaneously a wish (a disturbing motive) and a fear (a reactive motive).

Whitaker and Lieberman (1969) examined the process of the development of the group unconscious. They used the term *nuclear conflicts* to refer to conflicts from earlier life experiences that individuals bring to and manifest within the group. These nuclear conflicts differ from *group focal conflicts*, whereby individual and total group concerns become interdependent. Focal conflicts consist of shared desires, fears, and agreed-upon solutions. Both nuclear and focal conflicts are frequently unconscious. The group leader's job is to tailor the group interventions so that the group members become aware of and discuss these unconscious conflicts.

Another important principle of psychoanalytic theory that is applied to group therapy is the symbolic reenactment of the past in present relationships, a phenomenon known as *transference*. Transference, which is usually a distortion of present relationships with others that is caused by disturbed early formative relationships (frequently those with parents and siblings), can take various forms, depending on the object of the transference. The clue to the existence of transference is the existence of strong emotions by one member of the group toward another member or the leader of the group. Transference can be successfully examined in the group setting, assisting clients to gain insight into their feelings and behaviors through the process of consensual validation and feedback by the other group members. Reenactment provides the opportunity to work through past conflicts.

INTERPERSONAL/INTERACTIONAL MODEL

The **interpersonal model** of group psychotherapy is similar to the psychodynamic model, but it emphasizes peer interactions and interpersonal learning, rather than insight (Leszcz, 1992). Founded on the theories of Harry Stack Sullivan (1953), the model views clients' current emotions and behaviors as reflecting clients' past relationships with significant others, in particular, parental figures. This transference is evident in the client's one-to-one relationships with other members in the group, the client's relationship to the group as a whole, and the client's relationships in other group settings. Although the group focuses on the here and now of relationships, the group may replicate family dynamics.

The goal of interpersonal therapy is the reconstruction of the person's personality. Because people have a strong need for interpersonal security, anxiety is viewed as the chief disruptive force in interpersonal relationships. In groups, the members manifest their problems in relating to others, and the leader serves to protect the members from feeling insecure and to boost their self-esteem. Relief from anxiety is found in interactions that increase members' self-respect and self-esteem. Distortions in perceptions of current interpersonal relationships can occur because of earlier experiences. These distortions hinder mutual understanding. In interpersonal therapy groups, learning can occur when the group leader assists the process of consensual validation of group members' feelings, thoughts, behaviors, and interactions with one another.

Transactional analysis, originated by Berne (1961), is theoretically the closest to the interpersonal model. *Transactional analysis* views the client's interactions with others as being influenced by his or her adult, parent, and child ego states; these ego states are similar to Freud's ego, superego, and id, respectively (Gladfelter, 1992). Interactions among the group members in transactional analysis groups are analyzed on the basis of the ego states that clients display in their games, scripts, and transactions. Games are interchanges between people that result in bad feelings or blaming others. Scripts are life plans chosen early by the child ego state that may be maladaptive for the adult. Transactions are communicative interchanges between the ego states of two or more persons. People frequently change ego states in their interactions with others. This ability to switch ego state contributes to a healtheir adaptation to life, whereas rigidity in maintaining just one ego state can be associated with personality dysfunction.

COMMUNICATION/SYSTEMS MODEL

In the **communication/systems model** of group therapy, the group is considered as a whole. The group is viewed as more than the sum of its parts or individual members, with boundaries and change mechanisms taking on great importance. Systems theory applied to groups focuses on subgroups and boundaries and communications between these subgroups (Azarian, 1992).

Communication theory applied to group therapy considers both the content of messages of the group members and the method of transmission of these messages. Communication is both verbal and nonverbal, and messages can be misinterpreted if they are unclear. Communication contains both manifest elements and latent elements. The *manifest elements* are in the overt message; they are the feelings, thoughts, and opinions that are in the awareness of the sender. The *latent elements* are in the covert, or hidden, message and are the feelings and thoughts of which the sender is not aware. Therefore, there can be double message communications. The group leader is responsible for pointing out these double messages when they occur in the group and for teaching members the difference between clear and vague communication. The group leader also functions as a role model of clear and congruent communication.

Dysfunctional communication, unclear or confusing communication, is a result of not learning to communicate properly or of not taking responsibility for messages being sent (Marram, 1978). In groups, dysfunctional communication usually allows the sender to avoid responsibility for saying what he or she really wants to say or really means. The sender's avoidance of responsibility may manifest as blaming, projection of anger, denial of feelings, withdrawal, or other defensive behaviors. The group leader needs to confront this phenomenon. The timing and the participation of the other group members in this confrontation are important, because group members need to feel supported and secure if they are to change their dysfunctional patterns. The leader also models effective communication and works on building group members' self-esteem.

GROUP PROCESS/GROUP ANALYSIS MODEL

The **group process model** originated in the 1940s and its principles are used along with other individually focused theoretical models, such as the psychodynamic model or the interpersonal model, by most group practitioners. The group process framework sees groups as being in a constant state of flux, with the goal of the group being to find a state of equilibrium (Cartwright & Zander, 1960). Individual interactions in the group create tensions, and the group as a whole seeks ways to reduce these tensions. Group norms or acceptable ways of acting evolve from interactions between people and crystallize into the group culture.

According to the group process model, groups typically go through the following stages: the introductory phase, the established or working phase, and the termination phase. The main issues groups deal with during all these phases relate to dependence (the handling and distribution of power) and interdependence (members' feelings about closeness with others). Healthy groups are able to resolve anxieties concerning dependency and interdependency (authority and intimacy issues), whereas unhealthy groups cannot. Successful group leaders are able to mobilize the capacity of the group members to resolve these authority and intimacy issues without conflict. This process happens gradually as trust develops among the group members. If these issues of authority and intimacy are not at least partially resolved, the group is unable to move on to other tasks.

EXISTENTIAL/GESTALT MODEL

The application of existential and gestalt theoretical frameworks to group therapy began in the 1960s with the Human Potential Movement, and its main proponents were Fritz Perls (1951), Abraham Maslow (1962), and Carl Rogers (1961). These similar frameworks all have a here-and-now focus, with the goal of increasing people's awareness of their feelings. A person's feelings are thought to be suppressed by the person's own constraints or the constraining expectations of others. Self-actualization is a secondary goal of existential or gestalt therapy. A self-actualized person assumes responsibility for him- or herself and makes choices about feelings, thoughts, and behavior. Clients are free to define themselves and become self-actualized, but this process is impeded by their own self-imposed limitations caused by fear or emotional pain.

The **existential/gestalt model** of group therapy facilitates people's self-actualization processes by helping them become more aware of their full potential, their alternatives or choices, and their feelings and emotions. Although most types of groups have the goal of helping individual members take responsibility for their emotions and behaviors through the process of support and feedback, in existential/gestalt groups this is the preeminent goal. The group functions as a microcosm of the real world of social interactions for the members. After focusing on the here and now of the social interactions demonstrated in the group, individual members can apply what they learned to their personal social interaction problems outside the group.

According to these frameworks, insight into the "why" of behavior is less important than insight into the "what" of behavior. Dealing with personal problems through increased awareness is viewed as a growth process, not a corrective process. Individuals can deal adequately with their own life problems if they know what these problems are; they do not necessarily have to know why they exist. The group experience provides an environment in which people can identify with and accept the forming self through experiences of awareness.

BEHAVIORAL/COGNITIVE MODEL

Behavioral therapy also focuses on the "what" of behavior—that is, specific behaviors that present themselves in the here and now. The behavioral model further focuses on the motivation for these behaviors, or the reinforcers of the behaviors. Behaviors are viewed as adaptive or maladaptive, and maladaptive behaviors become the targets for change. Behavioral change is brought about through punishment of maladaptive acts and the positive reinforcement of adaptive behaviors. The goal of behavioral therapy is to change specific behaviors and determine how this change will be achieved.

The **behavioral model** of group therapy conceptualizes group membership as a reinforcer. The social climate of the group is seen as the source of positive social reinforcement. The group offers the members a feeling of belonging and allows interactions that allow members to be heard and appreciated by others. The ways in which other members and the group leader respond to the behavior of an individual member can be reinforcing or extinguishing and therefore the stimulus for change. For example, the positive response of group members to a member's behavior contributes to the reinforcement of that member's behavior. On the other hand, a negative response from any member contributes to extinguishing the behavior.

Cognitive therapy is similar to behavioral therapy in that it focuses more on changing behavior than on obtaining insight into the reasons for that behavior. This form of therapy examines the cognitions (thoughts) and related feelings that contribute to maladaptive behaviors. People's cognitions are believed to result from goals, standards, and values that are mainly learned from families and culture. These can become maladaptive when they become unrealistic rules of "shoulds," "oughts," and "musts" and internalized commands that are often projected onto others (Ellis, 1992).

In cognitive group therapy, clients are helped to change their thoughts, feelings, and behaviors through the use of confrontation and homework assignments. During the group therapy session, the members share their homework assignments, along with their problems, with the group, with the purpose of identifying their core dysfunctional beliefs. The other group members and the leader help the member identify these dysfunctional irrational beliefs and dispute them, helping the person to change them and the accompanying dysfunctional behaviors.

PSYCHODRAMA AND ROLE-PLAYING TECHNIQUES

Psychodrama and role playing are specific techniques used in group therapy that involve action rather than conversation, but they are not separate theoretical models. Psychodrama has its roots in the theater and is used by the group members to re-enact conflictual situations or interactions. The object is to gain an understanding of the behavior of oneself or the other person involved in the actual situation. Psychodrama is based on spontaneity, reality testing, catharsis, and role reversal. Alter egos are used in psychodrama. The purpose of the alter egos is to enact roles that require the client to explore the meaning of feelings and behaviors that maintain his or her present problems. Members of the group act out the conflictual situation while other members serving as alter-ego representatives ("doubles") stand beside them and indicate what they might be thinking or feeling. The individual involved in the actual situation frequently reverses roles in the psychodrama to gain a better understanding of the other person who was involved in the interaction (Moreno, 1946).

Role playing is similar to psychodrama. It uses role reversal but not alter egos. The members of the group must guess at what the actors in the role play are thinking, feeling, or trying to convey. The group as a whole discusses the interactions of the actors. These techniques work best when a member has experienced an actual situation that may serve as the basis of the psychodrama or the role play (Marram, 1978).

SUMMARY OF THEORETICAL FOUNDATIONS

This brief overview of the theoretical models of group therapy practice has attempted to provide a beginning understanding of the concepts that underlie the group dynamics and processes that occur in all groups, not just therapeutic groups. Which theory the clinician or group therapist uses depends on the goals and purposes of his or her group. For example, an outpatient support group for substance abusers will have quite different goals than an inpatient grief process group. Frequently, group therapists will use a combination of models, that is, an eclectic approach, to guide their work.

Even if they do not acknowledge using an eclectic approach, most group therapists use principles from various models. Dies (1992) discovered that the majority of therapists endorse concepts from various theoretical models, although they may prefer one model over the others. The majority of group therapists that Dies surveyed indicated the following as the most important issues in group therapy:

- Transference/countertransference
- Group resistance
- Here-and-now focus
- Underlying group process themes
- Boundary management cohesiveness
- Facilitation of feedback and self-disclosure
- Process versus content focus

These concepts come from the psychodynamic, interpersonal, communication/systems, and group process models.

What is most important is that the group therapist use some theoretical concepts and principles to guide his or her work, thereby providing a secure structure for the group. Otherwise, because of the complexity and rapidity of group interactions, the group therapist or leader can quickly lose control and the group may fail in its therapeutic mission, that is, for the members to be of benefit to each other.

THE NURSE'S ROLE

Nurses have the unique opportunity to work with clients in numerous health care settings. During the average hospital stay of only 1 to 2 weeks, nurses learn about clients' needs, disease process, and recovery from crises. Because most units offer many groups, nurses usually participate with clients in some aspect of this treatment modality. Staff nurses may be leaders of activity, psychoeducation, task, or support groups. They can also be therapists and co-therapists. The American Nurses Association (ANA) *Statement on Psychiatric–Mental Health Clinical Practice and Standards of Psychiatric–Mental Health Nursing Practice (1994)* specifies that nurses must provide, structure, and maintain a therapeutic environment and that advanced clinical expertise is required for functioning as a psychotherapist in individual and group treatment modalities.

EDUCATIONAL PREPARATION

Psychiatric nurses practicing as therapists (or psychotherapists) in group therapy need to have at least a master's degree in psychiatric–mental health nursing. Curricula at the master's level include psychodynamic education about group process as well as supervision of therapeutic groups. Preparation for the master's degree can lead to a clinical specialty in psychiatric–mental health nursing, and certification opportunities are also provided by the ANA. At this level of expertise, nurses can offer counseling in private practice and conduct outpatient groups.

Much overlap exists between the disciplines involved in inpatient psychiatry. Each professional offers a different perspective. For example, the social worker, who may be more aware than other professionals of rehabilitation opportunities in the community, provides the client with specifics about appropriate placement options for discharge. The occupational therapist may provide the most realistic appraisal of the client's functional abilities. The nurse, on the other hand, may be most aware of the client's physical conditions, medication requirements, and social skills. Because the nurse is often the coordinator of the assessments by other professionals, the presence of a nurse in group therapy is optimal. The nurse who is a group therapist may also be one of the nursing staff who works daily with all clients. Nurses also participate in groups as co-therapists. Because nurses have 24-hour responsibility for client care, their participation in group facilitates the continuity of care.

SUPERVISION

Supervision is one professional's guiding the practice of another professional. For example, a clinical nurse specialist, social worker, psychologist, or psychiatrist may supervise a nurse, or an experienced nurse may supervise a new nurse. In group therapy, supervision includes the ongoing evaluation of the leader's behavior, emotions, and interventions. The goal of this process is self-awareness through self-evaluation. Constructive criticism and feedback on performance are essential components of learning effective group leadership. All practitioners of group therapy need professional supervision to gain insight into their motives for their own interactions and to gain awareness of possible countertransference reactions. Supervision, then, is for both the novice and the expert group leader.

Supervision works best when the supervisor has no authority over the supervisee. Bonnivier (1992) described a peer supervision group established for nurses to explore their countertransference reactions to clients. The goals of the group were (1) to recognize countertransference reactions, which are unconscious by nature; (2) to explore and examine the basis and meaning of the reactions; and (3) to develop, collaboratively, interventions that would help the nurses behave therapeutically rather than angrily. After 1 year, the group of nurses felt that they could manage their countertransference therapeutically. As a result, the group became incorporated into nursing education on a yearly basis. The absolute requirement was that no one with administrative responsibilities over any of the members could participate in supervision. Hence, participants were free to examine their thoughts and feelings without fear of repercussions.

CO-THERAPY

Co-therapy is joint or dual leadership of a group. Sometimes an experienced therapist is the leader and the co-therapist is a less-experienced practitioner. This type of co-therapy is a strategy for training the new leader (Yalom, 1983). However, both therapists may share the leader role equally. Co-therapy is advantageous for those who like to work with others, to discuss each other's roles and participation within the group, and to explore the relationship they share with each other. More attention and interaction are available to clients when the leaders have distinctly different personalities. Clients witness the co-therapists actively solving problems and resolving conflicts. Ideally, such exposure provides clients role modeling of healthy, assertive, and successful relationships. When co-therapists are of different genders, clients can benefit optimally from the two therapists' resolution of gender-related issues, that is, identification with one sex and conflict resolution with the opposite sex. Most groups lend themselves to co-therapy.

GROUP THERAPY ON PSYCHIATRIC UNITS

Some of the purposes of group therapy in the hospital setting include encouraging social involvement, developing rapport between clients and staff, enabling clients to demonstrate support for each other and participate in mutual problem solving, and promoting the development of a sense of solidarity as a group of individuals in the hospital situation. Groups offer clients opportunities to explore new communication skills, make use of social contacts, obtain peer feedback on individual problems, and experience group support for evaluating behaviors. Clients sometimes accept confrontation or criticism better from other clients than from staff.

Styles of Group Leadership

Historically, the **group leadership** role was primarily filled by physicians or nurses. In the past 40 years, the role has been filled by nurses, social workers, psychologists, and psychiatrists. There are many styles of and theoretical approaches to conducting insight- or process-oriented groups, but, according to Rogers (1971), a client-centered philosophy is the basic foundation of all of them. Accordingly, the specific functions of the group leader are to

- Facilitate interactions within the group
- Respond to the feelings and meanings inherent in each member's statements
- Accept the group and its members
- Understand each person's verbal contribution
- Identify how those statements relate to the member

- Use self-disclosure and expression thoughtfully and professionally
- Provide feedback
- Avoid excessive planning or use of games or gimmicks
- Limit the use of interpretations

Rogers's style is a reflective, as opposed to authoritarian, style. Thus, rather than directing, confronting, and controlling the direction of the group, the leader encourages the expression of feelings and conveys emotional comfort. In contrast, a confrontive style might be used with groups of drug addicts or alcoholics whose defensive posture is detrimental to their recovery. The styles of group leadership are summarized in Table 23–3.

The group leader sets the tone of the group. He or she is responsible for providing structure in terms of the time and place of sessions, establishing rules for safe self-expression and confidentiality, and facilitating expression of feelings and participation by all members. The leader establishes a climate of comfort relatively free of tension and anxiety, balances the needs of the group against those of any member, and intervenes to promote safety and self-awareness (Pasquali et al., 1989).

Nurses as Group Leaders

Although nurses were involved with group therapies since the tuberculosis psychoeducation experiments, it was not until the 1960s that nursing education included group dynamics and process. Advanced education and training in group leadership were offered at the graduate nursing level. However, in the psychiatric units, nurses were often the only staff available to hold group meetings, regardless of their education or preparation. Thus psychiatric nurses have probably been doing group work for educational and communicative purposes longer than has been documented.

Ken Kesey's (1963) *One Flew Over the Cuckoo's Nest* is a negative demonstration of the nurse's role in group psychotherapy. Nurse Ratched is a malevolent, controlling, and domineering woman in a starched, white uniform. Her efforts to facilitate clients' self-disclosure are humiliating experiences for the clients, and group support is thwarted as she verbally threatens to reveal private material to the clients' families. Her tactics, far from being therapeutic, reveal unethical use of staff authority and a distinct lack of communication skills and group therapy training.

Yalom (1983) reported that a particular nurse-run inpatient group in 1974 provided clients with social learning experiences and open discussion of feelings that facilitated ward functioning. Clients reported that the group experience enhanced their use of other ward group activities. The negative aspect was the formality of the group, which was manifested in, among other things, the nurses' starched, white uniforms. Not surprisingly, nurses on most psychiatric units abandoned these white uniforms more than 20 years ago.

TABLE 23–3
Summary of Characteristics of Group Leadership

REFLECTIVE
► Facilitation
► Empathic listening
► Responsiveness
► Acceptance
► Identification of relevance of one member's statements to other member
► Thoughtful use of self-disclosure
► Ability to confront
► Provision of feedback
► Limited use of interpretation
► Avoidance of excessive planning, games, or gimmicks
AUTHORITARIAN
► Directiveness
► Confrontation
► Control of members' participation
► Control of choice of topics
► Planning methods for conduct of group sessions without allowing input from others

PROCESS AND CONTENT

Discussion about group sessions includes analysis of both process and content. **Process** refers to the manner in which clients talk about themselves and the way that the group responds. Analysis of group process provides assessment of the therapy's effects on individual group members. The assessment involves evaluation of individual clients' responses to each other, to the group as a whole, and to the leader. Group process can be described by the degree of the group's openness, cohesiveness, and responsiveness to particular individual concerns and the degree of consistency of individual behavior within the group. For example, a consistent tendency of older group members to act as parents or rescuers may influence the contributions of younger members who perceive them as parental figures. Questions that the leader may ask to evaluate group process include the following:

- Who started the group today?
- What happened when Ms. X. told her story?
- Did Mr. T. try to rescue as he always does?
- Did Mr. J. fall asleep?
- What precipitated Ms. Z.'s departure from the room?
- Who responded when Mr. Q. started crying?

Group process varies with each session and with the current moods of or events specific to individual members and to the group as a whole. Sometimes, the therapist may share his or her process comments with the group to stimulate insight or to teach group dynamics.

Content analysis is the evaluation of what was said during the group therapy session. Content includes overall themes of the group session. Examples of content themes are sadness, loneliness, leisure time activities, and relationship issues. The therapist's own content, as a group member, is included in this discussion. What is not said is often discussed, also. Topics may be avoided because they can evoke painful or conflict-ridden emotions.

Content and process are interrelated and are often discussed together. In a co-therapy situation, a helpful method for examining both is for one therapist to focus on process while the other focuses on content. Questions that could be asked include the following:

- Under what conditions did Ms. X. say what she said? And to whom?
- What was the person's response and what did that trigger in Ms. Z, Mr. Q., and Ms. S.?
- When Mr. J. left the room, what did Ms. X say, and how did the mood in the room change?

Like process, content varies within the group according to individual members' differences in moods, events, and relationships with each other.

In the psychiatric unit, some groups may lend themselves better than others to process and content discussions. That is, a group of people who are verbal, self-aware, and high functioning will talk and react, solve problems, and seek personal change. In contrast, less reaction to one another and problem solving occur in activity-oriented groups, in which clients are performing tasks and are moving at different paces. Certainly, the focus of the group determines the kind of activities that might occur in the session. Nevertheless, there is always information to assess and discuss about what was said, who said it and how, who did what activity, and what the themes of the session were.

APPLICATION OF THE NURSING PROCESS

The nursing process—assessing, diagnosing, planning, intervening, and evaluating the plan—is applied to individuals within a group as well as to the group as a whole. For example, 10 clients who have the same problem may be in one group. In this manner, specific interventions can be used for all of the members. Klose and Tinius (1992) developed a group for patients with low self-esteem, teaching them and having them practice specific strategies for enhancing self-esteem. The group's particular focus combined insight-oriented therapy and education, creating the opportunity for group members to provide constructive social interaction, trust, and support. Nursing diagnoses that might be applied to a whole group or to persons within a group are listed in Table 23–4.

Occasionally, an entire group can be viewed as the client and the nursing process applied. For example, the group may face a recently discharged member's suicide. The entire group may be avoiding or denying the reality of the event, and a nursing diagnosis such as ineffective coping or dysfunctional grieving might be considered. Similarly, a group for clients with schizophrenia may be given a diagnosis of altered health maintenance because all members are currently unable to procure and prepare food for themselves as a result of preoccupation with internal stimuli. A nursing diagnosis with plan and interventions can be applied to the group when all of the members support problematic or destructive behaviors by any one, several, or all members.

TABLE 23–4
Nursing Diagnoses that May Be Applied to a Group as a Whole or to Individual Members Within a Group

Altered Health Maintenance
Altered Role Performance
Anticipatory Grieving
Anxiety
Body Image Disturbance
Dysfunctional Grieving
High Risk for Self-Mutilation
Hopelessness
Ineffective Denial
Ineffective Family Coping: Compromised
Ineffective Family Coping: Disabling
Ineffective Individual Coping
Knowledge Deficit (of medication)
Noncompliance
Parental Role Conflict
Personal Identity Disturbance
Powerlessness
Self-Esteem Disturbance
Social Isolation

From North American Nursing Diagnosis Association. (1992). *NANDA nursing diagnoses: Definitions and classification, 1992–1993.* Philadelphia: Author.

GROUPS THAT FOCUS ON STRESS-RELATED ISSUES

Various types of groups exist to help the client deal with the stresses of life. The most common ones are task groups, teaching groups, self-awareness/personal growth groups, therapy groups, and social groups (Kneisel, 1992). These groups differ in their focus, their goals, and the functions of the leader and members. Table 23–5 identifies several types of groups.

Self-awareness groups focus on the interpersonal concerns (the here and now) of the members, with the goal of developing interpersonal strengths. Therapy groups are also member focused, but past experiences are also taken into consideration. The goal of therapy groups is to help the members gain self-understanding and find more satisfactory ways of relating to others. Social groups focus on enjoyment and mutual meeting of needs, the purpose being to allow members to find recreation, relaxation, and comfort. The goal of teaching groups is to impart information.

Although all types of groups are important, nurses are generally more interested in the groups in which they can use their professional skills to bring about educative or therapeutic effects on clients. Therefore, nurses are frequently involved in teaching, therapy, and support groups.

TASK GROUPS

Task groups focus on the performance of a specific task agreed on by the group. This task is usually important to the members of the group, and the group stays together only long enough to accomplish it. Sometimes these groups are conducted by occupational therapists, but

TABLE 23–5
Types of Groups, Their Purposes, and Examples

	PURPOSE OF GROUP	EXAMPLE
Task	Performance of particular task	Occupational therapy group; poetry group
Social	Recreation; comfort; mutual meeting of needs	Recreational outings, e.g., bowling
Teaching	Imparting of information	Medication group
Psychoeducational	Imparting of information; processing of emotional concerns	Dual-diagnosis (combination of psychiatric diagnosis and substance abuse) groups
Support/Therapeutic	Coping with particular stresses and concerns	Cancer support group; Alzheimer's caregiver support groups
Self-Help/Mutual Support	Peer support (no professional leader)	Overeaters Anonymous; Alcoholics Anonymous
Psychotherapeutic	Interpersonal concerns; present problems; past experiences; self-understanding; insight-oriented	Inpatient or outpatient groups
Symptom Management	Specific target (psychosis); coping strategies; stress management; not insight oriented	Schizophrenic group; exercise group; reminiscence group

nurses also lead groups that have specific purposes, such as collage making, poetry writing, or the planning of an outing.

TEACHING GROUPS

Medication groups, an example of teaching groups, are an important aspect of psychiatric care, usually provided by nurses or clinical pharmacists. Antipsychotics and antidepressants have unpleasant side effects that often result in clients' noncompliance with medication regimens. In group, members at varying stages of illness help each other by sharing coping strategies for managing side effects. They problem-solve and evaluate whether the side effects outweigh the benefits of the drugs for their illnesses. The group leader offers education about purposes, dosage, safe and unsafe side effects, metabolism, drug or food interactions, and the usual length of time necessary for the medication to start taking effect. Overall, groups encourage awareness of symptoms of illness, side effects of medications, and resources for obtaining information.

PSYCHOEDUCATIONAL GROUPS

Educative or teaching groups are those in which the nurse usually acts as the leader and imparts some health-related information. **Psychoeducational groups** are a variation of this in which the nurse imparts some information but also facilitates discussion of the related psychosocial issues. An example of this would be a group run by public health nurses that provides information on the treatment and management of sexually transmitted diseases but also encourages discussion of self-esteem and social issues related to these diseases.

Dual-diagnosis groups are becoming popular for people with psychiatric diagnoses who become involved with alcohol and substance abuse or addiction. The nurse leader is challenged to provide education and promote insight so that clients can acknowledge the abuse of substances as personally problematic.

SUPPORTIVE/THERAPEUTIC GROUPS

Supportive/therapeutic groups help members cope with the sources of stress in their lives and focus on existing strengths (La Salle & La Salle, 1991). This stress may be related to physical, psychological, or social problems. Support groups focus on thoughts, feelings, and behaviors. The group provides a safe environment for clients to share with others who are often in the same situation or dealing with the same stressors. Examples of these types of groups are cancer support groups, divorce support groups, and impaired health professional support groups. The nurse may act as the facilitator or initiator of these groups (Heiney & Wells, 1989; Swayze, 1991).

SELF-HELP/MUTUAL-HELP GROUPS

Self-help groups and mutual-help groups are peer support groups that are run by the members and have no professional leader. However, they usually do adhere to a prescribed structure. Alcoholics Anonymous (AA) and other substance abuse or codependency groups modeled on the twelve-step program are the best known of these mutual-help groups. Groups such as Overeaters Anonymous and Recovery Inc. are also becoming more prominent.

In general, self-help groups have arisen in populations that have conditions that cause them to exhibit some behaviors that are unacceptable to or stigmatized by society and for which effective treatment has not yet been found. The focus of self-help groups is not on insight into behavior or the reconstruction of personality, the traditional focuses of psychiatric practitioners. Instead, the focus is on controlling members' dysfunctional behavior, decreasing stress by giving advice and sharing coping strategies, and maintaining members' self-esteem and legitimacy in the face of societal pressure. In addition, self-help groups focus on socialization of members. The socialization process goes beyond meeting individual members' needs for social contact to include instillation of the perspectives and values of the entire group, which are usually more in accord with societal norms (Marram, 1978).

People abusing substances have turned to mutual-help groups to assist them with their recovery process. Mutual-help groups are associations that are voluntarily formed, are not professionally led, and operate through face-to-face supportive interaction focusing on a mutual goal. The first of the mutual-help groups was AA, founded officially in 1935. The early AA members developed what they called the Twelve Steps to guide the recovery process (Brown, 1985; Kurtz, 1979).

Alcoholics Anonymous has been viewed as relatively successful in helping people abusing alcohol to remain sober. Because it is nonprofessional, cost sparing, and an ongoing source of assistance, it is an invaluable resource to the community. Nurses frequently refer clients misusing substances to this type of group. AA meetings may be geared to special-interest groups (e.g., homosexual persons, professionals, or students).

Other Twelve Step programs have developed through adaptation of AA's approach. Narcotics Anonymous, Gamblers Anonymous, Debtors Anonymous, Cocaine Anonymous, Overeaters Anonymous, and Sex and Love Addicts Anonymous are examples. The Twelve Steps have also been applied to syndromes of compulsive behavior and other difficulties encountered in the children, partners, and close associates of substance abusers. Alanon, Codependents Anonymous, and Adult Children of Alcoholics are examples of these groups.

The proliferation of mutual-help groups is one of the important social developments of this century. The reason for this social development is not completely understood, but the structure is relatively straightforward. In general, Twelve Step meetings follow one of these general formats:

- Uninterrupted talk(s) by one or more speakers about "what it was like, what happened, and what it is like now"
- A discussion in which each person at the meeting has the opportunity to speak briefly
- Some combination of the preceding two options

The format and choice of particular step (of the Twelve Steps) of meetings vary according to the group's size, the region of the country in which the group meets, the ethnic and gender composition of the group, and other cultural characteristics of the members.

PSYCHOTHERAPEUTIC GROUPS

The biological basis for illness and symptoms provides a rationale for conducting groups made up of clients who suffer from the same ailments and problems. Having the same nursing diagnosis increases the likelihood that clients can be helpful to one another as they learn together to cope with their illness. An advantage to common-illness groups is that the rapid client turnover in the hospital provides ongoing membership of persons in different phases of the same illness. Denial becomes more difficult when people view the same symptoms in others.

Pollack (1990) began an inpatient group for people with bipolar disorder who were knowledgeable about their diagnosis, voluntarily took their medication, were sufficiently stabilized on their medication that they could attend meetings, and were motivated to attend meetings. The group met weekly, incorporating new members. Yalom's 11 therapeutic factors were the therapists' goals for this group (see Table 23–2). After 9 months, three goals emerged as most prominent: sharing information, coping with bipolar disorder, and improving interpersonal relationships. Clients recognized similar experiences, such as needing to be the center of attention, experiencing high energy levels or euphoric moods, and feeling the despair of depressive episodes. Skillful group leadership was required at these meetings because of the need for behavioral limits.

Other groups offered on the psychiatric unit might include groups for stress reduction, suicide prevention, intellectual discussion, occupational therapy, movement or dance therapy, current events, discharge issues, sexual health concerns, cooking, leisure activity, and entertainment.

SYMPTOM MANAGEMENT GROUPS

Group therapy is a helpful treatment method with schizophrenic clients. Kanas (1991) described a short-term approach of nine meetings. The therapeutic goals include teaching clients how to cope with their psychotic experiences and improve their interpersonal relationships. Members learn from one another's content and from the practice of interaction. The purposes of the group include providing safety, avoiding anxiety, promoting trust, and decreasing isolation and loneliness. This approach is used in conjunction with antipsychotic medication.

STRESS MANAGEMENT GROUPS

The basis of several groups is a biological approach to coping with stress. Relaxation groups teach slower breathing, deep muscle relaxation, elimination of distraction, and achievement of a calm mind and a peaceful mood. Exercise groups provide for the discharge of energy without demanding fine motor coordination. Exercise stimulates the whole body and can create a peaceful, relaxed, and satisfied mood. Similarly, music groups produce relaxation. Humor groups promote enjoyment of social interaction (Klein, 1986; McHale, 1989) and feelings of well-being (Ljungdahl, 1989; Siegel, 1986) while discharging excess physical and emotional tension (Freud, 1928; Goldstein, 1987).

GROUP THERAPY ACROSS THE LIFE SPAN

Table 23–6 summarizes the issues that may be addressed by group therapy across the life span.

TABLE 23–6

Group Therapy Across the Life Span

	ISSUES THAT ARE THE FOCUS OF GROUP WORK
Children	Social skills, emotional expression, behavioral expression of feelings, adult support, protection from unsafe environment
Adolescents	Peer relationships, sexual feelings, appropriate expression of feelings, social pressures, school performance, vocation and future plans, drugs, autonomy, relationships with parents
Adults	Gender support (for heterosexual and homosexual clients), parental roles, substance abuse, addiction, posttraumatic stress disorder (in veterans), victims of physical and/or sexual violence, incest survivors, dysfunctional relationships, marital discord, chronic illness
Elderly	Adjustment to aging, loneliness, widowhood, chronic illness, peer relationships, family relationships, financial adjustments, changes in housing, grieving of losses of friends and health, life review, preparation for end of life
Confined Elderly	Adjustment to health deterioration, adjustment to environment, loss of autonomy, change in family role, family relationships, caregiver relationships, grieving of losses, preparation for end of life, life review

CHILDHOOD

Emotional disturbances and psychiatric disorders in children often present as conduct and affective disorders (Barthel & Herrman, 1990). Assessment is frequently made through observations of children in group activities at school, on the hospital unit, with their peers, and with their families. Providing a safe environment for emotional expression is paramount in working with children. Developmental tasks must also be considered, so that feelings are expressed in age-appropriate activities. Some nonverbal group activities include play therapy, art therapy, movement or dance therapy, and sand tray therapy. Depending on the family, the therapist, the child, and the group, ages 8 to 10 years may be appropriate for verbal therapy groups. Childhood issues that might be amenable to group therapy include traumas such as accidents and natural disasters, grief over the death of a parent or other family member, and poor social adjustment. Many concerns, such as sexual abuse, neglect, battering, or parental substance and alcohol abuse, may be best managed in one-to-one therapy. However, successful group models exist for dealing with these problems.

Group therapy appears to be particularly useful in assisting children to improve their social skills. In a study of 102 elementary school children ages 8 to 10 years, Shechtman (1991) tested the hypothesis that small-group therapy would be effective in enhancing intimate friendships with same-sex peers. All of these children had been referred for counseling, and they were divided according to the similarity of their problems into control (no therapy) and experimental (group psychotherapy) groups. Recognizing the value of Yalom's therapeutic factors (see Table 23–2), the experimental group's therapy emphasized self-expression, support, freedom within stated limits, caring, and group cohesion. Enriching experiences included puppetry, drama, and social games. By the end of the study, the experimental group had demonstrated significant increases in the development of close relationships, supporting the hypothesis. Shechtman concluded that group therapy is a viable method for helping children to cope and feel secure, wanted, and loved in a society that can result in disruption, personal loss, and detachment in childrens' lives.

ADOLESCENCE

Adolescents are struggling with autonomy and independence from their parents and other authorities. As they establish their own identity, they are particularly vulnerable to peer pressure. Their problems are often reflective of social pressures and the concern they feel about their actions and physical appearance. Despite their needs for independence, they are dependent and require a great deal of emotional support from parents. Teenage issues include same- and opposite-sex peer relationships, sexually transmitted diseases, pregnancy, drug abuse, sexual abuse, aggression, social adjustment to school, depression, and suicide.

The combination of a strong desire for peer acceptance and rebellion toward authority makes adolescents optimal candidates for group therapy. Education groups, such as on prevention of infection by the human immunodeficiency virus (HIV), are effective with this age group. Alateen is effective for teenagers, particularly when alcoholic family members fail to support the adolescent. Peers coping with similar problems can be helpful and informative, strengthening one another's self-esteem. On the other hand, peers can also be cruel, scapegoating and rejecting each other. Group leadership skills are important with this age group to foster group cohesion, peer support, constructive behavior, and effective communication.

ADULTHOOD

Adults dealing with the stressors of modern life use a variety of support and therapy groups related to specific psychological or social concerns. Women's self-actualization groups and support groups began in the 1970s as part of the women's movement. Men's support groups are a more recent phenomenon, starting in the middle to late 1980s (Kipnis, 1991). These groups allow the members to deal with the general issues that are thought to be relevant to each gender and their social roles/expectations. Some of these groups are geared specifically toward homosexual persons.

There are also women's groups that address specific problems, such as incest and molestation or physical abuse. These groups may be mutual support groups modeled on the Twelve Step AA structure, or they may be leader-facilitated therapy groups (Delpo & Koontz, 1991; Kreidler & Carlson, 1991).

Pressures from social roles and transitions have spawned a variety of other types of support groups. For example, there are couples groups, multiple-family groups, parenting groups, new mothers groups, single parents groups, divorce groups, and bereavement groups. These groups are frequently short-term (10 to 12 sessions) and have a brief therapy/psychoeducational structure. Ongoing support and social groups, such as Parents Without Partners and Resolve (for infertility), are helpful when problems or concerns are not easily or quickly resolved.

Chronic medical conditions also frequently require ongoing support groups. Support groups for conditions such as cancer, HIV infection, acquired immunodeficiency syndrome, multiple sclerosis, Parkinson's disease, and ostomies help people to adapt to the physical and psychological changes associated with shared maladies. Members of these groups share emotions and adaptation strategies with each other in an effort to gain and give comfort and hope. Because family members also are affected by the medical and psychological conditions of their loved ones, there are support groups to address their concerns. Alzheimer's support groups and the Alliance for the Mentally Ill are but two examples of these family support groups.

OLDER ADULTHOOD

Persons over 65 years of age are considered elderly in American society. Because it is genetically and environmentally influenced, the aging process differs in each person. Regardless of individual differences, mental health may decline as health problems evolve. Participation in peer support groups, activity groups, religious or cultural organizations, volunteer centers, and senior citizens' centers may contribute to the maintenance of mental health.

Mental health problems of the elderly that may be amenable to group therapy include depression, social isolation, and grief. Grieving often occurs in response to adjustment to retirement, widowhood, loss of physical health and independence, loss of role in the family, and loss of family support. Inpatient and outpatient group therapy might focus on the maintenance of self-esteem through support and peer acceptance. Skills that might be taught in groups include problem solving, coping, and confrontation of negative beliefs (Grau, 1990).

Many elderly people must care for their spouses. Debilitating and progressive diseases take physical, emotional, and financial tolls on individuals and families. For example, elderly persons caring for a spouse with Alzheimer's disease suffer from more depression and anxiety than do noncaregiving spouses (Buffum, 1992). To assist families in caring for their loved ones and for their own mental health, local chapters of the Alzheimer's Association offer regular and frequent support groups. These groups are educational as well as supportive. For some members, these groups are useful because they provide time away and a social network of understanding new friends.

CONFINED ELDERLY

At retirement homes and nursing homes, groups provide residents with social opportunities. These include but are not limited to arts and crafts groups, day or weekend outings, hobby clubs, dances, dinners, newspaper publications, exercise clubs, and current events groups. Depending on the elders' level of functioning and motivation, the staff's creativity, and the financial resources of the facility, the possibilities are endless.

Zerhusen et al. (1991) studied depressed elderly residents in an intermediate care nursing home in Ohio. Their cognitive group therapy program consisted of a 10-week program that met for two 1-hour sessions each week. Leaders offered education about depression, information about cognitive therapy, and expectations about the group and the roles of the members. Behavior change was taught through planning desired activities, and cognitive change was taught by confronting members' negative thoughts and providing alternatives. Zerhusen et al. found significant differences between pre- and postintervention scores on the Beck Depression Inventory (BDI) in persons who attended the cognitive therapy group. No improvement in BDI scores was seen in clients who attended music therapy groups or in control groups.

The cognitively impaired elderly who reside in nursing homes or who attend senior day care centers also profit from group experiences. The focus of these groups is on the maintenance of self-esteem through supportive interaction. Often, this is done with reminiscence groups or with telling of humorous stories from the past. In cases of mild or nonprogressive impairment, groups can assist the individual to mourn loss of function and establish new goals in accord with decreased abilities (Grau, 1990).

VETERANS

Much of the group therapy research has come from Department of Veterans Affairs hospitals. Many of these hospitals are teaching hospitals associated with universities. Also, veterans of military service are often accustomed to working in groups and helping each other as buddies. Problems that veterans of wars have in common include adjustment to civilian life and post-traumatic stress disorder (PTSD) resulting from the trauma of combat or prisoner-of-war experiences. Currently, Vietnam War veterans use PTSD groups for support, spiritual development, management of anger, development of coping skills for living with others, and socialization.

Phases of treatment for PTSD include group therapy. According to Perconte (1988), therapeutic interventions in groups include education, supportive confrontation, communication training, social skills training, relaxation training, stress management, problem solving, and goal setting. Koller et al. (1992) emphasized the importance of timely integration and working through, in the group, of the traumatic experiences and pre- and postwar issues that are relevant to PTSD symptoms. New coping skills, correction of maladaptive behaviors, and support and understanding from group members are all emphasized in a treatment model that entails 16 weekly group sessions.

CURRENT RESEARCH ON GROUP THERAPIES/INTERVENTIONS

Nurses have begun to research the use of groups as part of their professional practice. They are examining the use of education groups, therapy groups, and support groups as interventions to help clients cope with physical and psychological conditions. The researchers either describe the process of using group interventions or evaluate the effectiveness of group interventions over other types of interventions. The accompanying Research Study display describes a study of the effectiveness of one nurse-created and -led group.

The descriptive studies of group process include a range of conditions. Krach and Zens (1988) researched the use of group techniques with incest perpetrators and described how the group dealt with these clients' needs for power and control. Delpo and Koontz (1991) reported the use of group therapy to address the inadequate parenting skills of mothers of incest victims. Urbancic (1989) described how the group process helped incest survivors to resolve their trauma. Gilbert (1988) studied the use of the group process to address the developmental tasks and age-related issues of preadolescent and adolescent sexually abused children. Staples

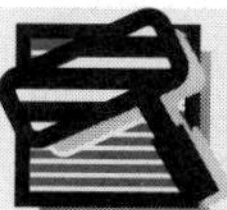

RESEARCH STUDY

A Self-Esteem Group at an Inpatient Psychiatric Hospital

Klose, P., & Tinius, T. (1992). *Journal of Psychosocial Nursing and Mental Health Services, 30*(7), 5–9.

Study Problem/Purpose

The purpose of the group was to facilitate clients' (a) acknowledgement of small accomplishments during hospitalization; (b) focusing on positive thoughts, feelings, and actions; (c) understanding of the effects of their emotions; and (d) thoughts about themselves in present and future situations.

Methods

An inpatient group of four to six patients, both men and women, ranging in age from 19 to 60 years, met for 45 minutes three times a week. The group was led by a nurse therapist and a coleader. Before the first session began, the therapist explained the group's purpose and the methods that would be used. The group was ongoing (number of weeks of attendance was not mentioned). Referral was by self or staff, and clients represented all diagnostic categories. Participation was voluntary, but commitment to attend was required. Clients who were hallucinating, delusional, manic, or in imminent danger of harming themselves or others were excluded.

The methods of therapy used were eclectic and included concepts from behavioral, interpersonal, and cognitive–behavioral psychotherapies, as well as therapist intuition.

Focus and Format of Group

Identification of one positive event, action, or thought within the past 12 days. A task was sometimes assigned, depending on the therapist's assessment. The focus was on the present rather than the past. Activities included structured exercises such as group art, poetry, pictures, music, and self-help strategies; leader participation; and discussion of outside material such as newspaper advice columns and magazines.

Anticipated Responses

It was expected that exercises would help clients reveal thoughts and feelings. Group interaction was expected to enable clients to provide feedback to each other. The group would provide members with emotional support for self-expression and for making changes. Clients would enjoy the positive focus. A goal was the group's creation of a holiday party for the entire unit.

Conclusions

Focusing on self-esteem was important. Clients were able to take a positive focus outside the group and the hospital. Clients with schizophrenia did not do well because of their disorganized thinking, impaired communication, lack of trust, short attention span, and difficulty in interpreting others' statements.

and Schwartz (1990) described their group therapy approach with anorexia nervosa clients. They found that the group process helped these clients change their narcissistic anorexic identity to a valuing of relationships with others. White (1987) studied the structure and usefulness of short-term psychiatric inpatient groups, describing the leadership skills needed to maintain an effective group. White (1988) also examined the use of groups for clients with long-term medical and psychosomatic problems; she found that these groups helped clients identify the underlying psychological issues related to these conditions.

In another type of descriptive study of the group process, the nursing model is applied to the understanding of the group process. For example, Forker and Billings (1989) used Martha Rogers's theory of unitary man to understand the group process in a community setting for aging clients. Another example is Laben et al.'s (1991) descriptive study of the application of Imogene King's goal attainment theory to group therapy work with juvenile offenders.

Group treatment evaluation studies by nurse researchers address the effectiveness of both therapy groups and support groups. Whitman and Gustafson (1989) found the use of support groups to be beneficial to families of oncology patients. Moores (1987) found a brief (six to eight sessions) psychoeducational group approach to have positive effects on anxiety disorder clients. Davis et al. (1992) studied the effect of a 10-week support group for grieving individuals and found that participation in the group decreased members' perceived levels of stress. Puskar (1990) determined that support groups for relocated corporate wives had a positive effect on decreasing the levels of anxiety and stress they experienced in relation to their relocation. Kane et al. (1992) compared the use of psychoeducational groups and the use of support groups in families of persons with chronic schizophrenia. They found that brief psychoeducational group interventions (four weekly sessions, each lasting 2 hours) provided to families by professionals during their relative's hospitalization were more effective at decreasing depression in the family members than were support groups of the same length. In addition, a majority of the family members preferred the psychoeducational groups over the support groups.

TABLE 23–7
Protocol for Planning and Evaluation of Nurse-Led Groups on Inpatient Units

- Title of group
- Staff involved in design, study of the group, and leadership of the group
- Purpose and goals of the group
- Theoretical foundations for the group
- Group composition: client population, content, methods
- Outcome measures: evaluation methods, frequency of evaluation, group process, and documentation of individual progress

Data from van Servellen, G., Poster, E., Ryan, J., et al. (1991). Nursing-led group modalities in a psychiatric inpatient setting: A program evaluation. *Archives of Psychiatric Nursing, 5,* 128–136.

One group of nurse researchers emphasized the importance of describing the purpose, process, and outcomes of groups led or co-led by nurses (van Servellen et al., 1991; van Servellen et al., 1992). Citing evidence from clinical practice and a review of the literature on nurse-led groups, they argued that there has been a lack of documentation of the specific aims and effectiveness of nurse-led groups. They proprosed a standardized protocol for reporting studies of nurse-led groups on inpatient psychiatric units; this format is presented in Table 23–7. Nursing research can enhance professional practice when documentation reflects accurately the efforts and outcomes of nurse-led groups.

CHAPTER SUMMARY

Group therapy began in the early 1900s with groups designed to provide education and emotional support. Pratt, Metzl, Adler, and Moreno were the pioneers of group therapy. Yalom's 11 therapeutic factors are the aims for most groups today. The types of group therapies vary and include process, psychoeducation, task, self-help, and support. Participants in group therapies include clients on psychiatric units as well as healthy clients desiring personal growth through the group process.

Theoretical perspectives on group therapy come from psychology, social psychology, and sociology. Group behavior theories describe and predict people's behavior in groups and group settings, whereas group therapy theories prescribe interventions that promote positive change in group members. Theories of group therapy include six models: psychodynamic/psychoanalytical, interpersonal/interactional, communication/systems, group process/analysis, existential/gestalt, and behavioral/cognitive. Different groups may be based on different perspectives; however, some groups are based on components of many theories. It is most important that the group therapist base his or her work on some theoretical foundation, lest the group lose its therapeutic mission.

Psychiatric nurses lead groups in many capacities. Advanced education and training are required for the role of therapist. Supervision and co-therapy are among the roles filled by the clinical specialist in psychiatric–mental health nursing. Staff nurses participate in and lead groups based on needs for education, support, recreation, task, or exercise. Of course, the nurse is involved in care planning for group therapy, applying nursing diagnoses to the group as well as to each member of the group. Other professionals who lead groups are psychiatrists, psychologists, social workers, occupational therapists, recreational therapists, and clinical pharmacists. Ideally, co-leaders have characteristics in common when conducting group therapy.

Many groups exist to help people with specific problems. Persons under stress may seek groups for support, education, and coping strategies. These persons may be suffering from cancer, HIV infections, multiple sclerosis, Parkinson's disease, or other conditions.

There are support and educational groups available for family caregivers of ill persons, such as the caregivers of persons with Alzheimer's disease or schizophrenia. Persons with substance abuse problems, veterans with PTSD, couples with parenting issues, or homosexual persons with relationship concerns can get relief from distress through group therapy. Most communities also provide group therapies for children, adolescents, and elderly. Some groups are of the self-help type, having no professional leaders.

Nursing research on group therapy focuses on the nature and content of groups offered to ill persons. The problems addressed by the groups examined in studies are varied, but usually nurses lead groups that are focused on particular health problems. While some researchers describe the groups, others look at outcomes. There is a need for group therapy research to be reported in a standardized format wherein purposes and specific outcomes are documented. Nursing practice will be enhanced when accurate documentation provides for replication of results.

Suggestions for Clinical Conference

1. Conduct a 1-hour, task-oriented group with your peers. Record your observations at the end of the session. Explore group process and content regarding (a) who took the leadership position and how the group members responded, (b) how conflicts were resolved, (c) how problems were solved, (d) the nature of each member's participation, and (e) members' satisfaction with the task accomplished.
2. Conduct two 1-hour groups with students assigned to the same clinical area. The group's purpose is to explore feelings about working in nursing, particularly in the current setting. Record your observations, feelings, and thoughts at the end of each session. Discuss each member's recordings in a postgroup meeting. Were there group themes for each session? Did members have similar or different feelings about each group session? Identify which of Yalom's therapeutic factors applied to your group sessions.
3. Attend a group on the psychiatric unit to which you are assigned. Identify the type and purpose of the group, the theoretical perspective(s) of the leader(s), the characteristics of the leader(s), and the outcomes of the group.
4. Compare two groups. For example, attend an Alanon meeting and an Alzheimer's disease family support group. How are the groups similar? How are they different? Identify the type of group (task, activity, psychoeducation, or process oriented) and the theoretical perspective.
5. Explain how you would evaluate the effectiveness of a group.
6. Attend two open meetings of an AA group that uses the Twelve Step program. Identify the twelve steps and discuss how this step-by-step approach was helpful to the attendees.

References

American Nurses Association. (1994). *A statement on psychiatric–mental health clinical nursing practice and standards of psychiatric–mental health clinical nursing practice*. Washington, DC: Author.

Azarian, Y. (1992). Contemporary theories of group psychotherapy: A systems approach to the group-as-a-whole. *International Journal of Group Psychotherapy, 42,* 177–203.

Bach, G. (1966). The marathon group: Intensive practice of intimate interaction. In H. M. Ruitenbeek (Ed.), *Group therapy today* (pp. 301–309). New York: Atherton.

Barthel, R., & Herrman, C. (1990). Psychiatric mental health nursing with children. In F. Gary & C. Kavanagh (Eds.), *Psychiatric mental health nursing* (pp. 801–861). Philadelphia: J. B. Lippincott.

Berne, E. (1961). *Transactional analysis in psychotherapy*. New York: Grove.

Bonnivier, J. (1992). A peer supervision group: Put countertransference to work. *Journal of Psychosocial Nursing and Mental Health Services, 30*(5), 5–8.

Bradford, L., Gibb, J., & Benne, K. (1964). *T-group theory and laboratory method: Innovations in re-education*. New York: Wiley.

Breuer, J., & Freud, S. (1957). In J. Strachey (Ed. and Trans.), Studies on hysteria. New York: Basic Books.

Brown, S. (1985). *Treating the alcoholic: A developmental model of recovery*. New York: Wiley.

Buffum, M. (1992). *Burden and humor: Relationships to mental health in spouse caregivers of Alzheimer's disease*. Ann Arbor, MI: University Microfilms International.

Cartwright, D., & Zander, A. (1960). *Group dynamics research and theory* (2nd ed.). New York: Elmsford, Row & Peterson.

Crenshaw, B. G. (1989). Groups and group therapy. In B. Johnson (Ed.), *Psychiatric–mental health nursing* (2nd ed., pp. 199–221). Philadelphia: J. B. Lippincott.

Davis, J., Hosiko, B., Jones, S., & Gosnell, D. (1992). The effect of a support group on grieving individuals' levels of perceived support and stress. *Archives of Psychiatric Nursing, 6,* 35–39.

Delpo, E., & Koontz, M. A. (1991). Group therapy with mothers of incest victims, Part I: Structure, leader attributes, and countertransference. *Archives of Psychiatric Nursing, 5,* 64–69.

Dies, R. (1992). Models of group psychotherapy: Sifting through confusion. *International Journal of Group Psychotherapy, 42,* 1–16.

Dreikurs, R. (1959). Early experiments with group psychotherapy: A historical review. In H. M. Ruitenbeek (Ed.), *Group therapy today* (pp. 18–27). New York: Atherton.

Ellis, A. (1992). Group rational–emotive and cognitive–behavioral therapy. *International Journal of Group Psychotherapy, 42,* 63–80.

Forker, J., & Billings, C. (1989). Nursing therapeutics in a group encounter. *Archives of Psychiatric Nursing, 3,* 108–112.

Freud, S. (1928). Humor. *International Journal of Psychoanalysis, 9,* 1–6.

Fromm, E. (1957, March 16). Man is not a thing. *Saturday Review,* pp. 9–11.

Gilbert, C. M. (1988). Sexual abuse and group therapy. *Journal of Psychosocial Nursing and Mental Health Services, 26*(5), 20.

Gladfelter, J. (1992). Redecision therapy. *International Journal of Group Psychotherapy, 42,* 319–333.

Goldberg, C. (1970). *Encounter: Group sensitivity training experience*. New York: Science House.

Goldstein, J. H. (1987). Therapeutic effects of laughter. In W. F. Fry & W. A. Salameh (Eds.), *Handbook of humor and psychotherapy* (pp. 1–19). Sarasota, FL: Professional Resources Exchange.

Grau, L. (1990). Psychiatric mental health nursing with the elderly. In F. Gary & C. Kavanagh (Eds.), *Psychiatric–mental health nursing* (pp. 862–897). Philadelphia: J. B. Lippincott.

Heiney, S., & Wells, L. (1989). Strategies for organizing and maintaining successful support groups. *Journal of Pediatric Oncology Nursing, 16,* 803–809.

Kanas, N. (1991). Group therapy with schizophrenic patients: A short-term, homogeneous approach. *International Journal of Group Psychotherapy, 41,* 33–48.

Kane, C., DiMartino, E., & Jimenez, M. (1990). A comparison of short-term psychoeducational and support groups for relatives coping with chronic schizophrenia. *Archives of Psychiatric Nursing, 4,* 343–353.

Kesey, K. (1963). *One flew over the cuckoo's nest.* New York: New American Library.

Kipnis, A. (1991). *Knights of armor.* Los Angeles: Jeremy Torcher.

Klein, A. (1986). Humor and death: You've got to be kidding. *American Journal of Hospice Care, 3*(4), 42–45.

Klose, P., & Tinius, T. (1992). A self-esteem group at an inpatient psychiatric hospital. *Journal of Psychosocial Nursing and Mental Health Services, 30*(7), 5–9.

Kneisel, C. (1992). Group process and group therapy. In H. Wilson & C. Kneisel (Eds.), *Psychiatric nursing* (4th ed, pp. 688–721). Redwood City, CA: Addison-Wesley.

Koller, P., Marmar, C., & Kanas, N. (1992). Psychodynamic group treatment of posttraumatic stress disorder in Vietnam veterans. *International Journal of Group Psychotherapy, 42,* 225–246.

Krach, P., & Zens, D. (1988). Incest: Nursing interventions for group therapy. *Journal of Psychosocial Nursing and Mental Health Services, 26*(10), 32–34.

Kreidler, M., & Carlson, R. (1991). Breaking the incest cycle: The group as a surrogate family. *Journal of Psychosocial Nursing and Mental Health Services, 29*(4), 28–32.

Kurtz, E. (1979). *Not God: A history of AA.* Center City, MN: Hazelden Educational.

Laben, J., Dodd, D., & Sneed, L. (1991). King's theory of goal attainment applied in group therapy for inpatient juvenile sexual offenders, maximum security state offenders, and community parolees, using visual aids. *Issues in Mental Health Nursing, 12,* 51–64.

LaSalle, P., & LaSalle, A. (1991). Small groups and their therapeutic force. In G. Stuart & S. Sundeen (Eds.), *Principles and practice of psychiatric nursing* (4th ed., pp. 809–826). St. Louis, MO: C. V. Mosby.

Leszcz, M. (1992). The interpersonal approach to group psychotherapy. *International Journal of Group Psychotherapy, 42*(1), 37–61.

Ljungdahl, L. (1989). Laugh if this is a joke. *Journal of the American Medical Association, 261,* 558.

Marram, G. (1978). *The group approach in nursing practice* (2nd ed.). St. Louis, MO: C. V. Mosby.

Maslow, A. (1962). *Toward a psychology of being.* Princeton, NJ: Van Nostrand.

McHale, M. (1989). Getting the joke: Interpreting humor in group therapy. *Journal of Psychosocial Nursing and Mental Health Services, 27*(9), 24–28.

Mintz, E. (1967). The extended-marathon groups. In H. M. Ruitenbeek (Ed.), *Group therapy today* (pp. 310–325). New York: Atherton.

Moores, A. (1987). Facing the fear. *Nursing Times, 83*(27), 44–46.

Moreno, J. (1946). Psychodrama and group therapy. *Sociometry, 9,* 249–253.

Mullan, H., & Rosenbaum, M. (1967). *Group psychotherapy.* New York: Free Press.

Pasquali, E., Arnold, H., & DeBasio, N. (1989). *Mental health nursing—A holistic approach* (3rd ed.). St. Louis, MO: C. V. Mosby.

Perconte, S. (1988, February). Stages of treatment in PTSD. *VA Practitioner,* pp. 47–57.

Perls, F. (1969). *Gestalt therapy verbatim.* Lafayette, CA: Real People Press.

Pollack, L. (1990). Improving relationships—Groups for inpatients with bipolar disorder. *Journal of Psychosocial Nursing and Mental Health Services, 28*(5), 17–22.

Pratt, J. H. (1906). The "home sanatorium" treatment of consumption. In H. M. Ruitenbeek (Ed.), *Group therapy today* (pp. 9–17). New York: Atherton.

Puskar, K. (1990). Relocation groups for corporate wives. *Administrative and Occupational Health Nursing Journal, 38*(1), 25–31.

Rogers, C. (1961). *Client-centered therapy.* Boston: Houghton Mifflin.

Rogers, C. (1971). Carl Rogers describes his way of facilitating encounter groups. *American Journal of Nursing, 7,* 275–279.

Ruitenbeek, H. (1969). New visions in group therapy. In H. M. Ruitenbeek (Ed.), *Group therapy today* (pp. 1–6). New York: Atherton.

Rutan, J. C. (1992). Psychodynamic group psychotherapy. *International Journal of Group Psychotherapy, 42,* 19–35.

Sandison, R. (1959). The role of psychotropic drugs in group therapy. *Bulletin of the World Health Organization, 21,* 505–515.

Shechtman, Z. (1991). Small group therapy and preadolescent same-sex friendship. *International Journal of Group Psychotherapy, 41,* 227–243.

Siegel, B. (1986). *Love, medicine and miracles.* New York: Harper & Row.

Staples, N. R., & Schwartz, M. (1990). Anorexia nervosa support group: Providing transitional support. *Journal of Psychosocial Nursing and Mental Health Services, 28*(2), 6–11.

Sullivan, H. S. (1953). *The interpersonal theory of psychiatry.* New York: Norton.

Swayze, S. (1991). Helping them cope: Developing self-help groups for clients with chronic illness. *Journal of Psychosocial Nursing and Mental Health Services, 29*(5), 35–37.

Urbancic, J. C. (1989). Resolving incest experiences through inpatient group therapy. *Journal of Psychosocial Nursing and Mental Health Services, 27*(9), 5–11.

van Servellen, G., Poster, E., Ryan, J. & Allen, J. (1991). Nursing-led group modalities in a psychiatric inpatient setting: A program evaluation. *Archives of Psychiatric Nursing, 5,* 128–136.

van Servellen, G., Poster, E., Ryan, J., Allen, J., & Randell, B. (1992). Methodological concerns in evaluating psychiatric nursing care modalities and a proposed standard group protocol format for nurse-led groups. *Archives of Psychiatric Nursing, 6,* 117–124.

Whitaker, D., & Lieberman, M. (1969). *Psychotherapy through the group process.* New York: Atherton.

White, E. M. (1987). Effective inpatient groups: Challenges and rewards. *Archives of Psychiatric Nursing, 1,* 422–429.

White, E. M. (1988). Use of medical support groups on a medical psychiatric unit. *Issues in Mental Health Nursing, 9,* 353–363.

Whitman, H. H., & Gustafson, J. P. (1989). Group therapy for families facing cancer crises. *Oncology Nursing Forum, 16,* 539–543.

Yalom, I. (1983). *Inpatient group psychotherapy.* New York: Basic Books.

Yalom, I. (1985). *The theory and practice of group psychotherapy* (3rd ed.). New York: Basic Books.

Zerhusen, J., Boyle, K., & Wilson, W. (1991). Out of the darkness: Group cognitive therapy for depressed elderly. *Journal of Psychosocial Nursing and Mental Health Services, 29*(9), 16–21.

CHAPTER 24

Milieu Therapy

JOHNNIE BONNER, M.S., R.N.

OUTLINE

CHAPTER OBJECTIVES

Upon completion of this chapter, you will be able to:

1. Discuss eight major components of milieu therapy.
2. Describe the client role in a therapeutic community.
3. Identify key components of the nurse's role in the therapeutic milieu.
4. Describe the use of nursing process in management of the therapeutic milieu.
5. Identify developmentally appropriate milieu interventions that address issues across the life span related to:
   a. responsibility
   b. autonomy
   c. safety

KEY TERMS

Milieu therapy
Therapeutic community
Therapeutic milieu

Milieu means environment; milieu therapy refers to the effective use of the social environment of treatment—staff, activities, and resources—to facilitate the client's highest level of function. Milieu therapy has played a significant role in the treatment of serious mental disorders since the 1950s. It has been defined as "psychosocial rehabilitation," and it integrates major biological, social, and behavioral concepts.

Classic milieu therapy focused on long-term treatment models. However, the advent of psychopharmacology in the 1950s shortened hospital stays and decreased relapse rates, playing a major role in deinstitutionalization. Recent socioeconomic and legislative changes have also stressed the importance of shorter hospital stays, cost-effective treatment, and access to care.

In spite of these trends, the major concepts of milieu therapy remain important: consistency of care, maintenance of therapeutic environments, and open communication between client and staff. This process requires the client to participate in decision making and unit activities (Gutheil, 1985). Therapeutic environments affect clients' thinking processes and behaviors, social interactions between staff and clients, the impact of a multidisciplinary staff, and the client–staff partnership (Kahn & White, 1989).

The milieu evolves on any unit, regardless of specific interventions. It may be therapeutic, neutral, or nontherapeutic; it is shaped by the staff's practices and attitudes, human nature, and group dynamics. Milieu therapy is managed by the structure of staff–client and staff–staff interactions. It is a dynamic and continuous process that involves commitment to maintain and promote therapeutic effects within a social context (Gutheil, 1985).

DEFINITIONS

The term ***therapeutic community*** is usually used to refer to the early milieu therapy approaches developed by Maxwell Jones and others in the 1940s and 1950s. In therapeutic communities, clients were encouraged to take responsibility for their own treatment, and traditional staff roles were blurred in a democratic power structure. The therapeutic community gave a new high value to the client's interaction with his or her environment. It also gave new decision-making and recommendation authority to staff, such as nurses, who worked closely with the client on a day-to-day basis (Garritson, 1988; Jones, 1953; LeCuyer, 1992).

Milieu therapy is the use of the total environment as the therapeutic agent (Greene, 1989). It is the use of people, resources, and events in the client's immediate environment to promote the client's optimal functioning, interpersonal growth, and adaptation to life outside the hospital (Garritson, 1988).

The term ***therapeutic milieu*** means "healing environment," and it is probably a more correct term than *milieu therapy* for describing the degree to which most treatment units apply the traditional principles of milieu therapy in the unit structure. The terms *therapeutic milieu* and *milieu therapy* are sometimes used interchangeably, though.

HISTORICAL ASPECTS OF MILIEU THERAPY

Throughout history, the care of the mentally ill has been influenced by societal, legislative, and economical factors (see Table 24–1). Early treatment was based on fear and consisted of confinement. Pinel and others revolutionized the treatment of people suffering from serious mental disorders, however. Their endeavors increased the public's awareness of maltreatment of the mentally ill and laid the foundation for moral treatment.

MORAL TREATMENT

Social awareness led to a movement to provide humane environments for mentally ill persons. Sentiment about the mentally ill evolved from the perception that they were dangerous animals to the perception of them as unfortunate human beings. Major advances in the care of the mentally ill accompanied the more progressive attitudes of the 1800s; the new model of care was called *moral treatment*. Turke, an English Quaker, founded the York Retreat, where he practiced moral therapy. His endeavors stemmed from concern for the deplorable conditions and treatment of the mentally ill. Moral therapy stressed the importance of physical and social environments as healing influences. Good nutrition, clean clothing, pleasant surroundings, kind treatment, and activity constituted early attempts to provide a healing environment (Garritson, 1988; LeCuyer, 1992). (See Chapter 1 for the history of psychiatric–mental health nursing.)

Some of the momentum of moral treatment was lost during the latter part of the nineteenth and early twentieth centuries. Socioeconomic and legislative concerns contributed to overcrowding and understaffing; growing interest in intrapsychic therapy took the focus off the treatment environment. These changes left many clients untreated or hopelessly institutionalized and regressed (LeCuyer, 1992; Tuck & Keels, 1992).

THERAPEUTIC COMMUNITIES

Some major developments in milieu therapy occurred just after the end of World War II. Pioneers like Maxwell Jones and others revolutionized treatment by intro-

TABLE 24–1
Events in the Development of Milieu Therapy

1. Moral treatment
2. World War II
3. "Therapeutic community" approach
4. "Short-stay hospitalization" approach

ducing the concept of the treatment setting as a therapeutic community. In this modality, staff worked *with* clients rather than working *on* them; activities and environments were distinguished as being either *therapeutic* or *nontherapeutic*. The treatment team attempted to eliminate nontherapeutic aspects of the treatment environment and enhance the therapeutic aspects. The structure of the unit was a basic part of treatment; the client was seen as an agent of change. Democratic participation of clients and all levels of staff in the decision-making process was expected and valued (LeCuyer, 1992; Tuck & Keels, 1992).

The idea of a therapeutic environment generated enthusiasm among mental health professionals. Early efforts centered on manipulating the milieu to achieve optimal levels of function among various populations of mentally ill clients. The concept of client participation in decision making and community meetings and client responsibility for unit activities is still relevant to today's treatment approaches.

IMPACT OF SOCIAL AND ECONOMIC CHANGES ON PSYCHIATRIC TREATMENT

Social, economic, and legislative changes continue to affect the health care delivery system. Recent changes stress the need for shorter hospital stay, community-based treatment, and access to adequate health care. Legislative issues focus on providing the least restrictive treatment and the right to treatment. Current demands on an already failing health care system are enormous. Mental health professionals are challenged to balance clients' enormous needs against limited funds and cost containment.

The evolution of milieu therapy has paralleled these changes. Today, milieu therapy is a viable modality for clients in both inpatient and community settings. The role of the psychiatric nurse has evolved with the changes within society. The nurse plays a major role on the interdisciplinary team that facilitates restorative rehabilitation of the acute or chronically mentally ill client.

COMPARISON OF TRADITIONAL AND SHORT-STAY TREATMENT GOALS

Contemporary units, with their acutely ill clients and short stays, still need to provide a therapeutic environment. Otherwise, antitherapeutic dynamics develop, staff stress escalates, and the milieu cannot support adaptation and wellness.

LeCuyer (1992) listed the three traditional treatment goals of milieu therapy as (1) resocialization, (2) ego development, and (3) prevention of regression. These goals were relevant and achievable in long-term treatment facilities. However, current treatment centers on providing quality care in a shorter hospital stay. Psychiatric nurses are challenged to develop more realistic goals that promote stabilization of acute conditions and minimize relapse. Specific nursing interventions include (1) promoting psychological growth, (2) facilitating adaptive coping behaviors, and (3) helping clients adjust to a chronic disorder (LeCuyer, 1992).

CONCEPTS AND PRINCIPLES OF MILIEU THERAPY

Five key variables in the planning and management of a milieu therapy program were described by Gunderson in 1978, and they continue to be quoted in the literature on contemporary applications. These variables are containment, support, validation, structure, and involvement. Other variables that have been added are negotiation, interaction, open communication, physical environment, and links with community and family (Gunderson, 1978; LeCuyer, 1992; Tuck & Keels, 1992).

CONTAINMENT

Containment deals with the safety, food, shelter, and medical care issues of a unit. It includes locked doors, seclusion, and restraints when necessary for clients to feel assured that their illness will not harm them, the hospital, or the staff (LeCuyer, 1992).

SUPPORT

Support includes the usual interventions that this term brings to mind: encouragement, attention, reassurance, praise, education, direction, and other techniques to enhance self-esteem and self-worth. A word of caution is warranted, however: If used indiscriminately, support can lead to regression and a sense of inadequacy, dependence, and inability to cope alone (LeCuyer, 1992).

VALIDATION

Validation is the affirmation of the client's individuality and is closely linked to respect, tolerance, and maintenance of dignity. Validating the client's individuality requires skill and sensitivity. The nurse provides validation through interventions such as allowing alone time, engaging in one-to-one interactions with the client, and viewing symptoms as meaningful communication (LeCuyer, 1992).

STRUCTURE

Structure includes written guidelines or expectations for conduct, a schedule of activities and therapies, the process for orienting new clients, and contingency plans for noncompliance with unit routines and expectations (Kahn & White, 1989). Structure also refers to all the mechanisms for providing staff–client, client–client, and staff–staff interactions, including formal therapies, community meetings, staff meetings, and treatment planning processes. The timing and frequency of interventions within the constraints of the client's length of stay and adaptation of the program to the client's developmental needs are also important aspects of structure (LeCuyer, 1992).

INVOLVEMENT

Involvement covers many issues in milieu therapy, beginning with the basic concept of the client's responsibility to participate actively in treatment, treatment planning, and decision making. Involvement is divided into levels and stages based on phases of illness and the capabilities of clients as they move through a program and adjust to their roles at their own rates (Kahn & White, 1989; Yurkovich, 1989). Clients' involvement in the community group through shared activities and group therapies, as opposed to individual treatment in isolation from others, is characteristic of milieu therapy. Teaching clients the skills of negotiation reinforces the need for them to participate actively in and be responsible for their care, rather than passively accepting care.

OPEN COMMUNICATION

Open communication within a therapeutic milieu requires some education for both staff and clients. Confidentiality is unit based: clients share information about each other to a greater degree than is done in other treatment settings. Both clients and staff must still respect client confidentiality, confining the shared information to the unit, to establish a safe place for therapy to occur (LeCuyer, 1992). Respect for privacy is not in conflict with therapeutic openness—some information can be restricted to sharing on a need-to-know basis. The point is that team members and clients need to understand the importance and value of open and honest sharing of information among each other, so that no one keeps secrets, withholds relevant treatment information, or plays people against each other. In a therapeutic milieu, openness to feedback is valued by the staff and clients as a means of making desired changes and striving toward maximum growth and effectiveness.

FAMILY AND COMMUNITY TIES

Family and community ties are important aspects of milieu therapy. Building, improving, or maintaining the client's links with his or her family and the community is encouraged. Every reasonable opportunity is used to reinforce the client's sense of responsibility and to improve his or her ability to cope and function outside the treatment setting. Inpatient or partial hospitalization is only part of treating the mentally ill. As the client moves back into the community, family involvement and support become critical aspects of health maintenance. Family involvement is a compassionate way to help the client and family deal with the crisis of acute illness and treatment. It also has an impact on the long-term outcome of therapy and the return to the community. Shorter hospital stays make it more vital than ever to have a treatment-continuum perspective and strong transitional links in the form of continuing outpatient and follow-up care.

PHYSICAL ENVIRONMENT

A patient's physical environment in and of itself can be therapeutic. The therapeutic environment supplements medication administration and psychotherapy by strengthening the patient's self-dignity and self-esteem, encouraging interaction with others, and promoting independent problem solving.

The Joint Commission on Accreditation of Healthcare Organizations (JCAHO, 1991) has established standards that promote cleanliness, safety, and comfort while enhancing the patient's social interactions with staff and other clients. These standards are based on client, staff, and institutional needs that are measured by clinical outcomes. Some of these standards involve personal items such as clean, well-fitting, and appropriate clothing, whereas others involve activities, such as those for self-care.

Regarding the therapeutic environment, the JCAHO recommendations include accessibility to certain areas and their characteristics. A sample list follows:

- Bathrooms
- Drinking water fountains or taps
- Facilities for handicapped clients and visitors
- Adequate living space
- Visiting or waiting rooms
- Facilities for partial hospitalization
- Private areas for telephone conversations
- Adequate furnishings and lighting
- Adequate ventilation
- Private, clean living accommodations
- Area for private personal hygiene and grooming
- Locked storage areas for personal items
- Laundry facilities
- A place for age-appropriate recreational activities

LIFE SPAN ISSUES AND SPECIAL POPULATIONS IN THE MILIEU

Developmental issues across the life span and the issues of special diagnostic populations must be considered by the nurse planning the day-to-day management of a therapeutic milieu. Recent literature discusses how the traditional milieu therapy approach may be adapted to treat children, adolescents, older populations, clients with schizophrenia, and clients with chemical addictions (Gold et al, 1992; Irwin et al, 1992; Kahn & White, 1989). Table 24–2 summarizes the methods.

TABLE 24–2

Milieu Elements and Interventions Across the Life Span

DEVELOPMENTAL SPAN	CONTAINMENT	SUPPORT	VALIDATION	STRUCTURE	INVOLVEMENT	OPEN COMMUNICATION	FAMILY AND COMMUNITY	PHYSICAL ENVIRONMENT
Childhood	Close supervision Time out Seclusion	Give attention Reassure Direct Redirect Praise Touch* Hug*	Be tolerant Show respect Affirm individuality Engage in 1-on-1 interaction Recognize that behavior has meaning	Schedule activities in short time periods	Allow choices Teach problem solving	Teach client to name feelings Encourage verbal expression of feelings Develop trust	Avoid abrupt separations	Age-sized furniture Client rooms easily observed Pleasant sensory stimulation
Adolescence	Flexible supervision Quiet time Seclusion Suicide alert	Give attention Reassure Encourage Educate Praise	Allow autonomy, alone time Show respect Engage in 1-on-1 interaction	Schedule activities and free time	Expect active participation in treatment Teach decision making	Avoid secrets Discourage manipulation Encourage verbal sharing with peers	Maintain strong school–unit collaboration	Group activity areas Quiet areas Music areas
Adulthood	Flexible supervision Quiet time Medication	Reassure Encourage Educate Praise Give feedback	Know that symptoms have meaning Show respect Alone time	Schedule activites and free time	Expect participation in treatment planning	Explain that confidentiality is unit based Encourage appropriate self-disclosure	Assist client with return to work	Group activity areas Quiet areas Attractive furniture
Older adulthood	Close supervision Suicide alert Medical care	Give attention Reassure Encourage Give direction Provide comfort measures	Maintain dignity Affirm individuality Show respect	Schedule activity with rest periods	Encourage social activity	Encourage client to share memories Encourage client to acknowledge loss and need to adapt	Assist with placement/home care decisions	Safe-mobility aides Many orientation cues

*Only with client's consent.

CHILDHOOD

Children who are treated in a variety of settings for a wide range of symptoms and diagnoses present with some common needs and deficits. An obvious one is the need for age-related safety and supervision. These requirements differ from adult needs on the basis of children's lack of judgment, immature cognitive development, impulsivity, and short attention span.

Irwin et al. (1992) developed a milieu therapy program that focused on the primary deficit among disturbed children: the inability to form meaningful, trusting relationships with peers and adults. The program fostered the formation of discriminating attachments: children were encouraged to select and work out treatment issues with a specific staff member. Limit setting and consequences for problem behaviors were handled within the context of these special relationships. The purpose of this strategy was to avoid the message that all adults are the same (Irwin et al., 1992).

Special attention was given to discharge rituals, so that the children could acknowledge their attachments and work through separation and abandonment issues. The transition from hospital to outpatient treatment was smoothed by having the child and family maintain some contact with hospital staff; separation was not abrupt (Irwin et al., 1992).

Behavioral interventions are important in treatment milieus for children. Children's short attention span requires putting a consequence as close as possible to the behavior it is intended to modify. Peer relationships and coping skills can be improved by implementing consequences for the entire group and therapy assignments after certain kinds of acting-out behavior (Irwin et al., 1992). The following case study illustrates the use of milieu therapy for child clients. See also Nursing Care Plan 24–1.

Case Study: Clients with Aggressive Behavior Toward Peers (Bobby and Ellen)

Bobby and Ellen are on a short-stay unit in which a milieu approach is used to treat children with severe behavior problems. Each has a problem with hitting others when he or she becomes frustrated. The treatment team is interpreting this behavior to them as a problem in relating to peers ("making and keeping friends"). Hitting is a common behavior among children, so the treatment team has clarified the expected conduct in Community Meeting: that the children will learn to express feelings with appropriate words, not hitting.

As the group left the unit classroom this morning, Bobby and Ellen each started pushing and hitting children next to them in line. Other children in the group also began yelling and pushing each other. The staff immediately implemented the preplanned group consequences and therapy activities for this type of behavior, with spontaneous adaptations to fit the situation. Interventions from the group plan can be incorporated into individual nursing care plans or master treatment plans where applicable. Written as a nursing care plan for the group, the strategy for consequences and activities is outlined in Nursing Care Plan 24–1.

Assessment. Aggressive behavior of individual clients creates a high risk for violence to others among the group as a whole.

ADOLESCENCE

Healthy adolescents normally share some of the needs of younger children across the developmental continuum; adolescents in treatment may have additional special problems with advanced or delayed development. Safety and supervision continue to be issues, and the possibility of sexual acting out increases.

School issues are an important aspect of treatment for all school-age groups. Both behavioral problems and educational needs must be addressed. Neuropsychological and psychoeducational testing are technological and theoretical advances in the school–hospital partnership. Structure varies with setting and local education systems, but a close collaboration between the classroom and the unit is vital in milieu therapy.

Traditionally, adolescents were hospitalized for as long as 2 or 3 years to deal with a perceived age-related resistance to change and trust. Future program evaluation will show the efficacy of the current practice of short-term hospitalization. Meanwhile, clinicians such as Gold et al. (1992) have concluded that short-stay treatment can be effective if the milieu focuses less on uncovering psychosocial issues than on developing effective coping methods and adaptation. A milieu-oriented adolescent treatment program can be adapted to the social and economic pressures of managed care and short-stay hospitalization. Such programs maintain family treatment, a multidisciplinary team, and a behavior-based milieu. The success of a short-stay program depends on the client's effective transition to outpatient treatment (Gold et al., 1992).

Developmentally, adolescents are sensitive to issues of autonomy, peer pressure, privileges, and responsibility. The treatment milieu often deals with these issues through a behavioral reinforcement and privilege system that ties progress to specific treatment goals (Gold et al., 1992).

OLDER ADULTHOOD

Suicide risk, cognitive and sensory deficits, physical changes, and health problems must be addressed in the therapeutic environment for the elderly. Behaviors such as wandering, severe withdrawal, agitation, verbal abusiveness, and aggressiveness can be manifestations of neurological or psychiatric disorders (Cassetta, 1993; Mellick et al., 1992). Clear communication may be difficult because of hearing, visual, and memory problems; nonverbal aspects of communication, including touch, need to be used purposefully to enhance communication and support.

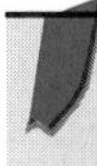

Nursing Care Plan 24–1 Application of Milieu Therapy to Children with Aggressive Behavior Toward Peers (Bobby and Ellen)

► **Nursing Diagnosis:** Ineffective Individual Coping related to inadequate skills for handling emotional discomfort.

OUTCOME IDENTIFICATION	NURSING ACTIONS	RATIONALES	EVALUATION
1. By [date], Bobby and Ellen will each process the event with a selected staff member and then with the community.	1a. Allow Bobby and Ellen to select their own staff member with whom to discuss their responses on the problem-solving tool.	1a. Selecting a staff member allows children to work through an issue within the context of a meaningful relationship. A written tool reinforces learning of the problem-solving process and impulse control.	*Goals met:* 1a. Bobby and Ellen each select a staff member and complete a written problem-solving tool.
	1b. Encourage Bobby and Ellen to process their tools together with staff supervision.	1b. Processing with a roommate is a manageable small step toward group processing and is also within the context of an established relationship.	1b. Bobby and Ellen read or discuss their own responses and listen to the responses of one other child.
	1c. Call a special community meeting and process the event as a group.	1c. Group processing helps build group cohesion and enhances clients' communication skills.	1c. Bobby and Ellen discuss what led to the event, how they felt, and what they did.
	1d. Return to regular schedule if most of the group is able to identify more appropriate coping responses.	1d. Expecting all the children in a group to reach this objective would be unrealistic; only a majority is needed for positive peer pressure.	1d. More than half of the children in the group verbally participate in sharing ideas about more appropriate behavior in such situations.

► **Nursing Diagnosis:** High Risk for Violence directed at others, related to aggressive acting out of feelings.

OUTCOME IDENTIFICATION	NURSING ACTIONS	RATIONALES	EVALUATION
1. By [date], Bobby and Ellen will each identify their feelings, the behavior they used, the consequences of the behavior, and more adaptive behavior alternatives for the situation.	1a. Bobby and Ellen use the problem-solving tool to write their feelings before, during, and after the event.	1a. The written tool structures and reinforces problem solving.	*Goals met:* 1a. Bobby and Ellen make an attempt to respond to all three areas, with staff prompting as needed.
	1b. Bobby and Ellen use the problem-solving tool to describe their behavior.	1b. Describing their own behavior helps children identify choices and consequences.	1b. Bobby and Ellen identify their own behavior versus blaming others.
	1c. Bobby and Ellen use the problem-solving tool to list alternative behaviors, including words.	1c. Listing alternative behaviors introduces children to new coping behaviors.	1c. Bobby and Ellen name at least one more adaptive behavior or choice of words.
	1d. Bobby and Ellen use the problem-solving tool to list the possible consequences of each behavior.	1d. Children are encouraged to consider how to elicit more positive consequences.	1d. Bobby and Ellen note how the behavior of others or consequences might be more positive, including their feelings about themselves.

In addition to the usual attention to the physical environment in terms of creating a pleasant atmosphere, a geropsychiatric unit has special safety considerations. Uncluttered, wide, well-marked passageways that are provided with support devices and resting places are needed within rooms and along corridors to accommodate weaker, slower, less agile clients. Boundaries to rooms and special areas need to be distinctly marked; for example, color changes assist orientation for the visually and cognitively impaired.

Pharmacological interventions, when used judiciously and after consideration of age-related physiological changes, can help geriatric clients cope with end-of-life issues with clearer thoughts and improved mood. This will enable them to have more satisfying social involvement with staff, family, and peers.

The interdisciplinary team approach and consistency in interventions can be effective for the elderly. The environment must be rich in orientation cues for cognitive challenges. Social involvement can be facilitated by providing structured interactions such as reminiscence groups or group leisure activities or comfortable group living areas where spontaneous socialization can occur.

Linkages with community resources are important for the elderly. A psychiatric hospitalization may or may not mark a point of change in living arrangements: effective discharge preparation requires that the treatment team, including the client and family, have mutual goals. The client and family may need to be educated about available community resources.

The following case study illustrates the use of milieu therapy with an elderly client. See also Nursing Care Plan 24–2.

Case Study: The Client with Adaptation Problems in the Aging Process (Mrs. Adams)

Mrs. Adams just had her 73rd birthday. Her children arranged her admission to a milieu-oriented geropsychiatric unit when they became alarmed because their usually cheerful, active Mom was sitting around crying for hours in her closed-up, unkept house. She was widowed 8 years ago, after a stable marriage of 35 years. She has comfortable relationships with her three married children, but she says she does not want to be a "burden" to them. She lives alone in the neighborhood where she has lived for more than 20 years. Mrs. Adams is a pleasant woman who used to have many women friends with whom she shared the experiences of raising children, seeing a husband through retirement, and puttering in her flower garden. She says, "I never was one to join a lot of clubs and such, or even go to church much after the kids lost interest in Sunday school. I was plenty busy taking care of my home and family."

Most of her friends have left the neighborhood; three of them died in the past 2 years, and last month the last of the group went to a nursing home. Mrs. Adams has not been able to shake off her gloomy feelings; even the flower garden doesn't cheer her up the way it used to, and the kitchen floor gets harder to mop every week.

Assessment. Client is experiencing multiple, cumulative losses and changes of aging; she is not using social support resources available to her.

THE CLIENT WITH SCHIZOPHRENIA

A unit for clients with schizophrenia can tailor milieu therapy principles to fit the current understanding of the biological and psychosocial aspects of schizophrenia. Assessment of the developmental needs of the client with schizophrenia requires thorough knowledge of the disorder: social and psychological development may not match chronological age in some areas (Kahn & White, 1989).

An intensely supportive holding environment can be provided for these clients, in which a graduated therapy program focuses on common client needs. A holding environment for clients with schizophrenia includes safety, structure, support, socialization, and self-understanding (see Table 24–3). Negative group dynamics, such as anxiety or overt psychotic behavior, require prompt intervention. Maintenance of a safe and healthy work environment for staff is an integral aspect of the therapeutic milieu (Kahn & White, 1989). See Chapter 12 for discussion of clients with schizophrenia.

THE CLIENT WITH A CHEMICAL ADDICTION

Treatment programs for clients with a chemical addiction often include key features of milieu therapy. After reviewing the recent literature on the treatment of alcoholism, Adelman and Weiss (1989) concluded that a milieu orientation is quite valuable in this area. Some features of milieu therapy that are particularly useful with clients with an addiction are intensive multimodal treatment, a peer-group-oriented approach, client participation in treatment planning, and interdisciplinary assessment and treatment (Adelman & Weiss, 1989).

One safety and trust issue that arises on chemical addiction units is the abuse of substances on the unit or during off-unit activities such as recreational or therapeutic-pass outings. The consequences of substance abuse need to be well defined at admission and consistently enforced to maintain an effective treatment milieu. Substance abuse is proved with objective data from laboratory drug screens or breath alcohol analyzer tests.

TABLE 24–3
Five Elements of a Holding Environment

1. Safety
2. Structure
3. Support
4. Socialization
5. Self-understanding

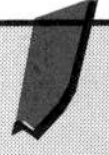

Nursing Care Plan 24–2 Application of Milieu Therapy to the Client with Adaptation Problems in the Aging Process (Mrs. Adams)

► **Nursing Diagnosis:** Grieving related to inadequate coping responses to multiple losses.

OUTCOME IDENTIFICATION	NURSING ACTIONS	RATIONALES	EVALUATION
1. By [date], Mrs. Adams and her family will gain awareness and understanding of her grief process.	1a. Provide brief family counseling.	1a. The family as well as the client needs support to deal with crisis of hospitalization and precipitating events.	*Goals met:* 1a. Mrs. Adams's family processes their concerns for her and how the decision to hospitalize was made. Possible guilt and fears about the future are addressed.
	1b. Encourage Mrs. Adams's family to participate in the unit's educational support group.	1b. Family members need education and support to understand the client's and their own responses to this life event.	1b. Mrs. Adams's family attends psychoeducational groups regularly. To identify potential problems, the nurse notes which members attend and the quality of their participation.
	1c. Encourage Mrs. Adams to participate actively in the unit's "Memories" and "Dealing with Loss" groups.	1c. Clients can process multiple losses with support.	1c. Mrs. Adams attends and participates in unit groups. She verbalizes her feelings and acknowledges others' responses.

► **Nursing Diagnosis:** Impaired Social Interaction related to resistance to forming new relationships and poor use of available resources.

OUTCOME IDENTIFICATION	NURSING ACTIONS	RATIONALES	EVALUATION
1. By [date], Mrs. Adams will demonstrate her ability to resume active social interactions.	1a. Expect Mrs. Adams to participate actively in community meetings and social activities on the unit.	1a. Clients respond to staff expectations regarding appropriate behavior in the new environment.	*Goals met:* 1a. Mrs. Adams attends activities regularly
	1b. Assess Mrs. Adams's strengths and weaknesses in social skills as you observe her interactions in the milieu.	1b. Clients demonstrate their level of functioning in the milieu.	1b. The nurse notes effective skills and identifies problem areas.
	1c. Use activity therapies to explore ways Mrs. Adams can adjust to the changes that accompany the aging process.	1c. These therapies can introduce new ways to cope with the changes of aging in a structured and supportive setting.	1c. Mrs. Adams's attempts to compensate for the changes of aging and activities she does not attempt or needs assistance with are noted.
2. By [date], Mrs. Adams and her family will develop an after-care plan for using resources that will allow Mrs. Adams to resume meaningful activity and social interactions.	2a. Teach Mrs. Adams and her family about the need for Mrs. Adams to secure new friends and meaningful socialization to help fill some of the voids left by the losses she has experienced.	2a. Client's support system has been shrinking through multiple losses without building new support. Because she now has only family to meet social needs, she feels like a burden to them.	2a. Mrs. Adams and family express awareness of her restricted social life and identify the benefits of change.

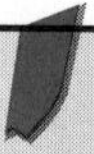

Nursing Care Plan 24–2 Application of Milieu Therapy to the Client with Adaptation Problems in the Aging Process (Mrs. Adams) (Continued)

OUTCOME IDENTIFICATION	NURSING ACTIONS	RATIONALES	EVALUATION
	2b. Include Mrs. Adams in outings to the local community seniors center.	2b. These activities educate clients about community resources in a meaningful way; they are more likely to return to a setting they have visited.	2b. Mrs. Adams identifies activities she enjoys and makes a commitment to continue them after discharge.
	2c. Educate Mrs. Adams and her family about community resources for seniors.	2c. Family members may need to expand their awareness of available resources to meet the client's social needs, so that the client can be less dependent on them.	2c. Mrs. Adams and family identify at least one other community activity for them to explore after discharge.

Clients with a chemical addiction often demonstrate some developmental deficits. Psychosocial growth may be arrested in approximately the same life span period as the substance abuse began. Coping skills can be incongruent with chronological age.

THE NURSE'S ROLE

Nurses have long had a very responsible role in the establishment, maintenance, and evaluation of the therapeutic environment of mental health facilities. Nurses are unique on the interdisciplinary team in terms of the large number of their ranks and the amount of time they spend with clients. Nurses also interact frequently and consistently with team members from every other discipline, whereas some team members only have sporadic contact with each other. Nurses have a daily, continuous, and constantly updated mechanism for communication: the shift-change report. Considering these circumstances, nurses have a vital opportunity and responsibility to be the mediator of the communication and decision-making processes that occur in the therapeutic milieu (see Table 24–4).

In addition, nurses are natural leaders in the creation and management of the therapeutic milieu. As valued members of the treatment team, nurses collaborate with the client, the other members of the team, and consultants to create and manage a therapeutic environment. Power, control, and authority issues within the milieu need to be handled within the team in the same respectful and professional manner in which they are handled with clients (Tuck & Keels, 1992).

TABLE 24–4
The Nursing Role in the Milieu

1. Create and manage the therapeutic environment.
2. Balance the needs of the group versus those of the individual client.
3. Support the dignity of all clients.
4. Assess the impact of the client on the milieu.
5. Assess the impact of the milieu on the client.
6. Monitor the impact of the staff's behavior on the milieu.
7. Collaborate in treatment decisions.
8. Mediate team communication.

Responsible decision making in milieu management requires that the nurse be knowledgeable of the concepts of milieu therapy and group process and the principles and techniques of interpersonal relationships (Tuck & Keels, 1992). Disciplines within the milieu treatment team cannot act in isolation from each other and still maintain effectiveness. Effective and exemplary communication is a vital foundation and serves as a learning model for clients. Team interaction and communication processes are extremely visible in the therapeutic milieu, and clients will model what is practiced long before or after they follow what is said.

Openness to feedback is required of both clients and staff if a milieu is to be managed effectively. To prevent or resolve staff conflicts that could disrupt the milieu, the nurse needs to be willing and able to practice self-awareness and critical self-assessment in a confident, nondefensive manner. The astute objectivity of a mentor or clinical supervision can be beneficial in this process (Tuck & Keels, 1992).

GENERALIST AND ADVANCED-PRACTICE ROLES

The nursing role described herein is primarily that of the generalist nurse. Additional responsibilities include being knowledgeable about the impact of the milieu on self-care activities and nursing actions and collaborating with the client, family, and other health care providers to optimize resources and facilitate growth (American

Nurses Association [ANA], 1994). The advanced-practice nurse's role in milieu therapy has all the responsibilities of the generalist and also staff development responsibilities such as education and clinical supervision. The advanced practitioner also provides consultation and psychotherapy, has prescriptive authority, participates in program planning, and develops research projects (ANA, 1994).

THE NURSING PROCESS

In the therapeutic milieu, nursing assessment, diagnosis, planning, intervention, and evaluation must reflect recognition of the collective needs of a group of clients and, simultaneously, consideration of the individual needs of a single client. Insight and competence are required to weigh individual needs against collective needs. The milieu therapy approach offers the flexibility and mechanisms for conflict resolution that the nurse needs to make therapeutic clinical judgments that best serve both the client and milieu (Tuck & Keels, 1992).

RESEARCH ON MILIEU THERAPY

The developmental process of a treatment unit begins with the philosophies and past experiences of the planners; a period of adjustments follows, based largely on trial and error. Features of milieu therapy are included in most units because multidisciplinary treatment teams consistently value the contribution of a therapeutic environment.

Research on milieu therapy has focused primarily on various applications rather than on client outcome. A milieu therapy program consists of many variables, making it difficult to study as a whole. However, researchers from numerous disciplines and theoretical frameworks have found the milieu-oriented unit to be a research-friendly setting. This is due in part to the consistency of goals and the methodical, thoughtful approaches to care that are used in an effective milieu (Kahn & White, 1989).

Two of the most frequently mentioned tools for research and program evaluation related to milieu therapy are Moos's Ward Atmosphere Scale and his Community-Oriented Program Environment scale (see the accompanying Research Abstract displays). These tools

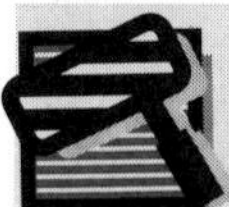

RESEARCH ABSTRACT

Planning and Evaluating Innovations in Nursing Practice by Measuring the Ward Atmosphere

Milne, D. L. (1986). *Journal of Advanced Nursing, 11*, 203–210.

Milne used the Ward Atmosphere Scale (WAS) to evaluate the effectiveness of some innovations in nursing practice that one unit implemented. In a baseline assessment, nurses and clients expressed an unfavorable view of the unit as providing little support and poor client involvement. After some planned program changes and staff training, results evaluated by the WAS indicated that both staff and clients saw the changes as improvements in the unit milieu.

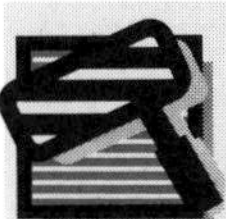

RESEARCH ABSTRACT

A Systematic Comparison of Feedback and Staff Discussion in Changing the Ward Atmosphere

James, I., Milne, D. L., & Firth, H. (1990). *Journal of Advanced Nursing, 15*, 329–336.

James et al. examined the use of feedback and discussion to improve a unit's therapeutic atmosphere. Using the Ward Atmosphere Scale, the staff indicated how the climate of the unit differed from the ideal climate they wanted. James et al. found that staff who both participated in discussion of the findings and received written feedback about the results were more likely to make positive changes in the unit milieu than were staff who only received written feedback and were not invited to discuss the findings.

RESEARCH ABSTRACT

Factors Related to Integrating Persons with Chronic Mental Illness into a Peer Social Milieu

Levin, S., & Brekke, J. S. (1993). *Community Mental Health Journal, 29*, 25–34.

In this recent study, Levin and Brekke considered how to predict how involved clients would become in a social network with peers on a treatment unit. The Community-Oriented Program Environment Scale was used as the assessment tool. Clients' perception of staff support and communication of clear expectations—two important elements of milieu therapy—were found to be better predictors of active social involvement than were clients' diagnosis and former social functioning ability. These results seem to validate the power of a therapeutic milieu to foster positive coping and behavior change.

measure staff and client perceptions of the elements of a milieu therapy program. Their 10 subscales are entitled Involvement, Support, Spontaneity, Autonomy, Practical Orientation, Personal Problem Orientation, Anger and Aggression, Order and Organization, Program Clarity, and Staff Control (Moos, 1974).

►CHAPTER SUMMARY

Milieu therapy refers to the social environment of treatment and may be defined as psychosocial rehabilitation. It encompasses the effective use of staff, activities, and resources to facilitate clients' highest level of function. Clients' participation in decision making and in self-care activities and maintenance of a therapeutic environment are emphasized.

Milieu therapy, or therapeutic community, has played a significant role in the treatment of serious mental disorders since the 1950s. Major concepts of milieu therapy, such as consistency of care, maintenance of therapeutic environments, and open communication between client and staff, remain important in current treatment settings. A milieu evolves on any unit with or without planning: it may be therapeutic, neutral, or nontherapeutic, depending on the staff's practices and attitudes.

Nurses have been natural leaders in the creation and management of therapeutic milieus in mental health facilities. Responsible decision making in milieu management requires knowledge of milieu therapy concepts, group process, and principles of interpersonal relationships. Balancing the collective needs of the group against the needs of a single client is a special aspect of nursing practice in the therapeutic milieu.

Adaptations of the milieu therapy approach are applicable across the life span and for all diagnostic populations. Because of the consistency of goals and the methodical, thoughtful approaches to care seen in effective milieu therapy, this form of therapy is research-friendly.

Suggestions for Clinical Conference

1. Observe clients' interactions in a community meeting and describe the behavior of clients in the early, middle, and late phases of hospitalization.
2. Ask a client to describe how other clients in the program have helped his or her treatment process.
3. Give examples that you have observed in the clinical setting of nursing staff using the following interventions:
   a. Setting limits
   b. Giving support for risk taking
   c. Coaching clients in practicing new behaviors
4. Using the steps of the nursing process, identify an actual or potential problem in the unit milieu and discuss effective problem solving for that issue with the interdisciplinary treatment team.
5. Discuss how a research tool such as the Ward Atmosphere Scale might be used in the clinical setting where you are rotating.

References

Adelman, S. A., & Weiss, R. D. (1989). What is therapeutic about inpatient alcoholism treatment? *Hospital and Community Psychiatry, 40*, 515–519.

Almond, R. (1974). *The healing community*. New York: Jason Aronson.

American Nurses Association. (1994). *A statement on psychiatric–mental health clinical nursing practice and standards of psychiatric–mental health clinical practice*. Washington, DC: American Nurses Publishing.

Bell, M. D., & Ryan, E. R. (1985). Where can therapeutic community ideals be realized? An examination of three treatment environments. *Hospital and Community Psychiatry, 36*, 1286–1291.

Cassetta, R. A. (1993, February). Playing a key role in the "Decade of the Brain." *The American Nurse*, p. 1.

Emrich, K. (1989). Helping or hurting? Interacting in the psychiatric milieu. *Journal of Psychosocial Nursing and Mental Health Services, 27*(12), 27–29.

Gabbard, G. O. (1988). A contemporary perspective on psychoanalytically informed hospital treatment. *Hospital and Community Psychiatry, 39*, 1291–1294.

Garritson, S. H. (1988). Milieu therapy. In H. S. Wilson & C. R. Kneisl (Eds.), *Psychiatric nursing* (3rd ed., pp. 829–849). Menlo Park, CA: Addison-Wesley.

Gold, I. M., Heller, C., & Ritorto, B. (1992). A short-term psychiatric inpatient program for adolescents. *Hospital and Community Psychiatry, 43*, 58–61.

Greene, J. A. (1989). Milieu therapy. In B. S. Johnson (Ed.), *Adaptation and growth: Psychiatric–mental health nursing* (2nd ed., pp. 171–182). Philadelphia: J. B. Lippincott.

Gunderson, J. (1978). Defining the therapeutic processes in psychiatric milieus. *Psychiatry, 41*, 327–335.

Gutheil, T. G. (1985). The therapeutic milieu: Changing themes and theories. *Hospital and Community Psychiatry, 36*, 1279–1285.

Irwin, M., Kline, P. M., & Gordon, M. (1992). Adapting milieu therapy to short-term hospitalization of children. *Child Psychiatry and Human Development, 21*, 193–201.

James, I., Milne, D. L., & Firth, H. (1990). A systematic comparison of feedback and staff discussion in changing the ward atmosphere. *Journal of Advanced Nursing, 15*, 329–336.

Joint Commission on Accreditation of Healthcare Organizations. (1991). Therapeutic environments. In *Consolidated standards manual*. Oakbrook Terrace, IL: Author.

Jones, M. (1953). *The therapeutic community*. New York: Basic Books.

Kahn, E. M., & White, E. M. (1989). Adapting milieu approaches to acute inpatient care for schizophrenic patients. *Hospital and Community Psychiatry, 40*, 609–614.

Kim, M. J., McFarland, G. K., & McLane, A. M. (Eds.). (1991). *Pocket guide to nursing diagnosis* (4th ed.). St. Louis: Mosby-Year Book.

LeCuyer, E. A. (1992). Milieu therapy for short-stay units: A transformed practice theory. *Archives of Psychiatric Nursing, 6*, 108–116.

Levin, S., & Brekke, J. S. (1993). Factors related to integrating persons with chronic mental illness into a peer social milieu. *Community Mental Health Journal, 29*(1), 25–34.

Mellick, E., Buckwalter, K. C., & Stolley, J. M. (1992). Suicide among elderly white men: Development of a profile. *Journal of Psychosocial Nursing and Mental Health Services, 30*(2), 29–34.

Moos, R. H. (1974). *Evaluating treatment environments: A social ecological approach*. New York: John Wiley & Sons.

Milne, D. L. (1986). Planning and evaluating innovations in nursing practice by measuring the ward atmosphere. *Journal of Advanced Nursing, 11*, 203–210.

Reighley, J. W. (Ed.). (1988). *Nursing care planning guides for mental health*. Baltimore: Williams & Wilkins.

Schultz, J. M., & Dark, S. L. (1986). *Manual of psychiatric nursing care plans* (2nd ed.). Boston: Little, Brown.

Tuck, I., & Keels, M. C. (1992). Milieu therapy: A review of the development of this concept and its implications for psychiatric nursing. *Issues in Mental Health Nursing, 13*(1), 51–58.

Yurkovich, E. (1989). Patient and nurse roles in the therapeutic community. *Perspectives in Psychiatric Care, 25*(3/4), 18–22.

C H A P T E R

Mental Health in the Home and Community

JANIE REHSCHUH GILKISON, M.S.N., R.N.
MELISSA BARKER NEATHERY, M.S.N., R.N.

OUTLINE

CHAPTER OBJECTIVES

Upon completion of this chapter, you will be able to:

1. Identify three types of alternative living centers.
2. Identify the roles of the nurse, consultant, clinician, and client educator in the community and home setting.
3. Identify significant historical events that affected the delivery of mental health services.
4. Identify the applications of community mental health services across the life span.

5. Develop a nursing care plan for partially hospitalized clients, clients residing in alternative living centers, homeless clients, clients receiving home health carre, and clients in community mental health centers.
6. Identify levels of intervention appropriate in a community mental health setting.

KEY TERMS

Case manager
Community mental health
Community mental health centers
Continuum of care
Deinstitutionalization
Foster care
Partial hospitalization

What is meant by *community mental health?* Originally, a person with a mental health problem received care in a familiar community atmosphere, but this system gave way to a system in which care was delivered by large bureaucracies. Because clients' needs far outweighed the means of the institutional system, however, a movement arose to return to community-based mental health care. Today, the term *community mental health services* refers to treatment that allows clients to continue functioning in their communities with as little disruption as possible. For example, clients can continue to perform duties at home while attending hospital programs during the day or can continue to attend school while living in a foster home. In contrast, inpatient psychiatric treatment curtails the client's normal functioning related to work, family, school, and hobbies.

Over the last 50 years, dramatic changes have been made in psychiatry and mental health services. Psychotropic medications have been developed and improved, and the community mental health movement has emerged, emphasizing community-based care and crisis intervention. These events have had a broad impact on the American mental health delivery system. The changes have affected the types of treatment available, the locations of delivery of care, and the numbers of clients served and have introduced a broader range of mental health professionals who provide services.

Health care consumers, health care providers, and third-party reimbursement agencies are now requiring more comprehensive mental health services, thus increasing the demands placed on community mental health systems. Community psychiatric nurses serve a wide range of people in a variety of settings. In this chapter, we discuss how community mental health is provided by partial hospitalization, home health care, alternative living centers, and community mental health centers. We explain how children, adolescents, adults, the elderly, the homeless chronically mentally ill, mentally retarded persons, persons with a chemical dependency, and others benefit from these programs. It is crucial to study how the community mental health nurse fills the roles of practitioner, administrator, consultant, and researcher in striving to meet society's increasing needs.

KEY CONCEPTS

A significant trend in community mental health is the emphasis on primary, secondary, and tertiary prevention of mental illness (Caplan, 1964). *Primary prevention* is the attempt to reduce the risk that people will develop mental illness. For example, a class lesson about the negative effects of illegal drug use may prevent some high school students from abusing chemical substances. *Secondary prevention* refers to nursing action that prevents the worsening of a mental disorder that has already manifested itself. It also reduces the duration of a disorder or illness. As an example, a nurse therapist who provides counseling to clients in bereavement helps them through the grief process more effectively so that emotional problems do not arise in the future. *Tertiary prevention* focuses on rehabilitation care that returns people to their highest degree of functioning. The problem may not be eliminated, but its effects are minimized. An example of tertiary care that prevents further disability is a nurse's teaching a young client with schizophrenia how to prepare meals and do other tasks in a group home.

Other key concepts relevant to community mental health nursing are after-care and extended care. *After-care* occurs after a hospitalization. Ideally, a client is not discharged without some plan for continued treatment. A client's after-care may include attending medication clinics, meeting weekly with a therapist, or attending a weekly support group. The goal of after-care is to help clients make the transition to a less restrictive form of treatment. *Extended care* encompasses after-care and refers to long-term treatment outside the hospital. Extended care can be provided by home health care or alternative living centers. Care is given as long as it is needed, but in the least restrictive environment possible.

HISTORY OF COMMUNITY MENTAL HEALTH

Dorothea Dix, a Boston school teacher, revolutionized mental health care in the mid-nineteenth century by eliminating inhumane treatment of the mentally ill through the improvement of state hospitals. Nearly a century later, the focus of care shifted from the institution to the community, because of the effectiveness of psychotropic medications and changing views on legislative and social issues.

The development of tranquilizers in the 1950s allowed clients to function without physical restraints and intense monitoring by institutional staff. Once stabilized on psychotropic medications, clients were more amenable to other interventions, such as education, social rehabilitation, and individual and group therapies.

Despite these advances, people realized the psychiatric hospital did not benefit clients, because although it provided custodial care, it did not provide rehabilitative care. Humanitarians and psychiatrists agreed that clients would be better off in the community and not isolated in the hospital. Concurrently, there was a public outcry about the expense of caring for institutionalized clients, and community treatment seemed to be more economical. As a result, the psychiatric hospital census decreased 60 percent by 1975.

In *Action for Mental Health,* published in 1961, the Joint Commission on Mental Illness and Health concluded that psychiatric services were not meeting the needs of the population. The Commission stressed the need for preventive services; comprehensive community-based care; improved access to mental health services for all segments of the population; increased education of mental health workers; support for research; and funding from federal, state, and local governments for the development of community mental health centers. The Community Mental Health Centers Act was amended in 1975 to broaden these services. President Jimmy Carter developed the President's Commission on Mental Health in 1977, which encouraged community-based programs; supported mental health research; recommended national mental health insurance; and provided funding for new programs for elderly, children, and minorities (Hadley, 1978). The Community Mental Health Systems Act was developed in 1980 to carry out the recommendations of the Commission, but it was repealed in 1981 as funding shifted from federal to state and local sources.

Unfortunately, **deinstitutionalization** did not go as smoothly and effectively as had been hoped. The hospitals released clients to communities that were not prepared for them. Instead of reducing mental illness, deinstitutionalization has been blamed for too-short, ineffective care leading to repeated episodes of illness. Because of deinstitutionalization, families have been pressured to care for their mentally ill relatives. Where have the mentally ill gone? It has been surmised that those who are not connected with community mental health services seek care in jails, homeless shelters, nursing homes, and private homes.

Today, community health care is supported by inadequate private and public funding that requires innovative treatment approaches to meet the enormous needs of psychiatric clients. Inadequate government funding further limits the extent to which the needs of the chronically mentally ill can be met. Community mental health nurses need to keep abreast of the rapidly changing policies and societal trends so that they may act effectively as client advocates in the legislative process.

PARTIAL HOSPITALIZATION

HISTORY AND DEVELOPMENT

One aspect of community-based psychiatry that has recently experienced a resurgence is **partial hospitalization,** also known as day treatment or day hospital. The resurgence of interest in partial hospitalization has been brought about by rekindled beliefs in the importance of preserving child, adolescent, and adult clients' positions in their family and community, minimizing the stigmatization of hospitalization, and lowering costs for both consumers and providers of mental health services.

Although currently in a phase of "reawakening," partial hospitalization programs have a long history and have gone through many developmental stages. The first distinct day hospital was developed in Russia and began operation in 1933. The program was described as a "day infirmary for the mentally ill" and was created to deal with a severe shortage of beds for inpatients, rather than out of any theoretical or philosophical position. It was intended to serve as a substitute for inpatient hospitalization. The history of partial hospitalization programs in the West began almost simultaneously, yet independently, in Canada and England in 1946 and 1947 (Luber, 1979). The development of these programs was fueled by the introduction of psychotropic medication, the development of group dynamics, the need for crisis intervention as a result of World War II, and the rapidly rising cost of hospital care (Goldman, 1990).

In the United States, day treatment programs were in operation as early as 1948 at the Yale University Clinic and the Menninger Clinic. Both of these programs were designed to be transitional treatment programs for clients who had been hospitalized on a full-time basis. The Yale University Clinic included an evening as well as a day hospital program (Turner, 1979). By the early 1950s, day hospital programs had been established in connection with state hospitals, state and county community mental health services, and the Veterans Administration hospital system. Between 1963 and 1972, partial hospitalization programs experienced growth in psychiatric hospitals and general hospital psychiatric services and in the construction of community mental health centers. This growth came about after the Mental Retardation Facilities and Community Mental Health Centers Construction Act was passed in 1963, making partial hospitalization a required service in federally funded projects (Luber, 1979). Today, the settings for partial hospitalization programs have expanded to include free-standing day treatment facilities and military settings. Along with the expansion of settings, a broadening of the range of clients served in partial hospitalization programs has occurred. Clients with acute illness or an acute exacerbation of a chronic illness are now considered appropriate for these programs. It must be noted, however, that clients must be mentally stable enough to participate in a program setting that does not provide 24-hour care. Many believe that two different and distinct programs are necessary to provide for acute and chronic clients. These programs can be differentiated as *active versus supportive treatment* or *day hospital versus day care programs* (Luber, 1979). Before the client populations appropriate for this level of treatment and the types of program designs possible can be discussed, it is important to understand the definitions of the different terms used.

DEFINITIONS

Block and Lefkovitz (1991) defined partial hospitalization as a "time-limited, ambulatory, active treatment program that offers therapeutically intensive, coordinated, and structured clinical services within a stable therapeutic milieu" (p. 1).

In 1988, the National Association of Private Psychiatric Hospitals and American Association of Partial Hospitalization stated,

> *Partial hospitalization is a method of treatment for some mentally ill persons of all ages. It is an ambulatory treatment approach that includes the major diagnostic, medical, psychiatric, psychosocial, and prevocational treatment modalities found in a comprehensive hospital program, yet it does not require 24 hour participation. It is designed for persons with serious mental disorders who require coordinated, intensive, comprehensive, and multidisciplinary treatment not provided in an outpatient clinic setting. By offering a medically supervised alternative, such programs provide a flexible alternative for those patients who need more than outpatient care, but less intense intervention than full 24 hour hospitalization.* (pp. 89–90)

The two organizations went on to say,

> *Partial hospitalization means an outpatient program specially designed for the diagnosis or active treatment of a serious mental disorder when there is a reasonable expectation for improvement or when it is necessary to maintain a patient's functional level and prevent relapse or full hospitalization.* (pp. 89–90)

PURPOSE

As the concept of partial hospitalization has developed, five major functions of this treatment modality have emerged:

1. An alternative to inpatient treatment
2. Transitional treatment
3. Rehabilitation
4. Maintenance of long-term clients
5. An alternative to or extension of outpatient treatment

An Alternative to Inpatient Treatment. When used as an alternative to inpatient treatment, partial hospitalization is geared to those clients who are so ill that if the partial hospitalization program were not available they would definitely need inpatient care. Although the clients using these programs have a wide range of diagnoses, the greatest treatment success occurs with depressive, psychosomatic, personality, and schizophrenic disorders.

Transitional Treatment. When used as a transitional treatment, partial hospitalization serves as a transition for clients who have been hospitalized in an inpatient setting and are not yet ready to be maintained in traditional outpatient care. The clients who benefit from a transitional level of treatment are those whose symptoms would be exaggerated by anxiety over impending discharge from an inpatient setting. Programs of this nature help clients reintegrate into the community and shorten inpatient lengths of stay. Clients with depressive and personality disorders most often use transitional treatment.

Rehabilitation. Partial hospitalization is used as a rehabilitation program primarily for clients with chronic mental disorders, most often schizophrenia. Resocialization and vocational training and placement are the main focuses of treatment level.

Maintenance of Long-Term Clients. Clients with chronic mental disorders may also be offered partial hospitalization as a means of maintenance. Treatment emphasizes activities and intervention that aid in relapse prevention.

An Alternative to or Extension of Outpatient Treatment. Partial hospitalization may also be used as an alternative to or extension of outpatient treatment. This level of care is used for clients who have been in outpatient treatment but, because of a relapse, need more intensive intervention than can be accomplished on an outpatient basis. Partial hospitalization is most often used to prevent a further exacerbation of symptoms that could necessitate an inpatient admission (Voineskos, 1976).

Advantages of Partial Hospitalization. The five major functions of partial hospitalization offer many advantages. Because treatment is not conducted on a 24-hours basis, it promotes the client's continued involvement in the community and in the family, allowing the client to maintain his or her social network. It enhances and encourages independence and responsibility for the self. The stigmatization of being in an inpatient facility is avoided. It is cost-effective for the consumer and the treatment providers. Finally, it is a flexible form of treatment that can be delivered during the day, in the evenings, or on weekends, again allowing the maximum level of independence and community involvement.

TYPES OF PROGRAMS

Partial hospitalization programs can be either free-standing or part of a psychiatric or general hospital. It is important that the partial hospital program associated with a hospital system be seen as a separate, identifiable entity that is part of the continuum of psychiatric services provided. It is vital that partial hospitalization programs have a tie with an inpatient program so that emergency inpatient admissions can be quickly accomplished when needed.

Partial hospitalization is based on a therapeutic milieu. It is this treatment modality that enhances client participation and fosters the socialization and group interaction skills needed to succeed in their environment outside of treatment. See Chapter 24 for a discussion of therapeutic community.

Therapies that should be offered in partial hospitalization programs include group, individual, and family therapy; patient education; psychodrama; substance abuse counseling; stress management; occupational therapy; and recreational therapy. By providing an array of therapies, partial hospitalization programs foster the development of new coping skills that clients can immediately apply to their life outside the treatment setting.

A multidisciplinary treatment approach is used in partial hospital programs. Psychiatrists, psychiatric nurses, social workers, expressive arts therapists, and recreational and occupational therapists are all important members of the treatment team. The combined efforts of the treatment team provide various types of interactions and treatment opportunities that maximize the therapeutic rewards for clients by helping them find their own particular formula for success.

As noted previously, one advantage of a partial hospital program is its flexibility. Day, evening, and weekend programming allows far-reaching participation at varied levels of intensity depending on clients' needs.

The type of partial hospitalization program used most often is the daytime program. Day treatment programs ideally offer 6 to 7 hours of scheduled treatment per day, 5 days per week. The number of hours per day can, however, be reduced to a minimum of 4 hours to serve the needs of a specialty population or if the program is being used as a "step down" from full-day treatment. Step-down options are made available to clients who have improved sufficiently to resume more active participation in their daily routines, be it attending school, going to work, or taking part in community activities. The step-down option is especially helpful in integrating treatment objectives into everyday life experiences. Evening treatment programs may be used as primary treatment programs, step-down programs, or a combination of the two. These programs should provide a minimum of 12 hours of scheduled activities a week, extending over a minimum of 3 days a week. Evening programs are specially designed for clients who are unable to be absent from work but need more intense treatment than can be provided in traditional outpatient therapy.

Like evening programming, weekend treatment is designed for clients who are able to or need to be more active with their commitments of regular daily life. The level of intensity is less than in day treatment programs, and treatment is more supportive in nature. Weekend programs should provide a minimum of 8 hours of scheduled programming over the span of the weekend.

Clients' lengths of stay and participation in any of these partial hospitalization programs depend on their condition and on the primary purpose of the program.

POPULATIONS SERVED

A unique strength of partial hospitalization is its appropriateness for a broad range of client populations and its effectiveness with an array of clinical conditions and varying degrees of pathology. Individualized treatment is combined with specialized programming for specific populations. The focus of a partial hospitalization program is based on the age and/or specialized needs of the population it is serving. Age-specific programs are designed for early childhood, preadolescence, adolescence, adulthood, and old age (see Table 25–1).

As mentioned, partial hospitalization programs can also be based on the special needs of client populations, rather than on age group. For example, programs serve clients dealing with chemical dependency, eating disorders, sexual trauma, and AIDS. Treatment program-

TABLE 25–1

Partial Hospitalization Across the Life Span

	COMMON DIAGNOSES	THERAPEUTIC MODALITIES
Early childhood (ages 2–5) Childhood (ages 6–9) Preadolescence (ages 10–12) Adolescence (ages 13–19)	Conduct disorders, chemical dependency, developmental delays, and pervasive personality disorders	Play therapy; chemical dependency education and prevention; problem solving; family living skills training; academics; individual, group, and family therapy
Adulthood (ages 18–60)	Depression, bipolar disorder, chemical dependency, anxiety disorder, personality disorder, schizophrenia	Individual, group, and family therapy; stress management; psychodrama; psychoeducation; family living skills training; men's and women's groups
Older adulthood (ages 60+)	Depression, mild to moderate dementia, adjustment disorder, paranoia	Individual, group, and family therapy; stress management; medication group; psychoeducation; community living skills training; occupational/recreational therapy; grief groups; coping with illness, disability, and loss

ming for these special client populations includes scheduled group, individual, and family therapy as well as patient education, coping skills groups, stress management, and other specific therapeutic activities based on respective needs.

THE NURSE'S ROLE

Partial hospitalization programs offer a wide range of opportunities for nursing involvement, from administrative, to clinical, to consultation/liaison services.

On an administrative level, nurses possess the organizational skills necessary to oversee the day-to-day operation of a partial hospitalization program. The nursing process is applied in a global sense to program assessment, planning, intervention, and evaluation. Nurses are adept at orchestrating all aspects of clients' care and coordinating the members of the treatment team. Nurses function as program coordinators and, with experience and graduate education, are placed in administrative roles as well. The responsibilities of the administrator role include budgeting, marketing, staff supervision, program development, program accreditation, and community involvement.

As clinicians, nurses bring to the treatment arena a well-rounded view of the client. Not only are they astute at assessing clients' psychiatric needs, but they also are able to identify and care for the clients' physical needs. Nurses act as individual and group therapists, patient educators, patient advocates, case managers, and as resources for community referrals. Nurses are valuable members of the treatment team and should be used to their maximum potential. The use of nursing diagnoses adds to the client's overall plan of treatment and suggests specific appropriate client interventions that can be provided by the entire treatment team. Evaluation of treatment goals is done on a continual basis. The educational preparation of the psychiatric nurses in partial hospitalization settings can range from an associate degree to a master's degree in psychiatric clinical nursing. The nurse needs a minimum of a master's degree to serve as the primary individual or group therapist.

The consultation/liaison role for nurses associated with partial hospitalization programs is an exciting one. The role has two distinct areas of responsibility. The first involves working with referring hospitals and/or agencies. Acting in this capacity, the nurse assesses clients for appropriateness of day treatment, liaisons with inpatient units if short-term hospitalization is needed for a day treatment client in crisis, and liaisons with agencies to coordinate and evaluate clients' follow-up care after discharge from day treatment.

The second responsibility of the consultation/liaison nurse is to provide consultation on the design, development, and startup of partial hospital programs. Nurses are excellent in this capacity because they possess a broad understanding of the requirements necessary for a viable program. Their areas of expertise include programming, staffing patterns, utilization review, case management, Joint Commission on Accreditation of Healthcare Organizations requirements, policies and procedures, budgeting, marketing, staff development, insurance and Medicaid/Medicare reimbursement, managed care contract negotiation, and community needs assessments. See Chapter 30 for more information on the role of the nurse in consultation liaison.

Partial hospitalization is an exciting area of community mental health nursing because of the diverse populations, clinical applications, and roles for nursing it involves. The growth of partial hospitalization programs will continue to occur, but along with growth will come the need for research on the application and efficacy of this modality, a need that nurses can help meet.

PSYCHIATRIC HOME HEALTH CARE

HISTORY AND DEVELOPMENT

One of the newest additions to the community psychiatry arena is psychiatric home health care. This treatment modality is a critical element in the continuum of mental health services. Psychiatric home health care began in the 1970s and has continued to gain momentum. As health care delivery costs have increased, home service has become apparent as yet another viable alternative to inpatient hospital admissions, a way to shorten inpatient stays, and a way to curb costs. Psychiatric home care was formally recognized as a reimbursable treatment alternative by the Health Care Financing Administration in 1979 (Pelletier, 1988).

DEFINITION

Psychiatric home health care is defined as services provided by mental health professionals to clients with a psychiatric diagnosis who require treatment in their home environment. Through teamwork, clients receive coordinated, comprehensive care aimed at keeping them active and functional without disrupting their familiar surroundings. The treatment team is multidisciplinary and consists of the psychiatrist, psychiatric nurses, mental health workers, social workers, and occupational and physical therapists. Psychiatric home health care can be the primary treatment modality or may be used as an adjunct to other outpatient treatment and services.

GOALS

The goals of psychiatric home health care may be divided into two categories: direct client care and community. Regarding direct client care, the goals of psychiatric home health care are to reduce the need for hospitalization or rehospitalization of clients in psychological crisis; increase clients' adjustment to the community and home; monitor medication compliance, effectiveness, and side effects; provide assistance through problem solving to families of persons with psychiatric or cognitive disorders; reinforce predischarge therapy and treatment; provide education to clients and their families regarding disease process, medication, diet, community resources, etc.; and provide in-home respite services to the clients' families (Pelletier, 1988).

Regarding the community, the goals of psychiatric home health care are to develop collaborative relationships with physicians, nurses, therapists, family members, and community agencies; provide ongoing community education; and act as a resource to the medical community, businesses, employee assistance programs, and insurance companies (Pelletier, 1988).

TYPES OF SERVICES

Psychiatric home health care is an adjunct to other services. It can be implemented for clients who are being discharged from inpatient treatment and can provide evening help to clients who attend day treatment. If psychiatric home health care is available, some clients are discharged from the hospital sooner than they would have been if it were not available. The psychiatric home health care option allows other clients to return to their own homes, rather than going to group homes or nursing homes.

The activities of psychiatric home health care include assessments and therapeutic interventions. The assessment phase begins after the referral is received. Referrals are made by physicians, therapists, hospitals, community agencies, outpatient clinics, families, or the clients themselves. Depending on the request of the referring party, assessments cover such areas as the home environment, the client's mental status and progress, the need for community referrals/resources, the level of family support, the client's compliance with prescribed treatment, and the beneficial or adverse effects of medication.

Therapeutic interventions include various types of psychotherapy, such as individual, marital, and family therapies. Also included are motivational therapies for dysfunctional depressed clients, social and coping skills training, stress management, crisis intervention, and psychiatric rehabilitation. Linking clients and their families to community support systems and psychoeducation regarding the disease processes, medications, and the signs and symptoms of adjustment and decompensation of the illness are additional therapeutic goals.

Family intervention is of the utmost importance and involves giving support by sharing the burden of care and providing family members a respite from caregiving. Periodic respite care allows families to focus on their own needs, temporarily eliminating the physical and emotional strain of caregiving.

Other services offered include meeting the client's personal care needs, providing companions to assist the client in re-entering the community, and helping the client keep follow-up appointments.

POPULATIONS SERVED

Persons with psychiatric conditions that might otherwise lead to hospitalization and persons who require follow-up care after hospital discharge are eligible for psychiatric home health care. The most frequently seen diagnoses are depression, bipolar disorder, schizophrenia, agoraphobia, anxiety disorder, and dementia. Clients of a wide range of ages can be served with this treatment modality, from children to the elderly.

Children who receive psychiatric home health care range in age from 2 to 12 years and usually have a diagnosis of attention deficit/hyperactivity disorder or pervasive personality disorder. The therapies most provided for children include family and play therapy.

The adolescent group includes clients ages 13 to 19. Bipolar disorder, depression, conduct disorder, schizophrenia, chemical dependency, and pervasive personality disorder are the diagnoses most often seen in adolescent clients receiving psychiatric home health care. Treatment for adolescents should include individual and family therapy.

Adults using psychiatric home health care range in age from 19 to 60 years and usually have a diagnosis of depression, schizoaffective disorder, or schizophrenia. Other diagnoses seen include reactive psychosis, borderline personality disorder, and posttraumatic stress disorder. The majority of adult clients suffer from a chronic psychiatric illness. Individual therapy is important for this population; family and marital therapy are also used when indicated.

Elderly clients receiving psychiatric home health care range in age from 60 years and over. Depression with psychosis and various forms of dementia are the diagnoses most often treated with psychiatric home health care. It should be noted that with this group of clients, particular attention must be paid to any medical illnesses that could be causing psychiatric illness or symptoms. Services provided for the elderly include individual therapy, family therapy, marital therapy, grief work with clients and families, ongoing physical and mental status assessments, legal assistance, meal provision, and assistance with housekeeping and home repairs. Psychiatric home health care is especially helpful with the elderly population. The following is an example of the multiple roles a psychiatric home health nurse might assume in caring for an elderly client.

Clinical Example 1

Willie was a 68-year-old single man who had both physical and mental health problems. Willie's diabetes had caused severe visual impairment. Although he was not totally blind, he had become increasingly fearful of total blindness and had begun experiencing high levels of anxiety and panic attacks. He was having difficulty maintaining his activities of daily living and could no longer make any but the simplest of decisions. Using cognitive therapy techniques and stress management skills taught by the psychiatric home health nurse, Willie was able to look more realistically at his situation. With further help from the psychiatric home health nurse, he improved his diabetes management, contacted a community agency for the blind, and was able to manage himself in his own home.

THE NURSE'S ROLE

There are many administrative and clinical opportunities for nurses in the psychiatric home health care field. A psychiatric home health program should be directed by a nurse with a master's degree in psychiatric nursing or one who has had broad experience working in an inpatient or outpatient psychiatric setting (Thobaben & Kozlak, 1990). The job responsibilities of the director include ensuring the delivery of high-quality care; marketing services to physicians, nurses, hospitals, and community agencies; developing referral bases with needed service providers; maintaining accreditation standards; budgeting, providing staff in-service education programs; and maintaining quality improvement standards.

The clinical or field nurse provides direct care to the clients and their families. This position requires extensive experience in acute inpatient settings and the ability to function independently in the field. In addition to providing therapeutic intervention, this nurse coordinates with the client's physician, interacts with the client's family, acts as the client's advocate, attends treatment team conferences, liaisons with community agencies and other referral sources, and attends discharge planning conferences. Psychiatric home health nurses must be adept at the following skills:

- Performing the mental status examination
- Assessing lethality
- Establishing the nurse–client relationship
- Managing assaultive behavior
- Observing emergency psychiatric symptoms
- Understanding pharmacology and psychopharmacology
- Assessing the client's physical status
- Forming collaborative relationships
- Implementing the nursing process
- Making nursing diagnoses

Some of the most frequently used nursing diagnoses in this treatment area are Social Isolation, Anxiety, Self-Care Deficit, Altered Thought Process, Potential for Violence, and Ineffective Individual Coping (Lesseig, 1987).

As psychiatric home health care programs continue to grow, so will the need for nursing research. Research should include studies of efficacy, cost containment, and broader use of the service.

COMMUNITY-BASED HOSPICE CARE

Death is a natural part of life and the final stage of human development. It is frequently a shared experience, depending on one's needs and dependency on others (Brescia, 1993). Most people would prefer to die from old age than from a terminal or debilitating illness. The terminally ill client often experiences feelings of anger, helplessness, pain, humiliation, guilt, and shame. Nursing care for the client and family coping with death involves promoting comfort, maintaining self-esteem, and empowering both the client and family in the necessary decisions that must be made as well as in the grief process.

The desire for independence, dignity, and control over one's care is the reason many clients prefer to remain at home during the last months of their lives. Home-based care is also a cost-effective treatment modality that enables the client and his or her family to be actively involved in decisions involving care. The nurse providing hospice care anticipates and provides the terminally ill client with continuous palliative care, rather than curative interventions (Amenta, 1985; Amenta & Bohnet, 1986). Most hospice clients are between 60 and 75 years of age (Mor & Masterson-Allen, 1987, 1990); approximately 1 percent are children (National Hospice Organization, 1988). Table 25–2 describes hospice care across the life span.

The success of hospice programs is rooted in the nurse–client relationship. This relationship enables the nurse to assess the client's and family's physical, spiritual, financial, and psychosocial needs. Included in this assessment are questions regarding the family's previous experience coping with death and the family's perception of the client's illness. The psychiatric nurse plays a key role in promoting the mental health of the family as well as of the terminally ill client.

THE NURSE'S ROLE

The generalist psychiatric nurse works with the hospice team to provide ongoing emotional support to clients and family members and to assess outcomes. Administration of psychotropic medications, crisis intervention, grief groups, and psychoeducational programs are critical components of client care. The role of the advanced-practice nurse may overlap that of the generalist as case manager, but the advanced-practice nurse may use additional interventions such as family, marital, or group psychotherapy and prescription of psychoactive agents. Additional comfort measures include administering analgesics, guiding the client in the use of image therapy, positioning, and keeping the bed linen dry and wrinkle free. The nurse may also provide additional psychosocial support by encouraging the client to express his or her feelings, by facilitating the grief process, and by providing emotional support and psychoeducation. Awareness of the client and family's cultural background and religious/belief system is necessary to facilitate the preparatory grieving and bereavement process.

In summary, home-based hospice care continues to be a primary treatment modality for clients and families faced with terminal illness. For an in-depth discussion of the issues of death and dying, see Chapter 8.

TABLE 25–2 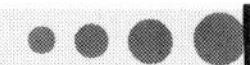

Hospice Care Issues Across the Life Span

	RESPONSE TO DEATH AND DYING	NURSING IMPLICATIONS
Childhood	Young children perceive death as separation, lacking a cognitive understanding of death. Factors that affect a child's reaction to death include ► Family Reactions ► Cultural-ethnic-religious influences ► Availability of emotional support	► Assess family and child's perception of illness (younger children may express feelings through behavior or other activities. ► Teach parents and child (age appropriate) about medications and other palliative measures. ► Assess child and family members' emotional, physical, social, and spiritual needs. ► Assess child's reaction to and perception of death. ► Encourage child and family to express the meaning of child's impending death. ► Facilitate the grief process. ► Instruct family and parents how to institute various comforting measures, such as pain medication, touching, hugging, music, and other relaxation measures. ► Encourage mobilization of social support systems.
Adolescence	Adolescents recognize that death is part of living, but they have difficulty accepting their own death.	► Encourage mobilization of support systems. ► Assess for self-destructive behaviors, such as substance abuse and suicidal behaviors. ► Encourage youth to express feelings. ► Encourage independence and self-care. ► Help youth deal with fears, anxiety, and anger. ► Encourage family to participate in grief process. ► Encourage social interactions with peers as long as possible. ► Provide comfort and relaxation measures.
Adulthood	Young adults may be struggling with leaving young children and spouse. Middle-aged adults may struggle with similar issues and concerns about body image if illness involves mutilation (e.g., mastectomy, colostomy, or prostatectomy).	► Assess client's and family's coping patterns. ► Assess past reactions to death. ► Assess understanding of impending death. ► Teach family members comfort and relaxation measures. ► Encourage self-care as long as possible. ► Encourage client to express feelings. ► Assess client's level of dangerousness, especially when depression or cognitive impairment is present.
Older Adulthood	Older adults often struggle with leaving a spouse but may be resigned to impending death, depending on age and resolution of developmental task of integrity, severity of pain, and physical disability.	► Assess coping patterns. ► Teach family members comfort and relaxation measures. ► Assess level of dangerousness, especially when depression or cognitive impairment is present.

Data from Mishne, J. M. (1986). *Clinical work with adolescents.* New York: Free Press; and Reighly, J. W. (1988). *Nursing care planning guides for mental health.* Baltimore: Williams & Wilkins.

COMMUNITY MENTAL HEALTH CENTERS

HISTORY

Community mental health centers are government-funded and -directed programs that attempt to address the needs of the mentally ill in the community. The Community Mental Health Centers Act of 1963 identified the essential and adequate mental health services of a community mental health center as outpatient services, partial hospitalization, emergency services, educational services, diagnostic services, and rehabilitative services. These services must be available and accessible to all community residents, regardless of their ability to pay. Although these guidelines have been amended over the years, health promotion, treatment, and rehabilitation continue to be the major areas of attention. The services provided by the community mental health center should reflect the needs of the community it serves. For example, some centers may have programs for Hispanic residents, clients with acquired immunodeficiency syndrome (AIDS), or pregnant teenagers.

TYPES OF SERVICES

Community mental health centers provide individual and family therapy, halfway house programs, partial hospitalization, and support groups. Halfway houses, or group homes, are discussed later in this chapter in the section on alternative living centers.

THE NURSE'S ROLE

Nurses function in a variety of capacities in the community mental health center. Some may have specific roles, such as assessing new clients (intake) or teaching sex education classes. Others have more generalized roles, such as case management, which involves following clients and families throughout treatment over a long period of time. Educating, discharge planning, and providing least restrictive care in the form of managing an alternative living center or making home visits are examples of preventive care provided by the community nurse. Nurses are valuable members of the mental health team because of their holistic approach to client care. Interdisciplinary team members such as social workers, psychiatrists, psychologists, mental health workers, and drug and alcoholism counselors collaborate to provide the most appropriate comprehensive treatment. Nurse managers and administrators collaborate to identify the needs of a community and to develop programs to meet those needs. Community needs are identified by administering consumer questionnaires and conducting interviews; holding community meetings; and studying statistics such as birth, crime, and morbidity rates (Flaskerud & van Servellen, 1985). Program development, implementation, and evaluation capitalize on nurses' creativity, ingenuity, and management skills. The following clinical example illustrates the role of two nurses in the development of an AIDS support group.

Clinical Example 2

Two nurses, one from a rural county mental health center and one from the county medical hospital, became aware of five reported cases of AIDS in their county, whereas there had been one the previous year and none the year before that. They distributed a survey and concluded from the results that the community was not aware of facts about the prevention of the spread of the disease. They developed a 2-hour program about the etiology, prevention, and treatment of AIDS based on empirical data. The presentation was given to school children and members of organizations such as the PTA, Lions Club, and church groups. They also made confidential laboratory services available for residents wishing to be tested. The CMHC nurse and a social worker held a weekly support group of AIDS patients and their families to help them deal with the fear, anxiety, guilt, and other emotions they were experiencing.

Nurse educators, consultants, and liaisons serve as the bridge between the CMHC and the community by (1) maximizing resources, (2) decreasing fragmentation of services, (3) increasing community awareness of mental health, (4) providing knowledge about primary prevention, and (5) treating mental health problems.

Schools, businesses, and organizations frequently enlist nurse consultants to help them cope with issues such as identifying suicide risk in teenagers, developing stop-smoking programs, or dealing with holiday stress. These interactions, in turn, provide information and recommendations that make the community mental health center services more applicable and accessible to the community. Nurse researchers are invaluable in studying community mental health trends and treatment effectiveness. Their research can change treatment strategies, validate the effectiveness of treatments, increase the community mental health center staff's understanding of the populations they serve, and assist the staff in procuring federal funding for primary prevention programs. The funding available for community mental health clinics is influenced by legislative and social factors. Nurses can influence the legislative process by actively participating in professional organizations and activities, becoming informed voters, and endorsing candidates' views on mental health issues. In addition, attendence at town meetings and active participation on community boards increase the public's understanding of mental illness and promote client advocacy.

Case Management

Case managers are community mental health center employees who develop long-term relationships with community mental health center clients. Case manager responsibilities include facilitating the client's access to services, protecting the client's legal rights, and counseling. The case manager thus helps the client live as independently as possible, by maintaining the client's psychosocial functioning and preventing regression or relapse (Gerhart, 1990). Nurse case managers apply the nursing process in the following ways:

1. They assess the client through intake calls; emergency assessments; individual and family interviews; and health and treatment histories, physical examinations, and laboratory services.
2. They diagnose through interpreting and prioritizing client's needs.
3. They plan for needed services, identifying client goals, collaborate with agencies and/or the CMHC team, and develop a nursing care plan.
4. They implement the care plan by mediating and coordinating access to other services, monitoring medications, providing therapy and/or education, advocating for the client, and involving the client's family in the treatment program.
5. They evaluate the client's status with regard to previous goals and outcomes; administer pretests and posttests; identify the client's current level of functioning on the basis of information from the client, family, and other mental health professionals and direct observation of the client in his or her home and work environment.

Gerhart (1990) identified the principles of case management as (1) providing individualized care, (2) using comprehensive and appropriate services, and (3) enhancing client autonomy and promoting continuity of care. All clients who use community mental health center services should be followed by a case manager. Some clients may require two weekly visits and home visits. Others may need only a phone call once a month. The intensity of case management depends on the severity of the client's illness; the number of services being used by the client; the number of people involved in the client's case, such as family members and school administrators; and the client's compliance with treatment. Case management is the crucial human relationship that allows the client to benefit from the CMHC services. The nurse and client should strive for mutual trust, open communication, and cooperation in the case management relationship; these qualities enable the activities described above to be effective. For case management to be of assistance, the client must attend scheduled sessions, attempt to carry out recommendations, openly discuss barriers to treatment, and state his or her expectations of the mental health system.

Medication Clinics

Some clients may need only medication management if they remain symptom free while taking adequate levels of prescribed medications. Others may use the medication clinics as an adjunct to other services. Nurses dispense, prescribe, and monitor the client's response to medication while providing individualized teaching. Clients are taught how, when, and why to take medications and to identify and report any desired or adverse reactions. Laboratory services are available to ensure appropriate blood levels of medications such as lithium or carbamazepine (Tegretol) and other hematological studies, such as complete blood count, white blood cell count, and renal and liver function tests. Drug screens can be conducted to evaluate whether the client is taking other prescribed or illicit drugs.

Educational Services

Community mental health centers often provide educational services and opportunities for clients, significant others, and communities. Nurse educators develop programs that focus on primary prevention and identify clients at risk. These programs target clients, families, and other health professionals. Examples of classes include medication management for clients taking lithium; relaxation and stress management for families of clients with schizophrenia; or for an entire community, the factors that increase the risk of contracting the human immunodeficiency virus. In addition, the nurse can serve as a consultant to various groups and provide information and recommendations on such topics as the signs and symptoms of depression and the risk factors for suicide in adolescents. Table 25–3 lists education programs provided by community mental health centers for some client populations.

The following case study illustrates the application of the nursing process in a community mental health center (see also Nursing Care Plan 25–1).

TABLE 25–3
Education Programs Provided by Community Mental Health Centers*

POPULATIONS	PROGRAMS
Child	Developmental assessments Referral to educational services Referral to psychiatric services Stress management
Adolescent	Teen parenting classes Individual and family therapy Vocational-educational counseling Referral for psychiatric chemical dependency services Psychological testing
Elderly	Respite care Senior centers Educational program for caregivers Medication management Referral for housing options Transportation coordination Referral to volunteer agencies Coordination of home health visits Referral to psychiatric services
Clients with acquired immune deficiency syndrome	Individual, marital, and family counseling Medication management Support groups for patients and families Patient, family, and community education Screening for the human immunodeficiency virus Crisis intervention
Chemical dependency	Referral to chemical dependency services Laboratory services Medication management Support groups (such as Alcoholics Anonymous, Narcotics Anonymous)

* This is not a comprehensive list, but samples of what a community mental health center may offer.

Case Study: The Client with Schizophrenia (Fred)

Fred was a 32-year-old man who was recently discharged from an inpatient psychiatric hospital where he had received treatment for his schizophrenia. He was to continue to live at home with his parents but was required to obtain follow-up services from the community mental health center. During assessment, he was fearful of the nurse, but he later shared that he felt the microwave oven sending him mental messages and saw foreign spies lurking in his closets and behind the furniture at home. He had poor eye contact, his speech was hesitant, he made periodic upward glances, and he was mildly anxious. Although his clothes were clean, his hair was unkempt. The nurse at the community mental health center developed the initial care plan for Fred on the basis of assessment.

ALTERNATIVE LIVING CENTERS

HISTORY AND PURPOSE

Alternative living centers provide residential and therapeutic care for clients who are unable to live independently or with their families. The goal of alternative

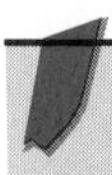

Nursing Care Plan 25–1 Nursing Care of the Client with Schizophrenia in a Community Mental Health Center (CMHC) (Fred)

Nursing Diagnosis: Self-Esteem related to inability to trust and withdrawal from contact with others

OUTCOME IDENTIFICATION	NURSING ACTIONS	RATIONALES	EVALUATION
1. By [date], Fred will attend sessions with the nurse and will tolerate the nurse's closeness and interest.	1a. Set up appointments that are convenient to Fred and his family. Meet Fred at these times and demonstrate an accepting attitude.	1a. When a nurse follows through with meetings, the client learns that the nurse is trustworthy. An accepting attitude promotes a positive self-esteem.	*Goals met:* Fred is able to tolerate the nurse's closeness and interest for up to 10 minutes by the third session. Fred attends three other CMHC activities this month. Fred begins to express his feelings through painting and clay.
	1b. Observe Fred's pattern of interaction and attendance.	1b. The nurse must assess and gather data on which to base interventions and goals.	
	1c. Encourage Fred to use a variety of media to express his feelings, such as painting, clay, and magazine pictures.	1c. The use of a variety of media may promote the client's self-expression in a nonthreatening manner.	
	1d. Provide positive reinforcement to Fred for talking.	1d. Reinforcement increases the probability that the client will talk more in the future.	
	1e. Discuss with Fred ways he might spend his day.	1e. Discussion helps the client develop problem-solving abilities.	
	1f. Give Fred information about other CMHC programs.	1f. This provides him with several community resources and support systems.	
	1g. Explore Fred's difficulty in trusting people and his progress in this area.	1g. Discussion identifies obstacles and facilitates problem solving. Identifying progress reinforces positive behaviors.	
	1h. Meet with Fred and his family to assess his ability to trust and socialize away from the CMHC.	1h. Meetings help to develop and reinforce the client's support system and provide data from the family. The nurse should meet with the family exclusively only when necessary, because the client may become suspicious and stop trusting the nurse.	

Nursing Diagnosis: Altered Thought Processes related to inability to evaluate reality

OUTCOME IDENTIFICATION	NURSING ACTIONS	RATIONALES	EVALUATION
1. By [date], Fred will learn to define and test reality and control behaviors negatively affected by thought disturbance.	1a. Support reality: remind Fred of session times and location, what was discussed last session, etc.	1a. Reinforcement and validation of reality helps the client learn to distinguish between reality and nonreality.	*Goal met:* Fred demonstrates reality testing, controls impulsive and socially inappropriate behaviors, and identifies adaptive ways to cope.

Nursing Care Plan 25–1 Nursing Care of the Client with Schizophrenia in a Community Mental Health Center (CMHC) (Fred) (Continued)

OUTCOME IDENTIFICATION	NURSING ACTIONS	RATIONALES	EVALUATION
	1b. Listen attentively and tell Fred when you do not understand what he is saying.	1b. Clarifying helps the nurse identify the thoughts of the client that are not reality based. It also helps the client develop more effective communication techniques.	
	1c. Help Fred identify hallucinations or delusions and subsequent feelings of anxiety.	1c. Talking about the hallucinations may decrease the client's fear of and/or embarrassment about them. It also provides data that may be used in assessment, goal, and intervention development.	
	1d. Validate reality by saying that you believe that Fred sees and hears hallucinations but that you do not see and hear the same things.	1d. Acknowledgment that the client is experiencing hallucinations helps the client feel validated but does not validate a false reality.	
	1e. Do not attempt to convince Fred that his hallucinations are false.	1e. Denying the existence of the client's hallucinations causes the client to feel threatened and discounted. Or the client may try to defend the existence of the hallucinations, making them stronger.	
	1f. Help Fred identify what is reality and what is hallucination.	1f. Helping the client identify hallucinations versus reality helps him or her make effective decisions and act in a more socially acceptable manner.	
	1g. Reinforce reality-based behaviors and beliefs.	1g. Reinforcement increases the probability that the client will display more reality-based behaviors and beliefs in the future.	

► **Nursing Diagnosis:** Knowledge Deficit regarding medication and community services

OUTCOME IDENTIFICATION	NURSING ACTIONS	RATIONALES	EVALUATION
1. By [date], Fred will identify medication name, schedule, and possible side effects.	1a. Teach Fred the name of the medication he is taking, his medication schedule, and possible side effects of the medication.	1a. The client will learn to take medications correctly, which will help to alleviate symptoms. Increased knowledge may also increase the client's independence and self-esteem.	*Goal met:* Fred is able to state the name of his medication, the importance of taking it, how to obtain it, the dosage, and what side effects to be aware of.

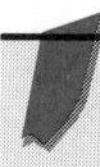

Nursing Care Plan 25–1 Nursing Care of the Client with Schizophrenia in a Community Mental Health Center (CMHC) (Fred) (Continued)

OUTCOME IDENTIFICATION	NURSING ACTIONS	RATIONALES	EVALUATION
	1b. Encourage Fred to ask questions and then answer them.	1b. Any incorrect information or beliefs may be addressed.	Fred reports a plan to maintain social activities. Fred attends outside activities and discusses his reaction to them.
2. By [date], Fred will take medications as prescribed.	2a. Teach Fred about the necessity of taking medications daily.	2a. Identifying the positive results of taking medications regularly increases compliance.	
	2b. Monitor Fred's blood levels as necessary.	2b. Monitoring blood levels ensures that the client is maintaining therapeutic levels in his or her system. Nontherapeutic levels may suggest a need for a dosage change or may indicate that the client is not taking the medications as ordered.	
3. By [date], Fred will use community resources.	3a. Discuss with Fred how he may obtain medication from the CMHC.	3a. Information facilitates the client's compliance.	
	3b. Plan for daily opportunities for positive activity.	3b. Helping the client to plan and follow through with positive activities promotes independence, socialization, and positive self-esteem in the client.	
	3c. Give Fred information on CMHC activities and services.	3c. The nurse should be a source of information that will increase the client's ability to follow through with positive behaviors.	
	3d. Arrange for transportation to these activities.	3d. Same as above.	

Nursing Diagnosis: Self-Care Deficit (Hygiene) related to lack of interest in body and appearance

OUTCOME IDENTIFICATION	NURSING ACTIONS	RATIONALES	EVALUATION
1. By [date], Fred will be maintaining good personal hygiene.	1a. Teach Fred the importance of good hygiene.	1a. The client may be helped to identify the positive consequences of behaviors.	*Goals met:* Fred demonstrates good personal hygiene at each session.
	1b. Teach Fred how to tend to personal hygiene: washing, laundry, bathing, combing hair, going to barber, etc.	1b. Teaching increases the probability that the client will carry out positive behaviors, increasing self-esteem.	Fred is able to discuss any difficulties he is having tending to hygiene.

Nursing Care Plan 25–1 Nursing Care of the Client with Schizophrenia in a Community Mental Health Center (CMHC) (Fred) (Continued)

OUTCOME IDENTIFICATION	NURSING ACTIONS	RATIONALES	EVALUATION
	1c. Ensure that Fred has needed materials: soap, towels, comb, etc.	1c. Providing the client with needed supplies increases the likelihood that he or she will follow through with positive behaviors, promoting a feeling of accomplishment, independence, and positive self-esteem.	
	1d. Reinforce when client attends session neatly groomed.	1d. Reinforcement increases the probability of similar actions in the future. The client feels validated when the nurse acknowledges his or her efforts.	
	1e. Meet with client's family to discuss and address any grooming difficulties.	1e. Additional data may be obtained from the family and their participation in the client's care reinforced.	

living centers is the normalization of clients. The structured facilities help clients achieve the highest level of functioning and independence possible while at the same time providing support and training. Community care for the mentally ill is not a recent concept. In the early 1400s, the nonviolent mentally ill were allowed to roam the countryside and had their needs met by people in the community (Scheerenberger, 1983). In the 1700s, local governments paid families to adopt mentally ill people and provide basic necessities. During the Industrial Revolution, the mentally ill and mentally retarded were kept in group settings as a source of cheap labor and entertainment. During the early 1900s, colonies of formerly institutionalized clients lived in group homes to work on a farm or in a factory. From this colony concept arose other living arrangements widely varied in structure, supervision, and setting (Novak & Heal, 1980).

POPULATIONS SERVED

Children and Adolescents

Foster care allows children and adolecents to live with families for years or until other treatment arrangements can be made, such as residential treatment, permanent adoption, or return to the original family if the reason the child was removed from the home has been corrected. Reasons for placing a youth in foster care include (1) the need for improved living conditions; (2) child abuse; (3) substance abuse; and (4) mental illness. The National Foster Care Association stated that all children and adolescents who need substitute care "should have the opportunity to live in a family, whatever their physical or mental abilities" (Aldgate, Maluccio, & Reeves, 1989, p. 19). Therefore, when a child is unable to live with his or her birth family, an organization, usually the Child Protective Services, places the child in the care of an approved foster family.

Sometimes children are removed from their family and placed in foster care while the parents develop better parenting skills, to obtain proper care, as a transition to sufficient living conditions or employment, or to receive treatment for mental illness or substance abuse. Other children and adolescents may live with foster families for many years and become emotionally attached.

Foster families are assessed and trained by the Child Protective Services or similar agency so as to provide stable and healthy environments. The role of foster parents includes providing physical care, emotional support, and socialization. In addition, children have access to treatment modalities such as long-term planning, experiential learning, and specialized schooling if needed (Aldgate et al., 1989).

Group homes allow as many as 10 children to live in an alternative homelike environment. Parental figures provide physical and emotional care to children and adolescents who live together like siblings to benefit from a safe family environment. A group home is an alternative to a home environment that lacks stability and safety. The goals of a group home are to (1) provide a stable, accepting, and nurturing substitute family; (2) to meet the children's educational needs; and (3) to provide group and experiential therapies.

Residential treatment centers provide psychosocial treatment and group living conditions for emotionally disturbed children. Sometimes, children who rebel against the single authority of parents respond more positively to group limits and pressures. Children who require residential treatment often demonstrate impulsivity, uncontrollable anger, antisocial behaviors, chemical dependency, or depression to the point that they are unable to function at home. Residential treatment centers vary greatly, but generally, they are not as restrictive as inpatient or partial hospitalization and provide more structure and therapy than group homes. Residential treatment centers provide 24-hour care for children and adolescents. Patients are sometimes able to attend their own school and activities and return to the programs for therapeutic groups, structure, and milieu. The goal of a residential treatment center is to promote a client's internal stability through peer structure, group process, routines, and adherence to a healthy value system (Wells, 1991).

Adults and Elderly

Cooperative apartments are typical apartment complexes that are owned and directed by private or public mental health centers. They enable clients to maintain independence and responsibility through paying rent and housekeeping. At the same time, support and structure are provided in the form of on-site supervision, counseling, social events, and educational programs. Most residents work or attend school part-time or full-time.

Foster homes for adults were originally defined as "the practice of placing unrelated, dependent adults in the care of private families" (Bogen, 1979, p. 5). They allow qualified people to have a client or clients live in their home (Bogen, 1979). In the early 1200s A.D., the "spiritually ill" pilgrimaged to Gheel, Belgium, for relief from mental illness. When Catholic churches were no longer able to house them, the families of Gheel accepted the "insane" into their homes and cared for them. This is the basis for today's foster care for adults, which targets the mentally ill, the mentally retarded, and the frail elderly (Sherman & Newman, 1988).

Whether they provide temporary or permanent housing, foster families must adhere to strict governmental guidelines regarding fire codes, sanitary food service, staff supervision, and client rights. These homes provide "family" environments, support services, supervision, and custodial or rehabilitative care for the mentally disabled clients (Sherman & Newman, 1988). Foster families have access to professional support services such as medical care for clients, therapy to help the client and family deal with emotional problems, and funding sources. Support groups for foster families are available to allow families to share experiences and information. A mental health center caseworker is usually assigned to each family.

Group homes (sometimes called "halfway houses") provide clients with homelike living arrangements. Five to 50 clients live together in a large house, sharing meals, chores, and rooms. Some group homes serve as transitional settings for clients discharged from the hospital after learning to cope with schizophrenia, depression, bipolar disorder, chemical dependency, or other psychiatric disorders. These environments foster self-confidence and independent living. In addition, they provide short- and long-term care that includes medication management, vocational programs, group therapy, and social skills training. Clients who are not appropriate for group homes include those with poor impulse control (difficulty adhering to rules) and suicidal or physically aggressive behaviors.

Mentally Retarded

Historically, mentally retarded people were cared for by their family in their houses and received little in the way of community support, or they were institutionalized and given custodial care but no training or rehabilitation.

Group homes and residential treatment communities help mentally retarded clients reach their highest level of functioning through independent living. Living with others in supervised settings gives the mentally retarded person a myriad of opportunities to learn the activities of daily living. Staffing of the home and the numbers of residents are determined by the severity of the clients' retardation and needs. For example, low-functioning clients who require assistance with bathing and eating live together in smaller numbers and require more staff 24 hours a day, whereas a larger number of high-functioning residents may live together and require less supervisory staff. Daily routines for the mentally handicapped are a key aspect of residential programs. Residential communities meet the physical, emotional, social, and intellectual needs of the residents. The following is a clinical example of a mentally retarded individual in a group home setting.

Clinical Example 3

Francie was a 38-year-old woman who had the developmental and intellectual capacities of an 8-year-old child. She loved music, hugs, and animals. Each day, her alarm went off at 8:00 A.M. She was able to get dressed, make her bed, and brush her teeth, but she required assistance in putting barrettes in her hair. With little direction, she set the table for breakfast with her eight other house residents and two house parents. The other members performed their assigned duties in preparing the morning meal. Together, they ate and cleaned up.

A van picked up her and five other residents at 9:30 and took her to work. She worked in a factory-like setting, partially funded by the community mental health center, where she put plastic forks in a "picnic pack" for a neighborhood fast-food restaurant. As she worked, she laughed, conversed, and occasionally became frustrated. She received refreshments and lunch and met daily with the supervisor/social worker and the nurse for a few minutes.

She rode home on the van at 3:30. From 4:00 to 4:45 each day, she and her housemates and house parents met for a "community meeting" in which they talked about how the day went and discussed issues related to their group life. Meal preparation began at 5:00 and the group ate together again at 6:00. Francie enjoyed pouring the beverages. After clean-up, she had leisure time where she enjoyed playing ping pong, listening to music, or playing with the house pets. At 8:30, she prepared for bed and was in bed by "lights off" at 9:30.

The community setting allowed Francie to expand her social environment. She felt important to the group and listened to people talk about dealing with the same struggles she had. The consistency in her home life, work, housemates, and chores provided repetition that enhanced her learning. Although there was some supervision, Francie was functioning at her most independent level.

THE NURSE'S ROLE

The nurse clinician working in alternative living centers provides therapies and assists in maintaining therapeutic milieus. As a therapist, the nurse assesses clients who have difficulty with impulse control, problem solving, depression, rebellion, anxiety, inappropriate anger, behavioral problems, and poor social skills. The nurse also provides client education through assertiveness training and activities of daily living, such as preparation of balanced meals and interventions to promote rest.

Nurses must be familiar with community resources and collaborate effectively with other health professionals in an effort to maximize health care to meet their client's emotional, physical, and psychosocial needs. As administrators, nurses use their managerial, clinical, creative, legal, and networking skills to develop and implement alternative living centers. By following federal and other organizational guidelines, nurses are supervising and running programs that provide needed services beyond the typical hospital setting. Nurses must take the lead in developing programs that facilitate independent living.

Balcerzak (1991) identified four factors that contribute to the development of an effective residential treatment program:

1. The nurse's courage to try things never done before as the basis of valid research and design effort
2. Interdisciplinary and interorganizational planning that focuses on the needs of multiproblem clients
3. The nurse's discontent with the status quo and concern about the quality of treatment
4. The establishment of the service's hours of operation, location, cost, and other infrastructure on the basis of the characteristics of the population being served and the agencies making referrals

Nurses need to inform the community and the mental and medical health professions of the innovative and exciting ways that clients are being served in the community.

COMMUNITY AND SOCIAL ISSUES: HOMELESSNESS

THE HOMELESS: PSYCHIATRY'S GREATEST CHALLENGE

The 30-year-old woman sobbing at the battered woman's shelter, the elderly man who is arguing aloud with himself on the subway, the skid row alcoholic who has covered himself with newspapers to keep warm, and the 16-year-old runaway are all common sights and examples of the homeless in America today. The homeless mentally ill are described as having slipped through the cracks of the community mental health system. They are not, or are very remotely, connected with community psychiatry services because of the difficulty in reaching them and lack of resources in which to serve them. Estimates of the number of homeless persons in the United States vary from 250,000 to 3 million, with 50 percent of them having mental illnesses (Rubenstein, 1990).

HISTORICAL OVERVIEW

The homeless mentally ill have been around since the beginning of America. Records from the Colonial Period mention the attempts to deal with the indigent insane and "wandering madmen" (Goldfinger & Chafetz, 1984). The deinstitutionalization of the late 1950s was based on the belief that the mentally ill could be better cared for in the community than in institutions. Although possible and feasible, deinstitutionalization was carried out without adequate planning and services. Because insufficient community services were in place, mentally ill patients were released into the streets. Today, political and social factors contribute to the phenomenon of the homeless mentally ill. This group is now more diverse than it has been at any other time in history, comprising children, families, adolescents, and elderly who have enormous psychosocial and physical needs.

MENTAL HEALTH ILLNESSES OF THE HOMELESS

The term *homeless mentally ill* has become synonymous with chronic mental illness. A large percentage of homeless persons suffer from schizophrenia and major affective disorders (depression and bipolar disorder). Chemical dependency is a major problem among the homeless, with an estimated 40 percent of residents in homeless shelters demonstrating symptoms of alcohol abuse (McCarty et al., 1991). Psychosocial stressors such as the loss of one's home, the lack of a support network, and uncertainty about meeting basic needs such as food, shelter, and medical care place the homeless at risk for emotional crisis.

HOMELESS FAMILIES

Poverty, family violence, unemployment, and emotional problems are factors that have increased the rate of homelessness among families. A vast number of homeless families are headed by single mothers and their children (Dail, 1988). A study of Boston homeless families revealed that two thirds of the mothers had personality disorders and the children had serious emotional, cognitive, and physical problems, including depression, failure to thrive, anxiety, and developmental lags (Bassuk et al., 1986). Children's problems are exacerbated by the chaos and disruptions associated with transiency and living in shelters.

HOMELESS ADOLESCENTS

Homelessness in adolescents is associated with runaway behavior. A large percentage of homeless youth have histories of runaway behaviors precipitated by family conflict. Caton and Schaffer (1984) found that in a sample of 118 homeless teens,

- The majority were depressed or exhibited antisocial behaviors
- Less than 2 percent met the criteria of schizophrenia
- 33 percent of the girls had a history of suicide attempts
- 50 percent of the girls and 75 percent of the boys had been expelled from school
- 70 percent admitted using drugs
- 50 percent had lived in an alternative living center

HOMELESS ADULTS

In a pioneer study, Arce and Vergare (1984) investigated mental illness among homeless adults and found that 85 percent demonstrated diagnosable mental illnesses based on criteria in the third edition of the *Diagnostic and Statistical Manual of Mental Disorders* (American Psychiatric Association, 1980) for schizophrenia, substance abuse, personality disorder, affective disorders, organic brain syndrome, and mental retardation. Deinstitutionalization, unemployment, stretched social welfare programs, lack of medical insurance, and noncompliance compound the mentally ill homeless person's plight. However, only 25 to 35 percent of homeless adults have been found to demonstrate mental illness severe enough to necessitate hospitalization (Roth & Bean, 1986; Fischer et al., 1986).

HOMELESS OLDER ADULTS

Elderly people make up a small percentage of the homeless population. Various studies estimate that 6 to 27 percent of homeless persons are over 60 years old (Kutza & Keigher, 1991). The majority of the elderly homeless population are men, but women are more likely to accept social services. The most common mental health problem in this age group is organic or alcohol-related dementia, which is manifested by confusion, disorientation, paranoia, and hallucinations (Kutza & Keigher, 1991). In a study of a shelter population, Lenehan et al. (1985) found that 90 percent of the elderly women exhibited psychiatric symptoms such as hallucinations, paranoia, phobias, and depression. Medical problems such as arthritis, hypertension, diabetes, fractures, pneumonia, and sensory deprivation compound the plight of the homeless elderly (Kutza & Keigher, 1991).

THE ROLE OF ALCOHOLISM AND DRUG ABUSE

Alcohol abuse affects 30 to 40 percent and drug abuse 10 to 15 percent of the homeless. Fischer et al. (1986) demonstrated that men were likely to report problems with alcohol and drugs, whereas women were more likely to report problems with mental illness. Chemical abuse and homelessness are related, but one does not always cause the other. Alcohol and drug abuse can lead to homelessness, or the stresses related to homelessness may lead to drug or alcohol use. Greater nursing challenges are presented when chemical dependence is compounded by other mental illnesses in the homeless. For example, a homeless alcoholic may also have schizophrenia (McCarty et al., 1991). The nurse must incorporate knowledge about many physiological and mental processes to assess, diagnose, plan for, and treat a person with concurrent disorders.

The current understanding of chemical dependency and its processes has influenced current treatment approaches. In the past, when public intoxication was declared a crime (1845), most homeless alcoholics were taken to drunk tanks at the local police department. However, in 1971, the Uniform Alcoholism and Intoxication Act encouraged local governments to establish community-based detoxification and alcohol treatment centers (McCarty et al., 1991). Treatment requires a holistic approach to address the addiction behavior as well as lack of housing, job skills, and social supports.

TYPES OF PROGRAMS

Shelters

Emergency shelters offer housing for brief stays (no longer than 2 weeks). National surveys show that these accommodations are usually open all year round and house an average of 53 people. Most are age or gender specific, that is, serve youth only, women only, or men only. Most shelters provide meals and showers costing an average of $14 to $30 per night. Counseling and referral services are available at most shelters. Some of them assist families with rent in order to prohibit evictions. Most of these shelters are funded by religious or volunteer organizations (Veragare & Arce, 1984). The transient nature of the homeless population makes it very difficult for shelters to provide long-term mental health services.

Community Support Programs

In 1977, the Community Support Program was the federal government's response to identifying an insufficient service system for the homeless mentally ill. Community Support Systems are networks of professionals who assist in meeting the needs of the homeless population. The goals of these systems are to (Levine et al., 1986)

1. Locate clients and reach out to inform them of available services, such as resources for shelter, food, clothing, income, and health care.
2. Assist clients in accessing the community mental health system.
3. Provide psychosocial and rehabilitative services.
4. Provide education and consultation to persons who interact with the homeless, such as landlords, employers, and members of the legal system.
5. Involve support systems such as businesses, neighborhoods, churches, and volunteer agencies.
6. Establish procedures for legal protection.

Drop-in Clinics

Drop-in services are often located in storefronts of areas frequently inhabited by homeless people. Many of them offer educational programs, self-help groups, referral services, food, housing, and counseling. Their main qualities are accessibility and informal affiliation.

BARRIERS TO TREATMENT

Socioeconomic changes such as "loss of low income housing, social service cutbacks, unemployment, and general economic trends" are obstacles to treatment of the homeless mentally ill (Jones, 1986, p. 95).

Health professionals may experience few reinforcements for working with the homeless mentally ill. Chafetz (1990) identified the following as the major reasons for withdrawal of the health caregiver from the homeless clientele:

1. The resource dilemma occurs when the needs of the client are so enormous and overwhelming that the care provider is unable to meet them or is only able to focus on the most immediate ones, such as food or shelter.
2. "Crisis of belief" occurs when a health provider has values and beliefs about health care that cannot be met and subsequently works without a philosophy that gives meaning and direction to daily work. For example, a nurse may believe that clients will follow through with recommendations and reach care plan goals. If, however, they do not carry out actions that could improve their condition and "sabatoges" their treatment, the nurse may become disillusioned and lose faith in the philosophy of care.
3. When inadequate resources are available to meet enormous client needs, feelings of helplessness and discouragement ensue among health care providers, further compromising their support systems.
4. Other workplace stressors include working with clients who exhibit hostile, angry, and threatening behaviors. These clients often have poor hygiene and other health-related problems such as tuberculosis and scabies.

THE NURSE'S ROLE

In working with the homeless population, the nurse must work corroboratively with many other health care professionals, such as social workers and physicians. Historically, nurses have developed and established services for the homeless, including the homeless mentally ill. Project Help and the Manhattan Bowery Project employ nurses to go to the shelters and the streets of New York City to link the homeless with community resources. Nurse practitioners, clinical specialists, public health nurses, and administrators provide on-site primary care, case management, and counseling for the homeless population. Nurses can also identify forces that contribute to homelessness and fragmentation of health care services. Nurses play key roles in social activism by serving on committees and foundations, lobbying for governmental policy changes and funding, and becoming political advocates.

The role of the nurse entails providing psychosocial care in a caring manner that minimizes stress and promotes health in homeless individuals. According to a study of Kinzel (1991), which identified the concerns of two homeless groups, "a recurring theme from the responses of the homeless was the need for interaction with a caring person" (p. 189). In fact, "the feeling that no one cares, . . . may lead to depression, hopelessness, and finally illness" (Kinzel, p. 181). The therapeutic relationship between the nurse and client helps the client to feel concerned for, cared about, and supported. To establish a therapeutic relationship, the nurse needs to be available, actively listen, provide feedback, meet the client's physiological and emotional needs, express concern, and meet with the client on a consistent basis (see Chapter 6 for a discussion of client interaction and assessment).

▶CHAPTER SUMMARY

The area of community mental health has far-reaching parameters that encompass various types of services. As more health care is delivered in the community, the need for these services will continue to expand. The result will be a wider range of roles for nurses. Historically, community mental health has evolved to meet the changing needs of our society, and it will continue to do so. As cost containment measures increase, so will the need to provide care to clients in the community. As our society ages, the elderly's need for care will grow. As the homeless population expands, the needs of various age groups must be identified and met. Care environments with the least restrictions will be in demand. Outpatient treatment will be the first line of defense in dealing with the needs of the mentally ill in the community. Through the evolution of community mental health services will come the increased need for nurses to provide care in the community. Community agencies, community mental health centers, partial hospitalization programs, home health care services, and alternative living centers all need nurses for their administrative, clinical, consultative, and research expertise. Community mental health nursing is an integral part of our health care system, providing care to clients of all ages, diagnoses, and economic levels.

Suggestions for Clinical Conference

1. Identify how community psychiatric nurses could be used in your community.
2. Identify community mental health needs in your area and how you could contribute to meeting those needs.
3. Identify community referral agencies in your area that do or could use community psychiatric nurses.
4. As a small-group activity, develop a partial hospitalization program for depressed high-functioning adults and a partial hospitalization program for mentally retarded adolescents.

References

Aldgate, J., Maluccio, A., & Reeves, C. (1989). *Adolescents in foster families*. Chicago: Lycem.

Amenta, M. (1985). Hospice in the United States: Multiple models and varied programs. *Nursing Clinics of North America, 20,* 269–279.

Amenta, M. (1991). Hospice services. In S. A. Baird, R. McCorkle, & M. Grant (Eds.), *Cancer nursing: A comprehensive textbook* (pp. 1033–1043). Philadelphia: W. B. Saunders.

Amenta, M., & Bohnet, N. (1986). *Nursing care of the terminally ill*. Boson: Little, Brown.

Arce, A. A., & Vergare, M. J. (1984). Identifying and characterizing the mentally ill among the homeless. In H. R. Lamb (Ed.), *The homeless mentally ill*. Washington, DC: American Psychiatric Association.

American Psychiatric Association. (1980). *Diagnostic and statistical manual of mental disorders* (3rd ed.). Washington, DC: Author.

Baird, S. V., McCorkle, R., & Grant, M. (1991). *Cancer nursing: A comprehensive textbook*. Philadelphia: W. B. Saunders.

Balcerzak, E. A. (1991). Toward the Year 2000: Strategies for the field of residential group care. *Residential Treatment for Children and Youth, 8,* 57–69.

Bassuk, E. L., and Rubin, L., & Lauriat, A. S. (1986). Characteristics of sheltered homeless families. *American Journal of Public Health, 76,* 1097–1101.

Block, B. M., & Lefkovitz, P. M. (1991). *Standards and guidelines for partial hospitalization*. Alexandria, VA: American Association of Partial Hospitalization.

Bogen, H. (1979). The history of adult foster home care. In K. H. Nash & D. J. Tesiny (Eds.), *Readings in foster care* (pp. 1–32). Albany, NY: School of Social Welfare, State University of New York at Albany.

Brescia, F. J. (1993). Specialized care of the terminally ill. In V. T. Devita, S. Hellman, & S. A. Rosenbery (Eds), *Cancer: Principles of oncology* (pp. 2501–2508). Philadelphia: J. B. Lippincott.

Caplan, G. (1964). *Principles of preventive psychiatry*. New York: Basic Books.

Caton, C., & Schaffer, D. (1984). *Runaway and homeless youth in New York City*. New York: Department of Psychiatry, Columbia University.

Chafetz, L. (1990). Withdrawal from the homeless mentally ill. *Community Mental Health Journal, 25,* 449–461.

Dail, P. W. (1988, May). *A psychosocial portrait of homeless women with children*. Paper presented at the American Psychological Association Conference on Reaching the Unreachable, Washington, DC.

Dail, P. W. (1990). The psychosocial context of homeless mothers with young children: Program and policy implications. *Child Welfare, 69,* 291–307.

Fischer, P. J., Shapiro, S., Breakey, W. R., Anthony, J. C., & Kramer, M. (1986). Mental health and social characteristics of the homeless: A survey of mission users. *American Journal of Public Health, 76,* 519–524.

Flaskerud, J. H., & van Servellen, G. M. (1985). *Community mental health nursing: Theories and methods*. Norwalk, CT: Appleton-Century-Crofts.

Gerhart, U.C. (1990). *Caring for the chronic mentally ill*. Itasca, IL: F. E. Peacock.

Goldfinger, S. M., & Chafetz, L. (1984). Developing a better service delivery system for the homeless mentally ill. In H. R. Lamb (Ed.), *The homeless mentally ill*. Washington, DC: American Psychiatric Association.

Goldman, D. L. (1990). Two pioneers of today's partial hospital and their ideas. *International Journal of Partial Hospitalization, 6,* 181–187.

Haldey, R. (1978). President's Commission sets national mental health goals. *American Nurse, 10*(1).

Herz, M. I., Endicott, J., Spitzer, R. L., et al. (1971). Day versus inpatient hospitalization: A controlled study. *American Journal of Psychiatry, 127,* 1371–1382.

Jones, B. E. (1986). Organizational barriers to serving the mentally ill homeless. In B. E. Jones (Ed.), *Treating the homeless: Urban psychiatry's challenge* (pp. 93–108). Washington, DC: American Psychiatric Press.

Kinzel, D. (1991). Self-identified health concerns of two homeless groups. *Western Journal of Nursing Research, 13,* 181–194.

Kutza, E. A., & Keigher, S. M. (1991). The elderly "new homeless": An emerging population at risk. *Social Work, 36,* 288–293.

Leighton, A. H. (1989). Global and specific approaches to prevention. In B. Cooper & T. Helgason (Eds.), *Epidemiology and the prevention of mental disorders*. London: Rutledge.

Leighton, A. H. (1990). Community mental health and information underload. *Community Mental Health Journal, 26,* 49–66.

Lenehan, G. P., McGinnis, D., O'Connell, D., & Hennessey, M. (1985). A nurse's clinic for the homeless. *American Journal of Nursing, 85,* 1237–1240.

Levine, I. S., Lezak, A. D., & Goldman, H. H. (1986). Community support system for the homeless mentally ill. In E. L. Bassuk (Ed.), *The mental health needs of homeless persons*. San Francisco: Jossey-Bass.

Lesseig, D. Z. (1987). Home care for psych problems. *American Journal of Nursing, 87,* 1317–1320.

Luber, R. F. (1979). The scope and growth of partial hospitalization. In R. F. Luber (Ed.), *Partial hospitalization: A current perspective* (pp. 3–20). New York: Plenum Press.

McCarty, D., Argeriou, M., Huebner, R. B., & Lubran, B. (1991). Alcoholism, drug abuse, and the homeless. *American Psychologist, 11,* 1139–1148.

Mishne, J. M. (1986). *Clinical work with adolescents.* New York: Free Press.

Mor, V., & Masterson-Allen, S. (1987). *Hospice care systems.* New York: Springer.

Mor, V., & Masterson-Allen, S. (1990). A comparison of hospice versus conventional care of the terminally ill patient. *Oncology, 4,* 85–91.

National Association of Private Psychiatric Hospitals and American Association of Partial Hospitalization. (1978). Definition of partial hospitalization. *The Psychiatric Hospital, 21*(2), 89–90.

National Hospice Organization. (February, 1988). National hospice reports seven percent growth in hospice programs. *Hospice News,* pp. 1–3.

Novak, A. R., and & Heal, L. W. (1980). *Integration of developmentally disabled individuals into the community.* Baltimore: Paul H. Brookes.

Pelletier, L. R. (1988). Psychiatric home care. *Journal of Psychosocial Nursing and Mental Health Services, 26*(3), 22–27.

Reighly, J. W. (1988). The child who is dying/terminal. In J. W. Reighly (Ed.), *Nursing care planning guides for mental health* (pp. 202–207). Baltimore: Williams & Wilkins.

Roth, D., & Bean, G. J. (1986). New perspective on homelessness: Findings from a statewide epidemiological study. *Hospital and Community Psychiatry, 37,* 712–719.

Rubenstein, E. (1990, May 14). How many homeless? *National Review,* p. 17.

Scheerenberger, R. C. (1983). *A history of mental retardation.* Baltimore: Paul H. Brookes.

Sherman, S. R., and & Newman, E. S. (1988). *Foster families for adults.* New York: Columbia University Press.

Thobaden, M., & Kozlak, J. (1990). Home health care's unique role in serving the elderly mentally ill. *Home Healthcare Nurse, 8*(4), 37–39.

Turner, S. M. (1979). Treatment orientation and program implications. In R. F. Luber (Ed.), *Partial hospitalization: A current perspective* (pp. 139–150). New York: Plenum Press.

Vergare, M. J., & Arce, A. A. (1984, May). *Mental illness in the homeless.* Paper presented at the annual meeting of the American Psychiatric Association, Los Angeles.

Voineskos, G. (1976). The neglected field of community psychiatry. *Canadian Medical Association Journal 114,* 320–324.

Wells, K. (1991). Placement of emotionally disturbed childrern in residential treatment: A review of placement criteria. *American Journal of Orthopsychiatry, 61,* 339–357.

CHAPTER 26

Psychopharmacological Therapy

DUANE F. PENNEBAKER, Ph.D., A.R.N.P., F.N.A.P., F.R.C.N.A.
JOY RILEY, D.N.Sc., R.N.,C.S.

OUTLINE

CHAPTER OBJECTIVES

Upon completion of this chapter, you will be able to:

1. Describe current knowledge about the brain and behavior as it relates to the clinical and pharmacokinetics of the major psychopharmaceutical agents.
2. Describe the clinical and pharmacokinetic properties of the major psychopharmaceutical agents and the use of these agents in the treatment of mental illness.

3. Apply knowledge about the pharmacokinetic properties of the major psychopharmaceutical agents to individualized patient care.
4. Explain the nurse's role in the administration of psychopharmacological agents within the treatment regime.
5. Describe the importance of client and family education in the use of psychopharmaceutical agents in the treatment of mental illness.
6. Comprehend the nurse's legal responsibilities and the ethical issues confronting the nurse in the use of psychopharmaceutical agents.

KEY TERMS

Akathesia
Akinesia
Cogwheeling
Dopaminergic pathway
Exponential kinetics
Extrapyramidal side effects
Linear kinetics
Neuroleptic malignancy syndrome
Neurotransmitters
Paradoxical reactions
Pharmacodynamics
Pharmacokinetics
Sedative
Serotonin syndrome
Steady state
Synaptic transmission
Tardive dyskinesia

The past 20 years of research in the neurosciences has dramatically increased our understanding of the biobehavioral aspects of mental illness, to the extent that the 1990s have been referred to as the *Decade of the Brain*. Historically, the advent of the first psychotropic medications in the 1950s significantly altered the treatment of the mentally ill. Part of the role of the psychiatric–mental health nurse has evolved in tandem with the unfolding success of psychotropic medications. The psychiatric–mental health nurse's knowledge of psychopharmacology and its associated therapeutic agents is a significant factor in contemporary practice. The psychiatric nurse has a critical role in assisting clients to incorporate psychopharmacological agents into their efforts to recover and maintain mental health and prevent negative sequelae and relapse. In addition, the psychiatric–mental health nurse is responsible for assessing the therapeutic effects of the drugs, monitoring adverse reactions, knowing therapeutic dosages, documenting administration, and educating the client and family members about the psychopharmacological agents being used in the treatment regimen. At the advanced-practice level in many states, psychiatric–mental health nurses also have prescriptive authority. This chapter presents an overview of current major concepts that relate brain and behavioral response to the major psychopharmacological agents used in the treatment of mental illness.

Recommended treatments and drug therapies are changed as new clinical and scientific findings are made available. In this chapter, we provide the most current information available at the time of this writing about the pharmatherapeutic agents covered herein. The information provided, however, is not intended to replace sound clinical judgment or individualized client care. Nurses are legally and ethically responsible for being familiar with information such as the action, dosage, adverse effects, and drug interactions of the medications they administer. The reader is advised to check product information before administering any drug, especially new or infrequently ordered drugs. Unless otherwise noted, all information concerning the pharmacokinetic and clinical properties of the psychopharmacological agents discussed in this chapter is based on adult oral dosages. It is assumed that the student has had as a prerequisite to the materials in this chapter introductions to pharmacology and the anatomy and physiology of the brain and central nervous system (CNS).

The authors thank Jean LaValley, M.N., A.R.N.P., for her contributions and critical review.

THE BRAIN AND BEHAVIOR

The brain is a unique mass of tissue consisting of approximately 10 billion neurons. These neurons coordinate all of a person's behavior by means of unceasing electrochemical activity (Gilman & Newman, 1992; Gomez & Gomez, 1990). The brain's high metabolic rate enables it to continually process, sort, analyze, integrate, store, and retrieve information from the environment. Because of its energy needs, the brain demands a constant supply of oxygen and glucose, approximately 20 percent of the body's total needs. These and small amounts of other nutrients (e.g., amino acids, vitamins, and minerals) are provided by a continuous supply of blood, 15 percent of the total cardiac output.

The brain stores energy mainly in the form of glucose, which is used to fuel the ion pumps that maintain a resting state or propagate impulses. However, it stores only enough to last about 30 seconds (Gilman & Newman, 1992; Gomez & Gomez, 1990). Thus, brain metabolism is quickly and severely altered when cerebral blood flow is compromised.

Behavior is the expression of brain function and represents a complex interplay between a person and the environment. Although certain characteristics of human behavior are universal in nature, many more are specific to the individual. Recent research indicates that genetics and neuroendocrine mechanisms may influence behavior; however, theories arising from this research remain controversial (see the Controversy display in Chapter 29).

NEUROANATOMICAL STRUCTURES RELEVANT TO BEHAVIOR

The brain can be divided into cortical and subcortical structures. The *cortical structures* (right and left cerebral hemispheres) make up the outer and largest portion of the brain and include the cerebral cortex, or gray matter; the underlying white matter; and the basal ganglia, hippocampus, and amygdala. The *subcortical structures* include the brain stem, which is made up of the midbrain, the pons, and the medulla; the cerebellum; and the diencephalon, which consists of the thalamus and the hypothalamus (see Fig. 2–4). Although each area performs highly specific functions, all areas are connected by an elegant network of nerve pathways that enables the brain to perform complex interactions and associations that result in appropriate psychomotor responses.

Cortical Structures

The Cerebral Cortex. The cerebral cortex, or surface layer, of the brain (also called the *gray matter*) is composed almost exclusively of nerve cell bodies. It is divided by gyri (ridges) and sulci (grooves), which greatly multiplies the surface area and potential for function. Localized areas of the cerebral cortex either have specific functions or serve as integration areas referred to as *association areas* (Kupferman, 1991). Association areas serve as intermediaries to assimilate and integrate multiple and diverse sensory stimuli from the specialized cortices. These areas enable the brain to generate complex responses involving more than one behavioral domain.

The Four Lobes and Their Functions. The cerebral hemispheres each have four lobes: frontal, parietal, temporal, and occipital (see Fig. 2–4). The *occipital lobes* are the primary visual areas. They receive impulses from the retina and interpret visual stimuli for recognition and identification. The occipital areas also connect with the areas of the cortex involved with perception, recall, and optically induced reflexes. The interactions between these cortices provide three-dimensional vision and recognition.

The *parietal lobes* perform a variety of sensory functions. The anterior portions are specialized in somatic sensation and perception. The more posterior parietal areas integrate visual and auditory stimuli useful for the sense of body position and movement in three-dimensional space.

The *temporal lobes* perform primary auditory processing and, on a basic level, detect sound and tone intensity. *Wernicke's area*, which is responsible for recognition and interpretation of words and letters for speech, is located here. Long-term memory storage areas are believed to be harbored in the temporal lobes, as is the ability to add affective perception to experience.

The *frontal lobes* are vital for cognition. Virtually all other areas of the brain provide information to and receive it from the frontal lobes. These are the areas of highest intellectual function, such as judgment, reasoning, and abstract thinking. The frontal lobes also organize more complicated motor responses and initiate complex voluntary and reflex movements. Psychomotor activity is also generated in the frontal lobes, including the inhibition of emotional impulses. *Broca's area*, located in the frontal temporal junction, is responsible for speech articulation and lies close to Wernicke's area. Interaction between the speech and hearing centers is the foundation of communication in humans.

The Association Cortices. Three main association areas lie between the primary functional cortices: the prefrontal motor association cortex, the limbic (affective) association cortex, and the sensory (parietal-temporal-occipital) association cortex (Kupferman, 1991). These association cortices enable a person to assimilate and integrate input from all sensory experiences and formulate effective response patterns such as assessment and problem solving followed by appropriate movement and speech. The *prefrontal association cortex* integrates sensory and intellectual information as well as correction in the planning of movement. The *limbic association cortex* adds affective tone to responses, and the *parietal-temporal-occipital association cortex* processes sensory information to enhance perception and language (Kupferman, 1991).

The Basal Ganglia. The basal ganglia are centralized collections of neuron cell bodies (nuclei) lying within the white matter (see Fig. 2–4). These nuclei include the caudate nucleus, the putamen, and the globus pallidus (Burt, 1993). Their principal function is the modulation of impulses for movement from the motor cortex to provide the smooth sequencing and execution of complex responses (Kupferman, 1991).

The Hippocampus and the Amygdala. The amygdala and the hippocampus are structures generally considered to be a part of the *limbic system*; they are often referred to as the *limbic lobe* (see Figs. 9–1 and 10–1). Other structures included in the limbic system are the parahippocampal gyrus and the cingulate gyrus. In general, the limbic system has a primary role in the behavioral responses of mood, memory, and learning. Dysfunction in these areas results in the inability to form new memory (Kolb & Wishaw, 1990).

The amygdala, located in the temporal lobes, is composed of many nuclei with connecting tracts to the hypothalamus, hippocampus, cerebral cortex, and thalamus (Kupferman, 1991). The amygdala is involved in short-term memory and its conversion to long-term memory (Kolb & Wishaw, 1990). In addition, the amygdala is believed to be involved in learning through assimilation and integration of information from different sensory modalities. In animal studies, direct stimulation of the amygdala has produced aggressive behavior, suggesting that this structure may play a major role in adding affective tone to human responses (Kolb & Wishaw, 1990; Kupferman, 1991).

Subcortical Structures

The Brain Stem. The brain stem, which connects the brain to the spinal cord and peripheral nervous system, is composed of the medulla, the pons, the midbrain, and the reticular formation. These structures have specialized neural and physiological regulating functions such as regulation of the heart, breathing patterns, and circadian rhythms. The brain stem also contains nuclei (clusters of nerve cell bodies) that secrete important neurotransmitters that influence brain activity and response. Biofeedback mechanisms that measure oxygen levels and blood pressure within the brain maintain the blood flow required for normal brain demands (Kelly & Dodd, 1991).

The *medulla* is the origin of adrenergic (adrenaline) pathways that project to the hypothalamus, the locus ceruleus, and the vagus nerve (Leonard, 1993). The *locus ceruleus*, a cluster of neurons located in the pons, is the source of noradrenergic (norepinephrine) pathways projecting to the spinal cord, cerebellum, and brain stem but largely converging in the thalamus and hypothalamus (see Fig. 10–1). The *reticular formation* is a diffuse network of nuclei known to integrate motor, sensory, and visceral functions (Sugarmen & Kinney, 1993), but more important, it is involved in regulation of arousal and consciousness. This network is responsive to the presence of norepinephrine, serotonin, acetylcholine, and dopamine—neurotransmitters that mediate brain function on the most basic level (Kelly & Dodd, 1991; Sugarmen & Kinney, 1993).

The *midbrain* lies between the pons and the diencephalon. Structures in the midbrain include the tectum, the tegmentum, the red nucleus, and the substantia nigra (Gilman & Newman, 1992; Kolb & Whishaw, 1990). These nuclei synthesize dopamine, a neurotransmitter important in movement. The tectum mediates whole-body movements in response to visual and auditory stimuli (Kolb & Whishaw, 1990). The ventral portion of the tegmentum is the origin of a network of fibers known as the *mesolimbic dopaminergic pathway*, which projects to the limbic system. Another set of fibers, the mesocortical **dopaminergic pathway**, projects to the cortex and hippocampal regions of the limbic system. The substantia nigra gives rise to another set of dopaminergic fibers, associating with the nigrostriatal pathway, between the striatum, the subthalamic nucleus, and the cortex (Leonard, 1993; Role & Kelly, 1991) (see Fig. 12–1).

The Cerebellum. The cerebellum lies dorsal to the pons and medulla and actually wraps around the brain stem (Kelly & Dodd, 1991). It resembles the cerebral cortex in that it has distinct lobes and a foliated surface. The cerebellum receives afferent somatosensory pathways from the spinal cord, efferent motor relays from higher cortical areas, and input about balance from the vestibular system of the inner ear (Kelly & Dodd, 1991). The body integrates all this information to plan and coordinate movement and posture.

The Diencephalon. The thalamus and the hypothalamus lie in the area called the *diencephalon*. It is the primary synaptic relay center of the brain for different sensory modalities, including somatic sensation, audition, and visual information. The *thalamus* distributes sensory information to the sensory cortex and also mediates motor functions by acting as a conduit for information from the cerebellum and the basal ganglia to the motor cortex.

The *hypothalamus* lies beneath the thalamus, with numerous afferent and efferent pathways to and from the other areas of the brain and the pituitary gland. The hypothalamus plays a vital role in the control of the endocrine system, the autonomic nervous system, and the limbic system through the release of hormones (see Fig. 2–4). Functions and activities regulated by the hypothalamus include temperature regulation, eating and drinking (appetite), metabolism, glucose utilization, blood pressure and fluid balance (osmolarity), sexual behavior, and emotional response.

NEUROPHYSIOLOGY AND BEHAVIOR

All behavior is generated and controlled by the nervous system. Nerve tissue is the most fragile of all tissue types and does not have regenerative and restorative abilities—injury to neurons within the brain and spinal cord is permanent. Protective bone structures such as the skull and the spinal column exist to prevent injury from external sources. Physiological mechanisms exist as well to shield the fragile brain tissue from chemical or mechanical injury. One of these mechanisms is a type of nerve cell called *glia*, or "nerve glue." Microglia and macroglia hold the conducting neurons in place and sequester extracellular potassium, thereby protecting neighboring neurons from inappropriate depolarization.

A particular type of glia, the astrocyte, wraps around penetrating capillaries and arterioles to stabilize them but, more important, to create a barrier between the blood vessels and the nervous tissue. This *blood–brain barrier* is impermeable to many substances that circulate in the blood stream yet are toxic to brain tissue. The blood–brain barrier prohibits molecules of low lipid solubility and strongly ionized agents from leaving the blood and entering the brain tissue (Benet et al., 1993). Most drugs do not cross this barrier, nor do large molecular bodies such as bacteria and blood cells, which would contaminate the neural tissue. Phagocytic microglia act as scavengers to remove by-products and other debris from the brain tissue and are the basis of scar formation in injured brain tissue.

Neurons

The most abundant type of nerve cell is the conducting neuron, which generates and transmits nerve impulses. *Dendrites* are projections from the neuron cell body that receive impulses from adjacent neurons. The *axon*, another projection from the cell body, is responsible for impulse propagation to other cells (see Fig. 2–3).

Synaptic Transmission

The propagation of electrochemical impulses from neuron to neuron is the basic mechanism for all nervous system activity. This process, known as *synaptic transmission*, is accomplished by the transfer of ionic charge along the cell membrane of the conducting neuron to the targeted receiving neuron. Ion channels (microscopic water-filled tunnels that perforate the cell membrane) open and close, depending on cellular demands, and allow ions such as sodium, potassium, and calcium to diffuse into or out of the cell. As ions flow across the cell membrane, the voltage charge increases to a critical threshold and an impulse is generated. This electrochemical impulse is called an *action potential*. As the action potential moves toward the end of the axon (terminal bouton), the voltage change triggers the release of neurochemicals called *neurotransmitters* from their storage vesicles into the extracellular space (synaptic cleft). These neurochemicals diffuse across the synaptic cleft and attach to specific receptor sites to initiate the impulse at the next neuron (see Fig. 2–4). After the impulse is transferred, some of the neurotransmitter remains in the synaptic cleft and is either broken down by enzymatic processes or reabsorbed into the presynaptic membrane by the process of reuptake. These processes of neurotransmitter degradation or reuptake can be altered by the action of psychotropic medications (Kandel, 1991b; Kolb & Wishaw, 1990). The psychopharmacological agent may increase or decrease the degradation or reuptake of the transmitter to alter its activity and "normalize" the transmitter levels. This regulation serves to alleviate the symptoms of mental illness.

Neurotransmitters

Neurotransmitters in the brain play an important role in normal function and survival. Many neurological diseases and virtually all medications that act on the nervous system influence the neurotransmitter systems in some way. Neurotransmitters have either excitatory or inhibitory abilities, and a few have both, depending on the nature of the postsynaptic membrane. Excitatory transmitters generate an action potential in the receiving neuron, whereas an inhibitory neurotransmitter dampens or stops the activity of the receiving neuron.

There are four classes of neurotransmitters: the biogenic amines, acetylcholine, the amino acids, and the peptides (see Table 26–1).

TABLE 26–1
Classes of Neurotransmitters

- Biogenic amines (monoamines)
  - Catecholamines
    - Dopamine
    - Norepinephrine
    - Epinephrine
  - Indoleamines
    - Serotonin
- Acetylcholine
- Amino acids
  - Glutamate
  - Aspartate
  - Glycine
  - Gamma-aminobutyric acid
- Peptides

Biogenic Amines

The first class of neurotransmitters is known as the biogenic amines, or monoamines. This class is divided into two subclasses: indoleamines and catecholamines. Serotonin is an indoleamine. Dopamine, norepinephrine, and epinephrine are catecholamines.

Indoleamines. *Serotonin*, also known as 5-hydroxytryptamine (5-HT), is hypothesized to play a significant role in states of consciousness, mood, depression, anxiety, and possibly schizophrenia (Leonard, 1993) (see Chapter 12). Serotonin is synthesized from the amino acid L-tryptophan. It is metabolized by monoamine oxidase (MAO) to yield 5-hydroxyindoleacetic acid, which can be assayed by 24-hour urine collection. Specialized nuclei, the upper and caudal raphe nuclei located within the pons, secrete serotonin to the serotonergic pathways and their target brain areas: the upper brain stem, the limbic system, and the hypothalamic-pituitary axis (Leonard, 1993) (see Fig. 9–1).

There are at least three different receptors and a number of subreceptors for serotonin. Lysergic acid, a commonly abused hallucinogen, is an agonist of serotonin in that it mimics serotonin's action at receptor sites. A relatively newer class of antidepressant medication, the selective serotonin reuptake inhibitors (SSRIs), acts by specifically blocking the reuptake of serotonin in the synapse thereby increasing levels of serotonin in the synaptic cleft (Kandel, 1991a; Kolb & Wishaw, 1990).

Catecholamines

Dopamine. The catecholamine dopamine is perhaps the single most important neurotransmitter, because it affects a large number of neurological functions. Dopamine is largely synthesized in the substantia nigra and the ventral tegmentum and is concentrated in the nigrostriatal and mesolimbic dopaminergic tracts (see Fig. 12–1). It is used particularly in the limbic system but also diffusely throughout the brain, and is believed to play a role in the initiation and execution of movement and regulation of emotional responses. Overactivity of dopamine is hypothesized to play a central role in many of the symptoms of schizophrenia (see Chapter 12 and Fig. 12–1). It also plays a role in the regulation of the endocrine system by alerting the hypothalamus to manufacture hormones for storage and release by the pituitary (Leonard, 1993).

Dopamine is synthesized from the amino acids phenylalanine and tyrosine and metabolized by MAO and catechol-*O*-methyltransferase (Leonard, 1993). There are currently six known postsynaptic dopamine receptors: D_1, D_{2a}, D_{2b}, D_3, D_4, and D_5 (Kandel, 1991b). Each of these receptors may exert different dopaminergic influences; thus, abnormalities in the dopaminergic system can cause various mental illnesses that respond to different treatments.

Norepinephrine and Epinephrine. Norepinephrine is believed to play a role in learning and memory. Neurons in the locus ceruleus and the lateral tegmentum produce norepinephrine and supply the noradrenergic pathways to the cerebral cortex, limbic system, brain stem, and spinal cord (see Fig. 10–1).

Norepinephrine is found to be depleted in clients with Alzheimer's disease and Korsakoff's syndrome, contributing to characteristic symptoms of compromised short-term and long-term memory and limited learning ability (Kolb & Whishaw, 1990) (see Chapter 13). Norepinephrine is also believed to play a role in mood stabilization, depression, drive, and motivation (Leonard, 1993). The most commonly prescribed class of antidepressants, the tricyclic antidepressants, act by increasing levels of norepinephrine in the limbic system. Norepinephrine and epinephrine are also secreted by the adrenal glands and play important roles in the arousal of the autonomic nervous system and the stress response (see Fig. 11–1).

Norepinephrine is synthesized from dopamine and is metabolized in the same manner; however, its distribution in the brain is not as widespread. There are four known norepinephrine receptors in the brain stem and midbrain: alpha-1, alpha-2, beta-1, and beta-2. These receptors appear to provide evidence that norepinephrine plays a role in blood pressure regulation and skeletal muscle flexion and that it influences the thalamus, hypothalamus, hippocampus, and cerebral cortex (Leonard, 1993).

Acetylcholine

Acetylcholine is believed to be the main transmitter responsible for intellectual functioning. It is heavily concentrated in the anterior thalamic nucleus, the septal nuclei, and the association pathways that connect all the primary and association areas with the frontal lobe (see Fig. 13–1). Acetylcholine transfers the impulses that convey calculations, problem analysis, recognition, learning, and recall. Acetylcholine levels have been found to be low or depleted in clients with Alzheimer's disease and other forms of dementia (Kolb & Whishaw, 1990). Acetylcholine is also critical to skeletal and cardiac muscle excitation: it is released at the motor end plate to initiate the contraction of the muscle fibers. Interference with acetylcholine at this peripheral location is the underlying pathology of myasthenia gravis, a neuromuscular disease characterized by gradual weakening and wasting of muscle.

Amino Acids

A third class of neurotransmitters is the amino acids. They include glutamate, aspartate, glycine, and gamma-aminobutyric acid (GABA). *Glutamate* and *aspartate* are excitatory in nature. They are rapid acting and serve as intermediate neurotransmitters to regulate ionic conditions along the axon membrane prior to the release of the other transmitters at the synaptic cleft. A receptor common to both glutamate and aspartate is the *N*-methyl-*D*-aspartate (NMDA) receptor. This specialized receptor records new experiences for learning and future use as memory. NMDA receptors are particularly sensitive to the effects of alcohol and are the first receptor sites to be destroyed in chronic alcohol use. Glutamate and aspartate also participate in the motor impulses initiated in the cerebellum and the spinal cord.

Glycine and GABA are inhibitory in nature. Glycine can be found mainly in the corticohypothalamic projection pathways through the reticular activating system in the brain stem. It serves as the impulse modulator for messages going to the spinal cord and the peripheral nervous system. GABA is synthesized from glutamate and is present in much higher concentrations throughout the brain than all of the other neurotransmitters described here. GABA pathways exist between the cortex and the basal ganglia and between the limbic system and the hypothalamic-pituitary axis (see Fig. 10–1). It serves as the brain's modulator and limits the effects of the excitatory neurotransmitters. GABA inhibits neuronal transmission by hyperpolarizing the receptor site to render it less sensitive to continual stimulation. GABA acts in the basal ganglia to regulate sensorimotor impulses for smooth and controlled movement. Low levels of brain GABA predispose a person to convulsions and disorganized sensorimotor function. The choreatic movements that characterize Huntington's chorea are believed to be associated with a decrease in GABA activity (Kolb & Whishaw, 1990). Benzodiazepines enhance GABA binding to receptor sites and are effective in treating anxiety. Anticonvulsants work in a similar manner to modulate hyperstimulation and prevent seizures.

Peptides

Another class of neurotransmitters, the peptides, are involved in the activation and regulation of response to stress and injury such as pain perception and reflex functions. Some families of neuroactive peptides are the opioid endorphins, neurohypophyseal hormones such as vasopressin and oxytocin, and other vasoactive substances that become active in the brain to cause inhibition, excitation, or both when applied to certain target neurons.

Neurotransmitter Action

Much of the current knowledge about mental illness, neurological diseases, and the medications that treat them is based on the understanding of the role of neurotransmitters in synaptic transmission. Recall that the process of synaptic transmission by the axons of neurons is accomplished by an increase in sodium and potassium permeability across the cell membrane. The flow of ions creates an action potential that travels to the end of the axon, where the voltage changes trigger the release of neurotransmitters from the presynaptic membrane into the synaptic cleft (Kandel, 1991b; Kolb & Wishaw, 1990) (see Fig. 2–4).

The neurotransmitter diffuses across the synaptic cleft to the postsynaptic receptor sites on the receiving neuron. The neurotransmitter attaches to each of these sites in a manner similar to a key fitting a lock: the chemical structure makes an exact or close fit with the receptor site. Once attached, the neurotransmitter activates the postsynaptic receptor by opening the ion channels, changing the membrane potential, and initiating another action potential at the next neuron (Kandel, 1991b; Kolb & Wishaw, 1990). An excitatory transmitter generates an action potential in the receiving neuron (depolarization), whereas an inhibitory neurotransmitter dampens or prohibits the activity of the receiving neuron (hyperpolarization).

Once the transmitter has performed its function, it must be removed to terminate its action; otherwise, the action potential is abnormally prolonged, inhibited, or exaggerated. The production and release of excess neurotransmitter or the excessive sensitivity of the receptor site to the action of the neurotransmitter also produce an exaggerated effect. For example, excessive norepinephrine secretion could be a cause of anxiety disorders (see Fig. 10–1). Conversely, deficient synthesis or insufficient release of the neurotransmitter, or decreased sensitivity of the receptor site could also produce abnormal results; for example, low dopamine levels could be a factor in depression (Kandel, 1991b; Kolb & Wishaw, 1990). The action of the neurotransmitters is ended by one of two mechanisms: reuptake or enzymatic deactivation. The postsynaptic potentials produced by almost all transmitter substances are terminated by *reuptake*, in which the transmitter is rapidly pumped from the synaptic cleft back into the presynaptic terminal bouton. *Enzymatic deactivation* is accomplished by enzymes (frequently MAO) that metabolize the transmitter. Acetylcholine, dopamine, and norepinephrine activity are terminated in this way (Kandel, 1991b; Kolb & Wishaw, 1990).

This description of synaptic transmission is greatly oversimplified. In reality, the surface of any individual neuron may have 2000 to 3000 receptor sites that may be highly specialized or perform a variety of functions.

Behavior is the manifestation of the combined action potentials emerging from the masses of neurons in the primary and association areas in response to a person's thoughts. It stands to reason that many behaviors and neurological symptoms of organic disorders are a manifestation of disruption to the transmission processes described earlier. Brain injury from trauma or hypoxia or abnormal cell formation in tumor growth interferes with normal neural function and metabolism. With aging, the brain undergoes changes more gradually (Moran & Thompson, 1988). Its plasticity is reduced as neurons die and glia become more rigid with scar tissue. The blood–brain barrier becomes increasingly permeable, which compromises neural tissue integrity. The overall brain metabolic rate slows, and mentation may become cloudy as transmitter activity becomes sluggish or levels become suboptimal. Brain water is decreased, which lessens the absorbability of neuropharmacological agents. All these factors have significant pharmacokinetic implications for the effective treatment of abnormal neural processes present with mental illness.

PHARMACOKINETIC CONCEPTS

Pharmacology is the scientific study of chemical formulations (drugs), including their sources, properties, uses, actions, and effects. Two areas of concern for the psychiatric–mental health nurse are pharmacodynamics and pharmacokinetics. **Pharmacodynamics** refers to the actual biochemical and physiological effects on living tissue that are caused by the interaction of drugs with tissue receptors. In other words, pharmacodynamic principles focus on what the drug does to the body. **Pharmacokinetics**, on the other hand, is the study of the absorption, distribution, metabolism, and elimination of drugs. In other words, it is concerned with what the body does to the drug.

Pharmacodynamic and pharmacokinetic concepts are important, because they provide the psychiatric–mental health nurse with an understanding of the important properties of psychopharmaceutical agents, their therapeutic properties, their potential adverse effects, their use in the treatment of mental illness, and their interactions between other pharmaceutical agents and the impact of these interactions on human responses. Of recent interest is the potential role that race and ethnicity play in the pharmacokinetics of psychotropic drugs (see Research Abstract display). Pharmacokinetic principles are emphasized in the pharmacodynamic discussions of the psychotropic drugs described in this chapter.

FACTORS THAT INFLUENCE DRUG INTENSITY AND DURATION

The first set of concepts is concerned with the general pharmacokinetic effects of psychopharmaceutical agents. There are four factors that influence the intensity and duration of drug effect: absorption, distribution, metabolism, and elimination.

Absorption. *Absorption* is the process by which drug molecules pass from the site of administration into the systemic circulation. Absorption is affected by route of administration (e.g., oral, intramuscular, or intravenous), drug formulation, and such factors as food and antacids in the case of oral administration (Benet et al., 1993; Correia & Castagnoli, 1989).

Distribution. *Distribution* is the movement of drug from the site of administration throughout the body and dilution in body fluids. The *volume of distribution* is an indicator of the degree of distribution a drug undergoes. A drug with low-volume is limited to intravascular space. Medium distribution means the drug appears in most extracellular fluid, and high distribution means drug concentration occurs inside cells and body fats. Factors that affect the body-fat-to-water ratio such as age, sex, and weight, also affect drug distribution (Benet et al., 1993; Correia & Castagnoli, 1989).

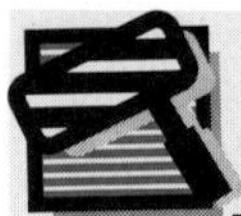

RESEARCH ABSTRACT

Ethnicity and Psychotropic Drugs.

Bond, W. S. (1991). *Clinical Pharmacy, 10,* 467–470.

Many studies have documented differential prescribing practices for psychotropic drugs with respect to the race of the client. Little, however, has been written about the pharmacokinetics and pharmacodynamics of these agents in clients of different races and ethnic backgrounds. Bond reviews the literature on research that compared or permitted comparisons for African American, Hispanic American, Asian American, and Caucasian subjects and makes recommendations based on the degree of confidence in the findings reported.

In general, the findings in the literature are lacking in confidence in most areas, as a result of small sample sizes, lack of control subjects and procedures, and inability to control for intervening variables. For example, it is noted that some studies comparing Caucasians with African Americans and Hispanic Americans with respect to therapeutic doses of antidepressant drugs are flawed because weight was not controlled, or they are otherwise inconclusive. Bond refrains from making any recommendations in this category of drugs.

Bond reports that Asian American clients require lower doses of antipsychotic drugs than do Caucasian, African American, or Hispanic American clients to maintain therapeutic effects. The reason for this seems to be increased absorption and reduced hepatic hydroxylation capacity, which result in higher serum concentrations. Bond recommends more research that takes into account body weight, surface area, and the influence of social habits. Claims have also been made for the use of lower doses of lithium in Asian American clients. Bond rejects this recommendation and suggests better controlled studies need to be undertaken before any conclusions can be made. On the other hand, survey data and pharmacokinetic studies provide convincing support for the use of lower initial doses of benzodiazepines in Asian American clients. Bond recommends that more pharmacokinetic and pharmacodynamic studies be done to increase our knowledge of the role that race and ethnicity play in the differential effects of psychotropic drugs.

Metabolism. *Metabolism* is the formation of active and inactive metabolites through conversion of a drug into a new, usually less active and more water-soluble compound and also by-products or waste products. The enzyme system responsible for metabolism of most drugs is located in the endoplasmic reticulum of the liver (known as the microsomal fraction). Other areas of metabolism are the epithelium of the gastrointestinal tract, the kidneys, the lungs, and the skin. The *first-pass effect* refers to the site of initial drug metabolism. As mentioned, the liver is the principle organ of drug metabolism. However, some drugs (e.g., clonazepam and chlorpromazine) are metabolized in the intestine. Thus the intestinal metabolism can contribute to the first-pass effect. First-pass effects, then, may limit the bioavailability of orally administered drugs such that alternate routes may need to be used to achieve the therapeutic blood levels desired (Benet et al., 1993; Correia & Castagnoli, 1989).

Elimination. *Elimination* is the removal of the drug, drug by-products, and inactive metabolites from the body, usually through urine or feces, perspiration, and respiration (Benet et al., 1993; Correia & Castagnoli, 1989).

STEADY STATE, HALF-LIFE, AND CLEARANCE

There are three other important concepts in the pharmacokinetics of drugs: steady state, half-life, and clearance.

Steady State. Steady state is the condition that occurs when the amount of drug removed from the body equals the amount being absorbed. The steady state is important because it represents the amount of drug thought to be required to achieve the desired therapeutic effects. Not all drugs have linear kinetics (a linear relationship between dose and plasma concentration) in steady state. **Linear kinetics** is a pharmacokinetic model in which a constant amount of a drug is eliminated in a set unit of time. It depicts the relationship between a drug's absorption and elimination necessary to achieve steady state. In linear kinetics, the drug half-life is *dose dependent*.

For certain drugs and for most drugs in large doses, however, the relationship is nonlinear. In this model, called *exponential kinetics*, the half-life of a drug is *independent of dose*. For example, this occurs with imipramine (Tofranil) in the elderly and in the long-term use of carbamazepine (Tegretol) or chlorpromazine (Thorazine). Caution is required, therefore, in increasing dosages into the upper range of acceptable prescribed dosages or in using these drugs in special populations such as the elderly or clients with concomitant illnesses—the likelihood of toxicity looms large (Benet et al., 1993; Correia & Castagnoli, 1989).

Half-life. A drug's *half-life* is the time in hours needed for the amount of drug in the body (as measured by plasma concentration) to decrease by one half, or 50 percent (Benet et al., 1993). The half-life of a drug is important for predicting the length of time necessary for the drug to be totally eliminated from the body. Drugs with long half-lives have slow rates of egress from the body. This information is useful; for example, when the physician is waiting for one antidepressant to be eliminated from the body before starting another. Such is the case when switching from treatment with an MAO inhibitor to an SSRI. For untoward effects to be avoided, drugs with short half-lives, such as the benzodiazepine triazolam (Halcion), may require tapering off of the dose rather than abrupt discontinuation (Benet et al., 1993; Correia & Castagnoli, 1989; Facts and Comparisons, 1993). The half-life of a drug is also important for determining the time required for achieving the stable concentration (or steady state) of a drug. In general, drugs require four to five half-lives to achieve steady state. Knowledge of a drug's half-life is also important for determining the frequency of dosing. Drugs with short half-lives require more frequent administration, whereas drugs with long half-lives can be administered in one daily dose.

Clearance. *Clearance* is the volume of blood in milliliters per minute from which all of the drug is removed per unit of time. Clearance determines the magnitude of the steady-state concentration and therefore the dosage required to achieve the desired steady state of a drug. Drugs that are efficiently eliminated by renal excretion and hepatic metabolism require a higher dosage regimen than do those that are inefficiently eliminated.

PROTEIN BINDING

Another important factor in understanding the pharmacokinetic properties of drugs is *protein binding*. Once a drug is absorbed into the vascular system, it is transported by protein molecules, usually albumin, to the site of action (Benet et al. 1993). The plasma proteins are generally unable to exit the vascular beds because of their molecular size. Similarly, protein-bound drugs are not able to exit unless they are freed from their binding sites. The stronger the binding site, the slower the freeing of drugs, resulting in a longer duration of action. As the drug is metabolized, more of the drug is released from the binding sites. Occasionally, two or more drugs compete for the same binding sites. When this occurs, the drug with the strongest affinity for the binding site displaces the other drug. When this interaction occurs, the displaced drug usually produces a toxic effect because a large concentration is free in the vascular bed (Benet et al., 1993; Correia & Castagnoli, 1989).

ACTIVE METABOLITES

Active metabolites play an important role in pharmacokinetics. With the exception of lithium, most of the psychopharmacological agents produce active metabolites during the process of metabolism. In general, the metabolites are more water soluble than the parent compound. The half-life of a metabolite is equal to, or longer than, that of its parent compound. The cyclic antidepressants, the antipsychotics, and some anxiolytics have major active metabolites. These drugs may require a longer time to reach a steady state. Hydroxylated and demethylated metabolites are generally pharmacologically active. Therefore, active metabolites complicate conclusions about the clinical effects of psychopharmaceutical agents based solely on serum levels and steady-state phenomena (Benet et al., 1993; Correia & Castagnoli, 1989).

PSYCHOPHARMACOLOGICAL THERAPEUTIC AGENTS

ANTIDEPRESSANTS

Depression is a common illness; it is estimated that 18 to 23 percent of women and 8 to 11 percent of men experience at least one serious depression in their lifetime (see Chapter 9). Untreated, depression can also be a dangerous illness: approximately 15 percent of clients with a primary affective illness (depression or manic-depressive illness) die by suicide (Bernstein, 1988). Historically, depression has been described as either endogenous or exogenous. Endogenous depressions were assumed to be the result of body-based changes and thus treatable with medication. Reactive or exogenous depressions were thought to occur in reaction to an environmentally caused event, such as the loss of a family member or a job. These depressions were "worked through" and not treated with medication. This dichotomy is currently generally rejected. The decision to use medication is now based on the severity of the presenting symptoms and *not* on presumed causality.

Antidepressants, as their name suggests, are medications prescribed to treat depression. In addition, antidepressants are used in the treatment of dysthmia, obsessive–compulsive disorder, panic attacks, anxiety, somatoform disorders, chronic pain, eating disorders, and childhood enuresis. Like the antipsychotics, most antidepressants have been categorized by their chemical structures. The newer antidepressants are being categorized by their chemical action. The clinical and pharmacokinetic parameters of the antidepressants are presented in Table 26–2.

Heterocyclics

The largest group of antidepressants can be described as *heterocyclic*, indicating their common structural characteristic: carbon rings. The most familiar type of antidepressants is a subgroup of the heterocyclic compounds called the tricyclic antidepressants or TCAs, so

TABLE 26-2
Clinical and Pharmacokinetic Parameters of Antidepressant Medications

GENERIC NAME	BRAND NAME	DOSAGE RANGE (MG/DAY)	HALF-LIFE (HOURS)	ONSET OF CLINICAL EFFECTS	ELIMINATION PERIOD AFTER LAST DOSE	AMINE BLOCKING ACTIVITY*
Tertiary Amines						
Amitriptyline	Elavil	75–200	31–46 (18–44 for nortriptyline)	2–4 weeks for all tertiary amines	≥2 weeks for tertiary amines	NE (2), 5HT (4)
Clomipramine	Anafranil	75–300	19–37			NE (2), 5HT (5)
Doxepin	Sinequan, Adapin	75–300	8–24 (desmethyline)			NE (1), 5HT (2)
Imipramine	Tofranil	75–200	11–25 (12–24 for desipramine)			NE (2), 5HT (4)
Trimipramine	Surmontil	75–200	7–30			NE (1), 5HT (1)
Secondary Amines						
Amoxapine	Asendin	150–300	8–30 (30 for 7-hydrox and 8-hydrox)	2–4 weeks for all secondary amines	2–4 weeks for all secondary amines	NE (3), 5HT (2), DA (2)
Desipramine	Norpramin	75–200	12–24			NE (4), 5HT (2)
Nortriptyline	Aventyl	75–150	18–44			NE (2), 5HT (3)
Protriptyline	Vivactyl	20–40	67–89			NE (4), 5HT (2)
Tetracyclic						
Maprotiline	Ludiomil	75–300	21–25	3–7 days 2–3 weeks	2 weeks	NE (3), 5HT (1)
Triazolopyridine						
Trazodone	Desyrel	50–600	4–9	1–4 weeks	2 weeks	5HT (3)
Bicyclics						
Fluoxetine	Prozac	20–80	2–5 days (7–9 days for norfluoxetine)	1–4 days	4 weeks	NE (1), 5HT (5)
Paroxetine	Paxil	20–50	5–21	Up to 8 weeks	2 weeks	NE (1), DA (1), 5HT (5)
Sertraline	Zoloft	50–200	24 N-desmethylsertraline (62–104 hours)	Up to 8 weeks	2 weeks	NE (1), DA (1), 5HT (5)
Aminoketone						
Bupropion	Welbutrin	200–300	8 days (4 weeks for active metabolites)	1–4 weeks	2 weeks	NE (1), 5HT (1), DA (1)

*NE = norepinepherine, DA = dopamine, 5HT = serotonin. 0 = none, 1 = very weak, 2 = weak, 3 = moderate, 4 = strong, 5 = strongest.

TABLE 26-3
Comparative Adverse Effects of Antidepressants

GENERIC NAME (BRAND NAME)	ANTICHOLINERGIC EFFECTS	SEDATION	ORTHOSTATIC HYPERTENSION
Tertiary Amines			
Amitriptyline (Elavil)	***	***	**
Clomipramine (Anafranil)	***	***	**
Doxepin (Tofranil)	**	***	**
Imipramine (Sinequan, Adapin)	**	**	***
Trimipramine (Surmontil)	**	**	**
Secondary Amines			
Amoxapine (Asendin)	***	**	*
Desipramine (Norpramin)	*	*	*
Nortriptyline (Aventyl)	**	**	*
Protriptyline (Vivactyl)	***	*	*
Tetracyclic			
Maprotiline (Ludiomil)	**	**	*
Triazolopyridine			
Trazodone (Desyrel)	*	**	**
Bicyclics			
Fluoxetine (Prozac)	*	0	*
Paroxetine (Palix)	*	0	*
Sertraline (Zoloft)	*	0	*
Aminoketone			
Bupropion (Welbutrin)	**	**	*

Incidence of side effects: *** = high, ** = moderate, * = some, 0 = none.

named because of the three carbon rings that characterize all the medications in this subclass. Maprotiline (Ludiomil) is considered a tetracyclic. Trazodone (Desyrel) is structurally unrelated to the tricyclics or tetracyclics but has many similar properties. Bupropion (Welbutrin) is also structurally unrelated to any other antidepressant; its mechanism of action is believed to be the facilitation of dopaminergic action, but the modus operandi is still unknown. Compared with classic TCAs, it is a weak blocker of the neuronal uptake of serotonin (Facts and Comparisons, 1993; Hollister, 1989).

Mechanism of Action. Until recently, the heterocyclics were thought to work by inhibiting the presynaptic reuptake of norepinephrine (a catecholamine) and serotonin (an indoleamine). Currently, however, several other hypotheses are being advanced. One approach focuses on the slower adaptive changes in norepinephrine and serotonin systems and the reregulation of an abnormal receptor–neurotransmitter relationship. It is thought that this reregulatory action speeds up the client's natural recovery process from a depressive episode by normalizing neurotransmission efficacy (Facts and Comparison, 1993). One specific reregulation hypothesis is the *down regulation theory*, which suggests that depression occurs concomitant with increased norepinephrine activity. According to this theory, antidepressants promote a down regulation of activity by decreasing beta-adrenergic receptor sensitivity to norepinephrine (Hollister, 1989). The mechanisms of action for trazodone and buproprion are poorly understood (Facts and Comparisons, 1993).

The heterocyclics are equally effective clinically, and many have similar metabolic pathways. These drugs are often divided into subgroups according to potency and secondary pharmacological properties, such as adverse reactions (Arana & Hyman, 1991; Hollister, 1989). As an example of grouping by *secondary properties*, the TCAs are grouped into secondary and tertiary amines. *Secondary amines* are considered activating antidepressants, whereas *tertiary amines* are considered sedating antidepressants. Thus, an activating secondary amine, desipramine (Norpramin), may be a useful choice for a client whose depression has retarded (slowed) his or her mental and physical activity, whereas imipramine, a commonly used tertiary sedating amine, may be a better choice for an agitated client who is not sleeping well.

Side Effects, Dosage, and Drug Interactions. Heterocyclic antidepressants usually take 2 to 4 weeks to have any significant antidepressant effect. Side effects, however, can occur within the first 24 hours and can continue throughout the drug course. A comparison of the relative degree of side effects for the antidepressants is presented in Table 26–3. Some side effects are to a client's benefit; for example, sedation is a benefit to a client suffering from insomnia. More frequently, however, side effects such as dry mouth, constipation, orthostatic hypertension, blurred vision, and impaired sexual arousal (erectile function and orgasm) are annoying at best and can seem debilitating at worst. To a person already suffering from depression these side effects can seem like too great a burden to bear. The nurse is in an excellent position to listen and offer hope by pointing out that the side effects will lessen and may disappear with time, whereas the antidepressant effects will increase.

It may take longer than 4 weeks to find the optimum dose of an antidepressant. Although 70 percent of clients respond positively to the first antidepressant prescribed, it is not unusual for a client to have to switch to another medication. This can be discouraging for the client. Again, the nurse can provide badly needed encouragement and perspective. All these medications can cause side effects to some degree in all clients (Arana & Hyman, 1991; Hollister, 1989). The associated symptoms of adverse effects of the antidepressants are presented in Table 26–4.

TABLE 26–4
Symptoms Associated with Adverse Effects of Tricyclics and Related Antidepressants

SYSTEM	COMMON ADVERSE EFFECTS	LESS COMMON ADVERSE EFFECTS
Cardiovascular	Orthostatic hypotension, tachycardia,	Palpitations
Central nervous	Drowsiness, weakness, fatigue, dizziness, tremors Maprotiline: headaches, restlessness Fluoxetine: headache, insomnia, anxiety Bupropion: agitation, headache, confusion, involuntary movements, ataxia, insomnia, seizures	Confusions, disturbed concentration, decreased memory, electrocardiographic changes
Neurological		Numbness, tingling, parasthesias of extremities, akathesia, ataxia, tremors, extrapyramidal side effects, neuropathy, seizures
Autonomic	Dry mouth, blurred vision, constipation, urinary retention Fluoxetine: excessive sweating	
Gastrointestinal	Maprotiline: nausea Trazodone: vomiting Fluoxetine: nausea, diarrhea, weight loss, dry mouth, anorexia Bupropion: nausea, vomiting, abdominal cramps, constipation, dry mouth	Vomiting, nausea, diarrhea, flatulence
Allergic		Skin rash, pruritis, urticaria, photosensitivity, itching, edema
Respiratory		Pharyngitis, rhinitis, sinusitis

Other possible side effects of heterocyclics include the following:

- Risk of seizure—all heterocyclics can lower the seizure threshold and must be used with caution in clients with a history of seizures. Moreover, maprotiline, clomipramine (Anafranil), and bupropion, even at therapeutic levels, have been associated with seizures in clients without a history of seizures.
- Cardiovascular risk—caution must be used when administering heterocyclics to clients with cardiovascular disease. In high doses, TCAs may produce arrhythmias, sinus tachycardia, and prolonged conduction time. Unlike other heterocyclics, trazodone has been associated with only minimal cardiovascular risks.
- Risk of overdose—heterocyclics can be lethal in an overdose, especially when combined with alcohol. Because the possibility of suicide is always a consideration with depressed clients, the potential lethality of heterocyclics can be a significant health problem.
- Priapism—this is defined as a persistent abnormal erection of the penis and has been reported in men taking trazodone. Therefore, trazodone must be prescribed with caution in men. The side effects should be carefully explained. The client should clearly understand the need to seek immediate attention should priapism or other sexual dysfunction occur.
- Metabolites—one of the breakdown products of the antidepressant amoxapine (Asendin) is loxapine (Loxitane). Because loxapine is an antipsychotic, it carries with it the risk of tardive dyskinesia (TD). Many prescribers are reluctant to prescribe amoxapine for this reason.

Possible drug interactions involving heterocyclics are the following:

1. Increased serum levels with concomitant use of fluoxetine (Prozac) or cimetidine (Tagamet)
2. Decreased therapeutic blood levels for some smokers
3. Increased pressor response to norepinephrine and intravenous epinephrine

Monamine Oxidase Inhibitors

Developed and prescribed in the early 1950s, the MAO inhibitors were the first effective antidepressants, as well as the first drugs that gave neuropharmacologists an opportunity to study the connection between neurotransmitters and mood (Bernstein, 1988). MAO is an enzyme that catalyzes the breakdown of various amines, including epinephrine, norepinephrine, serotonin, and dopamine. Inhibition of MAO results in an increased concentration of these amines in the synaptic cleft. Thus, the MAO inhibitor antidepressant effect is thought to result from the increased availability of CNS norepinephrine and serotonin (American Society of Hospital Pharmacists [ASHP], 1990). MAO inhibitors may be particularly useful with histrionic, hypochondriacal, or extremely obsessive or phobic clients and for clients with atypical depression (Arana & Hyman, 1991). The clinical and pharmacokinetic parameters are presented in Table 26–5.

There are two types of MAO currently described that display different preferences for substrates and inhibitors. *MAO-A* preferentially metabolizes norepinephrine and serotonin and has a selective sensitivity to the inhibitor clorgyline. *MAO-B* preferentially metabolizes phenylethylamine and benzylamine and has a selective sensitivity to the inhibitor selegiline (Eldepryl). The two MAO types appear to have distinct molecular structures and varying proportions of tissue distribution. For example, only MAO-A is contained in the intestinal mucosa, whereas MAO-B is contained in platelets and equal amounts of each in the liver and the brain (Baldessarini, 1993). The MAO inhibitors currently approved for use in the United States are relatively nonselective. However, in the treatment of depression, experimental MAO-A-type selective inhibitors may have advantages over the current nonselective agents (Baldessarini, 1993).

Side Effects, Dietary Precautions, and Drug Interactions. As Table 26–6 indicates, the side effects of MAO inhibitors are similar to those produced by the heterocyclics. The most troublesome common side effect is orthostatic hypotension. Furthermore, MAO inhibitors, when combined with tyramine-rich food or some medications, can also cause a hypertensive reaction, a potentially life-threatening condition. Tyramine is a monoamine present in some foods. A hypertensive reaction can be stimulated if the client ingests tyramine in food or takes some kinds of medications. Because MAO inhibitors prevent the body from breaking down this monoamine, tyramine can provoke the release of norepinephrine from endogenous stores in the body, causing an increase in blood pressure (Bernstein, 1988). Most hypertensive reactions are quite mild, with a 20 to 30 mm Hg rise in systolic blood pressure accompanied by headache, flushing, or sweating. An undetected severe reaction, although rare, can result in a cerebrovascular accident. The fear of a hypertensive crisis prevents many prescribers from using any medication in this class.

The general advice that can be given regarding dietary precautions with MAO inhibitor therapy is that any food subjected to fermentation during its processing or storage may be rich in tyramine and thus may present the risk of a hypertensive crisis. Foods that are very high in

TABLE 26–5
Clinical and Pharmacokinetic Parameters of Monoamine Oxidase Inhibitors

GENERIC NAME	BRAND NAME	DOSAGE RANGE (MG/DAY)	HALF-LIFE (HOURS)	ONSET (WEEKS)	DURATION (WEEKS)
Isocarboxazid	Marplan	30–50	?	1–4	2
Phenelzine	Nardil	45–90	?	4	2
Tranylcypromine	Parnate	30–60	1.5–3.2	2–21 days	3–5 days

TABLE 26–6
Symptoms Associated with Adverse Effects of Monoamine Oxidase Inhibitors

SYSTEM	COMMON ADVERSE EFFECTS	LESS COMMON ADVERSE EFFECTS
Cardiovascular	Orthostatic hypotension	Palpitations, tachycardia, peripheral edema
Central nervous	Dizziness, headache, confusion, fatigue, drowsiness	Akathesia, ataxia, neuritis, chills, vertigo, memory impairment, weakness, restlessness, hyperflexia, tremors
Gastrointestinal	Constipation, nausea, vomiting	Dysuria, diarrhea, urinary retention, incontinence
Miscellaneous	Dry mouth, blurred vision	Excessive sweating, nystagmus, weight gain

tyramine include cheeses such as Camembert, cheddar, Emmenthaler, and Stilton; meats such as fermented sausages (bologna, pepperoni, salami, and summer sausage); fish (especially herring); overripe fruits, such as avocados; and Chianti wine. Other foods that have vasopressors and should be used in moderation include beers, wines, chocolate, and coffee (Facts and Comparisons, 1993).

Some drugs must also be avoided. Phenylethylamine compounds, including amphetamines, phenylpropanolamine, ephredine, phenylephrine, and related stimulants; decongestants; and bronchodilators all may provoke severe reactions in clients treated with MAO inhibitors. The narcotic meperidine (Demerol) must be avoided. Persons taking MAO inhibitors must also avoid concomitant use of heterocyclics and SSRIs. There must be an antidepressant-free period when the client stops an MAO inhibitor before beginning another class of antidepressants and vice versa (Facts and Comparisons, 1993). Any nurse involved in client education is urged to consult a more detailed source. The list of foods and medicines to avoid can appear intimidating to both the prescriber and the client. This probably explains why MAO inhibitors are rarely initially prescribed as a first choice. However, it should be emphasized that these can be very useful medications, especially in clients with serious, difficult-to-treat depression. Many clients are willing to live with the proscriptions if they can experience relief from depression.

Selective Serotonin Reuptake Inhibitors

The SSRIs are the newest class of antidepressants and differ from the preceding classes of drugs in several important ways. As their name implies, these medications appear to affect only one neurotransmitter, serotonin. It is thought that they act by selectively inhibiting serotonin uptake, without significantly affecting norepinephrine uptake mechanisms (Bernstein, 1988; DeVane, 1992). Thus, their action appears to be more specific and their side effect profile more narrow. SSRIs currently available in the United States included fluoxetine, which has been available the longest; sertraline (Zoloft); and paroxetine (Paxil) (see Table 26–2).

The SSRIs have diverse structures. Paroxetine, for example, is a phenylpiperidine derivative, whereas sertraline is a naphthalenamine derivative. The efficacy of paroxetine and sertraline for the management of major depression has been established by controlled studies of 6 to 8 weeks principally in outpatient settings (DeVane, 1992; Facts and Comparisons, 1993). Paroxetine's metabolism through the microsomal enzyme P450IID6 suggests potential drug interactions and dosage adjustments. Caution should be used with the coadministration of paroxetine and other drugs metabolized by this isozyme, including MAO inhibitors, phenothiazines, and type IC antiarrhythmics (e.g., flecainide, encainide, and propafenone) or drugs that inhibit this enzyme (e.g., quinidine) (Facts and Comparisons, 1993).

SSRIs have a more rapid onset of action than do the other classes of antidepressants—1 to 3 weeks, rather than the 2 to 4 weeks suggested for the heterocyclics. Of note, fluoxetine has a significantly longer half-life than do most other antidepressants, which means that it will take much longer to clear out of the client's system on discontinuation of the medication (Facts and Comparisons, 1993). It has been recommended for all the SSRIs that an MAO inhibitor not be used concomitantly and that at least 5 weeks should lapse between discontinuation of an SSRI and initiation of therapy with an MAO inhibitor. Similarly, at least 2 weeks should be provided from the discontinuation of MAO inhibitor therapy and the initiation of therapy with an SSRI (Facts and Comparisons, 1993).

The side effect profile for SSRIs differs from those of the heterocyclics and MAO inhibitors. Common side effects include restlessness, insomnia, nausea, diarrhea, headache, dizziness, dry mouth, and tremor; ejaculatory delay may also occur in males (Bernstein, 1988; Facts and Comparisons, 1993). Unlike most other antidepressants, fluoxetine does not stimulate the appetite or cause carbohydrate craving. On the contrary, there is some evidence that SSRIs decrease appetite and can lead to weight loss. The SSRIs rarely appear to affect the electrocardiogram and have only minimal cardiovascular effects (Bernstein, 1988; DeVane, 1992).

The SSRIs appear to be much safer in overdose than other antidepressants and are not potentiated by alcohol. These features are attractive when one is prescribing to a population with a higher than average risk of suicide. Finally, the SSRIs need less dosage titration than do the heterocyclic and MAO inhibitor antidepressants. In general, this makes them easier to prescribe and easier to take.

A potential problem that can arise for clients taking medications that affect serotonin is called **serotonin syndrome**, a condition of serotonergic hyperstimulation (Sternbach, 1991). It can be caused by various combinations of medications, but it most commonly results from the combination of MAO inhibitors with serotonergic agents. These serotonergic agents include L-tryptophan (an amino acid precursor of serotonin) as well as fluoxetine, clomipramine, and paroxetine. The possibility of serotonergic syndrome provides additional rationale for the waiting period between antidepressant therapies involving MAO inhibitors.

The most frequent clinical features of serotonin syndrome are changes in mental status, restlessness, myoclonus, hyperreflexia, diaphoresis, shivering, and tremor. Obviously, though, these symptoms are not specific to serotonin syndrome. Careful observation of clients on medication and an understanding of serotonin syndrome enable the nurse to be alert to this possibility. The treatment of choice is to discontinue the involved medications and provide supportive measures (Sternbach, 1991).

LITHIUM

Lithium is a naturally occurring alkali metal that shares some characteristics with other monovalent cations, such as sodium and potassium, but not others. In 1949, Cade, in Australia, was the first to report the therapeutic effects of lithium in mania. However, lithium was not approved for use in the United States until 1970 because of reported severe and sometimes fatal cases from its uncontrolled use as a substitute for sodium chloride. Lithium is used to treat acute hypomanic or manic episodes and recurrent affective disorders. Table 26–7 presents the clinical and pharmacokinetic parameters of lithium. Seventy to ninety percent of clients with "typical" bipolar illness respond to lithium (Arana & Hyman, 1991). Although lithium has been shown to have mild antidepressant properties, it is not as effective as other antidepressants. Sometimes it is used to treat schizoaffective disorders, often in conjunction with an antipsychotic. Lithium also has nonpsychiatric uses. For example, clients taking lithium have an increased white blood cell count. This effect led to lithium's being used to improve the neutrophil count in clients with neutropenia secondary to chemotherapy for cancer or acquired immune deficiency syndrome (Facts and Comparisons, 1993). Lithium is useful in reducing drinking in alcoholics who display signs of depression or mania. In addition, lithium is frequently added to an antipsychotic agent to treat an otherwise treatment-resistant client.

Mechanism of Action. Although recognized as the drug of choice to treat manic–depressive illness, lithium's exact mechanism of action remains speculative. An important characteristic of lithium is its small gradient distribution across biological membranes. Although lithium can replace sodium in support of a single action potential, it cannot replace the action of sodium in the sodium pump and therefore cannot maintain membrane potentials (Baldessarini, 1993). Lithium's effect on transmembrane ion pumps can possibly alter the distribution of sodium, potassium, and calcium ions. However, these effects appear to occur at higher than therapeutic concentrations of lithium. Lithium has also been shown to effect neurotransmitter activity of serotonin and norepinephrine, resulting in a more stable system (Facts and Comparisons, 1993). The actual importance of this effect is uncertain (Baldessarini, 1993).

Other evidence suggests that lithium's effects are due to its action through a second-messenger system (Baldessarini, 1993; Hollister, 1989; Leonard, 1993). One second-messenger system involves lithium's inhibition of receptor-mediated activation of adenyl cyclase. Because this effect occurs at lithium levels outside the therapeutic concentration levels, it is an unlikely mechanism. However, the inhibition of adenyl cyclase may contribute to some of lithium's toxic effects, such as an increase in urine concentration and antithyroid effects. Another, more likely second-messenger system occurs at therapeutic concentrations of lithium. Lithium blocks the ability of neurons to restore normal levels of the membrane phospholipid phosphatidylinositol 4,5-biphosphate (PIP_2) after it is hydrolyzed after activation of receptors. PIP_2 is hydrolyzed into two second messengers: diacylglycerol and inositol 1,4,5-triphosphate (IP_3). IP_3 acts to release calcium from intracellular stores, which sets off a cascade of events in many cellular processes. Because the IP_3 cannot cross the blood–brain barrier, the brain must regenerate its own IP_3. Depletion of PIP_2 from cells may reduce the responsiveness of neurons to muscarinic cholinergic, alpha-adrenergic, or other stimuli. Thus, lithium could modulate the hyperactive neurons that contribute to the manic state (Arana & Hyman, 1991; Baldessarini, 1993).

Effects, Side Effects, and Compliance. When used to treat acute hypomanic or manic episodes, lithium can begin to be effective in 1 to 2 weeks, but it may take as long as several months to stabilize the mood fully. Antipsychotics and benzodiazepines are often used to manage the behavioral excitement and psychotic symptoms during the early stages of lithium therapy (Arana & Hyman, 1991; Leonard, 1993). Lithium is used for maintenance therapy, with the goal of decreasing the number, severity, and frequency of the affective episodes. Even

TABLE 26–7
Clinical and Pharmacokinetic Parameters of Bipolar Agents

BIPOLAR AGENTS	BRAND NAME	DOSAGE RANGE (MG/DAY)	HALF-LIFE (HOURS)	ONSET (WEEKS)	DURATION
Lithium carbonate	Lithium, Eskalith	Acute: 1800 Maintenance 900–1200	21–30	5–14 days	2 weeks
Carbamezepine	Tegretol	400–1200	25–65	Varies	6–12 hours

with regular lithium, some clients can experience symptoms, periods of distress, and unpleasant side effects.

About 20 to 30 percent of clients discontinue lithium therapy on their own (Arana & Hyman, 1991; Facts and Comparisons, 1993). The reasons vary. Some clients deny their need for lithium because they deny they have an illness. Some stop taking it after the episode has resolved, believing that prophylactic use of the medication is not necessary. Others like the feeling of being high during a manic episode, and others report that lithium decreases their creativity and productivity. Finally, some clients stop taking lithium because of its side effects. The nurse needs to assess clients' reasons for stopping medication before lecturing or educating them about compliance.

The common side effects of lithium can include polydipsia, polyuria, tremor, gastric irritation, diarrhea, fatigue, mental dullness, and weight gain. Many of these side effects appear only in the first days. However, though possibly transient and clinically benign, these side effects can be so bothersome to clients that they stop taking the drug. Often, propranolol (Inderal) is given to alleviate lithium-induced tremor. Clinically adverse cardiovascular reactions are rarely seen with lithium at therapeutic levels, although serious cardiovascular conditions can occur in overdose (Facts and Comparisons, 1993; Leonard, 1993).

A second category of side effects may result from either chronic administration of an inappropriately high dose or an acute overdose of lithium (see Table 26–8). These toxic reactions usually occur at serum levels higher than 2 mEq/L, although they can occur at lower levels, especially with elderly patients. Gastrointestinal symptoms may appear, followed by CNS depression, which can include somnolence, sluggishness, ataxia, dysarthria, seizures, increased muscle tone, and increased deep tendon reflexes. At serum levels of 3 mEq/L or higher, cardiovascular collapse can occur. Changes in a client's status in such areas as decreased serum sodium levels, use of diuretics, decreased renal function, and pregnancy can result in the accumulation of lithium and result in toxicity (Facts and Comparisons, 1993; Leonard, 1993).

Lithium is excreted almost entirely by the kidneys. Thus, effective regulation of lithium depends in part on the sodium and fluid balance of the body (Arana & Hyman, 1991); Baldessarini, 1993; Leonard, 1993). As an example, sodium depletion can lead to marked lithium retention and possible toxicity. Conversely, high levels of lithium can lead to sodium excretion. Because diuretics affect kidney action, they can also affect lithium levels. Thiazide diuretics commonly cause increased levels of lithium by decreasing clearance; this can happen quite quickly. Potassium-sparing diuretics may also cause moderate increases in lithium levels over time. Osmotic drugs and carbonic anhydrase inhibitors such as acetazolamide (Diamox) can decrease lithium levels by increasing excretion (Facts and Comparisons, 1993).

Long-term lithium therapy can have serious consequences for clients. It can cause a decrease in thyroid hormones (Arana & Hyman, 1991; Facts and Comparisons, 1993). Most clients can compensate for this initial decrease; about 5 percent develop signs of hypothyroidism and may need to take thyroid medication. Because hypothyroidism can be confused with depression, the clinician needs to keep both possibilities in mind.

The second serious adverse reaction that can occur with long-term lithium therapy is permanent structural changes in the kidneys. These changes result in chronic tubulointerstitial nephropathy. Because both the thyroid and kidney changes are potentially serious concerns, several guidelines need to be followed:

1. Thyroid and kidney screening tests must be performed before lithium is prescribed and then must be performed on a regular follow-up basis.
2. Regular lithium levels must be obtained.
3. The client should always be maintained on the lowest possible amount of lithium.
4. Because dehydration may increase kidney damage, adequate fluid intake must be maintained.

Nonsteroidal anti-inflammatory drugs (NSAIDs), such as ibuprofen, fenoprofen, etodolac, tolmetin, and piroxicam, can increase lithium levels (Facts and Comparisons, 1993). The exception is sulindac. Because NSAIDs are available over the counter, the possibility of this drug interaction is often missed by clinicians.

Finally, an encephalopathic syndrome, similar to neuroleptic malignant syndrome, has occurred in a few clients treated with an antipsychotic plus lithium. Al-

TABLE 26–8
Adverse Effects Associated with Lithium Therapy

PLASMA LEVEL (MEQ/L)	COMMON ADVERSE EFFECTS	LESS COMMON ADVERSE EFFECTS
<1.5	Initial treatment: fine hand tremors, polyuria, mild thirst, transient and mild nausea and discomfort Afterwards: fatigue, acne, electrocardiographic changes, hypothyroidism	Twitching, muscular weakness, restlessness, dry and thinning hair
1.5–2.0	Diarrhea, vomiting, nausea, drowsiness, muscle weakness, lack of coordination (may be early signs of toxicity)	
2.0–3.0	Giddiness, ataxia, blurred vision, tinnitus, vertigo, increasing confusion, slurred speech, blackouts, incontinence, fasciculation, myoclonic twitching, hyperlexia, hypertonia	
>3.0	Seizures, arrythmias, hypotension, peripheral vascular collapse, stupor, spasticity, coma	

though rare, the possibility of this syndrome increases the need to monitor clients for neurological toxicity (Facts and Comparisons, 1993).

Dosage and Toxicity. Lithium is available as a carbonate (pills, tablets, or Eskalith) and as a citrate (liquid). It is usually prescribed to be taken two or three times a day, although some prescribers believe once-daily dosing is effective. Lithium has a rather narrow range of effectiveness: too little lithium has little therapeutic value, but only a little too much can produce toxicity. Because of this narrow range, clients need to be well educated about signs of toxicity. It is for this reason also that clients on lithium are required to have serum lithium levels obtained. Initially, these are required frequently as the correct dosing regimen is sought. When stable, lithium levels are required every 1 to 3 months. The lithium level needs to be determined 12 hours after the client's last dose to be interpreted correctly. Although values may differ among laboratories, the usual therapeutic range is 0.5 to 1.5 mEq/L. When clients with manic–depressive illness do not respond to lithium or cannot tolerate it, other agents can be used (Arana & Hyman, 1991; Baldessarini, 1993; Bernstein, 1988).

Nonresponding Clients. Although lithium is considered the mainstay of pharmacological intervention for most clients with bipolar disorder, it is recognized that some clients with classic bipolar disorder and a significant number of clients with bipolar variants do not respond to lithium therapy. This subgroup of nonresponders may include those with rapid-cycling bipolar disorder (four or more affective episodes per year), schizoaffective disorder, or dysphoric or mixed mania (defined as a state that simultaneously has both manic and depressive elements); the elderly; and those with manias arising from CNS diseases and conditions caused by strokes, tumors, closed and open head injuries, and infections. It is also evident that some persons whose symptoms are controlled with lithium cannot tolerate its short- or long-term side effects.

ANTICONVULSANTS

The two most common medication alternatives to lithium for the treatment and prophylaxis of mania are carbamezepine and valproic acid (Depakene), both better known as anticonvulsants. Like lithium, both carbamazepine and valproic acid exert some antidepressant effect prophylactically, but they are not effective as primary agents in treating depression.

Carbamazepine

Carbamazepine is prescribed for a number of conditions, including convulsive disorder, trigeminal neuralgia, phantom limb pain, alcohol withdrawal, and restless leg syndrome (see Table 26–7). An unlabeled indication is neuronal diabetes insipidus (Facts and Comparisons, 1993). Carbamazepine has also been found to exert potent antimanic effects (DiSalver et al., 1993; Facts and Comparisons, 1993; Leonard, 1993). It has recently been used for treating intermittent explosive behavior disorder, which is associated with undiagnosed temporal lobe epilepsy. Although its mechanism of action is unknown, there has been a focus on carbamazepine's ability to inhibit kindling. *Kindling* is defined as increasing behavioral and convulsive responses occurring in reaction to the repetition of the same stimulus over time.

Side Effects, Toxicity, and Drug Interactions. As with lithium, screening blood tests are necessary. Carbamazepine can cause aplastic anemia and agranulocytosis (Facts and Comparisons, 1993; Leonard, 1993). Although the incidence of these reactions is low, a complete blood count, including platelets, reticulocytes, chemical screen, and electrolytes, is suggested before initiating treatment and should be repeated on a regular basis while the client continues on carbamazepine. In addition, regular testing is also required to check serum levels. The nurse can explain the rationale for this required blood study as well as provide encouragement around the sometimes frustrating need for regular venipuncture. The nurse can remind the client of the importance of reporting any signs and symptoms of possible hematological problems: fever, sore throat, mouth ulcers, easy bruising, petechiae, or purpural hemorrhage. Any rash needs to be reported immediately.

Initial treatment with carbamazepine may be associated with mild degrees of sedation, tremor, slurred speech, nausea, vomiting, vertigo, ataxia, and blurred vision (Facts and Comparisons, 1993; Leonard, 1993). The client is encouraged to take carbamazepine with food to decrease any nausea. Generally, these side effects lessen over time. If they persist or worsen, toxicity should be considered, the medication discontinued, and a serum level obtained.

Carbamazepine is a pharmacologically complicated drug, with several drug interactions that should be kept in mind. Besides inducing its own metabolism, it induces the metabolism of other drugs. For example, the concentration of antipsychotic medication (especially haloperidol [Haldol]) is decreased when carbamazepine is co-administered. This means that a client with previously well-controlled symptoms may experience a worsening of symptoms when carbamazepine is administered. The nurse can help clients monitor their symptoms during this initial period. Carbamazepine may reduce the effect of birth control pills and can cause birth defects. Both clients and their prescribers need to be aware that a higher dose of birth control pills may be required. Erythromycin can inhibit carbamazepine metabolism and lead to carbamazepine toxicity. Some additional medications that interact with carbamazepine metabolism and lead to toxicity are cimetidine, verapamil (Isoptil) and isoniazid (INH). Conversely, carbamazepine may increase the risk of isoniazid-induced hepatotoxicity (Facts and Comparisons, 1993).

Valproic Acid and Its Derivatives

This group includes valproic acid, its sodium salt valproate, and divalproex sodium (Depakote). Regardless of the form, the dosage is expressed as valproic acid equivalents. Valproic acid is prescribed as an anticonvulsant. Its mechanism of action is unclear, but it is thought to be a GABA-ergic drug. It, too, has been found to exert antimanic effects (DiSalver et al., 1993; Leonard, 1993).

As with lithium and carbamazepine, screening blood tests are necessary. Valproic acid has been reported to cause hepatic failure, although the incidence is low. Children younger than 2 years of age and clients on multiple anticonvulsants with severe seizure disorders accompanied by mental retardation appear to be the groups at greatest risk (Facts and Comparisons, 1993). Thus, liver function tests are suggested before valproic acid is begun. The nurse can review with the client the potential signs and symptoms of liver failure (malaise, weakness, lethargy, facial edema, anorexia, jaundice, and vomiting) as well as monitor for these signs and symptoms. A complete blood count including platelets is also recommended, because thrombocytopenia has been reported. These tests, along with valproic acid serum levels, need to be performed regularly while the client is on valproic acid.

Initial treatment with valproic acid may be associated with drowsiness, tremor, and nausea. Pure valproic acid is *very* poorly tolerated by clients; the enteric-coated preparation (Depakote) is preferred. Valproic acid's most significant drug interactions involve its effects on other anticonvulsants; otherwise, it has few significant drug interactions.

Overall, both valproic acid and carbamazepine are often better tolerated than lithium by clients (DiSalver et al., 1993; Leonard, 1993). Although both carbamazepine and valproic acid are prescribed as single-agent medications, it is not unusual to see either of them used in combination with lithium. As is true with lithium, both carbamazepine and valproic acid are dangerous in overdose. Because carbamazepine and valproic acid are anticonvulsants, neither should be stopped abruptly because that may precipitate status epilepticus. Other agents under consideration in the treatment of bipolar affective disorders include clonazepam (Klonopin), propranolol, clonidine (Catapres), bupropion, and verapamil.

ANTIPSYCHOTICS

The advent of antipsychotic medications in the early 1950s heralded a radical change in psychiatric care. Many clients who had been institutionalized indefinitely, often in inhumane conditions, were afforded symptom relief. The antipsychotic medications are divided into families based on their chemical structures. These structures also determine the mechanism of action of the medications. The clinical and pharmacokinetic parameters of the antipsychotics are presented in Table 26–9.

TABLE 26–9
Clinical and Pharmacokinetic Parameters of Antipsychotic Medications

GENERIC NAME	BRAND NAME	DOSAGE RANGE (MG/DAY)	ONSET (MINUTES)	DURATION OF ACTION (HOURS)	HALF-LIFE (HOURS)
Phenothiazines					
Apliphatic					
Chlorpromazine	Thorazine	30–800	30–60	4–6	10–20
Promazine	Sparine	40–1200	30–60	4–6	?
Triflupromazine	Vesprin	60–150	15–30	12	?
Piperidine					
Thioridazine	Mellaril	150-800	30–60	4–6	9–30
Mesoridazine	Serentil	30–400	30–60	4–6	?
Piperazine					
Acetophenazine	Tindal	60–120	30–60	4–6	?
Perphenazine	Trilafon	12–64	30–60	4–6	8–21
Prochlorperazine	Compazine	15–150	30–60	3–4	?
Fluphenazine	Prolixin	0.5–40	30–60	6–8	14–153 (3–10 days for active metabolites)
Trifluoperazine	Stelazine	2–40	30–40	4–6	?
Thioxanthene					
Chlorprothixene	Taractan	75–600	30–60	4–6	?
Thiothixene	Navane	8–30	slow	12–24	34
Butyrophenone					
Haloperidol	Haldol	1–15	erratic	24–72	12–38
Dihydroindolone					
Molindone	Moban	15–225	erratic	36	1.5
Dibenzoxazepine					
Loxapine	Loxitane	20–250	20–30	12	5–19
Dinenzodiazepine					
Clozapine	Clozaril	300–900			4–66
Diphenylbutylpiperidine					
Pimozide	Orap	1–10	varies	≥ 24	55 (mean)

Phenothiazine. The most commonly prescribed neuroleptics (antipsychotics) belong to the *phenothiazine* family. There are three distinct classes of this family. The *aliphatic phenothiazines* include chlorpromazine, promazine (Sparine), and triflupromazine (Vesprin) (Baldessarini, 1993). The aliphatic phenothiazines are relatively low in antipsychotic potency and high in sedation effects (DeVane, 1990). The *piperidine phenothiazines* include thioridazine (Mellaril) and mesoridazine (Serentil) (Baldessarini, 1993). These medications are of medium potency in antipsychotic actions, sedation, and extrapyramidal side effects (Baldessarini, 1993). The third class of phenothiazines are the *piperazines*. Commonly prescribed medications in this class include trifluperazine, fluphenazine (Prolixin), prochlorperazine (Compazine), and perphenazine (Trilafon) (Leonard, 1993). These medications are considered to be effective in controlling antipsychotic symptoms with little or no sedation, but they are more likely than more recently developed antipsychotics to cause extrapyramidal side effects (Baldessarini, 1993).

Butyrophenones. A second class of antipsychotic medications is the *butyrophenones*. The most commonly prescribed medication of this class is haloperidol. Haloperidol is considered similar in potency to the phenothiazine piperazines. It is also known to be related to extrapyramidal side effects, particularly acute dystonic reactions (DeVane, 1990).

Thioxanthenes. A third class of antipsychotics is the *thioxanthenes*, which include chlorprothixene (Taractan) and thiothixene (Navane). These medications are chemically similar to the phenothiazines and act in similar manners. Molindone (Moban), an indole, and loxapine are also commonly used antipsychotic medications.

Mechanism of Action

All antipsychotic medications just discussed act by blocking the actions of dopamine in the nigrostriatal area or the mesolimbic area of the brain (DeVane, 1990). A comparison of the degree of side effects of the various antipsychotics is presented in Table 26–10. It is currently believed that these medications have an affinity for the subtype of dopamine receptors known as D_2 receptors. The nigrostriatal area and the mesolimbic areas of the brain are rich in these receptors. The action in the mesolimbic area is believed to decrease the psychotic symptoms of hallucinations and delusions. Additional actions of these drugs include decreasing hostility and agitation, increasing organization in thought processes, and decreasing withdrawal behavior due to high anxiety and sensory overload associated with psychosis.

Side Effects

The action in the nigrostriatal area precipitates a set of side effects known as **extrapyramidal side effects**. These side effects include **akathesia**, a subjective feeling of restlessness (Table 26–11). Clients experiencing this side effect appear restless and move constantly. It is important to assess for akathesia, because it is often mistaken for agitation. The importance of assessment is indicated in the accompanying Research Abstract box.

TABLE 26–10
Comparative Adverse Effects of Antipsychotics

GENERIC NAME (BRAND NAME)	ANTICHOLINERGIC EFFECTS	SEDATION	EXTRAPYRAMIDAL SYMPTOMS	ORTHOSTATIC HYPERTENSION
Phenothiazines				
Apliphatic				
Chlorpromazine (Thorazine)	**	***	**	***
Promazine (Sparine)	***	**	**	**
Triflupromazine (Vesprin)	**	***	**	**
Piperidine				
Thioridazine (Mellaril)	***	***	*	**
Mesoridazine (Serentil)	***	***	*	**
Piperazine				
Acetophenazine (Tindal)	*	**	**	*
Perphenanzine (Trilafon)	*	*	**	*
Prochlorperazine (Compazine)	*	**	**	*
Fluphenazine (Prolixin)	*	*	**	*
Trifluoperazine (Stelazine)	*	*	**	*
Thioxanthene				
Chlorprothixene (Taractan)	**	***	**	**
Thiothixene (Navane)	*	*	**	*
Butyrophenone				
Haloperidol (Haldol)	*	*	*	*
Dihydroindolone				
Molindone (Moban)	*	**	*	0
Dibenzoxazepine				
Loxapine (Loxitane)	*	*	**	*
Dinenzodiazepine				
Clozapine (Clozaril)	*	*	0	*
Diphenylbutylpiperidine				
Pimozide (Orap)	**	*	***	*

Incidence of side effects: *** = high, ** = moderate, * = low, 0 = none.

TABLE 26–11
Extrapyramidal Side Effects from Antipsychotic Medications

	ACUTE DYSTONIA	AKATHISIA	AKINESIA	DYSKINESIA	DYSTONIA	TARDIVE DYSKINESIA
Manifestations	Painful and frightening to the client Rapid-onset oculogyric crisis Opisthotonos Torticollis	Subjective feelings of restlessness Tenseness or jumpiness Inability to sit still Rocking back and forth on feet Crossing legs frequently Inability to relax	Masklike face No swinging of arms Hesitancy of speech Decreased muscle strength Shuffling gait Pill-rolling motion Drooling	Involuntarily muscular activity shown by tic, spasm, tremor of face, arms, legs, and neck Resting tremor Rabbit syndrome	Tongue protrusion Rigidity Cogwheeling Complaints of feeling stiff or inability to move easily Numbness of limbs Hyperflexia Tight feeling in throat	Protrusion of tongue Chewing movement Puffing of cheeks Pelvic thrusting
Onset (days)	1–5	4–72	5–30	1–5	1–5	Months up to 2 or more years after treatment was begun
Treatment	Antiparkinsonian medications Symptoms disappear when antipsychotic is discontinued or dosage is reduced	Antiparkinsonian medications Symptoms disappear when antipsychotic is discontinued or dosage is reduced	Antiparkinsonian medications Symptoms disappear when antipsychotic is discontinued or dosage is reduced	Antiparkinsonian medications Symptoms disappear when antipsychotic is discontinued or dosage is reduced	Antiparkinsonian medications Symptoms disappear when antipsychotic is discontinued or dosage is reduced	No effective treatment Prevention is essential

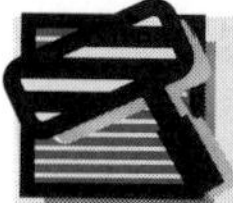

RESEARCH ABSTRACT

Identifying Akinesia and Akathisia: The Relationship Between Patient's Self-Report and Nurse's Assessment

Michaels, R., & Mumford, K. (1989). *Archives of Psychiatric Nursing, 3*, 97–101.

It is not uncommon for nurses to question the veracity of clients' reports of symptoms and subjective feelings during psychopharmacological therapy. Michaels and Mumford studied the relationship between patients' self-report and nurses' assessment of two important side effects of neuroleptic drugs: akinesia and akathisia. Akinesia was defined as a set of behaviors characterized by motor slowness and stiffness. Akathisia was defined as a subjective, distressing restlessness leading to the inability to relax. There is disagreement among researchers regarding the reliability of self-reports among psychiatric clients. On the other hand, some found clients' self-reports to be positively correlated with compliance and positive treatment outcomes.

Michaels and Mumford used a convenience sample of 96 community mental health center outpatients receiving neuroleptic drugs. Psychiatric–mental health nurses evaluated these subjects for akinesia and akathisia after training by a physician who was in the process of developing an evaluation tool. The subjects were also given a paper-and-pencil inventory that included self-report of akinesia and akathisia. The data were pulled from the inventory and clustered into scores for akinesia and akathisia. These scores were compared with those from the assessment tool. The patients' and the nurses' responses were positively correlated for akathisia ($r = .67$, $p < .001$) and akinesia ($r = .29$, $p < .05$). It was clear that there was closer correlation between patients and nurses on akathisia than akinesia.

On the basis of their findings, Michaels and Mumford recommend that (a) clients' self-reports of subjective distress during neuroleptic therapy should not be ignored and are believable; (b) assessment must include deliberate and active elicitation of symptom-specific subjective responses and systematic objective observations; and (c) an ongoing, supportive educative relationship is critical in sensitizing clinicians to the subtle symptoms of akinesia and akathisia. Observations and self-report work together to provide an accurate clinical picture and identification of these two side effects of neuroleptic therapy.

Parkinsonian-like extrapyramidal side effects include **akinesia**, which is slow or no movement. Manifestations of this side effect include hesitant speech; decreased blinking; and a slow, shuffling gait (Leonard, 1993). Clients display a masklike facial expression not unlike that of a client with Parkinson's disease. This side effect may contribute to an appearance of flattened affect. Closely allied to akinesia is dyskinesia, which is abnormal, involuntary movements. These movements may be spastic, ticlike, or tremorous. They are particularly noticeable in the hands, tongue, and nose.

Still another extrapyramidal side effect is dystonia—abnormal tension or muscle tone. Clients with dystonia often appear rigid and exhibit **cogwheeling**, a deep tremor of the muscles when a limb is moved while in a flaccid state (Baldessarini, 1993). Clients may also have acute dystonic reactions, which are rapid in onset and frightening. An acute dystonic reaction usually begins with a tightening of the jaw and thickening of the tongue. If untreated, acute dystonia may progress to impairment of the intercostal muscles and compromised respiration (Baldessarini, 1993). Other symptoms of acute dystonia are oculogyric crisis (eyes roll back), opisthotonos (neck contracts backward), and torticollis (neck contracts laterally) (Leonard, 1993).

Antiparkinsonian Agents. Extrapyramidal side effects are treated with a group of medications known as *antiparkinsonian agents* (Table 26–12). These agents include benztropine (Cogentin), diphenhydramine (Benadryl), and trihexyphenidyl (Artane), and their mechanism of action is anticholinergic. Amantadine (Symmetrel) is another commonly used antiparkinsonian agent, which acts by dopaminergic mechanisms (Schatzberg & Cole, 1987). Benztropine and diphenhydramine are both well absorbed and therefore act rapidly when administered intramuscularly, making them particularly useful in the treatment of acute dystonic reaction. Clients may be placed on these medications prophylactically, although whether this practice is safe and efficacious is controversial. Table 26–13 presents the symptoms associated with the adverse effects of the medications for extrapyramidal side effects.

Other side effects of antipsychotic medications include orthostatic hypotension, sedation, and endocrine and anticholinergic effects (Table 26–14). Endocrine effects are probably due to the action of the medication on the hypothalamus. Included in the metabolic changes are weight gain, abnormal blood glucose levels, amenorrhea, and galactorrhea. In addition, men may experience an inability to maintain erections and retrograde ejaculation, and women may experience inhibition of orgasm. Anticholinergic side effects include dry mouth, blurred vision, and constipation. The anticholinergic side effects, in particular, tend to decrease over time. However, all of these side effects should be kept in mind for the purposes of client education.

Another consequence of antipsychotic medications is **tardive dyskinesia**. Initially, tardive dyskinesia was thought to occur only after prolonged use of antipsychotics (Tanner, 1992), but current literature is showing an increased incidence of this side effect in short-term administration, particularly in the elderly (Kutcher et al., 1992). Tardive dyskinesia is irreversible and severely debilitating. In addition, there is no known treatment except to decrease antipsychotic medication to the absolute minimal level that will still afford symptom control. The most important factor in treating tardive dyskinesia is that the antipsychotic medication should never be abruptly stopped or the symptoms will quickly, and possibly irreversibly, exacerbate (Blair & Dauner, 1992). Therefore, it is imperative that the nurse distinguish these symptoms from those of extrapyramidal side effects. Tardive dyskinesia includes protrusion of the tongue, chewing movements, puffing of the cheeks, and pelvic thrusting.

Early detection of tardive dyskinesia is essential (Blair & Dauner, 1992; Leonard, 1993). The nurse is often involved in the routine screening and monitoring of clients for the presence of abnormal movements. Although standard neurological examinations can be used for this purpose, the Abnormal Involuntary Movement Scale, designed by the National Institute of Mental Health (NIMH), is more often used (see Table 26–15). The client should be screened before any antipsychotic is begun and then every 2 weeks to monthly. The NIMH form shows the areas to be screened and includes the examination procedure.

A rare but potentially fatal syndrome associated with antipsychotic medication is **neuroleptic malignancy syndrome**. The exact cause of this syndrome is unknown, but it may be associated with effects on the hypothala-

TABLE 26–12
Clinical and Pharmacokinetic Parameters of Extrapyramidal Side Effect Medications

GENERIC NAME	BRAND NAME	DOSAGE RANGE (MG/DAY)	HALF-LIFE (HOURS)	ONSET		DURATION (HOURS)
				ORAL	INTRAMUSCULAR	
Dopaminergic						
Amantadine	Symmetrel	100–300	9–37	4–48 hours*	NA	12–24
Anticholinergics						
Benztropine mesylate	Cogentin	0.5–6	?	1–2 hours	15 minutes	24
Biperiden	Akineton	2–16	18–24	60 minutes	15 minutes	6–10
Diphenhydramine	Benadryl	10–400	4–15	30–60 minutes	15–30 minutes	4–6
Procyclidine	Kemadrin	7.5–20	11–12	30–45 minutes	NA	4–6
Trihexyphenidyl	Artane	1–10	5.6–10	60 minutes	NA	6–12

*Response takes 2 weeks.

TABLE 26–13
Adverse Effects Associated with Antiparkinsonian Medications for Extrapyramidal Side Effects

SYSTEM	COMMON ADVERSE EFFECTS	LESS COMMON ADVERSE EFFECTS
Cardiovascular		Orthostatic hypotension, tachycardia, palpitations
Central nervous	Dizziness, drowsiness, blurred vision Amantadine: anxiety, confusion, irritability, difficulty concentrating	Confusion, headache, disorientation Amantadine: fatigue, insomnia, weakness, visual disturbances
Gastrointestinal	Dry mouth Amantadine: nausea, vomiting, anorexia, constipation	Amantadine: dry mouth, increased frequency of urination
Miscellaneous	Amantadine: urinary retention	Amantadine: skin rash, dyspnea

mus and medulla (Leonard, 1993). The symptomatology of neuroleptic malignancy syndrome is similar to that of malignant hyperthermia. This syndrome has a rapid onset and constitutes a medical emergency. Symptoms include hyperpyrexia (up to 107°F), that is, severe muscle rigidity that precipitates elevated blood creatinine phosphokinase and white blood cell counts (Schatzberg & Cole, 1987). Additional symptoms include changes in level of consciousness (agitation or delirium), elevated pulse and blood pressure, and profuse diaphoresis. Treatment includes symptomatic relief of the hyperpyrexia; dantrolene (Dantrium) to decrease muscle spasm, fever, and tachycardia; and bromocriptine (Parlodel) (Schatzberg & Cole, 1987).

Atypical Antipsychotics

A newer class of antipsychotics, the *atypical antipsychotics*, is currently being researched. One of these medications, clozapine (Clozaril), is on the market and has shown great potential with certain clients who have been refractory to traditional antipsychotic medications. This medication is believed to have an affinity for the D_1 receptor and is hypothesized to act on the newly found D_3, D_4, and D_5 receptors (Baldessarini, 1993; Leonard, 1993). These receptors are believed to be in very high concentration in the limbic system and to have little presence in the nigrostriatal system. Therefore, control of psychotic symptoms is limited, but the major action is for the treatment of ambivalence, which at times is virtually paralytic to the client with schizophrenia. Although there is limited documentation of extrapyramidal side effects or tardive dyskinesia, clozapine does produce a potentially fatal agranulocytosis. Therefore, clients on this medication must comply with routine blood monitoring. The cost of clozapine has prohibited its widespread use in the United States to date. However, this medication and others in its family have brought dramatic symptom relief to clients who would have been labeled treatment resistant.

ANXIOLYTICS

An anxiolytic is any medication used to treat anxiety. Whether and when to treat anxiety is often a difficult and controversial decision. Anxiety is a universal experience, a common response to daily stress and conflict (Arana & Hyman, 1991; Schatzberg & Cole, 1987). There is a spectrum of anxiety, ranging from mild to panic, which some might say is from "normal" to "pathological." How the clinician defines anxiety determines, in large part how, or whether, he or she treats

TABLE 26–14
Adverse Effects Associated with Antipsychotics

SYSTEM	COMMON ADVERSE EFFECTS	LESS COMMON ADVERSE EFFECTS	MECHANISM
Autonomic nervous	Dry mouth, blurred vision, constipation	Urinary retention, weight gain, dyspepsia, priapism, incontinence	Blockage of muscarinic cholinoceptors
	Orthostatic hypotension	Tachycardia, bradycardia, hypertension	Blockage of alpha-adrenoceptors
Central nervous	Sedation, extrapyramidal symptoms, headache		Blockage of dopamine receptors
	Tardive dyskinesia		Supersensitivity of dopamine receptors
Endocrine		Galactorrhea, changes in libido, impotence in men, amenorrhea	Blockage of dopamine receptors resulting in hyperprolactinemia
Hepatic	Jaundice at 2–4 weeks of medication		Unknown
Gastrointestinal	Nausea, vomiting	Diarrhea	Unknown
Ocular	Photophobia, blurred vision	Miosis	Unknown
Dermatological	Skin rashes, photosensitivity	Urticaria, petechiae, erythema, hyperpigmentation	Unknown
Respiratory		Nasal congestion	Unknown
Hemic/lymphatic		Clozapine: leukopinia, granulocytopenia; may cause agranulocytosis in up to 3% of clients	Unknown

TABLE 26–15

Abnormal Involuntary Movement Scale and Examination Procedure for Evaluating Tardive Dyskinesia

Instructions: Complete examination procedure before making ratings. Asterisk (*) denotes activated movements.

EXAMINATION PROCEDURE

Either before or after completing the Examination Procedure, observe the client unobtrusively, at rest (e.g., in waiting room). The chair to be used in this examination should be a hard, firm one without arms.

1. Ask the client whether there is anything in his or her mouth (gum, candy, etc.) and, if there is, to remove it.
2. Ask the client about the *current* condition of his or her teeth. Ask the client if he or she wears dentures. Do teeth or dentures bother the client *now*?
3. Ask the client whether he or she notices any movements in mouth, face, hands, or feet. If yes, ask the client to describe them and to what extent they *currently* bother the client or interfere with his or her activities.
4. Have the client sit in the chair with hands on knees, legs slightly apart, and feet flat on floor. (Look at entire body for movements while client is in this position.)
5. Ask the client to sit with hands hanging unsupported (if male, between legs; if female and wearing a dress, hanging over knees). (Observe hands and other body areas.)
6. Ask the client to open his or her mouth. (Observe tongue at rest within mouth.) Do this twice.
7. Ask the client to protrude his or her tongue. (Observe abnormalities of tongue movement.) Do this twice.

*8. Ask the client to tap his or her thumb with each finger, as rapidly as possible for 10 to 15 seconds, first with right hand, then with left hand. (Observe facial and leg movements.)

*9. Ask the client to stand up. (Observe the client's profile. Observe all body areas again, hips included.)

*10. Ask the client to extend both arms outstretched in front with palms down. (Observe trunk, legs, and mouth.)

*11. Have the client walk a few paces, turn, and walk back to chair. (Observe hands and gait.) Do this twice.

ABNORMAL INVOLUNTARY MOVEMENT SCALE (AIMS)

Movement Ratings: Rate highest severity observed. Rate movements that occur upon activation less than movements that occur spontaneously.

Codes:
0 = None
1 = Minimal; may be extreme normal
2 = Mild
3 = Moderate
4 = Severe

		(Circle one)				
Facial and Oral Movements	1. Muscles of facial expression, e.g., movements of forehead, eyebrows, periorbital area, cheeks; include frowning, blinking, smiling, grimacing.	0	1	2	3	4
	2. Lips and perioral area, e.g., puckering, pouting, smacking.	0	1	2	3	4
	3. Jaw, e.g., biting, clenching, chewing, mouth opening, lateral movements.	0	1	2	3	4
	4. Tongue. Rate only increase in movement both in and out of, NOT inability to sustain movement.	0	1	2	3	4
Extremity Movements	5. Upper (arms, wrists, hands, and fingers). Include choreic movements (i.e., rapid objectively purposeless, irregular, spontaneous), athetoid movements (i.e., slow irregular, complex, serpentine). Do NOT include tremor (i.e., repetitive, regular, rhythmic).	0	1	2	3	4
	6. Lower (legs, knees, ankles, and toes), e.g., lateral knee movement, foot tapping, heel dropping, foot squirming, inversion and eversion of foot.					
Trunk Movements	7. Neck, shoulders, hips, e.g., rocking, twisting, squirming, pelvic gyrations.	0	1	2	3	4

Global Judgments	8. Severity of abnormal movements.	None, normal	0
		Minimal	1
		Mild	2
		Moderate	3
		Severe	4
	9. Incapacitation due to abnormal movements.	None, normal	0
		Minimal	1
		Mild	2
		Moderate	3
		Severe	4
	10. Client's awareness of abnormal movements. Rate only client's report.	No awareness	0
		Awareness, no distress	1
		Aware, mild distress	2
		Aware, moderate distress	3
		Aware, severe distress	4
Dental Status	11. Current problems with teeth and/or dentures.	No	0
		Yes	1
	12. Does client usually wear dentures?	No	0
		Yes	1

(Adapted from Department of Health and Human Services, Public Health Service, Alcohol, Drug Abuse, and Mental Health Administration, National Institute of Mental Health.)

it. If the clinician decides the client's anxiety is "normal" and therefore should be tolerable, he or she may tell the client to go home and cope. If the client disagrees with the clinician's decision and believes the anxiety is unbearable, he or she may find another provider or self-medicate.

Anxiety manifests psychologically as anything from unease and irritability to a frightful feeling of doom. It can present physically in a variety of autonomic nervous system manifestations: tachycardia, palpitations, irregular heart rhythm, dizziness, tremor, excessive sweating, dry mouth, diarrhea, abdominal pain, or headache (Arana & Hyman, 1991). More commonly, it presents with a combination of physiological and psychological symptoms. Anxiety can underlie other psychiatric diagnoses (e.g., depression) as well as many medical conditions. Clearly, the diagnosis and assessment of anxiety are important and challenging initial tasks. Like other psychiatric conditions, anxiety can be treated with environmental, social, psychological, and other nonbiological interventions. These interventions should always be considered along with medication (see Chapter 10).

Current nomenclature divides anxiety disorders into three major subtypes: phobic disorders (agoraphobia, social phobia, and simple phobia), anxiety states (panic disorder, generalized anxiety disorder, and obsessive–compulsive disorder), and posttraumatic stress disorder (PTSD).

Benzodiazepine antianxiety agents are the most widely used and prescribed drugs in the world (Arana & Hyman, 1991; DeVane, 1990). Other classes of drugs that are used to treat anxiety include antidepressants, antihistamines, barbiturates, propanediols, beta blockers (e.g., propranolol), nonbenzos (e.g., buspirone), and the antipsychotic drugs (Table 26–16). Although the general use of antidepressants has already been discussed, their use in treating anxiety can be considered here. Clients with a history of anxiety are likely, even with optimal medication response, to require long-term pharmacological intervention. Because prolonged administration of benzodiazepines may be associated with drug dependence, it is particularly important to assess the particular type of anxiety disorder the client has. Some anxiety disorders, such as agoraphobia, panic disorder, and PTSD, often respond well to antidepressants. Buspirone appears useful in generalized anxiety disorder (Bernstein, 1988).

The antianxiety agents were introduced with the promise that they were effective, safe, and nonaddicting. Experience with the benzodiazepines and other antianxiety agents has shown otherwise. They can all produce tolerance, dependence, and withdrawal symptoms.

Benzodiazepines

Chlordiazepoxide (Librium), the first benzodiazepine, was marketed in 1960 and diazepam (Valium) 3 years after that. Benzodiazepines are highly effective for the alleviation of acute anxiety and retain at least a portion of their efficacy over time. They are remarkably safe in an overdosage situation, although the combination of a benzodiazepine with alcohol or another sedative–hypnotic agent can be hazardous. Overall, the safety record of benzodiazepines is unparalleled (Arana & Hyman, 1991; Greenblatt, 1992).

The anxiolytic potency of a benzodiazepine correlates with its affinity for benzodiazepine receptors. The benzodiazepines' ability to modulate the neurotransmitter activity of GABA is an important part of their action. Benzodiazepines raise the seizure threshold and increase the frequency and activity of brain waves. Other sedative–hypnotics, such as barbiturates, also produce these effects. Benzodiazepines, especially diazepam, cause skeletal muscle relaxation. Again, it appears that the GABA-ergic action of the benzodiazepines may at least partly account for the anticonvulsant and muscle relaxant effects. The benzodiazepines' effects on other organ systems appear to be minimal (DeVane et al., 1991; Nutt & Glue, 1989).

As with all CNS depressants, the most common unwanted effects of the benzodiazepines are drowsiness and ataxia. The elderly may be more vulnerable to these

TABLE 26–16
Clinical and Pharmacokinetic Parameters of Antianxiety Medications

GENERIC NAME	BRAND NAME	DOSAGE RANGE (MG/DAY)	HALF-LIFE (HOURS)	ONSET (MINUTES)	DURATION (HOURS)
Benzodiazepines					
Alprazolam	Xanax	0.75–4	12–15	15–60	
Chlordiazepoxide	Librium, et al.	15–100	5–30	15–45	Varies
Clorazepate	Tranxene	15–60	30–100	30–60	by age,
Diazepam	Valium, et al.	4–40	20–80	15–45	illness,
Halazepam	Paxipam	60–160	14	30–60	and
Lorazepam	Ativan	2–4	10–20	15–45	dosage
Oxazepam	Serax	30–120	5–20	15–90	
Prazepam	Centrax	20–60	30–100	?	
Other Drugs					
Buspirone	BuSpar	15–60	2–11	3–4 weeks	?
Chlormezanone	Trancopal	300–800	24	15–30	6
Diphenhydramine	Benadryl, et al.	75–200	2.4–4.3	30–60	4–10
Hydroxyzine	Atarax, Vistaril	50–100	3	15–30	4–6
Meprobamate	Miltown, Equinil	1200–1600	6–48	60	6–17

reactions, because they usually achieve higher blood and tissue drug levels for a given dose and also because the aging brain is more sensitive to the effects of sedatives (DeVane et al., 1991; Dubovsky et al., 1987).

Reports of **paradoxical reactions**, or disinhibition, are not infrequent. An increased tendency to express hostility, rage, or aggression, even in persons with no previous history of these feelings, has been reported with diazepam, alprazolam (Xanax), and chlordiazepoxide (Arana & Hyman, 1991). Benzodiazepines have well-known amnestic properties. Certainly, this effect can be used to the client's advantage. For example, benzodiazepines can be given during painful or unpleasant procedures in part because they cause anterograde amnesia. However, the untoward effects of this amnesia in regular doses of benzodiazepines must also be assessed.

Tolerance to the sedative effects of benzodiazepines develops; whether it also develops to the sleep-maintaining and antianxiety effects is unclear (Taniguchi & Westphal, 1986). Although benzodiazepine drugs have been used recreationally, most clients have not abused these drugs. The possibility of addiction must be kept in mind, though, because there are some exceptions (Dubovsky et al., 1987; Nutt & Glue, 1989). First, most prescribers believe that clients with substance abuse problems should not be prescribed these drugs. Second, if a client takes more of a benzodiazepine than is prescribed, this behavior needs to be carefully examined. Third, it should be recognized that the type of anxiolytic prescribed, the dosage used, and the duration of the agents effects all can affect the possibility of a problem in compliance. As an example, the shorter the half-life of the drug prescribed, the greater the risk of dependency and addiction (Bernstein, 1988).

Benzodiazepine withdrawal can lead to reactions much like those observed with other sedative–hypnotic compounds, such as barbiturates and alcohol. Whereas withdrawal reactions from cessation of benzodiazepine use were once thought to be rare, clinicians now believe that clients taking benzodiazepines for long periods, even at standard doses, are vulnerable to withdrawal reactions if the drug is discontinued abruptly. Therefore, clients need to consult with their prescriber and taper off the medication gradually.

Mild symptoms of withdrawal include insomnia, dizziness, headache, anorexia, tinnitus, blurred vision, and shakiness. These symptoms may also indicate a returning anxiety. If these symptoms begin to wane after several weeks, a withdrawal reaction seems unlikely.

Severe signs of benzodiazepine withdrawal may include hypotension, hyperthermia, neuromuscular rigidity, psychosis, and seizures. Short-acting benzodiazepines may cause a higher incidence of withdrawal symptoms.

Buspirone

Buspirone (BuSpar) is structurally and pharmacologically unrelated to the benzodiazepines. It has no direct effects on $GABA_A$ receptors, is not a CNS depressant, and lacks the sedative action of the benzodiazepines. It is speculated that buspirone exerts its anxiolytic effect by acting as a partial agonist at $5\text{-}HT_{1\alpha}$ receptors particularly in the hippocampus and other limbic structures. It also increases norepinephrine metabolism in the locus ceruleus. Buspirone does not appear to produce tolerance or dependence and has neither anticonvulsant nor muscle relaxant properties. The most common side effects are dizziness, nausea, headache, nervousness, lightheadedness, and excitement. Unlike any of the benzodiazepines, buspirone is effective only when taken regularly. It takes 1 to 2 weeks to show initial effects; maximal effectiveness may be reached after 4 to 6 weeks.

Antihistamines

Because of their sedative effects, drugs that block central and peripheral histamine receptors (primarily H_1) are sometimes used to calm anxious patients. Hydroxyzine (Vistaril) and diphenhydramine (Benadryl) are frequently prescribed examples of this class. Besides sedation, these medications also have antiemetic and antihistaminic properties. Unlike most antianxiety agents, antihistamines depress the seizure threshold and must be used with caution in clients with seizure disorders. They have more anticholinergic action than the benzodiazepines do, which limits their use, especially with the elderly.

Barbiturates

Benzodiazepines have largely replaced the once popular barbiturates. There are several reasons for this. First, benzodiazepines appear to be more effective than the barbiturates in treating anxiety. Second, a barbiturate overdose can be extremely serious. Third, barbiturates interact pharmacokinetically with a great number of agents.

Propranolol

Propranolol blocks beta-noradrenergic receptors in the peripheral sympathetic nervous system and probably centrally as well. Although drugs specific to beta-1 (cardiac) and beta-2 (pulmonary) receptors have recently been developed, propranolol itself blocks both receptors competitively and without discrimination. Propranolol has extensive effects on the cardiovascular system, the pulmonary bronchi, and carbohydrate and fat metabolism. Although propranolol is probably not as effective an antianxiety agent as other medications, clients who have many somatic complaints may find it useful. It should be noted propranolol has not been approved by the Food and Drug Administration (FDA) for the treatment of anxiety or any psychiatric condition (Facts and Comparisons, 1993). Propranolol is sometimes given to alleviate lithium-induced tremors.

Propanediols

The propanediols (e.g., meprobamate [Equanil]) were extremely popular in the 1950s, but controlled studies have failed to demonstrate their superiority over barbiturates in the treatment of anxiety. Neither class of drugs is used today.

Antipsychotics

The significant negative side effect profile of the antipsychotics makes them a poor choice to treat anxiety. Only when psychosis is the cause of anxiety should they be prescribed.

SEDATIVES AND HYPNOTICS

Almost 20 percent of clients who visit physicians complain of difficulty sleeping, and half of these clients are prescribed hypnotics. Insomnia is a symptom with diverse causes including medical, psychological, and situational. It is important to search for a specific treatable cause before prescribing a nonspecific therapy such as a hypnotic. The client's sleep behavior needs to be assessed and reviewed; nonpharmacological interventions, or sleep hygiene measures, should be implemented whenever possible (Greenblatt, 1992; Roth & Roehrs, 1992; Trevor & Way, 1989). Sleep hygiene measures are practices that promote sleep, such as drinking warm milk; taking a warm bath; reading; developing a regular routine for preparing for sleep; and avoiding food and fluids high in caffeine, such as chocolates, coffee, tea, and colas.

There are many substances, differing widely in their chemical structure, that can be considered sedative–hypnotics in that they all produce dose-dependent CNS depression (Arana & Hyman, 1991). The more commonly used agents are presented in Table 26–17 and the symptoms of adverse effects of their use are listed in Table 26–18. There can be cross-reactivity between these diverse compounds. For example, a client who has developed tolerance to a benzodiazepine not only will be tolerant to other benzodiazepines but will also be tolerant to barbiturates and other CNS depressants (Bernstein, 1988). Abrupt discontinuation of any of these medications is associated with a withdrawal syndrome. All clients, regardless of whether they have a history of drug abuse, who are regularly using small amounts of sedative–hypnotics may gradually develop tolerance and experience a withdrawal syndrome if the drug is suddenly stopped or significantly decreased. Note that the features of withdrawal syndrome (tremulousness, irritability, and sleep disturbance) may be mistaken for the original target symptoms. The nurse may be able to explore this in a careful interview.

In summary, it is important to remember (1) the need for careful evaluation before any medication is prescribed; (2) the importance of short-term use if these

TABLE 26–17
Clinical and Pharmacokinetic Parameters of Sedatives and Hypnotics

GENERIC NAME	BRAND NAME	DOSAGE RANGE (MG/DAY)		ONSET (MINUTES)	HALF-LIFE (HOURS)	DURATION OF ACTION (HOURS)
		Hypnotic	Sedative			
Nonbarbiturate						
Acetylcarbromal	Paxarel	—	250–500 bid or tid	15–60	?	
Chloral hydrate	Noctec	0.5–1g	250 tid	30–60	7–10	4–8
Ethchlorvynol	Placidyl	500	100–200 tid	15–60	10–20	5
Ethinamate	Valmid	—	500–1000	20	2.5	3–5
Glutethimide	Doriden	250–500	—	30	10–12	4–8
Methyprylon	Noludar	200–400	50–100 up to quid	45	3–6	5–8
Paraldehyde	Paral	10–30 ml	5–10 ml	10–15	3.4–98	8–12
Propiomazine	Largon	—	10–20			
Benzodiazepines						
Estazolam	Prosom	1–2	NA	30–60	10–24	
Flurazepam	Dalmane	15–30	NA	15–45	50–100	7–8
					(2–100 for metabolites)	
Quazepam	Doral	15	NA	45–120	25–41	
Temazepam	Restoril	15–30	NA	20–30	10–17	6–8
Triazolam	Halcion	0.125–0.5	NA	15–30	1.5–5.5	6–8
Barbiturates						
Long acting				≥60		10–12
Phenobarbital	Barbital, Luminal	100–320	30–120		53–118	
Mephobarbital	Mebural	—	90–400		11–67	
Intermediate acting				45–60		6–8
Amobarbital	Amytal	65–200	30–480		16–40	
Apropbarbital	Alurate	40–160	120		14–34	
Butabarbital	Butisol, Butratan	50–100	45–120		66–140	
Talbutal	Lotusate	120	60–80		15	
Short acting				10–15		3–4
Secobarbital	Seconal	100	—		15–40	
Pentobarbital	Nembutal	100	40–120		15–50	

TABLE 26–18
Adverse Effects Associated with Sedatives and Hypnotics

SYSTEM	COMMON ADVERSE EFFECTS	LESS COMMON ADVERSE EFFECTS
	Benzodiazepines	
Cardiovascular	Palpitations	Tachycardia
Central nervous	Sedation, lack of concentration, dizziness, drowsiness Estazolam: somnolence, asthenia	Tremors, apprehension, nervousness, confusion, headache, lethargy, weakness, paradoxical excitation, euphoria, coordination disorders
Gastrointestinal		Nausea, vomiting, heartburn, constipation, diarrhea
	Nonbarbiturates	
Cardiovascular		Hypotension
Central nervous	Dizziness, drowsiness	Ataxia, headache, paradoxical excitation, blurred vision Methyprylon: vertigo, nightmares
Gastrointestinal	Glutethimide: nausea, vomiting	Heartburn, constipation, diarrhea, flatulence, offensive breath, dry mouth
Dermatological	Glutethimide: skin rash	Skin rash, urticaria
	Barbiturates	
Cardiovascular		Hypotension, bradycardia, syncope
Central nervous	Somnolence, dizziness, drowsiness	Ataxia, confusion, hyperkinesia, paradoxical excitation, agitation, vertigo
Gastrointestinal		Nausea, vomiting, constipation, diarrhea
Dermatological		Skin rash, urticaria (with asthma)
Respiratory		Hypoventilation, apnea

medications are chosen; and (3) the importance of educating the client on sleep hygiene measures.

Benzodiazepines

Should a hypnotic (**sedative** or sleeping pill) be prescribed, the most likely choice would be a benzodiazepine. Currently, the FDA has designated flurazepam (Dalmane), temazepam (Restoril), triazolam (Halcion), and zolpidem tartrate (Ambien, a nonbenzodiazepine but within the same schedule) as hypnotics. It is likely that most, if not all, of the benzodiazepines used to treat anxiety could also induce sleep at the appropriate dosage. It is a corporate decision whether to market benzodiazepines as anxiolytics or hypnotics; FDA labeling approval is based almost entirely on information supplied by the manufacturer.

The two major concerns in choosing a benzodiazepine hypnotic are rapidity of onset and half-life. For clients who report difficulty falling asleep, the rate at which the drug achieves its hypnotic effect is important. Two benzodiazepines that have rapid onset are diazepam and flurazepam. Benzodiazepines with long half-lives decrease sleep latency (the time required to fall asleep), decrease early morning awakenings, diminish the number of awakenings, and usually increase the total amount of sleep. However, the tradeoff may be daytime drowsiness and related unwanted effects. Because long-acting drugs tend to accumulate with repeated use over time, their use must be assessed in terms of the benefits for the client (Arana & Hyman, 1991; Roth & Roehrs, 1992; Trevor & Way, 1989).

The second important consideration is half-life. Benzodiazepines with short half-lives do not accumulate, but they may cause rebound insomnia. Benzodiazepines decrease the length of sleep in stages 3 and 4; their effect on rapid-eye-movement (REM) sleep varies, depending on the client, the illness, and the type and dosage of the drug. Rebound insomnia may occur when a benzodiazepine with a short half-life is used on several consecutive nights.

Flurazepam is a long-acting drug that resemble diazepam. Its half-life of 40 to 250 hours means that the blood level on the eighth morning after a consecutive week of nightly flurazepam is likely to be four to six times that found on the first morning. A long half-life can have positive consequences: it may be useful for clients who are anxious, and rebound insomnia (sleep worse than pretreatment levels after drug withdrawal) is less likely with long-acting agents. Negative consequences may include a morning hangover (residual sedation and impaired cognitive and motor skills). In addition, potential interactions with other sedatives, including alcohol, may be prolonged.

Temazepam, with its shorter half-life, may reduce the hangover but increase rebound insomnia. Triazolam, the shortest-acting benzodiazepine with a half-life of 2 to 3 hours, has the benefit of little drug hangover, but it also has the problems associated with a short half-life (i.e., withdrawal syndrome) and the problem of waking while still intoxicated or amnestic.

Zolpidem has been recently released as a short-acting nonbenzodiazepine sleep agent that does not produce tolerance. Although zolpidem is technically not a benzodiazepine, the differences are subtle and thus claims to safety and efficacy need to be carefully evaluated over time.

Other Agents

The caveats mentioned regarding the prescription of barbiturates for anxiety apply equally to the prescription of hypnotics. Because of problems with tolerance, abuse, dependency, adverse effects, and rebound and the danger of overdose, barbiturates are rarely prescribed. Other agents formerly widely used and now much less frequently prescribed, for many of the same reasons, are chloral hydrate, glutethimide (Doriden), methaqualone (Quaalude), paraldehyde, and bromides.

Antihistamines

Sedating antihistamines, many of which are available over the counter, can be effective hypnotics for some adults. Diphenhydramine is probably the most commonly used drug in this class. It may suppress REM sleep, and REM rebound occurs following its discontinuation. Because of its anticholinergic effects, confusion and delirium can develop in susceptible clients, the elderly, and persons taking other drugs with anticholinergic activity.

PSYCHOPHARMACOLOGICAL THERAPY ACROSS THE LIFE SPAN

MEDICATION CONSIDERATIONS WITH THE ELDERLY

Although people age 65 or older make up 11 percent of the U.S. population, they receive approximately 25 percent of the prescriptions written for psychotropic medications and 22 percent of all written prescriptions. The elderly are more likely to be receiving multiple medications and are thus at greater risk for drug interactions; psychotropic medications place the elderly at particular risk for iatrogenic effects (Crismon, 1990; Gomez & Gomez, 1990). The use of psychotropics with the elderly has been an ongoing concern for many years (see Research Abstract displays on this and the following pages). Polytherapy that includes psychotropic drugs with anticholinergic action is the greatest precipitant of iatrogenic effects. When elderly clients experience changes in mental functioning, such as confusion, restlessness, irritability, depression, or psychosis, medications should be suspected as the cause. Age-related declines in a number of physiological systems are the underlying reasons for altered drug effects in the elderly (Crismon, 1990; Moran & Thompson, 1988). As a result, the total effective safe daily dose for the elderly is almost always *less* than in younger clients. The following are some of these age-related changes:

- Decreased renal blood flow, glomerular filtration, and renal tubular secretions of 50 percent by age 80, mean that medications may stay in the body longer.
- Gastric motility is decreased.
- An increased ratio of adipose tissue to lean body mass results in increased retention of fat-soluble drugs, including psychotropics such as sedatives, antidepressants, and antipsychotics.
- Many drugs are bound to plasma proteins, which are synthesized in the liver. With age, there may be fewer plasma binding sites and fewer drug-metabolizing enzymes, leading to prolonged, sustained serum drug concentrations. In addition, all psychotropic medications (except lithium) bind extensively to plasma albumin. Because albumin levels decrease with age, older clients may be more susceptible than middle-aged clients to toxic responses and may thus require smaller doses of medication.
- Decreased liver function limits drug metabolism and contributes to overdose drug accumulation and overdose.
- Cardiac output may decrease with age, delaying circulation time and thus affecting the distribution of drugs to tissue.

An adverse drug effect may be much more significant to an older person than a younger one. The postural hypotension and dizziness that can be produced by some psychotropics may be merely annoying to a younger person but they can predispose an older person to falling (Arana & Hyman, 1991).

Many psychotropic medications produce anticholinergic side effects such as blurred vision, dry mouth,

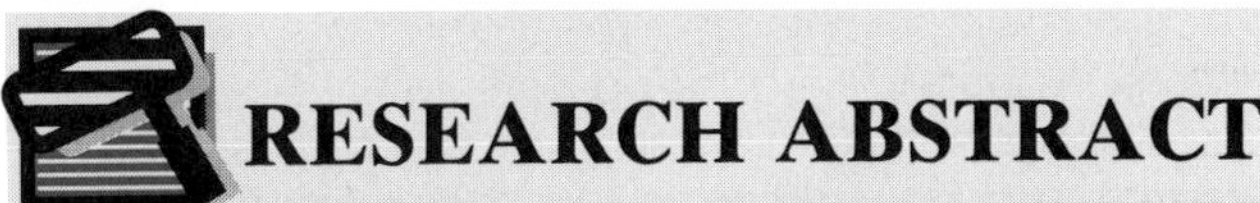

Drugging Elders

Huey, F. L. (1989). *Geriatric Nursing, 10*(16), 119.

The problems of psychotropic drug use and misuse with elderly clients in intermediate care facilities and nursing homes have a long history. In 1976, the Department of Health, Education and Welfare reported that psychoactive drugs were being prescribed for half the elders in skilled nursing facilities. More recently, it was reported antipsychotics are being prescribed for many elderly residents of intermediate care facilities who were not diagnosed as psychotic. Other studies corroborate these findings. It was discovered that antipsychotics were prescribed for 270 of 850 residents, although only 36 residents were diagnosed as psychotic. Half the residents were on psychoactive drugs. These drugs were often those known to produce problems for the elderly, such as amitriptyline and long-acting benzodiazepines. It seems the problem is persistent and will not go away. Why is this the case?

One suggestion is the increasing nursing workload. With client assignments skyrocketing, nurses have no time to deal with confusion, belligerence, and aggression in interactive ways that consume time and energy and can be overwhelming. Another factor is nurses' reluctance to coach physicians in appropriate psychotropic drugs and doses for elderly clients. The scenario, however, is that the elderly seem to be placed on the wrong drug or wrong dose and never taken off it. One solution is the use of geriatric nurse practitioners who have been shown to be careful about prescribing drugs to monitor medication regimens. Until that happens, nurses in nursing homes will continue to withhold PRN doses unless absolutely necessary.

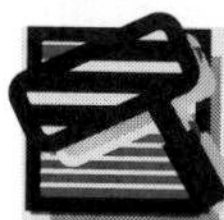

RESEARCH ABSTRACT

New Rules for Prescribing Psychotropics in Nursing Homes

Smith, D. A. (1990). *Geriatrics, 45*(2), 44–56.

Many older nursing home residents are prescribed psychotropic medications by their primary care physicians. Such use is not always appropriate, and geriatric psychiatrists are rare. The purpose of the federal Omnibus Budget Reconciliation Act (OBRA) of 1987 was to regulate the prescription of these drugs for elderly clients receiving Medicaid. Under the OBRA, some drugs, such as barbiturates and meprobamate, are expressly considered inappropriate for nursing home residents. Others, such as anxiolytics, are considered for short-term use only. Normal changing patterns of sleep in the elderly need not be treated with drugs. OBRA mandates routine blood testing for drug levels and reduces on the average of one half the maximum dose of selected antipsychotics allowed to the elderly. OBRA reviewers audit client records, looking for compliance with the regulations. The reviewers look for a decision to medicate a client that is based on a specific condition, not simply an annoying behavior, and evidence that nondrug therapy was tried first. They look for pretherapy lab work, proper dosages, routine drug levels, reassessment, drug holidays, detailed and accurate documentation, and continuing effort to get the client off psychotropic drugs altogether. Primary care physicians and other primary care providers need to become familiar with the new regulations and stay up-to-date with the medications they prescribe.

urinary retention, constipation, and tachycardia. Elderly clients, especially those with some underlying cognitive disorder, may also experience an acute toxic delirium secondary to these anticholinergic effects. Excessive sedation in the elderly is possible with most psychotropic medications. Oversedation may not only be mistaken for depression, but may also reduce the elderly person's contact with the surroundings, impair cognitive capacities, and decrease self-esteem. Signs of CNS depression may include ataxia, dysarthria, diplopia, blurred vision, confusion, dizziness, vertigo, nystagmus, muscle weakness, incoordination, somnolence, and (rarely) respiratory depression (Crismon, 1990; Meyers & Kalayam, 1989).

There is also an increased risk of cardiac effects from antipsychotics and heterocyclics. These risks include tachycardia, increased incidence of premature ventricular contractions, heart block, and atrial and ventricular arrhythmias. Alcohol and drug use must be carefully assessed in the elderly. The use of these agents significantly complicates prescribing for the elderly (Crismon, 1990; Meyers & Kalayam, 1989).

Antidepressants. Antidepressants with lower anticholinergic potential, such as amoxapine, desipramine, and trazodone are preferred to more strongly anticholinergic antidepressants, such as amitriptyline (Elavil). The MAO inhibitors are useful in that they lack anticholinergic effects, but they can produce significant hypotension (Arana & Hyman, 1991; Crismon, 1990; Meyers & Kalayam, 1989). The sedative effects of cyclic antidepressants may be useful in treating sleep disturbances, but they may be problematic in producing daytime drowsiness (Arana & Hyman, 1991; Meyers & Kalayam, 1989). The side effect profile of the SSRIs may make them particularly useful with the elderly (Crismon, 1990).

Lithium. Lithium can be used safely in the elderly, but it is generally used at lower dosages, maintaining blood levels in the 0.4 to 0.6 mEq/L range. Even these dosages may produce signs that appear toxic (Arana & Hyman, 1991; Crismon, 1990; Meyers & Kalayam, 1989). Diuretics must be cautiously co-administered because they can cause increased serum lithium levels or hypokalemia.

Sedative and Antianxiety Agents. Because the metabolism of benzodiazepines is slowed in the elderly, these drugs are likely to remain in the body at higher concentrations than they would under comparable conditions in a younger person. Thus, longer-acting benzodiazepines, such as diazepam and flurazepam are often avoided. Likewise, barbiturates with longer half-lives and meprobamate should also be avoided in the elderly. Regardless of the antianxiety or sedative changes, their effects on the elderly, especially on their mental status, must be regularly assessed (Crismon, 1990; Gomez & Gomez, 1990; Meyers & Kalayam, 1989).

Antipsychotics. Antipsychotics with greater hypotensive and anticholinergic effects, such as chlorpromazine, mesoridazine (Serentil), and thioridazine, should be avoided. Low doses of high-potency medication, such as haloperidol, trifluoperazine, and thiothixene, are preferred (Crismon, 1990; Meyers & Kalayam, 1989).

If extrapyramidal symptoms occur and cannot be treated by decreasing the dosage of the antipsychotic medication, conventional antiparkinsonian agents that are highly anticholinergic, such as benztropine or trihexyphenidyl, should be avoided in favor of an agent like amantadine (Crismon, 1990; Meyers & Kalayam, 1989).

MEDICATION CONSIDERATIONS WITH CHILDREN

The use of psychoactive drugs in children presents philosophical, legal, and diagnostic problems (Gadow, 1991). A nurse working with children who have been prescribed psychiatric medication needs to consider the following points:

- The emotional, behavioral, and social baselines against which psychiatric conditions in children are identified and treated are more fluid than those in adults. Variations of behavior within and between children and adolescents make diagnosis problematic.
- Research on the use of psychotropic medication in children is relatively sparse.
- There is warranted concern that medications may alter the normal psychological, behavioral, and physiological development of children and adolescents. There is also concern that medication administered in childhood may affect cognitive processes in adulthood.
- Conversely, there is equally warranted concern that children who would benefit greatly from treatment with medication will be denied this therapy because of the preceding considerations.
- Treating an adolescent with medication may present special challenges. Because adolescents often feel that adults are trying to control them, they may be particularly resistant to taking drugs prescribed by an authority figure. Therefore, a particularly important priority in working with an adolescent is the development of a trusting relationship.

Drug kinetics are different in children than in adults. For example, a child's liver represents a proportionally larger amount of the total body weight; children often metabolize agents more quickly (Gadow, 1991; Waters, 1990). A lower level of protein binding and lower percentage of total body adipose tissue result in smaller depots for drug storage, which means quicker onset of action and decreased duration of effect. Therefore, children may often require relatively higher and more frequent doses than adults, but they tend to develop fewer adverse effects (Waters, 1990). When unwanted reactions do occur, they are generally less severe and respond more readily to a decrease or discontinuation of the medication. Children should be systematically and repeatedly questioned about the development of untoward effects, because they volunteer this information less readily than adults (Gadow, 1991; Kutcher et al., 1992). Most of the untoward effects that children do develop are similar to those in adults.

Antipsychotics. Because most experience in and research on administering antipsychotics to children has involved chlorpromazine and thioridazine, these medications are often preferred. Haloperidol may be more effective in treating disruptive behavioral symptoms and may increase attention and concentration without decreasing mental alertness. On the other hand, there are reports that all antipsychotics impair learning. Because it seems likely that long-term use of antipsychotics increases the risk of tardive dyskinesia, the use of these agents in children must be particularly carefully weighed (Arana & Hyman, 1991; Gadow, 1991; Waters, 1990).

Antidepressants. Although the FDA has not approved the use of antidepressants in children younger than 12 years of age, the final decision to medicate rests with the physician and the parents. Because hepatic metabolism of tricyclic antidepressants is more rapid in children, they may require adult doses of antidepressants (Newcomb, 1991; Ryan, 1992). However, the nurse should closely observe as well as closely question young children who are taking antidepressants, because they may not report adverse effects and may develop serious toxicity at relatively low doses. More rapid metabolism may also mean that the therapeutic response may take longer in children than in adults. TCAs seizures caused by TCAs occur more frequently in children and adolescents than in adults (Waters, 1990). Amitriptyline and imipramine have been used to treat nocturnal enuresis. There have not been enough clinical trials with MAO inhibitors to determine either the efficacy or the safety of these agents for children.

Lithium. Although lithium has not been approved by the FDA for the treatment of manic–depressive illness in children, it has been used successfully to manage bipolar affective disorder. Because the renal clearance of lithium is higher in children than in adults, children and adolescents may require higher dosages to achieve therapeutic blood levels (Newcomb, 1991; Ryan, 1992).

THE NURSE'S ROLE

THE GENERALIST'S ROLE

Detailed knowledge of psychopharmacological agents is only part of the psychiatric–mental health nurse's responsibility in managing the use of these agents. Nurses are also ethically and legally responsible for making sure that clients have the information they need to achieve and maintain optimal health (American Nurses Association [ANA], 1994). The nurse is responsible for

- Evaluating the client's response to medications and documenting the response.
- Providing opportunities for the client to explore his or her feelings and concerns related to the medications.
- Collaborating with the client's prescriber to assess and plan the client's particular medication needs.
- Educating the client and his or her family about the expected effects, side effects, and food and drug interactions of the prescribed medication and how to deal with them (ANA 1994; Lund & Frank, 1991; Smith & Knice-Ambinder, 1989).

ROLE OF THE ADVANCED-PRACTICE NURSE

The role of the advanced-practice nurse in psychiatric–mental health nursing includes all the responsibilities of the generalist and also involves responsibilities based on additional expertise in and knowledge of the diagnosis and treatment of mental disorders (ANA, 1994). Educational preparation for the advanced role begins at the master's level and progresses through clinical experience, leading to certification as an advanced psychiatric–mental health practitioner. Concerning the use of pharmacological agents, the role of the certified psychiatric–mental health specialist may include prescriptive authority. The inclusion of prescriptive authority in the advanced-practice role is based on state nurse practice law, as well as state and federal regulations governing prescriptions. The advanced-practice psychiatric–mental health nurse applies neurobiological, psychopharmacological, and physiological knowledge to all aspects of the therapeutic process. Of particular importance is the use of this knowledge to diagnose mental disorders, to develop therapeutic strategies based on clinical indicators, and to treat mental disorders with pharmacological agents (ANA, 1994). In addition, advanced practice in psychiatric–mental health nursing includes educating other nurses and health care providers about psychopharmacological agents and consulting about their use and management.

COMPLIANCE

A major challenge to nurses in psychiatric–mental health practice is medication noncompliance (Lund & Frank, 1991). The result of clients' noncompliance with a medication regimen is often relapse and rehospitalization. Noncompliance relapse rates after treatment are estimated to be 50 percent in the first year and 70 percent in the second year after treatment (Sulliger, 1988). Client compliance is a complex and multifaceted challenge in psychiatric–mental health nursing practice. *Compliance* results when clients make informed choices that help them master the challenges they face with their illness (Smith & Knice-Ambinder, 1989). The nurse has a special responsibility to help clients make informed choices based on an understanding of their rights. Some guidelines for enhancing medication compliance are offered in Table 26–19.

In addition to the preceding responsibilities, the nurse needs to be mindful of a number of principles of medication use that are important to ensure the desired therapeutic effects. First, no person should be seen as only a medical client or only a psychiatric client. All clients should be given a complete workup that considers both medical and psychiatric causes for illness. For example, treating a medical condition such as hypothyroidism may cure a client's depression, while treating a psychiatric illness such as depression may improve a client's irritable bowel syndrome.

Second, nonpharmacological options should always be considered first. Crisis intervention, counseling, assistance in attaining financial help, diet, addiction treatment, and sleep hygiene measures are just some options to medication.

Third, medication alone is rarely indicated in the treatment of any psychiatric disorder; medication in combination with counseling is almost always more effective than medication alone. Psychiatric illnesses, including depression, can best be understood and treated by considering a biopsychosocial model.

Finally, the nurse should keep in mind the following points:

- The smallest possible effective dose should be used for the shortest effective period. This principle must be balanced against the knowledge that failure to use an adequate dosage and to continue medication long enough are significant contributors to treatment failures.
- The simpler the drug regimen, the higher the compliance. In most instances, a once-daily dosing schedule is possible. An obvious exception is lithium; most prescribers believe that its short half-life necessitates more frequent dosing.
- Polypharmacy should be avoided whenever possible. Combinations of psychoactive drugs generally are not more effective than a single drug (Arana & Hyman, 1991; Baldessarini, 1993; Bernstein, 1988). The more medications a client takes, the more side effects he or she experiences, making compliance more difficult.
- Overall, the safety of using most psychiatric medications during pregnancy and lactation has not been established, and the use of these medications must be carefully assessed by the prescriber and the client. Lithium is specifically contradicted during pregnancy, especially during the first trimester.

TABLE 26–19
Guidelines for Enhancing Medication Compliance

- Assist client in acquiring knowledge about medications, including actions, precautions, side effects, signs of toxicity, drug interactions, and food and drug interactions.
- Explore client's beliefs about medications and their effects.
- Explain nature of and time span for onset of therapeutic results.
- Help client develop strategies for dealing with common side effects and missed doses of medication.
- Relate medications to the target symptoms associated with client's illness.
- Explore with client any differing expectations regarding barriers and facilitators for medication compliance and medication effects.
- Provide written and verbal instructions to reinforce compliance.
- Develop strategies to help client incorporate medication taking into daily routine.
- Include family members or significant others in education about client's medications and illness and their own needs as caregivers.
- Explain complications that can result from use of alcohol and other drugs that can lead to establishment of a maladaptive pattern of coping.

LEGAL AND ETHICAL ISSUES

Patient Advocacy

The administration of psychotropic medications presents unique challenges to nurses. The medications themselves are often quite potent, and individual responses may be relatively unpredictable. To complicate the matter further, clients may have difficulty complying with the medication regimen, giving informed consent, recognizing and reporting therapeutic and adverse effects, and applying psychoeducational material. The first and foremost responsibility of psychiatric nurses is *client advocacy* (ANA, 1994). In terms of psychopharmacological intervention, client advocacy includes protection of the client from harm while ensuring the use of the least restrictive environment. This is particularly salient in ethical dilemmas created by the use of chemical restraints in some situations.

Controversies about the advertising, pricing, and unlabeled use of psychotropic medications can also present ethical dilemmas (see accompanying Controversy display).

CONTROVERSY

Issues in Psychopharmacological Therapy

Truth in Advertising

Truth in the advertising of psychotropic medication has become an issue over the past few years. Several of the newer compounds on the market have not lived up to their advanced billing. Some of the contradictions have occurred in reporting of addiction potential, indications for usage, and reported risks. Of particular concern is the increasing number of clients who are seeking and receiving treatment for mental health problems such as depression and anxiety outside of traditional psychiatry. At least partially responsible for this development is the high cost of psychiatric care and the severe limitations placed by many third-party payers on reimbursement for such care. Medical care providers whose practices do not include a large number of such clients are particularly vulnerable to misleading advertising. The extreme complexity of the actions of psychotropic medications, individual manifestations of mental disorders and medication responses, and medication monitoring make truth in the advertising of psychotropics an extremely controversial and ethical issue.

Unlabeled Use

Closely allied with the above controversy is the use of medications for purposes other than their governmentally approved uses, known as *unlabeled use*. Examples of unlabeled use include in some research settings' support of the efficacy of lithium for the treatment of some forms of unipolar depression and the promise of fluoxetine (Prozac) in the treatment of obsessive–compulsive disorder. Research evidence is also accumulating for the support of the use of serotonergic-reuptake blockers in decreasing alcohol consumption in some clients. Unless clients have access to such research centers, usually situated in university-affiliated medical centers in large cities, they have little access to these possible treatments.

Pricing

A third controversy is pricing. As with most medications, the cost of many psychotropic medications can be quite prohibitive. Third-party and government payers have become more stringent in reimbursement practices, which can make access to needed medications difficult. An added issue in psychiatry is that a great number of severely and persistently mentally ill persons are on some type of public assistance. Public assistance programs such as Medicare and Medicaid have stringent rules as to what medications they will pay for and will usually pay only when a medication has been prescribed by a physician. This is of particular relevancy in the development of clozapine (Clozaril) to treat previously medication-resistant schizophrenia. Clozapine specifically treats ambivalence and the chronic withdrawal/apathy that characterize many persons with chronic schizophrenia in the remittance phase and thus prohibit long-term adjustment. The cost of this medication is extremely prohibitive, in part because of the careful laboratory monitoring necessary to guard against the potential life-threatening side effects. A number of clients are being denied access to this potentially life-enhancing medication because the mental health system is unable to achieve some sort of resolution between public assistance and the pharmaceutical manufacturer.

Medication Administration

General principles of medication administration should be followed. These include ensuring the following:

Correct client
Correct medication
Correct dose
Correct route
Correct time (Sullivan, 1991)

The nurse should follow institutional protocol for medication administration procedures. As with any hospitalized client, documentation and reporting of procedures must be followed with the psychiatric client.

Right to Refuse

As mentioned, obtaining informed consent from the mentally ill client can be difficult. Many clients in these settings, perhaps because of their respective illnesses, their beliefs, or their fears, are reluctant to comply with medication administration. Except in unusual circumstances, a mentally ill client has the *right to refuse* medication. First, a client may have been involuntarily committed to the hospital because he or she was judged to be gravely disabled and harmful to himself or herself or others. States vary in their statutes regarding medicating these clients against their will, and it is imperative that the nurse be familiar with the laws of the state in

TABLE 26–20
Medications That Require That Postural Blood Pressure Be Taken

ANTIDEPRESSANTS	ANTIPSYCHOTICS	ALPHA-ANTAGONISTS
Amitriptyline (Elavil)	Acetophenazine (Tindal)	Doxepin (Sinequan) >150 mg/day
Imipramine (Tofranil)	Chlorpromazine (Thorazine)	Trifluoperazine (Stelazine) >5 mg/day
Protriptyline (Vivactyl)	Chlorprothixene (Taractan)	
Perphenazine and amitriptyline (Triavil)	Thioridazine (Mellaril)	
	Haloperidol (Haldol)	

which he or she works. In addition, in certain cases, a court may order clients to be medicated against their wishes. This usually happens to clients with long histories of noncompliance who have shown clear improvement when their symptomatology is under the control of medication. In clients without such legal support, however, exceptions may still need to be made. For example, in some cases, it may be believed that the client is so severely endangered by his or her behavior that a life-threatening crisis is imminent. It may be advisable for the nurse to collaborate and consult with the interdisciplinary team. If a decision is made to medicate a client against his or her will, it is imperative that documentation be clear, descriptive, and inclusive of other interventions that were tried.

The nurse also has a legal and ethical obligation to inform the client to the best of his or her ability to understand what a medication is, what symptoms it can be expected to treat, and its potential risks (ANA 1994; Smith & Knice-Ambinder, 1989). Information should be provided that will enable the client to recognize signs of symptom remittance as well as adverse effects. Clients should receive information about administration methods, any contraindications, and especially any adverse effects that could precipitate an emergency (such as the development of symptoms of tardive dyskinesia).

One of the challenges enjoyed by the psychiatric–mental health nurse is the development of creative psychoeducational strategies for medications. Common strategies include medication education groups, printed instructions, and self-medication programs. It is also crucial for the client's family or significant others to be involved in the educational process. A frequent problem cited by mental health advocacy groups is that families are often uninformed about the treatment itself and its risks and potential benefits. This process should also be documented (Lund & Frank, 1991; Smith & Knice-Ambinder, 1989).

Medication Monitoring

A final area of particular relevance in the legal and ethical administration of psychotropic medications is medication monitoring. The nurse must be thoroughly familiar with both the expected outcomes of the medication and the potential adverse effects. These include physical, affective, and behavioral sequelae. For instance, the nurse should know which medications will effect blood pressure (see Table 26–20 for a list). Many psychiatric settings use some sort of formalized system of symptom documentation, whether checklists for adverse effects or abbreviated mental status reports for affective and behavioral assessment. It is imperative that the nurse develop excellent assessment skills for this purpose.

CHAPTER SUMMARY

Recent advances in research on the brain have created a virtual explosion of knowledge of the relationship between the brain and human behavior. As a result, health care professionals' understanding of the neurobiological basis of many mental illnesses has been enhanced dramatically, and more efficacious pharmacological agents for the treatment of mental illness have been developed. This chapter has provided the reader with a review of areas of neuroanatomy and neurophysiology related to the pharmacokinetics of psychopharmacological agents used across the life span. Principles of pharmacokinetics and pharmacodynamics that are germane to an understanding of the psychopharmacological management of mental illness have been discussed. The nurse's roles in the use and administration of these agents and education of clients and their families have been described. The legal issues related to psychopharmacology and the ethical considerations in the management of the psychopharmacological treatment regimen have been highlighted.

Suggestions for Clinical Conference

1. Role-play one of your clients on medication and describe its effects, both positive and negative. Then discuss nursing interventions that could help the client and family cope with the drug's side effects and comply with therapy.
2. Review your clinical unit's policy concerning client refusal to take medications. Does it conform to legal and ethical standards? How is the client's freedom of choice supported and maintained? Interview a nurse on the unit about strategies he or she uses to assist clients with decisions about taking medications. Discuss whether these strategies conform with unit policy and with legal and ethical standards.
3. Differentiate the signs and symptoms of tardive dyskinesia, extrapyramidal side effects, and neuroleptic malignancy syndrome. Identify factors that place clients at risk for each. Then discuss nursing

interventions that can help clients prevent these side effects or remedy their severity.

4. Invite a clinical specialist nurse from the unit to talk about the nurse's role in psychopharmacological therapy. Discuss this role in relation to the American Nurses Association's *Standards of Psychiatric and Mental Health Nursing Practice* (1994).
5. Select a client you are working with who is taking medication. Explain what the client and his or her family need to know about the medication, and what teaching strategies you have been using to convey this information. Evaluate the effectiveness of your teaching at subsequent clinical conferences and discuss what should be done if the client is not complying with the medication regimen.

References

American Society of Hospital Pharmacists (1990). American Hospital Formulary Services drug information. Bethesda, MD: Author.

American Nurses Association (1994). *Standards of psychiatric and mental health nursing practice*. Kansas City, MO: Author.

Arana, G. W., & Hyman, S. E. (1991). *Handbook of psychiatric drug therapy* (2nd ed.). Boston: Little, Brown.

Baldessarini, S. J. (1993). Drugs and the treatment of psychiatric disorders. In A. Goodman, T. Rall, A. Neis, & P. Taylor (Eds.), *Goodman & Gilman's The Pharmacological Basis of Therapeutics* (8th ed., pp. 383–435). New York: McGraw-Hill.

Benet, L., Mitchell, J., & Sheiner, L. (1993). Pharmacokinetics: The dynamics of drug absorption, distribution and elimination. In A. Goodman, T. Rall, A. Neis, & P. Taylor (Eds.), *Goodman & Gilman's The Pharmacological Basis of Therapeutics* (8th ed., pp. 3–32). New York: McGraw-Hill.

Bernstein, J. (1988). *Drug therapy in psychiatry* (2nd ed.). Chicago: Year Book Medical Publishers.

Blair, D. T., & Dauner, A. (1992). Dangerous consequences: Induced tardive akathesia. *Journal of Psychosocial Nursing and Mental Health Services*, *30*(3), 41–43.

Bloom, F. E., & Lazerson, A. (1985). *Brain, mind, and behavior* (2nd ed.). New York: W. H. Freeman.

Burt, A. M. (1993). *Textbook of neuroanatomy*. Philadelphia: W. B. Saunders.

Cade, J. F. (1949). Lithium salts in the treatment of psychotic excitement. *Medical Journal of Australia*, *2*, 349–353.

Cohn, J., Katon, W., & Richelson, E. (1990). Choosing the right antidepressant. *Patient Care*, *24*, 88–116.

Correia, M. A., & Castagnoli, N. (1989). Drug transformation. In B. G. Katzung (Ed.), *Basic and clinical pharmacology* (4th ed., pp. 41–50). Norwalk, CT: Appleton & Lange.

Crismon, M. L. (1990). Psychotropic drugs in the elderly: Principles of use. *American Pharmacy*, *NS30*(12), 57–64.

DeVane, C. L. (1990). *Fundamentals of monitoring psychoactive drug therapy*. Baltimore: Williams & Wilkins.

DeVane, C. L. (1992). Pharmacokinetics of the selective serotonin reuptake inhibitors. *Journal of Clinical Psychiatry*, *53*(2), 13–20.

DeVane, C. L., Ware, M. R., & Lydiard, R. B. (1991). Pharmacokinetics, pharmacodynamics and treatment issues of benzodiazepines: Alprazolam, adinazolam and clonazepam. *Psychopharmacology Bulletin*, *27*, 463–473.

DiSalver, S. C., Swanan, A. C., Shoaib, A. M., & Bowers, T. C. (1993). The manic syndrome: Factors which may predict a patient's response to lithium, carbamezepine and valproate. *Journal of Psychiatry and Neuroscience*, *18*, 61–66.

Dubovsky, S. L., Katz, J. L., Scherger, J. E., & Uhde, T. W. (1987). Anxiolytics: When? Why? Which one? *Patient Care*, *21*(7), 60–81.

Facts and Comparisons. (1993). *Drug facts and comparisons* St. Louis, MO: Author.

Gadow, K. D. (1991). Clinical issues in child and adolescent psychopharmacology. *Journal of Consulting and Clinical Psychology*, *59*, 842–852.

Gilman, S., & Newman, S. W. (1992). *Manter and Gatz's essentials of clinical neuroanatomy and neurophysiology* (8th ed.). Philadelphia: F. A. Davis.

Gomez, G. E., & Gomez, E. G. (1990). The special concerns of neuroleptic use in the elderly. *Journal of Psychosocial Nursing and Mental Health Services*, *28*(1), 7–14.

Greenblatt, D. J. (1992). Pharmacology of benzodiazepine hypnotics. *Journal of Clinical Psychiatry*, *53*(6), 7–13.

Hollister, L. (1989). Antipsychotic agents. In B. G. Katzung (Ed.), *Basic and clinical pharmacology* (4th ed., pp. 345–367). Norwalk, CT: Appleton & Lange.

Kandel, E. (1991a). Disorders of thought: Schizophrenia. In E. Kandel, H. Schwartz, & T. Jessell (Eds.), *Principles of neural science* (3rd ed., pp. 853–867). New York: Elsevier.

Kandel, E. (1991b). Nerve cells and behavior. In E. Kandel, H. Schwartz, & T. Jessell (Eds.), *Principles of Neural Science* (3rd ed., pp. 18–32). New York: Elsevier.

Kelly, J. P., & Dodd, J. (1991). Anatomical organization of the nervous system. In E. Kandel, H. Schwartz, & T. Jessell (Eds.), *Principles of neural science* (3rd ed., pp. 273–282). New York: Elsevier.

Kolb, B. & Wishaw, I. Q. (1990). *Fundamentals of human neurophysiology* (3rd ed.) New York: W. H. Freeman.

Kupferman, I. (1991). Localization of higher cognitive and affective function. In E. Kandel, H. Schwartz, & T. Jessell (Eds.), *Principles of neural science* (3rd ed., pp. 823–838). New York: Elsevier.

Kutcher, S. P., Reiter, S., Gardner, D. M., & Klein, R. G. (1992). The pharmacotherapy of anxiety disorders in children and adolescents. *Psychiatric Clinics of North America*, *15*, 41–67.

Leonard, B. E. (1993). *Fundamentals of psychopharmacology*. West Sussex, England: John Wiley & Son.

Lund, V. E., & Frank, D. I. (1991). Helping the medicine go down: Nurses' and patients' perceptions about medication compliance. *Journal of Psychosocial Nursing and Mental Health Services*, *29*, 6–9.

Meyers, B. S., & Kalayam, B. (1989). Update in geriatric psychopharmacology. *Advances in Psychosomatic Medicine*, *19*, 114–137.

Moran, M. G., & Thompson, T. L. (1988). Changes in the aging brain as they affect psychotropics: A review. *International Journal of Psychiatry and Medicine*, *18*, 137–144.

Newcomb, P. (1991). Tricyclic antidepressants and children. *Nurse Practitioner*, *16*(5), 26–31.

Nutt, D. J., & Glue, P. (1989). Clinical pharmacology of anxiolytics and antidepressants: A psychopharmacological perspective. *Pharmacological Therapy*, *44*, 309–334.

Role, L. W., & Kelly, J. P. (1991). The brain stem: Cranial nerve nuclei and the monoaminergic system. In E. Kandel, H. Schwartz, & T. Jessell (Eds.), *Principles of Neural Science* (3rd ed., pp. 683–699). New York: Elsevier.

Roth, T., & Roehrs, R. (1992). Issues in the use of benzodiazepine therapy. *Journal of Clinical Psychiatry*, *53*(6), 14–18.

Ryan, N. D. (1992). The pharmacologic treatment of child and adolescent depression. *Psychiatric Clinics of North America*, *15*, 29–40.

Schatzberg, A. E., & Cole, J. O. (1987). *Manual of clinical psychopharmacology*. Washington, DC: American Psychiatric Press.

Smith, G. R., & Knice-Ambinder, M. (1989). Promoting medication compliance in clients with chronic illness. *Holistic Nursing Practice*, *4*, 70–77.

Sternbach, H. (1991). The serotonin syndrome. *American Journal of Psychiatry*, *148*, 705–713.

Sugarmen, R. A., & Kinney, C. F. (1993). Review of functional neuroanatomy. In N. Keltner & D. Folks (Eds.), *Psychotropic drugs* (pp. 8–25). St. Louis, MO: C. V. Mosby.

Sulliger, N. (1988). Relapse. *Journal of Psychosocial Nursing and Mental Health Services*, *26*(6), 20–23.

Sullivan, G. H. (1991). Five rights equal 0 errors. *RN*, *54*, 65–66, 68.

Taniguchi, G., & Westphal, J. R. (1986). Long-term benzodiazepine use in anxiety states. *Hospital Formulary*, *21*, 179–186.

Tanner, C. M. (1992). Tardive dyskinesia. In H. L. Klawans, C. G. Goetz & C. M. Tanner (Eds.), *Textbook of clinical neuropharmacology and therapeutics* (2nd ed., pp. 151–165). New York: Raven Press.

Trevor, A., & Way, W. (1989). Sedative–hypnotics. In B. G. Katzung (Ed.), *Basic and clinical pharmacology* (4th ed., pp. 264–277). Norwalk, CT: Appleton & Lange.

Waters, B. G. (1990). Psychopharmacology of the psychiatric disorders of childhood and adolescence. *Medical Journal of Australia*, *152*, 32–39.

CHAPTER

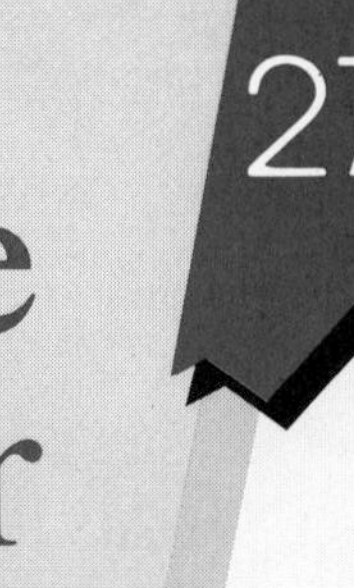

Electroconvulsive Therapy and Other Biological Therapies

DEBORAH ANTAI-OTONG, M.S., R.N.,C.S.

OUTLINE

Historical Aspects of Biological Therapies
- Psychosurgery
- Hydrotherapy: Continuous Bath and Cold Wet-Sheet Pack
- Convulsive Therapies
  - Insulin-Shock Therapy
  - Metrazol
  - Electroshock Therapy

Electroconvulsive Therapy
- Historical Aspects
- Major Indications
- Mechanism of Action: Neurobiological Theories
- Risks
- Contraindications
- Outpatient ECT
- Maintenance ECT

Life Span Issues
- The Use of ECT with Children and Adolescents
- The Use of ECT with Older Adults

The Nurse's Role in the Care of the Client Undergoing ECT
- Psychosocial Considerations
- ECT Protocols
- Ethical and Legal Considerations
  - Informed Consent

The Nursing Process
- Pretreatment Preparation

Other Biological Therapies
- Biological Cycles
- Light Therapy (Phototherapy)
- Sleep Cycle Alterations

Nursing Research on Biological Therapies

Chapter Summary

CHAPTER OBJECTIVES

Upon completion of this chapter, you will be able to:
1. Describe the evolution of biological therapies.
2. Develop a plan of care for a client undergoing ECT.
3. Analyze the relationship between client education and informed consent.
4. Discuss legal and ethical implication of biological therapies.
5. Recognize the relationship between biological therapies and human behavior.

KEY TERMS

Biological rhythms
Catatonia
Electroconvulsive therapy
Hydrotherapy
Insulin-shock therapy
Light therapy
Psychosurgery
Retino–hypothalamic–pineal axis
Seasonal affective disorder
Sleep-wake cycle

Somatic therapies, also called biological therapies, have evolved since the 1930s and are becoming increasingly helpful in enabling psychiatrists to understand the neurobiology of brain function. Numerous researchers have described the relationship between neurobiological and mental disorders. Historically, psychiatrists have explored numerous treatment modalities on the assumption that the biological and psychological components of mental illness affect human behavior. Psychiatry is shifting from primarily behavioral to primarily biological paradigms.

This shift emphasizes the role of neurobiological malfunction as a possible cause of mental illness. The science of neurobiology provides an approach to the treatment of mental illness that bridges the traditional boundary between soma (body) and psyche (mind) (Yodofsky & Hales, 1992).

The complexity of brain function and the brain's role in sustaining health and well-being are the bases of biological therapies. Somatic therapies used in the past include continuous baths, cold sheets, psychosurgery, and convulsive therapies. Some of these interventions were inhumane and their effectiveness questionable, but they were effective in calming clients. Technological advances have spawned new biological therapies, such as psychopharmacology, electroconvulsive therapy (ECT), light therapy, and sleep cycle alterations.

This chapter focuses on the impact of biological therapies on psychiatric–mental health nursing. The evolution of biological therapy, including insulin-shock therapy, psychosurgery, ECT, and newer biological therapies, is discussed. Other somatic therapies are discussed in Chapters 9 and 26. The terms *somatic therapy* and *biological therapy* are used interchangeably in this chapter.

HISTORICAL ASPECTS OF BIOLOGICAL THERAPIES

Somatic therapies evolved as researchers in the nineteenth century directed their energy toward improving ways to treat the mentally ill. The U.S. Congress's proclamation of the 1990s as the Decade of the Brain has renewed interest in biological therapies as viable treatment modalities. In issuing this proclamation, the Congress wished to draw attention to the growing number of people afflicted with disorders and disabilities that involve the brain (U.S. Congress, 1989). Technological advances in neurobiology have increased scientists' understanding of the brain's role in mental illness and other neurological disorders, such as Alzheimer's disease. As psychiatrists seek to understand the complexity of mental disorders and to develop innovative treatments for them, psychiatric–mental health nursing continues to play a vital role in reducing symptoms in the mentally ill.

PSYCHOSURGERY

Egas Moniz (1936), a Portuguese neurologist, introduced modern **psychosurgery** in the form of prefrontal lobotomy. In a prefrontal lobotomy, the nerve fibers that connect the thalamus with the frontal lobe of the brain are severed. Moniz surmised that the frontal lobe played a crucial role in the formation of mental illness and that by modifying various pathways or fibers joining the frontal lobes and thalamus, emotional and mental disturbance could be relieved. Initial surgical techniques involved drilling burr holes into the top or side of the skull and injecting alcohol at these sites; wires were then used to sever the front lobe. This procedure was blind in nature because the surgeon could not depict the surgical location. The American physicians Walter Freeman and James Watts introduced a modified version of this procedure in the United States the same year.

Psychosurgery never gained overwhelming popularity, and its use eventually waned because its effectiveness was questionable and was supported by little research. Charges of abuse by neurosurgeons and accusations that the technique was used for the purposes of social control and racial suppression added to the lack of acceptance of psychosurgery as a viable treatment for mental disorders. In addition, severe complications from this procedure consisted of motor dysfunction, seizures, and cognitive impairment (Kalinowsky & Hoch, 1950; Millon, 1969).

Historically, the nursing interventions required by clients undergoing prefrontal lobotomies were the same as those required by clients undergoing any neurosurgical procedure, including monitoring of neurological and vital signs, seizure activity, mental status changes, vomiting, and hemorrhaging. Major postoperative complications from psychosurgery included infection, seizures, and hemorrhaging (Kalinowsky & Hoch, 1950; Steele & Manfreda, 1959).

Since its advent almost 60 years ago, psychosurgery has been refined and restricted to specific destruction of modest regions of brain tissue. Major procedures include radioactive implants, cryoprobes, electrical coagulation, proton beams, ultrasonography, and bilateral cingulotomies (Henn, 1989). Currently, alteration of frontolimbic pathways that alter emotional disturbances, such as in chronic debilitating mental disorders that fail to respond to traditional treatment and chronic intractable depression, is the chief reason for psychosurgery. Overall, psychosurgery has been the least acceptable of the somatic therapies and has been used only as a last resort when clients fail to respond to other treatments.

HYDROTHERAPY: CONTINUOUS BATH AND COLD WET-SHEET PACK

Other procedures that were once used to control emotional and mental disturbances included two forms of **hydrotherapy**: the continuous bath and cold wet-sheet pack. The continuous bath was used to control agitation and erratic emotional disturbances and induce sleep. This procedure was used prior to bedtime and consisted of having the client lie on a hammock dangling in a continuous warm bath for extended periods. The client was constantly watched and assessed for signs of overheating, dizziness, convulsions, behavioral changes, and drowning (Steele & Manfreda, 1959).

Cold wet-sheet packs produced a sedative effect, promoting sleep and reducing agitation, anxiety, and irritability. This procedure consisted of removing the client's clothes, asking the client to void, and enclosing him or her in the wet-sheet pack. In a room that was dim and quiet to facilitate relaxation, the client was literally wrapped in at least two sheets that had been soaked in cold water and wrung out. A blanket was used to reduce chilling. The rationale behind the use of the cold wet-sheet pack was the constriction of blood vessels. Chilling for 5 to 10 minutes was intended to dilate blood vessels, thereby increasing cerebral flow and blood volume. The warmth subsequently produced a calming effect (Steele & Manfreda, 1959).

CONVULSIVE THERAPIES

The convulsive therapies were a major discovery during the twentieth century. A pioneer in convulsive therapies was Manfreda Sakel, a German psychiatrist who realized that a coma could be induced by administering large amounts of insulin. He noted that recovery from an insulin coma–produced calmness in clients who were formerly confused, delirious, and agitated. He therefore surmised that repeated doses of insulin could produce remission of schizophrenic symptoms. His work was soon embraced by the psychiatric community (Sakel, 1938).

Insulin-Shock Therapy

In **insulin-shock therapy** large doses of insulin were administered to induce marked hypoglycemia in clients. The hypoglycemic state produces a coma that may or may not induce a seizure. Insulin-shock therapy was used on clients with catatonia and paranoid forms of schizophrenia, but its exact psychotherapeutic effect was unknown. Major complications of this treatment modality were shock and death. Insulin-shock therapy lost its popularity years ago and disappeared from psychiatric treatment because of its questionable efficacy and potential danger.

Metrazol

Sakel's work stirred the interest of Ladislau von Meduna, a Hungarian neuropsychiatrist. Von Meduna postulated that schizophrenia and epilepsy rarely occurred simultaneously. Initially, Meduna injected camphor in oil intramuscularly to induce seizures, but because of the numerous side effects of this intervention, such as pain and unreliable response, he resorted to using pentylenetetrazol (Metrazol). Metrazol, a potent synthetic stimulant, was used to produce electrical stimulation of the brain and induce seizures. This treatment, like others, was not free of side effects. Major disadvantages were unreliable seizure activity, intense feelings of doom between injections, and loss of consciousness lasting approximately 3 to 30 seconds (Kalinowsky & Hoch, 1950). In spite of these side effects, treatment with metrazol gained popularity because it successfully induced remission of psychosis and depression. Its used declined with the emergence of electroshock therapy (EST).

Electroshock Therapy

Researchers continued to try to find the ideal approach to the treatment of mental and emotional illnesses. In 1938, Ugo Cerletti and Luciano Bini, Italian physicians, discovered that they could produce seizures with an electric current rather than a chemical stimulus. Cerletti (1950) surmised that seizures were biochemical drives that mobilized protective responses capable of improving adaptation and producing therapeutic results in the mentally ill. In 1938, Cerletti and Bini reported the first successful application of EST, or shock therapy, in a client with catatonic schizophrenia. Clients often experienced profound anxiety and fear during the interval between the application of EST and loss of consciousness. They were given drugs such as amobarbital and thiopental sodium to allay these feelings. Other common complications included lumbar and dorsal spine fractures (Cerletti, 1950; Steele & Manfreda, 1959).

EST became the dominant somatic therapy for mental disorders during the 1940s. However, several researchers observed that only a few clients with schizophrenia benefited from EST and only those who were acutely ill, agitated, or catatonic and those with affective symptoms found relief (Pacella et al., 1942).

The term *electroshock therapy* was later changed to ***electroconvulsive therapy***, or ECT, and modifications of this technique have emerged over the years, reducing its dangers. In 1940 Bennett, an American psychiatrist, improved ECT when he introduced a new method of anesthesia derived from the curare plant. He suggested that inducing paralysis during ECT reduced the risk of fractures. In 1951, succinylcholine was introduced to psychiatry and eventually became the most widely used muscle relaxant during this procedure.

ECT remained in favor among psychiatrists until the advent of psychotropics in the 1950s. Antidepressants and antipsychotics were the primary psychotropics, and they also curtailed the use of barbiturates, wet packs, and restraints. Recent years have seen a resurgence in the use of ECT, but controversy about its effectiveness remains (see Controversy display).

CONTROVERSY

Is Electroconvulsive Therapy Safe?

Electroconvulsive therapy (ECT) was introduced in the 1930s as an effective, yet controversial treatment for serious mental disorders. As we approach the twenty-first century, ECT remains a controversial treatment modality. Historically, its effectiveness has been questionable and unpredictable and has been likened to that of other radical treatment, such as the lobotomy. Early forms of ECT treatment subjected clients to profound anxiety and feelings of doom prior to losing consciousness from ECT.

Although the technique of ECT has been greatly refined since the 1930s, controversy over its use prevails for several reasons. One is continued fear about the application of electricity to the brain. Common fears associated with ECT include the fear of electrocution, brain damage, and permanent memory loss.

A second reason for the persistent controversy is that the public continues to perceive ECT as an inhumane and negative form of treatment, surmising that it is potentially damaging and unpredictable. The media reinforce this perception, portraying characters such as Frankenstein and other monsters as becoming violent and aggressive when their brains are aroused by electricity. Also, a movement in the 1960s and 1970s against ECT arose from the belief that mental disorders were caused primarily by maladaptive responses to the environment, rather than by biological factors.

As psychiatry moves into the twenty-first century, there has been a resurgence in the use of ECT and controversy over its use. Despite modifications in technique and improved proficiency, arguments over the safety and usefulness of ECT prevail. Some clients are adamantly against this treatment modality, asserting that it compromises their self-esteem and impairs their mental ability, whereas others claim that ECT is a life saver.

On the positive side, the efficacy of ECT has been well documented since its inception, and studies continue to show that it is an effective, cost-efficient treatment for some clients suffering from severe mental disorders.

ELECTROCONVULSIVE THERAPY

HISTORICAL ASPECTS

The misconception held by neuropsychiatrists early in the twentieth century that epilepsy and schizophrenia occurred simultaneously provided the rationale for the use of ECT. Its use climaxed in the 1940s and 1950s, when it was considered the treatment of choice for severe mental illness, such as schizophrenia and manic-type bipolar disorder. As mentioned, the use of ECT promptly declined with the advent of psychotropics in the 1950s. Today, ECT continues to be a controversial treatment modality. The controversy stems from the debate about whether its psychotherapeutic effect on the brain is worth its perceived invasiveness and brain-damaging aspects (Fink, 1991).

Black (1993) noted that ECT parallels psychosurgery as one of the least accepted forms of treatment. However, recent years have seen an increased acceptance of ECT as a safe, effective, and economical form of treatment. The effectiveness of ECT continues to be researched, and this intervention continues to gain approval for treating neurological disorders such as refractory parkinsonism and neuroleptic malignant syndrome (Rummans, 1993).

MAJOR INDICATIONS

Coffey and Weiner (1990) identified the major indications for ECT as major depression, psychosis, the need for a swift onset of action, and certain medical conditions. In 90 percent of cases, ECT is used to treat *major depression*. A number of researchers investigating its effectiveness contend that it is better than placebo in sustaining remission of depressive symptoms at least 80 percent of the time (Coffey & Weiner, 1990). The extent of improvement parallels the severity of illness (Hamilton, 1986). Other studies comparing the efficacy of antidepressants with that of ECT have revealed marked or comparable improvement in depressed clients (Coffey & Weiner, 1990).

Clients experiencing acute mania, delirium, and schizophrenia, particularly those with catatonia and affective symptoms, have exhibited a good response to ECT (Mukherjee et al., 1994; Rummans, 1993; Small et al., 1991). **Catatonia** refers to a complex syndrome manifested by either marked stupor and muscle rigidity or overactivity. This disorder is generally seen in clients with schizophrenia or affective disorders. ECT continues to be a controversial treatment for psychosis. Indications for ECT during psychotic episodes include ineffective response or contraindication to other therapies. In one study, some clients were found to show improvement when neuroleptics or antipsychotics were added to this treatment modality (Small, 1985).

One advantage of ECT is its ability to produce a rapid onset of action in severely depressed clients who need immediate treatment to alleviate life-threatening conditions such as suicidal risk, catatonia, or profound malnutrition and dehydration (Weiner & Coffey, 1987).

Welch (1991) delineated the following groups as good candidates for ECT, regardless of diagnosis:

1. Severely malnourished depressed clients at risk for medical complications
2. Medically ill clients with cardiac arrhythmias or coronary artery disease who cannot tolerate antidepressants or neuroleptics (e.g., elderly clients)
3. Psychotically depressed clients whose symptoms are not relieved by traditional antidepressant regimens
4. Clients who did not respond to medications during previous depressive episodes
5. Clients with catatonia, which may be a symptom of depression, schizophrenia, an endocrine disorder, or a brain lesion

Welch (1991) noted that in 50 percent of cases, untreated catatonia increases the likelihood of pulmonary complications, venous embolus, contractures, and impaired skin integrity. Table 27–1 summarizes the indications for ECT.

MECHANISM OF ACTION: NEUROBIOLOGICAL THEORIES

The efficacy of ECT has been linked with the production of grand mal seizures. The exact neurobiological effect of seizures elicited by ECT remains unknown. Current animal studies suggest that seizures elicited by ECT create alterations in neurochemical, neuroendocrine, and neurophysiological processes that are similar to those produced by antidepressants (Black, 1993). Fink (1990) postulated that ECT produces alterations in several neurotransmitter receptors, such as acetylcholine, norepinephrine, dopamine, and serotonin. This process is the same as that produced by long-term antidepressant use.

Neurophysiological theories suggest that certain regions in the brain are hyperactive during seizures and hypoactive after ECT. Dubovsky (1992) noted that the electrical stimulus generated by kindling or persistent stimulation calms hyperactive brain circuits. Other theories about the effectiveness of ECT suggest that it increases the levels of some neuropeptides that stabilize mood and modify regional cerebral blood flow (Fink, 1990). Table 27–2 summarizes the theories of the neurobiological effects of ECT.

Imaging technology is another avenue through which researchers are attempting to understand the effects of ECT on the brain. Imaging techniques include computerized tomography (CT), magnetic resonance imaging (MRI), regional cerebral blood flow, positron emission tomography, and single-photon emission computerized tomography. Findings are inconclusive that morphological changes do occur in the brain after a course of ECT (Coffey et al., 1991; Pande et al., 1990).

TABLE 27–1
Indications for ECT

PSYCHIATRIC	MEDICAL
Major depression (80%)	Catatonia secondary to medical conditions
Schizophrenia (10–20%)	Neuroleptic malignant syndrome secondary to neuroleptic use
Acute mania (3%)	Hypopituitarism Intractable seizure disorder Parkinsonism

Percentages are percentage of cases treated with electroconvulsive therapy.

Data from American Psychiatric Association Task Force on Electroconvulsive Therapy. (1990). *The practice of electroconvulsive therapy: Recommendations for psychiatric training and privileging.* Washington, DC: American Psychiatric Association.

RISKS

Technical advances in the study of ECT show decreasing risk of this therapy. Abrams (1992) described ECT as a low-risk procedure and stated that its safety is associated with a greater understanding of neurobiological processes and increased proficiency in monitoring. In addition, there is a lack of conclusive evidence that ECT produces brain damage or worsens dementia (Devanand et al., 1994; Weiner, 1984).

Initial risks, such as fractures, decreased with the advent of effective muscle relaxants and short-acting anesthetics, the use of supported oxygen perfusion, improvements in equipment, and increased competence in staff. As a result of these advances, the mortality rates have dropped tremendously. Recent reports indicate 2 deaths per 100,000 treatments (Kramer, 1985). Today, ECT is considered one of the safest somatic interventions that uses general anesthesia. Morbidity and mortality generally result from secondary complications from cardiovascular factors, such as arrhythmias, myocardial infarction, or hypertension (Dubovsky, 1992).

TABLE 27–2
Theories of the Neurobiological Effects of Electroconvulsive Therapy

NEUROCHEMICAL

- Dysregulates postsynaptic beta-adrenergic receptors
- Alters neurotransmitter sites (e.g., sites of acetylcholine, norepinephrine, dopamine, and serotonin)
- Increases cerebrospinal fluid calcium levels

NEUROPHYSIOLOGICAL

- Subdues kindling sites in brain
- Increases neuropeptide levels
- Affects cerebral blood flow

Clients with impaired cardiovascular and cerebral function have the greatest risk for adverse effects from ECT. Cardiovascular workload increases rapidly during the onset of the seizure or ECT, because of the sympathetic arousal. This stimulation generally persists throughout the seizure and is intensified by circulating catecholamines that peak after 3 minutes after the start of the seizure (Liston & Salk, 1990). When the seizure ceases, the parasympathetic response persists, producing transient hypotension and bradycardia. The client's baseline physiological function normally returns within 5 to 10 minutes (Welch, 1991). The major physiological responses to ECT are listed in Table 27–3.

The major cardiovascular complications from ECT are as follows:

- Acute myocardial infarction
- Coronary arrhythmias
- Myocardial rupture
- Cardiac arrest
- Congestive heart failure
- Hypertension

Cerebral responses to ECT arise from the tremendous amount of oxygen used during the procedure. The rate of oxygen consumption doubles during ECT, producing increased cerebral blood circulation, with a subsequent rise in intracranial pressure and increased permeability of the blood–brain barrier. These cerebral responses place the client at risk for neurological complications. Major neurological contraindications for ECT include space-occupying brain lesions, which have been related to decompensation and death. In spite of these risk factors, some clients with these lesions have been successfully treated with ECT. However, these clients usually had asymptomatic meningiomas or chronic subdural hematomas (Malek-Ahmado et al., 1990; Zwil et al., 1990).

CONTRAINDICATIONS

Most researchers contend that the contraindications for ECT have diminished since the advent of the use of brief pulse stimulation, rather than the traditional sine wave stimulus, to initiate a grand mal seizure. The principal advantage of the brief pulse stimulation is that it uses significantly less electrical energy than the sine wave stimulation does. Another factor that reduces cognitive impairment and adverse reactions to ECT is unilateral placement of electrodes on the nondominant hemisphere. The nondominant side in right-handed persons is the right side of the head (Abrams, 1992).

At one time, clients with various neurological conditions, such as space-occupying brain lesions, hydrocephalus, and arteriovenous malformations and clients recovering from stroke were considered absolutely contraindicated for ECT. Recent studies have shown that ECT can be administered safely and efficaciously to these clients, however (Cardno & Simpson, 1991; Escalona et al., 1991). At one time, pregnancy was also considered a contraindication for ECT, but recent studies indicate that severely depressed pregnant women, at risk for malnutrition and suicide, may be candidates for this therapy. However, these clients remain at risk for complications from ECT and need to be closely monitored (e.g., fetal cardiac monitoring and avoidance of excessive hyperventilation) during and after treatment. The usefulness of administering ECT to a pregnant client must outweigh the potential dangers of this procedure before it can be implemented (Dorn, 1985; Miller, 1994; Repke & Berger, 1984).

Table 27–4 lists the contraindications to ECT.

TABLE 27–3
Major Physiological Responses to Electroconvulsive Therapy

CARDIOVASCULAR

- 25% increase in heart rate occurs with induction of anesthesia.
- Vagal stimulation leads to transient bradycardia during and after administration of electrical stimulus.
- Heart rate increases at end of seizure.
- Increased blood pressure rate parallels heart rate.

CEREBRAL

- Seizure increases electroencephalographic activity.
- Transient memory and cognitive impairments occur, including disorientation, confusion, forgetfulness, retrograde and anterograde amnesia, and headaches.

TABLE 27–4
Contraindications to Electroconvulsive Therapy

- Intracranial lesions (e.g., tumors)
- Acute myocardial infarction or infarction within last 3 months
- Severe hypertension

OUTPATIENT ECT

The number of clients receiving ECT has risen in recent years. Treatment in outpatient settings is possible because ECT is a short, relatively safe, and well-tolerated procedure with a low risk for adverse reactions (Abrams, 1992). Outpatient ECT is usually coordinated by a registered nurse who engages the client and family in the education process that prepares them for treatment. Preparation for outpatient ECT is the same as that for inpatient treatment (Pileggi & Ryan, 1993).

MAINTENANCE ECT

In spite of its effectiveness in managing mood disorders, early relapse is common in ECT unless maintenance treatment is used. Good candidates for maintenance ECT are clients who have responded favorably as inpatients or those who have not responded to traditional medication regimens. The principal goal of maintenance ECT is to prevent relapse. Relapse is relatively common 6 months after ECT treatment; the relapse rate is 30 to 60 percent. An antidepressant or lithium has been used as an adjunct to ECT to sustain its therapeutic effects for about 6 months. Some researchers have challenged this notion, however, arguing that continuation of psychotropics may not be efficacious in clients who did not respond to antidepressants prior to ECT (Abrams, 1992; Penney et al., 1990; Sackheim et al., 1989).

Various psychotherapies have been surmised to enhance the effectiveness of ECT. Studies show that psychotherapy and psychotropics can reduce relapse between 6 and 12 months after ECT (Coffey & Weiner, 1990; Silver & Yudofsky, 1988). ECT is only one component of the treatment of depression. Psychiatric–mental health nurses can promote clients' health by actively working with them and their families to identify psychosocial factors that may precipitate depressive episodes. Collaborating with ECT team members allows nurses to mobilize resources and support the client at risk for relapse. Treatment approaches must incorporate psychosocial and biological therapies that meet clients' needs during vulnerable periods.

LIFE SPAN ISSUES

THE USE OF ECT WITH CHILDREN AND ADOLESCENTS

The use of ECT in children and adolescents is limited to the same conditions suggested for adult populations. Its uses is rare, and research supporting its efficacy is scarce. Guidelines for the administration of ECT to children 12 years of age or younger are delineated by the American Psychiatric Association Task Force on ECT (1990) and include the following:

1. It should be confined to those cases when other treatments are infeasible or unsafe.
2. Recommendation for ECT must come from two psychiatrists who are experienced in working with this population and are not involved in the case.
3. The anesthetist must also be adept in working with this age group.

Other suggestions include developing policies that parallel state and federal guidelines for the administration of ECT in this age group.

THE USE OF ECT WITH OLDER ADULTS

The management of mental disorders in the elderly has received increased attention in the past decade. Concern regarding the treatment of people 65 years of age and older arises from the enormous growth of this population group, which comprises 12 percent of the U.S. population. At the present growth rate, it is estimated that by 2000 this age group will comprise more than 40 million people (Kovar, 1982).

Another concern for the elderly is their vulnerability to a host of psychosocial and neurobiological stressors generated by the aging process. Psychosocial stressors include loss of health, loved ones, and financial security. The brain is affected by the aging process in that levels of neurotransmitters and precursors, such as dopamine and norepinephrine, are lowered, increasing the likelihood of depression. Lowered levels of these biochemicals are caused by altered neuroendocrine function of the thyroid and pituitary glands in the elderly (Adolfson et al., 1979; Lipton, 1976).

Depression in the elderly is often defined in terms of chronicity and disability. High mortality rates suggest the need for aggressive efforts to identify high-risk groups and accurately diagnose and treat mood disorders in the elderly client. These efforts may be compromised because of changes in drug metabolism and medical conditions that contraindicate the use of antidepressants.

ECT is considered a viable treatment option for the severely depressed older adult. Predictors of a hopeful outcome include neurovegetative symptoms such as sleep, appetite, and cognitive disturbances. Less favorable outcomes are predicted in the client with coexisting mental disorders such as dementia or somatization disorders. The *somatization disorders* refers to physical complaints, such as headaches, nausea, or vomiting, that have no physical or underlying general medical basis (APA, 1994; Coryell et al., 1985).

Major complications from ECT among the elderly fall into several categories: cardiovascular, respiratory, cognitive impairment, and falls (Burke et al., 1987). Clients 75 years of age and older who have coexisting medical conditions such as ventricular arrhythmias or recent myocardial infarctions present the greatest risk for serious complications from ECT. General anesthesia significantly increases the risk of cardiovascular complications in the elderly client who has experienced a myocardial infarction in the last 3 months, and ECT is contraindicated during this period (Miller et al., 1979). In spite of these risks, most elderly clients can benefit from the therapeutic effects of ECT.

The psychiatric nurse reduces these complications by collaborating with members of the treatment team. Collaboration is enhanced when the nurse

TABLE 27–5
Medication Interactions with Electroconvulsive Therapy

AGENTS THAT INCREASE SEIZURE ACTIVITY	AGENTS THAT DECREASE SEIZURE ACTIVITY	OTHER DRUG INTERACTIONS
Theophyllin Caffeine Lithium Tricyclic antidepressants Trazodone (Desyrel) Fluoxetine (Prozac) Bupropion (Wellbutrin) Antipsychotic agents	Benzodiazepines Anticonvulsants Barbiturate anesthetic Propofol anesthetic	Monoamine oxidase inhibitors (e.g., phenelzine) are potent pressor agents and either increase or decrease blood pressure* Lithium increases severity of post-ECT cognitive impairment and may increase length of hospital stay†

*Need to be discontinued 2 weeks before ECT.
†Needs to be discontinued a week before ECT, because it enhances action of neuromuscular blocking agent.

- Establishes a therapeutic relationship with the client and family.
- Participates in the pre-ECT evaluation process by gathering pertinent physical assessment data, such as blood pressure, heart and respiratory status, and present medications and medical conditions.
- Assesses current medications and treatment regimens; see Table 27–5 for a list of medications that interact with ECT.
- Documents, reports, and discusses these findings with the treatment team.

THE NURSE'S ROLE IN THE CARE OF THE CLIENT UNDERGOING ECT

PSYCHOSOCIAL CONSIDERATIONS

Clients and family members anticipating ECT frequently feel anxious, because they have misconceptions about the procedure or have had negative experiences with it. Common misconceptions about ECT are that it will result in electrocution, permanent brain damage, memory loss, and death. Several studies suggest that in spite of modifications in technique and pretreatment instructions, these misconceptions prevail (Benhow, 1988; Fox, 1993). Another study disputes this notion, suggesting that only a small percentage of clients actually dislike ECT and are unwilling to submit to more treatment (Freeman & Kendall, 1986).

Historically, nurses have supported clients' decisions about ECT, have provided education, and have assessed psychosocial and biological needs. Assessing and responding to the psychosocial needs of clients and families are responsibilities of the psychiatric–mental health nurse. Psychiatric nurses can allay fears and anxiety by providing environments that encourage expression of feelings, thoughts, and fears regarding the procedure. Various educational media are useful in describing the ECT process, including videos, tours of the facility, and discussion of the responsibilities of the ECT team (APA, 1990; Baxter et al., 1986).

ECT PROTOCOLS

Several organizations, including the American Nurses Association (ANA) (1994), the APA Task Force on Electroconvulsive Therapy (1990), and the Royal College of Nursing of the United Kingdom (1987), have developed protocols for ECT. The ANA defined the role of the nurse in the care of the client undergoing ECT as follows. The nurse

1. Provides educational and emotional support for the client and family
2. Assesses the client's baseline or pretreatment level of function
3. Prepares the client for the ECT process
4. Monitors and evaluates the client's response to ECT, shares it with the ECT team, and modifies treatment as needed (see Nursing Care Plan 27–1)

In 1987, the Royal College of Nursing of the United Kingdom formulated guidelines that delineated the nurse's role in the ECT process and suggested that nursing functions should include coordinating the process, attending educational programs on ECT, participating on interdisciplinary teams, and developing educational programs.

In 1990, the APA Task Force on Electroconvulsive Therapy made recommendations for the treatment, training, and privileging of psychiatrists and members of the ECT team. They recommended that nurses were responsible for

1. Educating clients and their families about ECT.
2. Organizing care, including tending to the treatment area to ensure that equipment (e.g., emergency equipment, monitoring devices, and ECT equipment) is available and working.
3. Carrying out various nursing interventions to ensure clients' safety and understanding before and after ECT.

Overall, the various ECT protocols emphasize the significance of nurses in teaching, ensuring safety, and providing emotional support for the client undergoing ECT.

ETHICAL AND LEGAL CONSIDERATIONS

Controversy over the advantages and disadvantages of ECT continues to be widespread among mental health advocates, clients, families, and mental health professionals. The persistent fears and myths affect the public's perception of this treatment modality that uses electricity to change behavior. Clients and their families need to be informed of the benefits and potential risks of all treatment, particularly somatic interventions. The informed-consent process is a mechanism that encourages dynamic interactions among clients, families, and health professionals. In these interactions, ethical considerations, legal issues, and psychosocial factors are addressed.

Informed Consent

Clients must be informed of the purpose of ECT and other somatic treatments and the benefits and risk factors associated with them. This information needs to be integrated into individualized treatment plans that encourage the client's, family's, and other health care professionals' active participation in the decision-making process. These interactions convey to clients and their families that they are respected and are essential for involving clients and families in decisions about treatment.

The term *informed consent* refers to a legal standard that claims the client has been given information that enables him or her to make an educated decision

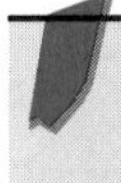

Nursing Care Plan 27–1 The Client Undergoing Electroconvulsive Therapy (Mrs. Moser)—Pretreatment

Nursing Diagnosis: Knowledge Deficit

OUTCOME IDENTIFICATION	NURSING ACTIONS	RATIONALES	EVALUATION
1. By [date], Mrs. Moser will understand the ECT procedure, including its purpose, benefits, and risks.	1. Have Mrs. Moser actively participate in the informed-consent process.	1. Enables client to make an informed decision.	*Goal met:* Mrs. Moser verbalizes her understanding of ECT and voluntarily participates in informed-consent process.
	2. Encourage Mrs. Moser to express her feelings, thoughts, and fears regarding ECT.	2. Enables client to cope with feelings and anxiety effectively.	

Nursing Diagnosis: Anxiety

OUTCOME IDENTIFICATION	NURSING ACTIONS	RATIONALES	EVALUATION
1. By [date], Mrs. Moser will experience minimal anxiety.	1. Approach Mrs. Moser in a calm, confident, and reassuring manner.	1. Allays anxiety by providing a calm environment.	*Goal met:* Mrs. Moser experiences minimal anxiety regarding procedure.
	2. Teach Mrs. Moser relaxation techniques.	2. Reduces anxiety.	
	3. Continuously assess Mrs. Moser's anxiety levels.	3. Provides information on clients response to stress/tension.	

whether to accept the treatment planned for him or her. The process of informed consent is an active process that begins, not ends, with the signing of the written consent form. It evolves between clients, families, and members of the ECT team throughout treatment (Abrams, 1992; Black, 1993). Three critical measures must exist within this process:

1. Voluntary consent
2. Competency of client
3. Information exchange

Furthermore, informed consent implies that the individual is competent and voluntarily submits to treatment after being presented adequate information about the procedure by the physician and other members of the ECT team.

Clients referred for ECT are initially evaluated by the physician for appropriateness. The decision for treatment is determined by the physician and client together, with the client actively participating in the informed-consent process. Client competency is an essential part of the informed-consent process, and nurses must be aware of hospital and state policy regarding involuntary treatment for an incompetent client. The presence of a life-threatening situation, along with a lack of appropriate treatment options, plays a major role in the decision to perform ECT on an incompetent client (Weiner, 1989). See Chapter 5 for an in-depth discussion of informed consent.

THE NURSING PROCESS

Assessment

Any procedure conducted under general anesthesia requires a medical and physical evaluation. In addition, the effects of ECT place enormous stress on the cardiovascular, respiratory, musculoskeletal, and neurological systems. Pretreatment diagnostic tests and examinations provide vital information about the client's physical and mental ability to undergo the procedure (Abrams, 1992; APA Task Force on Electroconvulsive Therapy, 1990).

Abrams (1992) suggested a number of pre-ECT procedures:

1. Thorough medical history
2. Physical examination
3. Routine blood and urine examinations (complete blood count, electrolytes, chemistries, and urinalysis)
4. Skull radiographs or use of imaging technique to rule out brain tumor (e.g., CT scan or MRI when a tumor is suspected)
5. Pseudokinesterase testing (the absence of this enzyme, which is responsible for catalyzing succinylcholine, a muscle relaxant used in ECT, increases the risk of apnea after ECT)

The electroencephalogram (EEG), brain CT, or MRI are not considered a good screening tool for ECT and should be used only when other diagnostic findings show structural changes.

Another concern of clients undergoing ECT is the interaction of ECT with a host of drugs. Most medications affect a person's seizure threshold and may need to be increased or decreased or stopped if the client is undergoing ECT. The use of psychotropics such as monamine oxidase inhibitors and lithium needs to be suspended 2 weeks prior to ECT (Runke, 1985).

Assessment of the client is enhanced by the use of a psychosocial assessment tool that elicits the following information:

- Duration of presenting symptoms
- Identification of present stressors
- Reasons for seeking treatment
- Current treatment, including medication and diet regimen
- Past treatment, including ECT, and response
- Level of dangerousness (e.g., presence of suicidal or homicidal ideations, intent, plan, or past attempts)
- Past psychiatric treatment
- Current or past substance misuse
- Present physical and mental status

Pretreatment Preparation

After the client is assessed to be appropriate for ECT, pretreatment preparation begins. Pretreatment nursing care varies, but it generally includes preparing the client both physically and psychologically for ECT. To prepare the client physically for the procedure, the nurse

- Assists the physician with the medical examination
- Educates the client and family on, for example, the preoperative protocol
- Instructs the client to take nothing by mouth at least 6 to 8 hours before treatment (clients receiving routine cardiovascular medications may be allowed to take these agents with sips of water several hours prior to treatment)
- Asks the client to remove dentures, eye glasses, or contact lenses
- Asks the client to void
- Confirms that the client's hair is shampooed and dry (and expecially that hair spray/creams are removed to reduce the risk of burns

Psychological preparation includes encouraging expression of feelings and thoughts regarding ECT and preoperative teaching (APA Task Force on Electroconvulsive Therapy, 1990; Royal College of Nursing, 1987).

The next part of pretreatment is premedication. Premedication normally consists of an intramuscular injection of an anticholinergic agent, such as atropine, to produce a mild tachycardia that will minimize the vagal stimulation produced by ECT and to reduce oral secretions. ECT induces a powerful vagal stimulation both during the procedure and promptly after it (Abrams, 1992; APA Task Force on Electroconvulsive Therapy, 1990).

Nursing Diagnoses

Major nursing diagnoses identified for clients undergoing ECT include the following:

- Knowledge Deficit
- Anxiety
- High Risk for Injury
- Decreased Cardiac Output
- Altered Thought Processes
- Self-Care Deficit
- Activity Intolerance
- High Risk for Aspiration

Planning

Treatment goals for the client undergoing ECT include the following:

1. The client makes an informed decision about ECT.
2. The client experiences minimal anxiety and fears about the procedure.
3. The client maintains vital signs within selected parameters during and after ECT.
4. The client remains free of injury.

Implementation

The ECT team generally consists of a psychiatrist, an anesthesia specialist, a registered nurse, and other nursing staff. The psychiatrist is normally responsible for coordinating the ECT team and managing medical treatment. The anesthesia specialist is responsible for providing anesthesia, maintaining a patent airway, and initiating emergency interventions if adverse reactions, such as cardiac arrhythmias or respiratory distress, occur.

The registered nurse is usually responsible for overseeing the general nursing care, including affirming that appropriate drugs are available and all emergency and resuscitation equipment is working properly, including oxygen and suction equipment. General nursing care prior to the procedure consists of (a) ensuring that the client is wearing comfortable attire to allow for placement of monitoring electrodes, (b) asking the client to void to minimize bladder distention and incontinence, (c) recording the client's vital signs, and (d) escorting the client to the treatment room. Reassurance and explanation throughout the treatment will allay the client's fears and anxiety.

After the client is assisted to the cart or stretcher, the nurse continues client education by explaining the placement of the blood pressure cuff and intravenous line. Later, the forehead or temples will be cleansed with alcohol or saline solution to reduce skin oils. Removal of skin oil assures proper electrode contact and minimizes skin burns (APA Task Force on Electroconvulsive Therapy, 1990; Burns & Stuart, 1991; Duffy & Conradt, 1989; Pileggi & Ryan, 1993). After the client is on the stretcher and the intravenous line is in place, the nurse continues to reassure the client by standing close by and explaining what is happening. The next step in preparation for ECT is electrode placement.

Recent modifications have been made in the location of the electrode placements. Historically, electrodes were placed bilaterally, but unilateral placement or stimulation has recently gained popularity. Bilateral ECT refers to placement on both sides of the head about 1 inch above the ear opening and outer seam of the eyelid. Unilateral ECT refers to electrode placement over the nondominant cerebral hemisphere, usually the right side of the head above the ear in right-handed persons, to facilitate EEG monitoring (Fig. 27–1). Additionally, the nondominant side of the brain possibly involves nonverbal responses and emotions rather than memory and language functions. Unilateral electrode placement is preferred because it reduces cognitive side effects, such as confusion, disorientation, and abnormal EEG changes (Abrams, 1992; APA Task Force on Electroconvulsive Therapy, 1990). Abrams (1992) asserted that the location of electrode placement is prompted by the variety of treatment.

Once the electrodes are in place, further monitoring is vital to the safe administration of ECT. This monitoring equipment used includes the following:

- Pulse oximeter (clipped to finger to monitor oxygen saturation)
- Blood pressure cuff (manual or automatic)
- Peripheral nerve stimulator (placed over ulnar nerve to assess muscle relaxation) (Abrams, 1992)

Administration of Anesthesia

The purposes of general anesthesia during ECT are as follows:

- To modulate the motor activity generated by the seizure activity
- To facilitate rapid induction and recovery
- To reduce adverse effects, such as musculoskeletal injury
- To expand the therapeutic effects of ECT

The major anesthetic agents used in ECT are short-acting anesthetics and muscle relaxants that are given intravenously shortly before induction of seizures or ECT. The neurobiological effects of ECT are closely monitored to appraise its effects and prolonged seizure activity. Seizure activity arises from application of controlled electrical stimulus to the scalp. The client's cardiovascular, respiratory, and systemic statuses are steadily monitored for adverse reactions (Abrams, 1992; APA Task Force on Electroconvulsive Therapy, 1990).

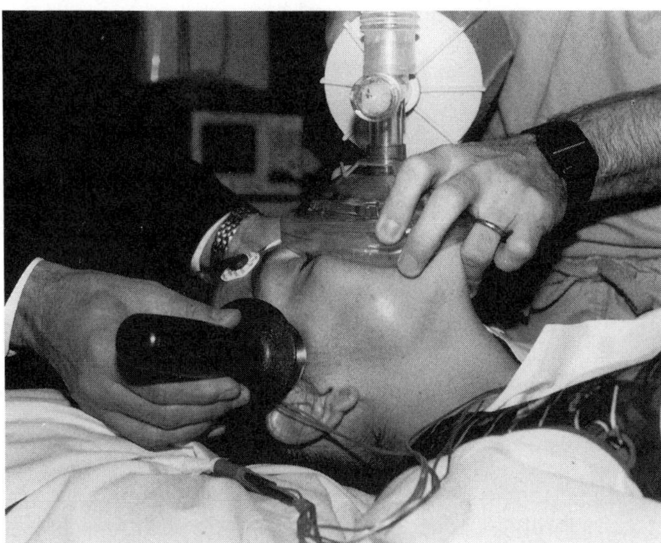

FIGURE 27–1
Unilateral electrode placement in ECT. The electrode is placed over the nondominant cerebral hemisphere above the ear (usually the right side of the head in right-handed persons). Unilateral placement reduces cognitive side effects.

Frequency of ECT Treatments

ECT is normally given three times a week until therapeutic response is achieved, approximately after 6 to 12 treatments, or 200 to 600 seizure seconds. The number of treatments administered is usually based on the following:

- Diagnosis
- Client's response to treatment
- Client's response to past treatment
- Severity of illness
- Quality of response

It is common for seriously ill clients to have two treatments per session, usually administered 1 to 2 minutes apart. Conditions that indicate two treatments include life-threatening mental disorders, such as severe depression with suicidal preoccupation, catatonic lethargy, and mania (Swartz & Mehta, 1986). Clients experiencing depression or psychotic disorders usually exhibit signs of improvement after several treatments and frequently reach maximum therapeutic response after 5 to 10 treatments (Abrams et al., 1991; Sackheim et al., 1991).

Evaluation

Nursing care for clients recovering from ECT is the same as for those recovering from general anesthesia. Initially, the client is placed in a supine position to facilitate drainage of secretions. Major systems assessed during the recovery period are the respiratory, cardiovascular, and neurological systems. Maintaining stability is the major goal of recovery (Schneider, 1981).

Once the client fully recovers from anesthesia, as evidenced by regained consciousness and stable vital and neurological signs within designated parameters, he or she may be discharged from the recovery area to the postrecovery area. The client needs continued reassurance, emotional support, and frequent reorientation to encourage full recovery from ECT.

After an ECT treatment, most clients experience confusion, transient memory or cognitive deficits, and headaches. Cognitive impairment is manifested by difficulty in recalling new information (anterograde amnesia) and in remembering events prior to treatment (retrograde amnesia) (Squire, 1986). Transient memory impairment may endure from minutes to hours, depending on the type, number, and spacing of treatments. Transitory memory deficits are normal responses to ECT and are not considered complications (Abrams, 1992). Clients who receive bilateral ECT are more likely

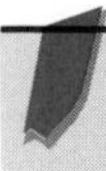

Nursing Care Plan 27–2 The Client Undergoing Electroconvulsive Therapy (Mrs. Moser)—Posttreatment

► **Nursing Diagnosis:** High Risk for Injury

OUTCOME IDENTIFICATION	NURSING ACTIONS	RATIONALES	EVALUATION
1. By [date], Mrs. Moser will undergo ECT safely and be free of injury. Vital and neurological signs will remain within specific parameters.	1. Monitor Mrs. Moser's neurological signs.	1. Provides information on physical status and response to treatment.	*Goal met:* Mrs. Moser remains free of injury. Her vital signs return to pretreatment level (stable). She is oriented to person, place, date, and time. She is taking fluids and diet and is free of nausea and vomiting. No seizure in activity observed. She denies suicidal ideations.
	2. Put siderails up and bed in low position.	2. Reduces falls and promotes safety.	
	3. Monitor changes or adverse reaction.	3. Provides information on physical status.	
	4. Maintain quiet environment.	4. Promotes rest and facilitates return to previous level of function.	
	5. Reorientate Mrs. Moser as needed.	5. Promotes cognitive function and orientation.	
	6. Observe Mrs. Moser for delirium or agitation.	6. Clients who have undergone ECT are at risk for these behaviors.	
	7. Offer Mrs. Moser oral fluids and diet as tolerated.	7. Promotes hydration/nutrition.	
	8. Maintain seizure precautions.	8. Reduces risk of injury.	
	9. Assess for symptoms of suicidality.	9. Depressed clients are at risk for this behavior. Promotes safety.	

to experience significant loss of old information than are those who receive unilateral ECT (Weiner et al., 1986).

Post-ECT agitated delirium is another adverse reaction and needs to be assessed and treated, usually with a benzodiazepine such as diazepam (Valium). Approximately 10 percent of clients develop delirium shortly after treatment. Symptoms of delirium include restlessness, disorientation, blank staring, confusion, and difficulty following instructions. Delirium normally lasts 10 to 45 minutes (Abrams, 1992). For further discussion of the symptoms of delirium, see Chapter 13.

The following are other adverse reactions to ECT:

- Mania
- Aspiration
- Ruptured bladder
- Nausea and vomiting
- Headache (generally occurs in one third of clients and is relieved by aspirin)

Clients recovering from ECT require close monitoring to assess for return to pre-ECT mental and physical states. Client education is an essential aspect of preparing the client and family for adverse reactions.

Case Study: Preparation of the Client for ECT (Mrs. Moser)

Mrs. Moser is 48 years old and has been unsuccessfully treated with an antidepressant for the past 3 months. Her depression has worsened in the past month. Her husband accompanies her to the ambulatory care area for outpatient ECT. She and her husband express concern about the procedure. Mrs. Moser's history is negative for present suicidal ideations or suicidal gestures in the past. She is dressed and groomed appropriately, but her mood is depressed. She is distant and her speech is in a monotone. Her husband is supportive and expresses an interest in his wife's care. Mrs. Moser is anxious about the procedure.

The nurse completes the assessment, including Mrs. Moser's understanding about ECT. The nurse reinforces instructions provided by the physician and encourages Mrs. Moser to express her feelings about the procedure. The Mosers admit they are very anxious about the procedure, but they understand its benefits and possible adverse reactions. Mrs. Moser signs the informed-consent form and reports she has not drunk or eaten since midnight, as instructed. She is instructed to put on a hospital gown and empty her bladder. She is given a preoperative injection and instructed to remain in bed with the side rails up. Mr. Moser is allowed to stay in the room until she is escorted to the ECT room.

See Nursing Care Plans 27–1 and 27–2.

OTHER BIOLOGICAL THERAPIES

BIOLOGICAL CYCLES

Major nursing interventions for the newer biological therapies are based on the client's presenting symptoms, duration of symptoms, level of dangerousness, and past treatment responses. Because most of the new biological interventions occur in the client's home, daily documentation is crucial to assessing client response and compliance.

All organisms are affected by environmental cues that modulate their biological rhythms; examples of these cues are the length of day (circadian rhythm) and the seasons. **Biological rhythms** are the innate pacemakers or timekeepers that mediate an organism's interpretation of its surroundings and its behavioral and biological responses. Biological rhythms are natural, expected, and vital to homeostasis and survival. Human cycles such as the light–dark, rest–activity, reproductive, and metabolic cycles are examples of biological rhythms that are affected by environmental cues (Jarrett, 1989). Aging and certain conditions, such as shift work, sleep deprivation, and jet lag, affect the stability of biological rhythms (Jarrett, 1989). The study of biological rhythms and regulation is called *chronobiology*.

The hypothalamus is the central regulator of the circadian cycle. Environmental cues are transmitted via neural pathways of the **retino–hypothalamic–pineal** axis. Furthermore, certain genetic influences arise from various components of this axis, such as c-*fos* in the suprachiasmatic nuclei (SCN) of the hypothalamus, that regulate the circadian oscillations of a number of body functions, such as temperature, sleep, and seasonal mood responses. The SCN is the primary pacemaker of the circadian system. It lies in the anterior hypothalamus directly above the optic chiasm, allowing it to receive visual input from the retina. Environmental cues are conveyed by the retina through the SCN to the pineal gland, where melatonin is produced. Melatonin is released during the night and is reduced by light (Culebras, 1992; Kupfermann, 1991; Wehr et al., 1987) (Fig. 27–2).

Conditions capable of activating the SCN include heat, dehydration, electrical stimulation, and light. The hormonal and metabolic components of the brain and body function according to a daily cycle 24 to 25 hours in length. For example, high corticosteroid secretion occurs in the morning and high melatonin secretion

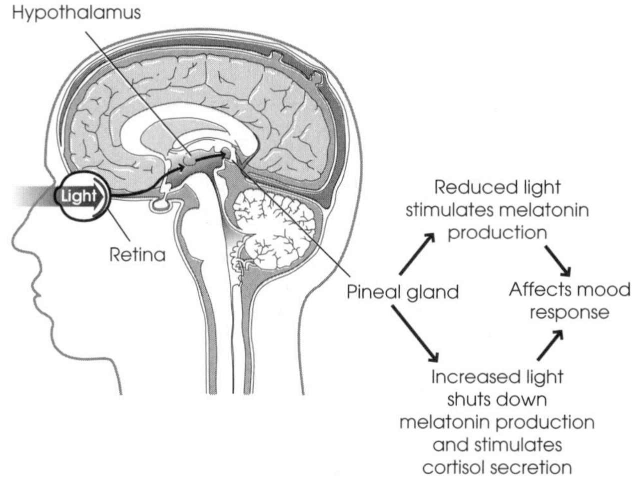

FIGURE 27–2
Retino–hypothalamic–pineal mechanism.

from the pineal gland occurs at night. Normally, the decreased light conveyed through the retina at the end of the day leads to production of melatonin in the pineal gland. Melatonin is influenced by solar light or wavelengths of light linked with circadion phase modulation (Terman & Schlager, 1990).

All biological cycles are influenced by seasonal changes linked to the timing of wavelength light, hormones and metabolism, available light, and components of the sleep-wake cycle. *Phase advancing* is a response to a light stimulus that is intentionally presented hours before the expected onset of solar or wavelength of environmental light. *Phase delaying* refers to a response elicited by a light stimulus presented hours later than expected.

New biological therapies are based on directing specific aspects of the circadian cycle to reduce symptoms of **seasonal affective disorder** (SAD). SAD is similar to a mood disorder but occurs during the fall and early winter months and remits in the spring. Symptoms often include hypersomnia, fatigue, irritability, increased appetite, hypomania, and atypical depression. (Rosenthal et al., 1984). Symptoms of SAD usually occur at the same time each year. Hypersomnia refers to the need for at least 1 additional hour of sleep during the winter months than in the summer months. This symptom may represent an underlying alteration in the phase-delayed circadian rhythm, differing from terminal insomnia, which usually manifests as a phase-advanced rhythm. Light therapy or phototherapy and sleep cycle alterations are examples of methods of manipulating the circadian cycle. See Chapter 9 for more information about seasonal affective disorder.

LIGHT THERAPY (PHOTOTHERAPY)

Light therapy is an accepted treatment modality for seasonal affective disorder (Avery et al., 1991; Lam et al., 1992). The effectiveness of light therapy is based on the premise that seasonal rhythms are affected by neuronal pathways that transmit light from the eye to the hypothalamus and ultimately to the pineal gland. Pineal melatonin secretion is altered by light. Light therapy suppresses nocturnal melatonin secretion, suggesting a relationship between seasonal changes and the mood of clients with SAD. Its effectiveness is linked with phase advancing and normalizing melatonin levels (Lewy et al., 1990; Rao et al., 1992; Wehr et al., 1987).

The typical process of light therapy consists of exposure to light that is about 200 lux, or 200 times stronger than usual indoor lighting. A lux is a unit of illumination equal to 1 lumen per square meter. The client is advised to establish a sleeping pattern (baseline)between 10:00 P.M. and 6:00 A.M. during the first week, during which no light treatment is given. Over the next few weeks, the client is exposed to several hours of light treatment. This normally consists of sitting 3 feet from the lights in either the morning or evening and looking at the lights every 1 or 2 minutes for 2 hours. Furthermore, the client is instructed to avoid exposure to natural morning light (Avery et al., 1991).

Dawn stimulation differs from traditional light therapy because it occurs earlier during the sleep cycle, with a gradual increase in exposure to dim light. In a recent study, Avery et al. (1993) compared the effects of dawn stimulation with placebo using a dimmer form of light therapy introduced by Terman and Schlager (1990). The findings supported earlier research that demonstrated the effectiveness of dawn stimulation in alleviating winter depression (Avery et al., 1993) (see Research Study display).

The exact mechanism of the psychotherapeutic effects of light therapy is unknown. The major disadvantage of this treatment is that its effectiveness is short-lived, usually lasting 2 to 4 days after treatment ends, and the rate of relapse is high (Kaplan & Boggiano, 1989).

Nursing care for the client undergoing light therapy consists of engaging the client in the informed-consent process and educating the client and his or her family about the protocol of light therapy. The protocol for light therapy varies.

The following is the protocol for dawn stimulation:

- Ask the client to sleep between the hours of 10:00 P.M. and 6:00 A.M.
- Ask the client to keep a daily log of sleeping patterns.
- The first week provides baseline information (no light therapy is used).
- Beginning with the second week, gradually expose the client to a 75-watt incandescent reflector flood light positioned 4 feet from the pillow.
- Gradually increase (2.2 log/lux/hour) dawn stimulation over a 2-hour period from 4:00 to 6:00 A.M. to a maximum of 250 lux.
- Instruct client to avoid sunlight before 8:00 A.M.
- Instruct client to avoid looking directly into the light (Avery et al., 1993).

The major side effects of light therapy include headaches; insomnia; agitation; eye strain; and, in clients with bipolar disorder, recurrent mania. These symptoms may emerge after the average 2-week course of therapy (Avery et al., 1993; Levitt et al., 1993). Clients need to be assessed throughout the course of treatment for these side effects, particularly for ocular side effects, because the eye is the site of entry for this form of treatment. Some question has been raised about the possibility of retinal damage from light therapy (Vanselow et al., 1991), but Waxler et al. (1992) disputed this notion, arguing that light therapy at 2000 lux is the equivalent of looking at the sky during early morning and dawn light. However, they suggested that a careful ophthalmological history be taken and an ophthalmologist be consulted if retinal damage is believed to be indicated. Manifestations of retinal damage include blurred vision, glare, or floaters in red blood cells in vitreous humor. Light therapy can be used as an adjunct to traditional biological therapies such as antidepressants or lithium.

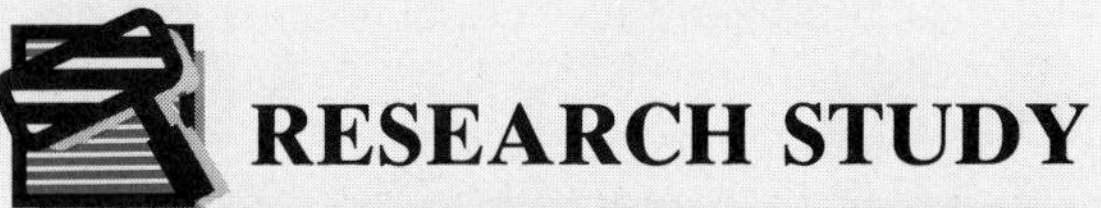

RESEARCH STUDY

Dawn Simulation Treatment of Winter Depression: A Controlled Study

Avery, D. H., Bolte, M. A., Dager, S. R., Wilson, L. G., Weyer, M., Cox, G. B., & Dunner, D. L. (1993). *American Journal of Psychiatry*, *150*, 113–117.

Purpose of Study

The purpose of the study was to determine whether dawn simulation was more effective than shorter, dimmer placebo dawn simulation in the treatment of winter depression.

Methodology

Twenty-two clients diagnosed with winter depression were randomly selected using a parallel design. Each subject was treated with either 1 week of 2-hour dawn simulation of up to 250 lux or 1 week of 30-minute dawn simulation of up to 0.2 lux. Subjects were told that they would either receive a dimmer or brighter light treatment. Scores on the Hamilton Rating Scale for Depression were obtained initially and during treatment. Scores from both groups were compared with an analysis of variance.

Findings

The 2-hour, 250-lux dawn simulation participants had significantly lower scores on the depression scale than did the placebo group.

Nursing Implications

Clients with winter depression can benefit from dawn simulation.

SLEEP CYCLE ALTERATIONS

Altering sleep cycles is based on the premise that certain mood disorders include alterations in the 24-hour circadian cycle. Sleepiness occurs at the low point of the body temperature in the circadian rhythm. Normally, sleeping occurs in two phases: rapid eye movement (REM) sleep and non-REM sleep. REM sleep is characterized by vivid dreaming and a consistently high level of brain activity. Non-REM, or slow-wave, sleep is characterized by diminished brain activity. Sleep deprivation is an example of an alteration in the sleep cycle. Clients experiencing depression usually have more REM sleep and are sensitive to the timing of lightness and darkness (McCarley, 1992).

Sleep deprivation is a biological therapy that consists of depriving clients of 1 hour of REM sleep. A typical sleep deprivation regimen occurs by advancing or delaying the time the client retires for bed. Varying the **sleep-wake cycle** facilitates re-establishment of normal sleeping patterns.

NURSING RESEARCH ON BIOLOGICAL THERAPIES

Historically, psychiatric–mental health nursing research has paralleled psychiatric paradigms. The Decade of the Brain has prompted a shift from a primarily psychological paradigm, based on interactions with the client, to the study of the impact of neurological processes on behavior. The increased interest in the science of neurobiology and advances in technological studies of the brain have resulted in expanded opportunities for psychiatric–mental health research by nurses.

The psychiatric nurse's role in research varies according to his or her interest, educational level, and expertise in the research process. Some nurses may be sole researchers or may collaborate with others to develop treatment research protocols. Other psychiatric nurses may prescribe or administer research medication or other biological therapies. Regardless of their role, nurses involved in research use the nursing process to assess client needs, formulate client outcomes and interventions, and evaluate and modify client responses to protocols. Manipulation of the circadian and sleep-wake cycles and light therapy are examples of biological therapies that nurses can use to modify distressful behaviors.

► CHAPTER SUMMARY

The emergence of biological therapies in the 1930s laid the foundation of many of today's interventions. One of the earliest and continually controversial therapies is ECT. Advances in neurobiology and diagnostic studies have increased the legitimacy of ECT for the treatment of specific client populations. Nurses play a vital role in educating and providing emotional comfort to clients undergoing ECT.

Newer biological therapies are innovative strategies that are designed to help clients suffering from SAD and sleep cycle disturbances. Numerous research and educational opportunities have emerged for nurses as a result of the advent of newer biological therapies.

Suggestions for Clinical Conference

1. Present a case study of a client undergoing ECT.
2. Present case histories of clients who were treated with ECT.
3. Divide into groups on the basis of your feelings and thoughts about ECT and debate controversial issues.
4. Have a psychiatric clinical nurse specialist discuss the role of the nurse in the informed-consent process.
5. Discuss the ethical and legal considerations related to somatic therapies.
6. Explain the nursing care of client undergoing light therapy.

References

Abrams, R. (1992). *Electroconvulsive therapy* (2nd ed.). New York: Oxford University Press.

Abrams, R., Swartz, C. M., & Vedak, C. (1991). Antidepressant effects of high-dose right unilateral electroconvulsive therapy. *Archives of General Psychiatry*, *48*, 746–748.

Adolfson, R., Gottries, C. G., & Roos, B. E. (1979). Post-mortem distribution of dopamine and homovanillic acid in human brain: Variations related to age and review of literature. *Journal of Neurotransmitters*, *45*, 81–105.

American Nurses Association. (1994). *A statement on psychiatric–mental health clinical nursing practice and standards of psychiatric–mental health clinical nursing practice*. Washington, DC: American Nurses Publishing.

American Psychiatric Association. (1994). *Diagnostic and statistical manual of mental disorders* (4th ed.). Washington, DC: Author.

American Psychiatric Association Task Force on Electroconvulsive Therapy. (1990). *The practice of electroconvulsive therapy: Recommendations for psychiatric training and privileging*. Washington, DC: American Psychiatric Association.

Avery, D. H., Bolte, M. A., Dager, S. R., Wilson, L. G., Weyer, M., Cox, G. B., & Dunner, D. L. (1993). Dawn stimulation treatment of winter depression: A controlled study. *American Journal of Psychiatry*, *150*, 113–117.

Avery, D. H., Khan, A., Dager, S. R., Cohen, S., Cox, G. B., & Dunner, D. L. (1991). Morning or evening bright light treatment of winter depression? The significance of hypersomnia. *Biological Psychiatry*, *29*, 117–126.

Baxter, L. R. J., Roy-Byrne, P., & Liston, E. H. (1986). Informing patients about electroconvulsive therapy: Effects of a videotape presentation. *Convulsive Therapy*, *2*, 25–29.

Benhow, S. M. (1988). Patients' views on electroconvulsive therapy on completion of course of treatment. *Convulsive Therapy*, *4*, 146–152.

Bennett, A. E. (1940). Preventing traumatic complications in convulsive shock therapy by curare. *Journal of the American Medical Association*, *114*, 322–324.

Black, J. L. (1993). ECT: Lessons learned about an old treatment with new technologies. *Psychiatric Annals*, *23*, 7–14.

Burke, W. J., Rubin, E. H., Zorumski, C. F., & Wetzel, R. D. (1987). The safety of ECT in geriatric psychiatry. *Journal of the American Geriatrics Society*, *35*, 516–521.

Burns, C. M., & Stuart, G. W. (1991). Nursing care in electroconvulsive therapy. *Psychiatric Clinics of North America, 14,* 971–988.

Cardno, A. G., & Simpson, C. J. (1991). Electroconvulsive therapy in Paget's disease and hydrocephalus. *Convulsive Therapy, 7,* 48–51.

Cerletti, U. (1950). Old and new information about electroshock. *American Journal of Psychiatry, 107,* 87–94.

Coffey, C. E., & Weiner, R. D. (1990). Electroconvulsive therapy: An update. *Hospital and Community Psychiatry, 41,* 515–521.

Coffey, C. E., Weiner, R. D., Djang, W. T., Figiel, G. S., Soady, S. A., Patterson, L. J., et al. (1991). Brain anatomical effects of electroconvulsive therapy: A prospective magnetic resonance imaging study. *Archives of General Psychiatry, 48,* 1013–1021.

Coryell, W., Pfohl, B., & Zimmerman, M. (1985). Outcome following electroconvulsive therapy: A comparison of primary and secondary depression. *Convulsive Therapy, 1,* 10–14.

Culebras, A. (1992). Update on disorders of sleep and the sleep-wake cycle. *Psychiatric Clinics of North America, 15,* 467–486.

Devanand, D. P., Dwork, A. J., Hutchinson, E. R., Bolwig, T. G., & Sackeim, H. A. (1994). Does ECT alter brain structure? *American Journal of Psychiatry, 151,* 957–970.

Dorn, J. B. (1985). Electroconvulsive therapy with fetal monitoring in a bipolar pregnant patient. *Convulsive Therapy, 1,* 217–221.

Dubovsky, S. L. (1992). Psychopharmacological treatment in neuropsychiatry. In S. C. Yudofsky & R. E. Hales (Eds.), *Textbook of neuropsychiatry* (2nd ed., pp. 663–701). Washington, DC: American Psychiatric Press.

Duffy, W. J., & Conradt, H. (1989). Electroconvulsive therapy. *AORN Journal, 50,* 806–812.

Escalona, P. R., Coffey, C. E., & Maus-Feldman, J. (1991). Electroconvulsive therapy in depressed patients with intracranial arachnoid cyst: A brain magnetic resonance study. *Convulsive Therapy, 7,* 133–138.

Fink, M. (1990). How does electroconvulsive therapy work? *Neuropsychopharmacology, 3,* 73–82.

Fink, M. (1991). Impact of the antipsychiatry movement on the revival of electroconvulsive therapy in the United States. *Psychiatric Clinics of North America, 14,* 793–801.

Fox, H. A. (1993). Patients fears and objection to electroconvulsive therapy. *Hospital and Community Psychiatry, 44,* 357–360.

Freeman, C. P. L., & Kendall, R. E. (1986). Patients' experience and attitudes towards electroconvulsive therapy. *Annals of the New York Academy of Sciences, 462,* 341–352.

Hamilton, M. (1986). Electroconvulsive therapy: Indications and contraindications. *Annals of the New York Academy of Science,* 149, 5–11.

Henn, D. (1989). Psychosurgery: Electroconvulsive therapy. In H. I. Kaplan & B. J. Sadock (Eds.), *Comprehensive textbook of psychiatry/V* (5th ed., pp. 1679–1680). Baltimore: Williams & Wilkins.

Jarrett, D. B. (1989). Chronobiology. In H. I. Kaplan & B. J. Sadock (Eds.), *Comprehensive textbook of psychiatry/V* (5th ed., pp. 125–131). Baltimore: Williams & Wilkins.

Kalinowsky, L. B., & Hoch, P. H. (1950). *Shock treatment and other somatic treatments in psychiatry.* New York: Grune & Stratton.

Kaplan, P., Boggiano, W. E. (1989). Anticonvulsants, noradrenergic drugs and other organic therapies. In H. I. Kaplan & B. J. Sadock (Eds.), *Comprehensive textbook of psychiatry/V* (5th ed., pp. 1681–1688). Baltimore: Williams & Wilkins.

Kovar, M. G. (1982). The public health impact of an increasing elderly population in the USA. *World Health Statistics Quarterly, 35,* 246–258.

Kramer, B. A. (1985). Use of ECT in California, 1977–1983. *American Journal of Psychiatry, 142,* 1190–1192.

Kupfermann, I. (1991). Hypothalamus and the limbic system: Motivation. In E. R. Kandel, J. H. Schwartz, & T. M. Jessel (Eds.), *Principles of neural science* (3rd ed., pp. 750–760). Norwalk, CT: Appleton & Lange.

Lam, R. W., Buchanan, A., Mador, J. A., & Corral, M. R. (1992). Hypersomnia and morning light therapy for winter depression. *Biological Psychiatry, 31,* 1062–1064.

Levitt, A. J., Joffe, R. T., Moul, D. E., Lam, R. W., Teicher, M. H., Lebegue, B., et al. (1993). Side effects of light therapy in seasonal affective disorders. *American Journal of Psychiatry, 150,* 650–652.

Lewy, A. J., Sack, R. L., & Singer, C. M. (1990). Bright light, melatonin, and biological rhythms in humans. In J. Montplaisir & R. Godbout (Eds.), *Sleep and biological rhythms* (pp. 99–112). New York: Oxford University Press.

Lipton, M. A. (1976). Age-differentiation in depression: Biochemical aspects. *Journal of Gerontology, 31,* 293–299.

Liston, E. H., & Salk, J. D. (1990). Hemodynamic responses to ECT after bilateral hematoma. *Convulsive Therapy, 6,* 160–164.

Malek-Ahmado, P., Becciro, J. B., McNeil, B. W., & Weddige, R. L. (1990). Electroconvulsive therapy and chronic subdural hematoma. Convulsive Therapy, *6,* 38–41.

McCarley, R. W. (1992). Human electrophysiology: Basic cellular mechanism and control of wakefulness and sleep. In S. C. Yudofsky & R. E. Hales (Eds.), *Textbook of neuropsychiatry* (2nd ed., pp. 29–55). Washington, DC: American Psychiatric Press.

Miller, L. J. (1994). Use of electroconvulsive therapy during pregnancy. *Hospital and Community Psychiatry, 45*(5), 444–450.

Miller, R., Silvay, G., & Lumb, X (1979). Anesthesia, surgery, and myocardial infarction. *Anesthesiology Review, 6,* 1402–1411.

Millon, T. (1969). *Modern psychopathology: A biosocial approach to maladaptive learning and functioning.* Philadelphia: W. B. Saunders.

Moniz, E. (1936). Prefrontal leucotomy in the treatment of mental disorder. *American Journal of Psychiatry, 93,* 1379–1385.

Mukherjee, S., Sackeim, H. A., & Schnur, D. B. (1994). Electroconvulsive therapy of acute manic episodes: A review of 50 years' experience. *American Journal of Psychiatry, 151*(2), 169–176.

Pacella, B. L., Barrerra, E. S., & Kalinowsky, L. (1942). Variations in the electroencephalogram associated with electroshock therapy in patients with mental disorders. *Archives of Neuro-Psychiatry, 47,* 367–384.

Pande, A. C., Grunhaus, L. J., Aisen, A. M., & Haskett, R. F. (1990). A preliminary magnetic resonance imagery study of ECT treated depressed patients. *Biological Psychiatry, 27,* 102–104.

Penney, J. F., Dinwiddie, S. H., Zorumski, C. F. & Wetzel, R. D. (1990). Concurrent and close temporal administration of lithium and ECT. *Convulsive Therapy, 6,* 139–145.

Pileggi, T. S., & Ryan, D. A. (1993). The role of nursing in electroconvulsive therapy. *Psychiatric Annals, 23,* 19–22.

Rao, M. L., Müller-Oerlinghausen, B., Mackert, A., Strebel, B., Stieglitz, R. D., & Volz, H. P. (1992). Blood serotonin, serum melatonin and light therapy in healthy subjects and inpatients with nonseasonal depression. *Acta Psychiatrica Scandinavica, 86,* 127–132.

Repke, J. T., & Berger, P. N. G. (1984). Electroconvulsive therapy in pregnancy. *Ob/Gynecology, 63*(Suppl.), 39–41.

Rosenthal, N. E., Sack, D. A., Gillin, J. C., Lewy, A. J., Goodwin, F. K., Davenport, Y., et al. (1984). Seasonal affective disorder: A description of the syndrome and preliminary findings of light therapy. *Archives of General Psychiatry, 41,* 72–80.

Royal College of Nursing. (1987). RCN nursing guidelines for ECT. *Convulsive Therapy, 3,* 158–160.

Rummans, T. A. (1993). Medical indications for electroconvulsive therapy. *Psychiatric Annals, 23,* 27–32.

Runke, B. (1985). Consensus panel backs cautious use of ECT for severe disorders. *Hospital and Community Psychiatry, 36,* 943–946.

Sackheim, H. A., Brown, R. P., Devanand, D. P., et al. (1989). Should tricyclic antidepressants or lithium be standard continuation treatment after ECT? An alternative view. *Convulsive Therapy, 5,* 180–183.

Sackheim, H. A., Devanand, D. P., & Prudic, J. (1991). Stimulus intensity, seizure threshold, and seizure duration: Impact on the efficacy and safety of electroconvulsive treatment. *Psychiatric Clinics of North America, 14,* 803–843.

Sakel, M. (1938). *The pharmacological shock treatment of schizophrenia.* New York: Nervous and Mental Disease Publishing Co.

Schneider, M. (1981). The recovery room as a special procedures unit. *AORN Journal, 34,* 490–498.

Silver, J. M., & Yudofsky, S. C. (1988). Psychopharmacology and electroconvulsive therapy. In J. Talbott, R. E. Hales, & S. C. Yudofsky (Eds.), *Textbook of psychiatry* (2nd ed., pp. 767–853). Washington, DC: American Psychiatric Press.

Small, J. G. (1985). Efficacy of electroconvulsive therapy in schizophrenia, mania, and other disorders. I. Schizophrenia. *Convulsive Therapy, 1,* 262–269.

Small, J. G., Milstein, V., & Small, I. F. (1991). Electroconvulsive therapy for mania. *Psychiatric Clinics of North America, 14*, 887–903.

Squire, L. R. (1986). Memory functions as affected by electroconvulsive therapy. *Annals of the New York Academy of Science, 462*, 307–314.

Steele, K. M., & Manfreda, M. L. (1959). *Psychiatric nursing* (6th ed.). Philadelphia: F. A. Davis.

Swartz, C. M., & Mehta, R. (1986). Double electroconvulsive therapy for resistant depression. *Convulsive Therapy, 2*, 55–57.

Terman, M., & Schlager, D. S. (1990). Twilight therapeutics, winter depression, melatonin and sleep. In J. Montpaisir & R. Godbout (Eds.), *Sleep and biological rhythms: Basic mechanisms and application to psychiatry* (pp. 113–128) New York: Oxford University Press.

U.S. Congress. (1989). Decade of the brain proclamation. Public Law 101-158 (HJ Res. 174). July 25, 1989, 130 STAT. 152–154.

Vanselow, W., Dennerstein, L., Armstrong, S., & Lockie, P. (1991). Retinopathy and bright light therapy [letter]. *American Journal of Psychiatry, 148*, 1266–1267.

Waxler, M., James, R. H., Brainard, G. C., Moul, D. E., Oren, D. A., & Rosethal, N. E. (1992). Retinopathy and bright light therapy [letter; comment] *American Journal of Psychiatry, 149*, 1610–1611.

Wehr, T. A., Skwerer, R. G., Jacobsen, F. M., Sack, D. A., & Rosenthal, N. E. (1987). Eye versus skin phototherapy of seasonal affective disorder. *American Journal of Psychiatry, 144*, 753–757.

Weiner, R. D. (1984). Does electroconvulsive therapy cause brain damage? *Behavioral and Brain Science, 7*, 1–54.

Weiner, R. D. (1989). Electroconvulsive therapy. In. H. I. Kaplan & B. J. Sadock (Eds.), *Comprehensive textbook of psychiatry/V* (5th ed., pp. 1670–1678). Baltimore: Williams & Wilkins.

Weiner, R. D., & Coffey, C. E. (1987). Electroconvulsive therapy in patients with severe medical illness. In A. Stoudemire & B. Fogel (Eds.), *Treatment of psychiatric disorders in medical-surgical patients* (pp. 113–134). New York: Grune & Stratton.

Weiner, R. D., Rogers, H. J., Davidson, J. R. T., & Squire, L. R. (1986). Effects of stimulus parameters on cognitive side effects. In S. Malitz & H. A. Sackheim (Eds.), *Electroconvulsive therapy: Clinical and basic research issues*. New York: Annals of the New York Academy of Sciences.

Welch, C. A. (1991). Electroconvulsive therapy in general hospital. In N. H. Cassem (Ed.), *Massachusetts General Hospital handbook of general hospital psychiatry* (3rd ed., pp. 269–280). St. Louis: Mosby-Year Book.

Yodofsky, S. C., & Hales, R. E. (1992). *Textbook of neuropsychiatry* (2nd ed.). Washington, DC: American Psychiatric Press.

Zwil, A. S., Bowring, M. A., Price, T. R. P., Goetz, K. L., Greenbarg, J. B., & Kane-Wagner, G. (1990). Prospective electroconvulsive therapy in the presence of intracranial tumor. *Convulsive Therapy, 6*, 299–307.

CHAPTER

Psychosocial Aspects of Nursing in Medical–Surgical Settings

DEBORAH ANTAI-OTONG, M.S., R.N.,C.S.

OUTLINE

CHAPTER OBJECTIVES

Upon completion of this chapter, you will be able to:

1. Analyze the relationship between biological and psychological factors in medical–surgical settings.
2. Recognize symptoms of psychosocial stress in clients who are medically ill.
3. Integrate psychosocial and physiological interventions in medical–surgical clients.
4. Discuss the psychological needs of the client across the life span.

KEY TERMS

Body image
Collaboration
Coping behaviors
Helplessness
Self-esteem
Spirituality
Stress

The client entering the hospital often experiences enormous **stress** generated by fear of the unknown, loss of privacy and autonomy, and a dependency on others. The client's response to his or her illness and hospitalization is affected by psychosocial, cultural, and biological factors. It is also influenced by developmental stage, personality traits, **coping behaviors,** support systems, and the nature of illness. Hospitalization can increase feelings of helplessness, anxiety, and stress. Clients surrender control over the time they eat, sleep, bathe, and perform activities of daily living. The capacity to handle stress is a complex process and the person's response to the stress of hospitalization may be unpredictable.

When coping with their fears and concerns, some clients may become demanding, angry, and uncooperative as a means of maintaining control over some aspect of their lives. When the nurse's perception of the client's situation differs from the client's, misunderstanding evolves. Understanding the meaning of the client's behaviors helps the nurse maximize and promote adaptive coping responses in the client in the medical–surgical setting.

Loss of individuality, increased feelings of **helplessness,** and dependency are elements of dehumanization. Nurses can provide humane care by approaching clients in an empathetic and caring manner. Therapeutic alliances foster autonomy and decrease feelings of powerlessness. Clients must be active participants in their care. Clients demand quality care that involves informed consent; some control over their environment; and safe, humane treatment. This chapter focuses on the stress generated by hospitalization in a nonpsychiatric setting and discusses the effects of biological and psychosocial factors on the medically ill in various clinical settings. In addition, it discusses ways in which every nurse can help clients identify their emotional responses to physical illness and develop adaptive coping skills.

CLIENTS' AND THEIR FAMILIES' PSYCHOSOCIAL RESPONSES IN THE MEDICAL–SURGICAL SETTING

Illness and hospitalization place tremendous stress on clients and their families. Anger, depression, and anxiety are common responses to illness. The 45-year-old man who is diagnosed with multiple sclerosis or the child hospitalized for a myringotomy experience similar feelings—fear of the unknown, sadness as a result of separation from significant others, and annoyance over the disruption in their lifestyle. Regardless of the source of these feelings, clients need emotional support, opportunities to express their feelings, and assistance in maintaining a sense of well-being. The nurse plays major roles in helping the client cope with illness and hospitalization.

Most clients have difficulty conforming to the daily hospital routine. The psychological trauma stems from changes related to major medical illnesses and treatment. In addition to the change in their daily routines, clients must cope with other major stressors, such as changes in personal and professional roles to which they have strong emotional ties. People's **self-esteem,** value systems, and sense of self-worth are linked to their roles. Debilitating, life-threatening, or chronic illnesses such as renal failure, diabetes, heart disease, and acquired immunodeficiency syndrome (AIDS) also threaten people's livelihood. Anger, depression, and demanding behaviors are normal reactions to these situations. Staff reactions frequently set the tone for client reactions. Understanding the need for clients to express their feelings and maintain some control and dignity is crucial to the effectiveness of treatment.

Like adults, children find hospitalization and illness highly stressful. Developmental stage, previous life experiences, family dynamics, and the history and seriousness of the illness play important roles in a child's response to stress. The earlier the illness, the greater risk of injury and emotional, social, and academic deficits (Mishne, 1986). Younger children tend to experience attachment and separation anxiety. Healthy child–parent relationships can buffer the deleterious effects of stress on infants. Separation, pain, loss of control, body image changes, and family dynamics influence the youth's response to hospitalization.

Childhood and adolescent illnesses place overwhelming stress on families, often resulting in immense parental guilt and emotional and physical strain. These responses increase the risk of overprotectiveness by parents and dependency in the chronically ill child. In addition, as the family attempts to cope with the child's illness and feelings, adaptive coping behaviors are taxed, generating anger, frustration, and depression and the likelihood of the complication of severe physical or emotional stress in the parents (Grey et al., 1991).

The nurse plays a key role in assessing and identifying the client at risk for maladaptive responses to illness and participating in crisis intervention. Demanding and angry clients are often labeled as problem clients because they disrupt the daily routine of the unit. All behavior has meaning and needs to be thoroughly assessed. Control and dependency factors tend to trigger intense feelings and behaviors.

Working in medical–surgical settings is often frustrating and stressful. Clients have numerous physical and emotional needs that require immediate or eventual attention. Numerous factors contribute to stressful work environments, such as increased workloads and sicker and more demanding clients and families. When faced with angry, demanding, depressed, suicidal, and dying clients, nurses need to use innovative treatment modalities that mobilize clients' adaptive coping responses and promote mental and physical health.

THE ANGRY CLIENT

Angry and demanding clients often generate feelings of helplessness and frustration in the nurse. These feelings can be effectively managed by recognizing the meaning of client responses and maintaining composure in the most stressful circumstances. Anger typically symbolizes underlying feelings of helplessness and should not be personalized.

Major interventions include approaching the client in a calm and firm manner, using direct eye contact and active listening skills. It is critical that the nurse be able to assess verbal and nonverbal cues to detect imminent physical aggression in the angry client. The likelihood of aggression increases when clients feel they are ignored or discounted. Hurried and unconcerned responses to the client may create or increase his or her feelings of anger, powerlessness, and dependency. Setting firm limits on how anger can be expressed is indicated if the client strikes out or throws things. Speaking in a firm, accepting, and caring tone is critical to minimizing acting-out behaviors. Normally, physical or verbal aggression indicates that the client is feeling out of control. Nurses can help the client regain control by remaining calm and accepting and using firm, consistent limit setting. In addition, the client's emotional needs can be assessed by encouraging verbalization of feelings and providing a safe environment that reduces stress and enhances adaptive coping skills (Antai-Otong, 1988a). Table 28–1 lists the Dos and Don'ts for coping with angry clients.

THE DEMANDING CLIENT

Demanding clients, like angry ones, often generate intense emotional reactions in the nurse. They are usually time conscious and self-absorbed and lack concern for others. Clients with chronic obstructive pulmonary disease (COPD) can be very demanding. These clients routinely experience intense anxiety, particularly during an extreme dyspneic period. Their lack of control over their illness, their fear of being unable to breathe, and the stimulant effects of bronchodilators increase their anxiety. As anxiety increases, feelings of dependency and helplessness and fears of dying ensue.

Major interventions for clients with COPD include encouraging activities that promote optimal ventilation; maintaining a calm, concerned approach; encouraging expression of feelings; and staying with client during periods of anxiety. Anxiety and demanding behaviors can be further reduced by encouraging the client to perform stress reduction and breathing exercises.

Overall, the nurse can help clients maintain control by speaking in a confident and caring voice to reduce escalation of negative responses. Keeping promises is critical to establishing trust and rapport. Managing demanding behavior requires active listening skills and patience to understand the meaning of the client's complaints and frustration. In addition, simple explanations of treatment procedures and daily routines and encouragement to participate in treatment reduces clients' fears and enhances their sense of control. Ignoring demanding clients or responding indifferently increases

TABLE 28–1
Dos and Don'ts for Coping with the Angry Client

WHAT TO DO	WHY
Keep your own emotions in check; speak in a calm, reassuring way.	Gaining control over your feelings lets you think rationally. Only then can you help the client. If you become angry, you'll probably incite the client even more.
Watch the client's body language.	The client's body language gives you clues to his or her potential for physical aggression. Pacing indicates agitation, for example; a clenched fist may mean imminent physical violence.
Let the client air feelings.	When the client airs his or her feelings, anger and tension decrease, enabling the client to deal with the situation rationally.
Determine the source of the client's anger.	Knowing the source of anger enables you to recognize that the anger is not directed toward you.
Involve the client in his or her treatment.	Involving the client in daily care decreases his or her feelings of helplessness and dependency.
Provide controls or limits as needed.	Setting limits on the client's behavior provides some controls. The client often welcomes these limits.
WHAT NOT TO DO	**WHY**
Don't shout or argue with the client. Avoid touching the client or invading the client's space.	Shouting, arguing, and touching the client can escalate anger. These behaviors prevent you from dealing effectively with the client and can make him or her become physically violent. Touching the client or invading his or her space can be threatening to the client and make him or her feel cornered. This may result in retaliation toward you.
Don't let the client stand between you and the door.	Maintain easy access to the door in case the client becomes violent and you need to get out quickly.
Don't patronize or talk down to the client.	Patronizing the client increases anger and potential for aggression.
Don't discount the client's feelings.	Dismissing the client's feelings interferes with establishing a therapeutic nurse–patient relationship.

their anxiety and fears (Antai-Otong, 1989). Maintaining therapeutic interactions is the key to establishing adaptive coping behaviors. Table 28–2 lists the Dos and Don'ts for coping with demanding clients.

THE DEPRESSED CLIENT

Feelings of helplessness and anger often precede depression. The prevalence of depression is 10 percent in the general population, and untreated depression places hospitalized clients at risk for complications and death (Wells et al., 1988). Absences of motivation, compliance, and hope are major issues for depressed clients (Beck et al., 1990; Cassem, 1991). The nurse progresses as follows in addressing the psychological responses of the depressed client.

First, recognizing the symptoms of depression in medical–surgical clients helps the nurse develop effective interventions that help clients learn adaptive coping behaviors (see Chapter 9 for a detailed discussion of depression). Depression is manifested by the following:

- Depressed or sad mood
- Changes in appetite, concentration, and sleeping patterns
- Social isolation
- A lack of interest or motivation

TABLE 28–2
Dos and Don'ts for Coping with the Demanding Client

DO	RATIONALE
Realize that the demanding client likely feels fearful, anxious, or angry and may even feel guilty.	You can then understand the client's demands. Also, it keeps you from taking what the client says personally.
Keep promises. If you say you'll be there in 20 minutes, be there.	Keeping promises increases the client's trust in you and decreases his or her fear of losing control.
Set limits. Reassure the client that you'll check on him or her regularly and be there immediately in an emergency. Strive for continuity of care.	Limit setting gives the client structure and decreases feelings of helplessness because he or she knows what to expect.
Listen to the client's complaints. If the client is frustrated by hospital procedures, let him or her express their concerns and then explain why things run as they do.	The client gains insight into his or her feelings.
DON'T	**RATIONALE**
Make excuses for not being immediately available to the client.	Demanding clients are self-absorbed. They won't feel sympathy for other clients.
Argue with the client.	The client will think you are losing control and will feel more anxious and angry.
Ignore call lights or respond to them *slowly*.	The client will feel more fearful and anxious, and he or she

- Expressed feelings of hopelessness
- Decreased libido and energy (American Psychiatric Association [APA], 1994)

Second, assessing the client's history and duration of depressive symptoms and identification of recent stressors or major lifestyle changes, such as recent losses or illness, is necessary. For example, the 50-year-old business executive who recently suffered a myocardial infarction is at risk for depression because of potential lifestyle changes. This client has generally worked more than 60 hours a week, and his life has centered primarily on building his career. His wife expresses concern that he refuses to talk to her or other family members and barely eats. He also admits to having thoughts of dying and feeling "less than a man" because he cannot take care of his family.

The assessment process involves gathering information from the client and from his or her family members who can provide invaluable information about the client's level of function and emotional state. Expressing their feelings and thoughts to the nurse helps clients and families understand the meaning and normality of their responses.

Third, assessing depressive symptoms is critical to reducing complications, such as associated impaired nutrition; biological complications, such as hypertension, hyperglycemia, and cardiac arrhythmias, related to noncompliance; and suicide. A psychiatric consultant liaison nurse (PCLN) should be consulted when a client is assessed to be suicidal and the nurse feels in need of assistance in formulating an effective treatment plan. See Chapter 30 for more information on the role of the PCLN and Chapter 16 for a detailed discussion of the suicidal client.

Overall, medical-surgical clients experiencing major role or lifestyle changes often feel helpless, hopeless, and depressed. Nurses can minimize these feelings and potential complications by assessing early depressive symptoms and reducing stress and suicidal risk (Antai-Otong, 1988b).

THE DYING CLIENT

Death and dying issues frequently arouse feelings of helplessness, anger, and frustration in the nurse. Exploring the meaning of these feelings can help the nurse understand the feelings of the dying client. Establishing rapport and conveying concern and empathy are vital to forming a therapeutic relationship. Death completes the cycle of the life span, and its certainty frequently generates feelings of hopelessness, guilt, and helplessness in the dying client, the client's family, and the nurses who care for them.

The client's response to death is influenced by coping skills, developmental stage, cultural, spiritual, psychosocial, and biological factors. Exploring one's early memories of these events is critical to understanding the client's feelings and attitudes about death and to self-awareness. Self-awareness strengthens healthy responses to dying clients. Crisis ensues when the dying client is unable to mobilize available resources to reduce anxiety and stress. Nurses can mobilize resources by collaborating with clients and families to ensure active participation in care to enhance independence and self-esteem.

The response to death and dying varies among children and adolescents. Their perception of death is influenced by the factors that affect adults' perception of death, that is, developmental stage and cultural, biological, and psychosocial influences. Some children may perceive death as magical and believe that the dead will eventually wake up and return to life. Many cartoon characters, such as the Road Runner, are splattered on the pavement and later jump up and spring back to life, reinforcing this perception. The child's perception of death needs to be explored. This process can be facilitated by play therapy, art, and support groups that encourage the child or adolescent to express feelings about death. Anxiety and fears often stem from fear of abandonment. Explanations can help the child understand death and facilitate the grief process (Furman, 1964; Mishne, 1986).

Overall, death and dying concerns generate various emotional reactions, including depression, helplessness, hopelessness, guilt, anger, and hostility. Some clients may even deny their feelings and experience difficulty grieving. Understanding the emotional reactions to and the effects of somatic interventions, such as chemotherapy, irradiation, dialysis, or life support systems, is important when caring for the dying patient.

An individualized care plan that incorporates psychosocial, biological, and spiritual components is critical to the care of the dying client. Emotional comfort and physical comfort are essential client outcomes. Assessing the needs of the dying client begins with identifying present stressors, present and past coping mechanisms, and available support systems.

Empathy and compassion are vital to psychosocial interventions and the grief process. Kubler-Ross's (1969) dynamic five stages of grief (Table 28–3) are useful in assessing the client and family's response to loss and death. Therapeutic interactions convey compassion, concern, and respect for the client's uniqueness. Active listening and therapeutic use of touch and silence are the basis of nursing interventions. Encouraging clients and their families to express their feelings and thoughts facilitates their grief process and helps them maintain their individuality (Saunders, 1969).

Focusing on the positive aspects of the client's life strengthens the client's self-esteem and coping mechanisms. Additional psychosocial interventions include encouraging the client to participate actively in care and increasing his or her social interactions. Participation in daily care fosters independence and a sense of control over some aspects of the client's life. Social interaction decreases feelings of alienation and despair. Nurses should seek out the client at regular intervals during each shift. In community settings, visiting nurses need to make regular visits to ensure that the client has access to nursing staff and to decrease the client's loneliness and depression. Support groups and structured community programs also enhance social interactions and self-worth.

TABLE 28–3
Kubler-Ross's Five Stages of Grief Applied to the Medical–Surgical Client

STAGE	CLIENT BEHAVIOR
Denial	Client refuses to acknowledge limits and comply with treatment.
Anger	Client is demanding, noncompliant, argumentative, and critical of his or her care and of others.
Bargaining	Client seeks new or questionable treatment modalities.
Depression	Client exhibits social withdrawal, agitation, impaired eating, sleep disturbance, and altered concentration patterns.
Acceptance	Client participates in care and verbalizes feelings; appetite, concentration, and sleeping patterns improve.

Biological Interventions

Biological interventions such as chemotherapy, radiation therapy, and surgery can increase clients' feelings of helplessness and anxiety, further compromising their ability to cope and adapt. Nurses need to assess these feelings and collaborate with other members of the treatment team to promote comfort and maintain clients' integrity and dignity. Providing pain medication and privacy, explaining all procedures, and involving the client in daily care are critical nursing interventions.

The client's emotional and biological stamina is often compromised by various biological interventions. One might wonder why some clients handle their illness better than others. Continued assessment of various attributes that allow different clients to deal with death and dying should shed some light on this question.

Spiritual Interventions

A significant factor that affects the coping process is **spirituality.** Spirituality is an aspect of client care that is often minimized or overlooked. It is defined as a dynamic phenomenon that enables clients to discover meaning and purpose in life, particularly during agonizing life events (Haase et al., 1992; Jourard, 1974). Spiritual and religious beliefs provide strength and hope (Reighley, 1988). Assessing spiritual needs involves obtaining personal data about the client's belief system, affirmation, coping behaviors, and psychosocial resources. Nurses can use spirituality to reinforce clients' coping mechanisms and facilitate the grieving. Grieving helps nurses connect with clients and appreciate their experience while exploring personal reactions to death and dying. Regular visits by the priest, minister, or

TABLE 28–4
Role of Spirituality in Coping

- Allows client to feel bonded with others and higher being.
- Provides client with sense of worth and affirmation.
- Generates resourceful energy.
- Helps client find significance and aim in life.
- Stems from client's belief system, values, and perception of illness and stressors.

Data from Haase, J. E., Britt, T., & Coward, D. D. (1992). Simultaneous concept analysis of spiritual perspective, hope, acceptance, and self-transcendence. *Image, 24,* 141–147.

rabbi need to be available to clients and families. Table 28–4 outlines the role of spirituality in coping.

The following case history portrays a client undergoing irradiation treatment and the nursing interventions that reinforce his coping behaviors and promote his emotional and physical comfort.

Clinical Example: The Dying Client (Mr. Jones)

The nurse greets Mr. Jones and his wife prior to his radiation therapy. He has had a "bad night," he says, describing it as painful and restless. The nurse approaches him in a caring and concerned manner, extending a hand, using good eye contact, and inquiring about pain medication. Mr. Jones says he does not feel like he needs pain medication, even though it was prescribed for him on a PRN basis. Further exploration of Mr. Jones's feelings about pain medication reveals that his reluctance to ask for pain medication is associated with the belief that it would make him less than a man to do so. He is a World War II veteran who prides himself as being strong and in control of his life.

The nurse spends about 10 minutes explaining that Mr. Jones's condition warrants using PRN pain medication and that he can control his pain by using it. The nurse further assures Mr. Jones that taking an analgesic is not a sign of weakness and that it has been ordered to relieve his pain. Encouraging Mr. Jones to take the medication alleviates his feelings of helplessness generated by the severe pain. He and his wife express appreciation for the nurse's thoughtfulness and time.

This clinical example shows how the nurse can use therapeutic interactions, such as compassion, active listening, education, and acceptance to maximize the coping behaviors, promote the comfort, increase the self-esteem, and maintain the integrity of the dying client.

SPECIFIC MEDICAL CONDITIONS IN THE MEDICAL–SURGICAL SETTING: LIFE SPAN ISSUES

Life span factors play a major role in people's adaptation and response to physical and emotional stressors. Medical–surgical conditions affect clients and families throughout the life span and can affect clients' developmental mastery. Understanding and integrating life span factors is critical to developing individualized care.

HOSPITALIZATION DURING CHILDHOOD AND ADOLESCENCE

Physical illness that occurs early in life poses more stress than does physical illness that occurs in later years. Long-term effects of childhood debilitating illnesses can disrupt psychosocial, biological, and academic development and generate family turmoil (Mishne, 1986).

The child or adolescent with a chronic or acute physical illness requires that the nurse use biological and psychosocial interventions to help the client and family cope with the tremendous stress. The emotional impact of physical illness is influenced by numerous factors, such as the nature and cause of the injury, the client's developmental stage, family dynamics, and the nature of the medical treatment.

Younger children tend to experience separation anxiety generated by hospitalization, unfamiliar people, pain, and distressful treatment modalities. They usually feel abandoned during hospitalization because special care often involves isolation to reduce infection. Because family members are the most significant people to the child, he or she may cry when family members leave. Helping the child and family cope with hospitalization is critical to restoration of mental and physical health.

Adolescents are struggling to gain independence, identity, and separation from their families. Hospitalization and chronic illness place them in a dependent position that increases their anxiety and feelings of powerlessness and inadequacy. Personal appearance, athletic abilities, and acceptance by peers are major components of the youth's self-concept. A threat to or change in **body image** can have a profound effect on the adolescent's self-image and concept. The physically ill adolescent may be faced with disfigurement, limitation in body movements, and poor academic performance, which intensify feelings of alienation and isolation among peers. Limited social interactions also threaten self-esteem and increase the risk of depression. Acceptance, positive affirmation, and support are vital to helping the adolescent adapt to serious and long-term illnesses.

The following are the major nursing interventions that promote the optimal level of function and restoration of health in the child and adolescent:

- Assessing developmental stage
- Explaining procedures and treatment
- Spending quality time to listen and assess the youth's concerns and emotional and physical status
- Encouraging expression of feelings and thoughts about present illness
- Encouraging age-appropriate level of participation in treatment

- Providing positive feedback and affirmation through encouragement and compliments
- Observing for symptoms of depression (change in appetite, apathy, sad or tearful mood, self-deprecating statements, and isolation)
- Encouraging parent–child interactions and participation in care
- Arranging for academic work to be brought to the hospital or for a teacher to work with student when possible

Families of hospitalized children and adolescents also experience tremendous stress because of the youth's condition. Families often experience guilt, anxiety, and fears about the child's condition. Moreover, they feel powerless and helpless, which is manifested in detachment, extreme anger, or overprotectiveness. Siblings often feel overlooked and resentful because of the attention given to the sick child's immense needs (Mishne, 1986). Fears of the unknown, financial strain, physical exhaustion, and intense guilt and anxiety often compromise the parent's coping skills and ability to adapt to the child's injuries or illness.

To help mobilize the family's resources and maximize their coping mechanisms, the nurse first establishes a therapeutic relationship that involves approaching the parents in a nonjudgmental and understanding manner, reassuring them that everything possible is being done to provide for the child's well-being. Next, the nurse actively involves the parents in the child's care. Explaining daily routines, providing client education, involving the parents in the child's care, and encouraging expression of feelings are critical components of supporting the family in crisis. The family and youth need to be informed of treatment procedures and progress and to feel supported throughout treatment. These interventions can decrease their feelings of powerless and helplessness, thereby strengthening the parent–child relationship and facilitating the adaptation process.

Emotional responses to physical illness vary among children, adolescents, and their families. Exploring the meaning of the client's responses helps the nurse develop an effective treatment plan that restores health and promotes optimal function.

HOSPITALIZATION DURING EARLY AND MIDDLE ADULTHOOD

Tremendous stress is generated during young adulthood, as the person struggles to master intimacy, understand his or her sexuality, and identify career goals. Physical illness that interferes with accomplishing these task places severe emotional stress on the young adult and impedes developmental progress. In this section, three medical conditions—spinal cord injury, AIDS, and renal failure—are discussed, because they place the individual and significant others at risk for severe emotional stress. In addition, they challenge nurses to explore personal reactions to demanding situations and to develop effective interventions that facilitate the development of adaptive coping skills in clients and themselves.

The Client with a Spinal Cord Injury

Spinal cord injuries often affect younger adults who are active and productive. Injuries range from transient numbness to permanent paralysis. Sensory and motor loss usually occur below the level of the spinal cord injury. The higher the injury, the greater the risk of serious complications. Major treatment goals during the acute phase include maintaining life support systems and preventing further spinal cord injury. Maximizing the client's level of function is a major treatment goal for the client with a spinal cord injury.

The psychological responses to spinal cord injuries are extensive and complex. Both biological and psychosocial factors affect client function. Intensive, long-term physical and psychological rehabilitation is required. Biological factors such as bladder and bowel control, immobility, skin care, sexuality, sensory deprivation, and change in body image and lifestyle evolve from acute to chronic concerns for clients and significant others (Ignatavicius et al., 1992).

Psychosocial factors affecting the client's response to the injury include the client's coping skills and available support systems. Psychosocial factors associated with loss in clients with spinal cord injuries include:

- Loss of mobility
- Increased dependency secondary to job loss or career
- Alterations in body image and self-concept
- Loss of control over body functions, such as sexuality, bladder, and bowel
- Potential loss of close interpersonal relationships

Understanding how the client copes involves assessing the impact of the injury on the client's livelihood. The client with a spinal cord injury suffers tremendous loss and grief, the resolution of which can be facilitated by using an accepting and understanding approach. Normal grief reactions include crying spells, depression, anger, and intense hostility toward loved ones and staff. Exploring the meaning of these behaviors helps nurses understand the extent of the client's emotional pain and coping skills.

The client who has lost personal body functions, such as bladder and bowel control, and who depends on others for care is likely to feel angry, helpless, and powerless. The client with a spinal cord injury tends to become very demanding in an effort to ward off these feelings and gain control of some aspects of his or her life. How the nurse responds to the client's intense emotional reactions is vital to the client's adaptation process. Demanding, hostile behavior should not be construed as a personal attack, but as a way the client attempts to cope with dramatic lifestyle and body image changes. Nurses need to (1) avoid personalizing clients' negative reactions, (2) explore the meaning of these reactions, and (3) collaborate with the client and significant others to help the client develop alternative adaptive coping skills.

The client's injuries also place enormous demands on significant others. The quality of the support systems available during this critical period of emotional and physical recovery is vital to health promotion. Nurses can assess the quality of significant relationships by observing family members' interactions with the client and participation in the client's care. Active involvement in the client's care promotes a sense of accomplishment and decreases feelings of inadequacy and helplessness in the client and family.

The Client with AIDS

AIDS and human immunodeficiency virus (HIV) infection challenges nurses to treat clients with an illness that involves complex psychosocial and neurobiological processes. Autopsy studies have shown that 80 percent of clients with AIDS had neurological changes and approximately half exhibited neurological disorders prior to their death (Dalakas et al., 1989). A number of clients with AIDS experience neurological and mental disorders such as dementias, delirium, and mood disorders arising from general medical conditions. Computed tomography scans show a progressive cortical dementia and diffuse cortical atrophy in the client with HIV or AIDS-related encephalopathy (Britton & Miller, 1984). In addition, the terminal nature of AIDS places tremendous psychosocial stress on, and requires enormous lifestyle changes of, the client and significant others. The psychosocial consequences of AIDS, like other life-threatening conditions, are multifaceted and include major lifestyle changes and losses, death and dying issues, and exposure to numerous medical interventions. Other potential psychosocial stressors include alienation from loved ones, social stigma, threat to self-integrity, and isolation. (See Chapter 13 for an in-depth discussion of cognitive disorders.)

Assessing AIDS clients' cognitive function and associated behaviors is an important aspect of care. Assessment of the progression and span of behavioral and mental status changes is a basic component of assessment of cognitive function (Antai-Otong, 1993). Cognitive changes reflect underlying general medical conditions such as dementias and delirium. The first step in assessing cognitive function is a comprehensive mental status examination. A mental status examination is an unstructured tool used to assess psychiatric and neurological function. This information may be gathered from the client, family, or significant others. Assessed in the mental status examination are attention, language, memory, and higher cortical function. The results of a mental status examination are used in conjunction with other diagnostic tests to determine a differential diagnosis of AIDS dementia. Table 28–5 lists the components of a mental status examination. Cummings's (1992) description of the mental status examination included the following:

- Attention (concentration and awareness)
- Memory (recent and remote recall of events)
- Language (spontaneous, reading and writing ability, and understanding)
- Executive function or higher cortical function (ability to abstract and judgment)

AIDS Dementia. AIDS dementia has a progressive degenerative course. Its symptoms include decreased concentration; memory, language, and motor difficulties; and the inability to abstract or the use of poor judgment. The degree of impairment reflects the nature of brain involvement. In fact, early neurological manifestations of AIDS dementia or encephalopathy are often subtle. Symptoms of early dementia include impaired concentration, irritability, mood changes, memory difficulties (recent recall), forgetfulness, apathy, and psychomotor slowing (Carne & Adler, 1986; Cummings, 1990; Pajeau & Román, 1992). Later symptoms suggest diffuse brain involvement and include the following:

- Delirium
- Delusions
- Hallucinations
- Severe headaches
- Fever
- Marked personality changes
- Severe cognitive involvement
- Motor signs (ataxia and spastic gait) (Navia et al., 1986)

TABLE 28–5
Components of the Mental Status Examination

1. General appearance
2. Level of functioning
3. Orientation
4. Attention (ability to attend matters at hand)
5. Language
6. Memory (immediate, short term, recent, and long term)
7. Higher cortical function (abstract vs. concrete thinking, judgment)
8. Perceptual impairment (hallucinations, delusions, and illusions)

Data from Antai-Otong, D. (1993). Cognitive and affective assessment of the geriatric patient. *MEDSURG Nursing, 2*, 70–74.

AIDS Delirium. AIDS delirium is an acute general medical condition manifested by disorientation, alterations in sensorium and attention, recent memory difficulties, motor restlessness or agitation, and perceptual distortions. Life-threatening symptoms of delirium include elevated blood pressure, pulse rates, and neurological changes (ataxia, nystagmus, and pupillary abnormality). This medical emergency is often misdiagnosed as a psychiatric disorder because it is accompanied by agitation, aggressive or violent behavior, and visual hallucinations. The symptoms of delirium must be assessed and reported as soon as possible, because delirium has a high mortality rate (Anderson, 1987; Murray, 1991; Weddington, 1982). See Table 13–9 for a detailed comparison of dementia and delirium.

Major nursing interventions center on medical stabilization and include the following:

- Reassuring the client and significant others
- Monitoring the client constantly (someone must be with the client at all times)
- Reorienting the client

The client may be treated with a combination of an anxiolytic and neuroleptic (an antipsychotic agent) to manage persistent agitation and aggressiveness. This combination lowers the need for high doses of neuroleptics and reduces the risk of extrapyramidal side effects (Adams, 1988). Nurses need to assess the client for desired and adverse reactions to these agents (see Chapter 26).

The complexity of the neurobiological and psychosocial components of AIDS increases clients' risk of depression and suicidal behaviors. Clients' responses must be assessed throughout treatment in efforts to identify and mobilize hospital and community resources that facilitate use of adaptive coping skills. Assessing and strengthening support systems are key to maximizing clients' emotional and physical resources.

The Client on Hemodialysis

Hemodialysis is a treatment that sustains the life of a client with chronic or acute renal failure, that is, cessation of renal function sufficient to maintain homeostasis. The focus of this discussion is on the client on hemodialysis who has chronic or end-stage renal failure. Other illnesses, such as diabetes mellitus, peripheral neuropathy, personality changes, and sexual dysfunction, frequently accompany renal diseases (Ignatavicus et al., 1992).

Renal failure, like other chronic illnesses, affects the client's livelihood. Psychosocial stressors related to hemodialysis include the following:

1. Loss of autonomy
2. Increased dependency
3. Major lifestyle and role changes
4. Major depression
5. Disturbances in body image
6. Impaired interpersonal relationships
7. Suicidal behaviors
8. Sexual dysfunction (Craven et al., 1987; Neu & Kjellstrand, 1985)

Reactions to dialysis vary among individuals. Some people are able to cope with a chronic debilitating condition, whereas others cannot. The client who can express his or her feelings, has strong social support, and is able to mobilize resources is advantaged. These factors affect the response to any illness, but they are especially important to clients with chronic illnesses. Anxiety and depression are common responses to end-stage renal or chronic renal failure.

Assessing clients' psychosocial and biological responses to dialysis is within the domain of nursing. Factors that affect the nurse–client relationship include the client's developmental stage, support system, perception of the illness, and role conflicts, and these factors need to be assessed throughout treatment.

Establishment of a therapeutic relationship is the basis of interventions that facilitate adaptive coping skills. It is important to develop an environment that fosters independence, enhances coping behaviors, strengthens support systems, and encourages expression of feelings. The client's active participation in care is crucial to maintaining his or her ability to cope with the chronic illness. Educating the client and family about hemodialysis, caring for the access (vascular entry for hemodialysis), dietary regimens, and skin care can allay anxiety and promote comfort. These interventions can help the client and family explore dependency issues and role changes and promote the client's self-esteem (Ulrich, 1989).

When the client fails to cope effectively with stress, maladaptive coping behaviors may emerge. Clients often use denial and other defense mechanisms to minimize the seriousness of their illness, increasing the risk of complications due to noncompliance. Clients must be assessed for symptoms of depression, persistent anxiety, suicidal behaviors, and substance abuse. When these symptoms are identified, psychiatric consultations are imperative to minimize the risk of self-destructive behaviors and alleviate the pain of depression and anxiety. Psychotropics may be ordered to manage depression and anxiety. Client education regarding expected and adverse responses to psychotropics is an important nursing intervention that promotes health and reduces the risk of ineffective coping patterns. See Chapters 9, 10, and 16 for in-depth discussions of depression, anxiety, and suicidal behavior, respectively.

One biological response to dialysis is chronic fatigue. The basis of this complication is a combination of psychological and neurobiological factors such as anemia, metabolic changes, stress, anxiety, and depression. Encouraging regular rest periods, administering medications (i.e., erythropoietin) to manage anemia, correcting metabolic imbalances, and modulating activities are useful in helping the client with fatigue and enhancing the client's quality of life (Jones, 1992; Wolcott et al., 1986).

Working with the client on hemodialysis requires integration of psychosocial and biological interventions that enhance coping and adaptive responses. Responses to chronic physical illness vary and are associated with the quality of support systems, the client's perception of the illness, and how the illness affects the client's lifestyle. Some clients accept their illness and cope effectively by mobilizing available resources. Others never accept their illness and stay in denial, compromising their health and increasing the risk of complications. Therapeutic interactions can help nurses identify adaptive and maladaptive coping behaviors. Interventions that increase self-esteem and strengthen adaptive coping skills are critical aspects of working with the client with a chronic physical illness.

HOSPITALIZATION DURING LATE ADULTHOOD

This life span discussion ends with a focus on a complex condition that primarily affects the older client, the cerebral vascular accident (CVA). A stroke, or CVA results from suspension of the circulation of the blood to the brain. CVAs are caused by blood clots, cerebral emboli, hypertension, narrowing or hardening of arteries that supply the brain, and cerebral aneurysm (Lishman, 1978).

Cassem (1991) asserted that direct brain injury causes

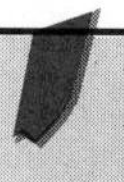

Nursing Care Plan 28–1 Psychosocial Aspects of Caring for the Client Who Has Experienced a CVA (Mrs. Jaycee)

Nursing Diagnosis: Ineffective Individual Coping related to adaptation to alterations in physical function.

OUTCOME IDENTIFICATION	NURSING ACTIONS	RATIONALES	EVALUATION
1. By [date], Mrs. Jaycee will adapt to and cope with limited physical function.	1a. Establish rapport with Mrs. Jaycee.	1a. Rapport conveys empathy and warmth.	*Goal met:* Therapeutic relationship with Mrs. Jaycee is established. Grief process is facilitated. Effective communication is established. Mrs. Jaycee is oriented as needed, especially during early phase of illness.
	1b. Assess Mrs. Jaycee's present/past coping behaviors.	1b–c. Strengths of previous coping patterns may be identified.	
	1c. Reorient Mrs. Jaycee as needed.		
	1d. Reassure Mrs. Jaycee that efforts will be made to help her communicate.	1d. Reassurance decreases anxiety and allows client to establish control over communication and care.	
	1e. Look directly at Mrs. Jaycee and use deliberate explanations and directions.	1e. Looking at client promotes understanding and enhances communication.	
	1f. Observe Mrs. Jaycee for signs of depression.	1f. Client is at risk for depression and grief reaction.	

Nursing Diagnosis: Self-care Deficit related to cognitive impairment.

OUTCOME IDENTIFICATION	NURSING ACTIONS	RATIONALES	EVALUATION
1. By [date], Mrs. Jaycee will participate in self-care activities.	1a. Assess Mrs. Jaycee's prestroke level of function (obtain this information from both Mrs. Jaycee and her family).	1a. Information about the client's baseline level of functioning is provided.	*Goal met:* Mrs. Jaycee and her family actively participate in her care. Family's initial attempts to do things for her that she was able to do for herself end after teaching begins. Mrs. Jaycee and her family are discharged to the rehabilitation program.
	1b. Encourage Mrs. Jaycee to participate in her daily care.	1b. Participation increases independence and restoration of function.	
	1c. Encourage Mrs. Jaycee's family to participate in her care.	1c. Family's sense of helplessness is decreased, and grief process is facilitated.	
	1d. Teach Mrs. Jaycee's family about the mental status changes in her.	1d–f. Teaching facilitates rehabilitation process, promoting control and restoration of health to highest level.	
	1e. Adhere to discharge/rehabilitation treatment plan.		
	1f. Stress the importance of firmness, consistency, and support.		

episodic changes in mood that eventually progress to major depression. Studies have shown that clients who experience injury to the left hemisphere and areas around the frontal lobe are vulnerable to severe depression (Robinson & Starkstein, 1990). In addition, two thirds of poststroke clients eventually manifest symptoms of severe depression, and the other one third manifest these symptoms by the sixth month. Clients with past and family histories of depression are also at risk for depression.

Major psychosocial stressors related to poststroke clients include the following:

1. Loss of ability to perform self-care (depending on the area and severity of brain damage)
2. Compromised coping skills
3. Difficulty adapting to limited or residual functioning
4. Personality changes and impaired intellectual function
5. Labile mood
6. Loss of effective communication skills

Neurobiological and psychosocial changes are expected outcomes in clients who have experienced a CVA. Family members are often overwhelmed by the client's increased dependency and neurobiological limitations. These feelings can be minimized by establishing therapeutic relationships with the client and family that provide emotional support, crisis intervention, and education about expected psychosocial and neurobiological changes and expectations.

Major client outcomes during the rehabilitation phase include the following:

- Attainment of an optimal level of function
- Development of adaptive coping behaviors
- Restoration of independence in self-care
- Adjustment to limited neurobiological function (client and family) (Ignatavicus et al., 1992)

The following case study illustrates the nursing process in the care of the client who has experienced a CVA. Also see Nursing Care Plan 28–1.

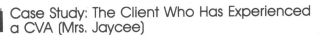

Case Study: The Client Who Has Experienced a CVA (Mrs. Jaycee)

Mrs. Jaycee is a 67-year-old woman who was a practicing pediatrician until a month ago, at which time she suffered a mild CVA. She is now actively involved in speech therapy. Her mood fluctuates from sad to normal but is mainly the former. Her family has been very supportive, but they are frustrated by her inability to cope with her illness. Her family reports that even though she is making tremendous progress, her mood is sad and depressed. They are concerned about her inability to cope. A request for consultation is sent to the psychiatric clinical specialist, who initially sees Mrs. Jaycee alone and later sees her with her spouse. Mrs. Jaycee communicates by writing notes and expresses frustration and a sense of loss because of her recent illness. She denies suicidal ideations, but she admits feeling depressed at times.

It is not uncommon for clients who have experienced a CVA to undergo mood changes, particularly depression. Mrs. Jaycee responds to individual psychotherapy that integrates grief work and other strategies that enable her to work through her sense of loss and increase her self-esteem and confidence. Later sessions with her spouse also enable him to deal with his grief and concern for his wife's well-being. After several months, Mrs. Jaycee is able to cope with her illness and gain the confidence for other aspects of her rehabilitation.

THE NURSE'S ROLE

THE GENERALIST NURSE

The medical–surgical generalist nurse plays several roles in helping clients cope with psychosocial stresses. The initial process involves the psychosocial assessment, which enables the nurse to assess present stressors, present and past coping behaviors, and available resources. Clients seen in the inpatient or ambulatory care setting experience similar stresses generated by fears of the unknown and alterations in self-esteem and body image.

The woman seeking a mammogram after finding a lump in her breast is just as stressed as the man who suffers acute chest pain. Inevitably, death and dying issues emerge in these circumstances. Medical–surgical staff nurses can help clients manage psychosocial stresses by using active listening skills and responding in a concerned and nonjudgmental manner. Nurse–client interactions provide opportunities to express feelings; assess verbal and nonverbal responses; and intervene to increase self-esteem, reduce feelings of helplessness, and promote an optimal level of function.

THE ADVANCED-PRACTICE NURSE

Clients experiencing various psychosocial reactions in medical–surgical settings may be seen by the PCLN. This advanced-practice nurse practitioner identifies the complex psychosocial responses of clients in medical–surgical settings. Major interventions include a complete psychosocial assessment, grief work, prescription of medication, crisis intervention, case management, and individual and family psychotherapy. In addition, the PCLN collaborates with the generalist nurse, the client and family, and the members of the health team in inpatient and community settings to mobilize the client's resources and promote an optimal level of function.

THE NURSING PROCESS

Assessment

Assessing the client's psychosocial needs begins with gathering data on the reason for seeking treatment, the nature and duration of symptoms, and past and present medications. Coping behaviors are assessed by inquiring how stress or similar events have been handled in the past. This information helps the nurse develop an innovative care plan to meet the client's present psychosocial needs.

Coping behaviors need to be assessed and strengthened throughout treatment. This includes identifying adaptive and maladaptive coping behaviors. Maladaptive coping responses include suicidal behaviors and substance abuse. It is helpful to inquire about present or past suicidal attempts, circumstances, and treatment when assessing the client's present coping behaviors. Furthermore, it is crucial to ask the client about present and past substance abuse or dependence, because times of stress increase the likelihood of relapse or increased abuse of drugs or alcohol.

Nursing Diagnoses

Major nursing diagnoses for clients experiencing psychosocial stressors include the following:

1. Ineffective Individual Coping
2. Self-Care Deficit
3. Alterations in Self-Image and Self-Esteem
4. Anxiety

Planning

Clients in medical–surgical settings experience tremendous stress. Coping with physical illness challenges them to face a number of issues, such as alterations in lifestyle, roles, and body image. Support systems are critical in helping them resolve crises generated by serious or life-threatening illnesses. Loss is a major concern for the client in the medical–surgical or rehabilitation setting. Nurses can facilitate the grief process by establishing therapeutic interactions that encourage expression of feelings and thoughts created by acute and chronic illnesses.

The following are the major client outcomes in medical–surgical settings:

1. Preservation of healthy physiological function
2. Reduction or cessation of the disease process
3. Strengthening of adaptive coping behaviors
4. Participation in the treatment and rehabilitation process

Implementation

Different illnesses require different biological interventions. For example, the elderly client who experiences a CVA requires neurological monitoring, and the spinal cord–injured client requires care for skin integrity.

Educating clients and families about the disease process, treatment modalities, and psychosocial responses is a major aspect of both the acute and rehabilitation phases. Support systems, community resources, and **collaboration** with nurses and other health professionals are vital to the success of managing acute and chronic medical conditions.

The major nursing interventions for clients in medical–surgical settings are as follows:

1. Establishment of rapport and therapeutic interactions with the client and family
2. Collaboration with the client, family, and interdisciplinary team to develop a comprehensive plan of care
3. Facilitation of the grief process
4. Reinforcement of the client's coping skills and mobilization of resources

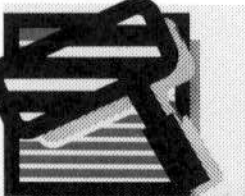

RESEARCH STUDY

Living with Dying: Coping with HIV Disease

McCain, N. L., & Gramling, L. F. (1992). *Issues in Mental Health Nursing, 13,* 271–284.

Purpose of Study

The purpose of this phenomenological study was to understand the experiences associated with living with HIV disease and to test a measure of stress and coping.

Methodology

The researchers interviewed 36 participants with HIV disease from a local infectious-disease clinic. In the tape-recorded interviews, participants were asked focused, open-ended questions about their thoughts, feelings, and behaviors associated with coping with the stress associated with HIV disease.

Findings

The researchers found a variety of experiences that paralleled the stages of the participants' disease, which ranged from the initial HIV-positive diagnosis, to AIDS, to impending death. The experiences were categorized as follows: living with dying, fighting the sickness, getting worn out. A number of these clients experienced depression, suicidal ideation, and grief, and some reported the benefits of having someone listen and encourage them to express their feelings about their illness.

Nursing Implications

The psychosocial impact of HIV disease is extensive and includes numerous losses, rejection, and stigmatization. Nurses play a major role in helping clients and their significant others in various settings cope with losses and death and dying issues. Clients and their significant others can benefit from active listening, psychotherapy, and appropriate community referrals.

Evaluation

Evaluation of the client's responses to treatment is a continuous process that is based on verbal and nonverbal feedback from clients, families, and members of the treatment team.

RESEARCH IN MEDICAL–SURGICAL SETTINGS

The psychosocial needs of clients in the medical–surgical setting are immense, and there is a growing trend to measure the cost-effectiveness and quality of such nursing care. Nurses can address these demands by collaborating in research to explore the effectiveness of interventions that enhance coping behaviors, increase self-esteem, and promote comfort and healing. Medical–surgical clients tend to experience intense anxiety and depression. The severity of these symptoms can be measured by using established research tools such as the Hamilton Anxiety and Depression Scales. Nursing interventions can reduce symptoms and behaviors generated by acute and chronic medical conditions. Outcomes can be determined by posttreatment scores and client feedback and responses. A research project can be developed by the staff nurse and psychiatric and other clinical specialists. See the Research Study display for an example of such a study.

►CHAPTER SUMMARY

Medical–surgical conditions affect clients and families throughout the life span and the individual responses to them are complex. Coping behaviors are taxed and compromised during illness and must be assessed on an ongoing basis so that support systems may be mobilized and coping behaviors reinforced when needed. Often during acute or crisis events, the client has to depend on the nurse for survival. This process lays the foundation of therapeutic interactions that foster dependence and, later, independence. The clients' psychological needs are immense and vary with developmental stage, the nature of the illness, personality traits, and coping skills. Clients' resources are maximized by assessing their special needs and collaborating with other team members to help clients meet them and attain their highest level of functioning.

Clients in medical–surgical settings have tremendous psychosocial and biological needs. Nursing interventions are based on developmental stage and psychosocial and biological needs. The discussion of various physical conditions emphasizes the complexity of adaptation and the significance of the therapeutic relationship in mobilizing resources to promote clients' health and restore them to an optimal level of functioning.

Suggestions for Clinical Conference

1. Present the case histories of several clients with chronic and acute medical conditions and identify these clients' psychosocial and biological needs.
2. Present nursing care plans for angry, demanding, depressed, and dying clients.
3. Role-play demanding, angry, and depressed clients.

References

Adams, F. (1988). Emergency intravenous sedation of the delirious medically ill patient. *Journal of Clinical Psychiatry, 49*(Suppl.), 22–26.

American Psychiatric Association. (1994). *Diagnostic and statistical manual of mental disorders* (4th ed.). Washington, DC: Author.

Anderson, W. H. (1991). The emergency room. In T. P. Hackett & N. H. Cassem (Eds.), *Massachusetts General handbook of psychiatry* (2nd ed., pp. 419–437). Littleton, MA; PSG.

Antai-Otong, D. (1988a). When your patient is angry. *Nursing, 18*(2), 44–45.

Antai-Otong, D. (1988b). When your patient is depressed. *Nursing, 18*(9), 70–72.

Antai-Otong, D. (1989). Dealing with demanding patients. *Nursing, 19*(1), 94–95.

Antai-Otong, D. (1993). Cognitive and affective assessment of the geriatric patient. *MEDSURG Nursing, 2*(1), 70–74.

Beck, A. T., Brown, G., Berchick, R. J., Stewart, B. L., & Steer, R. A. (1990). Relationship between hopelessness and ultimate suicide: A replication with psychiatric outpatients. *American Journal of Psychiatry, 147*(2), 190–195.

Britton C. B., & Miller, J. R. (1984). Neurological complications in acquired immunodeficiency syndrome (AIDS). *Neurology Clinics, 2,* 315–339.

Carne, C., & Adler, M. W. (1986). Neurological complications of human immunodeficiency virus infection. *British Medical Journal, 293,* 462–463.

Cassem, N. H. (1991). Depression. In N. H. Cassem (Ed.), *Massachusetts General handbook of psychiatry* (3rd ed., pp. 237–268). St. Louis, MO: Mosby Year Book.

Craven, J. L., Rodin, G. M., Johnson, L., & Kennedy, S. H. (1987). The diagnosis of major depression in renal dialysis patients. *Psychosomatic Medicine, 49,* 482–492.

Cummings, J. L. (1990). *Subcortical dementia*. New York: Oxford University Press.

Cummings, J. L. (1992, November). Using the mental status examination in neuropsychiatric diagnosis. *The Psychiatric Times: Medicine and Behavior,* pp. 20–21.

Dalakas, M., Wichman, A., & Sever, J. (1989). AIDS and the nervous system. *Journal of the American Medical Association, 261,* 2396–2399.

Furman, R. A. (1964). Health and the young child. In *The psychoanalytic study of the child* (Vol. 19, pp. 321–333). New York: International Universities Press.

Grey, M., Cameron, M. E., & Thurber, F. W. (1991). Coping and adaptation in children with diabetes. *Nursing Research, 40,* 144–149.

Haase, J. E., Britt, T., & Coward, D. D. (1992). Simultaneous concept analysis of spiritual perspective, hope, acceptance, and self-transcendence. *Image, 24,* 141–147.

Ignatavicius, D. J., Batterden, R. A., & Hausman, K. A. (1992). *Medical–surgical nursing*. Philadelphia: W. B. Saunders.

Jones, K. R. (1992). Risk of hospitalization for chronic hemodialysis patients. *Image, 24,* 88–94.

Jourard, S. (1974). *Health personality*. New York: Macmillan.

Kubler-Ross, E. (1969). *On death and dying*. New York: Macmillan.

Lishman, W. A. (1978). *Organic psychiatry*. Oxford, England: Blackwell Scientific Publications.

Mishne, J. M. (1986). *Clinical work with adolescents*. New York: Free Press.

Murray, G. B. (1991). Confusion, delirium, and dementia. In N. H. Cassem (Ed.), *Massachusetts General Hospital Handbook of General Hospital Psychiatry* (3rd ed., pp. 89–120). St. Louis: Mosby-Year Book.

Navia, B. A., Jordan, B. D., & Price, R. W. (1986). The AIDS dementia complex: I. Clinical features. *Annals of Nephrology*, 19, 517–524.

Neu, S., & Kjellstrand, C. M. (1985). Stopping long-term dialysis. *New England Journal of Medicine, 314,* 14–20.

Pajeau, A. K., and Român, G. C. (1992). HIV encephalopathy and dementia. *Psychiatric Clinics of North America, 15,* 455–466.

Rabins, P. V., Harvis, K., & Koven, S. (1985). High fatality rates of late-life depression associated with cardiovascular disease. *Journal of Affective Disorders, 9,* 165–167.

Reighley, J. W. (1988). *Nursing care plan guides for mental health*. Baltimore: Williams & Wilkins.

Robinson, R. G., & Starkstein, S. E. (1990). Current research in affective disorders following stroke. *Journal of Neuropsychiatry, 21,* 1–14.

Saunders, C. (1969). The moment of truth: Care of the dying person. In L. Pearson (Ed.), *Death and dying* (pp. 49–78). Cleveland, OH: Case Western Research University Press.

Ulrich, B. T. (1989). *Nephrology nursing: Concepts and strategies*. East Norwalk, CT: Appleton & Lange.

Weddington, M. W. (1982). The mortality of delirium: An unappreciated problem? *Psychosomatics, 23,* 241–249.

Wells, K. B., Golding, J. M., & Burman, M. A. (1988). Psychiatric disorders in a sample of the general population with and without chronic medical conditions. *American Journal of Psychiatry, 145,* 976–979.

Wolcott, D. L., Maida, C. A., Diamond, R., & Nissenson, A. R. (1986). Treatment compliance in end-stage renal disease patients on dialysis. *American Journal of Nephrology, 6,* 329–338.

Unit 3 Study Questions

See Appendix I for answers.

CHAPTER 21

1. M. M., a 15-year-old girl, is admitted to the acute psychiatric unit because of problems controlling her temper and striking her mother during a heated argument. Developmentally, what are her main stressors?
   a. Dealing with her need to control her temper.
   b. Learning how to develop adaptive coping behaviors.
   c. Dealing with issues associated with dependency.
   d. Staying out of trouble at school and with her parents.

2. As her nurse, you are responsible for gathering information to assist in making a provisional diagnosis. She has been shouting at other clients periodically during the past few days. What is the initial step in assessing this client?
   a. Keeping her calm.
   b. Approaching her in a calm, nonjudgmental manner.
   c. Inquiring about her hobbies and school activities.
   d. Setting limits and informing her that yelling is unacceptable.

3. Adolescents differ from adults in treatment because of the following reasons *except* that
   a. They are generally distrustful of adults.
   b. They usually do not seek treatment voluntarily.
   c. Their symptoms often reflect family conflict.
   d. They are not amenable to changing their behavior.

4. Self-disclosure is an important part of psychotherapy. What information places the nurse at greatest risk for negative consequences of self-disclosure?
   a. Sharing information about your family.
   b. Telling the client your first name.
   c. Sharing highly personal problems.
   d. Sharing your feelings about problems on the unit.

5. The success of psychotherapy is influenced by several qualities in the client and the nurse psychotherapist. Which behavior suggests that the client might terminate treatment prematurely?
   a. Substance abuse.
   b. Distrust.
   c. Poor insight.
   d. All of the above.

6. What single factor plays an important role in the success of psychotherapy?
   a. Self-disclosure.
   b. Therapeutic relationship.
   c. Keeping appointments.
   d. Insight into present problems.

CHAPTER 22

1. General systems theory can be applied to families. Which of the following represents an open system?
   a. H. is not allowed to play with neighborhood children his age.
   b. I. K. waits for her daughter at least 30 minutes before school ends.
   c. A. F. brings home a new friend who wants to play dolls.
   d. S. T. visits his mother every day.

2. Which system's theory concept allows exchange of energy and matter across boundaries?
   a. Feedback mechanism.
   b. Steady-state or equilibrium.
   c. Input mechanism.
   d. Hierarchy of subsystems.

3. Recognizing the couple dyad is the basis of effective family transactions. Which of the following represents pseudomutuality?
   a. After their child attempts suicide, the parents report that they have a perfect marriage.
   b. A child is admitted to the hospital for the fourth time in 2 weeks with asthma attack.
   c. The couple argues and resolves dispute over who will take the children to the soccer game.
   d. An adolescent expresses anger toward father when he is grounded for staying out late.

4. The *best* definition of congruent communication is
   a. Clear, direct, and honest.
   b. Conveys verbal cues.
   c. Confusing and contradictory.
   d. Contributes to maladaptive coping behaviors.

5. Functional families manage change by
   a. Perceiving it as a threat.
   b. Mobilizing resources within and outside the system.
   c. Minimizing resources to cope with stress.
   d. Decreasing permeability of boundaries.

CHAPTER 23

1. L. Q. is a 22-year old man newly diagnosed with schizophrenia who has been admitted for his first psychiatric hospitalization to your psychiatric unit. You are his nurse, and you find him suspicious, avoiding contact with peers, appearing preoccupied most of the time, and refusing to

answer your questions. Which group might be most therapeutic for this patient?

a. Men's group.
b. Medication class.
c. Exercise group.
d. Alcoholics Anonymous meeting.

2. The responsibilities of a group leader of group therapy include

a. Responsiveness to feelings.
b. Empathic understanding of each person's contribution.
c. Arrangements for meeting potential mates.
d. Provision of time extensions to each session, as needed.
e. a. and b.
f. c. and d.

3. Two weeks into hospitalization, L. Q. is assigned to a group focused on symptom management. In a postgroup meeting, the leaders described L. Q.'s effect on the group, the comments that members made, the unusual behaviors of two members, and the benefit to L. Q. What *best* describes this discussion?

a. Treatment planning.
b. Process and content.
c. Nursing care planning.
d. Group therapy evaluation.
e. Multidisciplinary rounds.

4. The group therapy approach that focuses on changing behavior by examining thoughts and related feelings that contribute to maladaptive behaviors *best* describes

a. Communication theory.
b. Group process theory.
c. Cognitive theory.
d. Psychodynamic theory.

CHAPTER 24

1. Indiscriminate use of support (too much) can lead to

a. Aggressive behavior, regression, and dependence.
b. Feelings of inadequacy, regression, and dependence.
c. Manipulation of staff and feelings of inadequacy.
d. Manipulation of staff and aggressive behavior.

2. Adolescents and chemically addicted clients benefit from the milieu therapy aspect of

a. Peer feedback and support.
b. Client responsibility for self.
c. Identification of consequences of maladaptive behavior.
d. All of the above.

3. A client tells you that you are the only staff member she can talk to, then mentions that something has been bothering her that she does not want everyone else to know. In formulating your response to the client, you will consider which of the following principles of milieu therapy?

a. This indicates therapeutic trust has been established.
b. Confidentiality is unit based in a therapeutic milieu.
c. Secret-keeping is a way to gain rapport with clients.
d. All of the above.

4. Characteristics of a therapeutic community include

a. Well-defined authority based on disciplinary specific expertise.
b. Relieving the client of the stress of treatment plan decisions.
c. Encouraging the client to separate from family and community responsibilities.
d. None of the above.

CHAPTER 25

1. Which of the following is in the order of least to most restrictive level of care?

a. Partial hospitalization, inpatient hospitalization, group home, residential treatment center, home care.
b. Home care, group home, residential treatment center, partial hospitalization, inpatient hospitalization.
c. Home care, partial hospitalization, inpatient hospitalization, group home, residential treatment center.
d. Partial hospitalization, home care, residential treatment center, group home, inpatient hospitalization.

2. Which is *not* a service for the homeless mentally ill?

a. Shelters.
b. Support programs.
c. Drop-in centers.
d. Home care.

3. Major events affecting deinstitutionalization included all of the following *except*

a. The success of psychotropic medications.
b. Joint Commission on Mental Illness and Health's *Action for Mental Health Report*.
c. Expense for caring for institutionalized patients.
d. Belief that the least restrictive measure of treatment was optimal.

4. The functions of partial hospitalization include all of the following *except*

a. An alternative to inpatient treatment.
b. Transitional treatment.
c. Long-term living arrangements.
d. Rehabilitation.

5. Psychiatric home health care focuses on direct client care and community programs.
   a. True.
   b. False.

6. Community mental health centers are directed and funded by
   a. Private business and industry.
   b. Government.
   c. Insurance providers.
   d. Non-profit organizations.

7. Case managers of the community mental health centers provide all of the following *except*
   a. Facilitating the client's access to services.
   b. Protecting the client's legal rights.
   c. Counseling.
   d. Administering medication.

8. Services for children include all of the following *except*
   a. Halfway houses.
   b. Foster care.
   c. Group homes.
   d. Residential treatment centers.

CHAPTER 26

1. The neurological blood–brain barrier is composed of
   a. Histaminic receptors in the stomach.
   b. Endothelial cells of the small intestine.
   c. Endothelial cells of the brain.
   d. Noradrenergic neurons in the brain.

2. Which of the following structures are considered part of the limbic system?
   a. The frontal lobes.
   b. The thalamus.
   c. The pons.
   d. The amygdala.

3. Parkinson's disease involves a depletion of which neurotransmitter in the basal ganglia of the brain?
   a. Norepinephrine.
   b. Dopamine.
   c. Gamma-aminobutyric acid.
   d. Glycine.

4. Which of the following structures associated with the reception of speech is located in the temporal lobe?
   a. Wernicke's area.
   b. Broca's area.
   c. Korsakoff's area.
   d. Hippocampus.

5. The concept of drug half-life time is important to determine
   a. The dosage necessary to achieve therapeutic effects.
   b. Toxicity.
   c. How often a drug needs to be administered.
   d. Side effects of a drug.

6. Which of the following is an important educational issue for client teaching with heterocyclic antidepressants?
   a. Foods containing tyramine should not be consumed.
   b. The effects should be immediate.
   c. Most side effects can be treated with an antiparkinsonian agent.
   d. It will take 2 to 4 weeks before a change in mood will become apparent.

7. Which of the following medications is specific to blocking the reuptake of serotonin?
   a. Fluoxetine (Prozac).
   b. Trazadone (Deseryl).
   c. Imipramine (Tofranil).
   d. Phenelzine (Nardil).

8. In the patient who is taking lithium carbonate, which of the following can affect serum levels?
   a. Lack of sleep.
   b. Osmotic diuretics.
   c. Asthma medications.
   d. Antihistamines.

9. A client experiencing akathisia most likely displays
   a. A tremor on resting.
   b. Orthostatic hypotension.
   c. Chewing, puffing movements around the mouth.
   d. Agitation and restlessness.

10. Pseudoparkinsonism is due to which of the following mechanisms?
   a. A sudden increase in serotonin in the limbic system.
   b. A depletion of gamma-aminobutyric acid in the striatum.
   c. An increase in norepinephrine in the temporal lobes.
   d. A depletion of dopamine in the basal ganglia nigrostriatum.

11. Which of the following is a significant consideration in the selection of a benzodiazepine for use in inducing sleep?
   a. Addiction potential.
   b. Interactions with food.
   c. Half-life.
   d. Effects on rapid-eye-movement sleep.

12. Which of the following is an important issue in using medications in the elderly?
   a. Aging alters the ability to metabolize and excrete medications.
   b. Older persons may have difficulty managing a number of medications at once.

c. Older persons have a higher rate of noncompliance.
d. Older persons are more susceptible to the cardiovascular effects of drugs.

CHAPTER 27

1. Which is the most appropriate use of somatic or biological therapies?
   a. Using light therapy to treat client with schizophrenia.
   b. Administering electroconvulsive therapy to client with obsessive-compulsive disorder.
   c. Using sleep-cycle alteration to treat client with seasonal affective disorder.
   d. Using dim light therapy for client withdrawing from alcohol.

2. E. B. is a 43-year-old woman who presents with symptoms of agitation, hypersomnia, and increased appetite over the past month. Her husband reports that she develops these symptoms every winter. As her nurse, which is the next *best* question to assess her present condition?
   a. Are you currently being treated for any major medical problems?
   b. What are your current medications?
   c. Have you ever been treated for these symptoms?
   d. Would you like to take something to calm you down?

3. Which of the following best defines E. B.'s symptoms?
   a. Bipolar disorder, depressed type.
   b. Seasonal affective disorder.
   c. Bipolar disorder, manic type.
   d. Seasonal anxiety disorder.

4. Informed consent can be best defined as
   a. Signing the consent form.
   b. A continuous educational process.
   c. The sole responsibility of the physician.
   d. Involving declaring someone competent.

5. A common side effect of electroconvulsive treatment is
   a. Permanent memory loss.
   b. Transient cognitive impairment.
   c. Loss of speech.
   d. Intermittent gastrointestinal disturbances.

CHAPTER 28

1. L. P. is admitted to the hospital with a diagnosis of acute back strain. She is demanding and frequently turns on the call light. The nurses expressed frustration and anger because the client criticizes them for taking too long to medicate her. What is the *best* approach to this client when she calls for pain medication?
   a. Take her the medication as soon as she can have it.
   b. Set limits with her, and explain the inappropriateness of her behavior.
   c. Explore her feelings about this hospitalization.
   d. Encourage her to talk about reasons for asking for pain medication.

2. Clients in medical-surgical settings are often overwhelmed by their illness. Which of the following indicates Ineffective Coping Behaviors?
   a. The client is talkative and willing to participate in treatment.
   b. The client elicits assistance from family members in daily care.
   c. The client asks the nurse to assist in routine care.
   d. The client expresses anger because the call light was not answered.

3. Childhood responses to medical illnesses are influenced by all *except*
   a. Developmental stage.
   b. Separation from parents.
   c. Nature of the illness.
   d. Change in role.

4. Adolescents with medical illness experience immense stress during hospitalization. Which is the best example of psychosocial stress for the medically ill adolescent?
   a. Fears of rejection by peers.
   b. Loss of health.
   c. Separation from parents.
   d. Fears of academic failure.

5. Clients who have had a stroke tend to become depressed. What is the best example of a depressed stroke client?
   a. Refuses to eat, isolates self, argumentative.
   b. Demanding and critical of staff.
   c. Argues with wife and uncooperative with staff.
   d. Frequently asks for assistance in managing daily care.

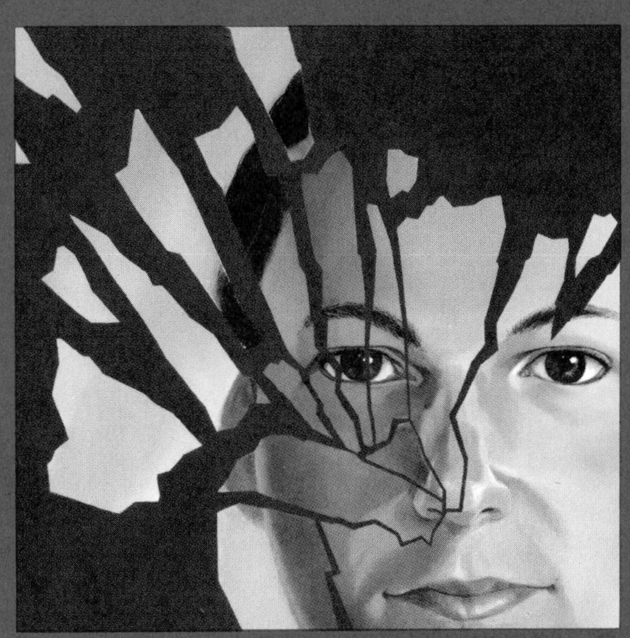

UNIT

4

Advanced Psychiatric Nursing Practice

CHAPTER

The Nurse's Role in the Behavioral–Biological Interface

DEBORAH ANTAI-OTONG, M.S., R.N.,C.S.
MARGARET BRACKLEY, PH.D., R.N.,C.S.

OUTLINE

CHAPTER OBJECTIVES

Upon completion of this chapter, you will be able to:

1. Identify major paradigms of mental disorders.
2. Integrate neurobiological and behavioral concepts into nursing practice.
3. Develop a plan of care using biological and behavioral interventions.

KEY TERMS

Genetic vulnerability
Hypothalamus
Kindling
Neuroendocrinology
Psychoneuroimmunology
Reinforcers
Twin studies

When the U.S. Congress proclaimed the 1990s to be the "Decade of the Brain," families of mentally ill clients welcomed this new perspective on mental disorders. In the past, parents and siblings were thought to be responsible for many mental illnesses as clinicians sought to explain those disorders solely in a behavioral context. As a consequence, family members have felt demoralized and blamed for their loved one's illnesses. Recently, however, neurobiological research findings have helped clinicians and researchers begin to understand the biological component in mental illness, particularly in terms of brain function and dysfunction, genetics, immunology, and endocrinology. The growth in biological knowledge has given clients, families, and mental health professionals hope for more effective treatment and possible cures for serious mental disorders (U.S. Congress, 1989).

Advances in neurobiology and neuroendocrinology parallel the sweeping technological findings of brain mapping, imaging, and scanning. Studies have demonstrated the underlying biological bases of schizophrenia, bipolar disorder, other affective disorders, and the aging process. In addition, the use of new psychopharmacological agents has produced remarkable results such as decreased side effects, decreased exacerbations, and increased compliance in clients with severe schizophrenia, depression, and anxiety disorders.

Many client symptoms or behaviors observed in people with mental illness are linked to underlying biological factors. Disturbances in mood, cognition, sensory-perceptual responses, impulse control, and social interactions are examples of behaviors that have been linked to biological abnormalities or disruption.

The purpose of this chapter is to explore major concepts of the biological–behavioral interface and its impact on psychiatric nursing practice. This chapter also identifies client outcomes from nursing interventions to meet the complex needs of the mentally ill.

HISTORY OF THE BIOLOGICAL–BEHAVIORAL DICHOTOMY

Recent expansion of neurobiological technology underscores the need to explain how both biological and behavioral factors relate to mental illness. The interrelatedness of biology and behavior is not a new concept. It has its beginnings as early as the fourteenth century, stemming from the works of Hippocrates, who explained the concept of mental illness as a process of the brain rather than a spiritual event. He surmised that the brain gave rise to pleasure, joy, sorrow, pain, and grief and contributed to disturbances in affect or mood. Although his early description of the tenuous balance of four humors (blood, phlegm, and yellow and black bile) and their relationship to mood disorders proved inaccurate, his premise that maladaptive behaviors arise from complex biological processes was correct.

In more recent times, Sigmund Freud contributed to neurobiology in the late 1800s through the phase of his work known as the *neurological phase*. During this period of his research, Freud sought to establish a relationship among neural mechanisms, behavior patterns, and cognitive distortions. Freud and others sought to understand psychopathology in relation to disturbances of specific areas of brain dysfunction. Ultimately, this work has led to the recent explosion of neurobiological research and discoveries.

The search for the ideal treatment of mental illness found a major breakthrough in the discovery of tranquilizers in the 1950s. These agents relieved clients with various symptoms of mental illness, such as intense anxiety, agitation, delusions, and hallucinations. Some of the tranquilizing agents uncovered during this era included the phenothiazines, such as chlorpromazine (Thorazine), the first of the medications that was effective in treating behavioral manifestations of schizophrenia. Other tranquilizers induced major behavioral and biological changes in the mentally ill, thus generating further clues to biological aspects of mental illness.

Newer psychotropics have emerged since the 1950s and have proved effective in the treatment of various mental disorders, such as schizophrenia and mood and addictive disorders (see Chapter 26). Over the past decade the effectiveness of these agents has increased because of improvements made in their ability to precisely target behavioral manifestations of the complex neurobiological processes, such as those located in the hypothalamus and other areas in the limbic system. Psychotropics are surmised to act on neurochemical mechanisms that in turn alter or interfere with behavioral patterns. Examples include the selective serotonergic reuptake blocking agents, such as fluoxetine (Prozac) and sertraline (Zoloft), which are used to treat major depression, and an atypical neuroleptic, clozapine, which is used to treat schizophrenia. Research and trial studies have drastically reduced the disabling side effects of some of these agents and provided hope and relief for clients and families.

MAJOR NEUROBIOLOGICAL MODELS

To understand the neurobiological models of mental illnesses and their implications for nursing, one must be familiar with the structure and function of the central nervous system (CNS) and its neurochemical processes. One also needs some basic knowledge of neuroendocrinology, psychoneuroimmunology, and genetics. Each of these models has widespread implications for behavioral and psychopharmacological interventions relevant to nursing practice.

THE CENTRAL NERVOUS SYSTEM

The CNS acts as the body's primary information processing center by gathering data about the internal and external environments. It is the most complex of the human systems, governing emotional and behavioral as well as biological processes. Highly developed networks of specialized cells work together to integrate a variety of stimuli to respond appropriately to internal and external needs.

Various conditions, such as mental illness, aging, and degenerative processes, affect brain function. Abnormalities in neurotransmitter production or absorption, neuroendocrine response, immunological responses, and genetic predisposition all may contribute to mental disorders. It has not been clearly established whether neurotransmitter and neuroendocrine abnormalities cause mental illness or vice versa; that is, underlying functional or structural disorders contributing to mental illness may cause neurotransmitter and neuroendocrine abnormalities.

Degenerative Processes. Degenerative processes may occur at any age, leading to cognitive and affective mental impairment. More importantly, these processes may be caused by underlying general medical conditions or their treatments. For example, many medications used to treat medical conditions contribute to depressed mood, and as many as 50 percent of persons who experience cerebral infarction (stroke) become severely and chronically depressed.

The brain shrinks with age; after 50 years of age, a considerable number of neurons are lost. Despite these neuronal changes, there is no definitive evidence of mental or cognitive decline associated with aging. Some researchers suggest that the brain adapts to aging by preserving an abundance of nerve cells rich in acetylcholine in transmitter pathways between the hippocampus and the cerebral cortex. These maturational changes are linked with higher cortical function (i.e., "wisdom"). Deterioration of these neurons is linked with degenerative processes such as those found in dementia associated with Alzheimer's disease and Parkinson's disease (Mesulam & Geula, 1991).

NEUROCHEMICAL PROCESSES

Neural regulation is based on a complex network of transmitter pathways that are sensitive to fluctuations of transmitter and hormonal balance. Neurotransmitters initially interact with receptor terminals of the postsynaptic cell membrane, resulting in either an inhibitory or excitatory response. The nature of the response is determined by the type of neurotransmitter and receptors. Norepinephrine, dopamine, acetylcholine, and serotonin are examples of excitatory transmitters, whereas amino acids such as gamma-aminobutyric acid have inhibitory effects (see Figs. 9–1, 10–1, and 12–1). Abnormal concentrations of these substances are associated with mental disorders such as depression, anxiety, addictive disorders, and schizophrenia. Antidepressants, neuroleptics, and other pharmacologic agents act on the neurotransmitters to increase or decrease their release and ultimately modify relative concentrations to improve the symptoms of the mental illness (see Chapter 26). Nurses must understand the neurochemical and systemic impact of the medications they administer, whether treating mental or concurrent medical illnesses. In this way, optimal responses will more often be achieved.

NEUROENDOCRINOLOGY

The neural and endocrine systems work together to support and maintain normal system function. These systems communicate through biofeedback mechanisms to establish a basis for all biological and behavioral responses. The neuroendocrine system is composed of the **hypothalamus**, pituitary gland, thyroid gland, adrenal glands, gonads, and pancreas. The hypothalamic-pituitary-adrenal (HPA) axis is particularly important in the response to threat or stress. Abnormalities in the HPA axis are known to contribute to, and are diagnostic of, functional psychosis and depressive and anxiety disorders (Coryell & Tsuang, 1992) (see Chapter 11 and Fig. 11–1). It is important for nurses to be aware of the endocrine-neural influences of mental disorders to better assess for and understand underlying pathology and potential treatment.

PSYCHONEUROIMMUNOLOGY

The immune system plays a key role in the development of infections and tumors when it is underactive, and of allergies and autoimmune diseases when it is overactive (Borysenko, 1987; Solomon, 1987). It is now becoming clear that the immune system plays a role in health and illness in the face of biological and psychosocial stress as well. The new field of **psychoneuroimmunology** is a developing body of knowledge concerned with the interconnections between the nervous system and the immune system.

Each cell in the human body contains a marker that identifies the cell as part of "self." Any material that does not contain this marker is identified as foreign antigen. The immune system serves the body by first detecting and protecting it from invasion of antigens, then by producing antibodies to destroy or neutralize the foreign body. The character of the antigen and the specific antibody are stored in memory of the immune cells, so that response to a next attack is more rapid and stronger. The immune system may be chronically activated as a stress response, or it may fail to recognize the self-marker and attack itself, as in autoimmune diseases.

The manner in which the immune system works has many implications for psychiatric nursing. Research has shown that negative life events and chronic stress affect health (Monroe & Simons, 1991). Recently, psychiatric illnesses, especially affective disorders (Hichie et al., 1990) and panic disorders (Brambilla et al., 1992), have been linked to immune dysfunction. Continued research in this area is critical. The National Institute of Nursing Research has called for research development in the areas of immunoincompetence and of interventions that bolster appropriate immune response.

GENETICS

Numerous research studies confirm the relationship between genetic and enzymatic defects and **genetic vulnerability** to mental illness. Genetic function is influenced by prenatal and environmental factors that activate intricate biochemical processes that affect behavior.

Twin, Adoption, and Family Studies. A number of researchers have attempted to explore the relationship between genetic factors and mental disorders using twin, adoption, and family studies. **Twin studies** are helpful in isolating genetic and environmental influences and determining preventive and precipitating factors. These studies usually include monozygotic (single ovum) and dizygotic (dual ova) twins. Adoption studies try to determine the impact of environmental factors on genetic expression. These studies generally examine and compare biological and adoptive parents of affected subjects and those of healthy biological and adoptive control subjects. Family studies contrast the occurrence of mental disorder among relatives of affected subjects and assess the relevance of heredity (Kaplan & Sadock, 1991).

Genetic theories regarding the cause of schizophrenia date back to Kraepelin in the early 1900s, who observed that bizarre behavior was commonly found in families of clients with schizophrenia. Twin, adoption, and family studies consistently link genetic factors, individual susceptibility, and psychosocial stressors with manifestations of schizophrenia; mental retardation; dementias; and affective, addictive, and other disorders (Jones & Murray, 1991; Lohr & Bracha, 1992; Prescott & Gottesman, 1993).

Environmental Factors. Genetic factors do not account for all variances between heredity and mental illness. Studies suggest that environmental factors are just as important as molecular-based genetic processes. Twin, adoption, and family studies tend to support this premise. Environmental factors include parental treatment, family structures, age spacing, and gender. These factors may buffer or protect genetically vulnerable clients (Goldsmith, 1983; Kendler et al., 1993; Parker et al., 1992), so that people with a predisposition to a particular mental illness may not develop it because of exposure to protective environmental factors.

Genetics and Addiction. A leading area of concern for nurses is identifying clients at risk for alcoholism and other addictions. One possible explanation for substance abuse is thought to lie in the mesolimbic-mesocortical areas in the brain, which activate dopamine and generate reward and reinforcement behaviors. A blend of biological and psychosocial factors places certain people at risk for addictive behaviors.

The role of genetic factors and alcoholism have generally been supported by twin, family, and adoption studies. Biological or gene markers are found in dopamine receptors. In addition, certain behaviors are commonly seen in clients who abuse substances (Arinami et al., 1993; Smith et al., 1992). Many people who have a genetic predisposition for substance abuse may adhere to cultural or religious principles that never allow substance use; therefore, addiction does not occur even though the person carries the vulnerability marker. Religious groups such as the Muslims and the Mormons that forbid the use of alcohol are believed to have fewer alcoholics than other religious groups. This finding does not mean that predisposition for addiction is not present in their genetic makeup. Researchers continue to explore the impact of genetics on mental illness and human behavior. The implications for finding clinical markers and detecting biological and psychosocial factors include searching for the cause of mental illness, identifying clients at risk, developing effective treatment, and preventing exposure to noxious factors that produce illness.

MAJOR BEHAVIORAL MODELS

Behavior represents an array of responses to internal and external stimuli. The behavioral approach to human activity assumes that behavior is influenced by specific interconnections between complex neural processes, heredity, environment, instinct, conditioning, and reinforcement. Behavior is directed toward meeting basic human needs. Most human behavior is voluntary and relates to avoiding negative experiences—behavior is not simply stimulus-response interactions. Behaviors are generally reinforced by rewards for doing the right thing or punishment for doing the wrong thing. Human responses are directed either at goal attainment, such as asking for another piece of cake, or at object avoidance, such as avoiding crowds or elevators. These responses are labeled either *approach* or *avoidance of stimuli.*

Reinforcers are used to modify maladaptive behavior and can be positive or negative. Reinforcers are personally determined. For example, it may be difficult to predict whether two people at a party where alcohol is served will drink: One may drink beer after beer, regardless of the morning-after consequences, whereas the other may avoid alcohol altogether. Reinforcers account for the difference. One person may have a biochemical predisposition to alcoholism and thus will gain reinforcement directly from the alcohol. The other may avoid alcohol because parental drunkenness resulted in his or her taking an oath not to drink. Or perhaps one agreed to serve as the designated driver at this party and will be rewarded by drinking at the next. Perhaps both have a heavy workload the next day and cannot face the consequences of drinking. Good job performance is the reinforcer in this example. It is evident that reinforcers are personal, complex, and learned and may be biochemical.

Behavior is observable and offers clues about the brain's functioning in relation to internal and external stimuli. Internal stimuli include complex biological changes or disturbances, personality traits, perception or temperament, and external factors may include developmental transitions or other psychosocial stressors.

Major behavioral theorists include Skinner, Bandura, and Walters (see Chapter 2).

INTEGRATION OF BRAIN FUNCTION AND BEHAVIOR

The interrelatedness of human behavior and brain function is complex. Neural processes that govern thirst, hunger, sex drive, aggression, and motivation are located in the hypothalamus and other areas of the limbic system. Internal and external stimuli are analyzed by the brain, and this process is the basis of perception. Perceptions generate neural signals that either inhibit or arouse cellular innervations. Motor commands arise from these signals. Complex nerve cell activity along the spinal cord governs motor and behavioral patterns. Lesions or alterations in the limbic system or sensory-perceptual mechanisms generate maladaptive behavioral patterns, such as those seen in psychosis. Psychosis is believed to arise from biochemical and anatomical abnormalities that are manifested by various behavioral responses, such as agitation, sensory-perceptual alterations, and social withdrawal.

Determining the origins and influences of human behavior is difficult, but researchers continue to demonstrate more conclusive, sometimes controversial, evidence of biological bases for mental illness (see the Controversy display). Determinants of various behavioral responses include psychosocial stress and neurobiological, genetic, and cultural factors. Appreciating the intricate link between psychosocial and neurobiological factors as causes of mental illness is critical to developing effective interventions, participating in research that integrates these concepts, and understanding the magnitude of technological advances.

KINDLING

Neurochemical changes are believed to be associated with psychosocial stressors. Kindling is an example of a neurobiological response that is activated by significant early stress and losses. ***Kindling*** refers to an underlying progression from stress-induced to spontaneous recurrence of depressive illness. Early losses and traumas are thought to increase sensitivity at some receptor sites by activating biochemicals that impair responsiveness and increase vulnerability to future mood disorders. In other words, in early life a psychosocial stressor, such as the death of a parent, may precipitate a depressive episode. The next time a major psychosocial stressor occurs, depression is experienced again. At some point after repeated recurrences, depressive episodes begin to occur spontaneously without a precipitating stressor. The basis of this premise is encoding of a "longstanding trait marker" to affective illness that increases susceptibility to stress (Post, 1992). Feelings of helplessness are marked in people who have experienced repeated trauma (Maier & Seligman, 1976).

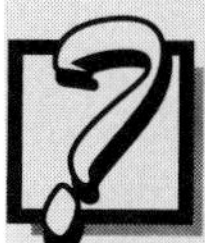

CONTROVERSY

A New Determinism: The Biological Determinants of Human Behavior

A growing body of research has developed supporting genetic links to human behavior, including alcoholism, violence, homosexuality, and bipolar disorder. The controversy of such research has gathered an ever-growing number of critics, who have charged that the suggestions of such connections are well ahead of the scientific research. In fact, there are few followup studies available to point to specific genes, and what studies are available provide contradictory findings. The popularization of such research has added to the debate. Research without substantiation has been widely disseminated by journalists without existing counterevidence and without reference to the well-known evidence for other influences on behavior such as social, cultural, and personal decision making. The critics say the idea that our behavior is determined before we were born is becoming part of our culture and has started showing up in court decisions and public policy. Critics worry that the idea of genetic essentialism, that is, that genetic constitution largely determines future behavior, will lead to things such as mandatory genetic screening of children, restrictive social controls, and a shift from blaming problems such as mental illness and poverty from society to the individual. This perspective takes what are known to be social and moral issues and places them squarely in the domain of technical problems to be solved by the biological sciences. The threat in this approach is the transformation of understanding ourselves as moral beings shaped by culture and society to essential biological beings. Such a transition would ignore all we have come to know about ourselves as human beings. Controversies over biology and behavior will continue as more research becomes available.

From Wheeler, D. L. (1992). An escalating debate over research that links biology and human behavior. *The Chronicle of Higher Education, 38*(42), A7–A8.

TRAUMA

Traumatic events across the life span are also tied to neurobiological and behavioral changes frequently seen in clients with borderline personality, posttraumatic stress disorder, depression, or dissociative identity disorder. Responses to trauma are generally behavioral and biological and are manifested in flashbacks, intrusive thoughts, numbing, startled reactions, and nightmares (American Psychiatric Association, 1994). Other behavioral responses to trauma include social isolation, irritability, and agitation.

Trauma also interferes with modulation of anxiety and aggression because of hyperarousal of the autonomic nervous system and sensitivity to feelings or environmental stimuli. Persistent, severe distress is associated with increased risk for certain cancers and immunosuppressive disorders, such as acquired immunodeficiency syndrome; biochemical changes in neurotransmitters; and endogenous opioid (endorphin) production and release. Studies suggest that during sustained stressful periods, immense quantities of neurotransmitters are secreted. With prolonged stimulation, depletion of neurotransmitters occurs, leading to receptor hyperstimulation (Anisman et al., 1981; Kraemer, 1985; van der Kolk, 1988). In other words, when the stress response is turned on too long or too often, or both, eventually it cannot be turned off. This area of research has potential for nursing practice in the area of preventive mental health care (Table 29–1).

Acute trauma or stress increases dopamine release and metabolism in certain brain centers, particularly the prefrontal cortex. Activated dopaminergic systems are presumed to be directly involved in mobilizing coping responses and playing a major role in the development of posttraumatic stress disorder (Antelman, 1988; Charney et al., 1993). This may explain why trauma leads to lifelong consequences in susceptible persons. It also validates the consideration of both psychosocial stressors and neurobiological responses in a holistic view of nursing.

Behavioral responses to depletion of certain neurotransmitters include social isolation, startle reactions, irritability, paranoia, and agitation. Serotonin is thought to modulate the activity of other neurotransmitters resulting in behavioral and emotional responses (Blier & de Montigney, 1985).

Adaptation to trauma is related to a number of factors (van der Kolk, 1987a), including

- Severity of stressor
- Genetic vulnerability
- Developmental stage
- Available support system
- History of trauma
- Ego function (personality traits)

Adaptation to stress is generally related to a person's coping behaviors. The severity of a stressor is determined by individual perception of the event.

The developmental stage during which the trauma is experienced influences the impact of the trauma. For instance, adults with adequate coping behaviors and support systems are likely to be less vulnerable to trauma than a child would be. Social systems during traumatic or stressful events act as buffers to sustain trust, security, and safety (Hendlin, 1984; van der Kolk, 1987b). The emotionally abused 1-year-old child is more likely to experience difficulty forming trusting and meaningful relationships through the remainder of the life span than is the battered housewife. Early traumatic experiences interfere with normal growth and development tasks such as learning trust, self-esteem, and autonomy, and influence adaptive responses throughout the life span.

Neurological damage has been detected in a number of abused children who have had no symptoms of head trauma. Psychosocial factors such as chaotic and abusive environments are associated with delayed or impaired CNS maturation, such as attention deficit disorder (Fish-Murray et al., 1987).

Bowlby (1973) believed that maturation of the CNS is affected by early attachments and relationships with primary caregivers and that abuse impairs emotional and intellectual development. He noted the affect of early emotional bonding and formation of endorphins or endogenous opiates. Endorphins play a major role in managing severe stress, producing calmness, and buffering one from emotional pain (van der Kolk et al., 1985). Understanding human response to trauma and other psychosocial stressors is critical to health maintenance. Hysterical seizures, abnormal electroencephalograms, and clients with multiple personality or dissociative identity disorder have been associated with neurological trauma (Brende, 1984). Interventions that modulate feelings, create trust, reduce anxiety, and promote a sense of control and power include various psychotherapies, cognitive-behavioral therapy, crisis intervention, stress management, and psychotropics. (See Chapters 8, 10, and 26 for a discussion of these interventions.)

TABLE 29–1
Biochemical and Behavioral Responses to Stress

BIOCHEMICAL RESPONSES	COGNITIVE APPRAISAL	POSSIBLE BEHAVIORAL RESPONSES
Forebrain		
Screens emotional responses to internal and external stimuli	Irrelevant stimuli	Ignored, no responses
Links hypothalamus to environment to activate proper neurochemical responses (i.e. autonomic nervous system, neuroendocrine)	Perceived danger, threat	Anxiety, sweating, restlessness, agitation, avoidance/social isolation, anger, aggression
Hypothalamus		
Acts as principal ganglion	Reappraisal of threat or danger	Calmness, decreased anxiety, fear, restlessness
Activates proper neurochemical responses, e.g., anterior pituitary to adrenal coA1ex		

PARADIGMS OF PSYCHIATRIC–MENTAL HEALTH NURSING

The recent explosion of knowledge in the area of neurobiology—involving advances in brain mapping, imaging, and scanning—has opened up a fascinating world concerning the human brain and behavior. Psychiatric nursing educators and clinicians will be challenged in their ability to integrate traditional psychiatric nursing and neurobiological concepts into nursing curricula and practice. Psychiatric nursing recently has struggled with integrating biological concepts into undergraduate and graduate curricula. A primary concern is a lack of recognition and the need to integrate the major neurobiological concepts with nursing science. McEnany (1991) stressed the complexity and urgency of integrating biological-behavioral concepts in regard to mental illness.

CLINICAL AND PRACTICE ISSUES

Recent discoveries in the field of neurobiology are revolutionizing the understanding and treatment of mental illness. Because psychiatric nurses work collaboratively for the most part, they cannot help but be affected by these advances and must continually be aware of new findings to communicate knowledgeably with other mental health professionals. In addition, having their clients' best interests in mind, nurses should incorporate recent findings into their practice. Obviously, nursing must not lose sight of its holistic tradition, taking all aspects of the client into consideration, including the spiritual, cultural, and psychosocial, as well as biological.

In spite of new discoveries regarding the role of neurobiology in understanding and treating mental illness, controversy and doubt over its relevancy to psychiatric nurses prevail. Peplau (1989) noted that specific mental disorders are difficult to explain as a "global or single entity" and determined that psychiatric nurses need to explore the basis of impaired behavioral patterns rather than biological aspects and focus on human responses to stress and societal changes. At the same time, Peplau strongly encouraged psychiatric nurses to value and appreciate the biological components of mental illness, as well as the psychosocial concepts such as caring. Application of biological interventions does not negate the effectiveness of other treatment modalities. In fact, psychosocial interventions such as psychoeducation, psychotherapy, relaxation, and cognitive therapy continue to be viable treatment options.

NURSING INTERVENTIONS

Historically, one of the major somatic interventions used by psychiatric nurses involved assessing the need for administering psychotropics to calm agitated clients experiencing hallucinations and delusions. Recent neurobiological findings have prompted the creation of new psychopharmacological agents that target specific areas in the brain to reduce symptoms and modify behaviors. Selective serotonin reuptake inhibitors such as fluoxetine and sertraline are examples of these new antidepressants. The use of electroconvulsive therapy is gaining renewed acceptance as an effective treatment modality for severe depression and various schizophenic disorders. Electroconvulsive and other somatic therapies also help severely depressed clients with psychomotor retardation, social withdrawal, and suicidal ideations. Other examples of biological therapies are rest–sleep manipulation for bipolar disorder, administration of full-spectrum lighting in seasonal affective disorder, and nutritional alterations in alcoholism.

Health promotion and primary prevention remain major nursing goals. These goals are consistent with proposed health care reform that vow to improve access to quality care. Prevention minimizes maladaptive behaviors and chronicity in high-risk clients and groups. The domain of psychiatric nurses lies in recognizing and assessing age-appropriate responses to developmental tasks, biological changes, and changes that define health and illness across the life span. Understanding the range of normal responses to stress helps nurses identify maladaptive responses and formulate outcomes and interventions that incorporate biological and behavioral concepts.

Client symptoms or behaviors allow the nurse to view the client's inner world that comprises biological and behavioral processes activated by internal and external stressors. Active listening and astute observation of verbal and nonverbal cues are key aspects of assessing client responses. For instance, the psychotic client may smile or talk inappropriately and have a disheveled appearance. These nonverbal cues link the nurse with complex neurobiological processes that affect the client's behavior and effective treatment modalities.

Major treatment modalities include using psychotherapy, behavior modification, and cognitive therapy; assessing the need for medications; and administering, prescribing, and monitoring client responses to psychotropics; and facilitating sleep–rest, light–dark, exercise–relaxation, and nutritional aspects of care. These interventions integrate biological and behavioral aspects of mental illness.

PSYCHIATRIC NURSING EDUCATION

The National League for Nursing has long stipulated that schools provide psychiatric nursing experiences as a requirement for accreditation. Core areas of curricula have focused on holistic concepts and health promotion and prevention, and major concepts have included caring for and meeting the psychosocial needs of clients (American Nurses Association [ANA], 1984; McBride, 1990; Pothier et al., 1990). A wealth of psychiatric nursing literature has permitted faculty to define the scope and character of this specialty. Over the years educators have become leaders in directing psychiatric nursing practice and generating specialization. These changes have paralleled the ANA specialization and expanding scope of practice.

A major task of psychiatric nurses in the 1990s is to define major biological and behavioral concepts and to integrate them into nursing practice. McBride (1990) suggested that this may be accomplished by balancing these concepts with care and collaborating with other disciplines to develop effective client outcomes.

Some educators and clinicians are already defining outcomes that integrate biological and behavioral concepts into nursing practice. Additionally, it is expected that undergraduate baccalaureate students are gaining knowledge of studies regarding the brain and neuroscience and their impact on human adaptation to stress.

The ANA has joined psychiatric nurses who advocate integrating biological and behavioral concepts into nursing practice. *A Statement on Psychiatric–Mental Health Nursing Practice and Standards of Psychiatric–Mental Health Clinical Nursing Practice* (ANA, 1994) addresses enormous changes in psychiatric nursing and the health care delivery system. The ANA stresses the impact of rapid evolution of biological sciences and advances in technology on psychiatric nursing practice. This statement establishes that neurobiological advances and development of interventions promise more effective response for the mentally ill. In addition, the ANA confirms the need for psychosocial and biological interventions, such as psychotherapy, cognitive therapy, psychoeducation, crisis intervention, and administration and prescription of psychotropics to help clients develop effective coping patterns.

THE NURSE'S ROLE

The general nurse and the advanced-practice nurse can use an array of biological and behavioral interventions to facilitate adaptive responses to internal and external stressors. Psychiatric nurses are faced with providing complex care that meets the needs of clients in inpatient, ambulatory, and community settings. These needs include psychosocial and biological factors that affect client behavior. Aggression, irritability, noncompliance, and social withdrawal are common behavioral responses to stress, which often arises from psychosocial and biological alterations.

THE GENERALIST NURSE

The generalist or psychiatric–mental health nurse works with clients, families, groups, and communities and uses the nursing process to assess adaptive and maladaptive responses. This nurse understands the relationship between underlying biological processes; develops interventions that promote health; facilitates and reinforces adaptive coping patterns; and assesses and prevents further disability. Specific interventions encouraging health promotion and maintenance include psychoeducation, administration of psychotropic medications and monitoring client response, milieu therapy, and crisis intervention. These interventions take place during various activities such as intake and screening and case management and in various settings such as community and mental health centers, day hospitals, home health settings, and homeless shelters (ANA, 1994). Biological and psychosocial interventions enable the generalist psychiatric–mental health nurse to alter or modify maladaptive responses seen in various mental disorders, such as psychosis and depression.

A combination of biological and psychosocial interventions can be used in caring for a client experiencing psychosis. The psychotic client experiences perceptual disturbances such as auditory hallucinations, which lead to suspiciousness and may result in irritability, social reclusiveness, and refusal to eat. Perceptual disturbances stem from neurobiological phenomena and result in behavioral responses to internal and external stimuli. The client may act on the command of the hallucinations and step in front of a car or refuse to eat because "someone poisoned the food." Assessing the nature of hallucinations is crucial to the safety of the client and the staff. Administering a neuroleptic such as haloperidol (Haldol) is a biological intervention that targets psychotic symptoms. The psychosocial intervention should be a calm, firm approach that conveys empathy and provides the client with structure and limit setting. These interventions can work together to increase the client's impulse control and thus reduce risk of violent, aggressive behaviors (see the Nursing Care Plan display).

Behavioral patterns can be adaptive or maladaptive. The depressed adolescent may use maladaptive behavioral patterns such as drinking alcohol, stealing, and quarreling to manage internal emotional pain and deal with psychosocial stressors of family pressures. Conversely, another adolescent may use adaptive responses and seek out family, friends, or clergy to verbalize feelings about a stressful situation. The nurse must operate on the premise that all behavior has meaning and can be clarified. Therefore, assessing behavioral responses to internal and external stimuli is a major nursing responsibility and involves collaborating with the client and other mental health professionals to develop effective interventions and outcomes.

THE ADVANCED-PRACTICE NURSE

The role of the advanced-practice psychiatric–mental health nurse encompasses those of the generalist in addition to providing direct clinical care, such as psychotherapy and prescriptive authority. Advanced educational and clinical preparation enable the psychiatric–mental health nurse specialist to assess complex problems and employ knowledge, skills, and clinical experience to modify maladaptive responses in various clinical settings (ANA, 1994).

Specific advanced psychiatric–mental health interventions include prescribing, administering, and evaluating client responses to various biological therapies

Nursing Care Plan 29-1 The Client Experiencing Sensory–Perceptual Disturbances (Psychosis): Biological–Behavioral Client Outcomes

► **Nursing Diagnosis:** Sensory–Perceptual Disturbances

OUTCOME IDENTIFICATION	NURSING ACTIONS	RATIONALES	EVALUATIONS
1. By [date], responds appropriately to internal/external stimuli.	1a. Establish rapport.	1a. Facilitates a trusting alliance and reduces anxiety and agitation.	*Goal met:* Client initially has difficulty trusting staff because of auditory hallucinations and persecutory delusions. Client experiences decreased hallucinations and delusions and agitation—no adverse responses noted except excessive sedation, which was decreased with dose reduction. Client's thoughts are coherent and anxiety is minimized. Client has minimally impaired self-care.
	1b. Assess the presence of hallucinations and/or delusions (i.e., smiling or nodding head inappropriately).	1b. Enables nurse to assess basis of client behavior and responses.	
	1c. Decrease environmental stimuli.	1c. Reduces anxiety and risk of aggression.	
2. By [date], verbalizes coherently to others.	2a. Give direct and concrete explanations.	2a. Decreases anxiety and increases coherence.	
	2b. Collaborate with client and family to establish a plan of care.	2b. Essential part of self-care/health promotion.	
	2c. Assist in self-care.	2c. Disturbed thoughts processes interfere with self-care.	
3. By [date], exhibits decreased agitation.	3. Administer neuroleptic and observe for desired and adverse responses.	3. Neuroleptics are important to reduce hallucinations/delusions and agitation and improve thought process.	

► **Nursing Diagnosis:** Impaired Social Interactions

OUTCOME IDENTIFICATION	NURSING ACTIONS	RATIONALES	EVALUATIONS
1. Initiates and interacts with others appropriately.	1. Designate staff for one-to-one relationships.	1. Decrease environmental stimuli and establish trusting relationships.	*Goal met:* Client is able to establish one-to-one alliance with several staff. Client continues to have difficulty interacting with some group members.
2. Verbalizes coherently with others.	2. Reinforce and validate clear communication.	2. Enables client to learn effective communication skills.	

such as psychotropics, electroconvulsive therapy, and phototherapy and integrating them with behavioral strategies. Furthermore, conducting research studies to assess client responses to behavioral and biological interventions is critical to evaluating and developing effective treatment.

Behavioral interventions offered by the advanced-practice nurse include cognitive therapy, progressive relaxation, guided imagery, psychotherapy, and psychoeducation. Various interventions depend on nurse–client collaboration that allows nurses to empower clients in understanding the basis of mental illness and creating interventions that can alleviate symptoms and promote quality life.

RELATED RESEARCH

Psychiatric nurses are in the midst of a neurobiological research explosion with numerous opportunities to de-

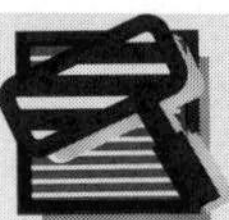

RESEARCH STUDY

Daily Light Exposure Among Psychiatric Inpatients

Loving, R. T., & Kripke, D. F. (1992). *Journal of Psychosocial Nursing, 30*(11), 15–19.

Study Problem/Purpose

To determine the light exposure of psychiatric inpatients.

Methods

Ten patients from an unlocked inpatient unit were randomly selected. The sample consisted of 8 men and 2 women ranging in age from 29 to 42 years, with a mean age of 35. Subjects met *Diagnostic and Statistical Manual of Mental Disorders, Third Edition, Revised* criteria for bipolar affective disorder, schizophrenia, atypical psychosis, major depression, and unspecified affective disorder. The patients were provided with a wristwatch converted to a Vitolog PMS-8 computer monitor. Illumination was recorded each minute for a 24-hour period.

Findings

Research findings indicated that light exposure for inpatient psychiatric patients was lower than the general population.

Implications

Nurses need to develop individualized interventions that increase light exposure for inpatient psychiatric patients.

fine and investigate client outcomes that integrate biological and behavioral concepts. Studies that compare the effectiveness of biological and behavioral interventions also can assist nurses in developing more effective interventions that meet complex needs of the mentally ill. Survival of psychiatric nursing as a specialty depends on the ability of educators, practitioners, and researchers to integrate biological and behavioral concepts into academic curricula and scope of practices. Evaluating student experiences that incorporate these concepts can generate data (see Research Study display) that direct students and practicing nurses.

►CHAPTER SUMMARY

Advances in neurobiological research help clinicians and researchers begin to understand the complexity of mental health and illness. The expansion of biological knowledge gives clients, families, and psychiatric nurses hope for more effective treatments and possible cures for serious mental disorders. The human experience arises from the complex interaction of the person's neurobiological mechanisms and the environment. The biological–behavioral interface of mental health and illness is complex and challenges nurses to integrate these concepts into practice, education, and research.

Suggestions for Clinical Conference

1. Present several case histories emphasizing relevant biological and behavioral concepts.
2. Invite a psychiatric–mental health advanced-practice nurse to present various psychopharmacological agents, emphasizing their major behavioral and biological effects.

References

American Nurses Association. (1984). *Distribution and utilization of psychiatric and mental health clinical nurse specialists in the United States*. Kansas City, MO: Author.

American Nurses Association. (1994). *Statement on psychiatric–mental health nursing practice and standards of psychiatric–mental health clinical nursing practice*. Washington, DC: American Nurses Publishing.

American Psychiatric Association (1994). *Diagnostic and statistical manual of mental disorders* (4th ed.). Washington, DC: Author.

Andreasen, N. C., Ehrhardt, J. C., Swayze, V. W. II, Alliger, R. J., Yuh, W. T., Cohen, G., & Ziebell, S. (1990). Magnetic resonance imaging of the brain in schizophrenia: The pathophysiologic significance of structural abnormalities. *Archives of General Psychiatry, 47*, 35–44.

Anisman, H. L., Ritch, M., & Sklar, L. S. (1981). Noradrenergic and dopaminergic interactions of escape behavior. *Psychopharmacology, 74*, 263–268.

Antelman, S. M. (1988). Time-dependent sensitization is the cornerstone for a new approach to pharmacotherapy: Drugs as foreign or stressful stimuli. *Drug Development (Research), 14*, 1–30.

Arinami, T., Itokawa, M., Komiyama, T., Mitsushia, H., Mari, H., Mifune, H., et al. (1993). Association between severity of alcoholism and the A1 allele of the dopamine D2 receptor gene TaqI A RFLP in Japanese. *Biological Psychiatry, 33*, 108–114.

Birmaher, B., Dahl, R. E., Ryan, N. D., Rabinovich, H., Ambrosini, P., al-Shabbout, M., et al. (1992). The dexamethasone suppression test in adolescent outpatients with major depressive disorder. *American Journal of Psychiatry, 149*(8), 1040–1045.

Blier, P., & de Montigney, C. (1985). Short-term lithium administration enhances serotonergic transmission. *European Journal of Pharmacology, 112*, 415–418.

Borysenko, M. (1987). Area review: Psychoneuroimmunology. *Annals of Behavioral Medicine, 9*(2), 3–10.

Bowlby, J. (1973). *Attachment and loss: Vol. 2. Separation*. New York: Basic Books.

Brambilla, F., Bellodi, L., Perna, G., Battaglia, M., Scivto, G., Diaferia, G., et al. (1992). Psychoimmunoendocrine aspects of panic disorder. *Neuropsychobiology, 26*, 12–22.

Brende, J. O. (1984). The psychophysiologic manifestation of dissociation: Electrodermal responses in a multiple personality patient. *Psychiatric Clinics of North America, 7*, 41–50.

Cannon, W. B. (1914). The emergency function of the adrenal medulla in pain and the major emotions. *American Journal of Physiology, 33*(3), 356–372.

Charney, D. S., Deutch, A. Y., Krystal, J. H., Southwick, S. M., & Davis, M. (1993). Psychobiologic mechanisms of posttraumatic stress disorder. *Archives of General Psychiatry, 50*(4), 294–305.

Coryell, W., & Tsuang, D. (1992). Hypothalamus-pituitary-adrenal axis by hyperactivity and psychosis: Recovery during an 8-year follow-up. *American Journal of Psychiatry, 149*(8), 1033–1039.

Fish-Murray, C. C., Koby, E. V., & van der Kolk, B. A. (1987). Evolving ideas: The effects on children's thoughts. In B. A. van der Kolk (Ed.), *Psychological trauma* (pp. 89–126). Washington, DC: American Psychiatric Press.

Goeders, N. E., & Smith, J. E. (1986). Reinforcing properties of cocaine in the medial prefrontal cortex: Primary action on presynaptic dopaminergic terminals. *Pharmacological Biochemical Behavior, 25*, 191–199.

Goldsmith, H. H. (1983). Genetic influences on personality from infancy to adulthood. *Child Development, 54*(2), 331–355.

Hendlin, H. (1984). Combat never ends: The paranoid adaptation to posttraumatic stress. *American Journal of Psychotherapy, 38*, 121–131.

Hichie, I., et al. (1990). Is there immune dysfunction in depressive disorder? *Psychological Medicine, 20*, 755–761.

Jones, P., & Murray, R. M. (1991). The genetics of schizophrenia in the genetic neurodevelopment. *British Journal of Psychiatry, 158*, 615–623.

Kaplan, H. I., & Sadock, B. J. (1991). *Synopsis of psychiatry: Behavioral Sciences, clinical psychiatry* (6th ed.). Baltimore: Williams & Wilkins.

Kendler, K. S., Kessler, R. C., Neale, M. C., Heath, A. C., & Eaves, L. J. (1993). The prediction of major depression in women: Toward an integrated etiologic model. *American Journal of Psychiatry, 150*(8), 1139–1145.

Kraemer, G. W. (1985). Effects of differences in early social experiences on primate neurobiological-behavioral development. In M. Reife & T. Field (Eds.), *The psychobiology of attachment and separation* (pp. 135–161). Orlando: Academic Press.

Lohr, J. B., & Bracha, H. S. (1992). A monozygotic mirror-image twin pair with discordant psychiatric illness: A neuropsychiatric and neurodevelopmental evolution. *American Journal of Psychiatry, 149*(8), 1091–1095.

Loving, R. T., & Kripke, D. F. (1992). Daily light exposure among psychiatric inpatients. *Journal of Psychosocial Nursing and Mental Health Services, 30*(11), 15–19.

Maier, S. F., & Seligman, M. E. P. (1976). Learned helplessness: Theory and evidence. *Journal of Experimental Psychology: General, 105*(1), 3–46.

McBride, A. B. (1990). Psychiatric nursing in the 1990s. *Archives of Psychiatric Nursing, 4*(1), 21–28.

McEnany, G. W. (1991). Psychobiology and psychiatric nursing: A philosophical matrix. *Archives of Psychiatric Nursing, 5*(5), 255–261.

Mesulam, M. M., & Geula, C. (1991). Acetylcholinesterase-rich neurons of the human cortex: Cytoarchitectonic and ontogenetic patterns of distribution. *Journal of Comprehensive Neurology, 306*(2), 193–220.

Monroe, S. M., & Simons, A. D. (1991). Diathesis-stress theories in the context of life stress research: Implications for the depressive disorders. *Psychological Bulletin, 110*(3), 406–425.

Parker, G. B., Barrett, E. A., & Hickie, I. B. (1992). From nurture to network: Examining links between parenting received in childhood and social bonds in adulthood. *American Journal of Psychiatry, 149*, 877–885.

Peplau, H. E. (1989). Future direction in psychiatric nursing from the perspective of history. *Journal of Psychosocial Nursing and Mental Health Services, 27*(2), 18–28.

Post, R. M. (1992). Transduction of psychosocial stress in the neurobiology of recurrent affective disorder. *American Journal of Psychiatry, 149*(8), 999–1010.

Pothier, P. C., Stuart, G. W., Puskar, K., & Babich, K. (1990). Dilemmas and direction for psychiatric nursing in the 1990s. *Archives of Psychiatric Nursing, 4*(5), 284–291.

Prescott, C. A., & Gottesman, H. S. (1993). Genetically mediated vulnerability to schizophrenia. *Psychiatric Clinics of North America, 16*(2), 245–267.

Selye, H. (1956). *The stress of life*. New York: McGraw-Hill.

Smith, S. S., O'Hara, B. F., Persico, A. M., Gorelick, D. A., Newlin, D. B., Vlahov D., et al. (1992). Genetic vulnerability to drug abuse: The D2 dopamine receptor TaqI B1 restriction fragment length polymorphism appears more frequently in polysubstance abusers. *Archives of General Psychiatry, 49*(9), 723–727.

Solomon, G. F. (1987). Psychoneuroimmunology: Interactions between central nervous system and immune system. *Journal of Neuroscience Research, 18*, 1–9.

U.S. Congress. (1989). Public Law 101-58 [HJ Res. 174]. Decade of the Brain—Proclamation 103 STAT. 152–154.

van der Kolk, B. A. (1987a). *Psychological trauma*. New York: American Psychiatric Press.

van der Kolk, B. A. (1987b). The trauma spectrum: The interaction of biological and social events in the genesis of trauma response. *Journal of Traumatic Stress, 1*, 273–290.

van der Kolk, B. A., Greenberg, M., Boyd, H., & Krystal, J. (1985). Inescapable shock, neurotransmitters and addiction to trauma: Towards a psychobiology of posttraumatic stress. *Biological Psychiatry, 20*, 314–325.

CHAPTER

30

Psychiatric Consultation-Liaison Nursing

SUSAN L. W. KRUPNICK, M.S.N., C.A.R.N., C.S.

OUTLINE

CHAPTER OBJECTIVES

Upon completion of this chapter, you will be able to:

1. Describe the historical development of psychiatric consultation-liaison nurse (PCLN) practice.
2. Define the traditional practice of PCLN within the health care delivery system.
3. Identify the expanding roles and functions of the PCLN within the changing health care delivery system.
4. Describe the goals of PCLN practice.
5. Identify the steps in the consultation process.
6. Differentiate between direct and indirect models of consultation.
7. Describe the types of consultation in PCLN practice.
8. Discuss the educational preparation, professional experience, and clinical supervision necessary for PCLN practice.
9. Discuss future trends and opportunities for PCLN practice.
10. Recognize the American Nurses Association's standards for practice.

KEY TERMS

Case management
Consultation
Entrepreneur
Intrapreneur
Liaison

Psychiatric consultation-liaison nurse (PCLN) practice is a subspecialty of advanced-nursing practice within the specialty of psychiatric–mental health nursing. The scope of PCLN practice is diverse and encompasses primary prevention, intervention, and rehabilitation strategies (American Nurses Association [ANA], 1990). This subspecialty emphasizes the assessment, diagnosis, and treatment of behavioral, cognitive, developmental, emotional, and spiritual responses of clients and families with actual or potential physical dysfunction. PCLN practice, by definition, includes consultation and liaison activities.

Consultation is an interactive process between a consultant, who has expertise, and a consultee, who is seeking advice. It is an interpersonal educational process in which the consultant collaborates with a person or a group that influences and participates in health care delivery and has requested assistance in problem solving (Blake, 1977). The recipient of PCLN consultation services may be the client, family members, or health care providers. The term ***liaison*** is used to describe the linkage of health care professionals to facilitate communication, collaboration, and building of partnerships between clients and themselves (Cassem, 1991; Robinson, 1987). The liaison process is commonly used to explicate the teaching, or educative, component of PCLN practice. The goals of consultation and liaison activities are mutually complementary and interdependent. The PCLN uses both processes in conjunction with specific theoretical knowledge, clinical expertise, and an ability to synthesize and integrate information to influence health care delivery systems.

HISTORY OF PCLN PRACTICE

Several significant forces have provided the impetus for the development of PCLN practice. These forces are multifaceted and include the general development of psychiatric–mental health nursing, the establishment and funding of psychiatric departments in university hospitals, and World War II, which ushered in the crisis intervention and brief psychotherapy models of treatment to address war-related mental health problems (Table 30–1). The development, introduction, and expansion of psychopharmacology and the use of psychotropic medications in the 1950s and 1960s increased the scope and impact of consultation-liaison services in the general hospital. The groundwork was established, and PCLN practice emerged as a subspecialty of psychiatric nursing during the early 1960s. During this period the nursing literature began to focus on the psychosocial assessment and management of the client with medical illness to foster therapeutic progress and positive outcomes (Brown, 1965; Dumas & Leonard, 1963; Elder, 1963). However, Betty Sue Johnson of Duke University Medical Center was the first clinical nurse specialist (CNS) to describe her role as a psychiatric nurse providing consultation services to nurses in the general hospital. In an article published in 1963, Johnson described the concept of cross-service consultation and the implementation of a nurse-to-nurse consultation model. The goal was to promote a higher level of client care in conjunction with maximizing the use of available nursing resources. The clinical consultant pool of nurses at Duke comprised head nurses, nursing supervisors, and instructors. Initially, they responded to requests from head nurses on medical–surgical units. The early PCLN work accomplished by these nursing pioneers focused on assessing and supporting the positive interpersonal

TABLE 30–1
Psychiatric Consultation-Liaison Nurse (PCLN) Specialty Evolution: A Chronological Overview

YEAR	EVENT
1960s	Beginning emergence of the psychiatric nursing consultation process
1963	Publication of an article by Betty Sue Johnson of Duke University discussing cross-service nursing consultation with psychiatric nurses
1970s	First publication of PCLN research
1971	Initiation of the University of Maryland graduate program in PCLN practice
1973	Initiation of the Yale University graduate program in PCLN practice
1974	Publication of the first PCLN text, *Liaison Nursing: Psychological Approach to Patient Care*, by Dr. Lisa Robinson of the University of Maryland
1980s	A decade of practice expansion and innovation
1982	Publication of *Psychiatric Liaison Nursing: The Theory and Clinical Practice* by Anita Lewis and Joyce Levy
1987	Development of the initial proposal of standards of PCLN practice by PCLN regional task forces
1990s	Transitions and formal organizational structuring
1990	Formation of PCLNs as a special interest group within the Psychiatric Mental Health Council of the American Nurses Association
1990	Publication of PCLN standards by the American Nurses Association
1992–1993	Organization of a national task force to develop a core curriculum for PCLN education
1993	Election of a governing board of the PCLN special interest group
1993	Celebration of 30 years of PCLN practice at the Annual National PCLN Conference and honoring of PCLNs with excellence awards
1994	Formal beginning of the International Society of Psychiatric Consultation-Liaison Nurses on March 25, 1994, in Baltimore

relationship skills employed by the staff members and building on them with subsequent consultations. The medical–surgical unit staff members understood that the PCLN would not assume responsibility for the client care problem but would assist and support them in problem solving and comprehending the emotional impact of illness, suffering, and recovery on the client (Johnson, 1963).

The evolution of PCLN practice continued, and the method of indirect intervention by employing consultee-centered consultation was being challenged. The next stage of PCLN practice development involved acknowledging the need for an advanced practitioner to have direct involvement with the client. Comprehensive assessment of a client's psychological and behavioral responses required active, direct intervention by the PCLN, using a client-centered consultation. This shift in the delivery of consultation services allowed PCLNs an opportunity to use their clinical expertise in direct assessment while collaborating with nursing staff members to formulate a holistic and relevant nursing care plan. In addition, with the expansion of consultation activity into direct care, the complexity and intensity of the emotional problems experienced by the medically ill client were illuminated. In response to this increasing awareness of complexity, the PCLNs acknowledged their need to acquire additional theoretical knowledge and clinical expertise in the realm of the consultation process and the psychophysiological approach to the care of medical–surgical clients.

PHILOSOPHY OF PCLN CLINICAL PRACTICE

The subspecialization of PCLN practice within psychiatric nursing is based on the synthesis, integration, and application of several theoretical models in nursing, psychiatry, psychology, and sociology. Specific models that are the foundations of PCLN practice include the consultation process, crisis intervention, systems theory, organizational behavior and dynamics, change process, problem-solving theory, cultural diversity, psychoneuroimmunology, and adult learning theory. The interrelationship of medical illness and its psychophysiological effects on hospitalized clients and their families is extremely complex and requires sophisticated, multidimensional assessment and intervention by advanced-practice nurses. PCLNs become involved in these complex client care situations to conduct assessments, provide therapeutic interventions, and enhance the clinical skills of the primary health care provider. PCLNs offer a broad range of services to clients and their support systems to reduce the incidence of distress, coping failure, and maladaptation in response to actual or potential physiologic dysfunction.

PREPARATION FOR PCLN PRACTICE

The PCLN is an advanced-practice nurse who has attained at least a master's degree in psychiatric–mental health nursing and has successfully completed a supervised graduate-level clinical program (ANA, 1990). Experience in the knowledge of medical–surgical and critical care nursing enhance the PCLN's credibility as a role model and the ability to assess and understand the complexities of acutely ill clients. Administrative experience in a middle management position, such as head nurse or nurse manager, assists the PCLN in comprehending the influence of health care organizations on clients and their family systems. In addition, managerial experience and administrative preparation can broaden the PCLN's knowledge of the politics and functioning of health care organizations (Lewis & Levy, 1982). Administrative preparation can assist the PCLN in gaining skills needed to participate in evaluating conditions, resources, and policies that are essential to the effective delivery of nursing care (Radke et al., 1990).

The personal and professional attributes that are hallmarks of successful PCLNs include an ability to be flexible, objective, creative, and resilient and to behave in a personally as well as professionally mature manner. PCLNs must acknowledge and manage intense levels of uncertainty and ambiguity while balancing their own emotional and physical wellness. PCLNs need to possess an ability to practice in an independent, autonomous manner while making linkages and coalitions within their institutions. In addition, they must be able to network within and outside their institutions to decrease their sense of isolation that can accompany autonomous practice situations in which the practitioner is privileged to sensitive and confidential information. PCLNs must engage in self-exploration and sharing of feelings to alleviate the daily effects of vicarious traumatization (McCann & Pearlman, 1990; Zerwekh, 1991).

EDUCATION AND CERTIFICATION

Formal graduate education and preparation of PCLNs began in the 1970s at the University of Maryland under the direction of Dr. Lisa Robinson (1972) and at Yale University with the leadership of Jill K. Nelson and Diane Schilke Davis (1979) (see Table 30–1). In preparation for moving into the mid 1990s and the twenty-first century, PCLN graduate education is now being addressed by a national PCLN core curriculum task force. The purpose of this task force is to develop a comprehensive core curriculum to adequately prepare PCLNs to meet the challenges of health care.

Certification by the ANA in the subspecialty of PCLN practice does not currently exist; however, certification as a CNS in psychiatric–mental health nursing is recommended as a requisite for PCLN practice and is necessary for third-party reimbursement (ANA, 1990). Professional certification combined with graduate nursing education may be used as qualification for second licensure as an advanced-practice nurse (Minarik, 1992). PCLNs function in advanced-practice roles and therefore must constantly address their own learning needs, especially in psychopharmacologic intervention.

TABLE 30–2

Roles of PCLNs: Specialties and Subspecialties of Current Practitioners

PSYCHIATRIC AND GENERAL CONSULTATION

- Acute confusional states
- Addictive diseases
- Adolescence/adolescent mental health
- Adult children of alcoholics
- Adult victims of domestic violence
- Alzheimer's caregivers
- Alzheimer's disease
- Behavioral medicine (mind–body)
- Bereavement/grief and loss counseling
- Child and adolescent bereavement
- Codependency
- Cognitive therapy
- Combat stress counseling
- Community mental health nursing
- Couples counseling
- Crisis intervention
- Cultural diversity
- Death and dying
- Dementia diagnosis and family training
- Depression
- Detoxification
- Developmentally impaired
- Dissociative disorder
- Dysfunctional family systems
- Eating disorders
- Ethics
- Families in crisis
- Generalized anxiety disorder
- Geropsychiatry/aging
- Homeless and unemployed
- Hospice/palliative care
- Hypnosis/relaxation/imagery
- Incest survivors and abuse
- Marriage and family counseling
- Milieu therapy
- Minority mental health
- Mood disorders
- Multigenerational family therapy
- Nephrology
- Nonviolent crisis intervention
- Panic disorders
- Parent–family dynamics
- Pediatrics
- Perinatal bereavement
- Phobias
- Postpartum depression
- Posttraumatic stress disorder
- Pregnancy loss
- Premenstrual syndrome (PMS) counseling
- Psychiatric triage and emergency care
- Psychoeducation for family members with a chronic mental illness
- Psychological trauma
- Relationship and marital therapy
- School health
- Self-actualization
- Sex therapy
- Sexual abuse
- Stepfamilies
- Stress management
- Suicide
- Therapeutic touch
- Time-limited psychotherapy
- Transsexualism
- Trauma/abuse
- Trauma psychology (individuals and organizations)
- Traumatic death
- Women's health

MEDICAL–SURGICAL CONSULTATION

- Advanced and terminal phase of illness counseling
- Aggressive/difficult patients (inpatient management)
- AIDS patients
- Biofeedback
- Cardiac comorbidity
- Cardiology
- Clients with automatic implantable cardioverter defibrillators
- Clients with pituitary tumors
- Coping with illness and hospitalization
- Critical care
- Cross-cultural nursing
- Diabetes
- Emotional response to physical illness
- Nurses' support group for transplantation
- Oncology
- Oncology: hospice
- Orthopedics
- Pain management
- Pain management in substance abusers
- Psychoneuroimmunology
- Pulmonary disease
- Rehabilitation
- Relaxation and guided imagery in hospitalized clients
- Renal failure
- Spinal cord injury
- Spouses of clients in intensive care units
- Support group for HIV and AIDS populations
- Transplantation (cardiac, liver, bone marrow, other)
- Trauma
- Trauma: critical incident stress debriefing
- Treatment planning

ADMINISTRATIVE/EMPLOYEE-RELATED CONSULTATION

- Administration
- Assertiveness training
- Career development
- Circadian disorders in shift workers
- Clinical ladder development
- Communication skills development
- Conflict management
- Continuing education program development
- Continuous quality improvement
- Critical incident stress debriefing
- Customer service in health care settings
- Employee advocacy
- Employee assistance
- Health care ethics
- Image enhancement
- Inservice education
- Management consultation
- Management/counseling for chemically dependent nurses
- Memorial service
- Nurse's resiliency building
- Nursing education/staff development
- Organizational change process
- Organizational communication
- Organizational development
- Peer assistance
- Recruitment and retention
- Research support
- Retreat and workshop development
- Staff stress management
- Staff support groups
- Team building
- Total quality management
- Work-related stress
- Worker's compensation

Data from International Directory of Psychiatric Consultation-Liaison Nurses, 1993–1994, 2nd edition.

(Many advanced-practice nurses have gained or are lobbying for prescriptive privileges.)

THE PCLN IN THE HEALTH CARE DELIVERY SYSTEM

EVOLUTION OF PRACTICE MODELS

The PCLN practice literature in the 1960s described how the early pioneers implemented the nurse-to-nurse consultation model in their practice (Johnson, 1963; Robinson, 1968) and became direct care providers of psychiatric services in general hospitals (Peterson, 1969). During this period, there was an increase in the number of publications that described a diversity in the method of clinical practice, from an autonomous position to a collaborative model between PCLNs and PCL physicians (Holstein & Schwab, 1965; Jackson, 1969). Several authors began to identify significant research interest in addressing the psychosocial needs of hospitalized clients (Dumas & Leonard, 1963; Elder, 1963; Elder & Diers, 1963; Peplau, 1964).

The 1970s ushered in a decade of proliferative role expansion (Table 30-2). The literature reflected this expansion into direct-care nurse consultation in general hospitals, as well as emergency services and nursing homes (Covert, 1979; Faast & Elstun, 1979; Forhan-Andrianos & Swain, 1979; Garant, 1977; Goldstein, 1979; Grace, 1974; Hedlund, 1978; Przepiorka & Bender, 1977; Severin & Becker, 1974). Some of the authors described collaborative practices in which the PCLN triaged clients in the emergency department prior to the PCL physician evaluating them. This ground-breaking practice portrayed a collaborative model between the client, nurse, and physician (Isscharoff et al., 1970). Barton and Kelso (1971) also described how the nursing perspective enhanced the functioning of a collaborative PCL team.

Additional articles published in the 1970s described specific practice sites, (e.g., the intensive care unit), or client populations (e.g., those with coronary disease or burns) for PCLN involvement (Baldwin, 1978; Davidson & Noyes, 1973; Pranulis, 1972). Several authors described their struggles and successes with establishing these positions and implementing the PCLN role on a neurosurgery pain service and a home care agency (Jones, 1978; Palermo, 1979). During the late 1970s and early 1980s the issue of evaluating PCLN practice and studying the referral process came to the forefront and was beginning to be addressed in the literature (Nelson & Davis, 1980). A change in clinical practice was emerging as the client–family situations became more complex. There was an increased level of sophistication needed by the PCLN to master these more complex and challenging consultations with somewhat diminishing resources.

This evolutionary process continued at a rapid rate during the 1980s with publication of more PCLN literature detailing specific roles, functions, and outcome evaluation of PCLN services. Advances in technology, diagnosis-related groups, and nursing shortages during the 1980s provided significant opportunities for the PCLN to be actively involved in developing strategies and programs to manage several sensitive clinical, organizational, and ethical situations that influenced the delivery of health care (Alexander, 1985; Barbiasz et al., 1982; Fife, 1986; Fife & Lemler, 1983; Samter et al., 1981). The PCLN is clearly a knowledgeable member of the interdisciplinary team in assessing the daily realities of a hospital or agency system. The complex and sometimes provocative clinical issues that several PCLN authors described in the 1980s have led to the tumultuous health care environment of the 1990s. These include but are not limited to unexpected surgical incidents, addiction issues in general hospital clients, cultural assessments and the impact on care, acquired immunodeficiency syndrome (AIDS), and keeping aging clients in their homes (Campinha-Bacote, 1988; Fincannon, 1988; Grant, 1988; Harper, 1989; Hathaway, 1987; Klebanoff & Casler, 1986; Palmateer, 1982).

Robinson (1987) illuminated the similarities and differences in medical and nursing PCL practice. PCLNs and PCL physicians share many theoretical beliefs and practices. This intersection of practice can foster a duplication of services as well as produce gaps in practice. The demands of cost reduction facing administrators and clinicians in health care institutions during the 1990s has produced an examination of all client services. PCLN and PCL physician services are being scrutinized for efficacy and efficiency. These efforts can lead to innovations in practice and necessary but creative work redesign. A well-integrated, interdisciplinary PCL department is necessary to successfully negotiate this tumultuous, rapidly changing health care system. These integrated, collaborative, interdisciplinary teams can focus on inpatient and outpatient care, with the ultimate goal of facilitating comprehensive client and family care while being fiscally responsible (Yoest, 1989). Meeting the psychosocial needs of clients and families in this rapidly changing health care arena has provided opportunities for PCLNs in advanced-practice roles to develop innovative approaches and nurse-managed programs (Abraham et al., 1991).

The 1990s has ushered in numerous challenges that confront the PCLN. The threat and effect of violence in the workplace that is generated by clients and family members is addressed in the PCLN practice literature. Additionally, PCLNs are often instrumental in developing therapeutic approaches to identifying and treating violence and the emotional aftermath (Kurlowicz, 1990; Murray & Snyder, 1991; Outlaw & Bond, 1992; Sheridan, 1993). Another important health care issue that PCLNs have made important contributions in is the area of ethical decision making in relation to level of care decisions that clients, family, and staff members are faced with daily (Broom, 1991; Hart, 1990). PCLN authors are detailing their work with clients with AIDS and the nurses who care for them (Kurlowicz, 1991; Strawn, 1991) and recognizing the addictive process in the health care professional (Krupnick, 1990).

The 1990s have produced some difficult times in the health care arena. PCLN have been affected by the phenomenon of "downsizing," or "rightsizing," which has resulted in job loss for some PCLNs. This unfortunate situation has produced opportunities for PCLNs to assist in improving work environments and diffusing work-related stress of those staff members who remain (Casey, 1989; Fishel, 1991; Guillory & Riggin, 1991; Kane, 1992; Tommasini, 1992).

The literature of the 1990s has also begun to reflect the research that PCLNs are conducting or participating in (discussed in a later section). Currently, there is some limited writing about subspecialization within PCLN practice, peer review for PCLNs to facilitate quality improvement and the future of advanced-nursing practice (Minarik, 1992; Moschler & Fincannon, 1992; Titlebaum et al., 1992).

ORGANIZATIONAL PLACEMENT OF THE PCLN

Traditional organizational placement for PCLN in a health care environment has been either in the department of nursing, usually psychiatric nursing, or within the department of psychiatry. Historically, it has been proposed that successful clinical relationships and alliances are best facilitated when the PCLN is in a staff position, not an administrative one. The belief is that placement of the PCLN in a nonhierarchical manner, with no administrative authority (which means no direct influence on the evaluation of staff performance), facilitates the consultant role. Therefore, the PCLN uses expert power rather than administrative, or line, "legitimate" power (Jimerson, 1986; Lewis & Levy, 1982). The movement of PCLNs into alternate practice settings such as psychiatric home care and consultants to long-term facilities continues to be an area of rapid expansion (Hellwig, 1993; Miller, 1993). These nurses are establishing themselves as **intrapreneurs** within workplaces and also as **entrepreneurs** in designing innovative practice programs as they function in independent contractor roles (Dibner & Murphy, 1991; Hazelton et al., 1993; Manion, 1990; Wolfson & Neidlinger, 1991).

In the health care arena, managed care and managed competition systems are becoming increasingly prevalent (Panzarino & Wetherbee, 1990; Papenhausen, 1990). Therefore, it is a natural transition for PCLNs to move into case manager roles. It is of utmost importance for these nurses to have a comprehensive understanding of the administrative role to traverse this transition smoothly. In addition, some nurse administrators are trying to protect their PCLNs by work redesign. One method has been to place the PCLN in an administrative position to insulate them from possible job loss by assigning them dual roles. Whether in a staff or a line position within the health care institution, the PCLNs scope of power rests in expert authority based on comprehensive and specialized knowledge. The issue of including curriculum content for CNSs about administration is beginning to be supported to adequately prepare them for the future transitions in nursing care delivery (Radke et al., 1990).

The movement to **case management systems** and other innovative models such as nurse-managed centers and collaborative nursing case management (ANA, 1988a; Mason et al., 1992; Togno-Armanasco et al., 1993) fits well with the theoretical knowledge and clinical expertise of the PCLN in an advanced-practice role. These nurses must competently negotiate organizational conflicts while effectively managing clinical situations and health care personnel to promote the successful implementation of case management systems, whether hospital wide or unit based (Krompotic, 1992; Sherman & Johnson, 1994).

THE CONSULTATION PROCESS

Each consultation is a unique experience that varies greatly from one situation to the next. Consultation and liaison processes, which are intertwined and represent a part of each consultation, are described in this section. Generally, consultation is an advisement process in which the consultant provides recommendations adapted to the special needs, problems, and situational constraints of the consultee (Rutherford, 1988; Stevens, 1978; Termini & Ciechoski, 1981). Caplan (1970) defined consultation as a process of communication between professionals that can be taught, applied, and analyzed systematically. The content of each consultation varies widely and is dependent on the specialized knowledge of the consultant. The skills and techniques are similar whether the focus is clinical or on process.

The consultation process involves four phases: entry, diagnosis, response-intervention, and closure and evaluation. The major steps in the consultative process are outlined in Table 30–3. The goals of the consultation process are to enhance the consultee's skill in managing a work-related problem and to facilitate the consultee's ability to master similar problems in the future.

PCLNs use several types of consultative activities. Lippitt and Lippitt's consultation model (1978) categorizes the various roles and corresponding activities used to actualize the consultation process (Table 30–4).

TABLE 30–3
Phases of the Consultation Process

1. **Entry:** Receiving a request for consultation or an invitation to participate
2. **Diagnosis:** Determining the need for and purposes of the consultation
3. **Response/Intervention:** Establishing a contractual agreement. Setting up an interaction between consultee and consultant to
   a. Seek and interpret information
   b. Identify the problem
   c. Carry out the prescriptive intervention
   d. Evaluate the intervention
4. **Closure and evaluation:** Termination of consultation process and consultee-consultant exploration of expectations

TABLE 30–4
Lippitt and Lippitt's Consultation Model

ROLE	ACTIVITIES
Advocate	► Proposes guidelines ► Persuades and directs in problem solving
Alternative identifier and linker	► Offers resources to the client ► Collaborates to assess the possible consequences of choices
Fact finder	► Collects data ► Stimulates thinking ► Provides information requested or needed by consultant
Informational expert	► Provides policy or practice decisions
Joint problem-solver	► Identifies options and alternatives ► Collaborates with consultee or team to solve problems
Objective observer/reflector	► Raises questions to be considered ► Clarifies questions
Process counselor	► Observes and monitors problem-solving process ► Raises issues ► Provides feedback
Trainer/educator	► Provides instruction to the consultee

Data from Lippitt, G., & Lippitt, R. (1978). *The consulting process in action.* San Diego: University Associates.

ENTRY: REQUEST FOR CONSULTATION

Initially, the consultant must identify *who* is initiating or requesting the consultation, for example, a nurse, physican, occupational or physical therapist, social worker, family member, client, or hospital administrator. The PCLN needs to consider the purpose and the timing of the consultation request: *What* is the reason for the consultation? *Why* has it been requested at this time? Does this request relate to discharge, or does it concern a newly admitted client? Has something, such as family member visitation, or someone, perhaps a care provider, changed recently? What else changed before the consultation was placed? The *who, what,* and *why now* are important areas to assess. Additionally, the affective, or emotional, tone of the communication by the consultee is equally important to understand and address. The consultant uses all these factors to determine the immediacy of the consultation request.

DIAGNOSIS: DETERMINING THE NEED FOR AND PURPOSES OF CONSULTATION

During the diagnosis stage of the consultation process, the consultant needs to ascertain the implications and appropriateness of this particular consultation request. The PCLN uses each consultation request as an opportunity to clarify and validate the psychological issues involved in the nursing care of clients. The PCLN provides an explanation of the PCLN role into each consultation. It is important to validate the involvement of PCLNs in the health care delivery team to facilitate making consultation alliances and use of services. Additionally, each consultation provides an opportunity for the PCLN to be a role model and develop a clearer perspective of the consultee, treatment team, nursing unit, and client-family system.

The information of who, what, and why now that was obtained during the entry phase must be used to facilitate the diagnosis phase, and consultants need to discover the "hidden agendas," or covert reasons of the consultee before engaging themselves in the response phase of consultation. An exploration of the differing perceptions as to the needs for and specific purpose of consultation must be illuminated so that the consultant can move into the response phase.

RESPONSE/INTERVENTION: ESTABLISHING A CONTRACTUAL AGREEMENT

The response or intervention phase involves the tasks of

1. Establishing a contractual agreement between the consultee and the consultant
2. Interacting between the consultee and the consultant to seek and interpret information for accurate problem identification
3. Designing the "prescriptive" intervention
4. Evaluating the intervention and revision of plan (when necessary)

Establishing a contractual agreement between the consultee and the consultant is a necessary part of the consultation process. All aspects of the nurse-to-nurse consultation process must be discussed and mutually agreed on by the consultee and the consultant. The decision-making process concerning the consultee's and the consultant's responsibilities and roles in the plan of care is the primary focus of the contractual agreement. The primary nurse or health care provider is responsible for contacting the consultant, collaborating with the consultant to negotiate the type and level of involvement necessary, and incorporating the consultant's recommendations into the care plan. The consultant collaborates with the consultee to develop a plan of care, then conducts and writes an assessment with recommendations on the consultation form. In addition, the consultant makes followup contact with the consultee for evaluation of the plan's effectiveness.

If this consultation is based on a fee for service, the issue of fees must be clearly defined, negotiated, and mutally agreed on. Some PCLN services are fee for service, and the consultee needs this information to be adequately informed about the fees that the client will be charged (Platt-Koch et al., 1990).

The consultant needs to enter the seeking and interpreting part of this stage of consultation with as few predetermined or set ideas as possible. It is important to keep an open mind while clarifying the nature of the request and listening for the explicit as well as the hidden agendas for consultation. Explicit as well as the hidden agendas for the consultation process need to be addressed for the consultation process to be complete and successful.

The issue that generated the consultation is initially conceptualized and defined by the consultee. The initial definition may be incomplete or inaccurate and become more crystallized throughout the information-seeking and interpretation stages. Exchanges between the consultee and the consultant assist in clarifying the client-family issues in relation to the needs and feelings of the consultee and how these issues intersect and impact each other. Lewis and Levy (1982) described the process of "diagnosing the total consultation." A comprehensive assessment of the client-family system, health care environment or unit, and the health care team must be addressed to obtain a complete analysis of the situation (Table 30–5).

TABLE 30–5
Components of Consultation, Assessment, and Diagnosis

1. **Consultation request:** Who is requesting the consult? When is the request for consult placed? What is the purpose of the consult?
2. **Consultee:** Who is the consultee (nurse, client, family, physician, physical therapist, or other)? What is *your* relationship with this consultee? How experienced is the consultee? Is the consultee experiencing work-related or personal stress that is impacting on this situation? Is this situation a *new* experience for this consultee or a repetitive pattern of consultation?
3. **Physician and health care team:** How does the physician view the problem? Is there conflict within the team? Is there any conflict with this patient and this physician? Does the physician value psychiatric nursing consultation? What is *your* relationship with this physician?
4. **Nursing staff members and the unit environment:** Is the unit a specialty setting (such as critical care, transplant, neonatal critical care)? Is the nursing staff experiencing significant stress from low staffing levels or cumulative patient losses? What type of leadership style does the nurse manager use? Is there a collaborative practice model on the unit between physicians and nurses or are the relationships strained or conflictual
5. **Family system:** Are any family members available to the client? Is the presence or absence of family members contributing to the distress? Are there family conflicts that are stressful for the client? Does the family have resources for support, or do they need additional support? What is this family's "usual" way of coping with health-related problems? What is the relationship between the family and the nursing and medical teams? How is the illness affecting the family system?
6. **Medical illness:** What are the most distressing signs and symptoms of the illness? What is the trajectory of the illness? How predictable or uncertain is the clinical course of this illness? Is the client's behavior possibly related to physiologic processes? Are treatments, tests and procedures, or medications contributing to the behavior?
7. **Chart review:** Has a psychosocial assessment been completed by nursing? Have there been numerous medical specialist consults with several changes in treatment? Has the client been moved from several units, (e.g., critical care unit to medical or surgical units back to the critical care unit)? Is this client assigned a primary nurse or case manager? Are there inconsistencies in assessment of the client's condition, and uncertainty of a clear plan?

The next task is to collaborate with the consultee in recommending strategies for problem solution. During this phase of response-intervention, the consultant and the consultee must determine the level and method of care to be provided by the PCLN. If the consultant is involved directly in the provision of care, individual roles, responsibilities, and accountability must be clearly negotiated and articulated by both consultation partners. In the direct consultation model, the PCLN assumes responsibility for interviewing the client and family, actively participates in the delivery of the psychosocial interventions, and collaborates in the evaluation of the care. In the indirect method, the consultant works with and through the health care professionals already involved in the client's and family members' care. Indirect consultation can be facilitated by using case conferences that are consult centered, scheduling time to focus on establishing mutual trust, and building alliances within the health care team. The PCLN uses indirect consultation to facilitate support for both the consultee and client-family system, with the goal of developing a mutually satisfying and workable plan of care (see Table 30–6 for a further description of subtypes of consultation using direct and indirect models of consultation). Several significant factors must be assessed before the PCLN can decide whether the direct or indirect consultation method is appropriate for the situation (see Table 30–7 for a guide in determining which method is appropriate for the situation).

Throughout the response-intervention phase, followup, reassessment, and evaluation of the outcomes based on the plan of care need to be negotiated, and both the consultee and the consultant need to be involved in making readjustments (see Table 30–8 for further clarification of duties in the consultation process). The PCLN discusses the recommendations with the consultee; however, a written consultation report is required so that all members of the health care team have access to relevant information concerning the plan of care. Institutions may differ in the consultation report format they use, but the following basic areas need to be included (Ingersoll & Jones, 1992):

- Purpose of the consultation and the identified problem
- Dates and activities throughout the consultation process
- Assessment of the present situation
- Specific interventions
- Recommendations on how to evaluate the outcomes of care
- Alternative plans for problem solving.

Followup progress notes describing interventions are necessary for an orderly transmission of relevant information.

CLOSURE OF CONSULTATION

The closure phase of the consultation process is just as important as the entry, diagnosis, and response phases. However, consultants periodically are remiss in establishing a formal closure phase that incorporates disengagement, termination, and, equally important, evaluation of the consultation process.

TABLE 30–6
Types of Consultation

TYPE	FOCUS	PURPOSE	PERSON OR GROUP PRIMARILY RESPONSIBLE TO	EXAMPLE
Client				
Direct	Consultant works with client and the client's family, environment, and community	To actively intervene with mental health needs of the client, such as death and dying, anger, change in body image, grief and loss	Client and family	Client who has undergone a traumatic hemipelvectomy and is dealing with a change in body image and functional ability and loss
Indirect	Consultant works with client and caregiver	To facilitate interventions by client caregiver	Health care provider	Health provider responds to family members who are dealing with a chronically critically ill family member and are making level of care decisions, which is increasing their anxiety level
Consultee				
Staff—direct	Consultant works with staff member	To deal with mental health needs of staff member, such as adjustment to new role, stress of workload, and exposure to multiple deaths in unit	Staff member	Staff member who is considering leaving nursing because of workload demands and negative impact of work-related stress on family system
Staff—indirect	Consultant works with manager regarding a staff member	To facilitate interventions by manager for a professional staff member's growth and to help manager work with other staff in relation to a staff member having performance-related issues.	Manager	Assisting a staff member to directly confront peer who does not assume his share of the workload, and decrease overinvolvement of colleagues
Intragroup—direct	Consultant works directly with a staff group on their issues	To actively intervene in coping and group dynamic issues of a group of staff members	Group of staff members	Group discussion with staff members who are dealing with the death of a long-term client
Intragroup—Indirect	Consultant works with a group of staff members to learn process for dealing with their own issues	To help a staff group learn to deal with group's mental health and group dynamics concerns	Group of staff members	Working with group of staff members to define group norms and role definitions
Intragroup—direct	Consultant works directly with two or more groups in relation to communication, collaboration, and conflict resolution	To actively intervene with two or more groups to develop or change patterns of communication, collaboration, or conflict resolution	Two or more groups	Physicians who desire research; nurses who desire clearly written protocols concerning the care of suicidal patients
Organizational or System				
Direct	Consultant works directly with administrators and managers on an administrative or organizational problem	To actively intervene in assessment, diagnosis, and change of organizational behavior	Administration manager	Provision of interventions needed for problems with absenteeism
Indirect	Consultant assists administrators and managers to develop proactive processes and programs to facilitate a mentally healthy organizational culture	To facilitate administrators and managers in the process of program development based on identified mental health needs of employees	Administration manager	Employee assistance programs, stress management programs

Adapted from Boyer, V. M., & Kirsch, J. C. (1991). Psychiatric consultant liaison nursing. In N. L. Keltner, L. H. Schwecke, & C. E. Bostrom (Eds.), *Psychiatric nursing: Psychotherapeutic management approach* (pp. 153–155). St. Louis: C. V. Mosby.

TABLE 30-7
Indications for Direct Versus Indirect Method of Consultation in Psychiatric Consultation-Liaison Nurse (PCLN) Practice

DIRECT	INDIRECT
▸ Problem identification is complex, unclear, and convoluted	▸ Problem identification is clear and straightforward
▸ Client request to speak with PCLN	▸ Consultee has established a "doable," effective plan and is requesting validation and support
▸ Special interest to PCLN or part of a specific program (e.g., trauma team, transplant team) that sees all these patients	▸ Consultee has adequate clinical skills and ability to establish and implement the recommended interventions
▸ Part or all the planned interventions are beyond the consultee's clinical expertise	▸ Consultee feels comfortable with plan and is not experiencing anxiety over situation
▸ PCLN is new to the health care system and direct consultation would increase visibility	▸ Identified problem is with consultee, not client focused
▸ Consultee is overwhelmed with anxiety or anger over situation	▸ Physician or team does not want client seen
▸ Alliances would be strengthened; systems networking would be enhanced	▸ Highly motivated consultee in agreement with plan
▸ Opportunity to model for consultee with a consultee-attended interview	▸ Consultee is user friendly and knowledgeable of PCLN role
▸ High-level resistance by consultee in relation to plan	▸ Low level of resistance by consultee in relation to plan
▸ Previously unsuccessful use of an indirect model with this consultee	▸ Previously successful use of an indirect model of consultation with this consultee

Ideally, termination and disengagement follow naturally the resolution of the identified problem or completion of the project. Before disengagement and termination, an evaluation of the consultation process is negotiated. The outcome of the consultation process and the process itself are reviewed between consultee and consultant. The evaluation process includes an assessment of the degree to which the desired or expected outcomes were achieved. A well-negotiated consultation includes time to explore whether the expectations of the consultee and the consultant were met. This is a good idea for both the novice and the expert PCLN. However, this may be the one aspect of the closure phase that can "fall between the cracks," even if the consultation process appears to be successful. The evaluation process can be a time for professional growth for both consultation partners. It is also anxiety producing for both partners in the consultation process. Truth telling and providing feedback about clinical practice and interpersonal style can be an emotional challenge for both of the consultation partners. Included in this evaluation process is a self-appraisal by the PCLN of his or her performance in the consultation process.

TABLE 30-8
Responsibilities of Consultee and Consultant

CONSULTEE	CONSULTANT
▸ Identifies client care problem	▸ Contacts primary nurse
▸ Contacts appropriate consultant(s)	▸ Collaborates with primary nurse to negotiate level of involvement
▸ Incorporates recommendations into the nursing care plan	▸ Writes assessment and recommendations on consultation form
▸ Communicates plan of care with client, family, and colleagues	▸ Makes followup contact with consultee for evaluation of effectiveness

Case Study: Direct, Client-Focused Consultation (Mr. Bradee)

Mr. Bradee is a 35-year-old married man. He is a construction worker who has been run over by a large quarry truck. He suffered an immediate traumatic hemipelvectomy at the accident site, and he and his leg were transported by medical helicopter to the trauma center. Mr. Bradee survived the initial trauma and was sent to the operating room. His wife was summoned to the hospital. When Mrs. Bradee arrived in the surgical intensive care unit (SICU), the staff nurses learned that she was 7 months pregnant.

Mr. Bradee's condition was very unstable the first 72 hours after the accident. He experienced two cardiac arrests, and Mrs. Bradee fainted twice in the SICU. The PCLN was consulted on the fourth day of hospitalization during multidisciplinary trauma rounds by the trauma nurse coordinator, SICU staff nurse, and trauma surgeon.

Consultation Request. The initial consultation request was for Mrs. Bradee, to assess her ability to cope with the client's potential death. A secondary request for consultation was to assist Mr. Bradee with the following issues:

- ▷ Mental status assessment for suspected delirium
- ▷ Pain control management
- ▷ Anxiety management
- ▷ Disturbed body image related to traumatic hemipelvectomy with surgical revision, colostomy, and fractured extremity

Assessment. The PCLN discussed the situation with the primary and associate nurses, the trauma nurse coordinator, and trauma service attending physician. After reviewing Mr. Bradee's medical record and interviewing Mrs. Bradee, the PCLN introduced herself briefly to the client, who was being administered a paralyzing agent, an amnestic benzodiazepine midazolam (Versed), and ventilator support. After completing an initial assessment, the PCLN negotiated with the health care team to remain involved as a direct provider to the wife and the client, if he survived.

Nursing Diagnoses

- Anxiety—Mr./Mrs. Bradee
- Body Image Disturbance—Mr. Bradee
- Grieving, Anticipatory—Mrs. Bradee

- Pain—Mr. Bradee
- Posttrauma Response—Mr. Bradee
- Powerlessness—Mr./Mrs. Bradee

Planning. The PCLN and primary nurse collaborated on additional consultant referrals to the maternal-child CNS and the social worker to secure immediate housing for the wife. PCLN involvement was maintained throughout Mr. Bradee's 3-month hospitalization. Initially, the PCLN focused on Mrs. Bradee and her parents. As the client's course became less tenuous after 2 weeks in the SICU, the PCLN provided direct care in collaboration with the trauma team members and SICU nursing staff.

Nursing Care Plan 30–1 identifies the desired outcomes for some of the nursing diagnoses listed earlier and delineates the nursing actions needed to achieve these outcomes, along with the rationales for these actions.

Implementation. The PCLN saw Mrs. Bradee for brief supportive sessions three or four times a week and collaborated with the social worker, the pain management team, and the pastoral counselor to facilitate Mr. Bradee's psychophysiological care. The maternal-child CNS remained involved—as Mrs. Bradee moved into the end of her eighth month of pregnancy, she began to feel an increased level of anxiety, abandonment, and isolation as the birth was becoming imminent.

When the nursing staff suggested giving Mrs. Bradee a baby shower to "normalize" her pregnancy experience, an exploration of the staff's need to be helpful and supportive was conducted by the PCLN and the SICU nurse manager. The decision was made to invite Mrs. Bradee's parents and friends from her home town (3 hours away). The baby shower was planned while Mr. Bradee's condition improved, so the party was held in his SICU room. Additionally, the maternal-child CNS did joint teaching with both Mr. and Mrs. Bradee to promote his inclusion in the pregnancy and childbirth education experience to facilitate a normal experience.

Mr. Bradee was transferred from the SICU to a general unit; within weeks, he was admitted to the rehabilitation unit. Mrs. Bradee went into labor and delivered a healthy daughter. The rehabilitation nursing staff, the PCLN, and the social worker arranged for Mr. Bradee to travel to the hospital where Mrs. Bradee had delivered to visit with his wife and daughter. Mr. Bradee was discharged to a long-term rehabilitation facility closer to his home with a positive feeling about his ability to adjust to his losses.

The strategies that the PCLN used throughout this consultation included the following:

- Providing immediate support for potential grief and mourning process by the wife
- Assessing, monitoring, and diminishing high levels of anxiety by the client and his wife
- Facilitating information sharing
- Interpreting information given to the client and his wife
- Planning cross-service referral and consultation to facilitate a normal childbearing experience and pain management
- Implementing a mental status examination and confusion management
- Reducing present or potential problems in self-esteem, body image, grief, and personal decision making, and quality of life

Evaluation. An evaluation of the initial plan in relation to outcomes was positive. The outcomes of the initial period of care (the first week) resulted in an increase in the amount of information shared with the family members, which significantly decreased their anxiety level. Cross-service consultation with the maternal-child CNS and PCLN support provided to Mrs. Bradee alleviated her fainting and confirmed a normal pregnancy with no apparent deleterious effect on the fetus. At the end of 1 month, Mr. Bradee's level of anxiety was diminishing, his pain control management was dramatically improved, and the team was considering ventilator weaning. The client's mental status was improving, and he was beginning to understand the impact of this traumatic event.

The PCLN collaborated with the primary nurse in planning for Mr. Bradee's transfer from the SICU, and this well-planned transfer was successful in alleviating the anxiety of the client and his family and in preparing the receiving unit's staff. This anticipatory guidance and planning served to diminish the client's anxiety response during his transfer.

Case conferences with the nursing staff in the SICU assisted the nurses in successfully dealing with the impact of vicarious traumatization. Additionally, these case conferences facilitated information sharing between the team members and the insurance nurse consultant, which facilitated comprehensive discharge planning for this client.

Case Study: Indirect, Consultee-Focused Consultation

Consultation Request. The PCLN received an urgent call from an assistant head nurse (AHN) in the medical intensive care unit (MICU) asking the PCLN to come to the unit immediately to discuss an "overwhelming situation." The PCLN had an established relationship with the AHN and realized that her assessment of situations was usually accurate and not exaggerated. The PCLN also recognized the urgency in the AHN's tone of voice. The PCLN went to the MICU to discuss the situation with the nurse. The AHN had been caring for a young woman who had attempted suicide several days earlier and now the MICU staff members were saying they felt like "air traffic controllers." The AHN reported that the overwhelming number of visitors were "interfering with the nursing care."

Assessment. The AHN was upset about all the client's nonrelated visitors. Throughout the AHN's description of this situation, it was apparent to the PCLN that she was extremely angry. The PCLN asked for validation of this assessment. The AHN said she was angry and up-

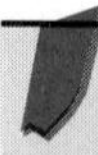

Nursing Care Plan 30–1 Direct Care Consultation Focused on Client (Mrs. and Mr. Bradee)

OUTCOME IDENTIFICATION	NURSING ACTIONS	RATIONALES	EVALUATION
Nursing Diagnosis: Anticipatory Grieving by Mrs. Bradee related to the uncertainty of her husband's survival			
1. Within 24 hours Mrs. Bradee will have her family supports at hospital to assist her in coping with uncertainty of husband's survival.	1a. PCLN will meet with Mrs. Bradee daily for support and crisis intervention.	1a. Mrs. Bradee required emotional support and assistance in problem solving during an intense crisis period in the early phase of this traumatic injury.	*Goal met:* Mrs. Bradee discussed fears of husband dying before their first baby is born. Mrs. Bradee activated her family and family support to have another adult with her every day.
	1b. Trauma team and critical care nurses meet with Mrs. Bradee to explore plans and possible outcomes.	1b. Mrs. Bradee needed clear communication from the multidisciplinary trauma team to clarify confusion and assist her in problem solving.	
	1c. Social worker will assist Mrs. Bradee in obtaining emergency housing.	1c. Mrs. Bradee needed to be housed close to the medical center to facilitate her daily involvement in Mr. Bradee's care.	
Nursing Diagnosis: Pain (acute) related to multiple orthopedic injuries and traumatic amputation			
1. Within 48 hours of admission to SICU, Mr. Bradee will have effective pain control.	1a. PCLN recommended pain management consultation after 72 hours of inadequate pain control.	1a. To clarify assessment by nurses and patient to improve pain management.	*Goal met:* Mr. Bradee had a fluctuating pain control pattern for 8 days. When his mental status improved, he was able to use patient-controlled analgesia appropriately and pain control was attained within 36 hours.
	1b. Streamlined pain medications with around-the-clock dosing instead of intermittent PRN dosing.	1b. To decrease negative effect of polypharmacy and intermittent, PRN dosing.	
	1c. Instruct Mr. Bradee in correct use of patient-controlled analgesia pump after mental status improves.	1c. Incorporating Mr. Bradee in his care and increasing his self-care concerning his pain will improve pain control.	
Nursing Diagnosis: Posttrauma Response			
1. Within 1 week, Mr. Bradee will have diminished nightmares of traumatic event, improved sleep pattern, and fewer intrusive thoughts of the accident.	1a. PCLN will see patient two or three times a week to begin debriefing from the accident.	1a. To allow Mr. Bradee sufficient time to process feelings to diminish deleterious effects of posttrauma response and alleviate development of posttraumatic stress disorder.	*Goal met:* Mr. Bradee was able to discuss his feelings of anger, disgust, and depression. Mr. Bradee made a successful transition to a rehabilitation facility without developing posttraumatic stress disorder.
	1b. Exploration of client and wife's feelings related to the accident and disruption in their family, social, and occupational spheres of life.	1b. To encourage discussion of feelings (anger, fear and depression) concerning significant body disruption and family function alterations.	

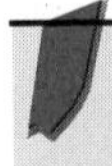

Nursing Care Plan 30–1 Direct Care Consultation Focused on Client (Mrs. and Mr. Bradee) (Continued)

OUTCOME IDENTIFICATION	NURSING ACTIONS	RATIONALES	EVALUATION
	1c. Multidisciplinary meetings to maintain a current, relevant plan of care to facilitate rehabilitation phase.	1c. To facilitate an effective discharge plan to minimize any distress related to discharge to a rehabilitation facility.	*Goal met:* Mr. Bradee's symptoms of posttrauma response were controlled by the time of discharge to the rehabilitation center.
	1d. Assist couple in normalizing posttrauma response vulnerability.	1d. To improve postaccident coping.	

set because "I want to protect the client's privacy but I can't." She became tearful and was clearly distressed about this situation. The PCLN decided that further exploration of her strong, angry response to this situation was necessary. Discussion revealed that she was handling this clinical situation in the absence of the head nurse, who was away for a couple of weeks, at the same time she was dealing with a personal tragedy. Her boyfriend's brother had attempted suicide and was in a persistent vegetative state, somewhat similar to the possible outcome of this young client.

Nursing Diagnoses

- Anxiety
- Coping, Defensive
- Powerlessness

Planning. The PCLN asked the AHN what would help her at this moment. She requested the PCLN's assistance in obtaining a list of who needed to visit this young woman. She also asked for some additional time to process her reaction to this particular situation.

Nursing Care Plan 30–2 identifies the desired outcomes for some of the nursing diagnoses listed earlier and delineates the nursing actions needed to achieve these outcomes, along with the rationales for these actions.

Implementation. Initially, the PCLN contacted another PCLN from the nearby children's medical center (where this young client had been followed) to facilitate information sharing with their staff members. These staff members had provided care to this client for several years and were upset to hear that the client had attempted suicide. Second, the PCLN spent time with the AHN listening to her describe the impact that this client's situation had on her. The PCLN made an agreement with the AHN to check with the MICU nurses daily to ascertain the level of anxiety over visitors. A case conference was planned to explore clinical issues, and a family meeting also occurred. A definitive visitor list was developed, and specific "point people" were determined to be "information disseminators" at the children's medical center.

The specific strategies that the PCLN used throughout this consultation included the following:

- Crisis intervention
- Values clarification
- Identification and resolution of ethical dilemmas
- Truth telling
- Advocacy

Evaluation. The AHN's level of anxiety and anger quickly diminished, and these feelings were replaced with guilt over her expressed anger. Within 24 hours the number of visitors had subsided and the staff members began to feel less overwhelmed and protective. The case conference illuminated the staff member's feelings of sadness, loss, shock, and being out of control. Networking with the PCLN at the other health care facility decreased some of the tension that had developed. The family meeting was successful in providing the family and team members with an opportunity to discuss options in a client whose outcome was determined to be "medically futile." The family decided on withdrawal of life support and reported feeling supported throughout this overwhelming ordeal. The AHN used some additional scheduled time with the PCLN to share her feelings about this overwhelming situation and discuss specific alternative strategies for future stressful events.

CONSULTATION PROCESS ISSUES

The consultation is not without some potential problems, specifically that of resistance to the consultation process itself (Miller, 1983). Transference and countertransference can also interfere with the consultation process. These consultation process issues can interfere with incorporation of the PCLN's recommendations into the plan of care.

Resistance is a covert or overt force that is oppositional in nature and may be generated from conscious or

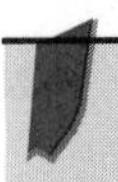

Nursing Care Plan 30–2 Indirect Care Consultation Focused on Consultee Assistant Head Nurse (AHN)

► Nursing Diagnosis: Anxiety

OUTCOME IDENTIFICATION	NURSING ACTIONS	RATIONALES	EVALUATION
1. Within 24 hours, the AHN's level of anxiety concerning the care of her young client will diminish.	1a. Explore with AHN feelings of anxiety in relation to visiting situation of client with suicide attempt.	1a. Identification of AHN's actual feelings of anxiety allowed her to redefine the situation and lessen her angry outburst.	*Goal met:* Client is able to identify feelings of anxiety and address competing situations that are increasing her anxiety.
	1b. Assist her in clarifying the interface of assuming leadership of the intensive care unit and responding to a personal tragedy that has similarities to the current situation.	1b. The AHN needed clarification and validation of her feelings to facilitate her problem-solving abilities.	

► Nursing Diagnosis: Coping, Defensive

OUTCOME IDENTIFICATION	NURSING ACTIONS	RATIONALES	EVALUATION
1. Within 48 hours, the AHN's ego integrity, self-concept, and tolerable emotional level will be maintained. 1. Within 48 hours the AHN will cope with a stressful situation in an adaptive problem-solving manner.	1a. Avoid direct confrontation of AHN's angry outburst.	1a. Direct confrontation can increase anger and defensive coping.	*Goal met:* AHN experiences less anger and hostility. AHN uses effective problem-solving strategies.
	1b. Examine the AHN's present coping behaviors and the consequences.	1b. Clarifying the underlying reasons for behavioral responses assists in understanding the consequences, thereby facilitating behavioral changes.	
	1c. Explore realistic interpretations and events with AHN and validate feelings.	1c. Establishing mutually agreed on goals and strategies helps promote behavioral changes and a concrete plan for continued personal growth for the AHN.	
	1d. Develop mutually agreed on goals to diminish AHN's increased defensiveness.		

► Nursing Diagnosis: Powerlessness

OUTCOME IDENTIFICATION	NURSING ACTIONS	RATIONALES	EVALUATION
1. Within 72 hours of incident, the AHN will be able to identify feelings of powerlessness and regain sense of control over feelings and behavioral responses.	1a. Determine the AHN's previous coping abilities and degree of mastery.	1a. Reminding the AHN of previous success enhances self-confidence, acknowledges options, and promotes self-control.	*Goal met:* AHN feels empowered and adequate. AHN uses resources to organize a workable plan and diminish feelings of being overwhelmed.
	1b. Assist the AHN to identify feelings of powerlessness and the specific factors that contribute to these feelings.	1b. Awareness of these feelings and their causes can promote positive coping.	

unconscious feelings. Resistance can be defined as behavior that protects a person from the psychological effects of change; it is not simply a rejection of ideas offered by the consultant. Resistance in the consultation process seems paradoxical because the relationship is engaged in voluntarily.

There are several reasons for the resistance that occurs in the consultation process. Even though consultees may seek assistance, they may believe that they should have solved the problem themselves. Therefore, it may be difficult for the consultees who feel inadequate to view a successful consultation as a positive, growth-producing experience. They may believe it is a personal defeat and become resistant to the consultant's ability to be successful, thereby "balancing the scales" and avoiding feelings of inadequacy because the consultant could not solve the problem either.

Resistance may also occur when consultees do not enter the consultation process in a completely voluntary manner. A supervisor or colleague may initiate or encourage the consultation process and then expect the "consultee" to use the consultant's services. Finally, resistance can develop when the consultees' workplace and personal issues become intertwined. A more complete description of specific resistance problems encountered in the consultation process is provided in Table 30–9.

There are several strategies that can be employed to manage resistance to the consultation process. Some interventions include the following:

- Provide accurate and complete information
- Treat each consultee as an individual and respectfully
- Include all the case providers in the planning process
- Allow time for exploration of feelings and the voicing of any objections to the proposed recommendations
- Consider group or unit norms and routines during the consultation process
- Provide feedback
- Remain open to questions and revisions concerning recommendations for care
- Design interventions that are within the expertise of the consultee

The PCLN can be most effective in alleviating resistance when considering all the possible reasons for the consultee's resistance.

The PCLN must carefully assess for the presence of transference and countertransference issues because they can influence all participants involved in the consultation process both positively and negatively (Marshall & Marshall, 1988). Transference can be a powerful force, involving the client's transfer of feeling and attitudes from his or her relationship with a significant other onto the nurse or therapist. Unresolved conflicts and unmet expectations may be reactivated by illness and the hospital experience.

Countertransference refers to the health care provider's emotional and behavioral response generated by specific qualities of the client. Clients and families may stimulate conflicts in the health care provider, including the PCLN involved in the consultation process. This can influence the delivery of psychological care. These

TABLE 30–9
Types of Consultee Resistance

TYPE OF CONSULTEE	DESCRIPTION OF BEHAVIOR
The eager consultee	This person experiences a great deal of anxiety about the situation and takes any recommendation(s) without determining whether it is appropriate to the particular situation
The "one-for-one" consultee	This assumes that the two people involved are on a reciprocal consultant–consultee basis. The consultee refers a case to the consultant as "payment" for a previous case consultation
The forgetful consultee	The consultee makes the initial request for consultation but then "forgets" and is remiss about appointments to discuss the situation, or forgets to read the consultation report and forgets the recommendations
The apologetic consultee	The consultant is asked to see the client; however, the consultee who requested the consult apologizes to the client and assures them that the consultant's assessment and recommendations need not be used
The expert consultee	The consultee already "knows" all the answers and is seeking agreement by the consultant. If disagreement occurs, the consultee may seek another opinion and not use the consultant again
The rejecting consultee	This consultee is angry at the client or family and tries to use the consultation process to punish the client

Data from Krakowski, A. J. (1975). Psychiatric consultation in the general hospital: An exploration of resistances. *Diseases of the Nervous System, 36,* 242–244.

feelings can be conscious or unconscious and can facilitate or interfere with the psychotherapeutic relationship.

PCLNs obviously are not immune to the effects of transference and countertransference. Therefore, they need to be actively involved in a consistent clinical supervision relationship to learn and incorporate problem-solving strategies to effectively manage their feelings. Clinical supervision affords PCLNs an opportunity to review their work with a senior clinician, a person with more experience and skill, to facilitate an objective self-evaluation process (Platt-Koch, 1986). The use of either individual clinical or peer group supervision can also enhance the PCLNs' ability to cope and adjust to this psychiatric specialty, which deals with clients' secrets and highly sensitive, potentially traumatizing physical and emotional material (Bonnivier, 1992). PCLNs are at high risk for "compassion fatigue" as well as the effects of secondary exposure to traumatic events and can become the victims of these emotionally charged situations. The issues of parallel process (Talbot, 1990), vicarious traumatization (McCann & Pearlman, 1990), or

TABLE 30–10
Guidelines for Self-Care Plan

INDIVIDUAL
▸ Personal—psychophysical health, social supports, life balance, spiritual connections, creative expression, self-awareness, plans for getting help, community activism, relaxation, humor
▸ Professional—boundaries/limit setting, plans for emergency coping, variety of tasks, adequate training, replenishment, active and consistent participation in clinical supervision
ENVIRONMENTAL
▸ Social—assessment and education of social supports
▸ Societal—educational strategies, coalition building, legislative reform social action
▸ Work environment—physical environment, articulated value system in concert with our value system, clear job tasks and personnel guidelines, supervisory and management support, collegial support

contact victimization (Courtois, 1988) all elaborate on the behavioral, cognitive, emotional, physical, and spiritual impact of health care providers caring for clients who are victims of atrocities and interpersonal violence.

PCLNs are requested to assist with several different types of intense and emotionally charged situations. Life-threatening illness and sudden and cumulative losses may contribute to the effects of disenfranchised grief for the consultee and the PCLN (Doka, 1989, 1993). The PCLN must develop a self-care strategic plan that involves individual, group, personal, and work-setting strategies to counterbalance these effects. A few recommendations are offered in Table 30–10.

THE LIAISON PROCESS

The liaison process facilitates the relationships among the client and his or her response and adjustment to illness and suffering, the consultee, and the health care environment. Liaison work involves preventive strategies and educative activities to support the partnership between the consultee and the consultant. PCLNs engage in several liaison process activities. (Table 30–11 lists activities that the PCLN engages in to foster the education and socialization of the nursing staff members.) The following clinical example is offered to illustrate the interface of consultation and liaison processes.

TABLE 30–11
Liaison Process Activities

Participating in discharge planning rounds on nursing units
Attending and participating in collaborative nursing and physician rounds
Unit-based educational programs
University teaching in nonpsychiatric programs concerning psychosocial issues
Teaching patient education programs
Facilitating support groups for health care professionals
Facilitating client–family support groups
Forming a journal club on units

Clinical Example

A unit-based CNS in the cardiothoracic SICU consulted the PCLN assigned to the SICU. The request was to discuss a particular client who was "uncooperative, unmotivated, and refusing to follow instructions." This client was a 60-year-old man who had undergone a lung transplantation. During the initial assessment by the PCLN, a mental status examination revealed that the client had severe delirium. The PCLN provided several recommendations in collaboration with the unit-based CNS. In addition, the PCLN recognized a persistent pattern of consult requests made in this particular SICU that reflected a need for teaching the staff about clients' behavior in the presence of delirium.

This consultation involved direct delivery of care to the client and assessment of the staff's need to learn how to assess the mental status of posttransplant clients. The PCLN and the CNS collaborated to design an educational program to meet this learning need. This collaborative effort produced a successful outcome by increasing the staff members' awareness and knowledge about postoperative delirium. Initially, the number of PCLN consult requests actually increased, and the problem identified was accurate for delirium instead of an "unmotivated or uncooperative" client.

PCLNs AND THE RESEARCH ROLE

The research aspect of any CNS role is quite important to promote advances in nursing practice. The research process is incorporated into the practice of PCLN. The actualization of this component of the role can sometimes be difficult. The PCLN who maintains accurate daily records and statistics of clinical consults and liaison activities is building a potential data base to provide information for clinical investigation and validation of clinical practice (Wu et al., 1994). However, several restraining factors may inhibit the PCLN from developing an accurate data base to facilitate the clinical research role. These restraining factors may include the following:

- Early stage of development of PCLN practice in the organization
- Organizational readiness
- No clear and easy method to organize, store, access, and retrieve records
- Organization that does not value or support the PCLN research role
- Lack of research mentor
- Overwhelming clinical workload

Many of these factors can be alleviated through networking with PCLNs and other advanced practitioners within and outside the organization. Coalitions can be built to develop a group model to facilitate research (Beavers et al., 1990). Additionally, developing collaborative relationships with doctoral-level nurse researchers at nearby universities can be a facilitative factor in developing collaborative research projects, especially for a novice researcher. PCLNs are in an excellent position to review and share relevant research findings with staff members. Also, PCLNs encourage, support, and consult with their nursing colleagues about research even if not directly involved in the project.

The research being done by PCLNs falls into two main categories: PCLN practice-related issues and PCLN outcome analysis. The first type addresses the types of clinical problems that PCLNs become involved in. A few examples include determining who calls for consultation and for what reasons (Wolff, 1978), assessing posttrauma response (Tanaka, 1988), assessing psychiatric morbidity following automatic implantable cardioverter-defibrillator implantation (Morris et al., 1991), assessing hope in the geriatric population (Farran & Popovich, 1990), and nurses' reports of psychiatric complications in patients with cancer (Pasacreta & Massie, 1990).

The second category of PCLN research is sometimes more challenging to develop and conduct because it directly examines and describes outcomes of PCLN practice. PCLN outcome-oriented research projects have investigated important areas of PCLN work such as consultee satisfaction with PCLN service (Newton & Wilson, 1990), the effect of PCLN consultation on the care of medical–surgical clients with sitters (Talley et al., 1990), the impact of a staff support group on the work environment of a specialty unit (Tommasini, 1992), and a description of nursing care hours of clients receiving varying amounts and types of consultation-liaison services (Mallory et al., 1993). This represents a small number of the present PCLN research projects in progress.

The next step is for PCLNs to share and communicate their findings at research conferences and in professional journals to continue building a research foundation to complement the strong clinical practice base of PCLN. Several important areas merit further research exploration by PCLNs, including the following examples:

- Cost analysis studies focusing on cost-effectiveness of PCLN service
- Employee access and utilization of PCLN services and their effect on staff emotional and physical well-being (i.e., absenteeism and illness)
- Impact of direct care intervention by a PCLN on client length of stay (i.e., decreased length of stay or nursing care hours)

This outcome-oriented research may be crucial to the survival of existing PCLN positions. Additionally, outcome-oriented research can be used to support and validate the creation of new roles and expansion of existing positions.

FUTURE TRENDS AND ISSUES

PCLN practice continues to evolve and be influenced by changes within the profession of nursing. Additionally, changes in psychiatry and reforms in the health care delivery system will significantly influence PCLN practice. The major forces that are influencing the health care delivery system include concerns for costs of service delivery and quality of life. In a period of fiscal restraint, the psychosocial aspects of health care are vulnerable yet more necessary. Achieving national health care reform will require effective, short-term, cost-managed psychological and psychotherapeutic strategies and participation of the client in managing health risk factors (Adams, 1992). PCLNs must continue to make themselves visible, accessible, and marketable in the health promotion sphere of health care.

PCLNs possess specific theoretical knowledge and clinical skills ideal for health care promotion, wellness programs, and human resource management. PCLNs can be instrumental in assisting organizations to identify and modify the culture of the organization (Caldwell, 1993). Organizational consultations can propel the PCLN into higher visibility positions. Participation by PCLNs on major organizational committees that have the legitimate power to positively impact client and family care, focus on quality improvement, and address the well-being of the organization's workforce is of the utmost importance. By this activity, PCLNs can help shape the organization's culture with respect to clients and families and a valuable asset, their employees (McGuire & Longo, 1993).

The future viability of the PCLN role is dependent on

- Outcome research that validates the positive impact of the PCLN in the health care arena
- Marketing to nursing and medical services in traditional and nontraditional settings
- Education of nurse colleagues to foster recognition and acknowledgement of the specific contributions of PCLN practice
- Third-party reimbursement and participation in political endeavors to educate consumers and lawmakers
- Continued political activity to lobby for expansion of prescriptive authority

The PCLN role continues to expand into several innovative specialty practice settings; as this occurs, the issue of accountability becomes extremely important. An autonomous, independent practitioner such as the PCLN needs the support and feedback offered by a peer review system (ANA, 1988b). Peer review is an organized procedure that can provide quality improvement and empowerment for practitioners. It is a formal, objective, systematic exchange among professional colleagues. A peer review model was developed specifically for PCLNs to ensure quality PCLN practice, foster member resilience, and create a support system to counterbalance the role isolation inherent in the autonomous practice of most PCLNs, thereby empowering this group of PCLNs (Titlebaum et al., 1992).

PCLNs have significant opportunities to be on the cutting edge of health care reform and strongly influence their own professional future by being proactive instead of reactive. Accessibility, accountability, and application of the PCLN role are specific areas that need focused attention to ensure the continued presence of the PCLN role in a cost-containing health care environment.

►CHAPTER SUMMARY

PCLN has emerged as a subspecialty within the specialty of psychiatric nursing. This subspecialty has evolved in response to an increased awareness and recognition of the psychophysiological interrelationship and the important role it plays in response to physical illness and recovery. Psychiatric–mental health consultation is defined as the provision of clinical expertise in relation to the delivery of psychological care in response to a specific request from health care providers (Lewis & Levy, 1982). The liaison process is the linkage of health care professionals to facilitate communication, collaboration, and building of partnerships between clients and health care providers. (Cassem 1991; Robinson 1987).

PCLN practice has expanded from the traditional indirect delivery model of psychosocial interventions in the general hospital setting. PCLNs now work in diverse health care settings in inpatient, outpatient, home care, and mobile mental health delivery programs. This wide variety of practice settings calls on the PCLNs' unique contributions and expertise through direct care delivery and organizational consultation. PCLNs are employing both intraprenurial and entrepreneurial skills as consultants to maintain their viability during this time of health care reform.

Suggestions for Clinical Conference

1. Discuss the extent to which the psychosocial dimension is incorporated into the plan of care for medical–surgical clients in the general hospital unit.
2. Write a PCLN assessment and intervention with a client who is agitated and disoriented in the surgical intensive care unit.
3. Identify and discuss several situations in which you would request the involvement of a PCLN.
4. Differentiate PCLN practice from primary nursing practice.

References

Abraham, I. L., Thompson-Heisterman, A. A., Harrington, D. P., Smullen, D. E., Onega, L. L., Droney, E. G., et al. (1991). Outpatient psychogeriatric nursing services: An integrative model. *Archives of Psychiatric Nursing, 5*(3), 151–164.

Adams, D. B. (1992). The future roles for psychotherapy in the medical-surgical arena. *Psychotherapy, 29*(1), 95–103.

Alexander, S. (1985). The consultation role of the psychiatric nurse clinician: From general health care to the industrial setting. *Occupational Health Nurse, 33,* 569–571.

American Nurses Association. (1990). *Standards of practice: Psychiatric consultation-liaison nursing.* Kansas City, MO: Author.

American Nurses' Association. (1988a). *Nursing case management.* Kansas City, MO: Author.

American Nurses' Association. (1988b). *Peer review guidelines.* Kansas City, MO: Author.

Baldwin, C. A. (1978). Mental health consultation in the intensive care unit: Toward greater balance and precision of attribution. *Journal of Psychosocial Nursing and Mental Health Services, 161,* 17–21.

Barbiasz, J., Blanford, K., Byrne, K., Horvath, K., Levy, J., Lewis, A., et al. (1982). Establishing the psychiatric liaison nurse role: Collaboration with the nurse administrator. *Journal of Nursing Administration, 12*(2), 14–18.

Barton, D., & Kelso, M. T. (1971). The nurse as a psychiatric consultation team member. *Psychiatry Medicine, 2,* 108–115.

Beavers, F. E., Gruber, M., & Johnson, B. (1990). A model for group research by master's degree RN's in advanced roles. *Clinical Nurse Specialist,4*(3), 130–136.

Blake, P. (1977). The clinical specialist as nurse consultant. *Journal of Nursing Administration, 7,* 33–36.

Bonnivier, J. F. (1992). A peer supervision group: Put countertransference to work. *Journal of Psychosocial Nursing and Mental Health Services, 30*(5), 5–8.

Broom, C. (1991). Conflict resolution strategies: When ethical dilemmas evolve to conflict. *Dimensions of Critical Care Nursing, 10*(6), 354–363.

Brown, E. (1965). Meeting patients' psychosocial needs in the general hospital. In J. Skipper & R. Leonard (Eds.), *Social interaction and patient care.* Philadelphia: J. B. Lippencott.

Caldwell, C. (1993). Accelerators and inhibitors to organizational change in a hospital. *Quality Review Bulletin, 19,* 42–46.

Campinha-Bacote, J. (1988). Culturological assessment—an important factor in psychiatric consultation-liaison nursing. *Archives of Psychiatric Nursing, 2*(4), 244–250.

Caplan, G. (1970). *The theory and practice of mental health consultation.* New York: Basic Books.

Casey, J. L. (1989). Counseling nurse managers. *Nursing Management, 20*(9), 52–53.

Cassem, N. H. (1991). *Massachusetts General Hospital: Handbook of general hospital psychiatry* (3rd ed.) St Louis: C. V. Mosby.

Courtois, C. (1988). *Healing the incest wound.* New York: W. W. Norton.

Covert, A. B. (1979). Community mental health nursing: The role of the consultant in the nursing home. *Journal of Psychosocial Nursing and Mental Health Services, 17*(7), 15–19.

Davidson, S., & Noyes, R. (1973). Psychiatric nursing consultation on a burn unit. *American Journal of Nursing, 73,* 1715–1718.

Dibner, L. A., & Murphy, J. S. (1991). Nurse entrepreneurs. *Journal of Psychosocial Nursing and Mental Health Services, 29*(5), 30–34.

Doka, K. J. (1989). *Disenfranchised grief: Recognizing hidden sorrow.* Lexington, MA: Lexington Books.

Doka, K. J. (1993). *Living with life-threatening illness: A guide for patients, their families, and caregivers.* New York: Lexington Books.

Dumas, R., & Leonard, R. (1963). The effect of nursing on the incidence of postoperative vomiting. *Nursing Research, 12,* 12–15.

Elder, R., & Diers, D. (1963). The patient comes to the hospital. *Nursing Forum 2,* 89–93.

Elder, R. (1963). What is the patient saying? *Nursing Forum, 2,* 25–37.

Faast, M., & Elstun, N. (1979). Psychiatric emergency service: A growing specialty. *Journal of Psychosocial and Mental Health Services, 16,* 13–19.

Farran, C. J., & Popovich, J. M. (1990). Hope: A relevant concept for geriatric psychiatry. *Archives of Psychiatric Nursing 4*(2), 124–130.

Fife, B. (1986). Establishing the mental health clinical specialist role in the medical setting. *Issues in Mental Health Nursing, 8,* 15–23.

Fife, B., & Lemler, S. (1983). The psychiatric nurse specialist: A valuable asset in the general hospital. *Journal of Nursing Administration, 13*(4), 14–17.

Fincannon, J. (1988). Meperidine addiction associated with amphotericin treatment in leukemia: Case study and staff reaction. *Archives of Psychiatric Nursing, 2*(5), 302–306.

Fishel, A. H. (1991). Psychiatric consultation: Improving the work environment. *Journal of Psychosocial Nursing and Mental Health Services, 29*(11), 31–34.

Forhan-Andrianos, A., & Swain, C. R. (1979). Interfacing the role of the psychiatric clinical nurse specialist with a hospital emergency room setting. *Journal of Psychosocial Nursing and Mental Health Services, 4,* 24–26.

Garant, C. A. (1977). The psychiatric liaison nurse: An interpretation of the role. *Supervisor Nurse, 8*(4), 75–78.

Goldstein, S. (1979). Psychiatric clinical specialist in the general hospital. *Journal of Nursing Administration, 9,* 34–37.

Grace, M. J. (1974). The psychiatric nurse specialist and medical/surgical patients. *American Journal of Nursing, 74*(3), 481–483.

Grant, S. M. (1988). The hospitalized AIDS patient and the psychiatric liaison nurse. *Archives of Psychiatric Nursing, 2*(1), 35–39.

Guillory, B., & Riggin, O. Z. (1991). Developing staff support model. *Clinical Nurse Specialist, 5*(3), 170–173.

Harper, M. (1989). Providing mental health services in the homes of the elderly. *Mental Health Nursing, 4*(2), 127–147.

Hart, C. A. (1990). The role of the PCLN's in the ethical decisions to remove life-sustaining treatments. *Archives of Psychiatric Nursing, 5*(6), 370–377.

Hathaway, G. I. (1987). The need for psychiatric nurse clinical specialists in geriatric long-term-care facilities. *Nursing Homes, 36*(4), 32–33.

Hazelton, J. H., Boyum, C. M., Frost, M. H. (1993). Clinical nurse specialist subroles: Foundations for entrepreneurship. *Clinical Nurse Specialist, 7*(1), 40–45.

Hedlund, N. (1978). Mental health nursing consultation in the general hospital. *Patient Counseling and Health Education, 1,* 85–88.

Hellwig, K. (1993). Psychiatric home care nursing: Managing patients in the community setting. *Journal of Psychosocial Nursing and Mental Health Services, 31*(12), 21–24.

Holstein, S., & Schwab, J. (1965). A coordinated consultation program for nurses and psychiatrists. *Journal of the American Medical Association, 194*(5), 491–493.

Ingersoll, G. L., & Jones, L. S. (1992). The art of the consultation note. *Clinical Nurse Specialist, 6*(4), 218–220.

Issacharoff, A., Goddahn, J., Schneider, D., Maysonett, J., & Smith, B. (1970). Psychiatric nurses as consultants in a general hospital. *Hospital and Community Psychiatry, 21*(11), 361–367.

Jackson, H. (1969). The psychiatric nurse as a mental health consultant in a general hospital. *Nursing Clinics of North America, 4*(3), 527–540.

Jimerson, S. S. (1986). Expanded practice in psychiatric nursing. *Nursing Clinics of North America, 21,* 527–535.

Johnson, B. S. (1963). Psychiatric nurse consultant in a general hospital. *Nursing Outlook, 2,* 728–729.

Jones, P. (1978). Psychiatric liaison nurse for neurosurgery: An innovative approach to management of chronic pain. *Journal of Neurosurgical Nursing, 10*(1), 160–165.

Kane, J. (1992). Allowing the novice to succeed: Transitional support in critical care. *Critical Care Quarterly, 15*(3), 17–22.

Klebanoff, N. A., & Casler, C. B. (1986). The psychosocial clinical nurse specialist: An untapped resource for homecare. *Home Healthcare Nursing, 4*(6), 36–40.

Krakowski, A. J. (1975). Psychiatric consultation in the general hospital: an exploration of resistances. *Diseases of the Nervous System, 36,* 242–244.

Krompotic, D. (1992). Successful implementation of case management. *Nursing Connections, 5*(2), 49–55.

Krupnick, S. (1990). Recognizing and avoiding negative addictions in your life. *Journal of Holistic Nursing Practice, 4*(4), 20–31.

Kurlowicz, L. H. (1991). Psychiatric consultation liaison nursing intervention with nurses of hospitalized AIDS patients. *Clinical Nurse Specialist, 5*(2), 124–129.

Kurlowicz, L. (1990). Violence in the emergency department. *American Journal of Nursing, 90,* 35–40.

Lewis, A., & Levy, J. S. (1982). *Psychiatric liaison nursing: The theory and clinical practice.* Reston, VA: Reston Publishing.

Lippitt, G., Lippitt, R. (1978). *The consulting process in action.* San Diego: University Associates.

Mallory, G. A., Lyons, J. S., Scherubel, J. P. & Reichelt, P. A. (1993). Nursing care hours of patients receiving varying amounts and types of C/L services. *Archives of Psychiatric Nursing, 7*(6), 353–360.

Manion, J. (1990). *Change from within: Nurse intrapreneurs as health care innovators.* Kansas City, MO: Author.

Marshall, R. J., & Marshall, S. V. (1988). *Transference–countertransference matrix.* New York: Columbia University Press.

Mason, T. H., Lazenby, R. B. & Fain, S. B. (1992). Nursing care centers: A collaborative effort. *Nursing Connections, 5*(2), 5–9.

McCann, L., & Pearlman, L. (1990). Vicarious traumatization: A framework for understanding the psychological effects of working with victims. *Journal of Traumatic Stress Studies, 3*(1), 131–149.

McGuire, T. P., & Longo, W. (1993). Evaluating your mission: A practical approach to developing and assessing a facility's organizational culture. *Quality Review Bulletin, 19,* 47–55.

Miller, L. E. (1983). Resistance to the consultation process. *Nursing Leadership, 6*(1), 10–15.

Miller, M. P. (1993). Planning and program development for psychiatric home care. *Journal of Nursing Administration, 23*(11), 35–41.

Minarik, P. (1992). Second license for advanced nursing practice? *Clinical Nurse Specialist, 6*(4), 221–222.

Morris, P. L., Badger, J., Chmielewski, C., Berger, E., & Goldberg, R. J. (1991). Psychiatric morbidity following implantation of the automatic implantable cardioverter defibrillator. *Psychosomatics, 32*(1), 58–63.

Moschler, L. B., & Fincannon, J. (1992). Subspecialization within psychiatric consultation liaison nursing. *Archives of Psychiatric Nursing, 6*(4), 234–238.

Murray, M. G., & Snyder, J. (1991). When staff are assaulted: A nursing consultation support service. *Journal of Psychosocial Nursing and Mental Health Services, 29*(7), 24–29.

Nelson, J., & Davis, D. (1980). Referrals to psychiatric liaison nurses: Changes in characteristics over a limited time period. *General Hospital Psychiatry, 23*(1), 41–45.

Nelson, J., & Davis, D. (1979). Educating the psychiatric liaison nurse. *Journal of Nursing Education, 18*(8), 14–20.

Newton, L., & Wilson, K. C. (1990). Consultee satisfaction with a psychiatric consultation liaison service. *Archives of Psychiatric Nursing, 4*(2), 114–123.

Outlaw, F. H., & Bond, M. (1992). Managing the violent addicted patient in the medical–surgical setting. *MEDSURG Nursing, 1*(1), 61–64.

Palermo, E. (1978). Mental health consultation in a home care agency. *Journal of Psychosocial Nursing and Mental Health Services, 16*(9), 21–23.

Palmateer, L. M. (1982). Consultation and liaison implications of awakening paralyzed during surgery: A syndrome of traumatic neurosis. *Journal of Psychosocial and Mental Health Services, 20*(11), 21–26.

Panzarino, P. J., & Wetherbee, D. G. (1990). Advanced case management in mental health: Quality and efficiency combined. *Quality Review Bulletin, 16*(11), 386–390.

Papenhausen, J. L. (1990). Case management: A model of advanced practice? *Clinical Nurse Specialist, 4*(4), 169–170.

Pasacreta, J., & Massie, M. J. (1990). Nurse's reports of psychiatric complications in patients with cancer. *Oncology Nursing Forum, 17*(3), 347–353.

Peplau, H. (1964). Psychiatric nursing skills and the general hospital patient. *Nursing forum, 3,* 28–37.

Peterson, S. (1969). The psychiatric nurse specialist in a general hospital. *Nursing Outlook, 17*(2), 56–58.

Platt-Koch, L., Gold, A., & Jacobsma, B. (1990). Setting up a fee for service program for psychiatric liaison nurses. *Clinical Nurse Specialist, 4*(14), 207–210.

Platt-Koch, L. M. (1986). Clinical supervision for psychiatric nurses. *Journal of Psychosocial Nursing and Mental Health Services, 26*(1), 7–15.

Pranulis, M. A. (1972). A factor affecting the welfare of the coronary patient. *Nursing Clinics of North America, 7,* 445–455.

Przepiorka, K. M., & Bender, L. S. (1977). Psychiatric nursing consultation in a university medical center. *Hospital and Community Psychiatry, 28*(10), 755–758.

Radke, K., McArt, E., Schmitt, M., & Walker, E. K. (1990). Administrative preparation of clinical nurse specialists. *Journal of Professional Nursing, 6*(4), 221–228.

Robinson, L. (1972). A psychiatric nursing liaison program. *Nursing Outlook, 20*(7), 454–457.

Robinson, L. (1987). Psychiatric consultation liaison nursing and psychiatric consultation liaison doctoring: Similarities and differences. *Archives of Psychiatric Nursing, 1*(2), 73–80.

Robinson, L. (1968). Liaison psychiatric nursing. *Perspectives in Psychiatric Care, 6*(2), 87–91.

Rutherford, D. E. (1988). Consultation: A review and analysis of the literature. *Journal of Professional Nursing, 4*(5), 339–344.

Samter, J., Scherer, M., & Shulman, D. (1981). Interface of psychiatric clinical specialists in a community hospital setting. *Journal of Psychosocial Nursing and Mental Health Services, 19*(1), 20–29.

Severin, N., & Becker, R. (1974). Nurses as psychiatric consultants in a general hospital emergency room. *Journal of Community Mental health, 10,* 261.

Sheridan, D. J. (1993). The role of the battered woman specialist. *Journal of Psychosocial Nursing and Mental Health Services, 31*(11), 31–37.

Sherman, J. J., & Johnson, P. K. (1994). CNS as unit-based case manager. *Clinical Nurse Specialist, 8*(2), 76–80.

Stevens, B. J. (1978). The use of consultants in nursing service. *Journal of Nursing Administration, 8,* 7–15.

Strawn, J. (1991). Psychosocial consequences of HIV infection. In J. Durham & T. Cohen (Eds.), *The person with AIDS in nursing perspectives.* New York: Springer.

Talbot, A. (1990). The importance of parallel processing in debriefing crisis counselors. *Journal of Traumatic Stress, 3*(2), 265–277.

Talley, S., Davis, D. S., Goicoechea, R., Brown, L., & Barber, I. (1990). Effect of psychiatric liaison nurse specialist consultation on the care of medical surgical patients with sitters. *Archives of Psychiatric Nursing, 4*(2), 114–123.

Tanaka, K. (1988). Development of a tool for assessing post-trauma response. *Archives of Psychiatric Nursing, 2*(6), 350–356.

Termini, M., & Ciechoski, M. A. (1981). The consultation process. *Issues in Mental Health Nursing, 3*(1/2), 77–89.

Titlebaum, H., Hart, C. A., & Romano-Egan, J. (1992). Interagency psychiatric consultation liaison nursing peer review and peer board: Quality assurance and empowerment. *Archives of Psychiatric Nursing, 6*(2), 125–131.

Togno-Armanasco, V. D., Hopkin, L. A., & Harter, S. (1993). *Collaborative nursing case management.* New York: Springer.

Tommasini, N. R. (1992). The impact of a staff support group on the work environment of a specialty unit. *Archives of Psychiatric Nursing, 6*(1), 40–47.

Wolff, B. (1978). Psychiatric nursing consultation: A study of referral process. *Journal of Psychosocial Nursing and Mental Health Services, 16,* 42–47.

Wolfson, B., & Neidlinger, S. H. (1991). Nurse entrepreneurship: Opportunities in acute care hospitals. *Nursing Economics, 9*(1), 40–43.

Wu, Y. W. B., Crosby, F., Ventura, M., & Finnick, M. (1994). In a changing world: Database to keep the pace. *Clinical Nurse Specialist, 8*(2), 104–108.

Yoest, M. A. (1989). The clinical nurse specialist on the psychiatric team. *Journal of Psychosocial Nursing and Mental Health Services, 27*(3), 27–32.

Zedeck, S. (Ed.). (1992). *Work, families, and organizations.* San Francisco: Jossey-Bass.

Zerwekh, J. V. (1991). At the expense of their souls. *Nursing Outlook, 39*(2), 58–61.

CHAPTER

31

Psychiatric Nursing Research

ROSE M. NIESWIADOMY, Ph.D., R.N.

OUTLINE

CHAPTER OBJECTIVES

Upon completion of this chapter, you will be able to:
1. Recall the steps in the scientific research process.
2. Identify the roles of psychiatric nurses in research.
3. Discuss the results of the some of the research studies across the life span that have been conducted by psychiatric nurses.
4. List barriers to research in psychiatric nursing.
5. Understand the need for quantitative and qualitative research in psychiatric nursing.
6. Describe the role of the National Institute of Mental Health in fostering psychiatric research.
7. Recognize future needs for psychiatric nursing research.

KEY TERMS

Client advocate
Critiquer of research findings
Data collector
Principal investigator
Qualitative research
Quantitative research
Utilizer of research findings

Nurses, like other health care providers, must define and promote their role in various health care settings, and research will help them accomplish this. As psychiatric nursing moves into the next century, clinicians need to be continually apprised of technological and biological advances in treating mental disorders in the changing health care system. A host of issues present themselves as potential topics for psychiatric nursing research, such as the following:

- The link between biological interventions and behavioral responses
- The impact of current health care trends (new health care payment systems, length of stay, and community-based care provisions) on mental health treatment
- Responses to demographic changes, such as increases in the number of elderly, people from varied cultural backgrounds, and the number of people with chronic illness
- Identification and assessment of high-risk populations and their needs
- Initiation and maintenance of preventive health care programs
- Continuous rehabilitative care of the chronically mentally ill

Psychiatric nursing has long trailed other nursing specialties in conducting research. Poster et al. (1992) attributed this disparity to several factors: (1) a lack of a psychiatric–mental health nursing coalition to help psychiatric nurses understand and employ research techniques; (2) a scarcity of nurses educationally and clinically prepared to conduct research; (3) a general lack of administrative support in the institutions where psychiatric nurses are employed; and (4) a negative perception of research among psychiatric nurses. The authors found that positive attitudes toward research among psychiatric nurses paralleled the level of education these nurses possessed. Additionally, conducting research was found to be an expectation of advanced-practice psychiatric nurses, whereas the generalist nurse faced more barriers to research, such as lack of administrative support and more focus on patient care.

Angela McBride (1990) wrote of the need to set a "research–practice agenda for the future," stressing that the future of psychiatric nursing depends on its ability to integrate behavioral, biological, and caring concepts in health promotion and disease prevention. These concepts were also supported by the American Nurses Association (ANA) in its *Statement on Psychiatric–Mental Health Clinical Nursing Practice and Standards of Psychiatric–Mental Health Clinical Nursing Practice* (1994). Overall, psychiatric nursing research must advance mental health, prevent mental illness, and foster treatment and rehabilitation of the mentally ill (McBride, 1990).

This chapter reviews further potential areas for psychiatric nursing research and briefly examines the research process.

Neurobiological Factors. As previously stated, integrating biological and behavioral concepts into psychiatric nursing practice, education, and research will become increasingly germaine as we move into the twenty-first century. Although explorations into the relationship between biological processes and behavioral responses is not new to medicine, nursing research in this area is still in its infancy. Historically, psychiatric nurses have been instrumental in research drug trials; there is a need to expand this role and explore further the behavioral changes brought about not only by psychotropic drugs but also by other biological interventions.

Stress and Coping. Stress often plays a major role in mental health. Research is needed to identify and help clients deal with distressful responses, including intense anxiety, grief reaction, depression, and maladaptive coping behaviors such as chemical addiction and suicide attempts. Research can help practitioners develop strategies to promote comfort and reduce symptoms of anxiety.

Developmental and Aging Issues. Research into stress and coping in school-age children has produced useful tools such as the Schoolagers Coping Strategy Inventory, which arose from an examination of the type, frequency, and effectiveness of children's coping behaviors (Ryan, 1989). Research showed that the effects of stressful events such as loss and intimidation can have lasting effects on children (Jacobson, 1994). Nursing research can explore these areas and provide guidance on how to help children reduce stress.

Research can offer unexpected solutions to common problems. For example, Melnyk's study (1994) reported how informational interventions can help children and their parents cope with hospitalization and home adjustment. Awareness of possible reactions in the hospitalized child helped parents cope with the child's illness so that they could support the child during various procedures by serving as a buffer and lessening the negative impact of the hospitalization and illness.

From reading and performing such research, nurses can learn to develop and enhance age-appropriate coping patterns and preventive interventions to promote adaptation and reduce mental illness in all age groups.

Psychosocial Factors. Stress and adaptation can be affected by the quality of the patient's support systems, socioeconomic and cultural milieu, and other psychosocial factors. A study (Ahijevych & Bernard, 1994) of 178 African American women found that the tools currently used to appraise health-promoting behaviors tend to be insensitive to diverse populations such as the economically disadvantaged and suggested a "middle-class bias" in current assessment instruments. Obviously, such findings indicate the need to explore better ways of assessment and health promotion among these patients. As American society becomes more diverse, psychiatric nurses must develop research studies that will lead to interventions sensitive to every segment of the population.

The remainder of this chapter reviews the basic steps in the research process and discusses specific implications for psychiatric nursing.

STEPS IN THE SCIENTIFIC RESEARCH PROCESS

The steps in the scientific research process are generally similar for each study. Although the number of steps varies according to sources in the literature, the steps are fairly consistent. These steps are summarized in Table 31–1.

IDENTIFY THE PROBLEM TO BE STUDIED

Determining a problem to be studied can be challenging. The most difficult part is narrowing the subject down to a workable topic. The study topic may be based on personal experiences, previous research, or the suggestions provided by others in the literature.

SURVEY THE LITERATURE ON THE TOPIC

Researchers do not want to "reinvent the wheel." Therefore, a review of the literature is necessary to determine what, if any, research has already been conducted on this particular topic. Other purposes of reviewing the literature are to help determine the study design and to discover if there are existing instruments available to measure the study variables (characteristics or attributes that differ among the people or objects that are being studied).

DEVELOP A STUDY FRAMEWORK

The goal of research is to build a scientific knowledge base. The theoretical or conceptual framework for a study helps provide a knowledge base into which the study results can be placed. Theory and research are intertwined: Research can be used to test and refine theories, but studies without a theoretical basis provide a set of isolated facts. Research that is conducted within the context of a theoretical framework is valuable in providing understanding of the study results. In other words, the researcher can better explain why the study findings turned out as they did.

TABLE 13–1
Steps in the Scientific Research Process

1. Identify the problem to be studied
2. Survey the literature on the topic
3. Develop a study framework
4. Formulate research questions or study hypothesis
5. Operationally define the study terms
6. Choose the design for the study
7. Select the study sample
8. Collect the data
9. Analyze the data
10. Communicate the study findings

FORMULATE RESEARCH QUESTIONS OR STUDY HYPOTHESIS

Research questions allow the investigator to focus on specific aspects of the study problem. If the study framework is strong enough to make a prediction about the study results, a hypothesis is used to state the study prediction. Hypotheses should be based on theories or previous research.

OPERATIONALLY DEFINE THE STUDY TERMS

The study variables should be operationally defined, which means that the means of measuring or observing the variables must be specified. If anxiety were one of the study variables, the exact way of measuring this concept should be specified; for example, anxiety may be measured by pulse rate.

CHOOSE THE DESIGN FOR THE STUDY

The plan for how a study will be conducted is called the *study design*. Designs can be broadly classified as experimental and nonexperimental. In an experimental study in nursing, the researcher usually carries out some type of intervention with a group of subjects and measures the outcomes. In nonexperimental studies, the researcher makes no interventions but rather collects data and records what has been observed.

SELECT THE STUDY SAMPLE

A set of persons or objects that are of interest to the researcher must be selected. This is usually done by choosing a large group of interest, called the *population,* and then selecting a subset of this large group to study. Researchers can choose random or nonrandom samples. Most groups that have been studied by nurses are nonrandom convenience samples because they were chosen from a group that was convenient or available. This type of sampling process is not the most scientific; however, less time and money are involved in this type of sampling process.

COLLECT THE DATA

The data are the facts or pieces of information that the researcher collects in a study. The researcher decides what data to collect and how to collect them; who will collect the data; and where and when the data will be collected. Data collection may be a time-consuming task, but it is often considered the most enjoyable part of the research process.

ANALYZE THE DATA

Many nurses fear the step of analyzing the data because they believe that they must be able to compute statistical formulas. However, in this day of the computer, data analysis has become quite simple. A researcher can input large amounts of data and receive almost instantaneous results. In addition, statisticians are now available to help with data analysis. After the data are analyzed, the researcher must try to interpret the findings. The results of the study are compared with the researchers' expectation that was stated in the hypothesis. Results are also compared with those of any similar studies in the literature. After the findings are interpreted, the researcher should suggest implications or changes that should be made in nursing practice, education, administration, and research as a result of the findings.

COMMUNICATE THE STUDY FINDINGS

Study results must be communicated to others before the research process is complete. There are a multitude of ways to communicate the results of nursing research, including oral presentations at research conferences, poster presentations, and publication of results in professional journals and other publications.

THE NURSE'S ROLE IN RESEARCH

Psychiatric nurses claim that they are unqualified to conduct research and believe that this relieves them of the responsibility of being involved in research. Although the role of principal investigator is important, it is by no means the only role nurses can play in research. Other roles include member of a research team, data collector, client advocate during a research study, critiquer of research findings, and utilizer of research findings.

PRINCIPAL INVESTIGATOR

The **principal investigator** of a research study is the person who has played the major role in the development and conduct of the research. Serving as a principal investigator requires special research preparation, generally obtained in a master's or doctoral program. As the number of nurses with advanced educational preparation in research has increased, the number of research studies has also increased. However, many one-of-a-kind studies have been conducted as part of the requirement for an advanced degree, with few replication studies conducted thereafter. These isolated bits of knowledge have provided only slight advancements in the body of psychiatric nursing knowledge. Nurse researchers must be willing to continue in their area of research after they complete their educational programs. The body of knowledge for psychiatric nurses will expand only as rapidly as there are nurses willing to conduct research studies.

MEMBER OF A RESEARCH TEAM

Each psychiatric nurse should consider becoming a member of a research team. The type of research preparation received in nursing school and the amount of clinical experience will dictate the nurse's ability to serve on a research team. Nurses with baccalaureate and higher degrees may be qualified for the role of coinvestigator. As nurses participate in research, it is quite likely that they will become interested in conducting their own studies.

DATA COLLECTOR

Data collectors are important to the success of a research project. Many research studies would never be completed without the assistance of data collectors. It is difficult for a principal investigator to do all the data collection that is required in a study.

Simmons-Alling (1990) pointed out the opportunity for the nurse, while collecting data, to educate consumers about risk factors in their daily lives. For example, the author wrote that while drawing blood the nurse can discuss with clients such topics as cholesterol screening, the benefits of exercise, the importance of nutritional habits, and appropriate responses to stress.

CLIENT ADVOCATE

The ethical aspects of a study are important. In the role of **client advocate,** the nurse can ensure that the rights of all prospective subjects and actual subjects are adequately protected. Nurses can answer questions about the study and make sure that the potential subjects fully understand the study before agreeing to participate. Nurses should also be available to subjects during the study if questions arise.

CRITIQUER OF RESEARCH FINDINGS

Nurses have to take responsibility for being informed about the most recent research findings in their areas of practice. When fulfilling the role of a **critiquer of research findings,** the nurse reviews and determines their applicability for nursing practice. The evaluation of research is not a simple task, but this skill can be attained by all nurses, to some degree. It is beyond the scope of this book to present critiquing guidelines. (For further information about critiquing, see Nieswiadomy [1992]). For nurses lacking in formal preparation in critiquing, self-instruction, attending workshops, and joining critiquing groups at work are methods to obtain this skill. Malone (1990) stated that "the bridge between research and clinical application is based on an informed staff" (p. 4).

UTILIZER OF RESEARCH FINDINGS

It is insufficient for the nurse to be informed about research findings; applicable findings should be integrated into the nurse's practice. As a **utilizer of research findings,** the nurse ensures that the latest knowledge is integrated into practice. However, nurses, just like all other people, are reluctant to accept change. Change is stressful and is frequently resisted. We want to do things "the way we have always done them."

Research findings are of little value if they are not used in practice. Nurses must be judicious in using the results of research studies, however. Therefore, it is extremely important that nurses know how to critique research results, as was mentioned in the previous section.

PUBLISHED RESEARCH

Research conducted by psychiatric–mental health nurses is not always easily identifiable in the literature. Because nurses in other specialty areas are also interested in mental health, the reader may be uncertain whether a particular study would qualify as psychiatric–mental health nursing research. If the research article concerns clients with a chronic mental illness, is published in a nursing journal, and was conducted by a nurse, the assumption can probably be made that the researcher is a psychiatric nurse.

McBride (1988) pointed out that nurses in the psychiatric specialty area have been more likely to study mental health than mental illness. Of the 400 psychiatric nursing references published between 1980 and 1989 that were reviewed by Fox (1992), fewer than 30 studies focused on chronic mental illness. Fox discussed 24 of these studies in a chapter in the *Annual Review of Nursing Research* published in 1992, and a list of them is found in Table 31–2.

Many published research studies that are classified as psychiatric–mental health nursing research are concerned with nurses themselves rather than clients. In Sills's classic research review article published in a 1977 issue of *Nursing Research,* the author indicated that one of the themes throughout the 1950s was a focus on the personality characteristics, preferences, attitudes, and evaluation of learning of psychiatric nurses. One half of the studies discussed in a book by Brooking entitled *Psychiatric Nursing Research,* published in England in 1986, focuses on nurses. Although research concerning nurses themselves is important, a greater emphasis in psychiatric–mental health nursing research should be placed on clients.

For more information on the research that was published in the literature from 1952 to 1976, refer to Sills's excellent 1977 article, which discusses all types of psychiatric nursing research published during that period. No other broad overview of psychiatric–mental health nursing research since 1976 is available in the literature. However, in 1992, Fox presented a review of research specific to chronic mental illness that was published between 1980 and 1989. She surveyed general nursing research journals, such as *Nursing Research* and *Western Journal of Nursing,* and psychiatric nursing specialty journals, such as the *Archives of Psychiatric Nursing, Issues in Mental Health Nursing,* the *Journal of Psychosocial Nursing and Mental Health Services,* and *Perspectives in Psychiatric Nursing.* She also reviewed issues of the *Community Mental Health Journal* and *Hospital and Community Psychiatry.* Research articles that were authored or coauthored by nurses (as determined by their published credentials) were included in the review.

The research was discussed under the following topics: community adjustment and intervention, recidivism, case management, client self-monitoring and patient education, verbal and nonverbal communication, violence and seclusion, medication compliance, rural service use, and cultural compatibility. Fox (1992) reported that there was an increasing trend for psychiatric nurses to conduct qualitative rather than quantitative research. These two types of research designs are compared later in this chapter.

RESEARCH ACROSS THE LIFE SPAN

The following section discusses research literature across the life span. An example is presented of a clinical study for each age group.

CHILDHOOD

The role of the nurse in child psychiatry has been minimal, according to McBride (1988), because there are few graduate programs in this subspecialty and fewer nurses are entering this clinical specialty area, funding levels for children and youth are low, child psychiatric nurses are underutilized, and there is a lack of research and publication by nurses in this area. Also, research with children has been hampered by the lack of reliable diagnostic tools (Simmons-Alling, 1990).

One indication that psychiatric nurses may be showing more interest in children and adolescents is demonstrated by the publication in 1987 of the first issue of the *Journal of Child and Adolescent Psychiatric–Mental Health Nursing.* It is hoped that more research will be conducted with children in the future. However, the difficulty of obtaining permission to conduct research with minors may limit research with this age group.

Jones and O'Brien (1990) described three unique child inpatient treatment techniques: (1) journal writing; (2) using clinical rounds with children; and (3) contracting for reduction in precaution levels. The child subjects

TABLE 31–2
Studies on Chronic Mental Illness: 1980–1989

Binder, B., & McCoy, S. (1983). A study of patients' attitudes toward placement in seclusion. *Hospital and Community Psychiatry, 34,* 1052–1053.
Chafetz, L. (1988). Recidivist clients: A review of pilot data. *Archives of Psychiatric Nursing, 2*(1), 14–20.
Davidhizer, R. (1982a). Compliance by persons with schizophrenia: A research issue. *Issues in Mental Health Nursing, 4,* 233–255.
Davidhizer, R. (1982b). Tool development for profiling the attitude of clients with schizophrenia toward their medication using Fishbein's expectancy value model. *Issues in Mental Helath Nursing, 4,* 343–357.
Davidhizer, R. (1984). Beliefs and values of the client with chronic mental illness regarding treatment. *Issues in Mental Health Nursing, 6,* 261–275.
Davidhizer, R., Austin, J., & McBride, A. (1986). Attitudes of patients with schizophrenia toward taking medication. *Research in Nursing and Health, 9,* 139–146.
Flaskerud, J. (1986a). Profile of chronically mentally ill psychotic patients in four community mental health centers. *Issues in Mental Health Nursing, 8*(2), 155–168.
Flaskerud, J. (1986b). The effects of culture-compatible intervention on the utilization of mental health services by minority clients. *Community Mental Health Journal, 22,* 127–141.
Flaskerud, J., & Koriz, F. (1982). Resources rural consumers indicate they would use for mental health problems. *Community Mental Health Journal, 18,* 107–119.
Goering, P., Waslenki, D., Farkas, M., Lancee, W., & Ballantyre, R. (1988). What difference does case management make? *Hospital and Community Psychiatry, 39,* 272–276.
Hardin, S. (1980). Comparative analyses of nonverbal interpersonal communication of schizophrenics and normals. *Research in Nursing and Health, 3,* 57–68.
Hicks, M. (1989). A community sojourn from the perspective of one who relapsed. *Issues in Mental Health Nursing, 10,* 137–147.
Jones, S., & Jones, P. K. (1987). Research in psychiatric and mental health nursing: The emergence of scientific rigor. *Archives of Psychiatric Nursing, 1*(3), 155–162.
Kucera-Bozarth, K., Beck, N., & Lyss, L. (1982). Compliance with lithium regimens. *Journal of Psychosocial Nursing and Mental Health Services, 20*(7), 11–15.
Kurucz, J., & Fallon, J. (1980). Dose reduction and discontinuation of antipsychotic medication. *Hospital and Community Psychiatry, 31,* 117–119.
McCandless-Glimcher, L., McKnight, S., Hamera, E., Smith, B., Peterson, K., & Plumber, A. (1986). Use of symptoms by schizophrenics to monitor and regulate their illness. *Hospital and Community Psychiatry, 37,* 929–933.
Morrison, E. (1989). Theoretical modeling to predict violence in hospitalized psychiatric patients. *Research in Nursing and Health, 12,* 31–40.
Pfieffer, S. (1990). An analysis of methodology in follow-up studies of adult inpatient psychiatric treatment. *Hospital and Community Psychiatry, 41,* 1315–1321.
Slavinsky, A., & Krauss, J. B. (1982). Two approaches to the management of long-term psychiatric outpatients in the community. *Nursing Research, 31,* 284–289.
Stickney, L., Hall, R., & Gardner, R. (1980). The effect of referral procedures on aftercare compliance. *Hospital and Community Psychiatry, 31,* 567–569.
Ulin, P. (1981). Measuring adjustment in chronically ill community mental health care. *Nursing Research, 30,* 229–235.
Whall, A., Engle, V., Edwards, A., Bobel, L., & Haberland, C. (1983). Development of a screening program for tardive dyskinesia: Feasibility issues. *Nursing Research, 32,* 151–156.
Youssef, F. (1984). Adherence to therapy in psychiatric patients: An empirical investigation. *International Journal of Nursing Studies, 21,* 51–59.
Youssef, F. (1987). Discharge planning for psychiatric patients: The effect of a family patient teaching program. *Journal of Advanced Nursing, 12,* 611–616

were asked to rate the interventions. Journal writings were seen as helpful in sorting out and expressing feelings. The youth rounds helped the child inpatients to set daily goals. Finally, contracting for a change in precautions was rated high in helping the child inpatients keep their promises. Jones and O'Brien (1990) indicated that these three interventions provided the psychiatric nurse the opportunity to take a more active role in patient treatment and promoted patient involvement in the treatment process.

Examples of additional nursing research articles focusing on this age group are found in Table 31–3.

ADOLESCENCE

Psychiatric nurses are increasingly conducting research with adolescents and publishing the results of these studies, although not as extensive as the research that is being conducted with adults. Again, it is important to

TABLE 31–3
Psychiatric Nursing Research Across the Life Span: Published Studies

CHILDHOOD
Effects of Methylphenidate Hydrochloride on the Subjective Reporting of Mood in Children with Attention Deficit Disorder. (In Walker, M. K., Sprague, R. L., Sleator, E. K., & Ullmann, R. K. [1988]. *Issues in Mental Health Nursing, 9,* 373–385.).
Children of Affectively Ill Parents. (In Buckwalter, K. C., Kerfoot, K. M., & Stolley, J. M. [1988]. *Journal of Psychosocial Nursing and Mental Health Services, 26,* 8–14.)
What Really Happened? Incidence and Factor Assessment of Abused Children and Adolescents. (In Polk-Walker, G. C. [1990]. *Journal of Psychosocial Nursing and Mental Health Services, 28,* 17–22.)
ADOLESCENCE
Suicidal and Nonsuicidal Coping Methods of Adolescents. (In Puskar, K., Hoover, C., & Miewald, C. [1992]. *Perspectives in Psychiatric Care, 28,* 15–20.)
Life Events, Problems, Stresses, and Coping Methods of Adolescents. (In Puskar, K. & Lamb, J. [1991]. *Issues in Mental Health Nursing, 12,* 267–281.)
Family Routines and Conduct Disorders in Adolescent Girls. (In Keltner, B., Keltner, N. L., & Farren, E. [1990]. *Western Journal of Nursing Research, 12,* 161–170.)
ADULTHOOD
The Effect of Staff Stress on Patient Behavior. (In Gray, S., & Diers, D. [1992]. *Archives of Psychiatric Nursing, 6,* 26–34.)
The Effect of a Support Group on Grieving Individuals' Levels of Perceived Support and Stress. (In Davis, J. M., Hoshiko, B. R., Jones, S., & Gosnell, D. [1992]. *Archives of Psychiatric Nursing, 6,* 35–39.)
Measurement of Locus of Control in Cocaine Abusers (In Oswald, L. M., Walker, G. C., Reilly, E. L., Krajewski, K. J., & Parker, C. A. [1992]. *Issues in Mental Health Nursing, 13,* 81–94.)
OLDER ADULTHOOD
Therapeutic Use of "Prizing" and Its Effect on Self-Concept of Elderly Clients in Nursing Homes and Group Homes. (In Williams-Barnard, C. L., & Lindell A. R. [1992]. *Issues in Mental Health Nursing, 13,* 1–18.)
Treating Depression in Well Older Adults: Use of Diaries in Cognitive Therapy. (In Campbell, J. M. [1992]. *Issues in Mental Health Nursing, 13,* 19–30.)
Disruptive Behaviors of a Cognitively Impaired Nursing Home Resident. (In Rossby, L., Beck, C., & Heacock, P. [1992]. *Archives of Psychiatric Nursing, 6,* 98–107.

mention the *Journal of Child and Adolescent Psychiatric–Mental Health Nursing.* The publication of this journal indicates psychiatric nurses' increased interest in this particular age group. However, obtaining permission to conduct research with this group of minors is difficult, as is the case with children.

Conrad (1992) examined the causes of adolescent suicide and the influence that suicide of others has on adolescent suicidal behavior. The sample consisted of 473 11th- and 12-grade students from a metropolitan area in the northeastern United States. Self-hurt behaviors were reported by 23 percent of the subjects and suicide attempts by 6.7 percent. The cause of suicide attempts, as reported by 40 percent of the subjects, was "too much pressure." It was found that 93 percent of the subjects who reported self-hurt behaviors knew a family member, friend, or schoolmate who had attempted or committed suicide. The author suggested that approximately one in three adolescents who report harming themselves at one time may later attempt suicide. The author also pointed out that when assessing suicidal intent, the nurse must be aware that adolescents may identify with peers who attempted or committed suicide.

Other examples of recently published research articles on this age group are found in Table 31–3.

ADULTHOOD

Most research in psychiatric–mental health nursing has been conducted with adults. This is the largest group of clients seen by psychiatric nurses.

Mackey et al. (1992) reported on the factors associated with long-term depression in victims of sexual assault. Of the 63 subjects, almost two thirds reported some degree of depression. More than one half of the sample reported a history of sexual abuse in childhood. Some of the factors associated with higher levels of depression were nondisclosure of the assault to significant others, the presence of children living with the victim, and pending civil lawsuit. Subjects who were presently sexually active were less likely to be depressed. The authors indicated that nurses must recognize depression as a common reaction to unresolved sexual trauma.

Examples of recently published research articles that address the adult client are found in Table 31–3.

OLDER ADULTHOOD

The geriatric population is a group in need of psychiatric–mental health nursing services (Fopma-Loy, 1989). Statistics indicate the great increase in the number of people 65 years of age and older. Although this group has needs for services similar to those of other adult groups, additional mental health services are needed because of the significant increase in emotional distress and behavioral and social dysfunction (Fopma-Loy, 1989). Depression and dementia are the most common mental health problems experienced by the aged.

Krach and Yang (1992) studied the functional status of older persons with chronic mental illness who were living in the home setting. Face-to-face interviews using the Older Adult Resources Survey were conducted with 100 subjects in their homes. Most subjects (53 percent) had psychiatric symptoms. Diagnoses included depression (42 percent), schizophrenia (22 percent), and bipolar disorder (13 percent). Subjects also listed many serious medical problems, including cardiovascular disease (92 percent), arthritis (45 percent), and urinary tract disorders (19 percent). Severe economic impairment was reported by 35 percent of the subjects, and 29 percent indicated that their social relationships were of poor quality.

Other examples of recently published research articles on the elderly client are found in Table 31–3.

BARRIERS TO PSYCHIATRIC RESEARCH

Baier (1988) identified some of the difficulties in studying clients with chronic mental illnesses. Clients with the same psychiatric diagnosis vary—much more so than clients with the same medical diagnosis—in their degree of impairment and response to treatment. Laboratory values may provide a fairly reliable source of evaluation for a medical condition, but no similar methods for evaluating psychiatric conditions are available.

There are ethical issues to be considered when conducting research with groups of people who may not be able to provide informed consent. Conducting research with clients experiencing psychological problems may be comparable to conducting research with children or mentally impaired older adults. The question arises as to whether these people are capable of understanding a research study for which they volunteer. It is also difficult to obtain permission of institutional review boards to study clients with mental illness.

Many clients are taking psychotropic medications, which may alter their responses to interventions that need to be tested. In addition, clinicians have difficulty in maintaining consistency of treatment conditions; as soon as it seems beneficial to change the treatment conditions, the clinician will do so. Thus, changes in treatment affect the validity of the study.

QUANTITATIVE AND QUALITATIVE RESEARCH IN PSYCHIATRIC–MENTAL HEALTH NURSING

Most nursing research studies have been quantitative rather than qualitative in nature. **Quantitative research** focuses on gathering numerical data and making generalizations across groups of people. **Qualitative research** focuses on the meaning of experiences to people and is not as concerned with generalizing study results.

Most research studies mentioned in this chapter have used quantitative methods. Qualitative studies may be distinguished from quantitative studies because the qualitative ones have small sample sizes (possibly as small as eight or nine subjects) and few statistics are used. In contrast, the quantitative studies will have larger sample sizes and statistics—often lots of statistics! Table 31–4 presents other characteristics of qualitative and quantitative research.

In the last decade nurses have increasingly come to view qualitative research methods as appropriate for the development of nursing knowledge. Nurses have always considered individualized nursing care to be extremely important, but their research has generally followed the scientific method, which searches for proof and verification of study results. The focus is on groups and on the generalizability of findings. Qualitative research focuses on the individual, and "truth" is whatever the individual says it is. An example of qualitative research is presented here.

TABLE 31–4
Quantitative and Qualitative Research Characteristics

QUANTITATIVE RESEARCH	QUALITATIVE RESEARCH
Hard science	Soft science
Focus: concise and narrow	Focus: complex and broad
Reductionistic	Holistic
Objective	Subjective
Reasoning: logistic, deductive	Reasoning: dialectic, inductive
Basis of knowing: cause-and-effect relationships	Basis of knowing: meaning, discovery
Tests theory	Develops theory
Control	Shared interpretation
Instruments	Communication and observation
Basic element of analysis: numbers	Basic element of analysis: words
Statistical analysis	Individual interpretation
Generalization	Uniqueness

From Burns, S., & Grove, S. K. (1993). *The practice of nursing research* (2nd ed., p. 27). Philadelphia: W. B. Saunders.

Dalton (1991) studied the "lived experience" of never-married women. A phenomenological study was conducted to explore the meaning of singleness to nine women who had never been married. A method of data analysis called *constant comparative analysis* revealed 13 categories or themes. One of these themes was called *trade-off* and compared the freedom and independence of being single with the loneliness and lack of companionship that accompanied this life state. Although some commonalities were found in the lived world of never-married women, it was determined that each woman was unique and the nurse must strive "to know her and care for her as a unique, existential human being" (Dalton, 1991, p. 77).

THE NATIONAL INSTITUTE OF MENTAL HEALTH

The National Institute of Mental Health (NIMH) has long considered psychiatric nursing to be one of the core mental health professional groups. However, the importance of nurses to the mission of this organization was greatly enhanced by the Task Force on Nursing that was appointed in 1985 by Dr. Shervert Frazier, the Director of NIMH. Members of the task force included well-known nurses such as Joyce Fitzpatrick, Kathryn Barnard, Jo Eleanor Elliott, and Ada Sue Hinshaw. The committee sought ways of increasing participation of nurses in the extramural activities of the NIMH, such as appointing nurses to advisory boards and increasing nurses' participation in grant-supported activities. The final report of the task force was presented in September 1987, and three major recommendations were made to NIMH: (1) prepare psychiatric nurses to be researchers; (2) support the ongoing research careers of psychiatric nurses; and (3) link psychiatric nurses with the existing system (McBride et al., 1992).

In regard to the first recommendation, the first NIMH institutional research training grant for psychiatric nursing was awarded in September 1989. The program emphasized geropsychiatric care (McBride et al., 1992). For the second recommendation, the support of ongoing research careers for psychiatric nurses has been fostered by several efforts. In October 1989, the NIMH cosponsored, with the National Institutes of Health, a conference entitled "Biological Psychiatry and the Future of Psychiatric–Mental Health Nursing." Several more research-building conferences for psychiatric nurses have been held since 1989. Additionally, funding for nursing research has increased a great deal, even though it is still low. Two research proposals submitted by nurse principal investigators were funded by the NIMH in 1985 to 1986 for a total of $98,138, whereas nine such proposals were funded in 1988 to 1989 for a total of $1,016,722 (McBride et al., 1992).

In regard to the third objective of the task force, McBride et al. (1992) discussed how nurses have become more linked to the NIMH system. In 1987, there were only four nurse members of the initial review groups (IRGs). This number increased to 10 nurses in 1990. For the first time, a nurse, Dr. Barbara Lowery, was appointed to chair an IRG (the Mental Health Behavior Research Review Committee).

TABLE 31–5
Research Questions for Psychiatric Nursing Across the Life Span

CHILDHOOD
1. What nursing intervention(s) are effective in raising the self-esteem levels of children who have experienced school failures?
2. Can a short assessment tool be developed to identify children at risk for physical abuse?
3. Do children with psychiatric diagnoses experience rejection by their peer group?
ADOLESCENCE
1. Does psychiatric nurses' knowledge of developmental stages influence their care of adolescents?
2. What factors are most influential in the suicidal ideation of adolescents?
3. Is there a correlation between the number and variety of coping responses used by adolescents and their ability to manage stressful life events?
ADULTHOOD
1. What factors are related to drug compliance in adults with a diagnosis of schizophrenia?
2. Is there a difference in the type and quality of care provided for adult psychiatric clients from different ethnic groups and social classes?
3. Does telephone followup by psychiatric nurses reduce recidivism rates of adult psychiatric clients?
OLDER ADULTHOOD
1. How are psychotropic medication side effects influenced by the interaction of age, nutritional status, and physical illness?
2. Is there a decrease in the depression levels of elderly clients who participate in a nurse-led reminiscing group?
3. What family characteristics are predictive of elder abuse?

FUTURE NEEDS FOR PSYCHIATRIC NURSING RESEARCH

Many nurse authors in psychiatric–mental health nursing have pointed out that this is the age of biological psychiatry (Lego, 1992; McKeon, 1990). Some psychiatric nurses argue that the art of psychiatric nursing will be diminished if the focus is shifted to biological issues. Others propose that the new evidence in psychobiology must be integrated but the psychosocial and interpersonal aspects that have been the foundation of practice should not be neglected. It seems appropriate that psychiatric nurses should become involved in neurobiological and psychopharmacological treatment research but not lose sight of the benefits of other treatment modalities. Comparisons should be made between client responses to drugs and those to other treatments. Nurses should examine mental health problems in a balanced way, integrating the relationships between the mind, the brain, and behavior (Babich & Tolbert, 1992; Lego, 1992; McEnany, 1991; Wolfe, 1994).

McBride (1986) called for the development of large data bases. She noted, for example, that if several institutions, rather than one, examined the influence of contacts with relatives and friends on the progress of psychiatric patients, a body of knowledge could be more readily developed.

Examples of research studies that are needed across the life span are presented in Table 31–5.

CHAPTER SUMMARY

Research has become an integral part of nursing. Every nurse should be familiar with the steps in the scientific research process. The roles of psychiatric nurses in research include those of (1) principal investigator; (2) member of a research team; (3) data collector; (4) client advocate; (5) critiquer of research findings; and (6) utilizer of research findings.

Much of the research in psychiatric–mental health nursing has focused on nurses. However, the greatest emphasis should be on clients. Research that has been conducted with clients across the life span has focused most often on adult clients, but more research is needed on the other age groups.

Quantitative research has been conducted more often than qualitative research. Quantitative research focuses on the use of numbers and is concerned with whether the findings can be generalized, whereas qualitative research is more concerned with individuals and the meaning of life experiences to these individuals.

The NIMH considers psychiatric nursing as one of the core mental health professional groups. There has been an increasing interest in psychiatric–mental health research at the NIMH, and funding levels for this type of research have increased at this agency. There is a great need for psychiatric–mental health nursing research. Nurses should become more involved in neurobiological and psychopharmacological treatment research, but they should not lose sight of the value of other treatment modalities.

Suggestions for Clinical Conferences

1. Identify research currently being conducted by or participated in by psychiatric–mental health nursing staff.
2. Discuss the role of generalist and advanced-practice nurses in clinical research.
3. Invite a psychiatric–mental health nurse researcher to discuss recent research findings and the associated nursing implications.

References

Ahijevych, K., & Bernard, L. (1994). Health-promoting behaviors of African-American women. *Nursing Research 43*(2), 86–89.

American Nurses Association. (1994). *A statement on psychiatric–mental health clinical nursing practice and standards of psychiatric–mental health clinical nursing practice.* Washington, DC: American Nurses Publishing.

Babich, K., & Tolbert, R. B. (1992). Professionally speaking: What is biological psychiatry? *Journal of Psychosocial Nursing and Mental Health Services, 30*(1), 33–38.

Baier, M. (1988). Why research doesn't yield treatment. *Journal of Psychosocial Nursing and Mental Health Services, 26*(5), 29–33.

Brooking, J. (1986). *Psychiatric nursing research.* Chichester, England: John Wiley.

Buckwalter, K. C., Kerfoot, K. M., & Stolley, J. M. (1988). Children of affectively ill parents. *Journal of Psychosocial Nursing and Mental Health Services, 26*(10), 8–14.

Burns, N., & Grove, S. K. (1993). *The practice of nursing research* (2nd ed.). Philadelphia: W. B. Saunders.

Conrad, N. (1992). Stress and knowledge of suicidal others as factors in suicidal behavior of high school adolescents. *Issues in Mental Health Nursing, 13,* 95–104.

Dalton, S. T. (1991). Lived experience of never-married women. *Issues in Mental Health Nursing, 12,* 69–80.

Davis, J. M., Hoshiko, B. R., Jones, S., & Gosnell, D. (1992). The effect of a support group on grieving individuals' levels of perceived support and stress. *Archives of Psychiatric Nursing, 6,* 35–39.

Fopma-Loy, J. (1989). Geropsychiatric nursing: Focus and setting. *Archives of Psychiatric Nursing, 3,* 183–190.

Fox, J. C. (1992). Chronic mental illness. In J. J. Fitzpatrick, R. L. Taunton, & A. K. Jacox (Eds.), *Annual review of nursing research* (Vol. 10, pp. 95–113). New York: Springer.

Gray, S., & Diers, D. (1992). The effect of staff stress on patient behavior. *Archives of Psychiatric Nursing, 6,* 26–34.

Jacobson, G. (1994). The meaning of stressful life experiences in nine- to eleven-year-old children: A phenomenological study. *Nursing Research 43*(2), 95–99.

Jones, R. N., & O'Brien, P. (1990). Unique interventions for child inpatient psychiatry. *Journal of Psychosocial Nursing and Mental Health Services, 28*(7), 29–31.

Jones, S. L. (1989). Bridging the gap between the nurse researcher and clinician. *Archives of Psychiatric Nursing, 3,* 181–182.

Krach, P., & Yang, J. (1992). Functional status of older persons with chronic mental illness living in a home setting. *Archives of Psychiatric Nursing, 6,* 90–97.

Lego, S. (1992). Biological psychiatry and psychiatric nursing in America. *Archives of Psychiatric Nursing, 6,* 147–150.

Mackey, T., Sereika, S. M., Weissfeld, L. A., Hacker, S. S., Zender, J. F., & Heard, S. L. (1992). Factors associated with long-term depressive symptoms of sexual assault victims. *Archives of Psychiatric Nursing, 6,* 10–25.

Malone, J. A. (1990). Schizophrenia research update: Implications for nursing. *Journal of Psychosocial Nursing and Mental Health Services, 28*(8), 4–9.

McBride, A. B. (1986). Present issues and future perspectives of psychosocial nursing theory and research. *Journal of Psychosocial Nursing and Mental Health Services, 24*(9), 27–32.

McBride, A. B. (1988). Coming of age: Child psychiatric nursing. *Archives of Psychiatric Nursing, 2,* 57–64.

McBride, A. B. (1990). Psychiatric nursing in the 1990s. *Archives of Psychiatric Nursing, 4*(1), 21–28.

McBride, A. B., Friedenberg, E. C., Babich, K. S., & Bush, C. T. (1992). Nursing research at NIMH: An update. *Archives of Psychiatric Nursing, 6,* 138–141.

McEnany, G. W. (1991). Psychobiology and psychiatric nursing: A philosophical matrix. *Archives of Psychiatric Nursing, 5*(5), 255–261.

McKeon, K. L. (1990). Introduction: A future perspective on psychiatric–mental health nursing. *Archives of Psychiatric Nursing, 4,* 19–20.

Melnyk, B. M. (1994). Coping with unplanned hospitalization: Effects of informational interventions on mothers and children. *Nursing Research, 43*(1), 50–55.

National Institute of Mental Health Task Force on Nursing. (1988). The state of psychiatric nursing. *Journal of Psychosocial Nursing and Mental Health Services, 26*(4), 38–40.

Nieswiadomy, R. M. (1992). *Foundations of nursing research* (2nd ed.), Norwalk, CT: Appleton & Lange.

Oswald, L. M., Walker, G. C., Reilly, E. L., Krajewski, K. J., & Parker, C. A. (1992). Measurement of locus of control in cocaine abusers. *Issues in Mental Health Nursing, 13,* 81–94.

Polk-Walker, G. C. (1990). What really happened? Incidence and factor assessment of abused children and adolescents. *Journal of Psychosocial Nursing and Mental Health Services, 28*(11), 17–22.

Poster, E. C., Betz, C. L., & Randell, B. (1992). Psychiatric nurses' attitudes toward and involvement in nursing research. *Journal of Psychosocial Nursing and Mental Health Services, 30*(10), 26–29.

Puskar, K., & Lamb, J. (1991). Life events, problems, stresses, and coping methods of adolescents. *Issues in Mental Health Nursing, 12,* 267–281.

Rossby, L., Beck, C., & Heacock, P. (1992). Disruptive behaviors of a cognitively impaired nursing home resident. *Archives of Psychiatric Nursing, 6,* 98–107.

Ryan, N. M. (1989). Stress-coping strategies identified from school-aged children's perspective. *Research in Nursing and Health, 12,* 111–122.

Sills, G. M. (1977). Research in the field of psychiatric nursing—1952–1977. *Nursing Research, 26,* 201–207.

Simmons-Alling, S. (1990). Genetic implications for major affective disorders. *Archives of Psychiatric Nursing, 4,* 67–71.

Walker, M. K., Sprague, R. L., Sleator, E. K., & Ullmann, R. K. (1988). Effects of methylphenidate hydrochloride on the subjective reporting of mood in children with attention deficit disorder. *Issues in Mental Health Nursing, 9,* 373–385.

Williams-Barnard, C. L., & Lindell, A. R. (1992). Therapeutic use of "prizing" and its effect on self-concept of elderly clients in nursing homes and group homes. *Issues in Mental Health Nursing, 13,* 1–18.

Wolfe, B. E. (1994). The use of challenge studies in behavioral nursing research. *Archives of Psychiatric Nursing, 8,* 145–149.

C H A P T E R

32

A Framework for Developing Psychiatric Nursing Skills

MARGARET BRACKLEY, Ph.D., R.N.,C.S.

OUTLINE

CHAPTER OBJECTIVES

Upon completion of this chapter, you will be able to:

1. Discuss possible roles of the psychiatric nurse in the twenty-first century.
2. Describe the leadership skills desired for psychiatric nurses.
3. Identify the trends and direction for research in psychiatric nursing.
4. Explore the impact of technology on psychiatric–mental health nursing practice.
5. Address the need for mental health promotion across the life span.

KEY TERMS

Assertiveness
Case management
Consumerism
Continuous quality improvement
Empowerment
Leadership
Nursing informatics
Vulnerability

All nurses, regardless of their area of practice, see clients with mental disorders. It makes no difference whether the nurse works in settings such as obstetrics, pediatrics, general medicine, or surgery or in the schools or community. Clients with mental disorders are seen in every setting, specialty, or situation, and they deserve to receive the same quality of care as the rest of the population. The American Nurses Association (ANA), in conjunction with psychiatric specialty organizations, including the American Psychiatric Nurses Association, the Society for Education and Research in Psychiatric–Mental Health Nursing (SERPN), and the Association of Child and Adolescent Psychiatric Nurses, set forth guidelines for basic mental health (Krauss, 1993). Clients with mental disorders should have health benefits equal to those of other citizens, including a wide range of services that are cost effective and allow for choice of health care provider.

Most of the mental health services are delivered by generalist health care providers, that is, registered nurses, school nurses, nurse practitioners, midwives, family practice physicians, internists, and pediatricians. Studies have shown that the 65 to 85 percent of mental health care provided by non–mental health specialists is lacking in recognition of and appropriate treatment and referral for mental disorders (Krauss, 1993). This situation must improve if all Americans are to have access to mental health services under health care reform. Krauss (1993) responded to these findings by calling for specific federally funded continuing education for these groups to teach mental health assessment, screening, methods for making appropriate referrals, and the use of consultation.

This chapter further defines the role of the psychiatric nurse in the twenty-first century, assesses the impact of technology and neurobiology on practice, and aligns psychiatric–mental health nursing to the national goals as outlined in *Healthy People 2000* (U.S. Department of Health and Human Services [USDHHS], 1990).

DEFINING THE ROLE OF PSYCHIATRIC NURSING IN THE TWENTY-FIRST CENTURY

The American Association of Colleges of Nursing (1986) issued a document on the essentials of professional nursing education and identified the three roles of the professional nurse as provider of care, coordinator of care, and member of a profession. This chapter discusses future trends in health care and the way in which these trends are predicted to influence roles in nursing. Preparation for psychiatric nurse career development in the year 2000 or thereafter must be instituted now if adequate members of nurses with the necessary characteristics for future practice are to be available.

PSYCHIATRIC NURSE AS A PROVIDER OF CARE

The psychiatric nurse as a provider of care is expected to be more involved in primary care and preventive services in community-based settings. Care of clients with chronic mental illness, dual diagnosis with substance abuse as one of the classifications, and violent and abusive behaviors will occur in hospital, community, and correctional facilities. The psychiatric nurse must be prepared to work more independently than in the past as a result of the change in settings for mental health care. It is also anticipated that increased skills in observation of the effects of biological treatments will be needed.

PSYCHIATRIC NURSE AS A COORDINATOR OF CARE

As the coordinator of care, the psychiatric nurse will work in conjunction with other disciplines on the mental health team. Role changes include a return to more active involvement in milieu management, **case management,** managed care systems, rehabilitation services, and other approaches. Because of the various innovative models of care delivery, more attention must be given to teaching nurses skills in critical thinking and self-learning strategies rather than those needed in traditional and perhaps outmoded systems of client care.

PSYCHIATRIC NURSE AS A MEMBER OF A PROFESSION

One characteristic of a profession is reliance on a body of knowledge that is distinct from other disciplines. The chapter on research (see Chapter 31) addresses this issue; however, research is not the only source of knowledge. Knowledge comes from personal experience, an ethical system, and the artistic aspect of caring (Watson, 1988). Psychiatric nurses must allow time for reflection and the development of knowledge.

Nursing students should also develop the characteristics of a professional by the end of their educational program. As a member of a professional group, nurses must invest time and energy in activities that promote the preservation of psychiatric nursing as well as resources for clients and their families. Membership in appropriate professional organizations is essential for meeting the goals of the specialty. Providing input into the political process, thus ensuring adequate resources not only for the nursing profession but also for underserved and stigmatized mental health consumer groups, is a professional responsibility. The Americans with Disabilities Act will help diminish some of the results of institutionalized stigma. Intensive education at all levels of society must be developed and implemented to address the stigma that the American culture associates with mental illness. Once this is eliminated, mental illness can be treated as any other illness.

LEADERSHIP SKILLS IN PSYCHIATRIC–MENTAL HEALTH NURSING

New nurses often ask what it takes to be a leader. The answer to this question lies in personal commitment and the willingness to take a risk. As members of a profession, nurses are expected to provide **leadership** within their potential sphere of influence. To lead is to show the way by going in advance, to guide or direct. Psychiatric–mental health nurses often lead by modeling acceptance of stigmatized groups. Historically, psychiatric nursing has often led the entire nursing profession in developing new roles like the role of the clinical nurse specialist (McBride, 1990). We have often led in reform of unjust practices, through groups such as the National Alliance for the Mentally Ill (NAMI) and the American Mental Health Association. Psychiatric–mental health nurses have also forged the way for mental health care reform, as for example, in the work of SERPN to identify competencies and skills for psychiatric–mental health nursing education and in nurse lobby groups that ensure adequate resources for mental health care reform.

Leadership skills are taught in basic programs of professional nursing. Nurses have the ability to influence various groups within health care. We try to influence clients and their families to adopt healthy lifestyles and habits. We influence our peers, colleagues in other disciplines, policymakers, and clients through the use of power. Schutzenhofer (1992) concluded that power must be learned early and well by students of nursing. Too often we have thought of power as a negative quality that others have used against us. We must reframe this thinking to view power, especially power that is shared with others, as the means of exerting positive pressure to bring about health care reform.

Collaboration with other disciplines is a leadership activity that will greatly increase our influence in health care. Schutzenhofer (1992) called for nurses to redefine ourselves as team players. We will be ahead in what some identify as the 1990s leadership style used by women, that is the leadership of collaboration instead of control. The power of one nurse is limited, whereas the power of many nurses in unison with other disciplines can direct health care change. Another way we can use power effectively is by influencing policymakers through lobbying efforts. In this manner, we can ensure that resources are made available to improve the quality of health care delivered.

CONCEPTS OF EMPOWERMENT

People in various settings and disciplines talk about **empowerment** in reference to federal workers, voters, consumers of health care, and many other examples. *To empower* simply means to invest with power or to authorize. We as nurses or voters are certainly authorized to provide good care or elect qualified representatives to government, so why should we discuss what we are already empowered to do? The truth is that "[we have not] educated nurses as full health caregiving professionals and have focused instead on how to prepare students to be institutional employees" (Watson, 1988).

As identified by Watson (1988), the traditional ways that schools of nursing have operated include the following:

- Treating students as objects
- Using mechanical or industrial terms, such as *products* and *aggregates*
- Focusing on cognitive–technical outcomes alone, thereby creating competency without compassion or caring
- Restricting teaching and learning to behavioral objectives, factual information, and techniques
- Tolerating power and dependence roles for teachers and learners
- Separating doing from knowing and being
- Tolerating accreditation processes that are in direct conflict with nursing's moral and scientific beliefs and educational philosophies and theories
- Fixating on entry into practice and a degree rather than how to educate thinking professional people in such a way as to prepare them for a role that is consistent with nursing's social, moral, and scientific mission to society

After defining the problem, Watson then suggested a "revolution" in nursing curricular practices. The National League for Nursing (NLN, 1988, 1989) has developed and published documents on curricular revolution in response to Watson's call. In this series, scholarly works are presented to increase the dialogue about the transition in nursing educational practices. The impetus behind the need for change is the failure of nursing schools to empower its graduates to develop and deliver the kind of caring that is the essential aspect of nursing (Watson, 1988).

Psychiatric–mental health nursing also has addressed the issue of transforming nursing education. SERPN (1994) developed a position paper on essential competencies and skills for generalist and advanced psychiatric–mental health nursing practice. The focus of this work is on holistic care for clients with mental illness that acknowledges the biological basis of mental illness and truly eliminates the destructive dualism of the mind–body split. Just as the NLN has suggested a curricular revolution, SERPN has identified the need to change the way we think about mental illness that will result in not only improved mental health care but empowerment of psychiatric–mental health nurses.

POLITICAL AND COMMUNICATION SAVVY

An essential aspect of empowerment is an understanding of the political process. The ANA (1993) has published a lobbying handbook to use at the local level to influence federal policy. Nurses, until recently, remained outside the political process. This lack of involvement may have been due to our military and religious roots or to the position of women in contemporary society. Historically, organized nursing separated itself from struggles for equality probably in an effort to be nonthreatening to physicians, hospital administrators, and clients. Even during the suffrage movement for women, nursing did not take an official stand (Reverby, 1987). As our practice began to be changed because of the pressure of other groups on legislators in the 1980s, nursing became involved in the political process. By this time women and minority rights had changed, and this may have influenced nurses to reevaluate their views on political involvement. Political activism has emerged in nursing as a positive force for change, and we are gaining skill in coalition building to truly effect the legislative and social change process.

To effectively influence the public or individuals, nurses need to have exceptional communication skills (see Chapter 6). Psychiatric nurses have always been interested and skilled in communication whether it involves listening to the client or family express feelings or being an advocate within large organizations and institutions. Awareness of one's own communication style, strengths, and weaknesses is essential. Caring about the effect of the messages one sends puts the responsibility on the sender for what the receiver of the message hears.

COLLABORATION, INTERDISCIPLINARY TEAMS, AND THE CONSUMER

As a member of the mental health team, the nurse can exhibit leadership skills by advocating for the patient and family while collaborating with both. The nurse, as Benner and Wrubel (1989) pointed out, acts as a cultural guide or interpreter of the mental health care facility. The nurse also serves in the "in-between" position in the group that includes the clients, family, and health care team. Bishop and Scudder (1990) identified this position as privileged, that is, a position in which the nurse can minister to the client's needs that demand extremely close contact, enter into the client's and family's experience of mental illness, and also act as an intermediary with all concerned participants in the care of this client. We also provide support and caring sometimes covertly, as we empower people to take charge of their lives.

Before the consumer movement that began in the 1970s, health professionals gave little thought to consumer concerns or demands. The general idea was that professionals knew what was best for the person with mental illness; consumers and families had few avenues to question the decisions made in this paternalistic fashion (Hatfield, 1990). Consumers of mental health now are included in clinical decisions (treatment planning) as well as programs that train mental health professionals. The client's perception of the care he or she received is made available to students through direct interactions or panel discussions.

Models of care that include consumers, advocates, significant others, and families are in their infancy. Most are based on redefining mental illness as illnesses with symptoms that need treatment (Hatfield, 1990). Consumers and families can provide insight into the nature of these symptoms and their management by sharing their experiences with students and practicing nurses. The nurse must understand these experiences to grasp the profound meanings consumers and families have gleaned from their day-to-day life. Various family theorists have tried to describe families, some with the motivation of assigning cause for psychopathology to families. Hatfield (1990) wrote, "It is our view that while each of the traditional theories of mental illness and the family provided new ways to label and describe families, they have contributed little to the understanding of these families" (p. 149).

When a family member is diagnosed with a mental illness, both the client and family experience a great deal of stress. Nurses, as members of the mental health team, often have the most direct contact with the client and their family because, as Virginia Henderson so aptly stated, the nurse is the "24-hour person" (1991). To best assess how families cope with this stressful situation, the nurse must identify the meaning the consumer and their family attaches to this stress and whether or not they believe they can cope with it. Nurses must never assume that the nurse's viewpoint is the same as that of the consumer and family.

The consumer of mental health care services is a vital member of the health care team. The perspective introduced by this client is one that no outside consultant can provide. Can an outside viewpoint describe the effects of psychoactive medications or what it is like to be placed in restraints? A client with brief reactive psychosis describes her feelings in the accompanying display.

Nurses play a major role in the care of seriously and persistently mentally ill clients. As new neurobiological treatments emerge, more nurses will be needed not only to monitor these therapies but to design new nursing interventions as well. Families and clients need psychoeducation so that they may participate in their care

THE CLIENT EXPERIENCING BRIEF REACTIVE PSYCHOSIS

I could hear someone saying they were only trying to help me. All I could feel was that I had to fight because I was tied down [restraints were being used] and being tortured [an intravenous catheter was being placed]. I whispered to my husband to help. He told me to stop fighting. I felt hopeless. After several days, I decided to escape or kill myself. Someone was poisoning me; I could feel myself slipping away [antipsychotic medication was started]. Then I heard your voice [nurse consultant's voice]. You told me I was in the hospital, and you explained it all to me. I began to have hope that this torture would end—that I would be rescued. [At this point the medication had become effective and the psychiatric consultation-liaison nurse had begun the consultation process.]

to the fullest extent possible. Mental health problems that do not fit into this category can be viewed as problems in living that need guidance and advice (Maxman, 1985). Nurses have always assumed a major role in providing anticipatory guidance during periods of transition, such as when a baby is born or a loved one dies. In addition, nurses traditionally have provided counseling in various health care settings and situations. This role of counselor will expand as the nation moves toward an emphasis on prevention of health problems.

ASSERTIVENESS AND CONFIDENCE IN CLINICAL SETTINGS

To provide health care in the ways previously discussed, the nurse needs to be assertive in the clinical setting and confident in the necessary competencies and skills. Helping and caring for others are the essential core of professional nursing. Often this core is viewed to be in conflict with assertive behaviors when goals are achieved through direct and effective communication of one's needs, desires, and wishes; however, **assertiveness** is essential to nursing in that the nurse acts as protector of, advocate for, and consultant to the client and the family.

Assertiveness skills can be learned by the nurse and in turn taught to others. The results of such learning and teaching are increased self-worth and decreased helplessness and hopelessness in the nurse. Preservation of self-respect and dignity is inherent in assertion behaviors.

INTEGRATING LEADERSHIP SKILLS IN NURSING CURRICULA

Nursing curricula contain both content and process. Educators have debated and written about what should be included as content in nursing programs, but until recently, little attention has been given to the process of educating nurses. A group of educators sponsored by the NLN has increased the dialogue about process in nursing education (NLN, 1988, 1989).

One factor that this group has identified as being counterproductive to the goals of creating nurses who are prepared to lead is the power relationship between faculty and student previously mentioned by Watson (1988). Nursing has set up its model of teaching in much the same way health care has set up its power relationships. The client has the least knowledge and power, the physician has the most, and nurses are somewhere in between—sometimes they are powerless, and sometimes they are powerful, depending on the situation. These relationships are based on one person as the elite expert and the other as the powerless unknowledgeable seeker. Students of nursing are treated as if they are powerless and lack basic knowledge.

Today's health care system requires that all involved persons become empowered to assume more responsibility for what they must do. Zander (1988) stated that the best way to empower nurses is through changing their roles to increase their authority. This empowerment must be initiated at the beginning of the educational program with more democratic relationships between faculty and students. If all of those involved in education view each other as learners with some more senior (faculty) than others (students), we can focus on human development of both rather than development of the curriculum (NLN, 1988).

Finally, we must look at the effect of nursing education on students, faculty, and health care in general. If we fail to nurture our students, what kind of nurses will they become? What does it do to faculty to maintain outmoded power relationships? Ultimately, a program can be judged only by the impact its graduates have had on the health of the community. To accomplish our goal of access to basic services, decreasing the disparities among all people and emphasizing the prevention of health problems, we must foster the empowerment of nurses, starting with the day they decide to become a nurse.

TRENDS AND DIRECTIONS FOR RESEARCH IN PSYCHIATRIC–MENTAL HEALTH NURSING

Several trends in psychiatric–mental health nursing have been identified, including biological psychiatry, family partnerships, consumerism, quality improvement, and the role of stress in illness. These areas also warrant further research. In addition, most authors agree that (1) there is a decrease in the number of nurses who select psychiatric–mental health nursing as a specialty; (2) the explosion of knowledge in the area of neurobiology will change psychiatric–mental health nursing practice; and (3) the setting and model of care will evolve into a new entity (Pothier et al., 1990).

THE DECADE OF THE BRAIN

In the 1980s, NAMI provided such a powerful argument for a focused effort to determine the cause of severe mental illness through brain science that Congress declared the 1990s to be the Decade of the Brain. Leaders in psychiatric–mental health nursing have tried to redefine the specialty role and responsibility as new knowledge has evolved relating to how the brain functions and what happens to a person's behavior when it malfunctions. The destructive mind–body split (see Chapter 12) has been replaced with a more helpful and hopeful integration of the human being. As Goodwin (1993) stated, "As framed today, the question is not 'disordered brain chemicals' versus 'environmental deprivation' but rather how biological vulnerability might contribute to a person's response to environmental inputs—and vice versa" (p. 32). Of the four mental health core disciplines—psychiatric nursing, psychiatry, social work, and psychology—nursing appears to have a solid biopsychosocial foundation upon which to address the interaction of vulnerable biological processes with environmental influences. Work in the area of psychoneuroimmunology has provided a foundation for nursing's value and belief of looking at the whole person within the environment (see Chapter 29).

BIOLOGICAL PSYCHIATRY

Babich (1992) stated that because of their education, nurses bridge the gap between biological and psychodynamic approaches to mental health and illness. The biological and genetic aspects of humans interplay with the environmental, cultural, educational, and developmental aspects to create a complex understanding of mental illness. For a detailed discussion of the biobehavioral interface, see the causative factors sections in previous chapters of this book.

Faced with new knowledge from the neurosciences, nurses must broaden their views of biobehavior. New ways of thinking about mental illness necessitate new approaches to nursing care. A cadre of nurses have been studying and writing about this problem. The numbers of such nurses must be increased through direct effort of the profession. Nurses in practice must become familiar with new knowledge and develop skills to ensure adequate care for their clients. Nursing interventions must be tested to determine their efficacy. The psychiatric–mental health nurse of the future will be concerned with the psyche and the soma. Specialty nurses will focus more on mental status, sleep-wake patterns, nutrition, medications, and environmental manipulation to put the client in the best position to heal in the way first described by Nightingale in the last century.

Nurses are in a better position to do this than some of the other core disciplines of mental health because of our firm foundation in the biopsychosociocultural model of nursing care. Babich (1992) has stated that most mental disorders have a biological basis. This knowledge allows for the discipline of nursing to realign psychiatric nursing into the mainstream of nursing, and with this alignment, old thinking about clients with serious, persistent mental illness must be confronted and changed. The need to stigmatize people with mental illness no longer exists if alterations in biology are the source of bizarre behavior.

PARTNERSHIPS IN HEALTH CARE: NURSES, CLIENTS, AND FAMILIES

A partner is one who is associated with another or others in an activity or a sphere of common interest. In the context of mental health care, the nurse enters into partnership with the client and family to work toward a common goal of alleviating troublesome symptoms and improving the quality of life for all involved. The most effective and efficient way of accomplishing this goal is to decide what each person's role and responsibility is in the partnership. For example, if the nurse is working with a suicidal client, a "no suicide" contract is negotiated in which each person is assured of the role and responsibility of the other. The client's responsibility is to report suicidal ideation in an agreed-on manner and to not act on the urge to commit suicide. The family's role and responsibility may be to ask the client about suicidal intent and to call the crisis intervention team in case of emergency. The nurse will provide the necessary education on suicide, help the client and family develop a plan for intervention, see the client as indicated, and provide emergency care if needed. In this manner, each person knows the role and responsibility of the others and can live day to day in the knowledge that all that can be done for the client is being done. All parties must keep their part of the contract, and the contract is subject to renegotiation whenever any of the parties requests it.

Families are a major source of strength in the lives of clients with mental illness. Nurses who work with the client and family together can tap into this strength. To work effectively, the nurse must share power and knowledge with the client and family. Families have found satisfaction in collaborating with mental health professionals who respect the family's role in caregiving for the person with mental illness (Hatfield, 1990). The nurse can increase in effectiveness by listening to the client and the family and learning about mental illness from them. From this dialogue, the nurse can glean information that can help in developing and implementing psychoeducation about topics the client and family may need clarified. In partnership, all parties can provide expertise and, in turn, each will benefit from the partnership and become more effective in alleviating symptoms and improving the quality of life for the client, the family, and the nurse.

On local, state, and national levels, nurses, clients, and families work in partnership to ensure that adequate resources are available for clients with serious mental illness. Prevention of mental health problems is included in this partnership and is addressed in the final section of this chapter.

CONSUMERISM

The *American Heritage Dictionary* (1992) defines a consumer as "one that acquires goods or services." **Consumerism** is "the movement seeking to protect and inform consumers by requiring such practices as honest packaging . . . and improved safety standards" (p. 405). The consumers of mental health services and their families have made policymakers and clinicians aware of their rights.

Consumers and their families had been quieter in the past when bad parenting, character flaws, and sinful behavior were thought to be the cause of mental illness (Flynn, 1993). Families feared judgment and censure if they dared to complain about the poor care and treatment their relatives received in institutions for the mentally ill. When biological bases for schizophrenia and bipolar disorder were discovered, families eagerly educated themselves and began to feel more justified in demanding improved treatment for their members.

Consumerism has had a profound effect on mental health services. The recent passage of Public Law 99-660 reflects its continued influence (Flynn, 1993). This law requires a variety of advocacy mechanisms to ensure quality care for the mentally ill, and it mandates the states to develop comprehensive living arrangements for people with serious mental illness. Advisory councils that oversee this effort for each state are required to have consumers and families appointed to them. These plans are to be reviewed by the National Institute of Mental Health (NIMH) for adequacy. The 102nd Congress went farther and made state block grants available to fund the developed plans (Flynn, 1993).

CONTINUOUS QUALITY IMPROVEMENT

In the past, quality assurance of care was left up to committees, which determined whether care met some agreed-on standard. If care was found to be flawed, steps were taken to improve it. It was assumed that the people delivering the care could not be trusted to ensure its quality; therefore, overseers brought in for periodic inspection were used to make sure that standards were met (Gilliam, 1988). This practice often resulted in attention to quality issues just before and after inspection; it was not expected that ongoing efforts would be made to improve quality. This situation was not conducive to professional practice.

Because mental health care did not attune itself to the needs of the consumer and those with health insurance quickly reached their policy limits, consumers of mental health services eventually became dependent on the state for their care. State services were usually underfunded and overburdened. Quality improvement in these institutions was more of a luxury rather than a necessity. The consumer and family suffered because of this situation.

A new approach to quality assurance has been injected into health care that has resulted in more emphasis on each nurse's responsibility for quality care. This method is revolutionary in its philosophy. The change has come about as a result of economic forces and consumer demands in this country. Couple that with impending health care reform and change is unavoidable. Gilliam (1988) wrote,

> *In the new age of health care, total quality will be the way one hospital differentiates itself from another. In the future, the prices people pay for a given level of service will be more or less equal, and the way to distinguish the services of one hospital from those of another will be based largely on quality and the value of those services. (p. 21)*

The same could be said for any health care service associated with a hospital. With health care reform, people who have traditionally gone to county, state, or federal facilities because of their inability to pay for private services will now have the means to choose their health care facility and provider. This change gives the consumer a tremendous amount of power. All service providers will have to compete for clients. No longer can agencies use overcrowding as a reason not to deliver prompt services. Providers who may have lacked compassion or "bedside manner" but were assured an abundance of clients because they were the major provider of public care may find themselves without people for whom to care. People will go where they get the quality of caring for which they have longed.

To avoid loss of clients, hospitals and other agencies have begun to look at ways to improve the quality of their care and thus the perception of their customers. Many have adopted a system that empowers the person directly involved in an activity to make changes to improve their work that will result in customer satisfaction, whether the customers are clients, physicians, nurses, or third-party payers of health services. Many have adopted **continuous quality improvement,** or total quality management, a method developed by Deming (1982), an American who consulted with the Japanese after World War II (his method is based on 14 points [Table 32–1]). Deming's recommendations for quality control were adopted and contributed to the fact that today Japanese goods are known for their durability and quality.

NAMI has published several reports that are of interest here. The first, *Care of the Seriously Mentally Ill: A Rating of State Programs* (Torrey, 1990), uses various indicators to evaluate each state's mental health services and is published every 2 years. The second is a

TABLE 32-1
Deming's 14 Points for Total Quality Management

Create constancy of purpose for service improvement
Adopt the new philosophy
Cease dependence on inspection to achieve quality
End practice of awarding business on price alone—make partners out of vendors
Constantly improve every process for planning, production, and service
Institute training and retraining on the job
Institute leadership for system improvement
Drive out fear
Break down barriers between staff areas
Eliminate slogans, exhortations, and targets for the work force
Eliminate numerical quotas for the work force and numerical goals for the management
Remove barriers to pride of workmanship
Institute a vigorous program of education and self-improvement for everyone
Put everyone to work on transformation

Data from Walton, M.K. (1986). *The Deming management method.* New York: Dodd, Mead & Co.

1992 study funded by NAMI on the use of jails to contain people with serious mental illness entitled *Criminalizing the Seriously Mentally Ill: The Abuse of Jails as Mental Hospitals* (Torrey, 1992). When NAMI families were surveyed, it was discovered that 40 percent of their relatives with mental illness had been jailed at one time or another because of symptoms of their illnesses (Flynn, 1993). By publishing these documents, NAMI educates the public and, as a result, citizens are prompted to support better funding for mental health care.

Continuous quality improvement places the responsibility for improving care to the mentally ill directly on the provider of services. The provider of services ranges from the housekeeper who ensures a safe, clean environment to the professional nurse who determines the needs for intervention for the client. No longer can either say it was not his or her job to worry about the client's experience. Each member of the health care team is expected to be concerned about the care delivered and to suggest and implement changes that improve its quality.

In 1994, the ANA (1994a, 1994b) identified standards of professional performance for psychiatric–mental health nursing. Standard I establishes that the psychiatric–mental health nurse must systematically evaluate the quality of care and effectiveness of practice. The rationale for this standard is that this specialty has its own body of knowledge derived from research and practice that provides the means and impetus to improve the care delivered. This standard will be measured by appropriate nursing activities based on each nurse's education, role, and work setting. Activities include identification of aspects of care that should be monitored, like consumer satisfaction, functional status, symptom management, health behaviors, and quality of life. Indicators will be monitored for effectiveness through use of the nurse process and working with multidisciplinary teams. Quality of care results will be documented and used by the nurse to make changes in personal practice, team activities, and the mental health care system.

Client and family satisfaction with services should be one of the quality indicators that is included in every aspect of care. As health care has moved out of hospitals and into community agencies and the home, clients and families have assumed more and more responsibility for the treatment of mental illness. Because professionals have less contact with clients and their families have more, both parties must actually be included in treatment planning if they are to be important members of the mental health care team. Therefore, satisfaction with treatment options and services is essential information for nurses to obtain.

THE ROLE OF STRESS, COPING, AND ADAPTATION

Stress is known to play a role in the development of some mental disorders. Chrousos and Gold (1992) reviewed the literature in stress and stress system disorders by looking at original articles of controlled studies with sound methodologies from the basic and human sciences. Dysregulation of the stress system results in numerous disorders. If the system activity increased, the results ranged from panic disorder, anorexia nervosa, addictions to alcohol or drugs, and premenstrual disorders. Decreased activity in the stress system resulted in Cushing's disease, seasonal and atypical depressions, obesity, inflammatory disorders, and post-traumatic stress disorders. The authors concluded that dysregulation of the stress system can lead to "a number of health problems of enormous impact to society" (p. 1249).

Nurses have long focused on mediating the effects of stress. Emphasis on recognizing stress and its effects has led to a large body of literature on stress reduction techniques. Benner and Wrubel (1989) discussed the phenomena of stress and coping and their relationships to health and illness. More rigorous study of nursing interventions for stress mediation and teaching of coping strategies should be the focus of nursing research in the future. The role of the stress response on immune function is of particular interest as identified by the National Institute of Nursing Research (1993) for its 5-year agenda for research funding.

THE IMPACT OF TECHNOLOGY ON PSYCHIATRIC–MENTAL HEALTH NURSING PRACTICE

TECHNOLOGY AND CARING

Caring is the essential activity of nursing. Some authors have dichotomized human caring and the use of technology. For example, Hall and Allen (1985) stated that the disease model and the health model nurses use cannot coexist in the same profession. They went so far as to suggest that the discipline of nursing be split into two professions, one called "healthing" and the other still to be called "nursing" if these models cannot be reconciled. Watson (1988) has warned of the tendency in nursing to dichotomize. Examples of dichotomies in nursing are research and practice, theory and practice, wellness and illness, and mind and body. When dichotomies are overused, common ground for agreement cannot be found.

We live in an age of technology, and this fact has influenced us in many ways. It behooves us to question the use of technology, but it seems unreasonable to eliminate it because the use of that technology can improve the caring aspect of the nursing profession. Some issues that arise with the use of technology are ethical, and some are practical.

NURSING INFORMATICS

Gorn (1983) defined informatics as computer science plus information science. ***Nursing informatics*** refers to the use of computer and information sciences to manage and process data, knowledge, and information in nursing practice and client care (Graves & Corcoran, 1989). Information is viewed as data, objective bits of fact, that are organized and interpreted. Informatics allows for the clustering and arranging of data so that information may be efficiently organized. Data can then be processed to yield useful information that can lead to meaning in clinical practice.

One possibility for using nursing informatics is in clinical decision making. Gottlieb (1989) addressed the various mental health specialties and diversity in their practice. This author stated that in the explosion of technology and information, some means of aiding human judgment in decision making is needed.

Three theories are described: information processing, decision rule, and social judgment. In information processing, cues, hypotheses, and information search units are used to test and reject hypotheses. Expert systems have been developed for use in the clinical areas. These are computers systems and artificial intelligence systems that can provide input to the clinician in decision making. Expert systems are only as good as the experts who provide data to them, however. This seems to be one way the mental health specialists could provide information to generalists for use in their decision making.

The other commonly used theory in mental health is the decision rule. The classifications systems of the *Diagnostic and Statistical Manual of Mental Disorders* and the North American Nursing Diagnosis Association (NANDA) are based on this theory, which uses decision analysis and decision trees to articulate the decision process. Risks and potential interventions are highlighted (Gottlieb, 1989). Inherent problems in using this theory are that mental health problems are complex and specific to the individual. Mistakes can be made, particularly if the cultural context is not taken into account.

Social judgment theory was not found to be useful with computers because it presents a problem and then asks for experts to weigh individual pieces of data as to their importance in solving the problem. Principal use of this method is to decide how information is used, not what decision was made. This method has not been widely used in psychiatric research (Gottlieb, 1989).

COMPUTERIZED DOCUMENTATION AND CONFIDENTIALITY

The use of computers for documentation in psychiatry, particularly psychiatric services within general hospitals, has lagged behind that in the other areas because of concerns expressed about confidentiality. The danger of access to computerized information and the known potential for computer "hackers" to find passwords for entrance into records has been foremost in these arguments. Because mental illness has been stigmatized, access to information that a person has been treated for mental illness has led to loss of jobs, marriages, and custody of children. Much adverse publicity has accompanied the release of information on politicians or celebrities who have been treated for depression, suicide attempts, or drug and alcohol addictions, so the real fear of discovery of mental illness has not been exaggerated.

CONTINUITY OF CARE AND ELIMINATING DUPLICATION OF SERVICES

There are many positive aspects to introducing computers into psychiatric–mental health nursing. The greatest benefit will be continuity of care from community-based programs to the hospital and back to the community. Many problems arise because of the lack of continuous quality care. Clients may find themselves being reassessed every time they move into a new setting, which may disturb their previous care and medication regimens. Sometimes services are duplicated, so the community-based service may have drawn blood samples and taken radiographs and the client incurs the unnecessary expense of repeating these tests when hospitalized. This duplication not only leads to increased costs but it also affects client trust in the system. Links between services could be facilitated by the increased use of computers.

Quality improvement indicators can be tracked with computers. Continuous care issues that arise when the client transfers from the hospital to the community can be monitored so that clients do not become lost to followup services. Linkages between systems can be facilitated through computer networks when clients and their families are included in the network. Nurses who have experience in collaborating with clients and their families can be instrumental in working out this linkage to ensure quality of services.

COMPUTER NETWORKS

Provider access to state-of-the-science information is possible through computer networks even in remote areas. Some of these, such as computer networks on information about psychoactive drugs, are already available. These networks can be helpful to clinicians in rural areas where specialists are unavailable, but the clinicians must not discount their own experience and knowledge when employing an information system.

Other uses for computers include researcher networks such as Internet and Bitnet. These networks are available for any subscriber and can link the work of many independent researchers with others with similar interests. Common problems can be addressed through network dialogue.

Computer networks for consumers and families have been used with increasing regularity in the last decade. Some nurses have been interested in the effects of such networks. People with human immunodeficiency virus (HIV) disease linked up early in the epidemic to discuss their condition and get up-to-date information about the current trends in treatment. Beginning interests in networks for people who have mental disorders are evident. Nurses can play a role in psychoeducation and learning from those who have these disorders by joining in computer networks and entering the interaction.

PROMOTION OF PSYCHIATRIC–MENTAL HEALTH ACROSS THE LIFE SPAN

Another factor that will influence nursing practice in the future is the addition of new groups at risk for mental illness. Traditional groups have been those with acute and chronic mental illnesses; new vulnerable groups are infants exposed to noxious substances (like cocaine) in utero, children and adolescents with behavior disorders and developmental disabilities, people with HIV disease and their families, substance abusers, women and children survivors of family violence, and the elderly with psychiatric problems. Nurses have focused on the needs of populations at risk for health deviations and have worked with communities for social change that would result in healthy citizens.

PREVENTION CONCEPTS

The NIMH developed a plan for prevention of mental disorders with a focus on current state of the science, training of mental health professionals in prevention, and future directions for prevention research. Shea (1991) submitted a report to the NIMH on the role of nursing in prevention research. In this report the author stated that nursing historically has been involved with integrating prevention of disease with the restoration of health, yet it was not identified by NIMH for its strengths and potential contributions to the national prevention effort.

The nursing profession is ready to provide leadership in meeting this challenge as evidenced by its interest in prevention, the number of people in the discipline who have specialized knowledge and skills in this area, and its support for nursing research at the national level. Identifying the potential nurses have for meeting the nation's need for prevention of mental disorders is but the tip of the iceberg of what the profession has to offer.

Concepts most associated with prevention are vulnerability, developmental processes that may lead to pathological outcomes, and epidemiological orientation (NIMH, 1991).

Vulnerability

Vulnerability refers to potential susceptibility of a person, family, or group to a health deviation. In evaluating vulnerability, the environment and a person's interaction with it should also be considered. For example, a person may have a high risk for developing depression because of characteristics of serotonin release or inhibition. However, if the environment interacts with the person so that loss is not experienced or appropriate interventions are provided when loss is experienced, depression may not occur.

Developmental Stage

Nurses have long been concerned with human development across the life span (Fawcett, 1986). Developmental theories, models, and interventions have been developed and implemented with various populations with some success. One area of concern for nurses has centered on adolescence as a stressful period of development. This age group experiences dramatic changes during puberty, including hormonal changes that greatly influence emotions and mood, establishes new roles with parents and peers, and deals with pressure to conform with peers. Some problems associated with adolescence are drug and alcohol abuse, pregnancy, and violence. For more information on disorders and behaviors across the life span, see the life span issues section of other chapters in this text. Nurses have begun to develop and test strategies to prevent long-lasting problems related to adolescent behaviors. Psychiatric nurses subspecialize in working with children and adolescents—many more are needed than the approximately 574 currently certified as specialists in this area.

Epidemiological Orientation

Nursing and epidemiology were developed concurrently (Shea, 1991). Florence Nightingale first described modern nursing as focused on health and illness. In a paper issued at the 1893 World's Fair, Nightingale wrote, "Sick nursing and health nursing . . . nursing proper is . . . to help the patient suffering from disease to live—just as health nursing is to keep or put the constitution of the healthy child or human being in such a state as to have no disease'' (Nightingale, 1894, p. 446). The use of statistical data to track health and illness was first employed by Nightingale, and nurses have followed her leadership in this practice. The discipline has used a biological, psychological, social, and cultural model of human beings that addresses the environment and the person–environment interaction as a source to define health and pathogical states.

PSYCHIATRIC NURSING'S ROLE IN MEETING NATIONAL HEALTH CARE GOALS

HEALTHY PEOPLE 2000

Healthy People 2000 (USDHHS) was developed and published by the federal government in 1990. The document responds to a call by the World Health Organization for each nation to set forth goals for the health of its population for the next decade. The United States was not the first nation to develop national health care goals; in fact, it was one of the last to do so. Goals were developed that are aimed at three broad areas:

- Increase the span of healthy life for Americans
- Reduce health disparities among Americans
- Achieve access to preventive services for all Americans

Twenty-two priority areas were identified in their order of importance to American health (Table 32–2). Included in these priorities are issues of interest to the psychiatric–mental health nurse, such as alcohol and drug use, mental health and mental disorders, and violent and abusive behaviors. Many of the other identified objectives have mental health implications as well.

Age-related objectives and objectives for special populations are also identified in *Healthy People 2000* (USDHHS). Special populations are of particular interest to those in psychiatric–mental health nursing because they include cultural minorities, people living in poverty, and people with disabilities. The last two groups are known to have large numbers of people with mental problems who are inadequately treated.

What is the psychiatric–mental health nurse's responsibility in relation to the goals of *Healthy People 2000?* The focus of the nation's goals are health promotion, health protection, preventive services, and surveillance and data systems. We have both specialist and generalist skills with which to respond to the goals and objectives for the nation's health. Nurses practicing in all areas of psychiatric–mental health should develop knowledge and skills needed to respond to people in stigmatized, impoverished, and isolated groups (Krauss, 1993). As a professional group we must educate ourselves as to the needs of citizens, then assume an active role in helping groups meet their goals for a healthy life.

Psychiatric–mental nursing has already directed its energy toward developing knowledge, skills, and models of care that can address the nation's goals. The ANA set forth goals for the development of new knowledge in relevant areas. More can be done to address the needs of people with serious, persistent mental illness. Outcomes of care must be assessed through rigorous methods, including comprehensive assessments of quality of life and patient satisfaction.

The NINR (1993) has also set forth an agenda for research that must be evaluated in light of the goals for the nation's health. Nurse scientists must rapidly move into areas of health promotion and disease prevention. Some of this is already established; examples include Pender's work on health promotion. More must be done in the area of mental health in particular.

TABLE 32–2
Priority Areas for America: *Healthy People 2000*

HEALTH PROMOTION
Physical activity and fitness
Nutrition
Tobacco
Alcohol and other drugs
Family planning
Mental health and mental disorders
Violent and abusive behaviors
Educational and community-based services
HEALTH PROTECTION
Unintentional injuries
Occupational safety and health
Environmental health
Food and drug safety
Oral health
PREVENTIVE SERVICES
Maternal and infant health
Heart disease and stroke
Cancer
Diabetes and chronic disabling conditions
Human immunodeficiency virus infection
Sexually transmitted diseases
Immunization and infectious diseases
Clinical preventive services
DATA SYSTEMS
Surveillance and data systems
AGE-RELATED OBJECTIVES
Infants–children–maternal care
Adolescents and young adults
Adults
Older adults
THE NATION'S HEALTH: SPECIAL POPULATIONS
People with low income
People in minority groups—Hispanics, African, and Asian Americans
People with disabilities
GOALS FOR THE NATION
Increase the span of healthy life for Americans
Reduce health disparities among Americans
Achieve access to preventive services for all Americans

Data from U.S. Department of Health and Human Services. (1990). *Healthy people 2000* (DHHS Publication No. DHS 91-50212). Washington, DC: U.S. Government Printing Office.

IDENTIFYING POPULATIONS AT RISK

One area for intensive effort is promotion of healthy, nonabusive environments for children. The school nurse should be involved not only with the school-age child but also with the day care centers that increasingly care for children from early infancy and later. Avance in San Antonio is one such program that combines child care with parent education for families at risk for health deviations. Mothers tend to be young, single, uneducated, and impoverished. Mothers and their children are nurtured through intensive community effort to help the family escape poverty and improve their quality of life.

Other examples may be drug awareness programs aimed at parents and children. These have had some success in reducing drug use in children. Community-based programs can best meet these needs for a comprehensive, holistic approach to health (Krauss, 1993). The nurse must recognize the interaction between the environment and behavior. The nurse must have the skills to work effectively with the community to address its needs.

Packaged health promotion programs are not helpful in this situation. For example, cholesterol screening may be viewed as a waste of time in an area where poverty prevents adequate nutrition. Even if the nurse can show the need for such a program, if the community perceives greater needs, the nurse will fail. Experienced nurses have always valued addressing the community's concerns first and then educating the group to additional areas for improvement.

CASE MANAGEMENT

Several models of nursing care delivery have been suggested to change the access, effectiveness, and choice in mental health care. Primary mental health care must be available to the population across the life span.

Case management is most often described as being the most promising of models (Krauss, 1993; Mundinger, 1984). Professional nurses are the most appropriate case managers for clients with mental disorders; however, they are underused, and case managers who are less well prepared are employed. Two specific reasons are cited most often to support using professional nurses more in the future: (1) the lack of general health care provided for the seriously, persistently mentally ill (Worley et al., 1990) and (2) the widespread use of psychoactive medications for treatment of most mental disorders (Pittman, 1989). Nurses, by virtue of their education, are grounded in a tradition of holistic care. Such an approach can eliminate the fragmented care prevalent today if assessment is based on the total client, family, and environment to determine the need for interventions (Pittman, 1989). Professional nursing care is often limited by policies made by those people more concerned with immediate cost savings than prevention of problems. Professional nurses must assert themselves to provide adequate, appropriate care for each client.

The case management model of care is potentially valuable in meeting the needs of people who have mental disorders (Lear et al., 1991). The two types of case management most often described in the literature are the "broker of services" model and the "therapeutic" case management model (Goering et al., 1988).

In the first model, the case manager focuses on determining which needs each client may have and then securing these services from a variety of sources. The case manager may come from various disciplines or be trained on the job in the skills required to broker services.

The second type of case manager acts as the client's and family's source of support. A therapeutic relationship is developed and maintained as a basis for on-going support. When the need for additional services is identified, the therapeutic case manager selects and oversees the provision of these services. Overall assessment and management remain with the case manager. This type of case management model has the following characteristics:

- A higher level of professional education is required.
- It takes intense effort and skill to develop and maintain the therapeutic relationship.
- The relationship is expected to last over a long period.

The therapeutic model would be more effective with people who are seriously and persistently mentally ill. The trust level among client, family, and case manager will gradually increase and strengthen over time. Professional nurses are well prepared to distinguish between exacerbation of mental disorders and development of new symptoms of other illnesses. Emergence of new symptoms is often ignored or overlooked by those less skilled in working with clients (Holmberg, 1988). For example, it has been shown that 46.2 percent of people with psychiatric illness have unmet needs for care of their physical disorders (Flynn, 1993).

Professional nurses are also knowledgeable in following clients in the community, whether the client is in a homeless shelter or in the home of their family. It takes the combination of psychiatric–mental health and community–home health nurses to deliver holistic, comprehensive, effective care to this population.

What nurses have not done is systematically study the effectiveness of nurses as care managers. This area of research is greatly needed if nurses are to be involved in care of the seriously, persistently mentally ill. All nurses in the psychiatric–mental health specialty can cite anecdotal information on the ineffectiveness of non–nurse case management models. We have seen people in the emergency centers who are exhibiting the effects of the broker-type case manager's failure to recognize dystonia or akathisia. We have seen people who are in acute pain from broken bones who are noted to have "delusions" of physical illness by their case managers. We have also seen emergency medical personnel who have failed to distinguish between delirium and dementia or have not recognized delirium tremens in psychiatric clients. These breakdowns in the system of care delivered to people with mental disorders must be eliminated, and professional nurses should be in the forefront of this effort.

PSYCHOEDUCATION AND ANTICIPATORY GUIDANCE

Anticipatory guidance and health care teaching are methods the professional nurse uses to reduce the risk of disease in vulnerable populations. Psychiatric–mental health nurses have thought of psychoeducation of clients and families during healthy periods as well as illness as one of their primary roles and responsibilities. Anticipatory guidance has been centered on stressful situational and developmental life events like natural disasters or child birth and adolescence. Examples of anticipatory guidance are given in many chapters throughout this textbook in the section on life span issues. Psychoeducation is most often used for specific health issues such as coping with rape and sexual assault and medication or social skills training.

The profession can have a positive impact on the nation's health through efforts that provide anticipatory guidance and psychoeducation for populations at risk. More research on the issues of the specific type of intervention needed during which period in the life span for which high-risk group should be conducted. For example, when do we provide education about topics such as alcohol and drug use, sexual behaviors, transitions during the life span, and psychopathology?

When prevention strategies fail, psychiatric–mental health nurses must be available to provide care to those experiencing addiction, teen pregnancy, and violence (both perpetrators and survivors). We must work with policymakers to address social problems that lead to increased failures in prevention for vulnerable groups.

PSYCHOACTIVE MEDICATION MANAGEMENT

Another set of knowledge and skills available through professional nurses is the management of clients who are taking psychoactive medication. Nurses have skills that help the client assume self-care responsibilities in terms of symptom management and adherence to the medication regimen that will prevent exacerbation of illness (Zander, 1988). Nurses are also experienced in working with families, who assume care for two thirds of clients discharged from psychiatric hospitals (Flynn, 1993).

►CHAPTER SUMMARY

Leaders in psychiatric–mental health nursing have speculated on what the specialty will need in terms of knowledge and skills for the next century. Some trends have been discussed in this chapter. The trend toward a real integration of the biological, psychological, sociological, and cultural aspects of human beings into a holistic entity that cannot be reduced into its parts has been predicted. Nurses in the specialty will provide holistic care in primary, secondary, and tertiary settings. Pothier (1990) stated that

> *The core of psychiatric nursing will still be the use of ourselves in therapeutic relationships, but the goal of our encounters will be to assist patients and their families in living and functioning better with chronic disorders, rather than emphasizing psychotherapy in the traditional sense. (p. 77)*

Leininger (1992) has predicted more emphasis on a "multicultural world." Common sense and theories of the dominant culture will not work. This author and theorist warned that knowledge and skills in transcultural health must predominate. Nurses must enter the world of the client and thereby come to know different cultural groups and their norms. We must not assume that Western psychiatric knowledge is valid in other cultures.

Pothier et al. (1990) identified the three trends in psychiatric nursing as (1) a decrease in the number of nurses entering the specialty; (2) the addition of neurobiological content; and (3) the change in setting and models of delivery of care. In light of these changes, drastic measures are needed to ensure adequate numbers of nurses prepared to deliver appropriate care to those in need. This group of authors recommended the formation of a consensus panel of leaders in the field to do the following:

1. Differentiate psychiatric nursing content for curricular development for education
2. Monitor accreditation for reflection of the change in psychiatric nursing care
3. Review standards of psychiatric nursing care and certification guidelines for inclusion of the new trends
4. Work with NANDA's Phenomenon Task Force to develop and test phenomena of concern to psychiatric nursing
5. Advocate that state boards of nursing reflect current knowledge and skills for psychiatric nursing rather than dictate curricular content
6. Encourage deans in schools of nursing to support psychiatric faculty developing ties with similar groups in other schools
7. Ask the deans to fund continuing education for psychiatric faculty to develop new knowledge and skills as it becomes available
8. Support the NIMH task force report on the need for nursing research in the specialty
9. Allow for professional role implementation by changing practice settings from inpatient to outpatient and nontraditional settings like homeless shelters and jails

Some of these recommendations have been or are now being implemented. The effort that is required to effect such broad changes is immense. We are on the brink of change, and such change brings out the best and the worst the profession has to offer. We have the strength of Florence Nightingale, Dorothea Dix, Clara Barton, Lillian Wald, Margaret Sanger and many other nurse heroes within our ranks. We must just step forward with a creative, innovative idea; take the risk of success or failure, but, above all, engage in the struggle to take our rightful place in psychiatric–mental health care.

Suggestions for Clinical Conferences

1. Ask experienced nurses to discuss changes in mental health care they have observed.
2. Have students attend a meeting of a mental health consumer group and discuss this experience with the other members of their student group.
3. Ask a nurse case manager to talk about this role.
4. Discuss the issues associated with the use of computerized information in mental health care.
5. Identify leadership skills in preceptor nurses.

References

American Association of Colleges of Nursing. (1986). *Essentials of college and university education for professional nursing*. Washington, DC: Author.

American Heritage Dictionary of the English Language (3rd ed.). (1992). New York: Houghton Mifflin.

American Nurses Assocation. (1993). *The grassroots lobbying book*. Washington, DC.

American Nurses Association. (1991). *Nursing's agenda for health care reform*. Washington, DC: Author.

American Nurses Association. (1994a). *Standards of psychiatric and mental health nursing practice*. Washington, DC: Author.

American Nurses Association. (1994b). *Statement on psychiatric–mental health nursing*. Washington, DC: Author.

Babich, K. (1992). What is biological psychiatry? *Journal of Psychosocial Nursing and Mental Health Services, 30*(1), 33–35.

Benner, B., & Wrubel, J. (1989). *The primacy of caring: Stress and coping in health and illness*. Menlo Park, CA: Addison-Wesley.

Bishop, A., & Scudder, J. (1990). *The practical, moral, and personal sense of nursing: A phenomenological philosophy of practice*. New York: SUNY Press.

Chrousos, G. P., & Gold, P. W. (1992). The concepts of stress and stress system disorders: Overview of physical and behavioral homeostasis. *Journal of the American Medical Association, 267*(9), 1244–1252.

Deming, W. E. (1982). *Out of the crisis*. Cambridge, MA: Massachusetts Institute of Technology Center for Advanced Engineering Study.

Fawcett, J. (1986). *Analysis and evaluation of conceptual models of nursing*. Philadelphia: FA Davis.

Flynn, L. M. (1993). Political impact of the family–consumer movement. *National Forum, 73*(1), 13–15.

Gilliam, T. R. (1988). Deming's 14 points and hospital quality: Responding to the consumer's demand for the best value health care. *Journal of Quality Assurance, 2*(3), 70–78.

Goering, P. N., Waslenki, D. A., Farkas, M., Lancee, W. J., & Ballantyne, R. (1988). What differences does case management make? *Hospital and Community Psychiatry, 39*, 272–276.

Goodwin, F. K. (1993). New directions for NIMH. *National Forum, 73*(1), 31–33.

Gorn, S. (1983). Informatics (computer and computer science): Its ideology, methodology, and sociology. In F. Machlup & U. Mansfield (Eds.), *The study of information: Indisciplinary messages*, (pp. 121–140). New York: Wiley.

Gottlieb, G. L. (1989). Diversity, uncertainty, and variations in practice: The behaviors and clinical decisionmaking of mental health care providers. In *The future of mental health services research*. (DHHS Publication No. ADM 89-1600). Washington, DC: U.S. Government Printing Office.

Graves, J. R., & Corcoran, S. (1989). An overview of nursing informatics. *Image: The Journal of Nursing Scholarship, 21*, 227–231.

Hall, B. A., & Allen, J. D. (1985). Sharpening nursing's focus by focusing on health. *Nursing & Health Care*, June, 315–320.

Hatfield, A. B. (1990). Incorporating the family's contribution to clinical training. In *Clinical training in serious mental illness* (DHHS Publication NO. ADM 90-1679). Washington, DC: U.S. Government Printing Office.

Henderson, V. A. (1991). *The nature of nursing: Reflections after 25 years*. New York: National League for Nursing.

Holmberg, S. (1988). Physical health problems of the psychiatric client. *Journal of Psychosocial Nursing*, 26 (5), P35–39.

Krauss, J. (1993). *Health Care Reform: Essential Mental Health Services*. Washington, DC: American Nurses' Association.

Lear, G., Morris, G., Parnell, M., & Wharne, S. (1991). Case management: Responding to need. *Nursing Times, 87*(50), 24–26.

Leininger, M. (1992). Psychiatric nursing and transculturalism: Quo vadis? *Perspectives in Psychiatric Care, 28*(1), 3.

Maxman, J. S. (1985). *The new psychiatry*. New York: Morrow.

McBride, A. B. (1990). Psychiatric nursing in the 1990's. *Archives of Psychiatric Nursing, 4*(1), 21–27.

Mundinger, M. O. (1984). Community-based care: Who will be the case managers? *Nursing Outlook, 32*(6), 294–295.

National Institute for Nursing Research. (1993). *Agenda for research*. Bethesda, MD: Author.

National League for Nursing. (1988). *Curriculum revolution: Mandate for change*. New York: Author.

National League for Nursing. (1989). *Curriculum revolution: Reconceptualizing nursing education*. New York: Author.

Nightingale, F. (1984). Sick nursing and health nursing. In J. S. Billingas & Henry Hurd (Eds.), *Hospitals dispensaries and nursing* (p. 446). Baltimore: John Hopkins Press.

Pittman, D. C. (1989). Nursing case management: Holistic care for the deinstitutionalized chronically mentally ill. *Journal of Psychosocial Nursing and Mental Health Services, 27*(11), 23–27.

Pothier, P. C. (1990). Toward a bio/psycho/social synthesis. *Archives of Psychiatric Nursing, 4*(2), 77.

Pothier, P. C., Stuart, G. W., Puskar, K. & Babich, K. (1990). Dilemmas and directions for psychiatric nursing in the 1990's. *Archives of Psychiatric Nursing, 4*(5), 284–291.

Reverby, S. (1987). A caring dilemma: Womanhood and nursing in historical perspective. *Nursing Research, 36*, 5.

Schutzenhofer, K. K. (1992). Essentials for nurses in the year 2000. *NursingConnections, 5*(1), 15–26.

Shea, C. A. (1991). Nursing and prevention research. Submitted to the Panel on Training in Prevention Research, National Institute of Mental Health National Conference on Prevention Research. Washington, DC: American Psychiatric Nurses Association.

Society for Education and Research in Psychiatric–Mental Health Nursing. (1994). *Position paper*. Pensacola, FL: Author.

Torrey, E. (1990). *Care of the seriously mentally ill: A rating of state programs*. Arlington, VA: National Alliance for the Mentally Ill.

Torrey, E. (1992). *Criminalizing the seriously mentally ill: The abuse of jails as mental hospitals*. Arlington, VA: National Alliance for the Mentally Ill.

United States Department of Health and Human Services. (1990). *Healthy people 2000* (DHHS Publication NO. PHS 91-50212). Washington, DC: U.S. Government Printing Office.

Watson, J. (1988). A case study: Curriculum in transition. In *Curriculum revolution: Mandate for change*. New York: National League for Nursing.

Worley, N. K., Drago, L., & Hadley, T. (1990). Improving the physical health–mental health interface: Could nurse managers make a difference? *Archives of Psychiatric Nursing, 4*(2), 108–113.

Zander, K. (1988). Nursing case management: Stragic management of cost and outcomes. *Journal of Nursing Administration, 18*(5), 23–30.

Unit 4 Study Questions

See Appendix I for answers.

CHAPTER 29

1. The "Decade of the Brain" refers to
   a. The focus during the 1950s on psychological aspects of mental disorders.
   b. The current focus on biological aspects of mental disorders.
   c. The period when Freud practiced.
   d. The decade of enormous mental relevance.

2. A major contributor to understanding the biological basis of mental illness is
   a. Freud.
   b. Cannon.
   c. Peplau.
   d. McBride.

3. The hypothalamus
   a. Is the brain center for emotions and various behavior.
   b. Regulates respiration and sleep.
   c. Is involved in controlling body movement and balance.
   d. Mediates sensory and motor impulses.

4. Major functions of behavior include all of the following *except*
   a. Directed toward meeting basic human needs.
   b. Simply a stimulus–response interaction.
   c. Represents various responses to internal and external demands.
   d. Aimed at goal attainment and avoidance.

CHAPTER 30

1. B. D., a 20-year-old male college student, was in a motor vehicle crash 6 months ago. Although his injuries were minor, his friend was killed. He complains to the primary nurse in the trauma clinic of inability to concentrate, insomnia, and thoughts that he is "going crazy." The nurse asks the psychiatric consultation-liaison nurse to perform a psychosocial assessment. The most important information for the PCLN to obtain is
   a. A complete physical and social history.
   b. A complete drug and alcohol history, including reports from a drug screen.
   c. A review of significant events of the past year.
   d. An exploration of how he coped with the motor vehicle accident and his friend's death.

2. The psychiatric consultation-liaison nurse (PCLN) is in the emergency department dealing with a victim of violence. The client has been medically stabilized and will be discharged. The first priority of the PCLN is to
   a. Encourage the client to express her feelings.
   b. Assess for physical trauma.
   c. Provide privacy and safety for the client during the interview.
   d. Help the client identify and mobilize resources and support systems.

3. The nurse is caring for M. L., a 70-year-old woman, with the following symptoms: temperature of 103.4°F, moderate dehydration, bilateral rales in the lower lobes of the lungs, disorientation to time and place, and severe agitation. The nurse contacts the psychiatric consultation-liaison nurse (PCLN) to assist in developing an appropriate, least-restrictive plan of care. The PCLN bases her recommendations on the understanding that
   a. The client is experiencing delirium secondary to the infectious process.
   b. The client is probably displaying early symptoms of Alzheimer's disease.
   c. Older people get confused often as a normal part of the aging process.
   d. A referral to a nursing home for continuing care will be necessary for this client.

4. A medical intensive care unit nurse is caring for O. S., who overdosed on sertraline (Zoloft), lorazepam (Ativan), and acetaminophen (Tylenol PM). The nurse contacts the psychiatric consultation-liaison nurse (PCLN) to assist in determining the client's level of care. O. S. is comatose and not responding to lifesaving and technological care. Which of the following actions are the first priority of PCLN intervention during the first several days of O. S.'s intensive care treatment?
   a. Complete a full psychiatric assessment.
   b. Get in touch with O. S.'s family, and try to involve them in immediate decision making.
   c. Observe and record vital signs frequently, including neurological symptoms.
   d. Determine whether O. S. may need long-term therapy after hospitalization for the overdose.

5. A. V. comes to the emergency department for an assessment of chest pain. As he is about to undergo an electrocardiogram, he says to the nurse, "I am so terribly afraid I am dying, even though I have had this pain before and the doctors can never find anything." Which of the following would be the *best* response for the nurse to make?
   a. "Our doctors here are the best. If there's something wrong, they'll find it."
   b. "Please be calm now so that your test will give us useful information."
   c. "You sound fearful. After the test is over, we can talk more about your feelings."
   d. "Do you think your pain is all in your head?"

CHAPTER 31

1. Which of the following statements is true concerning studies in psychiatric–mental health nursing?
   a. Most of these studies have used qualitative research designs.
   b. These studies are easily identifiable in the literature.
   c. Many of the studies have concerned nurses rather than clients.
   d. Psychiatric nurses have studied mental illness more than mental health.

2. Every psychiatric nurse is expected to carry out which of the following roles in research?
   a. Principal investigator.
   b. Member of a research team.
   c. Data collector.
   d. Critiquer of research findings.

3. Most research in psychiatric nursing has been conducted with which group of clients?
   a. Children.
   b. Adolescents.
   c. Adults.
   d. Elderly.

4. Future research in psychiatric nursing should focus on which of the following areas:
   a. Biological.
   b. Psychosocial.
   c. Interpersonal.
   d. All of the above.

5. Which of the following is a barrier to conducting nursing research with clients who have chronic mental illnesses?
   a. Clients with the same psychiatric diagnosis vary more in their impairment than do clients with the same medical diagnosis.
   b. The number of clients with chronic mental illnesses is decreasing each year.
   c. Nurses do not have access to client populations.
   d. Because of the large number of categories of mental illnesses, nurses are unsure about which client groups to study.

CHAPTER 32

1. When the document *Healthy People 2000* was developed, the impact for psychiatric mental health nursing included
   a. Integrating mental health into health care reform.
   b. Priority areas for research and practice.
   c. Role transformation.
   d. Essentials in mental health care.

2. R. P., age 23, was diagnosed with bipolar disorder 4 years ago. The case manager, a nurse, is concerned about R. V.'s lack of support from peers. To decrease R. V.'s isolation, the nurse refers her client to
   a. A singles club for young adults.
   b. A support group sponsored by the National Alliance for the Mentally Ill.
   c. A psychotherapist who specializes in young people with bipolar disorder.
   d. A church group for young adults.

3. The nurse meets with R. V. every week to assess the effectiveness of the medication and to provide counseling as the need arises. Which type of case manager is this nurse?
   a. Broker of services.
   b. Referral source.
   c. Therapeutic.
   d. Symptom.

4. The psychiatric–mental health nurse in the year 2030 will probably
   a. Be extinct.
   b. Have evolved into a social worker.
   c. Focus more on biobehavior.
   d. Be more like an administrator.

5. As members of a profession, nurses try to keep abreast of current trends in psychiatric nursing. To do this, nurses must
   a. Register for a new course at the local college every year.
   b. Join the professional organization and stay active in the local chapter.
   c. Read the local and state newspapers daily.
   d. Subscribe to at least three journals in the specialty.

Glossary

Absorption: process of movement of a drug from the site of administration to the vascular beds.

Abuse: actions and behaviors that result in serious physical injury, neglect, sexual abuse, and serious mental injury.

Acculturation: pertains to the process by which a given cultural group adapts to or takes on values, beliefs, and attitudes of another group.

Acting out: responding to a current situation as though it were the original one where discharge of drive tension was required; this involves immature responses in situations where higher level responses are now expected.

Action potential: the electrical impulse generated by ionic flow across the cell membrane.

Active listening: a dynamic process that requires using all senses to assess verbal and nonverbal messages.

Activity group therapy theory: groups that include physical activity, such as an exercise group and an occupational therapy outing or project.

Adaptation: sustaining homeostasis; the ability to mobilize resources and adjust to demands of internal and external environments.

Adrenoceptors: also called *adrenalceptors;* refers to the sites in effector nerve cells that are receptors for adrenaline as their neurotransmitter.

Adverse or side effects: any undesired, unintended, and noxious effect of a drug.

Advocacy: defending a cause or pleading a case in another's behalf.

Affect: the visible and audible manifestations of a person's feelings or mood.

Afferent: conducting or progressing toward a center or specific site of reference, as in an afferent nerve.

Against medical advice: an agreement between the physician and the client in which the client is allowed to be discharged but is informed that discharge is against the better judgment of the physician. The client agrees not to make the physician or hospital responsible for any harm that may occur as a result of the discharge.

Agonist: a drug that activates the functional properties of the receptor(s).

Agranulocytosis: an acute condition characterized by a dramatic decrease in the production of granulocytes resulting in neutropenia that leaves the body open to bacterial invasion. It is caused by drugs or chemicals that affect the bone marrow, resulting in depressed formation of granulocytes.

Akathisia: subjective feelings of restlessness and an inability to sit still resulting from dopamine blockade by certain neuroleptics; part of extrapyramidal side effects.

Akinesia: a condition characterized by the inability to make voluntary movements.

Al-Anon: an international self-help support organization composed of family members or friends of persons who have or have had a drug or alcohol problem.

Alcoholics Anonymous (AA): an international self-help support organization composed of persons who have a drinking (or drug) problem.

Alcohol withdrawal delirium: see Delirium tremens (DTs).

Alexithymia: difficulty in identifying inner mood states and giving names to inner feelings.

Alter: any personality fragment that has its own unique motif of perceptions regarding thoughts and relationships with self and others.

Alzheimer's disease: a condition characterized by progressive loss of memory, intellect, language, judgment, and impulse control. Neurofibrillary tangles and neuritic plaques are found in the cerebral cortex, particularly the hippocampus.

American Nurses Association (ANA) *Statement on Psychiatric–Mental Health Clinical Nursing Practice and Standards of Psychiatric and Mental Health Clinical Nursing Practice*: the ANA's statements of standards that specify that nurses must provide, structure, and maintain a therapeutic environment and that advanced-practice expertise is required for functioning as a psychotherapist in individual and group treatment modalities.

Anhedonia: inability to experience pleasure from activities that usually produce pleasurable feelings.

Anima: the feminine aspect of the male personality.

Animus: the masculine aspect of the female personality.

Anorexia nervosa: self-induced starvation resulting from fear of fatness; not due to true loss of appetite.

Antagonist: a drug that interferes with the action of an agonist.

Anticholinergic: an agent that antagonizes the action of acetylcholine, especially within the parasympathetic nervous system.

Anticonvulsants: drugs that suppress convulsions, used in the treatment of extrapyramidal side effects and bipolar disorders.

Antidepressants: a drug for the treatment of the symptoms of depression.

Antipsychotics: drugs used in the management of manifestations of psychotic disorders; also called *neuroleptics* or *major tranquilizers*.

Anxiety: an affect or emotion produced by stress or change accompanied by biological arousal, behavioral responses and elements of apprehension, impending doom, and tension.

Anxiolytics: drugs used for the relief of anxiety; also called *antianxiety agents* or *mild tranquilizers*.

Archetypes: primordial images that serve as the building blocks of the collective unconscious.

Arousal: mental stimulation or alertness that arises from the central and autonomic nervous system.

Assertiveness: clearly communicating needs, desires, or beliefs, directly and with self-confidence.

Asterixis: the inability of a person to maintain a fixed posture in space.

Asthenia: weakness.

Astrocyte: a star-shaped cell.

Ataxia: irregular coordination.

Athetoid: resembling athetosis; repetitive slow, twisting, involuntary movements of flexion, extension, pronation, and supination of the fingers and hands and sometimes the toes and feet.

Attachment theory: theory based on the classic works of Bowlby and Ainsworth that define attachment or bonding as an adaptive evolutionary and biological process of eliciting and maintaining physical closeness between a child and a mother or primary caregiver. This theory hypothesized that infant relationships with early caregivers were responsible for influencing future interactions and relationships.

Autism: a childhood mental disorder manifested by emotional aloofness, solitariness, inability to perform speech, highly repetitive play, and stereotypical movements such as rocking, rolling, and twirling.

Autonomy: freedom or independence of the individual or group.

Avoidant behaviors: refers to constricted social interaction with unfamiliar people or situations, subsequently leading to intense social impairment of interaction with others.

Axon: fibrous projection from the cell body that is responsible for impulse conduction and transmission.

Basal ganglia: five large nuclei located in the midbrain whose chief functions are regulating and mediating motor activity. This area is also thought to be the site of the development of side effects from short- and long-term neuroleptic treatment, such as extrapyramidal side effects and tardive dyskinesia.

Battering: violence or force experienced within an intimate relationship.

Behavioral and cognitive group therapy theory: the first focuses on the motivation for behavior in the form of reinforcers for the behavior. (Behavioral change occurs through the punishment of undesirable acts or the positive reinforcement of desirable alternative behaviors. The goal is changing specific behaviors.) The second focuses on changing behavior by examining thoughts and related feelings that contribute to maladaptive behaviors.

Beneficence: doing good; charitableness; liberality.

Binge: a period of uncontrolled eating in which a large amount of food is consumed, unrelated to physical hunger.

Bioethics: ethics applied to health care. See Ethics.

Blackouts: amnesia-like periods during drinking. The person seems to be functioning normally but later has no memory of what happened.

Blended families: stepfamilies or a mixture of families from other marriages.

Blood–brain barrier: the insulating sheath formed by astrocytes around capillaries in the brain that acts to form an impenetrable seal; prohibits many substances from directly entering the cerebral blood flow.

Body image: one's physical perception, sense of identity, strengths, and limitations.

Body image disturbance: refers to a distortion in the image of the body that is of near or actual delusional proportions; may include strong feelings of self-loathing projected onto the body, body parts, or perceived fat.

Body language: nonverbal communication or transmission of messages by way of physical gestures.

Boundary: rules defining who and how members participate in a subsystem or a relationship.

Brain lesion: a condition in which an abnormality is noted in the brain, such as a tumor and a hematoma; a potentially reversible dementia.

Bulimia nervosa: binge eating followed by self-induced vomiting, laxative or diuretic abuse, or starvation.

Case management: a model of comprehensive health care delivery that concentrates the responsibility for all care given to a client in one person or agency.

Case manager: a mental health professional who assesses, diagnoses, plans, implements, and evaluates clients and their treatments.

Catecholamines: any of the sympathomimetic amines, such as epinephrine, dopamine, and norepinephrine. These biochemicals play critical roles in the stress response.

Catharsis: healthy release of ideas and feelings that helps clients gain insight into conflicts and early developmental turmoil.

Cathexis: refers to concentration of psychic energy on a specific object such as an image, an idea, or a phenomenon.

Cations: positively charged ions.

Caudal: tail; toward the lower end of the body.

Character: behavioral patterns in which the learned personality traits of the person are manifested.

Cholinoceptors: refers to sites in effector cells that are receptors sensitive to choline.

Chorea: ceaseless occurrence of a wide variety of rapid, jerky but well coordinated movements, performed involuntarily.

Choreiform: movement that resembles chorea, a variety of involuntary jerky movements.

Chronobiology: field of science and medicine that explores the many bodily changes governed by the hours and the seasons; includes studies of cellular rhythms all the way through those of populations and ecosystems.

Circadian rhythms: biological cycles occurring over an approximate 24-hour period and influencing biochemical, biological, and behavioral processes.

Clarifying techniques: acts of clearing or making a message understandable.

Classical conditioning: a form of learning in which existing responses are attached to new stimuli by pairing those stimuli with those that naturally elicit the response; also referred to as *respondent conditioning*.

Clearance: a measure of the speed at which a drug leaves the body.

Client advocate: a person who tries to ensure that the rights of all prospective research subjects and actual subjects are adequately protected.

Codependence: a specific condition that is characterized by preoccupation and extreme dependency (emotionally, socially, and sometimes physically) on a person or object. Eventually, this dependency on another person becomes a pathological condition that affects the codependent individual in all other relationships.

Cognitive processes: higher cortical mental processes, including perception, memory, and reasoning, by which one acquires knowledge, solves problems, employs judgment, and makes plans.

Cogwheeling: refers to rigidity or rhythmic contractions noted on passive stretching of the muscles, as occurs in Parkinson's disease.

Collaboration: the act of working jointly with others to achieve a common goal. The mental health team is an example of collaboration.

Collective unconscious: that part of unconscious material that is universal in the human species, in contrast with the personal unconscious that is determined by individual personal experience; the collective unconscious contains symbolic access to archetypes.

Commitment: requirement of an unwilling person to be hospitalized based on "clear and convincing" evidence of imminent danger to the client or others.

Communication: transmission of feelings, attitudes, ideas, and behaviors from one person to another.

Communication and systems group therapy theories: the first theory considers both the content of messages of the group members and the process of transmission. Verbal and nonverbal behavior are confronted; there are manifest, latent, and double messages that the group leader presents. The second theory considers the group as a whole more than its individual members. It focuses on subgroups and boundaries and communication between the subgroups.

Community: a group of people who live in the same locality with common interests.

Community mental health centers: a community or neighborhood facility or a network of affiliated agencies that provides the coordinated delivery of mental health services to the population within that community or area.

Comorbity: coexistence of more than one psychiatric disorder.

Competency: ability to comprehend and make decisions; capability to be tried for a crime.

Compliance: the act of following directions or implementation by the client of the pharmaceutical therapeutic plan that has been established.

Compulsion: repetitive, ritualistic, unrealistic behaviors used to neutralize or prevent discomfort of stressful events or circumstances.

Confrontation: the act of pointing out contradictions or incongruencies between feelings, thoughts, and behaviors; specifically, pointing out parts of the assessment or treatment process that are contradictory or confusing.

Consultation: rendering of an expert opinion in response to a request.

Consumerism: a movement seeking to protect the rights of those acquiring a service (in this instance, mental health care) by requiring standards for effectiveness and safety.

Continuous quality improvement: a method of ensuring the adequacy of care developed by Deming and adopted by health care systems.

Continuum of care: provision of all levels of health care from the least restrictive to the most restrictive, including inpatient hospitalization, partial hospitalization, home care, outpatient therapy, supportive care, maintenance care, and preventive care.

Coping: an effort to reduce tension by minimizing, replacing, and resolving uncomfortable feelings such as anxiety, anger, frustration, and guilt.

Coping behaviors: coping mechanisms that enable one to manage stressful events effectively.

Countertransference: intense emotional reactions to clients stemming from the therapist's early childhood experiences.

Creutzfeldt-Jakob disease: syndrome of motor, sensory, and mental disturbances, with widespread degeneration and atrophy of the cerebral cortex, basal ganglia, and thalamus; the course of the disease is months to years.

Crisis: a turning point, or acute emotional turmoil, that stems from developmental, biological, situational, or psychosocial stressors that momentarily render the person's normal coping mechanisms inadequate.

Crisis intervention: short-term interventions that alleviate the impact of crisis-generated stress, enhance coping skills, and mobilize resources of affected clients.

Critiquer of research findings: a person who evaluates research findings and determines the usefulness of these findings for nursing practice.

Cultural relativism: emphasis on the unique aspects of each culture, without judgments.

Culture: pattern of learned shared behaviors, values, beliefs, and customs of a people transmitted through generations.

Data collector: a person who gathers information for a research study, such as obtaining information from research subjects.

Decade of the Brain: the U.S. Congress's proclamation that explains mental illness as a disease of the brain. It underscores the significance of technological advances in neurobiology and genetics and their impact on understanding of mental illness.

Decerebrate: a sign characterized by adduction and extension of the arms, pronated wrists, and flexed fingers. The legs are stiffly extended, with plantar flexion of the feet. This sign indicates upper brain stem damage and usually heralds neurological deterioration.

Decorticate: a sign characterized by adduction and flexion of the arms, with wrists and fingers flexed on chest. The legs are extended and internally rotated with plantar flexion of the feet. Most often, it results from cerebrovascular accident or head injury. It is a sign of corticospinal damage and is associated with a more favorable prognosis than decerebrate posture.

Defense mechanisms: unconscious self-protective processes that seek to protect the ego from intense feelings or affect and impulses.

Deinstitutionalization: caring for people outside the hospital who have been previously hospitalized for an extended period; caring for people in the community rather than in a state facility. A humanizing recommendation made by the Commission on Mental Illness (1961) that moved the care of the mentally ill from large state mental institutions to community mental health centers.

Delirium: a general medical condition that manifests as a psychiatric syndrome characterized by acute onset and impairment in cognition, perception, and behavior; also known as *acute confusion*.

Delirium tremens (DTs): now called *alcohol withdrawal delirium*. A medical diagnosis for a serious alcohol withdrawal syndrome that is characterized by delirium and autonomic hyperactivity occurring within 1 week of reduction or cessation of alcohol intake.

Delusion: a fixed false belief unchanged by logic. Types of delusions include paranoid thoughts ("The FBI is taping this conversation"), religious ("I am God"), grandiose ("I have special powers"), and nihilistic ("I feel like part of me is dead"). Other delusions include thought broadcasting (thinking that others hear one's thoughts), thought insertion (thinking someone can put thoughts into another's mind), and thought withdrawal (thinking that one's thoughts are being extracted from the mind).

Dementia: a condition manifested in the insidious development of memory and intellectual deficits, disorientation, and decreased cognitive functioning.

Dendrites: projections from neuronal cell bodies that receive impulse transmission from adjacent cells.

Depersonalization: a loss of personal identity accompanied by feeling unreal, strange, or emotional numbness.

Diplopia: double vision.

Disaster: a sudden unexpected calamitous event that leads to great loss, damage, or destruction.

Disease-prone behaviors: behaviors that sustain arousal of the sympathetic nervous system (e.g., inability to express feelings, overly appeasing).

Disengagement: implies that family boundaries are rigid or impermeable.

Dissociation: an unconscious defense mechanism that refers to a detachment or alteration in one's sense of reality, psychogenic amnesia, and perception of self and environment; used by a person to protect the self from being overwhelmed by anxiety, usually from a traumatic event. Memory and feeling related to an event are sealed off from conscious awareness.

Dissociative identity disorder: a disorder involving excessive use of dissociation so that the continuous development of personality throughout a person's life is seriously compromised or severely fragmented. This disorder usually results from trauma.

Distribution: the process of delivering a drug to the various tissues of the body.

Dopamine: a catecholamine neurotransmitter found in the brain; increased synaptic release is associated with schizophrenia and other psychotic disorders.

Dopaminergic: relating to nerve cells or fibers that employ dopamine as their neurotransmitter.

Drives: instinctual urges and impulses arising from biological and psychological needs.

Dyad: a two-person relationship, such as husband–wife and father–child.

Dyskinesia: a condition characterized by abnormal voluntary movement.

Dyspepsia: impairment of digestion, usually epigastric discomfort after a meal.

Dysphagia: difficulty swallowing.

Dysphoria: misery in various degrees; painful mood state based on self-abasement, sense of inadequacy, and worthlessness.

Dystonia: muscle spasms of head, neck, and tongue; a result of dopamine blockade from neuroleptic medications.

Dysuria: difficult or painful urination.

Eating disorder: a general term for abnormalities in behavior toward food growing out of fear of fatness and pursuit of excessive thinness.

Eclecticism: implies that the therapist is using two or more theories to meet client needs and to develop effective treatment.

Efferent: conducting or progressing away from a center or specific site of reference as in an efferent nerve.

Ego: the part of the mind that mediates between external reality and inner wishes and impulses.

Ego competency: the ability of the ego to do its job. Humans have a spectrum of levels of competency of the ego. The mentally ill have low levels of ego competency, whereas the mentally healthy have high levels of ego competency.

Ego-dystonic: refers to ego nonacceptibility of instinctual urges; such urges are prevented from reaching the ego for consideration.

Ego-syntonic: refers to ego acceptability of ideas or impulses so that the person is comfortable with personal peculiarities that are discomfiting to others.

Ego function: intrapsychic processes that enable people to mediate stress and adaptation using various defense mechanisms.

Electroconvulsive therapy: electrical current induction of seizures, primarily for the treatment of various mental disorders; used most frequently in depression.

Elimination: the removal of a drug or its byproducts from the body.

Elopement: clients who are absent from a psychiatric facility without following proper procedures for absence.

Empathy: refers to putting oneself into the psychological frame of reference of another. It conveys an understanding of the client's situation without becoming emerged or overwhelmed by the experience.

Empowerment: refers to a sense of inner strength, confidence, and self-worth; the investment of power or authority in a person or group.

Enabling: any behavior that encourages continued abuse by the addict of mood-altering chemicals or that protects the affected person from the consequences of abuse.

Encounter groups: intensive t-groups that provided a type of therapy to those generally interested in self-growth and group dynamics.

Enculturation: the process by which culture is learned and acquired by particular people.

Enmeshment: implies overinvolvement or a lack of separateness of family members.

Entrepreneurialism: The organizing, managing, and risk assumption of a business venture or enterprise.

Entropy: the tendency to increased randomness by the dissipation of energy; the running-down of a system.

Equifinality: the sameness of the end result starting from various points.

Eros: the instinct or drive for love.

Ethics: examination of moral judgments and decisions about conduct.

Ethnicity: a group classification in which members share a unique cultural heritage passed from generation to generation; involves customs, language, and religion; racial differences may or may not be germane to ethnic differences.

Ethnocentrism: pertains to looking at lifeways and values from one's own cultural perspective.

Evoked potentials: electrical activity produced at various levels of the central nervous system in response to sensory nerve stimulation.

Existential/gestalt group therapy theory: here-and-now awareness approach to group therapy, focusing on feelings; developed by Perls, Maslow, and Rogers. Feelings are thought to be suppressed because of the person's own constraints or the constraining expectations of others. The goal is self-actualization—the person is free to define oneself and can make choices about feelings, thoughts, and behavior.

Exponential kinetics: a pharmacokinetic model in which a constant fraction of a drug is eliminated in a set unit of time.

Extrapyramidal side effects: involuntary motor movements; side effects that result from dopamine blockade by neuroleptic medications.

Extrapyramidal symptoms: movement disorders that are caused by centrally acting antidopaminergic drugs such as the phenothiazines; included are dystonia, akathisia, akinesia, and Parkinson-like symptoms.

Family roles: expected patterns or specific behaviors within a social context.

Family structure: the manner in which a family adapts and maintains itself.

Fasciculation: a small, local, involuntary muscle contraction.

Fear of fatness: excessive fear of and preoccupation with the idea of becoming fat despite being normal in weight or even very thin.

Feedback mechanism: a process that permits exchange of energy and matter across various boundaries.

Fetal alcohol effects: a milder manifestation of intrauterine growth development than fetal alcohol syndrome resulting from fetal exposure to alcohol.

Fetal alcohol syndrome: a manifestation of intrauterine growth retardation caused by fetal exposure to alcohol that includes prenatal and postnatal growth retardation, central nervous system disorders, and abnormal craniofacial features.

First-pass effect: the process when a drug administered orally is first metabolized prior to reaching the systemic circulation whereby the amount of drug available is reduced.

Focal neurological signs: specific signs of neurological impairment, such as blurred vision and aphasia.

Focusing: the act of clarifying a perception or spotlighting a specific aspect of communication.

Foster care: a substitute family-like living situation provided by state or private agencies.

Galactorrhea: spontaneous or persistent secretion of milk, irrespective of nursing.

Gender: classification at birth, according to the appearance of the external genitalia, as male or female.

Genetic vulnerability: the relationship between genetic and enzymatic defects and vulnerability to mental illness. Genetic function is influenced by prenatal and environmental factors that activate intricate biochemical processes that affect behavior. A number of researchers have attempted to explore the relationship between genetic factors and mental disorders using twin, adoption, and family studies.

Granulocytopenia: fewer than the normal number of granular leukocytes in the blood; see Agranulocytosis.

Gray matter: the appearance of tissue in the central nervous system resulting from the presence of cell bodies.

Grief: a normal profound response to loss.

Group leadership: depending on the type of group, the director of the group is often one leader, or there may be two leaders—cotherapists. Style is unique to the leaders and may be authoritarian and confrontative or reflective.

Group process: sees groups as being in a constant state of flux, with the goal of the group being to find a state of equilibrium. As members introduce tension, the group as a whole seeks ways to reduce the tension. The group goes through an introductory phase, working phase, and termination phase as a group culture evolves.

Group therapy: a treatment modality for more than one person that provides therapeutic outcomes for each person and for the group as a whole.

Half-life: the amount of time required to reduce the original plasma concentration of a drug by half (50%).

Hallucinations: false sensory perceptions occurring when there is no external stimulus. Types of hallucinations include auditory (voices, sounds, music), visual (images), gustatory (unpleasant taste), tactile (touch), and olfactory (unpleasant smells).

Hardiness: a personality trait that enables people to maintain health and cope with stressful events.

Helplessness: a sense of powerlessness and lack of strength or effectiveness.

Hopelessness: a state of despondency and absolute loss of hope.

Huntington's disease: a genetically transmitted and progressive degenerative disease of the central nervous system; major neuropsychiatric manifestations include involuntary movements, psychosis, and depression.

Hyperhidrosis: a condition characterized by abnormal, excessive sweating.

Hyperkinesis: excessive motor functioning.

Hyperphagia: excessive amount of eating.

Hyperplexia: an abnormally increased or excessive network of nerves.

Hyperprolactinemia: increased levels of prolactin in the blood.

Hypersomnia: sleeping at least one additional hour during winter months as compared with summer months.

Hypnotic: an agent used to induce sleep.

Hypokinesis: slow, voluntary movement; decreased mobility.

Hypothalamus: combined with the pituitary gland, thyroid gland, adrenal glands, gonads, and the pancreas, the hypothalamus forms the major regulatory system and is involved in the biological aspects of behavior. The hypothalamic-pituitary-adrenal axis is important in understanding certain mental disorders. The hypothalamus regulates autonomic, endocrine, and visceral integration and is surmised to be the foundation of the limbic system and the brain center for emotions and certain behaviors such as eating, drinking, and sexuality. Information in the hypothalamus is modulated by ascending sensory pathways, hormones, and descending pathways of the cerebral cortex.

Iatrogenic effects: an unfavorable response or adverse condition produced by the treatment itself.

Id: the sum total of biological instincts, including sexual and aggressive impulses.

Idiosyncratic reaction: an unusual and unpredictable reaction to a drug occurring in a small portion of the population.

Impulsivity: the act of spontaneous action without thinking about consequences.

Incest: sexual intercourse with a blood relative or relative by adoption.

Inferiority complex: an exaggeration of feelings of inadequacy and insecurity resulting in defensiveness and neurotic behavior.

Infradian: biological variations with a frequency lower than circadian (rhythms that have longer, slower cycles than circadian rhythms).

Insight: self-awareness and understanding of the meaning and reasons of one's behavior or motives.

Insight-oriented groups or process-oriented groups: verbal group psychotherapy for high-functioning persons who can explore motives and feelings for behavior within themselves.

Insomnia: inability to fall asleep, difficulty staying asleep, and early-morning awakening.

Insulin coma shock: refers to administering large doses of insulin to induce marked hypoglycemia that produces a coma or seizure.

Internalized relationships: introjected impressions of early caregivers that determine the person's ability to adapt and reach optimal growth and health.

Interpersonal group therapy theory: based on Sullivan's views of the individual in relation to peers. The goal is the reconstruction of the individual's personality through interrelationships with peers based on early childhood relationships. Learning occurs when the group leader assists the process of consensual validation of interactions, feelings, thoughts, and behaviors of the group members toward each other.

Intrapreneurialism: The expansion of the traditional role as direct health care providers to that of creators of quality care products and services within an institution or organization.

Justice: appropriate execution of laws, to give every person their due, requires equality in dealing with each person.

Kindling: an underlying progression from stress-induced to spontaneous recurrence of depressive illness; an example of a neurobiological response that is activated by significant early stress and losses.

Korsakoff's syndrome: a psychosis that is usually based on chronic alcoholism and that is accompanied by disturbance of orientation, susceptibility to external stimulation and suggestion, falsification of memory, and hallucinations.

Language: a complex phenomenon and tool used to communicate.

Leadership: the ability to show others the way by going in advance; to act as a guide for others.

Lethality: level of dangerousness or injury.

Leukopenia: reduction in the number of leukocytes in the blood, usually fewer than $5000/mm^3$.

Lewy body: proteinaceous structures composed of a central core with radiating filaments, located in the substantia nigra in Parkinson's disease and in the cortex in diffuse Lewy body disease.

Liaison: the facilitation of the relationships between the client, the client's illness, the consultee, the health care team, and the environment.

Libidinal object constancy: the process by which the satisfactory or unsatisfactory attachments of infant and caregiver influence the infant's ability to experience a sense of continuity of an intrapsychic representation of the beloved object (caregiver).

Libido: the basic driving force of personality in Freud's system; it includes sexual energy but is not restricted to it.

Life expectancy: refers to the age at which a person born into a particular cohort is expected to die.

Life span: the maximum age that could be attained if a person were able to avoid or be successfully treated for all illness and accidents.

Light therapy: a biological treatment that increases exposure to artificial light whose intensity is equivalent to outdoor levels, more than 2000 lux. The aim of therapy is to suppress melatonin secretion and produce phase shifts of melatonin secretion.

Linear kinetics: a pharmacokinetic model in which a

constant amount of drug is eliminated in a set unit of time.

Love: affiliation and affection for self and other people.

Marathon groups: intensive 2- to 3-day group therapy designed for mentally healthy people interested in personal growth. The objectives are to explore and express honesty, intimacy, connectedness to others, and genuine communication.

Marital schism: a term used to describe intense marital conflict in which a parent attempts to enlist a child as an ally against the other parent.

Marital skew: severe marital discord arising from acceptance of maladaptive behaviors in one partner by the other partner.

Maturational crisis: refers to developmental stages marked by biological, psychosocial, and social transitions that generate characteristic disturbances in behavior and emotional responses.

Mental health: a relative state of well-being that enables persons, couples, families, and communities to adaptively respond to external and internal stressors.

Mental health movement: a movement that began more than 25 years ago focusing on humane treatment of the mentally ill, initially advocating release from state institutions to community mental health centers.

Mental health team: an interdisciplinary group of mental health staff who collaborate to assess, intervene, and evaluate client responses to treatment.

Mental illness: a condition manifested by disorganization and impairment of function that arises from various causes such as psychological, neurobiological, and genetic factors.

Metabolism: formation of active and inactive metabolites through conversion of a drug into a new, usually less active and more water-soluble compound.

Milieu therapy: use of the total environment as the therapeutic agent, including people, resources, and events, to promote optimal functioning, interpersonal growth, and enhanced adaptation to life outside the hospital.

Modeling: a form of learning in which a person learns by watching someone else perform a desired response.

Mood: the feeling of pleasure or displeasure by which a person experiences himself or herself and the world.

Moral treatment: humane treatment of the mentally ill; for example, releasing clients from mechanical restraints and improving physical care. Philippe Pinel and Benjamin Rush were instrumental in promoting this movement.

Multiple personality disorder: a severe disorder manifested by multiple amnestic episodes, severe behavioral changes, and distinctly different personalities residing in one person; synonymous with *dissociative identity disorder*.

Myelin: an insulating material that wraps around neuronal axons and acts to speed conduction of electrical impulses.

Myoclonus: shocklike contractions of a portion of a muscle, an entire muscle, or a group of muscles restricted to one area of the body or appearing synchronously or asynchronously in several areas.

Nar-Anon: an international self-help support organization composed of family members or friends of persons who have or have had a problem with drugs.

Narcotics Anonymous (NA): an international self-help support organization patterned after AA for persons who have a problem with drugs.

National Institute of Mental Health: a federally funded agency whose goals include developing and helping various states identify and use the most effective methods of prevention, diagnosis, and intervention of mental illnesses through research funding and staff development and education of mental health professionals to provide mental health treatment.

Negative symptoms: schizophrenic symptoms associated with structural brain abnormalities. Major negative symptoms include blunted affect, inability to experience pleasure, apathy, lack of feeling, and impaired attention. These symptoms tend to have an insidious and chronic course, and client response to neuroleptics is poor.

Negentropy: the counterforce to entropy; the evolving of more complete organization, complexity, and ability to transform resources.

Negligence: injury that is unintentional due to not taking the usual precautions expected in that instance.

Neuritic plaques: a patch or flat area of neurons.

Neurobiology: biology of the nervous system, particularly the brain.

Neuroendocrinology: the study of how the neural system and endocrine systems work together to maintain homeostasis. Communication between these systems is involved in biological and behavioral responses. Major organs of the neuroendocrine system are the hypothalamus; the pituitary, thyroid, and adrenal glands; the gonads; and the pancreas.

Neurofibrillary tangles: tangles of the neurofibril, which is the delicate threads running in every direction through the cytoplasm of the body of a nerve and extending into the axon and the dendrites of the cell.

Neuroleptic agent: a pharmacological agent that produces "antipsychotic effects" by inhibiting the reuptake of dopamine. Examples include haloperidol (Haldol), cloxapine (Clozaril), and fluphenazine (Prolixin).

Neuroleptic malignant syndrome: a rare syndrome caused by antipsychotic medications and characterized by muscle rigidity, high fever, altered consciousness, tachycardia, hypertension, and diaphoresis.

Neuroleptics: psychotropic medications; major tranquilizers; synonymous with *neuroleptic agent.*

Neuropathy: functional disturbances with noninflammatory etiology in the peripheral nervous system.

Neurotransmitter: a nervous system biochemical involved in facilitating the transmission of impulses across synapses between neurons. Examples include serotonin, norepinephrine, and dopamine.

Neurovegetative changes: psychophysiological functions such as sleep and eating patterns, energy level, sexual functioning, and elimination.

Normal-pressure hydrocephalus: a condition in which the cerebrospinal fluid pressure is normal or high normal, but excessive fluid exists in the ventricles of the brain.

Nursing informatics: the use of computers and information sciences to manage and process data, knowledge, and information in nursing practice and patient care.

Nystagmus: an involuntary, rapid rhythmic movement of the eyeball.

Object relations: emotional attachment for other persons or objects.

Obsession: intrusive, recurrent, and persistent thoughts, impulses, or images.

Oculogyric crisis: a syndrome characterized by hyperextension of the neck and upward fixation of the eyeballs.

Oliguria: diminished urine formation.

Open system: in systems theory, a term used to imply that members or parts are interrelated and responsive to each other's needs.

Operant conditioning: a type of learning in which responses are modified by their consequences. Reinforcement increases the likelihood of future occurrences of the reinforced response; punishment and extinction decrease the likelihood of future occurrences of the responses they follow.

Opisthotonos: severe muscular spasm characterized by the head and the heels being bent backward and the body bowed forward.

Orthostatic: relating to standing upright; in orthostatic hypertension, the blood pressure is normal while reclining but low while standing.

Paradoxical reaction: a response to a drug that is opposite to what would be predicted by the drug's pharmacology.

Paresthesia: unnatural tactile sensations, manifested by tingling, tickling, or creeping, having no physical basis.

Parkinson's disease: chronic condition marked by rigidity and tremor with intention; pathological changes are in the substantia nigra.

Partial hospitalization: a psychiatric treatment program for clients who require intensive hospital treatment but not on a full-time 24-hour-per-day basis. Partial hospitalization can include programs during the day and evening and on weekends.

Pattern(s): specific nuclear conflict or dynamic tendencies that is particularly typical of a person.

Pedophile: an adult who is sexually attracted to children.

Persona: a disguised or masked attitude useful in interacting with one's environment but frequently at variance with one's true identity.

Personal space: "comfort space" or "zone" in interpersonal relationships.

Personality: the characteristic and somewhat predictable traits influencing cognitive, affective, and behavioral patterns of human beings; an entity that has the following: (1) consistent and ongoing set of response patterns to given stimuli; (2) range of emotions available; (3) range of intensity of affect for each emotion; and (4) significant confluent history.

Pharmacodynamics: the study of biochemical and physiological actions and effects of drugs.

Pharmacokinetics: the study of a drug's absorption, distribution, metabolism, and elimination.

Pharmacology: the study of chemical formulations.

Philosophy: a view or theory on which one's actions may be based.

Phobia: an exaggerated or illogical fear of an event or object.

Photophobia: abnormal intolerance or sensitivity to light.

Physical dependence: a state occurring from drug use whereby tolerance has developed and withdrawal symptoms will occur when the usage of the substance is stopped.

Pick's disease: a rare, fatal degenerative disease of the nervous system, occurring mostly in middle-aged women; characterized by signs of severe frontal or temporal lobe dysfunction; symptomatology is similar to that of Alzheimer's disease.

Play therapy: an intervention tailored for children that gives them a symbolic way to express feelings, anxiety, aggression, and self-doubt.

Pleasure principle: a hypothetical mechanism that represents the claims of libido and functions to reduce the psychic tension deriving from the person's drive to act on unacceptable unconscious instincts.

Polyuria: an increasing volume of urine in a given period.

Positive symptoms: refers to schizophrenic symptoms with good premorbid functioning, acute onset, normal cognition, and positive response to neuroleptic treatment. Major positive symptoms include hallucinations, delusions, disorganized thinking and speech, and gross behavioral disturbances. These symptoms are surmised to be related to neurochemical abnormality rather than structural brain abnormality.

Potentially reversible dementia: a condition characterized by an acute onset, causing neurological symptoms and changes in level of consciousness. If treated in time, the condition may be reversed. See Delirium.

Priapism: persistent abnormal erection of the penis.

Primary appraisals: the initial response to a stressor.

Primary prevention: refers to measures or interventions to counteract circumstances or conditions that are potentially harmful. Additionally, these measures generate coping skills and reduce vulnerability to illness and promote health.

Principal investigator: a person who takes the major role in the development and conduct of a research study.

Probable irreversible dementia: progressive loss of intellectual functioning caused by permanent brain damage.

Process recording: an indepth evaluation of communication skills.

Progressive relaxation: a form of relaxation training that involves visualizing and progressively relaxing specific muscle groups from the scalp to the tips of the toes. This treatment reduces tension and stress.

Protein binding: the affinity of a drug to bind with plasma protein to form a drug–protein complex.

Pseudodementia: depression in the elderly that presents similar to a dementia.

Pseudomutuality: a transaction that infers a sense of relatedness and emotional connectedness; in reality, it represents shallow and empty relationships.

Psychic dependence (habituation): the compulsion to seek and use a chemical even though there are no apparent tolerance and withdrawal symptoms demonstrated.

Psychic organizers: the necessity for one particular affective behavior (i.e., crying, smiling) to be present before the emergence of a new one at a higher level. Such affective signals indicate that intrapsychic change or development is occurring.

Psychodrama: specific technique in group psychotherapy through dramatic means; developed by Jacob Moreno. Five aspects in the group setting include (1) the stage, which gives the patient the opportunity of expression; (2) the subject or client, who enacts a role emphasizing a past or present problem; (3) the director, who is the therapist and producer of the drama; (4) the staff of therapeutic aides (auxiliary egos), who are responsive to the producer and act as real or imagined persons in the patient's life; and (5) the audience, who are the rest of the group who act as a sounding board of public opinion.

Psychodynamic group therapy theory: based on the Freudian assumption that the id, the ego, and the superego are the psychological determinants of human behavior. Problems of people are conceptualized to center around unconscious conflicts and basic love–hate instincts. The group offers symbolic reenactment of the past in present relationships (transference and countertransference).

Psychoeducation: an individualized teaching plan that focuses on managing symptoms and course of illness, minimizing relapse, and altering the long-term debilitating effects of chronic mental illness.

Psychoeducation groups: educative or teaching groups that provide members with health-related information and opportunities to discuss the related psychosocial issues.

Psychogenic amnesia: a sudden disturbance in identity particularly related to significant personal information.

Psychogenic fugue: an identity and memory disturbance manifested by sudden travel and assumption of new identity.

Psychological autopsy: a process or mechanism to evaluate whether death was the result of suicide or an accident.

Psychomotor retardation: a slowing of physical and emotional reactions, including speech, affect, and movement.

Psychoneuroimmunology: the study of the role the immune system plays in health and illness in the face of biological or psychosocial stress. This field is developing knowledge about the interconnectedness of the nervous system and the immune system.

Psychophysiological disorder: denotes emotional states producing or exacerbating physical problems.

Psychosurgery: surgical or chemical alteration involving severing brain fibers with the purpose of modifying behavioral disturbance, thoughts, or mood.

Psychotherapy: a global process in which people seek professional help to resolve problems, promote personal growth, and reduce or eliminate maladaptive responses.

Psychotropics: various pharmacological agents used to affect behavior, mood, and feelings, such as antidepressant, antipsychotic, antimanic, and antianxiety agents.

Purge: a variety of methods used to counteract the fattening effects of a binge; may include self-induced vomiting or use of a cathartic, laxatives, diuretics, or amphetamines. Excessive exercise or fasting may also be used.

Qualitative research: research that focuses on the meaning of experiences to individuals rather than on the generalizability of study results.

Quantitative research: research that focuses on gathering numerical data, with the intent of generalizing the findings of the study.

Race: a subgroup of people possessing a definite combination of physical characteristics or genetic origin, the combination of which distinguishes the subgroup as different from other subgroups.

Reality principle: a hypothetical mechanism that represents outer world influence and functions to modify the pleasure principle.

Recovery: a term from the disease model of addiction indicating an ongoing process that begins with cessation of chemical use and continues with attainment of skills in living without the chemical.

Reflexes: localized spinal cord responses to stimuli that do not use the rest of the spinal cord; described as an arc.

Reinforcement: in classical conditioning, the process of following the conditioned stimulus with the unconditioned stimulus; in operant conditioning, the rewarding of desired responses.

Reinforcers: personal, complex, learned, and possibly biochemical rewards that are used to modify maladaptive behavior. Reinforcers can be positive, negative, or punishing and are personally determined.

Relapse: a process of becoming dysfunctional in sobriety that ends in a return to chemical use.

Repression: an unconscious process that removes anxiety-producing thoughts, desires, or memories from conscious awareness.

Role playing: a specific technique, similar to psychodrama, that uses role reversal. The members of the group must guess at what the actors in the role play are thinking, feeling, or trying to convey. The group as a whole discusses the interactions of the actors. Useful when a member of the group can take on the role of the person with whom he or she has an actual situational conflict or problem.

Ruminations: repetitive or continuous thinking about a particular subject that interferes with other thought processes.

Scapegoating: a form of displacement involving blaming a member for the actions of others.

Schema: strategies or ways of thinking comprising core beliefs and basic assumptions about how the world operates.

Schizophrenia: a group of chronic mental psychotic disorders manifested primarily by thought, affect, mood, social, and perceptual disturbances, such as hallucinations, delusions, withdrawal, and flat affect.

Seasonal affective disorder: recurrent depression that occurs during winter and remits in spring. Major symptoms include depressive mood, hypersomnia, tiredness, increased appetite, and craving for carbohydrates with subsequent weight gain.

Secondary appraisal: a response that arises with any form of perceived threat or harm if primary appraisals are ineffective or maladaptive.

Secondary prevention: refers to measures or interventions used to curtail disease processes.

Sedative: drugs used to calm nervousness, irritability, or excitement; these agents depress the central nervous system and tend to cause lassitude and reduced mental activity.

Self-awareness: recognition by the nurse of the nurse's personal attitudes, values, and beliefs and how these may affect the care of others.

Self-concept: one's belief and feeling about self.

Self-deprecatory ideas: negative thoughts about the self.

Self-destructive: behavior that tends to harm or destroy self.

Self-disclosure: exposing oneself to others; to make publicly known.

Self-esteem: one's feeling of self-worth and personal value; confidence and acceptance of oneself.

Self-healing: behaviors associated with emotional balance (e.g., spontaneity and healthy interpersonal skills).

Self-mutilation: the act of self-induced pain or tissue destruction void of the intent to kill oneself.

Separation anxiety: refers to anxiety that occurs when a child exhibits symptoms of panic or extreme fear of losing primary caregivers.

Serotonergic: the ability of nerve receptors to receive or reject serotonin as a chemical synaptic transmitter of impulses involved with wakefulness, feeling states, temperature and blood pressure regulation, and various other autonomic functions.

Serotonin syndrome: a condition characterized by serotonergic hyperstimulation that includes restlessness, myoclonus, hyperreflexia, diaphoresis, shivering, and tremor.

Sexual dysfunction: disturbance in sexual function that causes the person marked distress or interpersonal difficulty.

Sexual health: integration of aspects of sexual being in ways that enhance the self, communication with others, and love.

Sexual orientation: the personal experience of the sexual self as homosexual, heterosexual, or bisexual.

Sexual patterns: the person's experience of sexuality in his or her day-to-day routine.

Shadow: Carl Jung's term that refers to the unconscious.

Shame: the experience of the self in a painfully diminished sense. The self feels exposed both to itself and to anyone else present; contained in the experience of shame is the piercing awareness of ourselves as fundamentally deficient in some vital way as a human being.

Sick role: dependent, helpless, and ill behaviors often associated with control and maintenance of maladaptive relationships.

Sleep–wake cycle: one of the body's biological rhythyms normally determined by the day–night cycle.

Somatic preoccupation: an excessive focus on one's own body functioning.

Somatosensory: a sensation related to the body's superficial and deep parts as contrasted to specialized senses such as smell and sight.

Somnolence: sleepiness or unnatural drowsiness.

Special care units: a section of a nursing home (or hospital) that is dedicated to the care of clients with probable irreversible dementia.

Spirituality: receptiveness or devotion to religious values.

Splitting: an ego defense mechanism that precedes and determines some type of repression. In clients with borderline personality disorders, it encompasses the tendency to see things and people only one way (i.e., all good or all bad).

Standards: general recognition and conformity to established principles or rules.

Status epilepticus: rapid succession of seizures without regaining consciousness during the intervals. Such an event can overtax the system and cause death.

Status spongiosus: presence of coarse and fine vacuoles in all cortical layers.

Steady-state: the state whereby the amount of a drug eliminated from the body equals the amount being absorbed.

Stress: a stimulus or demand that generates disruption in homeostasis or produces a reaction.

Subculture: a group of people who are members of a larger group that shares values, beliefs, and customs that are not common to all members of the larger group.

Substance abuse: the continuation of use of a drug despite knowing one's social, occupational, psychological, or physical problems are caused by the use of the substance. This term is also one of the two diagnoses for chemical use used in the *Diagnostic and Statistical Manual of Mental Disorders* (4th edition).

Substance dependence: a cluster of cognitive, behavioral, and physiological symptoms that indicates that the person has impaired control of psychoactive substance use and continues use of the substance despite adverse consequences. One of the two diagnoses for chemical use used in the *Diagnostic and Statistical Manual of Mental Disorders* (4th edition). It must include several of nine different criteria.

Subsystems: smaller systems within larger systems.

Suicidal ideation: thoughts or ideas of suicide.

Suicide: the act of killing oneself.

Superego: the part of the personality structure that grows out of the ego and reflects early moral training and parental injunctions.

Support systems: refers to persons or endeavors that help people during stressful periods.

Switching: changing from one state of consciousness (reality) to another in an effort to cope with current conflict; usually occurs between "personalities" in multiple personality disorders (dissociative identity disorders).

Synaptic transmission: the process of nerve impulse transmission through the generation of action potentials from one neuron to another.

Synergy: the process of multiplication of energy; the concept that the whole is not just the sum of the parts but is something different from the parts because all the parts work together.

Systematic desensitization: behavioral therapy of reconditioning aimed at alleviating or removing the impact of a mental process, such as phobia.

T cells: viral- and tumor-fighting lymphocytes (also called *natural killer cells*) of the immune system.

T-groups: basic skills training groups that were specifically designed for providing experience of being in a group and understanding the group process. These training groups began in Bethel, Maine, in 1948 and 1949.

Tardive dyskinesia: a complex range of involuntary movements associated with long-term neuroleptic treatment. A chronic, progressive, and potentially fatal syndrome from dopamine blockade by neuroleptic medications. Major manifestations include choreiform movements of the face, tongue, upper and lower extremities, such as tongue movement or protrusion, lip sucking, chewing; other symptoms include chewing movements, puffing of cheeks, and pelvic thrusting.

Task group therapy theory: groups that focus on a specific task, usually agreed on by the group. The group stays together only long enough to complete the task.

Termination: the final phase of psychotherapy. This process involves exploring areas of accomplishment, goal attainment, and feelings generated by ending the relationship.

Tertiary prevention: refers to measures that minimize relapse and chronic disability, and restore client to optimal level of function.

Thanatos: the instinct toward death and self-destruction.

Theory: theory is an organized and systematic set of statements related to significant questions in a discipline. Theories describe, explain, predict, or prescribe responses, events, situations, conditions, or relationships. Theories consist of concepts that are related to each other.

Therapeutic alliance: refers to a trusting relationship that helps the client explore interpersonal and intrapersonal conflicts and gain insight into maladaptive behaviors.

Therapeutic communication: a healing or curative dialogue between people.

Therapeutic community: usually refers to the early milieu therapy approaches developed by Maxwell Jones and others in the 1940s and 1950s in which clients were encouraged to take responsibility for their own treatment, a new high value was given to the interaction of the client and his or her environment, and decision making and recommendation authority were given to the nursing staff.

Therapeutic milieu: a healing environment; also, probably the degree to which most treatment units apply the traditional principles of milieu therapy in the unit structure.

Therapeutic use of touch: refers to the healing powers of touch.

Tic: twitching; one or several involuntary muscle contractions most commonly involving the face, head, neck, or shoulder muscles.

Tolerance: occurs after repeated use of the drug requires more and more of the drug to achieve the same effect.

Tort law: law dealing with a person's decision to do another person wrong.

Torticollis: a contracted state of the cervical muscle, producing twisting of the neck and an unnatural position of the head.

Traits: human behaviors that are pervasive, distinctive, and enduring and characteristic of a particular person.

Transactional patterns: a set of patterned interactions among family members.

Transference: unconscious displacement or reenactment of feelings and attitudes from the client to the psychotherapist.

Trauma: an event that threatens to or does actually overwhelm a person's normal coping mechanism.

Tremens: includes all the symptoms of severe autonomic stimulation, including elevated vital signs, tremulousness, and agitation (i.e., delirium tremens [DTs]).

Tremor: involuntary shaking or trembling movement.

Triangulation: a term that describes a maladaptive triad transactional pattern.

Twin studies: researchers attempt to explore the relationship between genetic factors and mental disorders using these studies that usually include monozygotic or single ovum and dizygotic or two ova twins. Twin studies are helpful in isolating genetic and environmental influences and determining preventive and precipitating factors.

Type A personality: a constellation of personality traits, such as highly driven, time-conscious, and competitive behavior, associated with high risk for coronary disease.

Type B personality: a constellation of personality traits opposite from type A personality and manifested by "easy going, laid back, and reposed" behavior.

Ultradian: biological variations with a frequency higher than circadian, less than 24 hours (rhythms that have shorter, faster cycles than circadian rhythms). Biological rhythms refer to cyclic variations in biological and biochemical function, activity, and emotional state.

Urticaria: a vascular reaction in the upper dermis characterized by localized edema caused by increased permeability and dilation of the capillaries.

Utilizer of research findings: a person who integrates research findings into clinical practice.

Values: any consideration sufficient to support a belief; needs or desires of a person.

Vascular dementia: a probable irreversible dementia caused by many small strokes, or a large stroke.

Vertigo: disturbed equilibrium characterized by dizziness and lightheadedness.

Visual imagery: stress-reducing cognitive exercise that involves creating relaxing thoughts of positive or pleasant event or a place of serenity and calmness.

Vulnerability: the potential susceptibility of a person, family, or group to a health deviation.

Withdrawal: the substance-specific response of the body to the absence of a drug after it has become acclimated to this drug.

Yalom's therapeutic factors: the 11 beneficial aspects of groups, formerly called *curative factors*. They include the imparting of information, instillation of hope, universality, altruism, corrective recapitulation of the primary family group member, development of socializing techniques, imitative behavior, interpersonal learning, group cohesiveness, catharsis, and existential factors.

Zeitgeber: a synchronizer or periodic environmental stimulus that is the dominant factor in determining a rhythm.

APPENDIX I

Answers to Unit Study Questions

UNIT I

Chapter 1

1. b
2. a
3. b
4. c
5. c

Chapter 2

1. b
2. d
3. b
4. a
5. c
6. b
7. c
8. a
9. d
10. d
11. a

Chapter 3

1. c
2. a
3. c
4. c
5. b

Chapter 4

1. a
2. b
3. c
4. a
5. a

Chapter 5

1. b
2. c
3. d
4. a
5. c

Chapter 6

1. c
2. c
3. c
4. c

Chapter 7

1. a
2. a
3. a
4. c
5. d

Chapter 8

1. a
2. c
3. a
4. a
5. d

UNIT II

Chapter 9

1. b
2. b
3. d
4. b
5. c

Chapter 10

1. c
2. c
3. d
4. a
5. b

Chapter 11

1. a
2. a
3. d
4. b
5. a
6. a

Chapter 12

1. c
2. b
3. a
4. c
5. b

Chapter 13

1. b
2. c
3. b

Chapter 14

1. b
2. d
3. b
4. a
5. d
6. d
7. d
8. c

Chapter 15

1. c
2. d
3. a
4. d
5. a

Chapter 16

1. b
2. a
3. a
4. b
5. b
6. a

Chapter 17

1. c
2. b
3. a
4. d
5. c

Chapter 18

1. b
2. b
3. c
4. c
5. d

Chapter 19

1. b
2. c
3. d
4. c
5. d

UNIT III

Chapter 20

1. c
2. c
3. a
4. c
5. c

Chapter 21

1. c
2. b
3. d
4. c
5. d
6. b

Chapter 22

1. c
2. a
3. a
4. a
5. b

Chapter 23

1. c
2. e
3. b
4. c

Chapter 24

1. b
2. d
3. b
4. d

Chapter 25

1. b
2. d
3. b
4. c
5. a
6. b
7. d
8. a

Chapter 26

1. c
2. d
3. b
4. a
5. c
6. d
7. a
8. b
9. d
10. d
11. c
12. a

Chapter 27

1. c
2. c
3. b
4. b
5. b

Chapter 28

1. c
2. c
3. d
4. a
5. a

UNIT IV

Chapter 29

1. b
2. b
3. a
4. b

Chapter 30

1. d
2. c
3. a
4. b
5. c

Chapter 31

1. c
2. d
3. c
4. d
5. a

Chapter 32

1. b
2. b
3. c
4. c
5. b

APPENDIX II

Resources

DEPRESSION: SOURCES OF ADDITIONAL INFORMATION FOR CAREGIVERS AND CLIENTS

- Anxiety Disorders Association of America, 6000 Executive Blvd., Suite 200, Rockville, MD 20852
- Association for the Advancement of Behavior Therapy, 305 7th Avenue, New York, NY 10001
- Depression Awareness, Recognition, and Treatment (D/ART) Program, National Institute of Mental Health, 5600 Fishers Lane, Room 10-85, Rockville, MD 20857; phone: 800-421-4211. *Free brochure available in English and Spanish*
- National Alliance for the Mentally Ill, 2101 Wilson Blvd., Suite 302, Arlington, VA 22201; phone: 703-524-7600
- National Council on Child Abuse and Family Violence, 1155 Connecticut Avenue, NW, Suite 300, Washington, DC 20036
- National Coalition Against Domestic Violence, PO Box 34103, Washington, DC 20043; phone: 202-638-6388
- National Depressive and Manic-Depressive Association (NDMDA), Merchandise Mart, Box 3395, Chicago, IL 60654; phone: 312-446-9009
- National Foundation for Depressive Illness, 20 Charles Street, New York, NY 10014
- National Institute of Mental Health Panic Disorders Education—1-800-64-PANIC
- National Mental Health Association, 1021 Prince Street, Alexandria, VA 22314-2971; phone: 703-684-7722
- Schizophrenics Anonymous, 1209 California Road, Eastchester, NY 10709; phone: 914-337-2252

APPENDIX III

DSM-IV Classification*

NOS = Not Otherwise Specified.

An *x* appearing in a diagnostic code indicates that a specific code number is required.

An ellipsis (. . .) is used in the names of certain disorders to indicate that the name of a specific mental disorder or general medical condition should be inserted when recording the name (e.g., 293.0 Delirium Due to Hypothyroidism).

Numbers in parentheses are page numbers in the DSM-IV.

If criteria are currently met, one of the following severity specifiers may be noted after the diagnosis:

Mild
Moderate
Severe

If criteria are no longer met, one of the following specifiers may be noted:

In Partial Remission
In Full Remission
Prior History

Disorders Usually First Diagnosed in Infancy, Childhood, or Adolescence (37)

MENTAL RETARDATION (39)

***Note:** These are coded on Axis II.*

317 Mild Mental Retardation (41)
318.0 Moderate Mental Retardation (41)
318.1 Severe Mental Retardation (41)
318.2 Profound Mental Retardation (41)
319 Mental Retardation, Severity Unspecified (42)

LEARNING DISORDERS (46)

315.00 Reading Disorder (48)
315.1 Mathematics Disorder (50)
315.2 Disorder of Written Expression (51)
315.9 Learning Disorder NOS (53)

MOTOR SKILLS DISORDER

315.4 Developmental Coordination Disorder (53)

COMMUNICATION DISORDERS (55)

315.31 Expressive Language Disorder (55)
315.31 Mixed Receptive-Expressive Language Disorder (58)
315.39 Phonological Disorder (61)
307.0 Stuttering (63)
307.9 Communication Disorder NOS (65)

PERVASIVE DEVELOPMENTAL DISORDERS (65)

299.00 Autistic Disorder (66)
299.80 Rett's Disorder (71)
299.10 Childhood Disintegrative Disorder (73)
299.80 Asperger's Disorder (75)
299.80 Pervasive Developmental Disorder NOS (77)

ATTENTION-DEFICIT AND DISRUPTIVE BEHAVIOR DISORDERS (78)

314.xx Attention-Deficit/Hyperactivity Disorder (78)
.01 Combined Type
.00 Predominantly Inattentive Type
.01 Predominantly Hyperactive-Impulsive Type
314.9 Attention-Deficit/Hyperactivity Disorder NOS (85)
312.8 Conduct Disorder (85)
Specify type: Childhood-Onset Type/ Adolescent-Onset Type
313.81 Oppositional Defiant Disorder (91)
312.9 Disruptive Behavior Disorder NOS (94)

FEEDING AND EATING DISORDERS OF INFANCY OR EARLY CHILDHOOD (94)

307.52 Pica (95)
307.53 Rumination Disorder (96)
307.59 Feeding Disorder of Infancy or Early Childhood (98)

TIC DISORDERS (100)

307.23 Tourette's Disorder (101)
307.22 Chronic Motor or Vocal Tic Disorder (103)

* DSM-IV is an abbreviation for *Diagnostic and Statistical Manual of Mental Disorders, Fourth Edition.*

From American Psychiatric Association. (1994). *Diagnostic and statistical manual of mental disorders, fourth edition.* (pp. 13–24). Washington, DC: Author.

307.21 Transient Tic Disorder (104)
Specify if: Single Episode/Recurrent
307.20 Tic Disorder NOS (105)

ELIMINATION DISORDERS (106)

___._ Encopresis (106)
787.6 With Constipation and Overflow Incontinence
307.7 Without Constipation and Overflow Incontinence
307.6 Enuresis (Not Due to a General Medical Condition) (108)
Specify type: Nocturnal Only/Diurnal Only/Nocturnal and Diurnal

OTHER DISORDERS OF INFANCY, CHILDHOOD, OR ADOLESCENCE

309.21 Separation Anxiety Disorder (110)
Specify if: Early Onset
313.23 Selective Mutism (114)
313.89 Reactive Attachment Disorder of Infancy or Early Childhood (116)
Specify type: Inhibited Type/Disinhibited Type
307.3 Stereotypic Movement Disorder (118)
Specify if: With Self-Injurious Behavior
313.9 Disorder of Infancy, Childhood, or Adolescence NOS (121)

Delirium, Dementia, and Amnestic and Other Cognitive Disorders (123)

DELIRIUM (124)

293.0 Delirium Due to . . . [*Indicate the General Medical Condition*] (127)
___._ Substance Intoxication Delirium (129) (*refer to Substance-Related Disorders for substance-specific codes*)
___._ Substance Withdrawal Delirium (129) (*refer to Substance-Related Disorders for substance-specific codes*)
___._ Delirium Due to Multiple Etiologies (*code each of the specific etiologies*) (132)
780.09 Delirium NOS (133)

DEMENTIA (133)

290.xx Dementia of the Alzheimer's Type, With Early Onset (*also code 331.0 Alzheimer's disease on Axis III*) (139)
.10 Uncomplicated
.11 With Delirium
.12 With Delusions
.13 With Depressed Mood
Specify if: With Behavioral Disturbance
290.xx Dementia of the Alzheimer's Type, With Late Onset (*also code 331.0 Alzheimer's disease on Axis III*) (139)
.0 Uncomplicated
.3 With Delirium
.20 With Delusions
.21 With Depressed Mood
Specify if: With Behavioral Disturbance
290.xx Vascular Dementia (143)
.40 Uncomplicated
.41 With Delirium
.42 With Delusions
.43 With Depressed Mood
Specify if: With Behavioral Disturbance
294.9 Dementia Due to HIV Disease (*also code 043.1 HIV infection affecting central nervous system on Axis III*) (148)
294.1 Dementia Due to Head Trauma (*also code 854.00 head injury on Axis III*) (148)
294.1 Dementia Due to Parkinson's Disease (*also code 332.0 Parkinson's disease on Axis III*) (148)
294.1 Dementia Due to Huntington's Disease (*also code 333.4 Huntington's disease on Axis III*) (149)
290.10 Dementia Due to Pick's Disease (*also code 331.1 Pick's disease on Axis III*) (149)
290.10 Dementia Due to Creutzfeldt-Jakob Disease (*also code 046.1 Creutzfeldt-Jakob disease on Axis III*) (150)
294.1 Dementia Due to . . . [*Indicate the General Medical Condition not listed above*] (*also code the general medical condition on Axis III*) (151)
___._ Substance-Induced Persisting Dementia (*refer to Substance-Related Disorders for substance-specific codes*) (152)
___._ Dementia Due to Multiple Etiologies (*code each of the specific etiologies*) (154)
294.8 Dementia NOS (155)

AMNESTIC DISORDERS (156)

294.0 Amnestic Disorder Due to . . . [*Indicate the General Medical Condition*] (158)
Specify if: Transient/Chronic
___._ Substance-Induced Persisting Amnestic Disorder (*refer to Substance-Related Disorders for substance-specific codes*) (161)
294.8 Amnestic Disorder NOS (163)

OTHER COGNITIVE DISORDERS (163)

294.9 Cognitive Disorder NOS (163)

Mental Disorders Due to a General Medical Condition Not Elsewhere Classified (165)

293.89 Catatonic Disorder Due to . . . [*Indicate the General Medical Condition*] (169)
310.1 Personality Change Due to . . . [*Indicate the General Medical Condition*] (171)

Specify type: Labile Type/Disinhibited Type/Aggressive Type/Apathetic Type/Paranoid Type/Other Type/Combined Type/Unspecified Type

293.9 Mental Disorder NOS Due to . . . [*Indicate the General Medical Condition*] (174)

Substance-Related Disorders (175)

[a]*The following specifiers may be applied to Substance Dependence:*

With Physiological Dependence/Without Physiological Dependence
Early Full Remission/Early Partial Remission
Sustained Full Remission/Sustained Partial Remission
On Agonist Therapy/In a Controlled Environment

The following specifiers apply to Substance-Induced Disorders as noted:

[I]With Onset During Intoxication/[W]With Onset During Withdrawal

ALCOHOL-RELATED DISORDERS (194)

Alcohol Use Disorders

303.90 Alcohol Dependence[a] (195)
305.00 Alcohol Abuse (196)

Alcohol-Induced Disorders

303.00 Alcohol Intoxication (196)
291.8 Alcohol Withdrawal (197)
Specify if: With Perceptual Disturbances
291.0 Alcohol Intoxication Delirium (129)
291.0 Alcohol Withdrawal Delirium (129)
291.2 Alcohol-Induced Persisting Dementia (152)
291.1 Alcohol-Induced Persisting Amnestic Disorder (161)
291.x Alcohol-Induced Psychotic Disorder (310)
.5 With Delusions[I,W]
.3 With Hallucinations[I,W]
291.8 Alcohol-Induced Mood Disorder[I,W] (370)
291.8 Alcohol-Induced Anxiety Disorder[I,W] (439)
291.8 Alcohol-Induced Sexual Dysfunction[I] (519)
291.8 Alcohol-Induced Sleep Disorder[I,W] (601)
291.9 Alcohol-Related Disorder NOS (204)

AMPHETAMINE (OR AMPHETAMINE-LIKE)–RELATED DISORDERS (204)

Amphetamine Use Disorders

304.40 Amphetamine Dependence[a] (206)
305.70 Amphetamine Abuse (206)

Amphetamine-Induced Disorders

292.89 Amphetamine Intoxication (207)
Specify if: With Perceptual Disturbances
292.0 Amphetamine Withdrawal (208)
292.81 Amphetamine Intoxication Delirium (129)
292.xx Amphetamine-Induced Psychotic Disorder (310)
.11 With Delusions[I]
.12 With Hallucinations[I]
292.84 Amphetamine-Induced Mood Disorder[I,W] (370)
292.89 Amphetamine-Induced Anxiety Disorder[I] (439)
292.89 Amphetamine-Induced Sexual Dysfunction[I] (519)
292.89 Amphetamine-Induced Sleep Disorder[I,W] (601)
292.9 Amphetamine-Related Disorder NOS (211)

CAFFEINE-RELATED DISORDERS (212)

Caffeine-Induced Disorders

305.90 Caffeine Intoxication (212)
292.89 Caffeine-Induced Anxiety Disorder[I] (439)
292.89 Caffeine-Induced Sleep Disorder[I] (601)
292.9 Caffeine-Related Disorder NOS (215)

CANNABIS-RELATED DISORDERS (215)

Cannabis Use Disorders

304.30 Cannabis Dependence[a] (216)
305.20 Cannabis Abuse (217)

Cannabis-Induced Disorders

292.89 Cannabis Intoxication (217)
Specify if: With Perceptual Disturbances
292.81 Cannabis Intoxication Delirium (129)
292.xx Cannabis-Induced Psychotic Disorder (310)
.11 With Delusions[I]
.12 With Hallucinations[I]
292.89 Cannabis-Induced Anxiety Disorder[I] (439)
292.9 Cannabis-Related Disorder NOS (221)

COCAINE-RELATED DISORDERS (221)

Cocaine Use Disorders

304.20 Cocaine Dependence[a] (222)
305.60 Cocaine Abuse (223)

Cocaine-Induced Disorders

292.89 Cocaine Intoxication (223)
Specify if: With Perceptual Disturbances
292.0 Cocaine Withdrawal (225)
292.81 Cocaine Intoxication Delirium (129)
292.xx Cocaine-Induced Psychotic Disorder (310)
.11 With Delusions[I]
.12 With Hallucinations[I]
292.84 Cocaine-Induced Mood Disorder[I,W] (370)
292.89 Cocaine-Induced Anxiety Disorder[I,W] (439)
292.89 Cocaine-Induced Sexual Dysfunction[I] (519)
292.89 Cocaine-Induced Sleep Disorder[I,W] (601)
292.9 Cocaine-Related Disorder NOS (229)

HALLUCINOGEN-RELATED DISORDERS (229)

Hallucinogen Use Disorders

304.50 Hallucinogen Dependence[a] (230)
305.30 Hallucinogen Abuse (231)

Hallucinogen-Induced Disorders

292.89 Hallucinogen Intoxication (232)
292.89 Hallucinogen Persisting Perception Disorder (Flashbacks) (233)
292.81 Hallucinogen Intoxication Delirium (129)
292.xx Hallucinogen-Induced Psychotic Disorder (310)
.11 With Delusions[I]
.12 With Hallucinations[I]
292.84 Hallucinogen-Induced Mood Disorder[I] (370)
292.89 Hallucinogen-Induced Anxiety Disorder[I] (439)
292.9 Hallucinogen-Related Disorder NOS (236)

INHALANT-RELATED DISORDERS (236)

Inhalant Use Disorders

304.60 Inhalant Dependence[a] (238)
305.90 Inhalant Abuse (238)

Inhalant-Induced Disorders

292.89 Inhalant Intoxication (239)
292.81 Inhalant Intoxication Delirium (129)
292.82 Inhalant-Induced Persisting Dementia (152)
292.xx Inhalant-Induced Psychotic Disorder (310)
.11 With Delusions[I]
.12 With Hallucinations[I]
292.84 Inhalant-Induced Mood Disorder[I] (370)
292.89 Inhalant-Induced Anxiety Disorder[I] (439)
292.9 Inhalant-Related Disorder NOS (242)

NICOTINE-RELATED DISORDERS (242)

Nicotine Use Disorder

305.10 Nicotine Dependence[a] (243)

Nicotine-Induced Disorder

292.0 Nicotine Withdrawal (244)
292.9 Nicotine-Related Disorder NOS (247)

OPIOID-RELATED DISORDERS (247)

Opioid Use Disorders

304.00 Opioid Dependence[a] (248)
305.50 Opioid Abuse (249)

Opioid-Induced Disorders

292.89 Opioid Intoxication (249)
Specify if: With Perceptual Disturbances
292.0 Opioid Withdrawal (250)
292.81 Opioid Intoxication Delirium (129)
292.xx Opioid-Induced Psychotic Disorder (310)
.11 With Delusions[I]
.12 With Hallucinations[I]
292.84 Opioid-Induced Mood Disorder[I] (370)
292.89 Opioid-Induced Sexual Dysfunction[I] (519)
292.89 Opioid-Induced Sleep Disorder[I,W] (601)
292.9 Opioid-Related Disorder NOS (255)

PHENCYCLIDINE (OR PHENCYCLIDINE-LIKE)–RELATED DISORDERS (255)

Phencyclidine Use Disorders

304.90 Phencyclidine Dependence[a] (256)
305.90 Phencyclidine Abuse (257)

Phencyclidine-Induced Disorders

292.89 Phencyclidine Intoxication (257)
Specify if: With Perceptual Disturbances
292.81 Phencyclidine Intoxication Delirium (129)
292.xx Phencyclidine-Induced Psychotic Disorder (310)
.11 With Delusions[I]
.12 With Hallucinations[I]
292.84 Phencyclidine-Induced Mood Disorder[I] (370)
292.89 Phencyclidine-Induced Anxiety Disorder[I] (439)
292.9 Phencyclidine-Related Disorder NOS (261)

SEDATIVE-, HYPNOTIC-, OR ANXIOLYTIC-RELATED DISORDERS (261)

Sedative, Hypnotic, or Anxiolytic Use Disorders

304.10 Sedative, Hypnotic, or Anxiolytic Dependence[a] (262)
305.40 Sedative, Hypnotic, or Anxiolytic Abuse (263)

Sedative-, Hypnotic-, or Anxiolytic-Induced Disorders

292.89 Sedative, Hypnotic, or Anxiolytic Intoxication (263)
292.0 Sedative, Hypnotic, or Anxiolytic Withdrawal (264)
Specify if: With Perceptual Disturbances
292.81 Sedative, Hypnotic, or Anxiolytic Intoxication Delirium (129)
292.81 Sedative, Hypnotic, or Anxiolytic Withdrawal Delirium (129)
292.82 Sedative-, Hypnotic-, or Anxiolytic-Induced Persisting Dementia (152)
292.83 Sedative-, Hypnotic-, or Anxiolytic-Induced Persisting Amnestic Disorder (161)
292.xx Sedative-, Hypnotic-, or Anxiolytic-Induced Psychotic Disorder (310)
.11 With Delusions[I,W]
.12 With Hallucinations[I,W]

292.84 Sedative-, Hypnotic-, or Anxiolytic-Induced Mood Disorder[I,W] (370)
292.89 Sedative-, Hypnotic-, or Anxiolytic-Induced Anxiety Disorder[W] (439)
292.89 Sedative-, Hypnotic-, or Anxiolytic-Induced Sexual Dysfunction[I] (519)
292.89 Sedative-, Hypnotic-, or Anxiolytic-Induced Sleep Disorder[I,W] (601)
292.9 Sedative-, Hypnotic-, or Anxiolytic-Related Disorder NOS (269)

POLYSUBSTANCE-RELATED DISORDER

304.80 Polysubstance Dependence[a] (270)

OTHER (OR UNKNOWN) SUBSTANCE–RELATED DISORDERS (270)

Other (or Unknown) Substance Use Disorders

304.90 Other (or Unknown) Substance Dependence[a] (176)
305.90 Other (or Unknown) Substance Abuse (182)

Other (or Unknown) Substance–Induced Disorders

292.89 Other (or Unknown) Substance Intoxication (183)
Specify if: With Perceptual Disturbances
292.0 Other (or Unknown) Substance Withdrawal (184)
Specify if: With Perceptual Disturbances
292.81 Other (or Unknown) Substance–Induced Delirium (129)
292.82 Other (or Unknown) Substance–Induced Persisting Dementia (152)
292.83 Other (or Unknown) Substance–Induced Persisting Amnestic Disorder (161)
292.xx Other (or Unknown) Substance–Induced Psychotic Disorder (310)
.11 With Delusions[I,W]
.12 With Hallucinations[I,W]
292.84 Other (or Unknown) Substance–Induced Mood Disorder[I,W] (370)
292.89 Other (or Unknown) Substance–Induced Anxiety Disorder[I,W] (439)
292.89 Other (or Unknown) Substance–Induced Sexual Dysfunction[I] (519)
292.89 Other (or Unknown) Substance–Induced Sleep Disorder[I,W] (601)
292.9 Other (or Unknown) Substance–Related Disorder NOS (272)

Schizophrenia and Other Psychotic Disorders (273)

295.xx Schizophrenia (274)

The following Classification of Longitudinal Course applies to all subtypes of Schizophrenia:

Episodic With Interepisode Residual Symptoms (*specify if*: With Prominent Negative Symptoms)/Episodic With No Interepisode Residual Symptoms/Continuous (*specify if*: With Prominent Negative Symptoms)
Single Episode In Partial Remission (*specify if*: With Prominent Negative Symptoms)/Single Episode In Full Remission
Other or Unspecified Pattern

.30 Paranoid Type (287)
.10 Disorganized Type (287)
.20 Catatonic Type (288)
.90 Undifferentiated Type (289)
.60 Residual Type (289)
295.40 Schizophreniform Disorder (290)
Specify if: Without Good Prognostic Features/With Good Prognostic Features
295.70 Schizoaffective Disorder (292)
Specify type: Bipolar Type/Depressive Type
297.1 Delusional Disorder (296)
Specify type: Erotomanic Type/Grandiose Type/Jealous Type/Persecutory Type/Somatic Type/Mixed Type/Unspecified Type
298.8 Brief Psychotic Disorder (302)
Specify if: With Marked Stressor(s)/Without Marked Stressor(s)/With Postpartum Onset
297.3 Shared Psychotic Disorder (305)
293.xx Psychotic Disorder Due to . . . [*Indicate the General Medical Condition*] (306)
.81 With Delusions
.82 With Hallucinations
——.– Substance-Induced Psychotic Disorder (*refer to Substance-Related Disorders for substance-specific codes*) (310)
Specify if: With Onset During Intoxication/With Onset During Withdrawal
298.9 Psychotic Disorder NOS (315)

Mood Disorders (317)

Code current state of Major Depressive Disorder or Bipolar I Disorder in fifth digit:

1 = Mild
2 = Moderate
3 = Severe Without Psychotic Features
4 = Severe With Psychotic Features
Specify: Mood-Congruent Psychotic Features/Mood-Incongruent Psychotic Features
5 = In Partial Remission
6 = In Full Remission
0 = Unspecified

The following specifiers apply (for current or most recent episode) to Mood Disorders as noted:

[a]Severity/Psychotic/Remission Specifiers/[b]Chronic/[c]With Catatonic Features/[d]With Melancholic Features/[e]With Atypical Features/[f]With Postpartum Onset

The following specifiers apply to Mood Disorders as noted:

[g]With or Without Full Interepisode Recovery
[h]With Seasonal Pattern/[i]With Rapid Cycling

DEPRESSIVE DISORDERS

296.xx Major Depressive Disorder, (339)
.2x Single Episode[a,b,c,d,e,f]
.3x Recurrent[a,b,c,d,e,f,g,h]
300.4 Dysthymic Disorder (345)
Specify if: Early Onset/Late Onset
Specify: With Atypical Features
311 Depressive Disorder NOS (350)

BIPOLAR DISORDERS

296.xx Bipolar I Disorder, (350)
.0x Single Manic Episode[a,c,f]
Specify if: Mixed
.40 Most Recent Episode Hypomanic[g,h,i]
.4x Most Recent Episode Manic[a,c,f,g,h,i]
.6x Most Recent Episode Mixed[a,c,f,g,h,i]
.5x Most Recent Episode Depressed[a,b,c,d,e,f,g,h,i]
.7 Most Recent Episode Unspecified[g,h,i]
296.89 Bipolar II Disorder[a,b,c,d,e,f,g,h,i] (359)
Specify (current or most recent episode): Hypomanic/Depressed
301.13 Cyclothymic Disorder (363)
296.80 Bipolar Disorder NOS (366)
293.83 Mood Disorder Due to . . . [*Indicate the General Medical Condition*] (366)
Specify type: With Depressive Features/With Major Depressive–Like Episode/With Manic Features/With Mixed Features
___._ Substance-Induced Mood Disorder (*refer to Substance-Related Disorders for substance-specific codes*) (370)
Specify type: With Depressive Features/With Manic Features/With Mixed Features
Specify if: With Onset During Intoxication/With Onset During Withdrawal
296.90 Mood Disorder NOS (375)

Anxiety Disorders (393)

300.01 Panic Disorder Without Agoraphobia (397)
300.21 Panic Disorder With Agoraphobia (397)
300.22 Agoraphobia Without History of Panic Disorder (403)
300.29 Specific Phobia (405)
Specify type: Animal Type/Natural Environment Type/Blood-Injection-Injury Type/Situational Type/Other Type
300.23 Social Phobia (411)
Specify if: Generalized
300.3 Obsessive-Compulsive Disorder (417)
Specify if: With Poor Insight
309.81 Posttraumatic Stress Disorder (424)
Specify if: Acute/Chronic
Specify if: With Delayed Onset
308.3 Acute Stress Disorder (429)
300.02 Generalized Anxiety Disorder (432)
293.89 Anxiety Disorder Due to . . . [*Indicate the General Medical Condition*] (436)
Specify if: With Generalized Anxiety/With Panic Attacks/With Obsessive-Compulsive Symptoms
___._ Substance-Induced Anxiety Disorder (*refer to Substance-Related Disorders for substance specific codes*) (439)
Specify if: With Generalized Anxiety/With Panic Attacks/With Obsessive-Compulsive Symptoms/With Phobic Symptoms
Specify if: With Onset During Intoxication/With Onset During Withdrawal
300.00 Anxiety Disorder NOS (444)

Somatoform Disorders (445)

300.81 Somatization Disorder (446)
300.81 Undifferentiated Somatoform Disorder (450)
300.11 Conversion Disorder (452)
Specify type: With Motor Symptom or Deficit/With Sensory Symptom or Deficit/With Seizures or Convulsions/With Mixed Presentation
307.xx Pain Disorder (458)
.80 Associated With Psychological Factors
.89 Associated With Both Psychological Factors and a General Medical Condition
Specify if: Acute/Chronic
300.7 Hypochondriasis (462)
Specify if: With Poor Insight
300.7 Body Dysmorphic Disorder (466)
300.81 Somatoform Disorder NOS (468)

Factitious Disorders (471)

300.xx Factitious Disorder (471)
.16 With Predominantly Psychological Signs and Symptoms
.19 With Predominantly Physical Signs and Symptoms
.19 With Combined Psychological and Physical Signs and Symptoms
300.19 Factitious Disorder NOS (475)

Dissociative Disorders (477)

300.12 Dissociative Amnesia (478)
300.13 Dissociative Fugue (481)
300.14 Dissociative Identity Disorder (484)
300.6 Depersonalization Disorder (488)
300.15 Dissociative Disorder NOS (490)

Sexual and Gender Identity Disorders (493)

SEXUAL DYSFUNCTIONS (493)

The following specifiers apply to all primary Sexual Dysfunctions:

Lifelong Type/Acquired Type-Generalized Type/Situational Type Due to Psychological Factors/Due to Combined Factors

Sexual Desire Disorders

302.71 Hypoactive Sexual Desire Disorder (496)
302.79 Sexual Aversion Disorder (499)

Sexual Arousal Disorders

302.72 Female Sexual Arousal Disorder (500)
302.72 Male Erectile Disorder (502)

Orgasmic Disorders

302.73 Female Orgasmic Disorder (505)
302.74 Male Orgasmic Disorder (507)
302.75 Premature Ejaculation (509)

Sexual Pain Disorders

302.76 Dyspareunia (Not Due to a General Medical Condition) (511)
306.51 Vaginismus (Not Due to a General Medical Condition) (513)

Sexual Dysfunction Due to a General Medical Condition (515)

625.8 Female Hypoactive Sexual Desire Disorder Due to . . . [*Indicate the General Medical Condition*] (515)
608.89 Male Hypoactive Sexual Desire Disorder Due to . . . [*Indicate the General Medical Condition*] (515)
607.84 Male Erectile Disorder Due to . . . [*Indicate the General Medical Condition*] (515)
625.0 Female Dyspareunia Due to . . . [*Indicate the General Medical Condition*] (515)
608.89 Male Dyspareunia Due to . . . [*Indicate the General Medical Condition*] (515)
625.8 Other Female Sexual Dysfunction Due to . . . [*Indicate the General Medical Condition*] (515)
608.89 Other Male Sexual Dysfunction Due to . . . [*Indicate the General Medical Condition*] (515)
___._ Substance-Induced Sexual Dysfunction (*refer to Substance-Related Disorders for substance-specific codes*) (519)
Specify if: With Impaired Desire/With Impaired Arousal/With Impaired Orgasm/With Sexual Pain
Specify if: With Onset During Intoxication
302.70 Sexual Dysfunction NOS (522)

PARAPHILIAS (522)

302.4 Exhibitionism (525)
302.81 Fetishism (526)
302.89 Frotteurism (527)
302.2 Pedophilia (527)
Specify if: Sexually Attracted to Males/Sexually Attracted to Females/Sexually Attracted to Both
Specify if: Limited to Incest
Specify type: Exclusive Type/Nonexclusive Type
302.83 Sexual Masochism (529)
302.84 Sexual Sadism (530)
302.3 Transvestic Fetishism (530)
Specify if: With Gender Dysphoria
302.82 Voyeurism (532)
302.9 Paraphilia NOS (532)

GENDER IDENTITY DISORDERS (532)

302.xx Gender Identity Disorder (532)
.6 in Children
.85 in Adolescents or Adults
Specify if: Sexually Attracted to Males/Sexually Attracted to Females/Sexually Attracted to Both/Sexually Attracted to Neither
302.6 Gender Identity Disorder NOS (538)
302.9 Sexual Disorder NOS (538)

Eating Disorders (539)

307.1 Anorexia Nervosa (539)
Specify type: Restricting Type; Binge-Eating/Purging Type
307.51 Bulimia Nervosa (545)
Specify type: Purging Type/Nonpurging Type
307.50 Eating Disorder NOS (550)

Sleep Disorders (551)

PRIMARY SLEEP DISORDERS (553)

Dyssomnias (553)

307.42 Primary Insomnia (553)
307.44 Primary Hypersomnia (557)
Specify if: Recurrent
347 Narcolepsy (562)
780.59 Breathing-Related Sleep Disorder (567)
307.45 Circadian Rhythm Sleep Disorder (573)
Specify type: Delayed Sleep Phase Type/Jet Lag Type/Shift Work Type/Unspecified Type
307.47 Dyssomnia NOS (579)

Parasomnias (579)

307.47 Nightmare Disorder (580)
307.46 Sleep Terror Disorder (583)
307.46 Sleepwalking Disorder (587)
307.47 Parasomnia NOS (592)

SLEEP DISORDERS RELATED TO ANOTHER MENTAL DISORDER (592)

307.42 Insomnia Related to . . . [*Indicate the Axis I or Axis II Disorder*] (592)
307.44 Hypersomnia Related to . . . [*Indicate the Axis I or Axis II Disorder*] (592)

OTHER SLEEP DISORDERS

780.xx Sleep Disorder Due to . . . [*Indicate the General Medical Condition*] (597)
- .52 Insomnia Type
- .54 Hypersomnia Type
- .59 Parasomnia Type
- .59 Mixed Type

___.__ Substance-Induced Sleep Disorder (*refer to Substance-Related Disorders for substance-specific codes*) (601)
Specify type: Insomnia Type/Hypersomnia Type/Parasomnia Type/Mixed Type
Specify if: With Onset During Intoxication/With Onset During Withdrawal

Impulse-Control Disorders Not Elsewhere Classified (609)

312.34 Intermittent Explosive Disorder (609)
312.32 Kleptomania (612)
312.33 Pyromania (614)
312.31 Pathological Gambling (615)
312.39 Trichotillomania (618)
312.30 Impulse-Control Disorder NOS (621)

Adjustment Disorders (623)

309.xx Adjustment Disorder (623)
- .0 With Depressed Mood
- .24 With Anxiety
- .28 With Mixed Anxiety and Depressed Mood
- .3 With Disturbance of Conduct
- .4 With Mixed Disturbance of Emotions and Conduct
- .9 Unspecified

Specify if: Acute/Chronic

Personality Disorders (629)

Note: *These are coded on Axis II.*

301.0 Paranoid Personality Disorder (634)
301.20 Schizoid Personality Disorder (638)
301.22 Schizotypal Personality Disorder (641)
301.7 Antisocial Personality Disorder (645)
301.83 Borderline Personality Disorder (650)
301.50 Histrionic Personality Disorder (655)
301.81 Narcissistic Personality Disorder (658)
301.82 Avoidant Personality Disorder (662)
301.6 Dependent Personality Disorder (665)
301.4 Obsessive-Compulsive Personality Disorder (669)
301.9 Personality Disorder NOS (673)

Other Conditions That May Be a Focus of Clinical Attention (675)

PSYCHOLOGICAL FACTORS AFFECTING MEDICAL CONDITION (675)

316 . . . [*Specified Psychological Factor*] Affecting . . . [*Indicate the General Medical Condition*] (675)
Choose name based on nature of factors:
- Mental Disorder Affecting Medical Condition
- Psychological Symptoms Affecting Medical Condition
- Personality Traits or Coping Style Affecting Medical Condition
- Maladaptive Health Behaviors Affecting Medical Condition
- Stress-Related Physiological Response Affecting Medical Condition
- Other or Unspecified Psychological Factors Affecting Medical Condition

MEDICATION-INDUCED MOVEMENT DISORDERS (678)

332.1 Neuroleptic-Induced Parkinsonism (679)
333.92 Neuroleptic Malignant Syndrome (679)
333.7 Neuroleptic-Induced Acute Dystonia (679)
333.99 Neuroleptic-Induced Acute Akathisia (679)
333.82 Neuroleptic-Induced Tardive Dyskinesia (679)
333.1 Medication-Induced Postural Tremor (680)
333.90 Medication-Induced Movement Disorder NOS (680)

OTHER MEDICATION-INDUCED DISORDER

995.2 Adverse Effects of Medication NOS (680)

RELATIONAL PROBLEMS (680)

V61.9 Relational Problem Related to a Mental Disorder or General Medical Condition (681)
V61.20 Parent-Child Relational Problem (681)
V61.1 Partner Relational Problem (681)
V61.8 Sibling Relational Problem (681)
V62.81 Relational Problem NOS (681)

PROBLEMS RELATED TO ABUSE OR NEGLECT (682)

V61.21 Physical Abuse of Child (682) (*code 995.5 if focus of attention is on victim*)
V61.21 Sexual Abuse of Child (682) (*code 995.5 if focus of attention is on victim*)
V61.21 Neglect of Child (682) (*code 995.5 if focus of attention is on victim*)
V61.1 Physical Abuse of Adult (682) (*code 995.81 if focus of attention is on victim*)

V61.1 Sexual Abuse of Adult (682) (*code 995.81 if focus of attention is on victim*)

ADDITIONAL CONDITIONS THAT MAY BE A FOCUS OF CLINICAL ATTENTION (683)

V15.81 Noncompliance With Treatment (683)
V65.2 Malingering (683)
V71.01 Adult Antisocial Behavior (683)
V71.02 Child or Adolescent Antisocial Behavior (684)
V62.89 Borderline Intellectual Functioning (684)
***Note:** This is coded on Axis II.*
780.9 Age-Related Cognitive Decline (684)
V62.82 Bereavement (684)
V62.3 Academic Problem (685)
V62.2 Occupational Problem (685)
313.82 Identity Problem (685)
V62.89 Religious or Spiritual Problem (685)
V62.4 Acculturation Problem (685)
V62.89 Phase of Life Problem (685)

Additional Codes

300.9 Unspecified Mental Disorder (nonpsychotic) (687)
V71.09 No Diagnosis or Condition on Axis I (687)
799.9 Diagnosis or Condition Deferred on Axis I (687)
V71.09 No Diagnosis on Axis II (687)
799.9 Diagnosis Deferred on Axis II (687)

Multiaxial System

Axis I Clinical Disorders
Other Conditions That May Be a Focus of Clinical Attention
Axis II Personality Disorders
Mental Retardation
Axis III General Medical Conditions
Axis IV Psychosocial and Environmental Problems
Axis V Global Assessment of Functioning

Medication Reference for Psychiatric

from Nurse's Drug Handbook 1995 *by Barbara B. Hodgson, RH, Robert J. Kizior, BS, RPh., and Ruth T. Kingdon, RN, MSN. Philadelphia, W.B. Saunders Company.*

antianxiety

ACTION

Benzodiazepines are the largest and most frequently prescribed group of antianxiety agents. Exact mechanism unknown; may increase the inhibiting effect of gamma-aminobutyric acid (GABA) (inhibiting nerve impulse transmission) as well as other inhibitory transmitters by binding to specific benzodiazepine receptors in various areas of the CNS.

USES

Treatment of anxiety. Additionally, some benzodiazepines are used as hypnotics, anticonvulsants to prevent delirium tremors during alcohol withdrawal and as adjunctive therapy for relaxation of skeletal muscle spasms. Midazolam, a short-acting injectable form, is used for preop sedation, relieving anxiety for short diagnostic, endoscopic procedures.

PRECAUTIONS

CONTRAINDICATIONS: Hypersensitivity, renal or hepatic dysfunction, CNS depression, history of drug abuse, pregnancy, glaucoma, lactation, young children, within 14 days of MAO inhibitors, myasthenia gravis. **CAUTION:** Elderly or debilitated; pts w/COPD. Drugs should be withdrawn slowly.

INTERACTIONS

CNS depressants (e.g., alcohol, barbiturates, narcotics) may increase CNS effects of benzodiazepines (e.g., sedation).

SIDE EFFECTS

Drowsiness is the most common side effect; usually disappears w/continued use. Dizziness, hypotension occur frequently.

TOXIC EFFECTS/ADVERSE REACTIONS

Incidence of toxicity is very low when antianxiety drugs are taken alone. Confusion, hypersensitivity reactions, headache, stupor, paradoxical excitement, nausea and vomiting, blood dyscrasias, jaundice (hepatic dysfunction) are rare effects. These vary according to individual drug. IV administration may cause respiratory depression, apnea.

NURSING IMPLICATIONS

GENERAL: Provide restful environment and measures for comfort. Comply w/federal narcotic laws regarding Schedule IV drugs. Consider potential for abuse/dependence. For IV administration, have respiratory equipment available; keep pt recumbent. Most antianxiety drugs should not be mixed w/other drugs in a syringe. **INTERVENTION/EVALUATION:** Monitor B/P. Assess for therapeutic response (according to reason for use, e.g., seizure activity, anxiety, alcohol withdrawal) or paradoxical reaction. Take safety precautions for drowsiness, dizziness. **PATIENT/FAMILY TEACHING:** Avoid smoking; may interfere w/drug action. Do not drive or perform tasks requiring mental acuity until response to medication is controlled. Consult physician before taking other medications. Do not take alcohol. Medication must not be stopped abruptly. Inform other physicians, dentist of drug therapy.

ANTIANXIETY

Generic Name	Brand Name(s)	Uses	Dosage Range (mg/day)
alprazolam	Xanax	Anxiety Panic disorder	PO: 0.75-4
chlordiazepoxide	Librium Libritabs	Anxiety Alcohol withdrawal Preop	PO: 15-100
clonazepam	Klonopin	Anticonvulsant	PO: 1.5-20
clorazepate	Tranxene	Anxiety Alcohol withdrawal Anticonvulsant	PO: 15-60
diazepam	Valium	Anxiety Alcohol withdrawal Anticonvulsant Muscle relaxant	PO: 4-40
lorazepam	Ativan	Anxiety Preanesthetic	PO: 2-4
oxazepam	Serax	Anxiety	PO: 30-120

anticonvulsants

ACTION

Seizures consist of abnormal and excessive discharges from the brain. Anticonvulsants can prevent or reduce excessive discharge of neurons w/seizure foci or decrease the spread of excitation from seizure foci to normal neurons. Exact mechanism unknown. Anticonvulsants include the hydantoins, barbiturates, succinimides, oxazolidinediones, benzodiazepines, and several miscellaneous agents.

USES

Anticonvulsants are generally effective in the treatment of *absence (petit mal) seizures* (brief, abrupt loss of consciousness, some clonic motor activity ranging from eyelid blinking to jerking of entire body), *tonic-clonic (grand mal) seizures* (major convulsions, usually beginning w/spasm of all body musculature, then clonic jerking, followed by depression of all central function), and *complex partial seizures* (confused behavior, impaired consciousness, bizarre generalized EEG activity). Other types of seizures generally respond poorly to anticonvulsant therapy.

PRECAUTIONS

CONTRAINDICATIONS: Hypersensitivity, hepatic, renal, or thy-

nction, alcoholism, blood dyscrasias; diabetes mellitus, cardiac impairment, lactation. **CAUTIONS:** Pregnancy—risk benefit must eighed in relation to congenital abnormalities. Elderly, children, and ebilitated.

ANTICONVULSANTS

Generic Name	Brand Names(s)	Class	Uses	Dosage Range
carba-mazepine	Tegretol	Miscellaneous	Complex partial, tonic-clonic, mixed seizures, trigeminal neuralgia	Adults: 800-1200 mg/day Children: 400-800 mg/day
clonazepam	Klonopin	Benzodi-azepine	Petit mal, aki-netic, myo-clonic, ab-sence	Adults: 1.5-20 mg/day Children: 0.01-0.2 mg/kg/day
clorazepate	Tranxene	Benzodi-azepine	Partial seizures	Adults: 7.5-90 mg/day Children: 7.5-60 mg/day
diazepam	Valium	Benzodi-azepine	Adjunctive ther-apy status epi-lepticus	Adults: PO: 4-40 mg/day IM/IV: 5-30 mg Children: PO: 3-10 mg/day IM/IV: 1-10 mg
ethosuxim-ide	Zarontin	Succinimide	Absence seizures	Children: 20 mg/kg/day
felbamate	Felbatol	Miscellaneous	Partial seizures Lennox-Gustaut syndrome	Adults: 1200-3600 mg/day Children ≥14 yrs: 1200-3600 mg/day
gabapen-tum	Neurontin	Miscellaneous	Partial seizures	Adults: 900-1800 mg/day Children >12 yrs: 900-1800 mg/day
pheno-barbital	Luminal	Barbiturate	Tonic-clonic, partial, status epilepticus	Adults: PO: 100-300 mg/day IM/IV: 200-600 mg Children: PO: 3-5 mg/kg/day IM/IV: 100-400 mg
phenytoin	Dilantin	Hydantoin	Tonic-clonic, complex par-tial, auto-nomic sei-zures, status epilepticus	Adults: PO: 300-600 mg/day IV: 150-250 mg Status epilepti-cus: 15-18 mg/kg Children: PO: 4-8 mg/kg/day Status epilepti-cus: 10-15 mg/kg
primidone	Mysoline	Miscellaneous	Complex partial, partial, aki-netic, tonic-clonic	Adults: 0.75-2 Gm/day Children: 10-25 mg/kg/day
valproic acid	Depakene Depakote	Miscellaneous	Absence, multi-ple seizure types	Adults, children: 15-60 mg/kg/day

INTERACTIONS

Drug interactions are extensive; any other medication administered should be carefully checked for interaction w/anticonvulsants. Teach pts never to take medication w/o consulting physician. Effects are increased by CNS depressants; decreased w/tricyclic antidepressants, phenothiazine antipsychotics, antacids. Refer to individual monographs.

SIDE EFFECTS

Drowsiness, sedation, mild dizziness, gingival hyperplasia, anorexia, nausea, vomiting, hyperglycemia, and glycosuria.

TOXIC EFFECTS/ADVERSE REACTIONS

Visual disturbances, unusual excitement, confusion, skin disorders. Stevens-Johnson syndrome (headache, arthralgia, skin lesions w/other symptoms), liver damage, hirsutism, blood dyscrasias, enlarged lymph glands in neck and under arms.

NURSING IMPLICATIONS

GENERAL: Status epilepticus is a life-threatening emergency that requires immediate IV medication (diazepam is the drug of choice). *Never mix parenteral solutions w/other drugs or IV fluids—should be administered via slow IV push.* When discontinued, gradual reduction is recommended. Provide protection against injury. **INTERVENTION/EVALUATION:** Monitor B/P, pulse, respirations, serum drug levels. Assess neurologic status. Identify characteristics of seizures if they occur. **PATIENT/FAMILY TEACHING:** Therapy is usually several years to life. Take w/food or fluids to minimize GI irritation. Important to take as directed. Do not take other medications w/o consulting physician. Avoid alcohol. Do not drive or engage in activities requiring mental acuity until physician approves (seizures and response to drug are controlled). Carry identification card/bracelet indicating anticonvulsant therapy.

antidepressants

ACTION

Antidepressants are classified as tricyclic, monoamine oxidase (MAO) inhibitors, or miscellaneous. Depression may be due to reduced functioning of monoamine neurotransmitters in the CNS (decreased amount and/or decreased effects at receptor sites).

Antidepressants block metabolism, increase amount/effects of monoamine neurotransmitters (e.g., norepinephrine, serotonin [5-HT]) and act at receptor sites (change responsiveness/sensitivities of both pre- and postsynaptic receptor sites).

Miscellaneous, Tricyclics: Block reuptake of neurotransmitter at presynaptic nerve endings. Potency/selectivity varies w/these agents.

MAO inhibitors: Inhibit enzyme MAO, thus interfering w/degradation of monoamine neurotransmitters.

USES

Used primarily for the treatment of depression. Imipramine is also used for childhood enuresis, clomipramine is used only for obsessive-compulsive disorder (OCD). MAO inhibitors are rarely used as initial therapy except for pts unresponsive to other therapy or when other therapy is contraindicated.

PRECAUTIONS

CONTRAINDICATIONS: Pregnancy, lactation, children <16 yrs of age (exception: Imipramine to treat enuresis in children >6 yrs of age), hypersensitivity, liver dysfunction, renal dysfunction, glaucoma, elderly, CHF. **CAUTIONS:** Never use MAO inhibitors and tricyclic antidepressants together—can result in death. Effects of antidepressants can last 2-3 wks after discontinuation.

INTERACTIONS

Tricyclic antidepressants: Alcohol, CNS depressants may increase CNS, respiratory depression, hypotensive effects. Antithyroid agents may increase risk of agranulocytosis. Phenothiazines may increase sedative, anticholinergic effects. Cimetidine may increase concentration, toxicity. May decrease effects of clonidine, guanadrel. May increase cardiac effects w/sympathomimetics. May increase risk of hypertensive crisis, hyperpyretic, convulsion w/MAO inhibitors.

MAO inhibitors: Alcohol, CNS depressants may increase CNS depressant effects. Tricyclic antidepressants, fluoxetine, trazodone may cause serotonin syndrome. May increase effect of oral hypoglycemics, insulin, B/P may increase w/buspirone, Caffeine containing medications may increase cardiac arrhythmias, hypertension. May precipitate hypertensive crises w/carbamazepine, cyclobenzaprine, maprotiline, other MAO inhibitors. Meperidine, other opioid analgesics may produce immediate excitation, sweating, rigidity, severe hypertension or hypotension, severe respiratory distress, coma, convulsions, vascular collapse, death. May increase CNS stimulant, vasopressor effects. Tyramine, foods w/pressor amines (e.g., aged cheese) may cause sudden, severe hypertension.

SIDE EFFECTS

Tricyclic antidepressants: Dizziness, drowsiness, dry mouth, headache, weight gain, photosensitivity. *MAO inhibitors:* Dizziness, and orthostatic hypotension, blurred vision, constipation, difficulty w/urination, mild headache, weight gain, insomnia.

TOXIC EFFECTS/ADVERSE REACTIONS

Tricyclic antidepressants: Severe drowsiness, confusion, hallucinations, seizures, tachycardia or bradycardia, difficulty breathing. *MAO inhibitors:* Severe drowsiness or dizziness, hypertension or hypotension, tachycardia, difficulty sleeping, hallucinations, respiratory depression.

ANTIDEPRESSANTS

Generic Name	Brand Names(s)	Type	Amine Uptake Blockage	Dosage Range (mg/day)
amitriptyline	Elavil Endep	Tricyclic	Norepinephrine Serotonin	PO: 40-300
amoxapine	Asendin	Tricyclic	Norepinephrine Serotonin	PO: 100-600
bupropion	Wellbutrin	Miscellaneous	—	PO: 200-450
clomipramine	Anafranil	Tricyclic	Norepinephrine Serotonin	PO: 25-250
desipramine	Norpramin Pertofrane	Tricyclic	Norepinephrine Serotonin	PO: 25-100
doxepin	Adapin Sinequan	Tricyclic	Norepinephrine Serotonin	PO: 75-300
fluoxetine	Prozac	Miscellaneous	Serotonin	PO: 20-80
imipramine	Janimine Tofranil	Tricyclic	Norepinephrine Serotonin	PO: 30-300
maprotiline	Ludiomil	Miscellaneous	Norepinephrine	PO: 25-225
nortriptyline	Aventyl Pamelor	Tricyclic	Norepinephrine Serotonin	PO: 25-100
paroxetine	Paxil	Miscellaneous	Serotonin	PO: 20-50 mg/day
phenelzine	Nardil	MAO inhibitor	—	PO: 15-90
protriptyline	Vivactil	Tricyclic	Norepinephrine Serotonin	PO: 15-60
sertraline	Zoloft	Miscellaneous	Serotonin	PO: 50-200
tranylcypromine	Parnate	MAO inhibitor	—	PO: 30-60
trazodone	Desyrel	Miscellaneous	Sertonin	PO: 50-600
venlafaxine	Effexor	Miscellaneous	Norepinephrine Serotonin	PO: 75-375 mg/day

NURSING IMPLICATIONS

GENERAL: Closely supervise pts (potential for suicide increases when emerging from depression). Elderly should be observed carefully for increased response; small doses are usually indicated. **BASELINE ASSESSMENT:** Determine initial B/P. Assess pt and environment for support needed. **INTERVENTION/EVALUATION:** Monitor B/P. Assess mental status. Check bowel activity; avoid constipation. **PATIENT/FAMILY TEACHING:** Change positions slowly to avoid orthostatic hypotension. Take medication as ordered; do not stop taking or increase dosage. Avoid driving or performing tasks that require mental acuity until response to drug controlled. Extremely important to refrain from alcohol and other medications during therapy and for 2-3 wks thereafter. Omit foods rich in tyramine, such as products containing yeast, beer/wine, aged cheese (list of foods to avoid should be given); ingestion of such foods and antidepressant may cause hypertensive crisis. Inform other physicians or dentist of antidepressant therapy. Use protection from sunlight w/specific drugs. To the extent possible, drugs that cause drowsiness should be taken at bedtime, those causing insomnia should be taken in the morning.

antipsychotics

ACTION

Effects of these agents occur at all levels of the CNS. Antipsychotic mechanism unknown, but may antagonize dopamine action as a neurotransmitter in basal ganglia and limbic system. Antipsychotics may block postsynaptic dopamine receptors, inhibit dopamine release, increase dopamine turnover. These medications can be divided into the phenothiazines and nonphenothiazines (miscellaneous). In addition to their use in symptomatic treatment of psychiatric illness, some have antiemetic, antinausea, antihistamine, anticholinergic, and/or sedative effects.

USES

Antipsychotics are primarily used in managing psychotic illness (esp. those w/increased psychomotor activity). They are also used to treat manic phase of bipolar disorder, behavioral problems in children, nausea and vomiting, intractable hiccups, anxiety and agitation, as adjunct in treatment of tetanus, and to potentiate effects of narcotics.

PRECAUTIONS

CONTRAINDICATIONS: Alcoholism or other CNS depression, hepatic dysfunction, bone marrow depression, hypotension, glaucoma, cardiovascular disease, peptic ulcer, young children, hypersensitivity to any of the phenothiazines, pregnancy, lactation. **CAUTIONS:** Administer cautiously to elderly and debilitated pts; this group is more sensitive to effects and requires lower dosage. Drug should be withdrawn slowly; should be discontinued at least 48 hrs before surgery.

INTERACTIONS

Alcohol, CNS depressants may increase CNS, respiratory depression, hypotensive effects. Tricyclic antidepressants, MAO inhibitors may increase sedative, anticholinergic effects. Antithyroid agents may increase risk of agranulocytosis. Extrapyramidal symptoms (EPS) may increase w/EPS producing medications. Hypotensives may increase hypotension. May decrease levodopa effects. Lithium may decrease absorption, produce adverse neurologic effects.

SIDE EFFECTS

Orthostatic hypotension, drowsiness, blurred vision, constipation, nasal congestion, photosensitivity.

TOXIC EFFECTS/ADVERSE REACTIONS

Hyperpyrexia, depression, insomnia, convulsions, hypertension, adynamic ileus, laryngospasm, bronchospasm, urticaria, menstrual irregularities, impotence, urinary retention, blood dyscrasias, systemic lupus-like reaction, extrapyramidal reactions.

NURSING IMPLICATIONS

GENERAL: Do not mix parenteral solution w/other drugs in the same syringe; give deep IM injections. Have pt remain recumbent for at least 30 min, following parenteral dose, arise slowly and w/assistance. Avoid skin contact w/solutions (contact dermatitis). **BASELINE ASSESSMENT:** Determine initial B/P, pulse, respirations. Assess pt and environment for necessary supports. **INTERVENTION/EVALUATION:** Monitor B/P. Assess mental status, response to surroundings. Be alert to suicide potential as energy increases. Assure that oral medication is swallowed. Check bowel activity; avoid constipation. Promptly notify physician of extrapyramidal reactions (usually dose related; more frequent in female geriatric pts). **PATIENT/FAMILY TEACHING:** Take medication as ordered; do not stop taking or increase dosage. Do not drive or perform activities requiring motor skill until response has been controlled. Side effects usually subside after approximately 2 wks of therapy or can be eliminated/minimized by dosage adjustment. Avoid temperature extremes. Avoid alcohol, other medications. Inform other physicians, dentist of drug therapy. Change positions slowly to prevent orthostatic hypotension.

ANTIPSYCHOTICS

Generic Name	Brand Name(s)	Side Effects: Sedation	Side Effects: Hypotension	Side Effects: Anticholinergic	Side Effects: EPS	Dosage (mg/day)
chlorpromazine	Thorazine	High	High	Moderate	Moderate	30-800
clozapine	Clozaril	High	High	High	Low	25-900
fluphenazine	Prolixin	Low	Low	Low	High	0.5-50
haloperidol	Haldol	Low	Low	Low	High	1-100
loxapine	Loxitane	Moderate	Moderate	Low	High	20-100
mesoridazine	Serentil	High	Moderate	High	Low	30-400
molindone	Moban	Low	Low	Low	High	50-225
perphenazine	Trilafon	Low	Low	Low	High	12-64
pimozide	Orap	Moderate	Low	Moderate	High	1-10
risperidone	Risperdal	Low	Low	Low	Moderate	4-6
thioridazine	Mellaril	High	High	High	Low	150-800
thiothixene	Navane	Low	Low	Low	High	6-60
trifluoperazine	Stelazine	Low	Low	Low	High	4-40

EPS, extrapyramidal symptoms

sedative-hypnotics

ACTION

Sedatives decrease activity, moderate excitement, and have calming effects. Hypnotics produce drowsiness, enhance onset/maintenance of sleep (resembling natural sleep). Benzodiazepines are the most widely used agents (largely replace barbiturates): Greater safety, lower incidence of drug dependence. Benzodiazepines potentiate gamma-aminobutyric acid, which inhibits impulse transmission in the CNS reticular formation in brain. Benzodiazepines decrease sleep latency, number of awakenings and time spent in awake stage of sleep; increases total sleep time. Schedule IV drugs. See individual monographs for barbiturates.

USES

Treatment of insomnia, e.g., difficulty falling asleep initially, frequent awakening, awakening too early. For preop sedation.

PRECAUTIONS

CONTRAINDICATIONS: Hypersensitivity. Respiratory depression; respiratory diseases, porphyria, severe renal or hepatic dysfunction, history of alcohol or drug abuse, pregnancy, lactation, children. **CAUTIONS:** Elderly are more sensitive to adverse effects.

INTERACTIONS

Alcohol, narcotic analgesics, and other CNS depressants cause further CNS depressive effects. Combination w/CNS depressants should be avoided when possible.

SIDE EFFECTS

Drowsiness, dizziness, hangover, rebound insomnia due to altered REM, non-REM sleep stages.

TOXIC EFFECTS/ADVERSE REACTIONS

Hypersensitivity reactions: Rash, urticaria. Confusion, extreme drowsiness, diarrhea. Paradoxical excitation may occur, particularly in the elderly. Overdose: Respiratory depression, pulmonary edema, tachycardia and palpitations, marked hypotension, renal and hepatic damage, anoxia, cardiac collapse may proceed to coma and death. Potential for drug abuse and dependence, esp. w/barbiturates.

NURSING IMPLICATIONS

GENERAL: Provide environment conducive to sleep and pain relief. Put side rails up, lower bed, and put call light within reach. Assist in identifying cause of insomnia and encourage pt not to depend on medication. Comply w/federal narcotic laws regarding schedule IV drugs. Consider potential for abuse, dependence. Narcotics may need to be reduced when given w/hypnotics. **BASELINE ASSESSMENT:** Determine initial B/P, pulse, respirations, and sleep pattern. **INTERVENTION/EVALUATION:** Assure that pt has swallowed oral medication. Assess response to medication, sleep pattern. Monitor B/P, pulse, and respirations. **PATIENT/FAMILY TEACHING:** Instruct pt not to smoke or get up alone after taking hypnotic. Drowsiness may continue into next day; avoid driving or activities requiring mental acuity until response to drug controlled. Avoid alcohol. Consult physician before taking other medications. Take only as directed; do not increase dosage or abruptly discontinue (possible rebound insomnia).

HYPNOTICS

Generic Name	Brand Names(s)	Dosage Range
estazolam	ProSom	Adults: 1-2 mg before hs Elderly, Debilitated: 0.5-1 mg at hs
flurazepam	Dalmane	Adults: 15-30 mg before hs Elderly, Debilitated: Initially 15 mg, then based on pt response
quazepam	Doral	Adults: Initially 15 mg, may decrease to 7.5 mg in some pts Elderly, Debilitated: Initially 15 mg, then attempt to decrease dose after 1-2 nights
temazepam	Restoril	Adults: 15-30 mg before hs Elderly, Debilitated: Initially 15 mg, then based on pt response
triazolam	Halcion	Adults: 0.125-0.5 mg before hs Elderly, Debilitated: Initially 0.125 mg until response determined. Range: 0.125-0.25 mg
zolpidem	Ambien	Adults: 10 mg immediately before bedtime Elderly: 5 mg immediately before bedtime

hs, bedtime.

acetazolamide

ah-seat-ah-zole´ah-myd
(Dazamide, Diamox, AK-Zol)

acetazolamide sodium

(Diamox) [injection]

CANADIAN AVAILABILITY:
Acetazolam, Apo-Acetazolamide, Diamox

CLASSIFICATION

Carbonic anhydrase inhibitor

PHARMACOKINETICS

	ONSET	PEAK	DURATION
PO (tablets)	60-90 min	2-4 hrs	8-12 hrs
(capsules)	2 hrs	8-18 hrs	18-24 hrs
IV	2 min	15 min	4-5 hrs

Well absorbed from GI tract. Protein binding: 90%. Primarily excreted unchanged in urine. Half-life: 10-15 hrs.

ACTION

Reduces formation of hydrogen and bicarbonate ions from carbon dioxide and water by inhibiting, in proximal renal tubule, the enzyme carbonic anhydrase, thereby promoting renal excretion along w/potassium, bicarbonate, water. *Ocular effects:* reduces rate of aqueous humor formation, lowers intraocular pressure. *Renal, metabolic effects:* increases excretion of bicarbonate, sodium, potassium, water-producing alkaline diuresis. *Diamox only:* anticonvulsant; exact mechanism unknown.

USES

Treatment of open-angle (noncongestive, chronic simple) glaucoma. Used prior to surgery in correction of acute angle-closure (obstructive, narrow-angle) glaucoma. Used for prevention, treatment of high-altitude sickness. Adjunctive treatment of edema associated w/CHF, drug-induced edema, management of petit mal, or unlocalized seizures.

STORAGE/HANDLING

Store tablets, capsules, parenteral form at room temperature. Syrup suspension mixed w/acetazolamide is stable for 1 week at room temperature. After reconstitution, IV solution stable for 24 hrs.

PO/IV ADMINISTRATION

PO:

1. When oral liquid is needed, tablet may be crushed and mixed w/5 ml cherry, chocolate, raspberry, or other highly flavored carbohydrate syrup. Each tablet may be softened in 2 tsp hot water, then added to 2 tsp honey or syrup (mix just prior to administration). Drug will not dissolve in fruit juice.
2. Scored tablets may be crushed; do not crush or break extended-release capsules.
3. May give w/food if GI upset occurs.

IV:

NOTE: IM injection painful due to alkaline pH. IV preferred.

1. Reconstitute 500 mg vial w/5 ml sterile water for injection to provide solution containing 100 mg/ml.

INDICATIONS/DOSAGE/ROUTES

Glaucoma:
PO: Adults: 250 mg 1-4 times/day. **EXTENDED-RELEASE:** 500 mg 1-2 times/day usually given in morning and evening.

Secondary glaucoma, preop treatment of acute congestive glaucoma:
PO/IV: Adults: 250 mg q4h, 250 mg q12h; or 500 mg, then 125-250 mg q4h.
PO: Children: 10-15 mg/kg/day in divided doses.
IV: Children: 5-10 mg/kg q6h.

Edema secondary to CHF, drug therapy:
PO: Adults: Initially, 250-375 mg/day. (If pt fails to diurese, hold drug 1-2 days allowing kidneys to recover, then give drug intermittently.)
PO/IV: Children: 5 mg/kg/dose daily in morning.

Epilepsy:
PO: Adults, children: 375-1,000 mg/day in 1-4 divided doses.

Acute mountain sickness:
PO: Adults: 500-1,000 mg/day in divided doses. If possible, begin 24-48 hrs before ascent, continue at least 48 hrs at high altitude.

Usual elderly dosage:
PO: Elderly: Initially, 250 mg 2 times/day; use lowest effective dose.

PRECAUTIONS

CONTRAINDICATIONS: Hypersensitivity to sulfonamides, severe renal disease, adrenal insufficiency, hypochloremic acidosis. **CAUTIONS:** History of hypercalcemia, diabetes mellitus, gout, digitalized patients, obstructive pulmonary disease. **PREGNANCY/LACTATION:** Drug crosses placenta, unknown if distributed in breast milk. May produce skeletal anomalies, embryocidal effects at high doses. **Pregnancy Category C.**

INTERACTIONS

DRUG INTERACTIONS: May increase excretion of lithium; decrease excretion of quinidine, procainamide, methenamine. May increase digoxin toxicity (due to hypokalemia). **ALTERED LAB VALUES:** May increase ammonia, bilirubin, glucose, chloride, uric acid, calcium; may decrease bicarbonate, potassium.

SIDE EFFECTS

OCCASIONAL: Paresthesia in extremities/lips/mouth/anus; anorexia, polyuria, drowsiness, confusion. **RARE:** Nausea, vomiting, diarrhea, altered taste or smell, excessive thirst, headache, malaise, irritability, sedation, dizziness.

ADVERSE REACTIONS/TOXIC EFFECTS

Long-term therapy may result in acidotic state. Bone marrow depression may be manifested as aplastic anemia, thrombocytopenia, thrombocytopenic purpura, leukopenia, agranulocytosis, hemolytic anemia. Renal effects may include dysuria, crystalluria, renal colic/calculi.

NURSING IMPLICATIONS

BASELINE ASSESSMENT:

Glaucoma: Assess peripheral vision, acuity. Assess affected pupil for dilation, response to light. *Epilepsy:* Take history of seizure disorders (length, intensity, duration of seizures, presence of auras, LOC).

INTERVENTION/EVALUATION:

Monitor I&O, BUN, electrolytes (particularly serum potassium). Monitor pattern of daily bowel activity and stool consistency. Observe for signs of infection (fever, sore throat, unusual bleeding/bruising, fatigue) due to bone marrow depression. Monitor for acidosis (headache, lethargy progressing to drowsiness, CNS depression, Kussmaul's respiration).

PATIENT/FAMILY TEACHING:

Report presence of tingling or tremor in hands or feet, unusual bleeding/bruising, unexplained fever, sore throat, flank pain. Avoid tasks that require alertness, motor skills until response to drug is established.

---

alprazolam

ale-praz´oh-lam
(Xanax)

CANADIAN AVAILABILITY:

Apo-Alpraz, Novo-Alprazol, Xanax

CLASSIFICATION

Antianxiety: Benzodiazepine

PHARMACOKINETICS

Well absorbed from GI tract. Protein binding: 80%. Metabolized in liver. Primarily excreted in urine. Minimal removed by hemodialysis. Half-life: 11-16 hrs.

ACTION

Enhances action of inhibitory neurotransmitter gamma-aminobutyric acid (GABA). Depressant effects occur at all levels of CNS.

USES

Management of anxiety disorders associated w/depression, panic disorder.

PO ADMINISTRATION

1. May be given w/o regard to meals.
2. Tablets may be crushed.

INDICATIONS/DOSAGE/ROUTES

Anxiety disorders:

PO: Adults >18 yrs: Initially, 0.25-0.5 mg 3 times daily. Titrate to maximum of 4 mg daily in divided doses. **Elderly/debilitated/liver disease/low serum albumin:** Initially, 0.25 mg 2-3 times daily. Gradually increase to optimum therapeutic response.

Panic disorder:

PO: Adults: Initially, 0.5 mg 3 times/day. May increase at 3-4 day intervals at no more than 1 mg/day. **Range:** 1-10 mg/day.

Usual elderly dosage:

PO: Elderly: Initially, 0.125-0.25 mg 2 times/day; may increase in 0.125 mg increments until desired effect attained.

PRECAUTIONS

CONTRAINDICATIONS: Acute narrow-angle glaucoma, acute alcohol intoxication. **CAUTIONS:** Impaired renal/hepatic function. **PREGNANCY/LACTATION:** Crosses placenta; distributed in breast milk. Chronic ingestion during pregnancy may produce withdrawal symptoms, CNS depression in neonates. **Pregnancy Category D.**

INTERACTIONS

DRUG INTERACTIONS: Potentiated effects when used w/other CNS depressants, (including alcohol). **ALTERED LAB VALUES:** May produce abnormal renal function tests, elevate SGOT (AST), SGPT (ALT), LDH, alkaline phosphatase, serum bilirubin.

SIDE EFFECTS

FREQUENT: Drowsiness/lightheadedness (particularly elderly, debilitated), dry mouth, headache, constipation/diarrhea. **OCCASIONAL:** Nausea, confusion, insomnia, tachycardia, palpitations, nasal congestion, blurred vision. **RARE:** Paradoxical CNS excitement/restlessness in elderly/debilitated (generally noted during first 2 wks of therapy, particularly in presence of pain).

ADVERSE REACTIONS/TOXIC EFFECTS

Abrupt or too-rapid withdrawal may result in pronounced restlessness, irritability, insomnia, hand tremors, abdominal/muscle cramps, sweating, vomiting, seizures. Overdosage results in somnolence, confusion, diminished reflexes, coma.

NURSING IMPLICATIONS

BASELINE ASSESSMENT:

Offer emotional support to anxious pt. Assess motor responses (agitation, trembling, tension) and autonomic responses (cold, clammy hands, sweating).

INTERVENTION/EVALUATION:

For those on long-term therapy, liver/renal function tests, blood counts should be performed periodically. Assess for paradoxical reaction, particularly during early therapy. Assist w/ambulation if drowsiness, lightheadedness occur. Evaluate for therapeutic response: calm facial expression, decreased restlessness and/or insomnia.

PATIENT/FAMILY TEACHING:

Drowsiness usually disappears during continued therapy. If dizziness occurs, change positions slowly from recumbent to sitting position before standing. Avoid tasks that require alertness, motor skills until response to drug is established. Smoking reduces drug effectiveness. Sour hard candy, gum, or sips of tepid water may relieve dry mouth. Do not abruptly withdraw medication after long-term therapy. Avoid alcohol. Do not take other medications w/o consulting physician.

amantadine hydrochloride

ah-man´tih-deen
(Symadine, Symmetrel)

CANADIAN AVAILABILITY:
Symmetrel

CLASSIFICATION

Antiviral, antiparkinson.

PHARMACOKINETICS

Rapid, completely absorbed from GI tract. Widely distributed. Protein binding: 67%. Primarily excreted in urine. Minimal removed by hemodialysis. Half-life: 11-15 hrs (increased in elderly, decreased renal function).

ACTION

Antiviral action against influenza A virus believed to prevent uncoating of virus, penetration of host cells, release of nucleic acid into host cells. Antiparkinsonism due to increased release of dopamine. Virustatic.

USES

Prevention, treatment of respiratory tract infections due to influenza virus, Parkinson's disease, drug-induced extrapyramidal reactions.

PO ADMINISTRATION

Administer nighttime dose several hours before bedtime (prevents insomnia).

INDICATIONS/DOSAGE/ROUTES

Prophylaxis, symptomatic treatment respiratory illness due to influenza A virus:
NOTE: Give as single or in 2 divided doses.
PO: Adults (10-64 yrs): 200 mg daily. **Adults (>64 yrs):** 100 mg daily. **Children (9-12 yrs):** 100 mg 2 times/day. **Children (1-9 yrs):** 4.4-8.8 mg/kg/day (up to 150 mg/day).

Parkinson's disease, extrapyramidol symptoms:
PO: Adults: 100 mg 2 times/day. May increase up to 400 mg/day in divided doses.

Usual elderly dosage:
PO: Elderly: Based on renal function. Ccr 40-50 ml/min: 100 mg/day; Ccr 20 ml/min: 100 mg 3 times/wk.

Dosage in renal impairment:
Dose and/or frequency is modified based on creatinine clearance.

CREATININE CLEARANCE	DOSAGE
30-50 ml/min	200 mg first day; 100 mg/day thereafter
15-29 ml/min	200 mg first day; 100 mg on alternate days
<15 ml/min	200 mg every 7 days

PRECAUTIONS

CONTRAINDICATIONS: None significant. **CAUTIONS:** History of seizures, orthostatic hypotension, CHF, peripheral edema, liver disease, recurrent eczematoid dermatitis, cerebrovascular disease, renal dysfunction, those receiving CNS stimulants. **PREGNANCY/LACTATION:** Unknown if drug crosses placenta; distributed in breast milk. **Pregnancy Category C.**

INTERACTIONS

DRUG INTERACTIONS: Tricyclic antidepressants, antihistamines, phenothiazine, anticholinergics may increase anticholinergic effects. CNS stimulants may increase CNS stimulation. Hydrochlorothiazide, triamterene may increase concentration, toxicity. **ALTERED LAB VALUES:** None significant.

SIDE EFFECTS

FREQUENT: Nausea, dizziness, difficulty concentrating, insomnia. **OCCASIONAL:** Orthostatic hypotension, anorexia, constipation, irritability, headache, peripheral edema, confusion, depression, hallucinations, livedo reticularis (reddish-blue, net-like blotching of skin). **RARE:** Vomiting, dyspnea, skin rash, weakness, fatigue, urinary retention, slurred speech, eczematoid dermatitis.

ADVERSE REACTIONS/TOXIC EFFECTS

CHF, leukopenia, neutropenia occur rarely. Hyperexcitability, convulsions, ventricular arrhythmias may occur.

NURSING IMPLICATIONS

BASELINE ASSESSMENT:

Question history of allergies, especially to amantadine. When treating infections caused by influenza A virus, obtain specimens for viral diagnostic tests before giving first dose (therapy may begin before results are known).

INTERVENTION/EVALUATION:

Monitor I&O, renal function tests if ordered; check for peripheral edema. Evaluate food tolerance, vomiting. Assess skin for rash, blotching. Be alert to neurologic effects: headache, lethargy, confusion, agitation, blurred vision, seizures. Assess B/P at least twice daily. Determine bowel pattern, modify diet, or administer laxative as needed. Assess for dizziness. *Parkinsonism:* Assess for clinical reversal of symptoms (improvement of tremor of head/hands at rest, mask-like facial expression, shuffling gait, muscular rigidity).

PATIENT/FAMILY TEACHING:

Continue therapy for full length of treatment. Doses should be evenly spaced. Do not take any medications w/o consulting physician. Avoid alcoholic beverages. Do not drive, use machinery, or engage in other activities that require mental acuity if experiencing dizziness, confusion, blurred vision. Get up slowly from a sitting or lying position. Advise physician if no improvement in 2-3 days when taking for viral infection. Inform physician of new symptoms, especially blotching, rash, dizziness, blurred vision, nausea/vomiting. Take nighttime dose several hours before bedtime to prevent insomnia.

amitriptyline hydrochloride

a-me-trip′tih-leen
(Elavil, Endep)

FIXED-COMBINATION(S):

W/chlordiazepoxide, an antianxiety (Limbitrol); w/perphenazine, an antipsychotic (Etrafon, Triavil)

CANADIAN AVAILABILITY:

Apo-Amitriptyline, Elavil, Levate, Novotriptyn

CLASSIFICATION

Antidepressant: Tricyclic

PHARMACOKINETICS

Rapid, well absorbed from GI tract. Protein binding: 95%. Metabolized in liver, undergoes first pass metabolism. Primarily excreted in urine. Minimal removal by hemodialysis. Half-life: 10-26 hrs.

ACTION

Increases synaptic concentration of norepinephrine and/or serotonin (inhibits re-uptake by presynaptic membrane).

USES

Treatment of various forms of depression, often in conjunction w/psychotherapy.

STORAGE/HANDLING

Store parenteral form at room temperature. Protect from light (precipitate may form). Store tablets at room temperature. Protect Elavil tablets (10 mg strength only) from light.

PO/IM ADMINISTRATION

PO:

1. Give w/food or milk if GI distress occurs.

IM:

1. Give by IM only if oral administration is not feasible.
2. Crystals may form in injection. Redissolve by immersing ampoule in hot water for 1 min.
3. Give deep IM slowly.

INDICATIONS/DOSAGE/ROUTES

NOTE: May give entire daily oral dose at one time (preferably bedtime).

Inpatient:
PO: Adults: Initially, 75-100 mg daily in 1-4 divided doses. Gradually increase by 25-50 mg increments to maximum of 300 mg daily, then reduce slowly to minimum therapeutic level. **Elderly, adolescents:** Initially, 10 mg 3 times daily, plus 20 mg at bedtime. **Maintenance:** 40-100 mg/day.
IM: Adults: 20-30 mg 4 times daily.

Outpatient:
PO: Adults: Initially, 50-100 mg daily. May be gradually increased to 150 mg daily. **Elderly patients, adolescents:** 10 mg 3 times daily, plus 20 mg at bedtime. Maximum therapeutic effect should be achieved in 2-4 wks. Dosage should be gradually reduced to minimum therapeutic level.

Usual elderly dosage:
PO: Elderly: Initially, 10-25 mg at bedtime; increase at weekly intervals of 10-25 mg. **Range:** 25-150 mg/day.

PRECAUTIONS

CONTRAINDICATIONS: Acute recovery period following MI, within 14 days of MAO inhibitor ingestion. **CAUTIONS:** Prostatic hypertrophy, history of urinary retention or obstruction, glaucoma, diabetes mellitus, history of seizures, hyperthyroidism, cardiac/hepatic/renal disease, schizophrenia, increased intraocular pressure, hiatal hernia. **PREGNANCY/LACTATION:** Crosses placenta; minimally distributed in breast milk. **Pregnancy Category C.**

INTERACTIONS

DRUG INTERACTIONS: Alcohol, CNS depressants may increase CNS, respiratory depression, hypotensive effects. Antithyroid agents may increase risk of agranulocytosis. Phenothiazines may increase sedative, anticholinergic effects. Cimetidine may increase concentration, toxicity. May decrease effects of clonidine, guanadrel. May increase cardiac effects w/sympathomimetics. May increase risk of hypertensive crisis, hyperpyretic, convulsions w/MAO inhibitors. **ALTERED LAB VALUES:** May alter EKG readings, glucose.

SIDE EFFECTS

FREQUENT: Drowsiness, fatigue, dry mouth, blurred vision, constipation, delayed micturition, postural hypotension, excessive sweating, disturbed concentration, increased appetite, urinary retention. **OCCASIONAL:** GI disturbances (nausea, GI distress, metallic taste sensation). **RARE:** Paradoxical reaction (agitation, restlessness, nightmares, insomnia), extrapyramidal symptoms (particularly fine hand tremor).

ADVERSE REACTIONS/TOXIC EFFECTS

High dosage may produce cardiovascular effects (severe postural hypotension, dizziness, tachycardia, palpitations, arrhythmias) and seizures. May also result in altered temperature regulation (hyperpyrexia or hypothermia). Abrupt withdrawal from prolonged therapy may produce headache, malaise, nausea, vomiting, vivid dreams.

NURSING IMPLICATIONS

BASELINE ASSESSMENT:

For those on long-term therapy, liver/renal function tests, blood counts should be performed periodically.

INTERVENTION/EVALUATION:

Supervise suicidal-risk patient closely during early therapy (as depression lessens, energy level improves increasing suicide potential). Assess appearance, behavior, speech pattern, level of interest, mood. Monitor pattern of daily bowel activity and stool consistency. Monitor B/P, pulse for hypotension, arrhythmias. Assess for urinary retention by bladder palpation.

PATIENT/FAMILY TEACHING:

Change positions slowly to avoid hypotensive effect. Tolerance to postural hypotension, sedative and anticholinergic effects usually develop during early therapy. Maximum therapeutic effect may be noted in 2-4 wks. Photosensitivity to sun may occur. Dry mouth may be relieved by sugarless gum or sips of tepid water. Report visual disturbances. Do not abruptly discontinue medication. Avoid tasks that require alertness, motor skills until response to drug is established.

amoxapine

ah-mocks´ah-peen
(Asendin)

CANADIAN AVAILABILITY:

Asendin

CLASSIFICATION

Antidepressant: Tricyclic

PHARMACOKINETICS

Rapid, well absorbed from GI tract. Protein binding: 92%. Metabolized in liver, undergoes first-pass metabolism. Primarily excreted in urine. Minimal removal by hemodialysis. Half-life: 8-30 hrs.

ACTION

Increases synaptic concentration of norepinephrine and/or serotonin (inhibits re-uptake by presynaptic membrane).

USES

Treatment of neurotic, endogenous depression, and mixed symptoms of anxiety, depression.

PO ADMINISTRATION

Give w/food or milk if GI distress occurs.

INDICATIONS/DOSAGE/ROUTES

NOTE: May give entire daily dose at one time (preferably bedtime).
PO: Adults: Initially, 50 mg 2-3 times/day. May gradually increase to 200-300 mg/day by end of first wk of therapy. If therapeutic response does not occur by end of 2 wks, may increase dose to maximum 400 mg/day for outpatients. Hospitalized patients w/no history of seizures may receive up to 600 mg daily in divided doses.

Usual elderly dosage:
PO: Elderly: Initially, 25 mg, then increase at 25 mg increments q3days for hospitalized pts; q7days for outpts. **Range:** 50-150 mg/day. **Maximum:** 300 mg/day.

PRECAUTIONS

CONTRAINDICATIONS: Acute recovery period following MI, within 14 days of MAO inhibitor ingestion. **CAUTIONS:** Prostatic hypertrophy, history of urinary retention or obstruction, glaucoma, diabetes mellitus, history of seizures, hyperthyroidism, cardiac/hepatic/renal disease, schizophrenia, increased intraocular pressure, hiatal hernia. **PREGNANCY/LACTATION:** Crosses placenta; is distributed in breast milk. **Pregnancy Category C.**

INTERACTIONS

DRUG INTERACTIONS: Alcohol, CNS depressants may increase CNS, respiratory depression, hypotensive effects. Antithyroid agents may increase risk of agranulocytosis. Phenothiazines may increase sedative, anticholinergic effects. Cimetidine may increase concentration, toxicity. May decrease effects of clonidine, guanadrel. May increase cardiac effects w/sympathomimetics. May increase risk of hypertensive crisis, hyperpyretic, convulsions w/MAO inhibitors. **ALTERED LAB VALUES:** May alter ECG readings, glucose.

SIDE EFFECTS

FREQUENT: Drowsiness, fatigue, dry mouth, blurred vision, constipation, delayed micturition, postural hypotension, excessive sweating, disturbed concentration, increased appetite, urinary retention. **OCCASIONAL:** GI disturbances (nausea, GI distress, metallic taste sensation). **RARE:** Paradoxical reaction (agitation, restlessness, nightmares, insomnia), extrapyramidal symptoms (particularly fine hand tremor).

ADVERSE REACTIONS/TOXIC EFFECTS

High dosage may produce cardiovascular effects (severe postural hypotension, dizziness, tachycardia, palpitations, arrhythmias) and seizures. May also result in altered temperature regulation (hyperpyrexia or hypothermia). Abrupt withdrawal from prolonged therapy may produce headache, malaise, nausea, vomiting, vivid dreams.

NURSING IMPLICATIONS

BASELINE ASSESSMENT:

For those on long-term therapy, liver/renal function tests, blood counts should be performed periodically.

INTERVENTION/EVALUATION:

Supervise suicidal-risk patient closely during early therapy (as depression lessens, energy level improves increasing suicide potential). Assess appearance, behavior, speech pattern, level of interest, mood. Monitor pattern of daily bowel activity and stool consistency. Monitor B/P, pulse for hypotension, arrhythmias. Assess for urinary retention by bladder palpation.

PATIENT/FAMILY TEACHING:

Change positions slowly to avoid hypotensive effect. Tolerance to postural hypotension, sedative and anticholinergic effects usually develops during early therapy. Therapeutic effect may be noted within 1-2 wks. Photosensitivity to sun may occur. Dry mouth may be relieved by sugarless gum or sips of tepid water. Report visual disturbances. Do not abruptly discontinue medication. Avoid tasks that require alertness, motor skills until response to drug is established.

benztropine mesylate

benz´row-peen
(Cogentin)

CANADIAN AVAILABILITY:
Apo-Benztropine, Cogentin, PMS Benztropine, Bensylate

CLASSIFICATION

Anticholinergic, Antiparkinson

PHARMACOKINETICS

	ONSET	PEAK	DURATION
PO	1 hr	—	24 hrs
IM	15 min	—	24 hrs

Well absorbed from GI tract.

ACTION

Suppresses central cholinergic activity, may inhibit reuptake/storage dopamine, thus prolonging its action.

USES

Treatment of Parkinson's disease, drug-induced extrapyramidal reactions, except tardive dyskinesia.

INDICATIONS/DOSAGE/ROUTES

Idiopathic parkinsonism:
PO/IM: Adults: Initially, 0.5-1 mg/day at bedtime up to 6 mg/day.

Postencephalitic parkinsonism:
PO/IM: Adults: 2 mg/day as single or divided dose.

Drug-induced extrapyramidal symptoms:
PO/IM: Adults: 1-4 mg 1-2 times/day.

Acute dystonic reactions:
IV: Adults: 1-2 mg, then 1-2 mg orally 2 times/day to prevent recurrence.

Usual elderly dosage:
PO: Elderly: Initially, 0.5 mg 1-2 times/day, may increase by 0.5 mg every 5-6 days. **Maximum:** 6 mg/day.

PRECAUTIONS

CONTRAINDICATIONS: Angle-closure glaucoma, GI obstruction, paralytic ileus, intestinal atony, severe ulcerative colitis, prostatic hypertrophy, myasthenia gravis, megacolon, children <3 yrs. **CAUTIONS:** Treated open-angle glaucoma, autonomic neuropathy, pulmonary disease, esophageal reflux, hiatal hernia, heart disease, hyperthyroidism, hypertension. **PREGNANCY/LACTATION:** Unknown if drug crosses placenta; distributed in breast milk. **Pregnancy Category C.**

INTERACTIONS

DRUG INTERACTIONS: Alcohol, CNS depressants may increase sedation. Amantadine, anticholinergics, MAO inhibitors may increase effects. Antacids, antidiarrheals may decrease absorption, effects. **ALTERED LAB VALUES:** None significant.

SIDE EFFECTS

NOTE: Elderly (>60 yrs) tend to develop mental confusion, disorientation, agitation, psychotic-like symptoms. **FREQUENT:** Drowsiness, dizziness, muscular weakness, dry mouth/nose/throat/lips, urinary retention, thickening of bronchial secretions. Sedation, dizziness, hypotension more likely noted in elderly. **OCCASIONAL:** Epigastric distress, flushing, visual disturbances, hearing disturbances, paresthesia, sweating, chills.

ADVERSE REACTIONS/TOXIC EFFECTS

Children may experience dominant paradoxical reaction (restlessness, insomnia, euphoria, nervousness, tremors). Overdosage in children may result in hallucinations, convulsions, death. Hypersensitivity reaction (eczema, pruritus, rash, cardiac disturbances, photosensitivity) may occur. Overdosage may vary from CNS depression (sedation, apnea, cardiovascular collapse, death) to severe paradoxical reaction (hallucinations, tremor, seizures).

NURSING IMPLICATIONS

BASELINE ASSESSMENT:

If pt is undergoing allergic reaction, obtain history of recently ingested foods, drugs, environmental exposure, recent emotional stress. Monitor rate, depth, rhythm, type of respiration; quality and rate of pulse. Assess lung sounds for rhonchi, wheezing, rales.

INTERVENTION/EVALUATION:

Be alert to neurologic effects: headache, lethargy, mental confusion, agitation. Monitor children closely for paradoxical reaction. Assess for clinical reversal of symptoms (improvement of tremor of head/hands at rest, mask-like facial expression, shuffling gait, muscular rigidity).

PATIENT/FAMILY TEACHING:

Avoid tasks that require alertness, motor skills until response to drug is established. Dry mouth, drowsiness, dizziness may be an expected response of drug. Avoid alcoholic beverages during therapy. Sugarless gum, sips of tepid water may relieve dry mouth. Coffee or tea may help reduce drowsiness.

bromocriptine

brom-oh-crip´teen
(Parlodel)

CANADIAN AVAILABILITY:
Parlodel

CLASSIFICATION

Antiparkinson, prolactin inhibitor

PHARMACOKINETICS

	ONSET	PEAK	DURATION
PO	1-2 hrs	—	4-5 hrs
	(growth hormone decrease)		
PO	2 hrs	8 hrs	24 hrs
	(prolactin decrease)		

Minimal absorption from GI tract. Protein binding: 90-95%. Metabolized in liver. Excreted in feces via biliary secretion. Half-life: 15 hrs.

ACTION

Directly inhibits prolactin release from anterior pituitary. Stimulates presynaptic and postsynaptic dopamine receptors. Suppresses secretion, reduction of elevated growth hormone concentration.

USES

Treatment of hyperprolactinemia conditions (amenorrhea w/or w/o galactorrhea, prolactin secreting adenomas, infertility). Formerly used for prevention of lactation or when mother elects not to breast-feed; recommendation for this use was voluntarily withdrawn by manufacturer, August 1994. Treatment of Parkinson's disease, acromegaly.

PO ADMINISTRATION

1. Pt should be lying down before administering first dose.
2. Give after food intake (decreases incidence of nausea).

INDICATIONS/DOSAGE/ROUTES

Hyperprolactinemia:
PO: Adults, elderly: Initially, 1.25-2.5 mg/day. May increase by 2.5 mg/day at 3-7 day intervals. **Range:** 2.5-15 mg/day.

Parkinson's disease:
PO: Adults, elderly: Initially, 1.25 mg 2 times/day. Increase by 2.5 mg/day every 14-28 days. **Range:** 10-40 mg/day.

Acromegaly:
PO: Adults, elderly: Initially, 1.25-2.5 mg/day at bedtime for 3 days. May increase by 1.25-2.5 mg/day every 3-7 days. **Range:** 20-30 mg/day. **Max:** 100 mg/day.

PRECAUTIONS

CONTRAINDICATIONS: Pregnancy, peripheral vascular disease, severe ischemic heart disease, uncontrolled hypertension, hypersensitivity to ergot alkaloids. **CAUTIONS:** Impaired hepatic/cardiac function.

INTERACTIONS

DRUG INTERACTIONS: Disulfiram reaction may occur w/alcohol. Estrogens, progestins may decrease effects. Phenothiazines, haloperidol, MAO inhibitors may decrease prolactin effect. Hypotensive agents may increase hypotension. Levodopa may increase effects. **ALTERED LAB VALUES:** May elevate BUN, SGOT (AST), SGPT (ALT), CPK, alkaline phosphatase, uric acid.

SIDE EFFECTS

NOTE: Incidence of side effects is high, especially at beginning of therapy or w/high dosage. **FREQUENT:** Nausea, constipation, hypotension noted by dizziness, lightheadedness, anorexia, headache, abdominal cramps, vomiting, nasal stuffiness, constipation or diarrhea, peripheral vasoconstriction (Raynaud's phenomenon). **RARE:** Confusion, muscle cramping, visual hallucinations.

ADVERSE REACTIONS/TOXIC EFFECTS

Visual or auditory hallucinations noted in parkinsonism syndrome. Long-term, high-dose therapy may produce reversible pulmonary infiltrates, pleural effusion, thickening of pleura.

NURSING IMPLICATIONS

BASELINE ASSESSMENT:

Determine baseline, stability of vital signs. Evaluation of pituitary (R/O tumor) should be done prior to treatment for hyperprolactinemia w/amenorrhea/galactorrhea and infertility. Pregnancy test.

INTERVENTION/EVALUATION:

Assist w/ambulation if dizziness is noted after administration. Monitor B/P for evidence of hypotension, particularly during early therapy. Assess for therapeutic response (decrease in engorgement, decreases in parkinsonism symptoms). Monitor for constipation.

PATIENT/FAMILY TEACHING:

Take w/food. To reduce lightheadedness, rise slowly from lying to sitting position and permit legs to dangle momentarily before standing. Avoid sudden posture changes. Avoid tasks that require alertness, motor skills until response to drug is established. Must use contraceptive measures (other than oral) during treatment. Report any watery nasal discharge to physician. Do not suddenly discontinue the drug. Avoid alcohol.

bupropion

byew-pro´peon
(Wellbutrin)

CLASSIFICATION

Antidepressant

PHARMACOKINETICS

Rapidly absorbed from GI tract. Crosses blood-brain barrier. Protein binding: 85%. Extensive first-pass metabolism in liver to active metabolite. Primarily excreted in urine. Half-life: 14 hrs.

ACTION

Weakly blocks neuronal re-uptake of serotonin, norepinephrine.

USES

Treatment of depression, particularly endogenous depression, exhibited as persistent and prominent dysphoria (occurring nearly every day for at least 2 wks) manifested by 4 of 8 symptoms: change in appetite, change in sleep pattern, increased fatigue, impaired concentration, feelings of guilt/worthlessness, loss of interest in usual activities, psychomotor agitation/retardation, or suicidal tendencies.

PO ADMINISTRATION

Avoid bedtime dosage (decreases risk of insomnia).

INDICATIONS/DOSAGE/ROUTES

NOTE: Reduce dosage in renal/hepatic impairment, elderly.
PO: Adults: Initially, 75 mg 3 times/day or 100 mg 2 times/

day. May increase to 100 mg 3 times/day no sooner than 3 days after initial dosage. Do not exceed dose increase of 100 mg/day in 3-day period. **Maximum daily dose:** 150 mg 3 times/day. Do not exceed any single dose of 150 mg.

Usual elderly dosage:
PO: Elderly: Initially, 50-100 mg/day. May increase by 50-100 mg/day every 3-4 days.

PRECAUTIONS

CONTRAINDICATIONS: Those w/seizure disorder, current or prior diagnosis of bulimia or anorexia nervosa, concurrent use of MAO inhibitor. **EXTREME CAUTION:** History of seizure, cranial trauma; those currently taking antipsychotics, antidepressants. **CAUTIONS:** Impaired renal, hepatic function. **PREGNANCY/LACTATION:** Unknown if drug crosses placenta or is distributed in breast milk. **Pregnancy Category B.**

INTERACTIONS

DRUG INTERACTIONS: Alcohol, tricyclic antidepressants, lithium, trazodone may increase risk of seizures. May increase risk of acute toxicity w/MAO inhibitors. **ALTERED LAB VALUES:** May decrease WBCs.

SIDE EFFECTS

FREQUENT: Agitation, dry mouth, constipation, headache/migraine, weight loss/anorexia, excessive sweating, dizziness, tremor, sedation, insomnia, nausea. **OCCASIONAL:** Blurred vision, weight gain, tachycardia, confusion. **RARE:** Rash, diarrhea, cardiac disturbances (hyper/hypotension, palpitations), fatigue.

ADVERSE REACTIONS/TOXIC EFFECTS

Increased risk of seizures w/increase in dosage greater than 150 mg/dose, in those w/history of bulimia or seizure disorders, of discontinuing agents that may lower seizure threshold.

NURSING IMPLICATIONS

BASELINE ASSESSMENT:

For those on long-term therapy, liver/renal function tests should be performed periodically.

INTERVENTION/EVALUATION:

Supervise suicidal-risk patient closely during early therapy (as depression lessens, energy level improves, increasing suicide potential). Assess appearance, behavior, speech pattern, level of interest, mood. Monitor pattern of daily bowel activity, stool consistency. Monitor B/P, pulse for hypotension, arrhythmias.

PATIENT/FAMILY TEACHING:

Full therapeutic effect may be noted in 4 wks. Avoid alcohol (increases risk of seizure). Avoid tasks that require alertness, motor skills until response to drug is established. Dry mouth may be relieved by sugarless gum/sips of tepid water.

buspirone hydrochloride

byew´spear-own
(BuSpar)

CANADIAN AVAILABILITY:
Buspar

CLASSIFICATION

Antianxiety

PHARMACOKINETICS

Rapidly completely absorbed from GI tract. Undergoes extensive first-pass metabolism. Protein binding: 95%. Metabolized in liver to active metabolite. Primarily excreted in urine. Half-life: 2-3 hrs.

ACTION

Unknown. Binds to serotonin, dopamine receptors.

USES

Short-term relief (up to 4 wks); management of anxiety disorders.

PO ADMINISTRATION

1. Give w/o regard to meals.
2. Tablets may be crushed.

INDICATIONS/DOSAGE/ROUTES

PO: Adults: 5 mg 2-3 times daily. May increase in 5 mg increments/day at intervals of 2-4 days. **Maintenance:** 15-30 mg/day in 2-3 divided doses. Do not exceed 60 mg/day.

Usual elderly dosage:
PO: Elderly: Initially, 5 mg 2 times/day. May increase by 5 mg every 2-3 days. **Maximum:** 60 mg/day.

PRECAUTIONS

CONTRAINDICATIONS: Severe renal/hepatic impairment, MAO inhibitor therapy. **CAUTIONS:** Renal/hepatic impairment. **PREGNANCY/LACTATION:** Unknown if drug crosses placenta or is distributed in breast milk. **Pregnancy Category B.**

INTERACTIONS

DRUG INTERACTIONS: Alcohol, CNS depressants may increase sedation. MAO inhibitors may increase B/P. **ALTERED LAB VALUES:** May increase SGOT (AST), SGPT (ALT).

SIDE EFFECTS

FREQUENT: Dizziness, drowsiness, headache, nausea, lightheadedness, fatigue (particularly at dosage higher than 20 mg/day), insomnia and/or nervousness (particularly at very high dosage). **OCCASIONAL:** Paresthesia, excitement, tremors, dry mouth, tinnitus, nasal congestion, sore throat, redness/itching of eyes, abdominal distress, diarrhea/constipation, musculoskeletal aches/pains. **RARE:** Nightmares, blurred vision, tachycardia, palpitations.

ADVERSE REACTIONS/TOXIC EFFECTS

No evidence of tolerance or psychologic and/or physical dependence, no withdrawal syndrome. Overdosage may produce severe nausea, vomiting, dizziness, drowsiness, abdominal distention, excessive pupil contraction.

NURSING IMPLICATIONS

BASELINE ASSESSMENT:

Offer emotional support to anxious pt. Assess motor responses (agitation, trembling, tension) and autonomic responses (cold, clammy hands, sweating).

INTERVENTION/EVALUATION:

For those on long-term therapy, liver/renal function tests, blood counts should be performed periodically. Assist w/ambulation if drowsiness, lightheadedness occur. Evaluate for therapeutic response: calm, facial expression, decreased restlessness and/or insomnia.

PATIENT/FAMILY TEACHING:

Improvement may be noted in 7-10 days, but optimum therapeutic effect generally takes 3-4 wks. Drowsiness usually disappears during continued therapy. If dizziness occurs, change positions slowly from recumbent to sitting position before standing. Avoid tasks that require alertness, motor skills until response to drug is established. Avoid alcohol and other CNS depressants (unless ordered by physician). Do not discontinue drug abruptly.

carbamazepine

car-bah-maz´eh-peen
(Epitol, Tegretol)

CANADIAN AVAILABILITY:
Apo-Carbamazepine, Mazepine, Tegretol

CLASSIFICATION

Anticonvulsant

PHARMACOKINETICS

Slowly, completely absorbed from GI tract. Protein binding: 75-90%. Metabolized in liver to active metabolite. Primarily excreted in urine. Half-life: 25-65 hrs (decreased w/chronic use).

ACTION

Decreases synaptic transmission by blocking or inhibiting sodium channels.

USES

Management of generalized tonic-clonic seizures (grand mal), complex partial seizures (temporal lobe, psychomotor), mixed seizures; treatment of trigeminal neuralgia (tic douloureux).

STORAGE/HANDLING

Store oral suspension, tablets at room temperature.

PO ADMINISTRATION

1. Give w/meals to reduce risk of GI distress.
2. Shake oral suspension well.

INDICATIONS/DOSAGE/ROUTES

NOTE: When replacement by another anticonvulsant is necessary, decrease carbamazepine gradually as therapy begins w/low replacement dose. When transferring from tablets to suspension, divide total tablet daily dose into smaller, more frequent doses of suspension.

Seizure control:
PO: Adults, elderly, children >12 yrs: Initially, 200 mg 2 times/day. Increase dosage up to 200 mg/day at weekly intervals until response is attained. **Maintenance:** 800-1200 mg/day. Do not exceed 1,000 mg/day in children 12-15 yrs, 1,200 mg/day in pts >15 yrs. **Children 6-12 yrs:** Initially, 100 mg 2 times/day. Increase by 100 mg/day until response is attained. **Maintenance:** 400-800 mg/day. Give dosage 200 mg or greater/day in 3-4 equally divided doses. **Syrup: Children 6-12 yrs:** Initially, 50 mg 4 times/day. Increase dosage slowly (reduces sedation risk).

Trigeminal neuralgia:
PO: Adults, elderly: 100 mg 2 times/day on day 1. Increase by 100 mg q12h until pain is relieved. **Maintenance:** 200-1200 mg/day. Do not exceed 1200 mg/day.

PRECAUTIONS

CONTRAINDICATIONS: History of bone marrow depression, history of hypersensitivity to tricyclic antidepressants. **CAUTIONS:** Impaired cardiac, hepatic, renal function. **PREGNANCY/LACTATION:** Crosses placenta; distributed in breast milk. Accumulates in fetal tissue. **Pregnancy Category C.**

INTERACTIONS

DRUG INTERACTIONS: May decrease effect of steroids, anticoagulants. May increase metabolism of anticonvulsants, barbiturates, benzodiazepines, valproic acid. Tricyclic antidepressants, haloperidol, antipsychotics may increase CNS depressant effects. Cimetidine may increase concentration, toxicity. May decrease effects of estrogens, quinidine. Diltiazem, erythromycin, propoxyphene, verapamil may increase toxicity. May increase metabolism of isoniazid (hepatotoxicity). Isoniazid may increase concentration, toxicity. MAO inhibitors may cause hypertensive crises, convulsions. **ALTERED LAB VALUES:** May increase BUN, glucose, protein, SGOT (AST), SGPT (ALT), alkaline phosphatase, bilirubin, cholesterol, HDL, triglycerides. May decrease calcium, T_3, T_4, T_4 index.

SIDE EFFECTS

OCCASIONAL: Drowsiness, dizziness, nausea, vomiting, visual abnormalities (spots before eyes, difficulty focusing, blurred vision), dry mouth/pharynx, tongue irritation, headache, water retention, increased sweating, constipation/diarrhea.

ADVERSE REACTIONS/TOXIC EFFECTS

Toxic reactions appear as blood dyscrasias (aplastic anemia, agranulocytosis, thrombocytopenia, leukopenia, leukocytosis, eosinophilia), cardiovascular disturbances (CHF, hypo/hypertension, thrombophlebitis, arrhythmias), dermatologic effects (rash, urticaria, pruritus, photosensitivity). Abrupt withdrawal may precipitate status epilepticus.

NURSING IMPLICATIONS

BASELINE ASSESSMENT:

Seizures: Review history of seizure disorder (intensity, frequency, duration, LOC). Provide safety precautions; quiet, dark environment. CBC, platelet count, serum iron determinations, urinalysis, BUN should be performed before therapy begins and periodically during therapy.

INTERVENTION/EVALUATION:

Seizures: Observe frequently for recurrence of seizure activity. Assess for clinical improvement (decrease in intensity/frequency of seizures). Monitor for therapeutic serum level (3-14 mcg/ml). Assess for clinical evidence of early toxic signs (fever, sore throat, mouth ulcerations, easy bruising, unusual bleeding, joint pain). *Neuralgia:* Avoid triggering tic douloureux (draft, talking, washing face, jarring bed, hot/warm/cold food or liquids).

PATIENT/FAMILY TEACHING:

Do not abruptly withdraw medication following long-term use (may precipitate seizures). Strict maintenance of drug therapy is essential for seizure control. Drowsiness usually disappears during continued therapy. Avoid tasks that require alertness, motor skills until response to drug is established. Report visual abnormalities. Blood tests should be repeated frequently during first 3 mos of therapy and at monthly intervals thereafter for 2-3 yrs.

carbidopa/levodopa

car´bih-dope-ah/lev´oh-dope-ah
(Sinemet)

CANADIAN AVAILABILITY:
Sinemet

CLASSIFICATION

Antiparkinson

PHARMACOKINETICS

Carbidopa: Rapid, completely absorbed from GI tract. Widely distributed. Protein binding: 36%. Excreted primarily in urine. Half-life: 1-2 hrs. *Levodopa:* Converted to dopamine. Excreted primarily in urine. Half-life: 1-3 hrs.

ACTION

Carbidopa: Inhibits peripheral decarboxylation of levodopa. *Levodopa:* Stimulates dopaminergic receptors in basal ganglia improving balance of cholinergic/dopaminergic activity, improving modulation of voluntary nerve impulse transmission to motor cortex.

USES

Treatment of idiopathic Parkinson's disease (paralysis agitans), postencephalitic parkinsonism, symptomatic parkinsonism following injury to nervous system by carbon monoxide poisoning, manganese intoxication.

PO ADMINISTRATION

1. Scored tablets may be crushed.
2. May be given w/o regard to meals.
3. Do not crush sustained-release tablet; may cut in half.

INDICATIONS/DOSAGE/ROUTES

PARKINSONISM:

Not receiving levodopa:
PO: Adults: 25/100 mg tablet 3 times/day or 10/100 mg tablet 3-4 times/day. May increase by 1 tablet every 1-2 days up to 8 tablets/day.

Usual elderly dosage:
PO: Elderly: Initially, 25/100 2 times/day, gradually increased as necessary.
SUSTAINED RELEASE: Adults: 1 tablet 2 times/day no closer than 6 hrs between doses. **Range:** 2-8 tablets at 4-8 hr intervals. May increase dose at intervals not less than 3 days.

Receiving only levodopa:
NOTE: Discontinue levodopa at least 8 hrs prior to carbidopa/levodopa. Initiate w/dose providing at least 25% of previous levodopa dosage.
PO: Adults (<1500 mg levodopa/day): 1 tablet (25/100 mg) 3-4 times/day.
PO: Adults (>1500 mg levodopa/day): 1 tablet (25/250 mg) 3-4 times/day.
SUSTAINED RELEASE: Adults: 1 tablet 2 times/day.

Receiving carbidopa/levodopa:
SUSTAINED RELEASE: Adults: Provide about 10% more levodopa; may increase up to 30% more at 4-8 hr dosing intervals.

PRECAUTIONS

CONTRAINDICATIONS: Narrow-angle glaucoma, those on MAO inhibitor therapy. **CAUTIONS:** History of MI, bronchial asthma (tartrazine sensitivity), emphysema; severe cardiac, pulmonary, renal, hepatic, endocrine disease; active peptic ulcer, treated open-angle glaucoma. **PREGNANCY/LACTATION:** Unknown if drug crosses placenta or is distributed in breast milk. May inhibit lactation. Do not nurse. **Pregnancy Category C.**

INTERACTIONS

DRUG INTERACTIONS: Anticonvulsants, benzodiazepines, haloperidol, phenothiazines may decrease effect. MAO inhibitors may increase risk of hypertensive crises. Selegiline may increase dyskinesias, nausea, orthostatic hypotension, confusion, hallucinations. **ALTERED LAB VALUES:** May increase alkaline phosphatase, SGOT (AST), SGPT (ALT), LDH, bilirubin, BUN.

SIDE EFFECTS

FREQUENT: Nausea, anorexia, dizziness, orthostatic hypotension, bradycardia, akinesia (temporary muscular weakness; lasts 1 min to 1 hr; also known as "on-off" phenomenon). **OCCASIONAL:** Dry mouth, blurred vision, nervousness, constipation, decreased sweating, mydriasis (pupil dilation), loss of taste, urinary hesitancy and/or retention, headache, dizziness, drowsiness, confusion. **RARE:** Palpitations, tachycardia.

ADVERSE REACTIONS/TOXIC EFFECTS

High incidence of involuntary choreiform, dystonic, dyskinetic movements may be noted in pts on long-term therapy. Mental changes (paranoid ideation, psychotic episodes, depression) may be noted. Numerous mild to severe CNS, psychiatric disturbances may include reduced attention span, anxiety, nightmares, daytime somnolence, euphoria, fatigue, paranoia, hallucinations.

NURSING IMPLICATIONS

BASELINE ASSESSMENT:

Instruct pt to void before giving medication (reduces risk of urinary retention).

INTERVENTION/EVALUATION:

Be alert to neurologic effects: headache, lethargy, mental confusion, agitation. Monitor for evidence of dyskinesia (difficulty w/movement). Assess for clinical reversal of symptoms (improvement of tremor of head/hands at rest, mask-like facial expression, shuffling gait, muscular rigidity).

PATIENT/FAMILY TEACHING:

Avoid tasks that require alertness, motor skills until response to drug is established. Dry mouth, drowsiness, dizziness may be an expected response of drug. Avoid alcoholic beverages during therapy. Sugarless gum, sips of tepid water may relieve dry mouth. Coffee/tea may help reduce drowsiness.

chloral hydrate

klor′al-high′drate
(Noctec, Aquachloral Supprettes)

CANADIAN AVAILABILITY:

Noctec, Novochlorhydrate

CLASSIFICATION

Sedative, hypnotic

PHARMACOKINETICS

	ONSET	PEAK	DURATION
PO	30-60 min	—	4-8 hrs
Rectal	30-60 min	—	4-8 hrs

Readily absorbed from GI tract. Protein binding: 35-41%. Metabolized in liver, erythrocytes to active metabolite. Excreted in urine. Half-life: 7-10 hrs.

ACTION

Unknown. CNS depressant by action of active metabolite.

USES

Short-term treatment of insomnia (up to 2 wk). Also used for routine sedation, preop sedation, EEG testing, prevention/suppression of alcohol-withdrawal symptoms.

PO/RECTAL ADMINISTRATION

PO:

1. May be given w/o regard to meals.
2. Capsules may be emptied and mixed w/food.
3. Mix syrup form with 1/2 glass (4 oz) water, fruit juice, ginger ale.

RECTAL:

1. If suppository is too soft, chill for 30 min in refrigerator or run cold water over foil wrapper.
2. Moisten suppository w/cold water before inserting well up into rectum.

INDICATIONS/DOSAGE/ROUTES

Hypnotic:
PO/RECTAL: Adults: 500 mg-1 Gm 15-30 min before bedtime, or 30 min before surgery. **Elderly:** 250 mg at bedtime. **Children:** 50 mg/kg to maximum 1 Gm per single dose.

Sedative:
PO/RECTAL: Adults: 250 mg 3 times/day after meals. **Children:** 8.3 mg/kg 3 times/day.

Alcohol withdrawal:
PO/RECTAL: Adults: 500 mg-1 Gm q6h. Do not exceed 2 Gm daily.

EEG evaluation:
PO/RECTAL: Children: 20-25 mg/kg.

PRECAUTIONS

CONTRAINDICATIONS: Marked hepatic, renal impairment, severe cardiac disease, presence of gastritis. *Oral form:* Esophagitis, gastritis, gastric/duodenal ulcer. **CAUTIONS:** History of drug abuse, mental depression. **PREGNANCY/LACTATION:** Crosses placenta; small amount distributed in breast milk. Withdrawal symptoms may occur in neonates born to women who receive chloral hydrate during pregnancy. May produce sedation in nursing infants. **Pregnancy Category C.**

INTERACTIONS

DRUG INTERACTIONS: Alcohol, CNS depressants may increase effects. May increase effect of warfarin. IV furosemide given within 24 hrs following chloral hydrate may alter B/P, cause diaphoresis. **ALTERED LAB VALUES:** None significant.

SIDE EFFECTS

Generally well tolerated w/only mild and transient effects. **OCCASIONAL:** Gastric irritation (nausea, vomiting, flatulence, diarrhea), allergic skin rash, sleepwalking, disorientation, paranoid behavior. **RARE:** Residual hangover, headache, paradoxical CNS hyperactivity/nervousness in children, excitement/restlessness in elderly (particularly noted when given in presence of pain).

ADVERSE REACTIONS/TOXIC EFFECTS

Overdosage may produce somnolence, confusion, slurred speech, severe incoordination, respiratory depression, coma. Tolerance and psychological dependence may occur by second wk of therapy. Abrupt withdrawal of drug after long-term use may produce weakness, facial flushing, sweating, vomiting, tremor.

NURSING IMPLICATIONS

BASELINE ASSESSMENT:

Assess B/P, pulse, respirations immediately before administration. Raise bedrails. Provide environment conducive to sleep (backrub, quiet environment, low lighting).

INTERVENTION/EVALUATION:

Assess sleep pattern of pt. Assess elderly/children for paradoxical reaction. Evaluate for therapeutic response to insomnia: a decrease in number of nocturnal awakenings, increase in length of sleep.

PATIENT/FAMILY TEACHING:

Do not abruptly withdraw medication after long-term use. Avoid tasks that require alertness, motor skills until response to drug is established. Tolerance/dependence may occur w/ prolonged use of high doses.

chlordiazepoxide

klor-dye-az-eh-pox´eyd

(Libritabs)

chlordiazepoxide hydrochloride

(Librium, Lipoxide)

FIXED-COMBINATION(S):

W/clidinium bromide, an anticholinergic (Librax); w/estrogen (Menrium); w/amitriptyline hydrochloride, an antidepressant (Limbitrol)

CANADIAN AVAILABILITY:

Apo-Chlordiazepoxide, Librium, Medilium, Novopoxide

CLASSIFICATION

Antianxiety: Benzodiazepine

PHARMACOKINETICS

	ONSET	PEAK	DURATION
IV	1-5 min	—	15 min-1 hr

Well absorbed from GI tract; slow, erratic after IM administration. Protein binding: 96%. Metabolized in liver to active metabolite. Excreted in urine. Half-life: 5-30 hrs.

ACTION

Enhances action of inhibitory neurotransmitter gamma-aminobutyric acid (GABA). Depressant effects occur at all levels of CNS.

USES

Management of anxiety disorders, acute alcohol-withdrawal symptoms; short-term relief of symptoms of anxiety, preop anxiety, tension.

STORAGE/HANDLING

Store unreconstituted parenteral form at room temperature. Refrigerate diluent; do not use if hazy or opalescent. Prepare immediately before administration; discard unused portions. Do not mix w/infusion fluids.

PO/IM/IV ADMINISTRATION

PO:

1. Give w/o regard to meals.
2. Tablets may be crushed (do not crush combination form).
3. Capsules may be emptied and mixed w/food.

Parenteral form: Do not exceed 300 mg over a 6-hr period or 300 mg/24 hrs.

IM:

1. Do not use IV preparation for IM injection (produces pain at injection site).
2. Add 2 ml of diluent provided to 100 mg ampoule to yield 50 mg/ml. Add diluent carefully to minimize air bubbles. Agitate gently to dissolve.
3. Inject deep IM slowly into upper outer quadrant of gluteus maximus.

IV:

1. Do not use IM diluent solution for IV injection (air bubbles form during reconstitution of diluent).
2. Dilute each 100 mg ampoule w/5 ml of 0.9% NaCl or sterile water for injection administration to yield 20 mg/ml. Agitate gently until dissolved.
3. Use Y tube or 3-way stopcock to control infusion rate.
4. Administer 100 mg or fraction thereof over at least 1 min.
5. A too-rapid IV may produce hypotension, respiratory depression.

INDICATIONS/DOSAGE/ROUTES

NOTE: Use smallest effective dose in elderly or debilitated, those w/liver disease, low serum albumin.

Mild to moderate anxiety:

PO: Adults: 5-10 mg 3-4 times/day. **Elderly/debilitated:** 5 mg 2-4 times/day. Do not exceed 10 mg/day initially. **Children >6 yr:** 5 mg 2-4 times/day. Do not exceed 10 mg/day initially.

Severe anxiety:

PO: Adults: 20-25 mg 3-4 times/day.

IM/IV: Adults: Initially, 50-100 mg, then 25-50 mg 3-4 times/day. **Elderly:** 25-50 mg 3-4 times/day.

Preoperative:

IM/IV: Adults: 50-100 mg 1 hr before surgery. **Elderly/debilitated, children 12-18 yr:** 25-50 mg 1 hr before surgery.

Alcohol withdrawal:

PO: Adults: 50-100 mg followed by repeated doses until agitation is controlled. Do not exceed 300 mg/day.

IM/IV: Adults: Initially, 50-100 mg. May repeat in 2-4 hrs, if necessary.

PRECAUTIONS

CONTRAINDICATIONS: Acute narrow-angle glaucoma, acute alcohol intoxication. **CAUTIONS:** Impaired kidney/liver function. **PREGNANCY/LACTATION:** Crosses placenta; distributed in breast milk. May increase risk of fetal abnormalities if administered during first trimester of pregnancy. Chronic ingestion during pregnancy may produce withdrawal symptoms, CNS depression in neonates. **Pregnancy Category D.**

INTERACTIONS

DRUG INTERACTIONS: Alcohol, CNS depressants may increase CNS depressant effect. **ALTERED LAB VALUES:** None significant.

SIDE EFFECTS

FREQUENT: Pain w/IM injection; drowsiness, ataxia, dizziness, confusion noted w/oral dose, particularly in elderly, debilitated. **OCCASIONAL:** Skin rash, edema, GI disturbances. **RARE:** Paradoxical CNS hyperactivity/nervousness in children, excitement/restlessness in elderly (generally noted during first 2 wk of therapy, particularly noted in presence of uncontrolled pain).

ADVERSE REACTIONS/TOXIC EFFECTS

IV route may produce pain, swelling, thrombophlebitis, carpal tunnel syndrome. Abrupt or too-rapid withdrawal may result in pronounced restlessness, irritability, insomnia, hand tremors, abdominal/muscle cramps, sweating, vomiting, seizures. Overdosage results in somnolence, confusion, diminished reflexes, coma.

NURSING IMPLICATIONS

BASELINE ASSESSMENT:

Assess B/P, pulse, respirations immediately before administration. Pt must remain recumbent for up to 3 hrs (individualized) after parenteral administration to reduce hypotensive effect. Assess autonomic response (cold, clammy hands, sweating) and motor response (agitation, trembling, tension). Offer emotional support to anxious pt.

INTERVENTION/EVALUATION:

Assess motor responses (agitation, trembling, tension) and autonomic responses (cold, clammy hands, sweating). Assess children, elderly for paradoxical reaction, particularly during early therapy. Assist w/ambulation if drowsiness, ataxia occur. For those on long-term therapy, liver/renal function tests, blood counts should be performed periodically.

PATIENT/FAMILY TEACHING:

Discomfort may occur w/IM injection. Drowsiness usually disappears during continued therapy. If dizziness occurs, change positions slowly from recumbent to sitting before standing. Avoid tasks that require alertness, motor skills until response to drug is established. Smoking reduces drug effectiveness. Do not abruptly withdraw medication after long-term therapy.

chlorpromazine

klor-pro´mah-zeen
(Thorazine)

chlorpromazine hydrochloride

(Thorazine)

CANADIAN AVAILABILITY:
Chlorpromanyl, Largactil, NovoChlorpromazine

CLASSIFICATION

Antipsychotic

PHARMACOKINETICS

	ONSET	PEAK	DURATION
PO	30-60 min	—	4-6 hrs
Ext.-release	30-60 min	—	10-12 hrs
IM	Rapid	—	—
IV	Rapid	—	—
Rectal	>60 min	—	3-4 hrs

Variably absorbed after oral administration; well absorbed after IM administration. Protein binding: >90%. Metabolized in liver to some active metabolites. Excreted in urine, eliminated in feces. Half-life: 30 hrs.

ACTION

Blocks postsynaptic dopaminergic receptors in brain. Possesses strong alpha-adrenergic blocking, anticholinergic effects.

USES

Management of psychotic disorders, manic phase of manic-depressive illness, severe nausea or vomiting, preop sedation, severe behavioral disturbances in children. Relief of intractable hiccups, acute intermittent porphyria.

STORAGE/HANDLING

Store at room temperature (including suppositories), protect from light (darkens on exposure). Yellow discoloration of solution does not affect potency, but discard if markedly discolored or if precipitate forms.

PO/IM/IV/RECTAL ADMINISTRATION

PO:

1. Dilute oral concentrate solution w/tomato, fruit juice, milk, orange syrup, carbonated beverages, coffee, tea, water. May also mix w/semisolid food.

IM:

NOTE: After parenteral administration, pt must remain recumbent for 30-60 min in head-low position w/legs raised to minimize hypotensive effect.

1. Inject slow, deep IM. If irritation occurs, further injections may be diluted w/0.9% NaCl or 2% procaine hydrochloride.
2. Massage IM injection site to reduce discomfort.

IV:

NOTE: Give by direct IV injection or IV infusion.

1. Direct IV used only during surgery to control nausea and vomiting.
2. For direct IV, dilute w/0.9% NaCl to concentration not exceeding 1 mg/ml.
3. Administer direct IV at rate not exceeding 1 mg/min for adults and 0.5 mg/min for children.
4. IV infusion used only for intractable hiccups.
5. For IV infusion, add chlorpromazine hydrochloride to 500-1000 ml of 0.9% NaCl.

RECTAL:

1. If suppository is too soft, chill for 30 min in refrigerator or run cold water over foil wrapper.
2. Moisten suppository w/cold water before inserting well up into rectum.

INDICATIONS/DOSAGE/ROUTES

NOTE: Replace parenteral w/oral as soon as possible.

Outpatient: mild psychotic disorders, acute anxiety:
PO: Adults: 30-75 mg/day in 2-4 divided doses.
IM: Adults: 25 mg initially. May repeat in 1 hr.

Outpatient: moderate to severe psychotic disorders:
PO: Adults: 25 mg 3 times/day. Increase twice weekly by 20-25 mg until therapeutic response is achieved. Maintain dosage for 2 wk, then gradually reduce to maintenance level.

Hospitalized: acute psychotic disorders:
PO: Children: 0.55 mg/kg q4-6h.
IM: Adults: 25 mg. May give an additional 25-50 mg in 1 hr if needed. Gradually increase over several days to maximum 400 mg q4-6h.
RECTAL: Adults: 50-100 mg 3-4 times/day. **Children:** 1.1 mg/kg q6-8h (severe cases).

Nausea, vomiting:
PO: Adults: 10-25 mg q4-6h.
RECTAL: Adults: 50-100 mg q6-8h. **Children:** 1.1 mg/kg q6-8h.
IM: Adults: 25 mg. Give additional 25-50 mg q3-4h if hypotension does not occur. **Children:** 0.55 mg/kg q6-8h.

Porphyria:
PO: Adults: 25-50 mg 3-4 times/day.
IM: Adults: 25 mg 3-4 times/day.

Intractable hiccups:
PO: Adults: 25-50 mg 3 times/day. If symptoms continue, administer by IM or slow IV infusion.

Preop:
PO: Adults: 25-50 mg 2-3 hrs before surgery. **Children:** 0.55 mg/kg.
IM: Adults: 12.5-25 mg 1-2 hrs before surgery. **Children:** 0.55 mg/kg.

Usual elderly dosage (nonpsychotic):
PO: Elderly: Initially, 10-25 mg 1-2 times/day. May increase by 10-25 mg/day every 4-7 days. **Maximum:** 800 mg/day.

PRECAUTIONS

CONTRAINDICATIONS: Severe CNS depression, comatose states, severe cardiovascular disease, bone marrow depression, subcortical brain damage. **CAUTIONS:** Impaired respiratory/hepatic/renal/cardiac function, alcohol withdrawal, history of seizures, urinary retention, glaucoma, prostatic hypertrophy, hypocalcemia (increases susceptibility to dystonias). **PREGNANCY/LACTATION:** Crosses placenta; distributed in breast milk. **Pregnancy Category C.**

INTERACTIONS

DRUG INTERACTIONS: Alcohol, CNS depressants may increase CNS, respiratory depression, hypotensive effects. Tricyclic antidepressants, MAO inhibitors may increase sedative, anticholinergic effects. Antithyroid agents may increase risk of agranulocytosis. Increased risk of extrapyramidal symptoms (EPS) w/EPS-producing medications. Hypotensives may increase hypotension. May decrease levodopa effects. Lithium may decrease absorption, produce adverse neurologic effects. **ALTERED LAB VALUES:** May produce false-positive pregnancy test, phenylketonuria (PKU). EKC changes may occur, including Q and T wave disturbances.

SIDE EFFECTS

FREQUENT: Hypotension, dizziness, and fainting occur frequently after parenteral form is given, occasionally thereafter, and rarely w/oral dosage. **OCCASIONAL:** Drowsiness during early therapy, dry mouth, blurred vision, lethargy, constipation or diarrhea, nasal congestion, peripheral edema, urinary retention. **RARE:** Ocular changes, skin pigmentation (those on high doses for prolonged periods).

ADVERSE REACTIONS/TOXIC EFFECTS

Extrapyramidal symptoms appear dose related (particularly high dosage), and divided into 3 categories: akathisia (inability to sit still, tapping of feet, urge to move around), parkinsonian symptoms (mask-like face, tremors, shuffling gait, hypersalivation), and acute dystonias: torticollis (neck muscle spasm), opisthotonos (ridigity of back muscles), and oculogyric crisis (rolling back of eyes). Dystonic reaction may also produce profuse sweating, pallor. Tardive dyskinesia (protrusion of tongue, puffing of cheeks, chewing/puckering of the mouth) occurs rarely (may be irreversible). Abrupt withdrawal after long-term therapy may precipitate nausea, vomiting, gastritis, dizziness, tremors. Blood dyscrasias, particularly agranulocytosis, mild leukopenia may occur. May lower seizure threshold.

NURSING IMPLICATIONS

BASELINE ASSESSMENT:

Avoid skin contact w/solution (contact dermatitis). *Antiemetic:* Assess for dehydration (poor skin turgor, dry mucous membranes, longitudinal furrows in tongue). *Antipsychotic:* Assess behavior, appearance, emotional status, response to environment, speech pattern, thought content.

INTERVENTION/EVALUATION:

Monitor B/P for hypotension. Assess for extrapyramidal symptoms. Monitor WBC, differential count for blood dyscrasias. Monitor for fine tongue movement (may be early sign of tardive dyskinesia). Supervise suicidal-risk pt closely during early therapy (as depression lessens, energy level improves, increasing suicide potential). Assess for therapeutic response (interest in surroundings, improvement in self-care, increased ability to concentrate, relaxed facial expression).

PATIENT/FAMILY TEACHING:

Full therapeutic response may take up to 6 wk. Urine may darken. Do not abruptly withdraw from long-term drug therapy. Report visual disturbances. Sugarless gum or sips of tepid water may relieve dry mouth. Drowsiness generally subsides during continued therapy. Avoid tasks that require alertness, motor skills until response to drug is established. Avoid alcohol.

clomipramine hydrochloride

klow-mih´prah-meen
(Anafranil)

CANADIAN AVAILABILITY:

Anafranil

CLASSIFICATION

Antidepressant: Tricyclic

PHARMACOKINETICS

Well absorbed from GI tract. Protein binding: 96-97%. Metabolized in liver, undergoes first-pass metabolism. Primarily excreted in urine. Minimal removal by hemodialysis. Half-life: 21-31 hrs.

ACTION

Increases synaptic concentration of norepinephrine and/or serotonin (inhibits re-uptake by presynaptic membrane).

USES

Treatment of obsessive-compulsive disorder manifested as repetitive tasks producing marked distress, time-consuming, or significantly interfering w/social or occupational behavior.

PO ADMINISTRATION

Give w/food or milk if GI distress occurs.

INDICATIONS/DOSAGE/ROUTES

Obsessive compulsive disorder:

PO: Adults: Initially, 25 mg/day. Gradually increase over 2 wks to 100 mg/day in divided doses. May further increase over several weeks to 250 mg/day in divided doses. After titration, may give as single bedtime dose (reduces daytime sedation). **Children >10 yrs:** Initially, 25 mg/day. Gradually increase over 2 wks to 3 mg/kg or 100 mg/day in divided doses (whichever is less). May then increase over several weeks up to 3 mg/kg or 200 mg (whichever is less). **Maintenance:** Lowest effective dose.

PRECAUTIONS

CONTRAINDICATIONS: Acute recovery period following MI, within 14 days of MAO inhibitor ingestion. **CAUTIONS:** Prostatic hypertrophy, history of urinary retention or obstruction, glaucoma, diabetes mellitus, history of seizures, hyperthyroidism, cardiac/hepatic/renal disease, schizophrenia, increased intraocular pressure, hiatal hernia. **PREGNANCY/LACTATION:** Crosses placenta; minimally distributed in breast milk. May produce neonatal withdrawal. **Pregnancy Category C.**

INTERACTIONS

DRUG INTERACTIONS: Alcohol, CNS depressants may increase CNS, respiratory depression, hypotensive effects. Antithyroid agents may increase risk of agranulocytosis. Phenothiazines may increase sedative, anticholinergic effects. Cimetidine may increase concentration, toxicity. May decrease effects of clonidine, guanadrel. May increase cardiac effects w/sympathomimetics. May increase risk of hypertensive crisis, hyperpyretic, convulsions w/MAO inhibitors **ALTERED LAB VALUES:** May alter EKG readings, glucose.

SIDE EFFECTS

FREQUENT: Drowsiness, fatigue, dry mouth, blurred vision, constipation, sexual dysfunction (42%: ejaculatory failure, 20%: impotence), weight gain (18%), delayed micturition, postural hypotension, excessive sweating, disturbed concentration, increased appetite, urinary retention. **OCCASIONAL:** GI disturbances (nausea, GI distress, metallic taste sensation), asthenia, aggressiveness, muscle weakness. **RARE:** Paradoxical reaction (agitation, restlessness, nightmares, insomnia), extrapyramidal symptoms (particularly fine hand tremor), laryngitis, seizures.

ADVERSE REACTIONS/TOXIC EFFECTS

High dosage may produce cardiovascular effects (severe postural hypotension, dizziness, tachycardia, palpitations, arrhythmias) and seizures. May also result in altered temperature regulation (hyperpyrexia or hypothermia). Abrupt withdrawal from prolonged therapy may produce headache, malaise, nausea, vomiting, vivid dreams. Anemia has been noted.

NURSING IMPLICATIONS

BASELINE ASSESSMENT:

For those on long-term therapy, liver/renal function tests, blood counts should be performed periodically.

INTERVENTION/EVALUATION:

Supervise suicidal-risk pt closely during early therapy (as depression lessens, energy level improves, increasing suicide potential). Assess appearance, behavior, speech pattern, level of interest, mood. Monitor pattern of daily bowel activity and stool consistency. Monitor B/P, pulse for hypotension, arrhythmias. Assess for urinary retention by bladder palpation.

PATIENT/FAMILY TEACHING:

Change positions slowly to avoid hypotensive effect. Tolerance to postural hypotension, sedative, and anticholinergic effects usually develops during early therapy. Maximum therapeutic effect may be noted in 2-4 wks. Photosensitivity to sun may occur. Dry mouth may be relieved by sugarless gum, sips of tepid water. Report visual disturbances. Do not abruptly discontinue medication. Avoid tasks that require alertness, motor skills until response to drug is established. Avoid alcohol.

clonazepam

klon-nah´zih-pam
(Klonopin)

CANADIAN AVAILABILITY:

Rivotril

CLASSIFICATION

Anticonvulsant

PHARMACOKINETICS

Well absorbed from GI tract. Protein binding: 85%. Metabolized in liver. Excreted in urine. Half-life: 18-50 hrs.

ACTION

Enhances presynaptic inhibition, suppresses spread of seizure activity.

USES

Adjunct in treatment of Lennox-Gastaut syndrome (petit mal variant epilepsy), akinetic, and myoclonic seizures, absence seizures (petit mal).

PO ADMINISTRATION

1. Give w/o regard to meals.
2. Tablets may be crushed.

INDICATIONS/DOSAGE/ROUTES

Anticonvulsant:
NOTE: When replacement by another anticonvulsant is necessary, decrease clonazepam gradually as therapy begins w/ low-replacement dose.
PO: Adults, elderly: 1.5 mg daily. Dosage may be increased in 0.5-1 mg increments at 3-day intervals until seizures are controlled. Do not exceed maintenance dose of 20 mg daily. **Infants, children <10 yrs, or <66 lbs:** 0.01-0.03 mg/kg daily in 2-3 divided doses. Dosage may be increased in up to 0.5 mg increments at 3-day intervals until seizures are controlled. Do not exceed maintenance dose of 0.2 mg/kg daily.

PRECAUTIONS

CONTRAINDICATIONS: Significant liver disease, narrow-angle glaucoma. **CAUTIONS:** Impaired kidney/liver function, chronic respiratory disease. **PREGNANCY/LACTATION:** Crosses placenta, may be distributed in breast milk. Chronic ingestion during pregnancy may produce withdrawal symptoms, CNS depression in neonates. **Pregnancy Category C.**

INTERACTIONS

DRUG INTERACTIONS: Alcohol, CNS depressants may increase CNS depressant effect. **ALTERED LAB VALUES:** None significant.

SIDE EFFECTS

FREQUENT: Drowsiness, ataxia, behavioral disturbances (especially in children) manifested as aggressiveness, irritability, agitation. **OCCASIONAL:** Skin rash, ankle/facial edema, nocturia, dysuria, change in appetite/weight, dry mouth, sore gums, nausea, blurred vision, dry mouth. **RARE:** Paradoxical CNS hyperactivity/nervousness in children, excitement/restlessness in elderly (particularly noted in presence of uncontrolled pain).

ADVERSE REACTIONS/TOXIC EFFECTS

Abrupt withdrawal may result in pronounced restlessness, irritability, insomnia, hand tremors, abdominal/muscle cramps, sweating, vomiting, status epilepticus. Overdosage results in somnolence, confusion, diminished reflexes, coma.

NURSING IMPLICATIONS

BASELINE ASSESSMENT:

Review history of seizure disorder (frequency, duration, intensity, level of consciousness). Implement safety measures and observe frequently for recurrence of seizure activity.

INTERVENTION/EVALUATION:

Assess children, elderly for paradoxical reaction, particularly during early therapy. Assist w/ambulation if drowsiness, ataxia occur. For those on long-term therapy, liver/renal function tests, blood counts should be performed periodically. Evaluate for therapeutic response: a decrease in intensity/frequency of seizures.

PATIENT/FAMILY TEACHING:

Drowsiness usually diminishes w/continued therapy. Avoid tasks that require alertness, motor skills until response to drug is established. Smoking reduces drug effectiveness. Do not abruptly withdraw medication after long-term therapy. Strict maintenance of drug therapy is essential for seizure control. Avoid alcohol.

clorazepate dipotassium

klor-az´eh-payt
(Traxene)

CANADIAN AVAILABILITY:

Novoclopate, Tranxene

CLASSIFICATION

Antianxiety, anticonvulsant

PHARMACOKINETICS

Rapidly, well absorbed from GI tract. Widely distributed. Protein binding: 97%. Metabolized in stomach and liver (first-pass metabolism) to active metabolites. Excreted in urine. Half-life: metabolite: 48-96 hrs.

ACTION

Enhances action of inhibitory neurotransmitter gamma-aminobutyric acid (GABA). Depressant effects occur at all levels of CNS. Suppresses spread of seizure activity.

USES

Management of anxiety disorders, short-term relief of anxiety symptoms, partial seizures, acute alcohol withdrawal symptoms.

PO ADMINISTRATION

1. Give w/o regard to meals.
2. Tablets may be crushed.
3. Capsules may be emptied and mixed w/food.

INDICATIONS/DOSAGE/ROUTES

NOTE: When replacement by another anticonvulsant is necessary, decrease clorazepate gradually as therapy begins w/ low-replacement dose.

Anxiety:
PO: Adults: 30 mg daily in divided doses. **Elderly, debilitated:** 7.5-15 mg in divided doses or single bedtime dose. **Daily dose range:** 15-60 mg.

Partial seizures:
PO: Adults, children >12 yrs: Initially, up to 7.5 mg 3 times daily. Do not increase dosage more than 7.5 mg/wk or exceed 90 mg/day.

Alcohol withdrawal:
PO: Adults: Day 1: 30 mg followed by 30-60 mg in divided doses. **Day 2:** 45-90 mg in divided doses. **Day 3:** 22.5-45 mg in divided doses. **Day 4:** 15-30 mg in divided doses, then gradually reduce to 7.5-15 mg daily.

PRECAUTIONS

CONTRAINDICATIONS: Acute narrow-angle glaucoma, acute alcohol intoxication. **CAUTIONS:** Impaired renal/hepatic function. **PREGNANCY/LACTATION:** May cross placenta; distributed in breast milk. Chronic ingestion during pregnancy may produce withdrawal symptoms, CNS depression in neonates. **Pregnancy Category C.**

INTERACTIONS

DRUG INTERACTIONS: Alcohol, CNS depressants may increase CNS depressant effect. **ALTERED LAB VALUES:** None significant.

SIDE EFFECTS

FREQUENT: Drowsiness. **OCCASIONAL:** Dizziness, GI disturbances, nervousness, blurred vision, dry mouth, headache, confusion, ataxia, skin rash, irritability, slurred speech. **RARE:** Paradoxical CNS hyperactivity/nervousness in children, excitement/restlessness in elderly/debilitated (generally noted during first 2 wks of therapy, particularly noted in presence of uncontrolled pain).

ADVERSE REACTIONS/TOXIC EFFECTS

Abrupt or too-rapid withdrawal may result in pronounced restlessness, irritability, insomnia, hand tremors, abdominal/muscle cramps, sweating, vomiting, seizures. Overdosage results in somnolence, confusion, diminished reflexes, coma.

NURSING IMPLICATIONS

BASELINE ASSESSMENT:

Anxiety: Assess autonomic response (cold, clammy hands, sweating), and motor response (agitation, trembling, tension). Offer emotional support to anxious pt. *Seizures:* Review history of seizure disorder (intensity, frequency, duration, LOC). Observe frequently for recurrence of seizure activity. Initiate seizure precautions.

INTERVENTION/EVALUATION:

For those on long-term therapy, liver/renal function tests, blood counts should be performed periodically. Assess for paradoxical reaction, particularly during early therapy. Assist w/ambulation if drowsiness, dizziness occur. Evaluate for therapeutic response: *Anxiety:* A calm facial expression; decreased restlessness. *Seizures:* A decrease in intensity or frequency of seizures.

PATIENT/FAMILY TEACHING:

Do not abruptly withdraw medication following long-term use (may precipitate seizures). Strict maintenance of drug therapy is essential for seizure control. Drowsiness usually disappears during continued therapy. If dizziness occurs, change positions slowly from recumbent to sitting position before standing. Avoid tasks that require alertness, motor skills until response to drug is established. Smoking reduces drug effectiveness. Avoid alcohol.

---

clozapine

klow´zah-peen
(Clozaril)

CANADIAN AVAILABILITY:

Clozaril

CLASSIFICATION

Antipsychotic

PHARMACOKINETICS

Rapid, almost completely absorbed from GI tract. Widely distributed. Protein binding: 95%. Extensively metabolized by first-pass liver metabolism. Primarily excreted in urine. Half-life: 8-12 hrs.

ACTION

Interferes w/binding of dopamine at dopaminergic receptors. Binds primarily to nondopaminergic sites (e.g., alpha-adrenergic, serotonergic, cholinergic).

USES

Management of severely ill schizophrenic pts who fail to respond to other antipsychotic therapy.

PO ADMINISTRATION

May give w/o regard to meals.

INDICATIONS/DOSAGE/ROUTES

Schizophrenic disorders:
PO: Adults: Initially, 25 mg 1-2 times/day. May increase by 25-50 mg/day over 2 wks until dose of 300-450 mg/day achieved. May further increase dose by 50-100 mg/day no

more frequently than 1-2 times/wk. **Range:** 200-600 mg/day. **Maximum:** 900 mg/day.

Usual elderly dosage:
PO: Elderly: Initially, 25 mg/day. May increase by 25 mg/day. **Maximum:** 450 mg/day.

PRECAUTIONS

CONTRAINDICATIONS: Myeloproliferative disorders, history of clozapine-induced agranulocytosis or severe granulocytopenia, concurrent administration w/other drugs having potential to suppress bone marrow function, severe CNS depression, comatose state. **CAUTIONS:** History of seizures, cardiovascular disease, impaired respiratory, hepatic, renal function, alcohol withdrawal, urinary retention, glaucoma, prostatic hypertrophy. **PREGNANCY/LACTATION:** Crosses placenta; distributed in breast milk. **Pregnancy Category C.**

INTERACTIONS

DRUG INTERACTIONS: Alcohol, CNS depressants may increase CNS depressant effects. Bone marrow depressants may increase myelosuppression. Lithium may increase risk of seizures, confusion, dyskinesias. **ALTERED LAB VALUES:** None significant.

SIDE EFFECTS

FREQUENT: Drowsiness, salivation, constipation, dizziness, tachycardia. **OCCASIONAL:** Nausea, sweating, dry mouth, headache, hypotension, GI upset, weight gain. **RARE:** Visual disturbances, diarrhea, rash, urinary abnormalities.

ADVERSE REACTIONS/TOXIC EFFECTS

Most common symptoms include altered state of consciousness, CNS depression (drowsiness, coma, delirium), cardiac arrhythmias, hypotension, respiratory depression, increased salivation, seizures. Blood dyscrasias, particularly agranulocytosis, mild leukopenia may occur.

NURSING IMPLICATIONS

BASELINE ASSESSMENT:

Obtain baseline WBC and differential count before initiating treatment and WBC count every week during treatment and every week for 4 wks after treatment is discontinued. Assess behavior, appearance, emotional status, response to environment, speech pattern, thought content.

INTERVENTION/EVALUATION:

Monitor B/P for hypotension. Assess for extrapyramidal symptoms. Monitor WBC, differential count for blood dyscrasias. Monitor for fine tongue movement (may be early sign of tardive dyskinesia). Supervise suicidal-risk pt closely during early therapy (as depression lessens, energy level improves, increasing suicide potential). Assess for therapeutic response (interest in surroundings, improvement in self-care, increased ability to concentrate, relaxed facial expression).

PATIENT/FAMILY TEACHING:

Do not abruptly withdraw from long-term drug therapy. Report visual disturbances. Sugarless gum or sips of tepid water may relieve dry mouth. Drowsiness generally subsides during continued therapy. Avoid tasks that require alertness, motor skills until response to drug is established. Avoid alcohol.

desipramine hydrochloride

deh-sip´rah-meen
(Norpramin, Pertofrane)

CANADIAN AVAILABILITY:

Norpramin, Pertofrane

CLASSIFICATION

Antidepressant: Tricyclic

PHARMACOKINETICS

Rapid, well absorbed from GI tract. Protein binding: 90-92%. Metabolized in liver. Primarily excreted in urine. Half-life: 12-27 hrs.

ACTION

Increases synaptic concentration of norepinephrine and/or serotonin (inhibits re-uptake by presynaptic membrane), producing antidepressant effect. Strong anticholinergic activity.

USES

Treatment of various forms of depression, often in conjunction w/psychotherapy.

PO ADMINISTRATION

Give w/food or milk if GI distress occurs.

INDICATIONS/DOSAGE/ROUTES

Depression:
PO: Adults: Initially, 75-150 mg daily as single daily dose, or in divided doses. Gradually increase to lowest effective therapeutic level. Do not exceed 300 mg daily.

Usual elderly dosage:
PO: Elderly: Initially, 75 mg/day in divided doses. May gradually increase to 150-200 mg/day. **Maximum:** 300 mg/day.

PRECAUTIONS

CONTRAINDICATIONS: Acute recovery period following MI, within 14 days of MAO inhibitor ingestion. **CAUTIONS:** Prostatic hypertrophy, history of urinary retention or obstruction, glaucoma, diabetes mellitus, history of seizures, hyperthyroidism, cardiac/hepatic/renal disease, schizophrenia, increased intraocular pressure, hiatal hernia. **PREGNANCY/LACTATION:** Crosses placenta; minimally distributed in breast milk. **Pregnancy Category C.**

INTERACTIONS

DRUG INTERACTIONS: Alcohol, CNS depressants may increase CNS, respiratory depression, hypotensive effects. Antithyroid agents may increase risk of agranulocytosis. Phenothiazines may increase sedative, anticholinergic effects.

Cimetidine may increase concentration, toxicity. May decrease effects of clonidine, guanadrel. May increase cardiac effects w/sympathomimetics. May increase risk of hypertensive crisis, hyperpyrexia, convulsions w/MAO inhibitors. Phenytoin may decrease concentrations. **ALTERED LAB VALUES:** May alter ECG readings, glucose.

SIDE EFFECTS

FREQUENT: Drowsiness, fatigue, dry mouth, blurred vision, constipation, delayed micturition, postural hypotension, excessive sweating, disturbed concentration, increased appetite, urinary retention. **OCCASIONAL:** GI disturbances (nausea, GI distress, metallic taste sensation). **RARE:** Paradoxical reaction (agitation, restlessness, nightmares, insomnia), extrapyramidal symptoms (particularly fine hand tremor).

ADVERSE REACTIONS/TOXIC EFFECTS

High dosage may produce cardiovascular effects (severe postural hypotension, dizziness, tachycardia, palpitations, arrhythmias) and seizures. May also result in altered temperature regulation (hyperpyrexia or hypothermia). Abrupt withdrawal from prolonged therapy may produce headache, malaise, nausea, vomiting, vivid dreams.

NURSING IMPLICATIONS

BASELINE ASSESSMENT:

For those on long-term therapy, liver/renal function tests, blood counts should be performed periodically.

INTERVENTION/EVALUATION:

Supervise suicidal-risk pt closely during early therapy (as depression lessens, energy level improves, increasing suicide potential). Assess appearance, behavior, speech pattern, level of interest, mood. Monitor pattern of daily bowel activity and stool consistency. Monitor B/P, pulse for hypotension, arrhythmias. Assess for urinary retention by monitoring I&O and by bladder palpation.

PATIENT/FAMILY TEACHING:

Change positions slowly to avoid hypotensive effect. Tolerance to postural hypotension, sedative, and anticholinergic effects usually develops during early therapy. Maximum therapeutic effect may be noted in 2-4 wks. Photosensitivity to sun may occur. Dry mouth may be relieved by sugarless gum, or sips of tepid water. Do not abruptly discontinue medication. Report visual disturbances. Avoid tasks that require alertness, motor skills until response to drug is established. Avoid alcohol.

diazepam

dye-az´eh-pam

(Valium, Valrelease)

CANADIAN AVAILABILITY:

Apo-Diazepam, Meval, Novodipam, Valium, Vivol

CLASSIFICATION

Antianxiety: Benzodiazepine **(Schedule IV)**

PHARMACOKINETICS

	ONSET	PEAK	DURATION
IV	1-5 min	—	15-60 min

Well absorbed from GI tract. Widely distributed. Protein binding: 98%. Metabolized in liver to active metabolite. Excreted in urine. Half-life: 20-70 hrs (increased in elderly, liver dysfunction).

ACTION

Enhances action of inhibitory neurotransmitter gamma-aminobutyric acid (GABA). Depressant effects occur at all levels of CNS. Enhances presynaptic inhibition, suppresses spread of seizure activity. Inhibits spinal polysynaptic pathways. Directly depresses motor nerve, muscle function.

USES

Short-term relief of anxiety symptoms, preanesthetic medication, relief of acute alcohol withdrawal. Adjunct for relief of acute musculoskeletal conditions, treatment of seizures (IV route used for termination of status epilepticus).

STORAGE/HANDLING

Store tablets, extended-release capsules, oral/parenteral solutions at room temperature.

PO/IM/IV ADMINISTRATION

PO:

1. Give w/o regard to meals.
2. Dilute oral concentrate w/water, juice, carbonated beverages; may also be mixed in semisolid food (applesauce, pudding).
3. Tablets may be crushed.
4. Do not crush or break capsule.

Parenteral form: Do not mix w/other injections (produces precipitate).

IM:

1. Injection may be painful. Inject deeply into deltoid muscle.

IV:

1. Give by direct IV injection.
2. Administer directly into a large vein (reduces risk of thrombosis/phlebitis). If not possible, administer into tubing of a flowing IV solution as close to the vein insertion point as possible. Do not use small veins (e.g., wrist/dorsum of hand).
3. Administer IV rate not exceeding 5 mg/min. For children, give over a 3-min period (a too-rapid IV may result in hypotension, respiratory depression).
4. Monitor respirations q5-15 min for 2h. May produce arrhythmias when used prior to cardioversion.

INDICATIONS/DOSAGE/ROUTES

NOTE: Use smallest effective dose in those w/liver disease, low serum albumin.

Anxiety:
PO/IM/IV: Adults: 2-10 mg 2-4 times/day. **Elderly/debilitated:** 2.5 mg 2 times/day. **Children >6 mo:** 1 to 2.5 mg 3-4 times/day.

Preanesthesia:
IV: Adults, elderly: 5-15 mg 5-10 min prior to procedure.

Alcohol withdrawal:
PO: Adults, elderly: 10 mg 3-4 times during first 24 hrs, then reduce to 5-10 mg 3-4 times/day as needed.
IM/IV: Adults, elderly: Initially, 10 mg, followed by 5-10 mg q3-4h.

Musculoskeletal spasm:
PO: Adults: 2-10 mg 2-4 times/day. **Elderly:** 2-5 mg 2-4 times/day.
IM/IV: Adults: 5-10 mg q3-4h.

Seizures:
PO: Adults: 2-10 mg 2-4 times/day. **Elderly, debilitated:** 2.5 mg 2 times/day.
IM/IV: Adults: 5-10 mg, repeated at 10-15 min intervals to total of 30 mg. **Elderly, debilitated:** 2-5 mg, increase gradually as needed.

PRECAUTIONS

CONTRAINDICATIONS: Acute narrow-angle glaucoma, acute alcohol intoxication. **CAUTIONS:** Impaired kidney/liver function. **PREGNANCY/LACTATION:** Crosses placenta; distributed in breast milk. May increase risk of fetal abnormalities if administered during first trimester of pregnancy. Chronic ingestion during pregnancy may produce withdrawal symptoms, CNS depression in neonates. **Pregnancy Category D.**

INTERACTIONS

DRUG INTERACTIONS: Alcohol, CNS depressants may increase CNS depressant effect. **ALTERED LAB VALUES:** None significant.

SIDE EFFECTS

FREQUENT: Pain w/IM injection, drowsiness, fatigue, ataxia (muscular incoordination). **OCCASIONAL:** Slurred speech, orthostatic hypotension, headache, hypoactivity, constipation, nausea, blurred vision. **RARE:** Paradoxical CNS hyperactivity/nervousness in children, excitement/restlessness in elderly/debilitated (generally noted during first 2 wks of therapy, particularly noted in presence of uncontrolled pain).

ADVERSE REACTIONS/TOXIC EFFECTS

IV route may produce pain, swelling, thrombophlebitis, carpal tunnel syndrome. Abrupt or too-rapid withdrawal may result in pronounced restlessness, irritability, insomnia, hand tremors, abdominal/muscle cramps, sweating, vomiting, seizures. Abrupt withdrawal in pts w/epilepsy may produce increase in frequency and/or severity of seizures. Overdosage results in somnolence, confusion, diminished reflexes, coma.

NURSING IMPLICATIONS

BASELINE ASSESSMENT:

Assess B/P, pulse, respirations immediately before administration. Pt must remain recumbent for up to 3 hrs (individualized) after parenteral administration to reduce hypotensive effect. *Anxiety:* Assess autonomic response (cold, clammy hands, sweating), and motor response (agitation, trembling, tension). Offer emotional support to anxious pt. *Musculoskeletal spasm:* Record onset, type, location, duration of pain. Check for immobility, stiffness, swelling. *Seizures:* Review history of seizure disorder (length, intensity, frequency, duration, LOC). Observe frequently for recurrence of seizure activity. Initiate seizure precautions.

INTERVENTION/EVALUATION:

Monitor IV site for swelling, phlebitis (heat, pain, red streaking of skin over vein, hardness to vein). Assess children, elderly for paradoxical reaction, particularly during early therapy. Assist w/ambulation if drowsiness, ataxia occur. For those on long-term therapy, liver/renal function tests, blood counts should be performed periodically. Evaluate for therapeutic response: a decrease in intensity/frequency of seizures; a calm, facial expression, decreased restlessness; decreased intensity of skeletal muscle pain.

PATIENT/FAMILY TEACHING:

Discomfort may occur w/IM injection. Drowsiness usually diminishes w/continued therapy. Avoid tasks that require alertness, motor skills until response to drug is established. Smoking reduces drug effectiveness. Do not abruptly withdraw medication after long-term therapy. Strict maintenance of drug therapy is essential for seizure control. Avoid alcohol.

diphenhydramine hydrochloride

dye-phen-high´dra-meen
(Benadryl, Benylin)

FIXED-COMBINATION(S):

W/calamine, an astringent, and camphor, a counter-irritant (Caladryl)

CANADIAN AVAILABILITY:

Allerdryl, Benadryl, Insomnal

CLASSIFICATION

Antihistamine

PHARMACOKINETICS

	ONSET	PEAK	DURATION
PO	15-30 min	1-4 hrs	4-6 hrs
IM/IV	<15 min	1-4 hrs	4-6 hrs

Well absorbed following oral, parenteral administration. Widely distributed. Protein binding: 98-99%. Metabolized in liver. Primarily excreted in urine. Half-life: 1-4 hrs.

ACTION

Prevents, antagonizes most histamine effects (e.g., urticaria, pruritus). Anticholinergic effects cause drying of nasal mucosa. Antidyskinetic effect related to central inhibition of acetylcholine, sedative effect. Antiemetic, antitussive through central effect.

USES

Treatment of allergic reactions, parkinsonism, prevention and treatment of nausea, vomiting, vertigo due to motion sickness; antitussive, short-term management of insomnia. Topical form used for relief of pruritus, insect bites, skin irritations.

STORAGE/HANDLING

Store oral, elixir, topical, parenteral form at room temperature. Powder slowly darkens on exposure to light (does not alter effectiveness).

PO/IM/IV ADMINISTRATION

PO:

1. Give w/o regard to meals. Scored tablets may be crushed. Do not crush capsules or film coated tablets.

IM:

1. Give deep IM into large muscle mass.

IV:

NOTE: Compatible w/most IV infusion solutions.
1. May be given undiluted.
2. Give IV injection over at least 1 min.

INDICATIONS/DOSAGE/ROUTES

Allergic reaction, parkinsonism, treatment of motion sickness:
PO: Adults: 25-50 mg 3-4 times/day q4-6h. **Elderly:** Initially, 25 mg 2-3 times/day. May increase as needed. **Children >20 lbs:** 5 mg/kg/24 hrs in divided doses 4 times/day.
IM/IV: Adults: 10-50 mg. **Maximum daily dose:** 400 mg. **Children >20 lbs:** 5 mg/kg/24 hrs 4 times/day.

Prevention of motion sickness:
PO: Adults: 25-50 mg 30 min before exposure to motion. Give subsequent doses q4-6h.

Nighttime sleep aid:
PO: Adults: 50 mg 20 min before bedtime.

Cough:
PO: Adults: 25 mg q4h.
SYRUP: Adults: 10-20 ml 3-4 times/day. **Children:** 5-10 ml 3-4 times/day.

Pruritus relief:
TOPICAL: Adults: Apply to affected area 3-4 times/day.

PRECAUTIONS

CONTRAINDICATIONS: Acute asthmatic attack, those receiving MAO inhibitors. **CAUTIONS:** Narrow-angle glaucoma, peptic ulcer, prostatic hypertrophy, pyloroduodenal or bladder neck obstruction, asthma, COPD, increased intraocular pressure, cardiovascular disease, hyperthyroidism, hypertension, seizure disorders. **PREGNANCY/LACTATION:** Crosses placenta; detected in breast milk (may produce irritability in nursing infants). Increased risk of seizures in neonates, premature infants if used during third trimester of pregnancy. May prohibit lactation. **Pregnancy Category B.**

INTERACTIONS

DRUG INTERACTIONS: Alcohol, CNS depressants may increase CNS depressant effects. MAO inhibitors may increase anticholinergic, CNS depressant effects. Anticholinergics may increase anticholinergic effects. **ALTERED LAB VALUES:** May suppress wheal and flare reactions to antigen skin testing unless antihistamines are discontinued 4 days prior to testing.

SIDE EFFECTS

FREQUENT: Drowsiness, dizziness, muscular weakness, dry mouth/nose/throat/lips, urinary retention, thickening of bronchial secretions. Sedation, dizziness, hypotension more likely noted in elderly. **OCCASIONAL:** Epigastric distress, flushing, visual disturbances, hearing disturbances, paresthesia, sweating, chills.

ADVERSE REACTIONS/TOXIC EFFECTS

Children may experience dominant paradoxical reactions (restlessness, insomnia, euphoria, nervousness, tremors). Overdosage in children may result in hallucinations, convulsions, death. Hypersensitivity reaction (eczema, pruritus, rash, cardiac disturbances, photosensitivity) may occur. Overdosage may vary from CNS depression (sedation, apnea, cardiovascular collapse, death) to severe paradoxical reaction (hallucinations, tremor, seizures).

NURSING IMPLICATIONS

BASELINE ASSESSMENT:

If pt is undergoing allergic reaction, obtain history of recently ingested foods, drugs, environmental exposure, recent emotional stress. Monitor rate, depth, rhythm, type of respiration and quality and rate of pulse. Assess lung sounds for rhonchi, wheezing, rales.

INTERVENTION/EVALUATION:

Monitor B/P, esp. in elderly (increased risk of hypotension). Monitor children closely for paradoxical reaction.

PATIENT/FAMILY TEACHING:

Tolerance to antihistaminic effect generally does not occur; tolerance to sedative effect may occur. Avoid tasks that require alertness, motor skills until response to drug is established. Dry mouth, drowsiness, dizziness may be an expected response of drug. Avoid alcoholic beverages during antihistamine therapy. Sugarless gum, sips of tepid water may relieve dry mouth. Coffee or tea may help reduce drowsiness.

disulfiram

dye-sul´fi-ram
(Antabuse)

CANADIAN AVAILABILITY:

Antabuse

CLASSIFICATION

Alcohol deterrent

PHARMACOKINETICS

Slowly absorbed from GI tract. Metabolized in liver. Primarily excreted in urine. Up to 20% of dose remains in body for at least 1 week.

ACTION

Inhibits enzyme aldehyde dehydrogenase, responsible for breakdown of ethanol metabolite acetaldehyde. Increased acetaldehyde responsible for disulfiram reaction after alcohol ingestion.

USES

Adjunct in management of selected chronic alcoholic pts who want to remain in state of enforced sobriety.

PO ADMINISTRATION

1. Scored tablets may be crushed.
2. Give w/o regard to meals.

INDICATIONS/DOSAGE/ROUTES

NOTE: Pts must abstain from alcohol for at least 12 hrs before initial dose is administered.
PO: Adults, elderly: Initially, administer maximum of 500 mg daily given as a single dose for 1-2 wks. **Maintenance:** 250 mg daily (normal range: 125-500 mg). Do not exceed maximum daily dose of 500 mg.

PRECAUTIONS

CONTRAINDICATIONS: Severe heart disease, psychosis. **CAUTIONS:** Alcoholic disease.

INTERACTIONS

DRUG INTERACTIONS: Alcohol within 14 days results in disulfiram-alcohol reaction. Oral anticoagulant effect may increase. May increase concentration, toxicity of phenytoin. Isoniazid may increase CNS effects. Metronidazole may increase toxicity. **ALTERED LAB VALUES:** May increase cholesterol concentrations. May decrease VMA concentrations.

SIDE EFFECTS

Experienced during first 2 wks of therapy: mild drowsiness, fatigue, headache, metallic or garlic aftertaste, allergic dermatitis, acne eruptions. Symptoms disappear spontaneously w/continued therapy or w/reduced dosage.

ADVERSE REACTIONS/TOXIC EFFECTS

Disulfiram-alcohol reaction to ingestion of alcohol in any form: flushing/throbbing in head and neck, throbbing headache, nausea, copious vomiting, diaphoresis, dyspnea, hyperventilation, tachycardia, hypotension, marked uneasiness, vertigo, blurred vision, confusion. Can produce death.

NURSING IMPLICATIONS

INTERVENTION/EVALUATION:

Do not give w/o pt's knowledge. Fully inform pt of consequences of alcohol ingestion. Therapy cannot be started until a minimum of 12 hrs has elapsed since pt's last ingestion of alcohol.

PATIENT/FAMILY TEACHING:

Avoid cough syrups, vinegars, fluid extracts, elixirs because of their alcohol content. Even external application of liniments, shaving or body lotion may precipitate a crisis. Effects of medication may occur several days after discontinuance.

---

doxepin hydrochloride

dox´eh-pin
(Adapin, Sinequan)

CANADIAN AVAILABILITY:

Sinequan, Triadapin

CLASSIFICATION

Antidepressant: Tricyclic

PHARMACOKINETICS

Rapid, well absorbed from GI tract. Protein binding: 80-85%. Metabolized in liver to active metabolite. Primarily excreted in urine. Half-life: 11-23 hrs.

ACTION

Increases synaptic concentration of norepinephrine and/or serotonin (inhibits re-uptake by presynaptic membrane). Has strong anticholinergic activity.

USES

Treatment of various forms of depression, often in conjunction w/psychotherapy. Treatment of anxiety.

PO ADMINISTRATION

1. Give w/food or milk if GI distress occurs.
2. Dilute concentrate in 8-oz glass of water, milk, orange, grapefruit, tomato, prune, pineapple juice. Incompatible w/carbonated drinks.

INDICATIONS/DOSAGE/ROUTES

Mild to moderate depression/anxiety:
PO: Adults: 25 mg 3 times/day (75 mg/day). **Usual therapeutic range:** 75-150 mg/day. Alternately, 150 mg/day as single dose at bedtime.

Severe depression/anxiety:
PO: Adults: 50 mg 3 times/day. Gradually increase to 300 mg/day, if needed.

Emotional symptoms accompanying organic brain disease:
PO: Adults: 25-50 mg/day.

Usual elderly dosage:
PO: Elderly: Initially, 10-25 mg at bedtime. May increase by 10-25 mg/day every 3-7 days. **Maximum:** 75 mg/day.

PRECAUTIONS

CONTRAINDICATIONS: Acute recovery period following MI, within 14 days of MAO inhibitor ingestion. **CAUTIONS:** Prostatic hypertrophy, history of urinary retention/obstruction, glaucoma, diabetes mellitus, history of seizures, hyperthyroidism, cardiac/hepatic/renal disease, schizophrenia, increased intraocular pressure, hiatal hernia. **PREGNANCY/LACTATION:** Crosses placenta; distributed in breast milk. **Pregnancy Category C.**

INTERACTIONS

DRUG INTERACTIONS: Alcohol, CNS depressants may increase CNS, respiratory depression, hypotensive effects. Antithyroid agents may increase risk of agranulocytosis. Phenothiazines may increase sedative, anticholinergic effects. Cimetidine may increase concentration, toxicity. May decrease effects of clonidine, guanadrel. May increase cardiac effects w/sympathomimetics. May increase risk of hypertensive crisis, hyperpyretic, convulsions w/MAO inhibitors. **ALTERED LAB VALUES:** May alter ECG readings, glucose.

SIDE EFFECTS

FREQUENT: Drowsiness, fatigue, dry mouth, blurred vision, constipation, delayed micturition, postural hypotension, excessive sweating, disturbed concentration, increased appetite, urinary retention. **OCCASIONAL:** GI disturbances (nausea, GI distress, metallic taste sensation). **RARE:** Paradoxical reaction (agitation, restlessness, nightmares, insomnia), extrapyramidal symptoms (particularly fine hand tremor).

ADVERSE REACTIONS/TOXIC EFFECTS

High dosage may produce cardiovascular effects (severe postural hypotension, dizziness, tachycardia, palpitations, arrhythmias) and seizures. May also result in altered temperature regulation (hyperpyrexia or hypothermia). Abrupt withdrawal from prolonged therapy may produce headache, malaise, nausea, vomiting, vivid dreams.

NURSING IMPLICATIONS

BASELINE ASSESSMENT:

For those on long-term therapy, liver/renal function tests, blood counts should be performed periodically.

INTERVENTION/EVALUATION:

Supervise suicidal-risk pt closely during early therapy (as depression lessens, energy level improves, increasing suicide potential). Assess appearance, behavior, speech pattern, level of interest, mood. Monitor pattern of daily bowel activity, stool consistency. Monitor B/P, pulse for hypotension, arrhythmias. Assess for urinary retention by bladder palpation. Avoid alcohol.

PATIENT/FAMILY TEACHING:

Change positions slowly to avoid hypotensive effect. Tolerance to postural hypotension, sedative and anticholinergic effects usually develops during early therapy. Therapeutic effect may be noted within 2-5 days, maximum effect within 2-3 wks. Photosensitivity to sun may occur. Dry mouth may be relieved by sugarless gum, sips of tepid water. Report visual disturbances. Do not abruptly discontinue medication. Avoid tasks that require alertness, motor skills until response to drug is established.

estazolam

es-tah´zoe-lam
(ProSom)

CLASSIFICATION

Sedative-hypnotic

PHARMACOKINETICS

Well absorbed from GI tract. Crosses blood-brain barrier. Protein binding: 93%. Metabolized in liver. Primarily excreted in urine. Half-life: 10-24 hrs.

ACTION

Enhances action of inhibitory neurotransmitter gamma-aminobutyric acid (GABA). Depressant effects occur at all levels of CNS.

USES

Short-term treatment of insomnia (up to 6 wks). Reduces sleep-induction time, number of nocturnal awakenings; increases length of sleep.

PO ADMINISTRATION

1. Give w/o regard to meals.
2. Tablet may be crushed.

INDICATIONS/DOSAGE/ROUTES

NOTE: Use smallest effective dose in those w/liver disease, low serum albumin.

Insomnia:

PO: Adults >18 yrs: 1-2 mg at bedtime. **Elderly/debilitated:** 0.5-1 mg at bedtime.

PRECAUTIONS

CONTRAINDICATIONS: Acute narrow-angle glaucoma, acute alcohol intoxication. **CAUTIONS:** Impaired renal/hepatic function. **PREGNANCY/LACTATION:** Crosses placenta; may be distributed in breast milk. Chronic ingestion during pregnancy may produce withdrawal symptoms, CNS depression in neonates. **Pregnancy Category X.**

INTERACTIONS

DRUG INTERACTIONS: Alcohol, CNS depressants may increase CNS depressant effect. **ALTERED LAB VALUES:** None significant.

SIDE EFFECTS

FREQUENT: Drowsiness, sedation, rebound insomnia (may occur for 1-2 nights after drug is discontinued), dizziness, confusion, euphoria. **OCCASIONAL:** Weakness, anorexia, diarrhea. **RARE:** Paradoxical CNS excitement, restlessness (particularly noted in elderly/debilitated).

ADVERSE REACTIONS/TOXIC EFFECTS

Abrupt or too-rapid withdrawal may result in pronounced restlessness, irritability, insomnia, hand tremors, abdominal/muscle cramps, sweating, vomiting, seizures. Overdosage results in somnolence, confusion, diminished reflexes, coma.

NURSING IMPLICATIONS

BASELINE ASSESSMENT:

Assess B/P, pulse, respirations immediately before administration. Raise bedrails. Provide environment conductive to sleep (backrub, quiet environment, low lighting).

INTERVENTION/EVALUATION:

Assess sleep pattern of pt. Assess elderly/debilitated for paradoxical reaction, particularly during early therapy. Evaluate for therapeutic response: a decrease in number of nocturnal awakenings, increase in length of sleep.

PATIENT/FAMILY TEACHING:

Smoking reduces drug effectiveness. Do not abruptly withdraw medication following long-term use. Rebound insomnia may occur when drug is discontinued after short-term therapy. Do not use during pregnancy.

ethosuximide

eth-oh-sucks´ih-myd
(Zarontin)

CANADIAN AVAILABILITY:

Zarontin

CLASSIFICATION

Anticonvulsant

PHARMACOKINETICS

Rapid, completely absorbed from GI tract. Protein binding: low. Metabolized in liver. Primarily excreted in urine. Half-life: adults: 56-60 hrs; children: 30-36 hrs.

ACTION

Increases seizure threshold, reduces synaptic response in nerve transmission, suppressing paroxysmal spike, wave pattern noted w/absence (petit mal) seizures.

USES

Management of absence (petit mal) seizures, as adjunct w/phenytoin and phenobarbital, in treatment of mixed seizures (absence seizures w/tonic-clonic seizures).

STORAGE/HANDLING

Store capsules, syrup at room temperature.

PO ADMINISTRATION

Give w/o regard to meals.

INDICATIONS/DOSAGE/ROUTES

Seizures:

PO: Adults, children >6 yrs: Initially, 500 mg daily in divided doses. **Children 3-6 yrs:** 250 mg daily given as single dose. **Maintenance:** Increase daily dose by 250 mg q4-7days until control is achieved. **Usual maintenance dose:** 20 mg/kg daily. Do not exceed 1.5 Gm daily, given in divided doses.

PRECAUTIONS

CONTRAINDICATIONS: Hypersensitivity to succinimides. **EXTREME CAUTION:** Hepatic/renal disease. **PREGNANCY/LACTATION:** Unknown if drug crosses placenta or is distributed in breast milk. **Pregnancy Category C.**

INTERACTIONS

DRUG INTERACTIONS: Alcohol, CNS depressants may increase CNS depression. Tricyclic antidepressants, antipsychotics may decrease seizure threshold effects, increase CNS depression. May decrease concentration of haloperidol (may change pattern/frequency of epileptiform seizures). **ALTERED LAB VALUES:** None significant.

SIDE EFFECTS

FREQUENT: GI disturbances (nausea, anorexia, vague gastric upset, cramps, weight loss, diarrhea, abdominal and epigastric distress). **OCCASIONAL:** Headache, hiccups, dizziness, drowsiness, irritability, tiredness.

ADVERSE REACTIONS/TOXIC EFFECTS

Psychiatric/psychologic disturbances (sleep disturbances, nightmares, aggressiveness, inability to concentrate) may be noted. Blood dyscrasias, systemic lupus erythematosus occur rarely. Abrupt withdrawal may precipitate status epilepticus. Skin eruptions appear as hypersensitivity reaction.

NURSING IMPLICATIONS

BASELINE ASSESSMENT:

Review history of seizure disorder (intensity, frequency, duration, LOC). Initiate seizure precautions. Liver function tests, CBC, platelet count should be performed before therapy begins and periodically during therapy.

INTERVENTION/EVALUATION:

Observe frequently for recurrence of seizure activity. Monitor for therapeutic serum level (40-100 mcg/ml). Assess for clinical improvement (decrease in intensity or frequency of seizures).

PATIENT/FAMILY TEACHING:

Do not abruptly withdraw medication following long-term use (may precipitate seizures). Strict maintenance of drug therapy is essential for seizure control. Drowsiness usually disappears during continued therapy. Avoid tasks that require alertness, motor skills until response to drug is established.

felbamate

fell-bah'mate
(Felbatol)

CLASSIFICATION

Anticonvulsant

PHARMACOKINETICS

Well absorbed from GI tract. Binds to plasma proteins (22-25%). Excreted in urine. Food does not affect absorption. Half-life: 20-23 hrs.

ACTION

Exact mechanism unknown. May reduce seizure spread, may increase seizure threshold. Possesses weak inhibitory effects on GABA-receptor and benzodiazepine receptor binding.

USES

Monotherapy and adjunctive therapy in treatment of partial and secondary generalized seizures in adults; adjunctive therapy in treatment of partial and generalized seizures associated w/Lennox-Gastaut syndrome in children.

PO ADMINISTRATION

1. Scored tablets may be crushed.
2. May give w/food to avoid or reduce GI upset.

INDICATIONS/DOSAGE/ROUTES

Monotherapy:
PO: Adults, elderly, children >14 yrs: Initially, 1,200 mg/day in divided doses 3-4 times daily. Increase dosage in 600 mg increments every 2 wks to 2,400 mg/day based on clinical response and thereafter to 3,600 mg/day if clinically indicated.

Conversion to monotherapy:
PO: Adults, elderly, children >14 yrs: 1,200 mg/day in divided doses 3-4 times daily and reduce concurrent antiepileptic drug (AED) by one third at initial felbamate therapy. At week 2, increase felbamate dosage to 2,400 mg/day while reducing AED up to an additional third of its original dosage. At week 3, increase felbamate dosage up to 3,600 mg/day and continue to reduce AED as clinically indicated.

Adjunctive therapy:
PO: Adults, elderly, children >14 yrs: Add 1,200 mg/day in divided doses 3-4 times daily while reducing present AEDs by 20%. Increase felbamate by 1,200 mg/day increments at weekly intervals to 3,600 mg/day.

Children w/Lennox-Gastaut syndrome (adjunctive therapy):
PO: Children 2-14 yrs: Add 15 mg/kg/day in divided doses 3-4 times daily while reducing present AED by 20%. Increase felbamate by 15 mg/kg/day increments at weekly intervals to 45 mg/kg/day.

PRECAUTIONS

CONTRAINDICATIONS: None significant. **CAUTIONS:** Previous hypersensitivity reaction to carbamates. **PREGNANCY/LACTATION:** Unknown whether drug crosses placenta; detected in breast milk. **Pregnancy Category C.**

INTERACTIONS

DRUG INTERACTIONS: May increase carbamazepine, phenytoin, valproate serum concentrations. Carbamazepine, phenytoin may increase clearance of felbamate. **ALTERED LAB VALUES:** None significant.

SIDE EFFECTS

Side effects appear mild and transient. **OCCASIONAL: (Monotherapy):** Anorexia, nausea, insomnia, headache. **(Adjunctive therapy):** Anorexia, nausea, insomnia, headache, dizziness, somnolence. **RARE:** Rash, photosensitivity.

ADVERSE REACTIONS/TOXIC EFFECTS

Abrupt withdrawal may precipitate seizure status. May cause aplastic anemia.

NURSING IMPLICATIONS

BASELINE ASSESSMENT:

Review history of seizure disorder (intensity, frequency, duration, level of consciousness). Initiate safety measures. Unnecessary to routinely monitor clinical laboratory parameters (unprecedented safety profile).

INTERVENTION/EVALUATION:

Observe frequently for recurrence of seizure activity. Assess for clinical improvement (decrease in intensity/frequency of seizures).

PATIENT/FAMILY TEACHING:

Do not abruptly withdraw medication following long-term use (may precipitate seizures). Strict maintenance of drug therapy is essential for seizure control. Avoid tasks that require alertness, motor skills until response to drug is established. Avoid sunlight until sensitivity established. Carry ID card/bracelet indicating anticonvulsant therapy.

fluoxetine hydrochloride

flew-ox´eh-teen
(Prozac)

CANADIAN AVAILABILITY:

Prozac

CLASSIFICATION

Antidepressant

PHARMACOKINETICS

Well absorbed from GI tract. Crosses blood-brain barrier. Protein binding: 94%. Metabolized in liver to active metabolite. Primarily excreted in urine. Half-life: 2-3 days; metabolite: 7-9 days.

ACTION

Selectively inhibits serotonin (5-HT) uptake in CNS enhancing serotonergic function.

USES

Outpatient treatment of major depression exhibited as persistent, prominent dysphoria (occurring nearly every day for at least 2 wk) manifested by 4 of 8 symptoms: change in appetite, change in sleep pattern, increased fatigue, impaired concentration, feelings of guilt or worthlessness, loss of interest in usual activities, psychomotor agitation or retardation, or suicidal tendencies. Treatment of obsessive-compulsive disorder (OCD).

PO ADMINISTRATION

Give w/food or milk if GI distress occurs.

INDICATIONS/DOSAGE/ROUTES

NOTE: Use lower or less frequent doses in those w/renal, hepatic impairment, elderly, those w/concurrent disease or on multiple medications.

Depression, OCD:

PO: Adults: Initially, 20 mg each morning. If therapeutic improvement does not occur after 2 wk, gradually increase dose to maximum 80 mg/day in 2 equally divided doses in morning, noon. **Elderly:** Initially, 10 mg/day. May increase by 10-20 mg q2wks. Avoid administration at night.

PRECAUTIONS

CONTRAINDICATIONS: Within 14 days of MAO inhibitor ingestion. **CAUTIONS:** Impaired renal or hepatic function. **PREGNANCY/LACTATION:** Not known whether drug crosses placenta or is distributed in breast milk. **Pregnancy Category B.**

INTERACTIONS

DRUG INTERACTIONS: Alcohol, CNS depressants antagonize CNS depressant effect. May displace highly protein-bound medications from protein binding sites (e.g., oral anticoagulants). MAO inhibitors may produce serotonin syndrome **ALTERED LAB VALUES:** None significant.

SIDE EFFECTS

FREQUENT: Headache, nervousness, insomnia, drowsiness, excessive sweating, anxiety, tremor, anorexia, nausea, diarrhea, dry mouth. **OCCASIONAL:** Dizziness, fatigue, constipation, rash, pruritus, vomiting, back pain, visual disturbances.

ADVERSE REACTIONS/TOXIC EFFECTS

Overdosage may produce seizures, nausea, vomiting, excessive agitation, restlessness.

NURSING IMPLICATIONS

BASELINE ASSESSMENT:

For those on long-term therapy, liver/renal function tests, blood counts should be performed periodically.

INTERVENTION/EVALUATION:

Supervise suicidal-risk pt closely during early therapy (as energy level improves, suicide potential increases). Assess appearance, behavior, speech pattern, level of interest, mood. Assist w/ambulation if dizziness occurs. Monitor stool frequency and consistency. Assess skin for appearance of rash.

PATIENT/FAMILY TEACHING:

Change positions slowly to avoid hypotensive effect. Maximum therapeutic response may require 4 or more wks of therapy. Photosensitivity to sun may occur. Dry mouth may be relieved by sugarless gum, or sips of tepid water. Report visual disturbances. Do not abruptly discontinue medication. Avoid tasks that require alertness, motor skills until response to drug is established. Avoid alcohol.

---

fluphenazine decanoate

flew-phen´ah-zeen

(Prolixin)

fluphenazine enanthate

(Prolixin)

fluphenazine hydrochloride

(Prolixin, Permitil)

CANADIAN AVAILABILITY:

Apo-Fluphenazine, Modecate, Moditen, Permitil

CLASSIFICATION

Antipsychotic

PHARMACOKINETICS

Variably absorbed after oral administration; well absorbed after IM administration. Protein binding: >90%. Metabolized in liver to active metabolites. Primarily excreted in urine. Half-life: 33 hrs.

ACTION

Blocks postsynaptic dopaminergic receptors in brain. Produces weak anticholinergic, sedative, antiemetic effects, strong extrapyramidal activity.

USES

Management of psychotic disturbances (schizophrenia, delusions, hallucinations).

STORAGE/HANDLING

Store oral and parenteral form at room temperature. Yellow discoloration of solution does not affect potency, but discard if markedly discolored or if precipitate forms.

PO/IM ADMINISTRATION

PO:

1. Mix oral concentrate w/water, 7-Up, carbonated orange drink, milk, V-8, pineapple, apricot, prune, orange, tomato, grapefruit juice.
2. Do not mix oral concentrate w/caffeine (coffee, cola), tea, apple juice because of physical incompatibility.

IM:

NOTE: Pt must remain recumbent for 30-60 min in head-low position w/legs raised, to minimize hypotensive effect.

1. Use a dry 21-gauge needle, syringe for administering fluphenazine decanoate or enanthate (wet needle and syringe turn solution cloudy).
2. Inject slow, deep IM into upper outer quadrant of glu-

teus maximus. If irritation occurs, further injections may be diluted w/0.9% NaCl or 2% procaine hydrochloride.

3. Massage IM injection site to reduce discomfort.

INDICATIONS/DOSAGE/ROUTES

Psychotic disorders:

PO: Adults: Initially, 0.5-10 mg/day fluphenazine HCl in divided doses q6-8h. Increase gradually until therapeutic response is achieved (usually under 20 mg daily); decrease gradually to maintenance level (1-5 mg/day). **Elderly:** Initially, 1-2.5 mg/day.

IM: Adults: Initially, 1.25 mg, followed by 2.5-10 mg/day in divided doses q6-8h.

Chronic schizophrenic disorder:

IM: Adults: Initially, 12.5-25 mg of fluphenazine decanoate q1-6wk, or 25 mg fluphenazine enanthate q2wk.

Usual elderly dosage (nonpsychotic):

PO: Elderly: Initially, 1-2.5 mg/day. May increase by 1-2.5 mg/day q4-7 days. **Maximum:** 20 mg/day.

PRECAUTIONS

CONTRAINDICATIONS: Severe CNS depression, comatose states, severe cardiovascular disease, bone marrow depression, subcortical brain damage. **CAUTIONS:** Impaired respiratory/hepatic/renal/cardiac function, alcohol withdrawal, history of seizures, urinary retention, glaucoma, prostatic hypertrophy, hypocalcemia (increased susceptibility to dystonias). **PREGNANCY/LACTATION:** Crosses placenta; distributed in breast milk. **Pregnancy Category C.**

INTERACTIONS

DRUG INTERACTIONS: Alcohol, CNS depressants may increase CNS, respiratory depression, hypotensive effects. Tricyclic antidepressants, MAO inhibitors may increase sedative, anticholinergic effects. Antithyroid agents may increase risk of agranulocytosis. Extrapyramidal symptoms (EPS) may increase w/EPS-producing medications. Hypotensives may increase hypotension. May decrease levodopa effects. Lithium may decrease absorption, produce adverse neurologic effects. **ALTERED LAB VALUES:** May produce false-positive pregnancy test, PKU. EKG changes may occur, including Q and T wave disturbances.

SIDE EFFECTS

FREQUENT: Hypotension, dizziness, and fainting occur frequently after first injection, occasionally after subsequent injections, and rarely w/oral dosage. **OCCASIONAL:** Drowsiness during early therapy, dry mouth, blurred vision, lethargy, constipation or diarrhea, nasal congestion, peripheral edema, urinary retention. **RARE:** Ocular changes, skin pigmentation (those on high doses for prolonged periods).

ADVERSE REACTIONS/TOXIC EFFECTS

Extrapyramidal symptoms appear dose related (particularly high dosage); divided into 3 categories: akathisia (inability to sit still, tapping of feet, urge to move around); parkinsonian symptoms (mask-like face, tremors, shuffling gait, hypersalivation); and acute dystonias—torticollis (neck muscle spasm), opisthotonos (rigidity of back muscles), and oculogyric crisis (rolling back of eyes). Dystonic reaction may also produce profuse sweating, pallor. Tardive dyskinesia (protrusion of tongue, puffing of cheeks, chewing/puckering of the mouth) occurs rarely (may be irreversible). Abrupt withdrawal after long-term therapy may precipitate nausea, vomiting, gastritis, dizziness, tremors. Blood dyscrasias, particularly agranulocytosis, mild leukopenia (sore mouth/gums/throat) may occur. May lower seizure threshold.

NURSING IMPLICATIONS

BASELINE ASSESSMENT:

Avoid skin contact w/solution (contact dermatitis). Assess behavior, appearance, emotional status, response to environment, speech pattern, thought content.

INTERVENTION/EVALUATION:

Monitor B/P for hypotension. Assess for extrapyramidal symptoms. Monitor WBC, differential count for blood dyscrasias. Monitor for fine tongue movement (may be early sign of tardive dyskinesia). Supervise suicidal-risk pt closely during early therapy (as depression lessens, energy level improves, increasing suicide potential). Assess for therapeutic response (interest in surroundings, improvement in self-care, increased ability to concentrate, relaxed facial expression).

PATIENT/FAMILY TEACHING:

Full therapeutic effect may take up to 6 wk. Urine may darken. Do not abruptly withdraw from long-term drug therapy. Report visual disturbances. Sugarless gum or sips of tepid water may relieve dry mouth. Drowsiness generally subsides during continued therapy. Avoid tasks that require alertness, motor skills until response to drug is established. Avoid alcohol.

flurazepam hydrochloride

flur-a´zah-pam
(Dalmane)

CANADIAN AVAILABILITY:

Apo-Flurazepam, Dalmane, Novoflupam

CLASSIFICATION

Sedative-hypnotics **(Schedule IV)**

PHARMACOKINETICS

	ONSET	PEAK	DURATION
PO	15-45 min	—	7-8 hrs

Well absorbed from GI tract. Crosses blood-brain barrier. Widely distributed. Protein binding: 97%. Metabolized in liver to active metabolite. Primarily excreted in urine. Half-life: 2.3 hrs; metabolite: 40-114 hrs.

ACTION

Enhances action of inhibitory neurotransmitter gamma-aminobutyric acid (GABA). Depressant effects occur at all levels of CNS.

USES

Short-term treatment of insomnia (up to 4 wk). Reduces sleep-induction time, number of nocturnal awakenings; increases length of sleep.

PO ADMINISTRATION

1. Give w/o regard to meals.
2. Capsules may be emptied and mixed w/food.

INDICATIONS/DOSAGE/ROUTES

PO: Adults: 15-30 mg at bedtime. **Elderly/debilitated/liver disease/low serum albumin:** 15 mg at bedtime.

PRECAUTIONS

CONTRAINDICATIONS: Acute narrow-angle glaucoma, acute alcohol intoxication. **CAUTIONS:** Impaired renal/hepatic function. **PREGNANCY/LACTATION:** Crosses placenta; may be distributed in breast milk. Chronic ingestion during pregnancy may produce withdrawal symptoms, CNS depression in neonates. **Pregnancy Category C.**

INTERACTIONS

DRUG INTERACTIONS: Alcohol, CNS depressants may increase CNS depressant effect. **ALTERED LAB VALUES:** None significant.

SIDE EFFECTS

FREQUENT: Drowsiness, dizziness, ataxia, sedation. Morning drowsiness may occur initially. **OCCASIONAL:** Dizziness, GI disturbances, nervousness, blurred vision, dry mouth, headache, confusion, skin rash, irritability, slurred speech. **RARE:** Paradoxical CNS excitement/restlessness (particularly noted in elderly/debilitated).

ADVERSE REACTIONS/TOXIC EFFECTS

Abrupt or too-rapid withdrawal may result in pronounced restlessness and irritability, insomnia, hand tremors, abdominal/muscle cramps, sweating, vomiting, seizures. Overdosage results in somnolence, confusion, diminished reflexes, coma.

NURSING IMPLICATIONS

BASELINE ASSESSMENT:

Assess B/P, pulse, respirations immediately before administration. Raise bed rails. Provide environment conducive to sleep (back rub, quiet environment, low lighting).

INTERVENTION/EVALUATION:

Assist w/ambulation. Assess for paradoxical reaction, particularly during early therapy. Evaluate for therapeutic response: a decrease in number of nocturnal awakenings, increase in length of sleep duration.

PATIENT/FAMILY TEACHING:

Smoking reduces drug effectiveness. Do not abruptly withdraw medication after long-term use. Avoid alcohol.

fluvoxamine

flu-vocks'ah-meen
(Luvox)

CLASSIFICATION

Antidepressant

ACTION

Selectively inhibits serotonin (5-HT) uptake in CNS enhancing serotonergic function.

USES

Treatment of depression, obsessive compulsive disorder (OCD).

INDICATIONS/DOSAGE/ROUTES

Depression, OCD:
PO: Adults, elderly: Initially, 50-100 mg/day (50 mg may decrease incidence of nausea). **Maintenance:** 100-300 mg/day.

SIDE EFFECTS

FREQUENT: Nausea, somnolence, asthenia, headache, dry mouth, insomnia. **OCCASIONAL:** Abdominal pain, dizziness, nervousness, tremor, vomiting, dyspepsia.

gabapentin

gah-bah-pen'tin
(Neurontin)

CLASSIFICATION

Anticonvulsant

PHARMACOKINETICS

Well absorbed from GI tract (not affected by food). Widely distributed. Crosses blood-brain barrier. Protein binding: $<3\%$. Primarily excreted unchanged in urine. Removed by hemodialysis. Half-life: 5-7 hrs (increased in decreased renal function, elderly).

ACTION

Exact mechanism unknown. May be due to increased GABA synthesis rate, increased GABA accumulation, or binding to as yet undefined receptor in brain tissue.

USES

Adjunctive therapy in treatment of partial seizures and partial seizures w/secondary generalization in adults.

PO ADMINISTRATION

1. May be given w/o regard to meals; may give w/food to avoid or reduce GI upset.
2. If treatment is discontinued or anticonvulsant therapy is added, do so gradually over at least 1 week (reduces risk of loss of seizure control).

INDICATIONS/DOSAGE/ROUTES

Seizure control:

NOTE: Maximum time between doses should not exceed 12 hrs.

PO: Adults, elderly: 900-1800 mg/day given in divided doses q8h. May titrate to effective dose rapidly: *Day 1:* 300 mg (give at bedtime). *Day 2:* 300 mg q12h. *Day 3:* 300 mg q8h.

Renal function impairment:

Based on creatinine clearance:

CREATININE CLEARANCE	DOSAGE
>60 ml/min	400 mg q8h
30-60 ml/min	300 mg q12h
15-30 ml/min	300 mg daily
<15 ml/min	300 mg every other day
Hemodialysis	200-300 mg after each 4 hr hemodialysis

PRECAUTIONS

CONTRAINDICATIONS: None significant. **CAUTIONS:** Renal impairment. Discontinue/add anticonvulsant therapy gradually (reduces loss of seizure control). Children <18 yrs of age. **PREGNANCY/LACTATION:** Unknown whether it is distributed in breast milk. **Pregnancy Category C.**

INTERACTIONS

DRUG INTERACTIONS: None significant. **ALTERED LAB VALUES:**p May decrease WBCs.

SIDE EFFECTS

FREQUENT: Ataxia, dizziness, fatigue, nystagmus, somnolence. **OCCASIONAL:** Increased weight, dyspepsia, myalgia, tremor, nervousness, rhinitis, pharyngitis, blurred vision, nausea, vomiting.

ADVERSE REACTIONS/TOXIC EFFECTS

Abrupt withdrawal may increase seizure frequency. Overdosage may result in double vision, slurred speech, drowsiness, lethargy, diarrhea.

NURSING IMPLICATIONS

BASELINE ASSESSMENT:

Assess type, onset, duration, intensity, and frequency of seizures. Routine laboratory monitoring of blood serum levels unnecessary for safe use.

INTERVENTION/EVALUATION:

Provide safety measures as needed. Assess for seizure activity.

PATIENT/FAMILY TEACHING:

Take gabapentin only as prescribed; do not abruptly stop taking drug because seizure frequency may be increased. Do not drive, operate machinery, or perform activities requiring mental acuity due to potential dizziness, somnolence. Avoid alcohol. Carry identification card/bracelet to note anticonvulsant therapy.

haloperidol

hal-oh-pear´ih-dawl

(Haldol)

CANADIAN AVAILABILITY:

Apo-Haloperidol, Haldol, Novoperidol, Peridol

CLASSIFICATION

Antipsychotic

PHARMACOKINETICS

Readily absorbed from GI tract. Protein binding: 92%. Extensively metabolized in liver. Primarily excreted in urine. Half-life: *oral:* 12-37 hrs; *IM:* 17-25 hrs, *IV:* 10-19 hrs.

ACTION

Competitively blocks postsynaptic dopamine receptors, increases turnover of brain dopamine producing tranquilizing effect. Has anticholinergic, alpha-adrenergic blocking activity.

USES

Management of psychotic disorders, control of tics, vocal utterances in Tourette's syndrome. Used in management of severe behavioral problems in children, short-term treatment of hyperactivity in children.

STORAGE/HANDLING

Store all preparations at room temperature. Discard if precipitate forms, discoloration occurs.

PO/IM ADMINISTRATION

PO:

1. Give w/o regard to meals.
2. Scored tablets may be crushed.

IM:

Parenteral administration: Pt must remain recumbent for 30-60 min in head-low position w/legs raised to minimize hypotensive effect.

1. Prepare IM injection using 21-gauge needle.
2. Do not exceed a maximum volume of 3 ml per IM injection site.
3. Inject slow, deep IM into upper outer quadrant of gluteus maximus.

INDICATIONS/DOSAGE/ROUTES

NOTE: Increase dosage gradually to optimum response, then decrease to lowest effective level for maintenance. Replace parenteral therapy w/oral therapy as soon as possible.

Moderate symptoms:

PO: Adults, elderly: Initially, 0.5-2 mg 2-3 times/day; may titrate up to 100 mg/day. **Maintenance:** Lowest effective dose.

Severe symptoms:

PO: Adults, elderly: Initially, 3-5 mg 2-3 times/day; may titrate up to 100 mg/day. **Maintenance:** Lowest effective dose.

Usual parenteral dosage:
IM: Adults, elderly: 2-5 mg; may repeat at 1-8 hr intervals. Give oral dose 12-24 hrs after last parenteral dose administered.

Usual elderly dosage (nonpsychotic):
PO: Elderly: Initially, 0.25-0.5 mg 1-2 times/day. May increase by 0.25-0.5 mg q4-7days. **Maximum:** 50 mg/day.

Usual pediatric dosage:
PO: Children (3-12 yrs): Initially, 0.5 mg/day. May increase by 0.5 mg q5-7 days. Total daily dose given in 2-3 doses/day. **Psychotic disorders:** 0.05-0.15 mg/kg/day. **Nonpsychiatric disorders, Tourette's disorder:** 0.05-0.075 mg/kg/day.

PRECAUTIONS

CONTRAINDICATIONS: Coma, alcohol ingestion, Parkinson's disease, thyrotoxicosis. **CAUTIONS:** Impaired respiratory/hepatic/cardiovascular function, alcohol withdrawal, history of seizures, urinary retention, glaucoma, prostatic hypertrophy, elderly. **PREGNANCY/LACTATION:** Crosses placenta; distributed in breast milk. **Pregnancy Category C.**

INTERACTIONS

DRUG INTERACTIONS: Alcohol, CNS depressants may increase CNS depression. Epinephrine may block alpha-adrenergic effects. Extrapyramidal symptom (EPS) producing medications may increase EPS. Lithium may increase neurologic toxicity. **ALTERED LAB VALUES:** None significant.

SIDE EFFECTS

OCCASIONAL: Orthostatic hypotension, mild, transient leukopenia, dry mouth, blurred vision, lethargy, constipation or diarrhea, peripheral edema, urinary retention, nausea.

ADVERSE REACTIONS/TOXIC EFFECTS

Extrapyramidal symptoms appear to be dose related and may be noted in first few days of therapy. Marked drowsiness and lethargy, excessive salivation, fixed stare may be mild to severe in intensity. Less frequently seen are severe akathisia (motor restlessness), and acute dystonias: torticollis (neck muscle spasm), opisthotonos (rigidity of back muscles), and oculogyric crisis (rolling back of eyes). Tardive dyskinesia (protrusion of tongue, puffing of cheeks, chewing/puckering of the mouth) may occur during long-term administration or following drug discontinuance, and may be irreversible. Risk is greater in female geriatric pts. Abrupt withdrawal following long-term therapy may provoke transient dyskinesia signs.

NURSING IMPLICATIONS

BASELINE ASSESSMENT:

Assess behavior, appearance, emotional status, response to environment, speech pattern, thought content.

INTERVENTION/EVALUATION:

Supervise suicidal-risk pt closely during early therapy (as depression lessens, energy level improves, causing increased suicide potential). Monitor B/P for hypotension. Assess for peripheral edema behind medial malleolus (sacral area in bedridden pts). Assess stool consistency and frequency. Monitor for rigidity, tremor, masklike facial expression, fine tongue movement. Assess for therapeutic response (interest in surroundings, improvement in self-care, increased ability to concentrate, relaxed facial expression).

PATIENT/FAMILY TEACHING:

Full therapeutic effect may take up to 6 wks. Do not abruptly withdraw from long-term drug therapy. Report visual disturbances. Sugarless gum or sips of tepid water may relieve dry mouth. Drowsiness generally subsides during continued therapy. Avoid tasks that require alertness, motor skills until response to drug is established. Avoid alcohol.

hydroxyzine hydrochloride

high-drox´ih-zeen
(Atarax, Vistaril)

hydroxyzine pamoate

(Vistaril)

CANADIAN AVAILABILITY:
Apo-Hydroxyzine, Atarax, Novohydroxyzin

CLASSIFICATION

Antihistamine

PHARMACOKINETICS

	ONSET	PEAK	DURATION
PO	15-30 min	—	—

Well absorbed from GI tract, after IM administration. Metabolized in liver. Primarily excreted in urine. Half-life: 20-25 hrs (increased in elderly).

ACTION

Prevents, antagonizes most histamine effects (e.g., urticaria, pruritus). Anticholinergic effects cause drying of nasal mucosa. Suppresses activity in subcortical area of CNS. Diminishes vestibular stimulation and depresses labyrinthine function. May act on CTZ in medulla.

USES

Relief of anxiety, tension; pruritus caused by allergic conditions, preop and postop sedation, control of muscle spasm, nausea and vomiting.

STORAGE/HANDLING

Store oral solution/suspension, parenteral form at room temperature.

PO/IM ADMINISTRATION

PO:

1. Shake oral suspension well.
2. Scored tablets may be crushed.
3. Do not crush or break capsule.

IM: Note: Significant tissue damage, thrombosis, gangrene may occur if injection is given SubQ, intra-arterial, or IV injection.

1. IM may be given undiluted.
2. Use Z-track technique of injection to prevent SubQ infiltration.
3. Inject deep IM into gluteus maximus or midlateral thigh in adults, midlateral thigh in children.

INDICATIONS/DOSAGE/ROUTES

Anxiety, tension:
PO: Adults, elderly: 25-100 mg 3-4 times/day. **Children >6 yrs:** 50-100 mg/day in divided doses. **Children <6 yrs:** 50 mg/day in divided doses.
IM: Adults, elderly: 25-100 mg q4-6h, as needed. **Children:** 0.5 mg/kg.

Nausea, vomiting:
IM: Adults, elderly: 25-100 mg. **Children:** 1.1 mg/kg.

Pruritus:
PO: Adults, elderly: 25 mg 3-4 times/day. **Children >6 yrs:** 50-100/day in divided doses. **Children <6 yrs:** 50 mg/day in divided doses.

Agitation due to alcohol withdrawal:
IM: Adults, elderly: 50-100 mg. May be repeated q4-6h, as needed.

PRECAUTIONS

CONTRAINDICATIONS: None significant. **CAUTIONS:** None significant. **PREGNANCY/LACTATION:** Unknown if hydroxyzine crosses placenta or is distributed in breast milk. **Pregnancy Category C.**

INTERACTIONS

DRUG INTERACTIONS: Alcohol, CNS depressants may increase CNS depressant effects. MAO inhibitors may increase anticholinergic, CNS depressant effects. **ALTERED LAB VALUES:** May cause false positives w/17-hydroxy corticosteroid determinations.

SIDE EFFECTS

Side effects are generally mild and transient. **FREQUENT:** Drowsiness, dry mouth, marked discomfort w/IM injection. **OCCASIONAL:** Dizziness, ataxia (muscular incoordination), weakness, slurred speech, headache, agitation, increased anxiety. **RARE:** Paradoxical CNS hyperactivity/nervousness in children, excitement/restlessness in elderly/debilitated pts (generally noted during first 2 wks of therapy, particularly noted in presence of uncontrolled pain).

ADVERSE REACTIONS/TOXIC EFFECTS

Hypersensitivity reaction (wheezing, dyspnea, tightness of chest).

NURSING IMPLICATIONS

BASELINE ASSESSMENT:

Anxiety: Offer emotional support to anxious pt. Assess motor responses (agitation, trembling, tension) and autonomic responses (cold, clammy hands, sweating). *Antiemetic:* Assess for dehydration (poor skin turgor, dry mucous membranes, longitudinal furrows in tongue).

INTERVENTION/EVALUATION:

For those on long-term therapy, liver/renal function tests, blood counts should be performed periodically. Monitor lung sounds for signs of hypersensitivity reaction. Monitor serum electrolytes in those w/severe vomiting. Assess for paradoxical reaction, particularly during early therapy. Assist w/ambulation if drowsiness, lightheadedness occur.

PATIENT/FAMILY TEACHING:

Marked discomfort may occur w/IM injection. Sugarless gum, sips of tepid water may relieve dry mouth. Drowsiness usually diminishes w/continued therapy. Avoid tasks that require alertness, motor skills until response to drug is established.

imipramine hydrochloride

ih-mip´prah-meen
(Janimine, Tofranil)

Imipramine pamoate

(Tofranil-PM)

CANADIAN AVAILABILITY:
Api-Imipramine, Impril, Novopramine, Tofranil

CLASSIFICATION

Antidepressant: Tricyclic

PHARMACOKINETICS

Rapidly, well absorbed from GI tract. Widely distributed. Protein binding: 89-95%. Metabolized in liver, undergoing first-pass effect. Primarily excreted in urine. Half-life: 11-25 hrs.

ACTION

Increases synaptic concentration of norepinephrine and/or serotonin (inhibits re-uptake by presynaptic membrane). Antienuretic effect due to anticholinergic action.

USES

Treatment of various forms of depression, often in conjunction w/psychotherapy. Treatment of nocturnal enuresis in children >6 yrs.

STORAGE/HANDLING

Parenteral form takes on yellow or reddish hue when exposed to light. Slight discoloration does not affect potency but marked discoloration is associated w/potency loss.

PO/IM ADMINISTRATION

PO:

1. Give w/food or milk if GI distress occurs.
2. Do not crush or break film-coated tablets.

IM:

1. Give by IM only if oral administration is not feasible.

2. Crystals may form in injection. Redissolve by immersing ampoule in hot water for 1 min.
3. Give deep IM slowly.

INDICATIONS/DOSAGE/ROUTES

Depression:
PO: Adults: Initially, 75-100 mg daily. Dosage may be gradually increased to 300 mg daily for hospitalized pts, 200 mg for outpatients, then reduce dosage to effective maintenance level (50-150 mg daily). **Elderly:** Initially, 10-25 mg/day at bedtime. May increase by 10-25 mg q3-7days. **Range:** 50-150 mg. **Adolescents:** 30-40 mg daily in divided doses to maximum of 100 mg/day.
IM: Adults: Do not exceed 100 mg/day, administered in divided doses.

Childhood enuresis:
PO: Children >6 yrs: 25 mg 1 hr before bedtime.

PRECAUTIONS

CONTRAINDICATIONS: Acute recovery period following MI, within 14 days of MAO inhibitor ingestion. **CAUTIONS:** Prostatic hypertrophy, history of urinary retention or obstruction, glaucoma, diabetes mellitus, history of seizures, hyperthyroidism, cardiac/hepatic/renal disease, schizophrenia, increased intraocular pressure, hiatal hernia. **PREGNANCY/LACTATION:** Crosses placenta; distributed in breast milk. **Pregnancy Category C.**

INTERACTIONS

DRUG INTERACTIONS: Alcohol, CNS depressants may increase CNS, respiratory depression, hypotensive effects. Antithyroid agents may increase risk of agranulocytosis. Phenothiazines may increase sedative, anticholinergic effects. Cimetidine may increase concentration, toxicity. May decrease effects of clonidine, guanadrel. May increase cardiac effects w/sympathomimetics. May increase risk of hypertensive crisis, hyperpyretic, convulsions w/MAO inhibitors. Phenytoin may decrease concentrations. **ALTERED LAB VALUES:** May alter ECG readings, glucose.

SIDE EFFECTS

FREQUENT: Drowsiness, fatigue, dry mouth, blurred vision, constipation, delayed micturition, postural hypotension, excessive sweating, disturbed concentration, increased appetite, urinary retention. **OCCASIONAL:** GI disturbances (nausea, metallic taste sensation). **RARE:** Paradoxical reaction (agitation, restlessness, nightmares, insomnia), extrapyramidal symptoms (particularly fine hand tremor).

ADVERSE REACTIONS/TOXIC EFFECTS

High dosage may produce cardiovascular effects (severe postural hypotension, dizziness, tachycardia, palpitations, arrhythmias) and seizures. May also result in altered temperature regulation (hyperpyrexia or hypothermia). Abrupt withdrawal from prolonged therapy may produce headache, malaise, nausea, vomiting, vivid dreams.

NURSING IMPLICATIONS

BASELINE ASSESSMENT:

For those on long-term therapy, liver/renal function tests, blood counts should be performed periodically.

INTERVENTION/EVALUATION:

Supervise suicidal-risk pt closely during early therapy (as depression lessens, energy level improves, causing increased suicide potential). Assess appearance, behavior, speech pattern, level of interest, mood. Monitor pattern of daily bowel activity and stool consistency. Monitor B/P, pulse for hypotension, arrhythmias. Assess for urinary retention by bladder palpation.

PATIENT/FAMILY TEACHING:

Change positions slowly to avoid hypotensive effect. Tolerance to postural hypotension, sedative, and anticholinergic effects usually develop during early therapy. Therapeutic effect may be noted within 2-5 days, maximum effect within 2-3 wks. Photosensitivity to sun may occur. Dry mouth may be relieved by sugarless gum, or sips of tepid water. Report visual disturbances. Do not abruptly discontinue medication. Avoid tasks that require alertness, motor skills until response to drug is established. Avoid alcohol.

---

lithium carbonate

lith´ee-um
(Lithane, Eskalith, Lithotabs)

lithium citrate

(Cibalith-S)

CANADIAN AVAILABILITY:
Carbolith, Duralith, Lithane, Lithizine

CLASSIFICATION

Antimanic

PHARMACOKINETICS

Rapid, complete absorption from GI tract. Protein binding: none. Primarily excreted unchanged in urine. Half-life: 18-24 hrs (increased in elderly).

ACTION

Alters ion transport at cellular sites in body tissue. Cations necessary in synthesis, storage, release, reuptake of neurotransmitters involved in producing antimanic, antidepressant effects.

USES

Prophylaxis, treatment of acute mania, manic phase of bipolar disorder (manic-depressive illness).

STORAGE/HANDLING

Store all forms at room temperature.

PO ADMINISTRATION

1. Preferable to administer w/meals or milk.

2. Do not crush, chew, or break extended-release or film-coated tablets.

INDICATIONS/DOSAGE/ROUTES

NOTE: During acute phase, therapeutic serum lithium concentration of 1-1.4 mEq/L is required. Desired level during long-term control: 0.5-1.3 mEq/L.

Acute manic phase:
PO: Adults: Initially, 1.8 Gm (or 20-30 mg/kg) lithium carbonate or 30 ml lithium citrate/day, in 2-3 divided doses. **Elderly:** 600-900 mg/day.

Long-term control:
PO: Adults: 900 mg-1.2 Gm lithium carbonate or 15-20 ml lithium citrate, daily, in 2-4 divided doses.

Usual elderly dosage:
PO: Elderly: Initially, 300 mg 2 times/day. May increase by 300 mg/day at weekly intervals. **Maintenance:** 900-1200 mg/day.

PRECAUTIONS

CONTRAINDICATIONS: Severe cardiovascular disease, severe renal disease, severe dehydration/sodium depletion, debilitated patients. **CAUTIONS:** Cardiovascular disease, thyroid disease, elderly. **PREGNANCY/LACTATION:** Freely crosses placenta; distributed in breast milk. **Pregnancy Category D.**

INTERACTIONS

DRUG INTERACTIONS: May increase effects of antithyroid medication, iodinated glycerol, potassium iodide. NSAIDs may increase concentration, toxicity. May decrease absorption of phenothiazines. Phenothiazines may increase intracellular concentration, increase renal excretion, extrapyramidal symptoms (EPS), delirium, mask early signs of lithium toxicity. Diuretics may increase concentration, toxicity. Haloperidol may increase EPS, neurologic toxicity. Molindone may increase risk of neurotoxic symptoms. **ALTERED LAB VALUES:** May increase blood glucose, calcium, immunoreactive parathyroid hormone.

SIDE EFFECTS

HIGH INCIDENCE: Polyuria (increased urination), polydipsia (excessive thirst) due to reversible diabetes insipidus. **FREQUENT:** Dry mouth, lethargy, fatigue, muscle weakness, headache, GI disturbances (mild nausea, anorexia, diarrhea, abdominal bloating), fine hand tremor, and inability to concentrate. **RARE:** Muscle hyperirritability (hyperactive reflexes, twitching), vertigo, hypothyroidism.

ADVERSE REACTIONS/TOXIC EFFECTS

Serum lithium concentration of 1.5-2.0 mEq/L may produce vomiting, diarrhea, drowsiness, incoordination, coarse hand tremor, muscle twitching, ECG T-wave depression, mental confusion. Serum lithium concentration of 2.0-2.5 mEq/L may result in ataxia, giddiness, tinnitus, blurred vision, clonic movements, severe hypotension. Acute toxicity characterized by seizures, oliguria, circulatory failure, coma, death.

NURSING IMPLICATIONS

BASELINE ASSESSMENT:

Serum lithium levels should be tested every 3-4 days during initial phase of therapy, every 1-2 mo thereafter, and weekly if there is no improvement of disorder or adverse effects occur.

INTERVENTION/EVALUATION:

Lithium serum testing should be performed as close as possible to 12th hour after last dose. Besides serum lithium concentration levels, clinical assessment of therapeutic effect or tolerance to drug effect are necessary for correct dosing level management. Assess behavior, appearance, emotional status, response to environment, speech pattern, thought content. Monitor serum lithium concentrations, differential count, urinalysis, creatinine clearance. Assess for increased urine output, persistent thirst. Report polyuria, prolonged vomiting, diarrhea, fever to physician (may need to temporarily reduce or discontinue dosage). Monitor for signs of lithium toxicity. Supervise suicidal-risk pt closely during early therapy (as depression lessens, energy level improves, and suicide potential increases). Assess for therapeutic response (interest in surroundings, improvement in self-care, increased ability to concentrate, relaxed facial expression).

PATIENT/FAMILY TEACHING:

Take as directed; do not discontinue except on physician's advice. Do not engage in activities requiring alert response until effects of drug are known. Thirst, frequent urination may occur. A fluid intake of 2-3 quarts liquid per day and maintenance of a normal salt intake are necessary during initial phase of treatment to avoid dehydration. Thereafter, 1-1.5 L fluid intake daily is necessary. GI disturbances generally disappear during continued therapy. Thyroid function tests should be performed every 6-12 mo in elderly pts (increased incidence of goiter, hypothyroidism). Therapeutic improvement noted in 1-3 wks. Avoid alcohol and over-the-counter drugs. Consult physician regarding contraception.

lorazepam

lor-az´ah-pam
(Alzapam, Ativan)

CANADIAN AVAILABILITY:

Apo-Lorazepam, Ativan, Novolorazepam

CLASSIFICATION

Antianxiety

PHARMACOKINETICS

	ONSET	PEAK	DURATION
IM	15-30 min	—	12-24 hrs
IV	1-5 min	—	12-24 hrs

Well absorbed after oral, IM administration. Widely distributed. Protein binding: 85%. Metabolized in liver. Primarily excreted in urine. Half-life: 10-20 hrs.

ACTION

Enhances action of inhibitory neurotransmitter gamma-aminobutyric acid (GABA). Depressant effects occur at all levels of CNS. Enhances presynaptic inhibition, suppresses spread of seizure activity. Inhibits spinal polysynaptic pathways. Directly depresses motor nerve, muscle function.

USES

Management of anxiety disorders associated w/depressive symptoms. Parenteral form used preoperatively to provide sedation, relieve anxiety, and produce anterograde amnesia.

STORAGE/HANDLING

Refrigerate parenteral form. Do not use if precipitate forms or solution appears discolored. Avoid freezing.

PO/IM/IV ADMINISTRATION

PO:

1. Give w/food.
2. Tablets may be crushed.

IM:

1. Give deep IM into large muscle mass.

IV:

1. Dilute w/equal volume of sterile water for injection, 0.9% NaCl injection, or 5% dextrose injection.
2. To dilute prefilled syringe, remove air from half-filled syringe, aspirate equal volume of diluent, pull plunger back slightly to allow for mixing, and gently invert syringe several times (do not shake vigorously).
3. Give by direct IV injection or into tubing of free-flowing IV infusion (0.9% NaCl, 5% dextrose) at rate of infusion not to exceed 2 mg/min.
4. Direct IV injection should be made w/repeated aspiration to ensure prevention of intra-arterial administration (produces arteriospasm; may result in gangrene).

INDICATIONS/DOSAGE/ROUTES

Anxiety:
PO: Adults: 1-2 mg daily in 2-3 evenly divided doses. **Elderly:** Initially, 0.5-1 mg/day. May increase gradually.

Insomnia due to anxiety:
PO: Adults: 2-4 mg at bedtime. **Elderly:** 0.5-1 mg at bedtime.

Preop:
IM: Adults, elderly: 0.05 mg/kg given 2 hrs before procedure. Do not exceed 4 mg.
IV: Adults, elderly: 0.044 mg/kg (up to 2 mg total) 15-20 min before surgery.

PRECAUTIONS

CONTRAINDICATIONS: Acute narrow-angle glaucoma, acute alcohol intoxication. **CAUTIONS:** Impaired kidney/liver function. **PREGNANCY/LACTATION:** May cross placenta; may be distributed in breast milk. May increase risk of fetal abnormalities if administered during 1st trimester of pregnancy. Chronic ingestion during pregnancy may produce fetal toxicity, withdrawal symptoms, CNS depression in neonates. **Pregnancy Category D.**

INTERACTIONS

DRUG INTERACTIONS: Alcohol, CNS depressants may increase CNS depressant effect. **ALTERED LAB VALUES:** None significant.

SIDE EFFECTS

FREQUENT: Drowsiness, dizziness, incoordination. Morning drowsiness may occur initially. **OCCASIONAL:** Blurred vision, slurred speech, hypotension, headache. **RARE:** Paradoxical CNS restlessness, excitement in elderly/debilitated (generally noted during first 2 wks of therapy, particularly noted in presence of uncontrolled pain).

ADVERSE REACTIONS/TOXIC EFFECTS

Abrupt or too-rapid withdrawal may result in pronounced restlessness, irritability, insomnia, hand tremors, abdominal/muscle cramps, sweating, vomiting, seizures. Overdosage results in somnolence, confusion, diminished reflexes, coma.

NURSING IMPLICATIONS

BASELINE ASSESSMENT:

Offer emotional support to anxious pt. Pt must remain recumbent for up to 8 hrs (individualized) after parenteral administration to reduce hypotensive effect. Assess motor responses (agitation, trembling, tension) and autonomic responses (cold, clammy hands, sweating).

INTERVENTION/EVALUATION:

For those on long-term therapy, liver/renal function tests, blood counts should be performed periodically. Assess for paradoxical reaction, particularly during early therapy. Assist w/ambulation if drowsiness, lightheadedness occur. Evaluate for therapeutic response: a calm facial expression, decreased restlessness and/or insomnia.

PATIENT/FAMILY TEACHING:

Drowsiness usually disappears during continued therapy. If dizziness occurs, change positions slowly from recumbent to sitting position before standing. Avoid tasks that require alertness, motor skills until response to drug is established. Smoking reduces drug effectiveness. Do not abruptly withdraw medication after long-term therapy. Do not use alcohol or CNS depressants. Contraception is recommended for long-term therapy. Notify physician at once if pregnancy is suspected.

---

loxapine hydrochloride

lox´ah-peen
(Loxitane)

loxapine succinate

(Loxitane)

CANADIAN AVAILABILITY:
Loxapac

CLASSIFICATION

Antipsychotic

PHARMACOKINETICS

	ONSET	PEAK	DURATION
PO (sedation)	20-30 min	1.5-3 hrs	12 hrs
IM (sedation)	15-30 min	—	12 hrs

Well absorbed after oral, IM administration. Metabolized in liver to active metabolite. Primarily excreted in urine. Half-life: 12-19 hrs.

ACTION

Blocks dopamine at postsynaptic receptor sites in brain. Has strong alpha blocking, anticholinergic effects.

USES

Symptomatic management of psychotic disorders.

STORAGE/HANDLING

Store oral, parenteral form at room temperature. Yellow discoloration of solutions does not affect potency, but discard if markedly discolored.

PO/IM ADMINISTRATION

NOTE: Give by oral or IM route.

PO:

1. Give w/o regard to meals.
2. Dilute oral concentrate w/orange or grapefruit juice.

IM:

1. Inject slow, deep IM into upper outer quadrant of gluteus maximus.

INDICATIONS/DOSAGE/ROUTES

PO: Adults: 10 mg 2 times/day. Increase dosage rapidly during first week to 50 mg, if needed. **Usual therapeutic, maintenance range:** 60-100 mg daily in 2-4 divided doses. **Maximum daily dose:** 250 mg.
IM: Adults: 12.5-50 mg q4-6h.

Usual elderly dosage (nonpsychotic):
PO: Elderly: Initially, 5-10 mg 1-2 times/day. May increase by 5-10 mg q4-7days.
IM: Elderly: 12.5-25 mg q48h. May increase by 12.5 mg up to 50 mg.

PRECAUTIONS

CONTRAINDICATIONS: Severe CNS depression, comatose states. **EXTREME CAUTION:** History of seizures. **CAUTION:** Cardiovascular disorders, glaucoma, history of urinary retention, prostatic hypertrophy. **PREGNANCY/LACTATION:** Crosses placenta; distributed in breast milk. **Pregnancy Category C**

INTERACTIONS

DRUG INTERACTIONS: Alcohol, CNS depressants may increase CNS depression. Antacids, antidiarrheals may decrease absorption. Extrapyramidal symptom (EPS) producing medications may increase risk of EPS. **ALTERED LAB VALUES:** None significant.

SIDE EFFECTS

FREQUENT: Transient drowsiness, dry mouth, constipation, blurred vision, nasal congestion. **OCCASIONAL:** Diarrhea, peripheral edema, urinary retention, nausea, mild/transient postural hypotension, tachycardia.

ADVERSE REACTIONS/TOXIC EFFECTS

Extrapyramidal symptoms frequently noted are akathisia (motor restlessness, anxiety). Less frequently noted are akinesia (rigidity, tremor, salivation, mask-like facial expression, reduced voluntary movements). Infrequently noted are dystonias: torticollis (neck muscle spasm), opisthotonos (rigidity of back muscles), and oculogyric crisis (rolling back of eyes). Tardive dyskinesia (protrusion of tongue, puffing of cheeks, chewing/puckering of mouth) occurs rarely but may be irreversible. Risk is greater in female elderly pts. Grand-mal seizures may occur in epileptic pts (risk higher w/IM administration).

NURSING IMPLICATIONS

BASELINE ASSESSMENT:

Assess behavior, appearance, emotional status, response to environment, speech pattern, thought content.

INTERVENTION/EVALUATION:

Supervise suicidal-risk pt closely during early therapy (as depression lessens, energy level improves, and suicide potential increases). Monitor B/P for hypotension. Assess for peripheral edema behind medial malleolus (sacral area in bedridden pts). Assess stool consistency and frequency. Monitor for rigidity, tremor, mask-like facial expression (especially in those receiving IM injection). Assess for therapeutic response (interest in surroundings, improvement in self-care, increased ability to concentrate, relaxed facial expression).

PATIENT/FAMILY TEACHING:

Full therapeutic effect may take up to 6 wks. Report visual disturbances. Sugarless gum or sips of tepid water may relieve dry mouth. Drowsiness generally subsides during continued therapy. Avoid tasks that require alertness, motor skills until response to drug is established. Avoid alcohol, CNS depressants, over-the-counter medications. Describe signs and symptoms of extrapyramidal involvement and tardive dyskinesia for pt to report immediately.

maprotiline hydrochloride

mah-pro´tih-leen
(Ludiomil)

CANADIAN AVAILABILITY:

Ludiomil

CLASSIFICATION

Antidepressant

PHARMACOKINETICS

Slowly, completely absorbed from GI tract. Widely distributed. Protein binding: 88%. Metabolized in liver to active metabolites. Primarily excreted in urine. Half-life: 27-58 hrs; metabolite: 60-90 hrs.

ACTION

Blocks reuptake of norepinephrine by presynaptic neuronal membranes. May change beta-adrenergic receptor sensitivity and enhance response to alpha adrenergic, serotonergic stimulation. Has moderate anticholinergic activity.

USES

Relief of depressive-affective (mood) disorders, including depressive neurosis, major depression. Also used for depression phase of bipolar disorder (manic-depressive illness).

PO ADMINISTRATION

1. Give w/food or milk if GI distress occurs.
2. Do not crush or break enteric-coated tablets.
3. Scored tablets may be crushed.

INDICATIONS/DOSAGE/ROUTES

Mild to moderate depression:
PO: Adults: 75 mg/day to start, in 1-4 divided doses. **Elderly:** 50-75 mg/day. In 2 wks, increase dosage gradually in 25 mg increments until therapeutic response is achieved. Reduce to lowest effective maintenance level.

Severe depression:
PO: Adults: 100-150 mg/day in 1-4 divided doses. May increase gradually to maximum 225 mg/day.

Usual elderly dosage:
PO: Elderly: Initially, 25 mg at bedtime. May increase by 25 mg q3-7days. **Maintenance:** 50-75 mg/day.

PRECAUTIONS

CONTRAINDICATIONS: Acute recovery period following MI, within 14 days of MAO inhibitor ingestion. **CAUTIONS:** Prostatic hypertrophy, history of urinary retention or obstruction, glaucoma, diabetes mellitus, history of seizures, hyperthyroidism, cardiac/hepatic/renal disease, schizophrenia, increased intraocular pressure, hiatal hernia. **PREGNANCY/LACTATION:** Crosses placenta; distributed in breast milk. **Pregnancy Category C.**

INTERACTIONS

DRUG INTERACTIONS: Alcohol, CNS depressants may increase effect. MAO inhibitors may increase risk of hypertensive crisis, severe convulsions. Sympathomimetics may increase cardiovascular effects (arrhythmias, tachycardia, severe hypertension). **ALTERED LAB VALUES:** None significant.

SIDE EFFECTS

FREQUENT: Drowsiness, fatigue, dry mouth, blurred vision, constipation, delayed micturition, postural hypotension, excessive sweating, disturbed concentration, increased appetite, urinary retention. **OCCASIONAL:** GI disturbances (nausea, GI distress, metallic taste sensation). **RARE:** Paradoxical reaction (agitation, restlessness, nightmares, insomnia), extrapyramidal symptoms (particularly fine hand tremor).

ADVERSE REACTIONS/TOXIC EFFECTS

Higher incidence of seizures than w/tricyclic antidepressants (esp. in those w/no previous history of seizures). High dosage may produce cardiovascular effects (severe postural hypotension, dizziness, tachycardia, palpitations, arrhythmias) and seizures. May also result in altered temperature regulation (hyperpyrexia or hypothermia). Abrupt withdrawal from prolonged therapy may produce headache, malaise, nausea, vomiting, vivid dreams.

NURSING IMPLICATIONS

BASELINE ASSESSMENT:

For those on long-term therapy, liver/renal function tests, blood counts should be performed periodically.

INTERVENTION/EVALUATION:

Supervise suicidal-risk pt closely during early therapy (as depression lessens, energy level improves, increasing suicide potential. Assess appearance, behavior, speech pattern, level of interest, mood. Monitor bowel activity; avoid constipation. Monitor B/P, pulse for hypotension, arrhythmias. Assess for urinary retention.

PATIENT/FAMILY TEACHING:

Change positions slowly to avoid hypotensive effect. Tolerance to postural hypotension, sedative and anticholinergic effects usually develops during early therapy. Therapeutic effect may be noted within 3-7 days, maximum effect within 2-3 wks. Wear protective clothing, use sunscreen to protect skin from ultraviolet or sunlight. Dry mouth may be relieved by sugarless gum or sips of tepid water. Report visual disturbances. Do not abruptly discontinue medication. Avoid tasks that require alertness, motor skills until response to drug is established.

mesoridazine besylate

mess-oh-rid´ah-zeen
(Serentil)

CANADIAN AVAILABILITY:

Serentil

CLASSIFICATION

Antipsychotic

PHARMACOKINETICS

Variably absorbed from GI tract. Protein binding: >90%. Metabolized in liver to some active metabolites. Primarily excreted in urine. Half-life: 20-40 hrs.

ACTION

Blocks postsynaptic dopaminergic receptors in brain. Possesses strong alpha-adrenergic blocking, anticholinergic effects.

USES

Symptomatic management of psychotic disorders, treatment of hyperactivity, uncooperativeness associated w/mental deficiency, chronic brain syndrome; as adjunctive treatment of alcohol dependence, management of anxiety/tension associated w/neurosis.

STORAGE/HANDLING

Store oral, parenteral form at room temperature. Yellow discoloration of solution does not affect potency, but discard if markedly discolored or if precipitate forms.

PO/IM ADMINISTRATION

PO:

1. Dilute oral solution w/water, orange, grape juice.

IM:

NOTE: Pt must remain recumbent for 30-60 min in head-low position w/legs raised, to minimize hypotensive effect.

1. Inject slow, deep IM into upper outer quadrant of gluteus maximus. If irritation occurs, further injections may be diluted w/0.9% NaCl or 2% procaine hydrochloride.
2. Massage IM injection site to reduce discomfort.

INDICATIONS/DOSAGE/ROUTES

NOTE: Increase dosage gradually to optimum response, then decrease to lowest effective level for maintenance. Replace parenteral therapy w/oral therapy as soon as possible.

Usual parenteral dosage:
IM: Adults, children >12 yrs: 25 mg given as single dose. May repeat in 30-60 min, if needed. **Maximum dose:** 200 mg/day.

Psychotic disorders:
PO: Adults, children >12 yrs: Initially, 50 mg 3 times/day. **Maintenance:** 100-400 mg/day.

Hyperactivity:
PO: Adults, children >12 yrs: 25 mg 3 times/day. **Maintenance:** 75-300 mg/day.

Alcohol dependence:
PO: Adults, children >12 yrs: 25 mg twice/day. **Maintenance:** 50-200 mg/day.

Anxiety/tension:
PO: Adults, children >12 yrs: 10 mg 3 times/day. **Maintenance:** 30-150 mg/day.

Usual elderly dosage (nonpsychotic):
PO: Elderly: Initially, 10 mg 1-2 times/day. May increase by 10-25 mg/day every 7-10 days. **Maximum:** 250 mg/day.

PRECAUTIONS

CONTRAINDICATIONS: Severe CNS depression, comatose states, severe cardiovascular disease, bone marrow depression, subcortical brain damage. **CAUTIONS:** Impaired respiratory/hepatic/renal/cardiac function, alcohol withdrawal, history of seizures, urinary retention, glaucoma, prostatic hypertrophy. **PREGNANCY/LACTATION:** Crosses placenta, distributed in breast milk. **Pregnancy Category C.**

INTERACTIONS

DRUG INTERACTIONS: Alcohol, CNS depressants may increase CNS, respiratory depression, hypotensive effects. Tricyclic antidepressants, MAO inhibitors may increase sedative, anticholinergic effects. Antithyroid agents may increase risk of agranulocytosis. Extrapyramidal symptoms (EPS) may increase w/EPS producing medications. Hypotensives may increase hypotension. May decrease levodopa effects. Lithium may decrease absorption, produce adverse neurologic effects.

SIDE EFFECTS

FREQUENT: Hypotension, dizziness and fainting occur frequently after first injection, occasionally after subsequent injections, and rarely w/oral dosage. **OCCASIONAL:** Drowsiness during early therapy, dry mouth, blurred vision, lethargy, constipation or diarrhea, nasal congestion, peripheral edema, urinary retention. **RARE:** Ocular changes, skin pigmentation (those on high doses for prolonged periods).

ADVERSE REACTIONS/TOXIC EFFECTS

Extrapyramidal symptoms appear dose-related (particularly high dosage), and is divided into three categories: akathisia (inability to sit still, tapping of feet, urge to move around), parkinsonian symptoms (mask-like face, tremors, shuffling gait, hypersalivation), and acute dystonias: torticollis (neck muscle spasm), opisthotonos (rigidity of back muscles), and oculogyric crisis (rolling back of eyes). Dystonic reaction may also produce profuse sweating, pallor. Tardive dyskinesia (protrusion of tongue, puffing of cheeks, chewing/puckering of the mouth) occurs rarely (may be irreversible). Abrupt withdrawal following long-term therapy may precipitate nausea, vomiting, gastritis, dizziness, tremors. Blood dyscrasias, particularly agranulocytosis, mild leukopenia (sore mouth/gums/throat) may occur. May lower seizure threshold.

NURSING IMPLICATIONS

BASELINE ASSESSMENT:

Avoid skin contact w/solution (contact dermatitis). Assess behavior, appearance, emotional status, response to environment, speech pattern, thought content.

INTERVENTION/EVALUATION:

Monitor B/P for hypotension. Assess for extrapyramidal symptoms. Monitor WBC, differential count for blood dyscrasias. Monitor for fine tongue movement (may be early sign of tardive dyskinesia). Supervise suicidal-risk pt closely during early therapy (as depression lessens, energy level improves, increasing suicide potential). Assess for therapeutic response (interest in surroundings, improvement in self-care, increased ability to concentrate, relaxed facial expression).

PATIENT/FAMILY TEACHING:

Full therapeutic effect may take up to 6 wks. Urine may become pink, reddish brown. Do not abruptly withdraw from long-term drug therapy. Report visual disturbances. Sugarless gum or sips of tepid water may relieve dry mouth. Drowsiness generally subsides during continued therapy. Avoid tasks that require alertness, motor skills until response to drug is established. Do not use alcohol or other CNS depressants. Use sunscreen, protective clothing for possible photosensitivity.

methadone hydrochloride

meth´ah-doan
(Dolophine)

CLASSIFICATION

Opioid analgesic **(Schedule II)**

PHARMACOKINETICS

	ONSET	PEAK	DURATION
PO	30-60 min	0.5-1 hr	4-6 hrs
SubQ	10-15 min	—	4-6 hrs
IM	10-15 min	—	4-6 hrs

Well absorbed after IM injection. Protein binding: 80-85%. Metabolized in liver. Primarily excreted in urine. Half-life: 15-25 hrs.

ACTION

Binds w/opioid receptors within CNS, altering processes affecting pain perception, emotional response to pain.

USES

Relief of severe pain, detoxification and temporary maintenance treatment of narcotic abstinence syndrome.

STORAGE/HANDLING

Store oral, parenteral form at room temperature. Do not use if solution appears cloudy or contains a precipitate.

PO/SubQ/IM ADMINISTRATION

PO:

1. May give w/o regard to meals.
2. Dilute syrup in ½ glass H_2O (prevents anesthetic effect on mucous membranes).

SubQ/IM:

NOTE: IM preferred over SubQ route (SubQ produces pain, local irritation, induration).

1. Administer slowly.
2. Those w/circulating impairment experience higher risk of overdosage because of delayed absorption of repeated administration.

INDICATIONS/DOSAGE/ROUTES

Pain:

PO/SubQ/IM: Adults: 2.5-10 mg q3-4h as necessary. **Elderly:** 2.5 mg q8-12h.

Detoxification:

NOTE: Refer to local FDA-approved methadone programs.
PO: Adults: 15-40 mg/day until suppression of withdrawal symptoms. **Maintenance:** 20-100 mg/day.

PRECAUTIONS

CONTRAINDICATIONS: Hypersensitivity to narcotics, diarrhea due to poisoning, delivery of premature infant, during labor. **EXTREME CAUTION:** Impaired renal, hepatic function, elderly/debilitated, supraventricular tachycardia, cor pulmonale, history of seizures, acute abdominal conditions, increased intracranial pressure, respiratory abnormalities. **PREGNANCY/LACTATION:** Crosses placenta; distributed in breast milk. Respiratory depression may occur in neonate if mother received opiates during labor. Regular use of opiates during pregnancy may produce withdrawal symptoms in neonate (irritability, excessive crying, tremors, hyperactive reflexes, fever, vomiting, diarrhea, yawning, sneezing, seizures). **Pregnancy Category C.**

INTERACTIONS

DRUG INTERACTIONS: Alcohol, CNS depressants may increase CNS, respiratory depression, hypotension. MAO inhibitors may produce severe, fatal reaction (reduce dose to 1/4 usual dose). Effects may be decreased w/buprenorphine. **ALTERED LAB VALUES:** May increase amylase, lipase.

SIDE EFFECTS

NOTE: Effects are dependent on dosage amount, route of administration. Ambulatory pts and those not in severe pain may experience dizziness, nausea, vomiting more frequently than those in supine position or having severe pain. **FREQUENT:** Sedation, decreased respirations, nausea, vomiting/constipation, lightheadedness, dizziness, sweating. **OCCASIONAL:** Euphoria/dysphoria, urinary retention.

ADVERSE REACTIONS/TOXIC EFFECTS

Overdosage results in respiratory depression, skeletal muscle flaccidity, cold, clammy skin, cyanosis, extreme somnolence progressing to convulsions, stupor, coma. *Antidote:* 0.4 mg naloxone (Narcan). Tolerance to analgesic effect, physical dependence may occur w/repeated use.

NURSING IMPLICATIONS

BASELINE ASSESSMENT:

Pt should be in recumbent position before drug is administered by parenteral route. Assess onset, type, location, duration of pain. Obtain vital signs before giving medication. If respirations are 12/min or lower (20/min or lower in children), withhold medication, contact physician. Effect of medication is reduced if full pain recurs before next dose.

INTERVENTION/EVALUATION:

Monitor vital signs 15-30 min after SubQ/IM dose, 5-10 min after IV dose (monitor for decreased B/P and/or respirations, change in rate or quality of pulse). Oral medication is one-half as potent as parenteral. Assess for adequate voiding. Monitor stools; avoid constipation with increased fluids, bulky foods, and exercise. Initiate deep breathing and coughing exercises, particularly in those w/impaired pulmonary function. Assess for clinical improvement and record onset of relief of pain. Provide support to pt in detoxification program; monitor for withdrawal symptoms.

PATIENT/FAMILY TEACHING:

Discomfort may occur with injection. Change positions slowly to avoid orthostatic hypotension. Avoid tasks that require alertness, motor skills until response to drug is established. Tolerance/dependence may occur w/prolonged use of high doses. Do not take alcohol or other CNS depressants.

molindone hydrochloride

mole-in´doan
(Moban)

CLASSIFICATION

Antipsychotic

PHARMACOKINETICS

	ONSET	PEAK	DURATION
PO	—	—	36 hrs

Rapidly absorbed from GI tract. Widely distributed. Protein binding: 90-99%. Metabolized in liver to active metabolite. Primarily excreted in urine.

ACTION

Decreases dopamine activity. Occupies dopamine receptors in reticular activating, limbic systems in brain.

USES

Symptomatic management of schizophrenic disorders.

PO ADMINISTRATION

1. Give w/o regard to meals.
2. Give oral concentrate alone or mix w/water, milk, fruit juice, or carbonated beverages.

INDICATIONS/DOSAGE/ROUTES

Management of schizophrenia:
PO: Adults: Initially, 50-75 mg/day in 3-4 divided doses. Increase to 100 mg/day in 3-4 days, if needed.

Maintenance (mild symptoms):
PO: Adults: 5-15 mg 3-4 times/day.

Maintenance (moderate symptoms):
PO: Adults: 10-25 mg 3-4 times/day.

Maintenance (severe symptoms):
PO: Adults: Up to 225 mg may be needed.

Usual elderly dosage (nonpsychotic):
PO: Elderly: Initially, 5-10 mg 1-2 times/day. May increase by 5-10 mg every 4-7 days. **Maximum:** 112 mg/day.

PRECAUTIONS

CONTRAINDICATIONS: Severe CNS depression, comatose states. **CAUTIONS:** Severe cardiovascular disorders, history of seizures. **PREGNANCY/LACTATION:** Unknown whether drug crosses placenta or is distributed in breast milk. **Pregnancy Category C.**

INTERACTIONS

DRUG INTERACTIONS: Alcohol, CNS depression producing medications may prolong CNS effects. Anticholinergics, antihistamines, MAO inhibitors, maprotiline, tricyclic antidepressants may increase anticholinergic, sedative effects. Extrapyramidal symptoms (EPS) may increase in severity, frequency w/EPS producing medications. May cause neurotoxic symptoms w/lithium. **ALTERED LAB VALUES:** May alter BUN, RBCs, glucose values. May increase prolactin concentration, WBCs.

SIDE EFFECTS

FREQUENT: Transient drowsiness, dry mouth, constipation, blurred vision, nasal congestion. **OCCASIONAL:** Diarrhea, peripheral edema, rash, urinary retention, nausea, mild/transient postural hypotension, tachycardia. **RARE:** Skin pigmentation, ocular changes.

ADVERSE REACTIONS/TOXIC EFFECTS

Frequently noted extrapyramidal symptom is akathisia (motor restlessness, anxiety). Occurring less frequently is akinesia (rigidity, tremor, salivation, mask-like facial expression, reduced voluntary movements). Infrequently noted are dystonias: torticollis (neck muscle spasm), opisthotonos (rigidity of back muscles), and oculogyric crisis (rolling back of eyes). Tardive dyskinesia (protrusion of tongue, puffing of cheeks, chewing/puckering of mouth) occurs rarely but may be irreversible. Risk is greater in female geriatric pts. Potentially fatal neuroleptic malignant syndrome (NMS) requires immediate discontinuation of the drug.

NURSING IMPLICATIONS

Baseline Assessment:

Assess behavior, appearance, emotional status, response to environment, speech pattern, thought content.

Intervention/Evaluation:

Supervise suicidal-risk pt closely during early therapy (as depression lessens, energy level improves, increasing suicide potential). Monitor B/P for hypotension. Assess for peripheral edema behind medial malleolus (sacral area in bedridden pts). Monitor stools; avoid constipation. Assess for extrapyramidal symptoms (see above), hyperthermia, altered mental status or level of consciousness, and autonomic instability (NMS); evaluate for evidence of tardive dyskinesia. Assess for therapeutic response (interest in surroundings, improvement in self-care, increased ability to concentrate, relaxed facial expression).

Patient/Family Teaching:

Full therapeutic effects may take up to 6 wks. Report visual disturbances. Sugarless gum or sips of tepid water may relieve dry mouth. Drowsiness generally subsides during continued therapy. Avoid tasks that require alertness, motor skills until response to drug is established. Avoid alcohol and CNS depressants.

naloxone hydrochloride

nay-lox´own
(Narcan)

CANADIAN AVAILABILITY:

Narcan

CLASSIFICATION

Opioid antagonist

PHARMACOKINETICS

	ONSET	PEAK	DURATION
IV	1-2 min	—	1-4 hrs
IM	2-5 min	—	1-4 hrs
SubQ	2-5 min	—	1-4 hrs

Well absorbed after IM, SubQ administration. Metabolized in liver. Primarily excreted in urine. Half-life: 60-100 min.

ACTION

Displaces opioid analgesics from receptors. Competitively inhibits opioid analgesic action effects.

USES

Reversal of narcotic-induced respiratory depression, diagnostic tool in suspected acute narcotic overdosage, treatment of asphyxia neonatorum.

STORAGE/HANDLING

Store parenteral form at room temperature. Use mixture within 24 hrs; discard unused solution.

IM/IV ADMINISTRATION

IM:

1. Give in upper, outer quadrant of buttock.

IV:

1. May dilute 1 mg/ml with 50 ml sterile water for injection to provide a concentration of 0.02 mg/ml.
2. The 0.4 mg/ml and 1 mg/ml for injection used for adults, the 0.02 mg/ml concentration used for neonates.
3. For continuous IV infusion, dilute each 2 mg of naloxone with 500 ml of 5% dextrose in water or 0.9% NaCl, producing solution containing 0.004 mg/ml.

INDICATIONS/DOSAGE/ROUTES

Respiratory depression:

SubQ/IM/IV: Adults, elderly: 0.1-0.2 mg at 2-3min intervals until adequate alertness and ventilation are achieved. **Children:** 0.005-0.01 mg q2-3min. Repeated doses may be required at 1-2 hr intervals.

Narcotic overdosage:

IV: Adults, elderly: Initially, 0.4-2 mg. May repeat at 2-3 min intervals until desired response is obtained.

Asphyxia neonatorum:

IV: Neonates: 0.01 mg/kg injected into umbilical vein. Repeat at 2-3 min intervals until desired response is obtained.

PRECAUTIONS

CONTRAINDICATIONS: Respiratory depression due to nonopiate drugs. **CAUTIONS:** Opiate-dependent pt, cardiovascular disorders. **PREGNANCY/LACTATION:** Unknown whether drug crosses placenta or is distributed in breast milk. **Pregnancy Category B.**

INTERACTIONS

DRUG INTERACTIONS: Reverses analgesic/side effects, may precipitate withdrawal symptoms of butorphanol, nalbuphine, pentazocine, opioid agonist analgesics. **ALTERED LAB VALUES:** None significant.

SIDE EFFECTS

None significant (little or no pharmacologic effect in absence of narcotics).

ADVERSE REACTIONS/TOXIC EFFECTS

Too-rapid reversal of narcotic depression may result in nausea, vomiting, tremulousness, sweating, increased B/P, tachycardia. Excessive dosage in postop pts may produce significant reversal of analgesia, excitement, tremulousness. Hypotension or hypertension, ventricular tachycardia and fibrillation, pulmonary edema may occur in those w/cardiovascular disease.

NURSING IMPLICATIONS

BASELINE ASSESSMENT:

Maintain clear airway. Obtain weight of children to calculate drug dosage.

INTERVENTION/EVALUATION:

Monitor vital signs esp rate, depth, and rhythm of respiration during and frequently after administration. Carefully observe pt after satisfactory response (duration of opiate may exceed duration of naloxone resulting in recurrence of respiratory depression). Assess for increased pain w/reversal of opiate.

nortriptyline hydrochloride

knor-trip´teh-leen
(Aventyl, Pamelor)

CANADIAN AVAILABILITY:

Aventyl

CLASSIFICATION

Antidepressant: Tricyclic

PHARMACOKINETICS

Rapid, well absorbed from GI tract. Protein binding: 92%. Metabolized in liver, undergoes first-pass metabolism. Primarily excreted in urine. Minimal removal by hemodialysis. Half-life: 18-44 hrs.

ACTION

Increases synaptic concentration of norepinephrine and/or serotonin (inhibits reuptake by presynaptic membrane).

USES

Treatment of various forms of depression, often in conjunction w/psychotherapy.

PO ADMINISTRATION

Give w/food or milk if GI distress occurs.

INDICATIONS/DOSAGE/ROUTES

PO: Adults: 75-100 mg/day in 1-4 divided doses until therapeutic response achieved. Reduce dosage gradually to effective maintenance level. **Elderly:** Initially, 10-25 mg at bedtime. May increase by 25 mg q3-7days. **Maximum:** 75 mg/day.

PRECAUTIONS

CONTRAINDICATIONS: Acute recovery period following MI, within 14 days of MAO inhibitor ingestion. **CAUTIONS:** Prostatic hypertrophy, history of urinary retention or obstruction, glaucoma, diabetes mellitus, history of seizures, hyperthyroidism, cardiac/hepatic/renal disease, schizophrenia, increased intraocular pressure, hiatal hernia. **PREGNANCY/LACTATION:** Crosses placenta; distributed in breast milk. **Pregnancy Category C.**

INTERACTIONS

DRUG INTERACTIONS: Alcohol, CNS depressants may increase CNS, respiratory depression, hypotensive effects. Antithyroid agents may increase risk of agranulocytosis. Phenothiazines may increase sedative, anticholinergic effects. Cimetidine may increase concentration, toxicity. May decrease effects of clonidine, guanadrel. May increase cardiac effects w/sympathomimetics. May increase risk of hypertensive crisis, hyperpyretic convulsions w/MAOIs. **ALTERED LAB VALUES:** May alter ECG readings, glucose.

SIDE EFFECTS

FREQUENT: Drowsiness, fatigue, dry mouth, blurred vision, constipation, delayed micturition, postural hypotension, excessive sweating, disturbed concentration, increased appetite, urinary retention. **OCCASIONAL:** GI disturbances (nausea, GI distress, metallic taste sensation). **RARE:** Paradoxical reaction (agitation, restlessness, nightmares, insomnia), extrapyramidal symptoms (particularly fine hand tremor).

ADVERSE REACTIONS/TOXIC EFFECTS

High dosage may produce cardiovascular effects (severe postural hypotension, dizziness, tachycardia, palpitations, arrhythmias) and seizures. May also result in altered temperature regulation (hyperpyrexia or hypothermia). Abrupt withdrawal from prolonged therapy may produce headache, malaise, nausea, vomiting, vivid dreams.

NURSING IMPLICATIONS

BASELINE ASSESSMENT:

For those on long-term therapy, liver/renal function tests, blood counts should be performed periodically.

INTERVENTION/EVALUATION:

Supervise suicidal-risk pt closely during early therapy (as depression lessens, energy level improves, increasing suicide potential). Assess appearance, behavior, speech pattern, level of interest, mood. Monitor stools; avoid constipation w/increased fluids, bulky foods. Monitor B/P, pulse for hypotension, arrhythmias. Assess for urinary retention including output estimate and bladder palpation if indicated.

PATIENT/FAMILY TEACHING:

Change positions slowly to avoid hypotensive effect. Tolerance to postural hypotension, sedative and anticholinergic effects usually develops during early therapy. Therapeutic effect may be noted in 2 or more wks. Photosensitivity to sun may occur. Use sunscreens, protective clothing. Dry mouth may be relieved by sugarless gum, or sips of tepid water. Report visual disturbances. Do not abruptly discontinue medication. Avoid tasks that require alertness, motor skills until response to drug is established.

oxazepam

ox-az´eh-pam
(Serax)

CANADIAN AVAILABILITY:

Apo-Oxazepam, Novoxapam, Serax

CLASSIFICATION

Antianxiety: Benzodiazepine

PHARMACOKINETICS

Well absorbed from GI tract. Protein binding: 97%. Metabolized in liver. Primarily excreted in urine. Half-life: 5-15 hrs.

ACTION

Enhances action of inhibitory neurotransmitter gamma-aminobutryic acid (GABA). Depressant effects occur at all levels of CNS.

USES

Management of acute alcohol withdrawal symptoms (tremulousness, anxiety on withdrawal). Treatment of anxiety associated w/depressive symptoms.

PO ADMINISTRATION

1. Give w/o regard to meals.
2. Capsules may be emptied and mixed w/food.

INDICATIONS/DOSAGE/ROUTES

NOTE: Use smallest effective dose in elderly, debilitated, those w/liver disease, low serum albumin.

Mild to moderate anxiety:
PO: Adults: 10-15 mg 3-4 times/day.

Severe anxiety:
PO: Adults: 15-30 mg 3-4 times/day.

Alcohol withdrawal:
PO: Adults: 15-30 mg 3-4 times/day.

Usual elderly dosage:
PO: Elderly: Initially, 10 mg 2-3 times/day. May gradually increase up to 30-45 mg/day.

PRECAUTIONS

CONTRAINDICATIONS: Acute narrow-angle glaucoma. **CAUTIONS:** Impaired renal/hepatic function. **PREG-**

NANCY/LACTATION: May cross placenta; may be distributed in breast milk. Chronic ingestion during pregnancy may produce withdrawal symptoms, CNS depression in neonates. **Pregnancy Category C.**

INTERACTIONS

DRUG INTERACTIONS: Potentiated effects when used w/ other CNS depressants, including alcohol. **ALTERED LAB VALUES:** None significant.

SIDE EFFECTS

FREQUENT: Mild, transient drowsiness at beginning of therapy. **OCCASIONAL:** Dizziness, headache. **RARE:** Paradoxical CNS hyperactivity/nervousness in children, excitement/restlessness in elderly/debilitated (generally noted during first 2 wks of therapy, particularly noted in presence of uncontrolled pain).

ADVERSE REACTIONS/TOXIC EFFECTS

Abrupt or too-rapid withdrawal may result in pronounced restlessness, irritability, insomnia, hand tremors, abdominal/muscle cramps, sweating, vomiting, seizures. Overdose results in somnolence, confusion, diminished reflexes, coma.

NURSING IMPLICATIONS

BASELINE ASSESSMENT:

Offer emotional support to anxious pt. Assess motor responses (agitation, trembling, tension) and autonomic responses (cold, clammy hands, sweating).

INTERVENTION/EVALUATION:

For those on long-term therapy, liver/renal function tests, blood counts should be performed periodically. Assess for paradoxical reaction, particularly during early therapy. Assist w/ambulation if drowsiness, lightheadedness occur. Evaluate for therapeutic response: A calm facial expression, decreased restlessness and/or insomnia.

PATIENT/FAMILY TEACHING:

Drowsiness usually disappears during continued therapy. If dizziness occurs, change positions slowly from recumbent to sitting position before standing. Avoid tasks that require alertness, motor skills until response to drug is established. Smoking reduces drug effectiveness. Do not abruptly withdraw medication after long-term therapy.

paroxetine hydrochloride

pear-ox'eh-teen
(Paxil)

CLASSIFICATION

Antidepressant

PHARMACOKINETICS

Well absorbed from GI tract. Widely distributed. Highly bound to plasma proteins (95%). Metabolized in liver; excreted in urine. Half-life: 24 hrs.

ACTION

Selectively blocks uptake of neurotransmitter, serotonin, at CNS neuronal presynaptic membranes, thereby increasing availability at postsynaptic neuronal receptor sites. Resulting enhancement of synaptic activity produces antidepressant effect.

USES

Treatment of major depression.

PO ADMINISTRATION

1. Give w/food or milk if GI distress occurs.
2. Scored tablet may be crushed.
3. Best if given as single morning dose.

INDICATIONS/DOSAGE/ROUTES

NOTE: Reduce dosage in elderly, pts w/severe renal, hepatic impairment. Dose changes should occur at 1 wk intervals.

Depression:
PO: Adults: Initially, 20 mg/day, usually in morning. Dosage may be gradually increased in 10 mg/day increments to 50 mg/day. **Elderly, debilitated, those w/severe hepatic, renal impairment:** Initially, 10 mg/day. Do not exceed maximum 40 mg/day.

PRECAUTIONS

CONTRAINDICATIONS: Within 14 days of MAO inhibitor therapy. **CAUTIONS:** Severe renal, hepatic impairment. History of mania, seizures, those w/metabolic or hemodynamic disease, history of drug abuse. **PREGNANCY/LACTATION:** May impair reproductive function. Distributed in breast milk. **Pregnancy Category B.**

INTERACTIONS

DRUG INTERACTIONS: MAO inhibitors may cause serotonergic syndrome (excitement, diaphoresis, rigidity, hyperthermia, autonomic hyperactivity, coma). Cimetidine may increase concentrations; phenytoin may decrease concentrations. **ALTERED LAB VALUES:** May increase liver enzymes.

SIDE EFFECTS

FREQUENT: Nausea, somnolence, headache, dry mouth, weakness, constipation/diarrhea, dizziness, insomnia, ejaculatory disturbance, sweating, tremor. **OCCASIONAL:** Decreased appetite, nervousness, anxiety, flatulence, paresthesia, decrease in libido, abdominal discomfort, urinary frequency, yawning. **RARE:** Palpitations, vomiting, blurred vision, taste change, confusion.

ADVERSE REACTIONS/TOXIC EFFECTS

None significant.

NURSING IMPLICATIONS

BASELINE ASSESSMENT:

Assess appearance, behavior, speech pattern, level of interest, mood. Assess for history of drug abuse.

INTERVENTION/EVALUATION

For those on long-term therapy, liver/renal function tests, blood counts should be performed periodically. Supervise suicidal-risk pt closely during early therapy (as depression lessens, energy level improves, increasing suicide potential). Assess appearance, behavior, speech pattern, level of interest, mood.

PATIENT/FAMILY TEACHING:

Therapeutic effect may be noted within 1-4 weeks. Dry mouth may be relieved by sugarless gum or sips of tepid water. Do not abruptly discontinue medication. Avoid tasks that require alertness, motor skills until response to drug is established. Inform physician if intention of pregnancy or if pregnancy occurs. Avoid alcohol.

pentobarbital

pent-oh-bar´bih-tall
(Nembutal)

pentobarbital sodium

(Nembutal Sodium)

CANADIAN AVAILABILITY:
Nembutal, Nova-Rectal, Novopentobarb

CLASSIFICATION

Sedative-hypnotic **(Schedule II)**

PHARMACOKINETICS

	ONSET	PEAK	DURATION
PO	15-60 min	30-60 min	1-4 hrs
IM	10-25 min	—	—
IV	1 min	—	15 min
Rectal	15-60 min	—	1-4 hrs

Variably absorbed after oral, parenteral administration. Rapidly, widely distributed. Protein binding: 60-70%. Metabolized in liver. Primarily excreted in urine. Half-life: 15-50 hrs.

ACTION

CNS depressant producing all levels from mild sedation, hypnosis to deep coma.

USES

Treatment of insomnia (up to 2 wks), preop sedation, routine sedation; parenteral form to control status epilepticus, acute seizure episodes, facilitate intubation procedures, control agitated behavior in psychosis, provide hypnosis for general, spinal, regional anesthesia.

STORAGE/HANDLING

Store capsules, elixir, parenteral form at room temperature. Refrigerate suppositories. Discard parenteral solution if precipitate forms or solution becomes cloudy.

PO/IM/IV/RECTAL ADMINISTRATION

PO:

1. Give w/o regard to meals.
2. Elixir may be given w/water, milk, or fruit juice.

PARENTERAL FORM: Do not mix w/acidic solutions (produces precipitate).

IM:

1. Do not inject more than 250 mg or 5 ml in any one IM injection site.
2. Inject IM deep into gluteus maximus or lateral aspect of thigh.

IV:

1. Administer IV at rate not greater than 50 mg/min (a too rapid IV may produce severe hypotension, marked respiratory depression).
2. Monitor vital signs q3-5min during and q15min for 1-2 hrs after administration for excessive narcosis (deep unconsciousness, amnesia).
3. Inadvertent intra-arterial injection may result in arterial spasm w/severe pain, tissue necrosis. Extravasation in subcutaneous tissue may produce redness, tenderness, tissue necrosis. If either occurs, treat w/injection of 0.5% procaine solution into affected area, apply moist heat.

RECTAL:

1. Moisten suppository w/cold water before inserting well up into rectum.

INDICATIONS/DOSAGE/ROUTES

NOTE: Reduce dosage in elderly, debilitated, impaired liver function.

Hypnotic:
PO: Adults: 100-200 mg at bedtime.
IM: Adults: 150-200 mg. **Children:** 2-6 mg/kg or 125 mg/m^2. Do not exceed 100 mg.
RECTAL: Adults: 120 or 200 mg at bedtime. **Children 12-14 yrs:** 60-120 mg. **Children 5-12 yrs:** 60 mg. **Children 1-4 yrs:** 30-60 mg. **Children 2 mo-1 yr:** 30 mg.

Sedation:
PO: Adults: 20-40 mg 2-4 times daily.
PO/RECTAL: Children: 2-6 mg/kg daily in 3 divided doses.

Preanesthetic:
PO: Children 10-12 yrs: Average dose: 100 mg.
IM: Adults: 150-200 mg. **Children >10 yrs:** 5 mg/kg.
RECTAL: Children <10 yrs: 5 mg/kg.

Seizures, intubation procedures:
IV: Adults: Initially, 100 mg. Wait 1 min to determine full IV effect. Small doses may then be given up to total 200-500 mg.

PRECAUTIONS

CONTRAINDICATIONS: History of porphyria, bronchopneumonia. **CAUTIONS:** Uncontrolled pain (may produce paradoxical reaction), impaired liver function. **PREGNANCY/LACTATION:** Readily crosses placenta; distributed in breast milk. Produces respiratory depression in neonate during labor. May produce postpartum hemorrhage, hemorrhagic disease in newborn. Withdrawal symptoms may occur in neonates born to women who receive barbiturates during last trimester of pregnancy. **Pregnancy Category D.**

INTERACTIONS

DRUG INTERACTIONS: May decrease effects of glucocorticoids, digoxin, metronidazole, oral anticoagulants, quinidine, tricyclic antidepressants. Alcohol, CNS depressants may increase effect. May increase metabolism of carbamazepine. Valproic acid decreases metabolism, increases concentration, toxicity. **ALTERED LAB VALUES:** May decrease bilirubin.

SIDE EFFECTS

FREQUENT: Drowsiness, sedation, residual "hangover" effect, lethargy, irritability, nausea, anorexia, muscle aches and pains, gastric distress. **OCCASIONAL:** Paradoxical CNS hyperactivity/nervousness in children, excitement/restlessness in elderly (generally noted during first 2 wks of therapy, particularly noted in presence of uncontrolled pain).

ADVERSE REACTIONS/TOXIC EFFECTS

Abrupt withdrawal after prolonged therapy may produce effects ranging from markedly increased dreaming, nightmares and/or insomnia, tremor, sweating, vomiting, to hallucinations, delirium, seizures, status epilepticus. Skin eruptions appear as hypersensitivity reaction. Blood dyscrasias, liver disease, hypocalcemia occur rarely. Overdosage produces cold, clammy skin, hypothermia, severe CNS depression, cyanosis, rapid pulse, Cheyne-Stokes respirations. Toxicity may result in severe renal impairment.

NURSING IMPLICATIONS

BASELINE ASSESSMENT:

Assess B/P, pulse, respirations immediately before administration. *Hypnotic:* Raise bed rails, provide environment conducive to sleep (back rub, quiet environment, low lighting). *Seizures:* Review history of seizure disorder (frequency, duration, intensity, level of consciousness). Observe frequently for recurrence of seizure activity. Initiate seizure precautions.

INTERVENTION/EVALUATION:

Assess sleep pattern of pt. Assess elderly/debilitated for paradoxical reaction, particularly during early therapy. Evaluate for therapeutic response: *Insomnia:* Observe for decrease in number of nocturnal awakenings, increase in length of sleep duration time. *Seizures:* Observe for decrease in number, frequency of seizures.

PATIENT/FAMILY TEACHING:

Drowsiness usually diminishes w/continued therapy. Do not abruptly withdraw medication following long-term use. Avoid tasks that require alertness, motor skills until response to drug is established. Tolerance/dependence may occur w/ prolonged use of high doses. Avoid alcohol and CNS depressants. Do not use during pregnancy, nursing.

perphenazine

per-fen´ah-zeen
(Trilafon)

FIXED-COMBINATION(S):

W/amitriptyline, a tricyclic antidepressant (Etrafon, Triavil)

CANADIAN AVAILABILITY:

Apo-Perphenazine, Trilafon

CLASSIFICATION

Antipsychotic

PHARMACOKINETICS

Well absorbed from GI tract. Widely distributed. Protein binding: >90%. Metabolized in liver to active metabolite. Primarily excreted in urine.

ACTION

Blocks postsynaptic dopaminergic receptors in brain. Possesses strong alpha-adrenergic blocking, anticholinergic effects.

USES

Management of psychotic disorders, control of nausea, vomiting, intractable hiccups.

STORAGE/HANDLING

Store oral, parenteral form at room temperature. Yellow discoloration of solution does not affect potency, but discard if markedly discolored or if precipitate forms.

PO/IM/IV ADMINISTRATION

PO:

1. Do not mix oral concentrate w/caffeine (coffee, cola, tea), apple juice because of physical incompatibility.
2. Mix each 5 ml oral concentrate w/60 ml water, 7-Up, carbonated orange drink, milk, V-8, pineapple, apricot, prune, orange, tomato, grapefruit juice.

NOTE: Parenteral Administration: Pt must remain recumbent for 30-60 min in head-low position w/legs raised, to minimize hypotensive effect.

IM:

1. Inject slow, deep IM into upper outer quadrant of gluteus maximus. If irritation occurs, dilute further injections w/0.9% NaCl or 2% procaine hydrochloride.
2. Massage IM injection site to reduce discomfort.

IV:

NOTE: Give by fractional IV injection or IV infusion.

1. For fractional IV, dilute each 5 mg (1 ml) w/9 ml 0.9% NaCl, producing final concentration of 0.5 mg/ml.
2. Do not give more than 1 mg per injection at slow rate at not less than 1-2 min intervals.
3. For IV infusion, dilute further and give at rate of 0.5 mg or less/min.

INDICATIONS/DOSAGE/ROUTES

NOTE: Decrease dose gradually to optimum response. Decrease to lowest effective level for maintenance. Replace parenteral therapy w/oral therapy as soon as possible.

Hospitalized psychotic:
PO: Adults, children >12 yrs: 8-16 mg 2-4 times/day. **Extended release:** 8-32 mg 2 times/day.
IM: Adults, children >12 yrs: 5 mg q6h, as needed.

Nonhospitalized:
PO: Adults, children >12 yrs: 4-8 mg 3 times/day. **Extended release:** 8-16 mg 2 times/day.

Severe nausea, vomiting, intractable hiccups:
IM: Adults: 5 mg.
IV: Adults: Up to 5 mg.

Usual elderly dosage (nonpsychotic):
PO: Elderly: Initially, 2-4 mg/day. May increase by 2-4 mg/day every 4-7 days. **Maximum:** 32 mg/day.

PRECAUTIONS

CONTRAINDICATIONS: Severe CNS depression, comatose states, severe cardiovascular disease, bone marrow depression, subcortical brain damage. **CAUTIONS:** Impaired respiratory/hepatic/renal/cardiac function, alcohol withdrawal, history of seizures, urinary retention, glaucoma, prostatic hypertrophy, hypocalcemia (increases susceptibility to dystonias). **PREGNANCY/LACTATION:** Crosses placenta; distributed in breast milk. **Pregnancy Category C.**

INTERACTIONS

DRUG INTERACTIONS: Alcohol, CNS depressants may increase CNS, respiratory depression, hypotensive effects. Tricyclic antidepressants, MAO inhibitors may increase sedative, anticholinergic effects. Antithyroid agents may increase risk of agranulocytosis. Extrapyramidal symptoms (EPS) may increase w/EPS producing medications. Hypotensives may increase hypotension. May decrease levodopa effects. Lithium may decrease absorption, produce adverse neurologic effects. **ALTERED LAB VALUES:** May produce false-positive pregnancy test, phenylketonuria (PKU). EKG changes may occur, including Q and T wave disturbances.

SIDE EFFECTS

FREQUENT: Hypotension, dizziness, fainting occur frequently after parenteral form is given and occasionally thereafter but rarely w/oral dosage. **OCCASIONAL:** Marked photosensitivity. Drowsiness during early therapy, dry mouth, blurred vision, lethargy, constipation/diarrhea, nasal congestion, peripheral edema, urinary retention. **RARE:** Ocular changes, skin pigmentation (those on high doses for prolonged periods).

ADVERSE REACTIONS/TOXIC EFFECTS

Extrapyramidal symptoms appear dose related (particularly high dosage) and are divided into 3 categories: akathisia (inability to sit still, tapping of feet, urge to move around), parkinsonian symptoms (mask-like face, tremors, shuffling gait, hypersalivation), and acute dystonias: torticollis (neck muscle spasm), opisthotonos (rigidity of back muscles), and oculogyric crisis (rolling back of eyes). Dystonic reaction may also produce profuse sweating, pallor. Tardive dyskinesia (protrusion of tongue, puffing of cheeks, chewing/puckering of the mouth) occurs rarely (may be irreversible). Abrupt withdrawal following long-term therapy may precipitate nausea, vomiting, gastritis, dizziness, tremors. Blood dyscrasias, particularly agranulocytosis, mild leukopenia may occur. May lower seizure threshold.

NURSING IMPLICATIONS

BASELINE ASSESSMENT:

Avoid skin contact w/solutions (contact dermatitis). *Antiemetic:* Assess for dehydration (poor skin turgor, dry mucous membranes, longitudinal furrows in tongue). *Antipsychotic:* Assess behavior, appearance, emotional status, response to environment, speech pattern, thought content.

INTERVENTION/EVALUATION:

Monitor B/P for hypotension. Assess for extrapyramidal symptoms. Monitor WBC, differential count for blood dyscrasias. Monitor for fine tongue movement (may be early sign of tardive dyskinesia). Supervise suicidal-risk pt closely during early therapy (as depression lessens, energy level improves increasing suicide potential. Assess for therapeutic response (interest in surroundings, improvement in self-care, increased ability to concentrate, relaxed facial expression). For antiemetic use: monitor I&O and food tolerance.

PATIENT/FAMILY TEACHING:

Full therapeutic effect may take up to 6 wks. Urine may turn pink or reddish-brown. Do not abruptly withdraw from long-term drug therapy. Report visual disturbances. Sugarless gum or sips of tepid water may relieve dry mouth. Drowsiness generally subsides during continued therapy. Avoid tasks that require alertness, motor skills until response to drug is established. Avoid alcohol and CNS depressants. Wear protective clothing, sunscreens in sunlight.

phenelzine sulfate

fen´ell-zeen
(Nardil)

CANADIAN AVAILABILITY:

Nardil

CLASSIFICATION

Antidepressant: MAO inhibitor

PHARMACOKINETICS

Well absorbed from GI tract. Metabolized in liver. Primarily excreted in urine.

ACTION

Inhibits monoamine oxidase enzyme (assists in metabolism of sympathomimetic amines) at CNS storage sites. Increased levels of epinephrine, norepinephrine, serotonin, dopamine at neuron receptor sites, producing antidepressant effect.

USES

Management of atypical, nonendogenous, neurotic depression associated w/anxiety, phobic, hypochondriacal features in those not responsive to other antidepressant therapy.

PO ADMINISTRATION

Give w/food if GI distress occurs.

INDICATIONS/DOSAGE/ROUTES

Depression:
PO: Adults <60 yrs: 15 mg 3 times daily. Increase rapidly to 60 mg daily until therapeutic response noted (2-6 wks). Thereafter, reduce dose gradually to maintenance level. **Elderly:** Initially, 7.5 mg. May increase by 7.5-15 mg q3-4 days. **Maintenance:** 15-60 mg/day in 3-4 divided doses.

PRECAUTIONS

CONTRAINDICATIONS: Pts >60 yrs, debilitated/hypertensive pts, cerebrovascular/cardiovascular disease, foods containing tryptophan/tyramine, within 10 days of elective surgery, pheochromocytoma, CHF, history of liver disease, abnormal liver function tests, severe renal impairment, history of severe/recurrent headache. **CAUTIONS:** Impaired renal function, history of seizures, parkinsonian syndrome, diabetic pts, hyperthyroidism. **PREGNANCY/LACTATION:** Crosses placenta; unknown whether distributed in breast milk. **Pregnancy Category C.**

INTERACTIONS

DRUG INTERACTIONS: Alcohol, CNS depressants may increase CNS depressant effects. Tricyclic antidepressants, fluoxetine, trazodone may cause serotonin syndrome. May increase effect of oral hypoglycemics, insulin. B/P may increase w/buspirone. Caffeine containing medications may increase cardiac arrhythmias, hypertension. May precipitate hypertensive crises w/carbamazepine, cyclobenzaprine, maprotiline, other MAO inhibitors. Meperidine, other opioid analgesics may produce immediate excitation, seating, rigidity, severe hypertension or hypotension, severe respiratory distress, coma, convulsions, vascular collapse, death. May increase CNS stimulant effects of methylphenidate. Sympathomimetics may increase cardiac stimulant, vasopressor effects. Tyramine, foods w/pressor amines (e.g., aged cheese) may cause sudden, severe hypertension. **ALTERED LAB VALUES:** None significant.

SIDE EFFECTS

FREQUENT: Postural hypotension, restlessness, GI upset, insomnia, dizziness, headache, lethargy, weakness, dry mouth, peripheral edema. **OCCASIONAL:** Flushing, increased perspiration, rash, urinary frequency, increased appetite, transient impotence. **RARE:** Visual disturbances.

ADVERSE REACTIONS/TOXIC EFFECTS

Hypertensive crisis may be noted by hypertension, occipital headache radiating frontally, neck stiffness/soreness, nausea, vomiting, sweating, fever/chilliness, clammy skin, dilated pupils, palpitations. Tachycardia or bradycardia, constricting chest pain may also be present. Antidote for hypertensive crisis: 5-10 mg phentolamine IV injection.

NURSING IMPLICATIONS

BASELINE ASSESSMENT:

Periodic liver function tests should be performed in those requiring high dosage undergoing prolonged therapy. MAO inhibitor therapy should be discontinued for 7-14 days prior to elective surgery.

INTERVENTION/EVALUATION:

Assess appearance, behavior, speech pattern, level of interest, mood. Monitor for occipital headache radiating frontally and/or neck stiffness/soreness (may be first signal of impending hypertensive crisis). Monitor blood pressure diligently for hypertension. Discontinue medication immediately if palpitations or frequent headaches occur.

PATIENT/FAMILY TEACHING:

Antidepressant relief may be noted during first wk of therapy; maximum benefit noted in 2-6 wks. Report headache, neck stiffness/soreness immediately. To avoid orthostatic hypotension, change from lying to sitting position slowly and dangle legs momentarily before standing. Avoid tasks that require alertness, motor skills until response to drug is established. Avoid foods that require bacteria or molds for their preparation or preservation or those that contain tyramine, e.g., cheese, sour cream, beer, wine, pickled herring, liver, figs, raisins, bananas, avocados, soy sauce, yeast extracts, yogurt, papaya, broad beans, meat tenderizers, or excessive amounts of caffeine (coffee, tea, chocolate), or over-the-counter preparations for hay fever, colds, weight reduction. Avoid alcohol.

phenobarbital

feen-oh-bar´bih-tall
(Barbita, Sulfoton)

phenobarbital sodium

(Luminal)

FIXED-COMBINATION(S):
W/phenytoin sodium, an anticonvulsant (Dilantin w/Phenobarbital Kapseals)

CLASSIFICATION

Anticonvulsant, hypnotic

PHARMACOKINETICS

	ONSET	PEAK	DURATION
PO	20-60 min	—	—
IM	10-15 min	—	4-6 hrs
IV	5 min	30 min	4-6 hrs

Well absorbed after oral, parenteral administration. Rapidly, widely distributed. Protein binding: 20-45%. Metabolized in liver. Primarily excreted in urine. Half-life: 53-118 hrs.

ACTION

CNS depressant producing all levels from mild sedation, hypnosis to deep coma. *Anticonvulsant:* Elevates seizure threshold for motor cortex to electrical/chemical stimulation.

USES

Management of generalized tonic-clonic (grand mal) seizures, partial seizures, control of acute convulsive episodes (status epilepticus, eclampsia, febrile seizures). Relieves anxiety, provides preop sedation.

STORAGE/HANDLING

Store oral, parenteral form at room temperature. Do not use oral liquid or parenteral form if solution is cloudy or contains precipitate.

PO/IM/IV ADMINISTRATION

PO:

1. Give w/o regard to meals. Tablets may be crushed. Capsules may be emptied and mixed w/food.
2. Elixir may be mixed w/water, milk, fruit juice.

IM:

PARENTERAL FORM: Do not mix w/acidic solutions (forms precipitate). May be diluted w/normal saline, 5% dextrose, lactated Ringer's, Ringer's.

1. Do not inject more than 5 ml in any one IM injection site (produces tissue irritation).
2. Inject IM deep into gluteus maximus or lateral aspect of thigh.

IV:

1. Administer at rate not greater than 60 mg/min (too rapid IV may produce severe hypotension, marked respiratory depression).
2. Monitor vital signs q3-5min during and q15min for 1-2 hrs after administration.
3. Inadvertent intra-arterial injection may result in arterial spasm w/severe pain, tissue necrosis. Extravasation in subcutaneous tissue may produce redness, tenderness, tissue necrosis. If either occurs, treat w/injection of 0.5% procaine solution into affected area, apply moist heat.

INDICATIONS/DOSAGE/ROUTES

NOTE: When replacement by another anticonvulsant is necessary, decrease phenobarbital over 1 wk as therapy begins w/low replacement dose.

Anticonvulsant:
NOTE: Administration may be necessary for 2-3 wks before full therapeutic response is noted.
PO: Adults, elderly: 100-300 mg/day, preferably at bedtime. **Children:** 3-5 mg/kg/day.

Prevention of febrile seizures:
PO: Children: 3-4 mg/kg/day.

Status epilepticus, acute seizures:
IM/IV: Adults, elderly: 200-600 mg. **Children:** 100-400 mg. Administer until seizure stops or 20 mg/kg is reached.

Sedation:
PO: Adults, elderly: 30-120 mg daily, usually given in 2-3 divided doses. **Children:** 6 mg/kg/day in 3 divided doses.

Hypnotic:
PO/IM/IV: Adults, elderly: 100-320 mg.

Preop sedation, antianxiety:
IM: Adults, elderly: 100-200 mg. **Children:** 16-100 mg given 60-90 min before surgery.

PRECAUTIONS

CONTRAINDICATIONS: History of porphyria, bronchopneumonia. **EXTREME CAUTION:** Nephritis, renal insufficiency. **CAUTIONS:** Uncontrolled pain (may produce paradoxical reaction), impaired liver function. **PREGNANCY/LACTATION:** Readily crosses placenta; distributed in breast milk. Produces respiratory depression in neonates during labor. May cause postpartum hemorrhage, hemorrhagic disease in newborn. Withdrawal symptoms may appear in neonates born to women receiving barbiturates during last trimester of pregnancy. Lowers serum bilirubin concentration in neonates. **Pregnancy Category D.**

INTERACTIONS

DRUG INTERACTIONS: May decrease effects of glucocorticoids, digoxin, metronidazole, oral anticoagulants, quinidine, tricyclic antidepressants. Alcohol, CNS depressants may increase effect. May increase metabolism of carbamazepine. Valproic acid decreases metabolism, increases concentration, toxicity. **ALTERED LAB VALUES:** May decrease bilirubin.

SIDE EFFECTS

FREQUENT: Drowsiness, sedation, irritability, headache, restlessness, ataxia (muscular incoordination), joint aches, vertigo, anorexia, nausea, gastric distress. **OCCASIONAL:** Paradoxical CNS hyperactivity/nervousness in children, excitement/restlessness in elderly (generally noted during first 2 wks of therapy, particularly noted in presence of uncontrolled pain).

ADVERSE REACTIONS/TOXIC EFFECTS

Abrupt withdrawal after prolonged therapy may produce effects ranging from markedly increased dreaming, nightmares and/or insomnia, tremor, sweating, vomiting, to hallucinations, delirium, seizures, status epilepticus. Skin eruptions appear as hypersensitivity reaction. Blood dyscrasias, liver disease, hypocalcemia occur rarely. Overdosage produces cold, clammy skin, hypothermia, severe CNS depression, cyanosis, rapid pulse, Cheyne-Stokes respirations. Toxicity may result in severe renal impairment.

NURSING IMPLICATIONS

BASELINE ASSESSMENT:

Assess B/P, pulse, respirations immediately before administration. Liver function tests, blood counts should be performed before therapy begins and periodically during therapy. *Hypnotic:* Raise bed rails, provide environment conducive to sleep (back rub, quiet environment, low lighting). *Seizures:* Review history of seizure disorder (length, presence of auras, level of consciousness). Observe frequently for recurrence of seizure activity. Initiate seizure precautions.

INTERVENTION/EVALUATION:

Assess elderly, debilitated, children for evidence of paradoxical reaction, particularly during early therapy. Evaluate for therapeutic response: Decrease in length, number of seizures. Monitor for therapeutic serum level (10-30 mcg/ml).

PATIENT/FAMILY TEACHING:

Drowsiness may gradually decrease/disappear w/continued use. Do not abruptly withdraw medication following long-term use (may precipitate seizures). Avoid tasks that require alertness, motor skills until response to drug is established. Tolerance/dependence may occur w/prolonged use of high doses. Strict maintenance of drug therapy is essential for seizure control. Avoid alcohol and other CNS depressants. Notify physician promptly of pregnancy.

---

phenytoin

phen´ih-toy-in
(Dilantin)

phenytoin sodium

(Dilantin)

FIXED-COMBINATION(S):

W/phenobarbital, a barbiturate (Dilantin w/Phenobarbital)

CANADIAN AVAILABILITY:

Dilantin

CLASSIFICATION

Anticonvulsant

PHARMACOKINETICS

Slow, variably absorbed after oral administration; slow but complete absorption following IM administration. Widely distributed. Protein binding: >90%. Metabolized in liver. Primarily excreted in urine. Half-life: 22 hrs.

ACTION

Anticonvulsant: Stabilizes neuronal membranes, limits spread of seizure activity. Decreases sodium, calcium, ion influx in neurons. Decreases post-tetanic potentiation and repetitive after-discharge. *Antiarrhythmic:* Decreases abnormal ventricular automaticity (shortens refractory period, QT interval, action potential duration).

USES

Management of generalized tonic-clonic seizures (grand mal), complex partial seizures (psychomotor), cortical focal seizures, status epilepticus. Ineffective in absence seizures, myoclonic seizures, atonic epilepsy when used alone. Treatment of cardiac arrhythmias due to digitalis intoxication.

STORAGE/HANDLING

Store oral suspension, tablets, capsules, parenteral form at room temperature. Precipitate may form if parenteral form is refrigerated (will dissolve at room temperature). Slight yellow discoloration of parenteral form does not affect potency, but do not use if solution is not clear or if precipitate is present.

PO/IV ADMINISTRATION

PO:

1. Give w/food if GI distress occurs.
2. Do not chew/break capsules. Tablets may be chewed.
3. Shake oral suspension well before using.

IV:

NOTE: Give by direct IV injection. Do not add to IV infusion (precipitate may form).

1. Severe hypotension, cardiovascular collapse occurs if rate of IV injection exceeds 50 mg/min for adults. Administer 50 mg >2-3 min for elderly. In neonates, administer at rate not exceeding 1-3 mg/kg/min.
2. IV injection very painful (chemical irritation of vein due to alkalinity of solution). To minimize effect, flush vein w/sterile saline solution through same IV needle/catheter following each IV injection.
3. IV toxicity characterized by CNS depression, cardiovascular collapse.

INDICATIONS/DOSAGE/ROUTES

NOTE: Pts who are stabilized on 100 mg 3 times daily may receive 300 mg once daily w/extended release medication. When replacement by another anticonvulsant is necessary, phenytoin should be decreased over 1 wk as therapy is begun w/low dose of replacement drug.

Seizure control:

PO: Adults, elderly: Initially, 100 mg 3 times daily. May be increased in 100 mg increments q2-4wks until therapeutic response achieved. **Usual dose range:** 300-400 mg daily. **Maximum daily dose:** 600 mg daily (300 mg for extended release). **Children:** Initially, 5 mg/kg daily in 2-3 equally divided doses. **Usual maintenance dose:** 4-8 mg/kg. **Maximum daily dose:** 300 mg daily.

Status epilepticus:

IV: Adults, elderly: 150-250 mg, then 100-150 mg in 30 min, if needed. **Children:** 250 mg/m^2.

Arrhythmias:

IV: Adults, elderly: 100 mg at 5 min intervals until arrhythmias disappear or undesirable effects occur.

Management of arrhythmias:

PO: Adults, elderly: 100 mg 2-4 times daily.

PRECAUTIONS

CONTRAINDICATIONS: Seizures due to hypoglycemia, hydantoin hypersensitivity. *IV route only:* Sinus bradycardia, sinoatrial block, second- and third-degree heart block, Adam-Stokes syndrome. **EXTREME CAUTION:** *IV route only:* Respiratory depression, myocardial infarction, CHF, damaged myocardium. **CAUTIONS:** Impaired hepatic/renal function, severe myocardial insufficiency, hypotension, hyperglycemia. **PREGNANCY/LACTATION:** Crosses placenta; is distributed in small amount in breast milk. Fetal hydantoin syndrome (craniofacial abnormalities, nail/digital hypoplasia, prenatal growth deficiency) has been reported. There is increased frequency of seizures in pregnant women due to altered absorption of metabolism of phenytoin. May increase risk of hemorrhage in neonate, maternal bleeding during delivery. **Pregnancy Category D.**

INTERACTIONS

DRUG INTERACTIONS: May decrease effect of glucocorticoids. Alcohol, CNS depressants may increase CNS depression. Antacids may decrease absorption. Amiodarone, anticoagulants, cimetidine, disulfiram, isoniazid, sulfonamides may increase concentration, effects, toxicity. Fluconazole, ketoconazole, miconazole may increase concentration. Lidocaine, propranolol may increase cardiac depressant effects. Valproic acid may increase concentration, decrease metabolism. May increase xanthine metabolism. **ALTERED LAB VALUES:** May increase alkaline phosphatase, GGT, glucose.

SIDE EFFECTS

Effects are dose related and generally occur w/larger doses. **FREQUENT:** Drowsiness, lethargy, irritability, headache, restlessness, joint aches, vertigo, anorexia, nausea, gastric distress, gingival hyperplasia (w/prolonged therapy). **OCCASIONAL:** Morbilliform rash, hypertrichosis (hair growth).

ADVERSE REACTIONS/TOXIC EFFECTS

Abrupt withdrawal may precipitate status epilepticus. Blood dyscrasias, lymphadenopathy, osteomalacia (due to interference of vitamin D metabolism) may occur. Phenytoin blood concentration of 25 mcg/ml (toxic) may produce ataxia (muscular incoordination), nystagmus (rhythmic oscillation of eyes), double vision. As level increases, extreme lethargy to comatose states occur.

NURSING IMPLICATIONS

BASELINE ASSESSMENT:

Anticonvulsant: Review history of seizure disorder (intensity, frequency, duration, level of consciousness). Initiate seizure precautions. Liver function tests, CBC, platelet count should be performed before therapy begins and periodically during therapy. Repeat CBC, platelet count 2 wks after therapy begins, and 2 wks after maintenance dose is given.

INTERVENTION/EVALUATION:

Observe frequently for recurrence of seizure activity. Assess for clinical improvement (decrease in intensity/frequency of seizures). Monitor EKG for cardiac arrhythmias. Assess B/P, EKG diligently w/IV administration. Assist w/ambulation if drowsiness, lethargy, vertigo occurs. Monitor for therapeutic serum level (10-20 mcg/ml).

PATIENT/FAMILY TEACHING:

Pain may occur w/IV injection. To prevent gingival hyperplasia (bleeding, tenderness, swelling of gums) encourage good oral hygiene care, gum massage, regular dental visits. CBC should be performed every month for 1 yr after maintenance dose is established and q3mo thereafter. Urine may appear pink, red, or red-brown. Report sore throat, fever, glandular swelling, skin reaction (hematologic toxicity). Drowsiness usually diminishes w/continued therapy. Do not abruptly withdraw medication following long-term use (may precipitate seizures). Strict maintenance of drug therapy is essential for seizure control, arrhythmias. Avoid tasks that require alertness, motor skills until response to drug is established. Avoid alcohol.

pimozide

pim´oh-zied
(Orap)

CANADIAN AVAILABILITY:

Orap

CLASSIFICATION

Antipsychotic

PHARMACOKINETICS

Poorly absorbed from GI tract. Undergoes first-pass effect. Widely distributed. Metabolized in liver to active metabolite. Primarily excreted in urine. Half-life: 55 hrs.

ACTION

Inhibits dopamine receptors in CNS, interrupting impulse movement. Produces strong extrapyramidal, moderate anticholinergic, sedative effects.

USES

Suppression of severely compromising motor and phonic tics in those w/Tourette's disorders who have failed to respond adequately to standard treatment.

PO ADMINISTRATION

May give w/o regard to meals.

INDICATIONS/DOSAGE/ROUTES

Tourette's disorder:
PO: Adults: Initially, 1-2 mg/day in divided doses. Increase every other day. **Maintenance:** <0.2 mg/kg/day or 10 mg/day, whichever is less. **Maximum:** 0.2 mg/kg/day or 10 mg/day.

PRECAUTIONS

CONTRAINDICATIONS: Congenital QT syndrome, history of cardiac arrhythmias, administration w/other drugs that prolong QT interval, severe toxic CNS depression, comatose states. **CAUTIONS:** History of seizures, cardiovascular disease, impaired respiratory, hepatic/renal function, alcohol withdrawal, urinary retention, glaucoma, prostatic hypertrophy. **PREGNANCY/LACTATION:** Unknown whether drug crosses placenta or is distributed in breast milk. **Pregnancy Category C.**

INTERACTIONS

DRUG INTERACTIONS: Alcohol, CNS depressants may increase CNS depressant effect. Methylphenidate, pemoline may mask signs of tics. Anticholinergics may increase anticholinergic effects. Tricyclic antidepressants, phenothiazines, quinidine may increase risk of cardiac arrhythmias. Extrapyramidal symptom producing medications (EPS) may increase anticholinergic, CNS depressant, and EPS effects. **ALTERED LAB VALUES:** None significant.

SIDE EFFECTS

FREQUENT: Drowsiness, salivation, constipation, dizziness, tachycardia. **OCCASIONAL:** Nausea, sweating, dry mouth, headache, hypotension, GI upset, weight gain. **RARE:** Visual disturbances, diarrhea, rash, urinary abnormalities.

ADVERSE REACTIONS/TOXIC EFFECTS

Extrapyramidal reactions occur frequently but are usually mild and reversible (generally noted during first few days of therapy). Motor restlessness, dystonia, hyperreflexia occur much less frequently. Persistent tardive dyskinesia has occurred. Those on long-term maintenance may experience transient dyskinetic signs following abrupt withdrawal.

NURSING IMPLICATIONS

BASELINE ASSESSMENT:

Obtain baseline EKG. Potassium level should be checked and corrected if necessary.

INTERVENTION/EVALUATION:

EKG should be periodically monitored. Assess for extrapyramidal symptoms. Monitor WBC, differential count for blood dyscrasias. Monitor for fine tongue movement (may be early sign of tardive dyskinesia). Assess for therapeutic response (decreased tic activity).

PATIENT/FAMILY TEACHING:

Do not exceed prescribed dose. Do not abruptly withdraw from long-term drug therapy. Report visual disturbances. Drowsiness generally subsides during continued therapy. Avoid tasks that require alertness, motor skills until response to drug is established. Avoid alcohol and CNS depressants.

primidone

pri´mih-doan
(Mysoline)

CANADIAN AVAILABILITY:

Apo-Primidone, Mysoline, Sertan

CLASSIFICATION

Anticonvulsant

PHARMACOKINETICS

Rapid, completely absorbed from GI tract. Widely distributed. Protein binding: 0-20%. Metabolized in liver to active metabolite (phenobarbital). Primarily excreted in urine. Half-life: 3-23 hrs; metabolite: 75-126 hrs.

ACTION

Elevates seizure threshold for motor cortex to electrical/chemical stimulation.

USES

Management of partial seizures w/complex symptomatology (psychomotor seizures), generalized tonic-clonic (grand mal) seizures.

PO ADMINISTRATION

1. Give w/o regard to meals.
2. Shake oral suspension well before administering (may be mixed w/food).
3. Tablets may be crushed.

INDICATIONS/DOSAGE/ROUTES

NOTE: When replacement by another anticonvulsant is necessary, decrease primidone gradually as therapy begins w/low replacement dose.

Anticonvulsant:

PO: Adults, elderly, children >8 yrs: 100-125 mg daily for 3 days at bedtime, then 100-125 mg 2 times/day for days 4-6, then 100-125 mg 3 times/day for days 7-9, then maintenance of 250 mg 3 times/day. **Children <8 yrs:** 50 mg at bedtime for 3 days, then 50 mg 2 times/day for days 4-6, then 100 mg 2 times/day for days 7-9, then maintenance of 125-250 mg 3 times/day.

PRECAUTIONS

CONTRAINDICATIONS: History of porphyria, bronchopneumonia. **EXTREME CAUTION:** Nephritis, renal insufficiency. **CAUTIONS:** Uncontrolled pain (may produce paradoxical reaction), impaired liver function. **PREGNANCY/LACTATION:** Readily crosses placenta; is distributed in breast milk in substantial quantities. Produces respiratory depression in the neonate during labor. May cause postpartum hemorrhage, hemorrhagic disease in newborn. Withdrawal symptoms may occur in neonates born to women who receive barbiturates during last trimester of pregnancy. Lowers serum bilirubin concentrations in neonates. **Pregnancy Category D.**

INTERACTIONS

DRUG INTERACTIONS: May decrease effects of glucocorticoids, digoxin, metronidazole, oral anticoagulants, quinidine, tricyclic antidepressants. Alcohol, CNS depressants may increase effect. May increase metabolism of carbamazepine. Valproic acid decreases metabolism, increases concentration, toxicity. **ALTERED LAB VALUES:** May decrease bilirubin.

SIDE EFFECTS

FREQUENT: Drowsiness, sedation, muscular incoordination. **OCCASIONAL:** Irritability, headache, restlessness, dizziness, ataxia (muscular incoordination), joint aches, vertigo, mood changes, anorexia, nausea, gastric distress.

ADVERSE REACTIONS/TOXIC EFFECTS

Abrupt withdrawal after prolonged therapy may produce effects ranging from markedly increased dreaming, nightmares and/or insomnia, tremor, sweating, vomiting, to hallucinations, delirium, seizures, status epilepticus. Skin eruptions may appear as hypersensitivity reaction. Blood dyscrasias, liver disease, hypocalcemia occur rarely. Overdosage produces cold, clammy skin, hypothermia, severe CNS depression followed by high fever, coma.

NURSING IMPLICATIONS

BASELINE ASSESSMENT:

Review history of seizure disorder (intensity, frequency, duration, level of consciousness). Observe frequently for recurrence of seizure activity. Initiate seizure precautions.

INTERVENTION/EVALUATION:

For those on long-term therapy, liver/renal function tests, blood counts should be performed periodically. Assist w/ ambulation if dizziness, ataxia occur. Assess children, elderly for paradoxical reaction (particularly during early therapy). Assess for clinical improvement (decrease in intensity/frequency of seizures). Monitor for therapeutic serum level (5-12 mcg/ml).

PATIENT/FAMILY TEACHING:

Do not abruptly withdraw medication following long-term use (may precipitate seizures). Strict maintenance of drug therapy is essential for seizure control. Drowsiness usually disappears during continued therapy. If dizziness occurs, change positions slowly from recumbent to sitting position before standing. Avoid tasks that require alertness, motor skills until response to drug is established. Avoid alcohol.

protriptyline hydrochloride

pro-trip´teh-leen
(Vivactil)

CANADIAN AVAILABILITY:

Triptil

CLASSIFICATION

Antidepressant: Tricyclic

PHARMACOKINETICS

Well absorbed from GI tract. Widely distributed. Protein binding: 92%. Metabolized in liver (undergoes first-pass effect). Primarily excreted in urine. Half-life: 67-89 hrs.

ACTION

Increases synaptic concentration of norepinephrine and/or serotonin (inhibits reuptake by presynaptic membrane).

USES

Treatment of various forms of depression, often in conjunction w/psychotherapy.

PO ADMINISTRATION

1. Give w/food or milk if GI distress occurs.
2. Do not break or chew tablets.

INDICATIONS/DOSAGE/ROUTES

Depression:
PO: Adults: Initially, 15-40 mg daily, given in 1-4 divided doses. Increase dosage gradually to 60 mg daily, then reduce dosage to lowest effective maintenance level. **Adolescents:** Initially, 5 mg 3 times daily.

Usual elderly dosage:
PO: Elderly: Initially, 5-10 mg/day. May increase by 5-10 mg/day q3-7days. **Maintenance:** 10-20 mg/day.

PRECAUTIONS

CONTRAINDICATIONS: Acute recovery period following MI, within 14 days of MAO inhibitor therapy. **CAUTIONS:** Prostatic hypertrophy, history of urinary retention/obstruction, glaucoma, diabetes mellitis, history of seizures, hyperthyroidism, cardiac/hepatic/renal disease, schizophrenia, increased intraocular pressure, hiatal hernia. **PREGNANCY/LACTATION:** Crosses placenta; is distributed in breast milk. **Pregnancy Category C.**

INTERACTIONS

DRUG INTERACTIONS: Alcohol, CNS depressants may increase CNS, respiratory depression, hypotensive effects. Antithyroid agents may increase risk of agranulocytosis. Phenothiazines may increase sedative, anticholinergic effects. Cimetidine may increase concentration, toxicity. May decrease effects of clonidine, guanadrel. May increase cardiac effects w/sympathomimetics. May increase risk of hypertensive crisis, hyperpyretic convulsions w/MAO inhibitors. **ALTERED LAB VALUES:** May alter EKG readings, glucose.

SIDE EFFECTS

FREQUENT: Drowsiness, fatigue, dry mouth, blurred vision, constipation, delayed micturition, postural hypotension, excessive sweating, disturbed concentration, increased appetite, urinary retention. **OCCASIONAL:** GI disturbances (nausea, GI distress, metallic taste sensation). **RARE:** Paradoxical reaction (agitation, restlessness, nightmares, insomnia), extrapyramidal symptoms (particularly fine hand tremor).

ADVERSE REACTIONS/TOXIC EFFECTS

High dosage may produce cardiovascular effects (severe postural hypotension, dizziness, tachycardia, palpitations, arrhythmias) and seizures. May also result in altered temperature regulation (hyperpyrexia/hypothermia). Abrupt withdrawal from prolonged therapy may produce headache, malaise, nausea, vomiting, vivid dreams.

NURSING IMPLICATIONS

BASELINE ASSESSMENT:

For those on long-term therapy, liver/renal function tests, blood counts should be performed periodically.

INTERVENTION/EVALUATION:

Supervise suicidal-risk patient closely during early therapy (as depression lessens, energy level improves, increasing suicide potential). Assess appearance, behavior, speech pattern, level of interest, mood. Monitor stools; avoid constipation. Monitor B/P, pulse for hypotension, arrhythmias. Closely monitor for cardiac disturbances in elderly pts receiving more than 20 mg daily. Assess for urinary retention by bladder palpation.

PATIENT/FAMILY TEACHING:

Change positions slowly to avoid hypotensive effect. Tolerance to postural hypotension, sedative and anticholinergic effects usually develops during early therapy. Therapeutic effect may be noted within 2-5 days, maximum effect within 2-3 weeks. Photosensitivity to sun may occur; use sunscreens, wear protective clothing. Dry mouth may be relieved by sugarless gum, sips of tepid water. Report visual disturbances. Do not abruptly discontinue medication. Avoid tasks that require alertness, motor skills until response to drug is established. Avoid alcohol and other CNS depressants.

quazepam

quay´zah-pam
(Doral)

CLASSIFICATION

Sedative-hypnotic **(Schedule IV)**

PHARMACOKINETICS

Well absorbed from GI tract. Widely distributed. Protein binding: >95%. Metabolized in liver to active metabolite. Primarily excreted in urine. Half-life: 39 hrs.

ACTION

Enhances action of inhibitory neurotransmitter gamma-aminobutyric acid (GABA). Depressant effects occur at all levels of CNS.

USES

Short-term treatment of insomnia (up to 4 wks). Reduces sleep-induction time, number of nocturnal awakenings; increases length of sleep.

PO ADMINISTRATION

Give w/o regard to meals.

INDICATIONS/DOSAGE/ROUTES

Hypnotic:
PO: Adults: 15 mg at bedtime until pt responds; then decrease to 7.5 mg in some pts. **Elderly/debilitated/liver disease/low serum albumin:** 7.5-15 mg at bedtime, attempt to decrease dose after 2 nights.

PRECAUTIONS

CONTRAINDICATIONS: Acute narrow-angle glaucoma, acute alcohol intoxication. **CAUTIONS:** Impaired renal/hepatic function. **PREGNANCY/LACTATION:** Crosses placenta; may be distributed in breast milk. Chronic ingestion during pregnancy may produce withdrawal symptoms, CNS depression in neonates. **Pregnancy Category X.**

INTERACTIONS

DRUG INTERACTIONS: Alcohol, CNS depressants may increase CNS depressant effect. **ALTERED LAB VALUES:** None significant.

SIDE EFFECTS

FREQUENT: Drowsiness, dizziness, ataxia, sedation. Morning drowsiness may occur initially. **OCCASIONAL:** GI disturbances, nervousness, blurred vision, dry mouth, headache, confusion, skin rash, irritability, slurred speech. **RARE:** Paradoxical CNS excitement/restlessness (particularly noted in elderly/debilitated).

ADVERSE REACTIONS/TOXIC EFFECTS

Abrupt or too-rapid withdrawal may result in pronounced restlessness and irritability, insomnia, hand tremors, abdominal/muscle cramps, sweating, vomiting, seizures. Overdosage results in somnolence, confusion, diminished reflexes, coma.

NURSING IMPLICATIONS

BASELINE ASSESSMENT:

Provide environment conducive to sleep (back rub, quiet environment, low lighting). Provide protective measures, e.g., raise bed rails, place call light within easy reach.

INTERVENTION/EVALUATION:

Evaluate for therapeutic response (a decrease in number of nocturnal awakenings, increase in length of sleep duration time). Assess for paradoxical reaction, esp. during early therapy and in elderly, debilitated. Provide assistance w/ambulation, including daytime if drowsiness continues.

PATIENT/FAMILY TEACHING:

Smoking reduces drug effectiveness, increases risk of fire by falling asleep w/lighted cigarette. Do not take alcohol or other CNS depressants w/this drug. Notify physician promptly of pregnancy. Do not abruptly withdraw medication following long-term use.

risperidone

ris-pear'ih-doan
(Risperdal)

CLASSIFICATION

Antipsychotic

PHARMACOKINETICS

Well absorbed from GI tract (unaffected by food). Extensively metabolized in liver to active metabolite. Protein binding: 90% (metabolite: 77%). Primarily excreted in urine. Half-life: 3-20 hrs; metabolite: 21-30 hrs (increased in elderly).

ACTION

Exact mechanism unknown. Action may be due to dopamine and serotonin receptor antagonism.

USES

Management of manifestations of psychotic disorders.

PO ADMINISTRATION

May take w/o regard to food.

INDICATIONS/DOSAGE/ROUTES

Antipsychotic:

PO: Adults: Initially, 1 mg 2 times/day for 1 day; then, 2 mg 2 times/day for 1 day; then, 3 mg 2 times/day for 1 day. Further adjustments of 1 mg 2 times/day made at at least 1 wk intervals. Maximum effect in range of 4-6 mg/day. **Elderly, debilitated, pts w/severe liver, renal impairment, risk of hypotension:** Initially, 0.5 mg 2 times/day for 1 day; then, 1 mg 2 times/day for 1 day; then, 1.5 mg 2 times/day for 1 day. Further adjustments made at at least 1 wk intervals.

PRECAUTIONS

CONTRAINDICATIONS: Hypersensitivity to risperidone. **CAUTIONS:** Cardiac pts (e.g., history of MI, ischemia, CHF, conduction abnormality); pts w/cerebrovascular disease, dehydration, hypovolemia, use of antihypertensives. History of seizures. Safety in children unknown. May mask signs of drug overdose, intestinal obstruction. **PREGNANCY/LACTATION:** Unknown whether drug crosses placenta or is excreted in breast milk. Recommend against breast feeding. **Pregnancy Category C.**

INTERACTIONS

DRUG INTERACTIONS: May decrease effects of levodopa, dopamine agonists. Carbamazepine may decrease concentration. Clozapine may increase concentration. **ALTERED LAB VALUES:** May increase creatine phosphokinase, uric acid, triglycerides, SGOT (AST), SGPT (ALT), prolactin. May decrease potassium, sodium, protein, glucose. May cause ECG changes.

SIDE EFFECTS

FREQUENT: Extrapyramidal symptoms (EPS), insomnia, agitation, anxiety, stuffy nose. **OCCASIONAL:** Somnolence, constipation, nausea, dyspepsia, vomiting. **RARE:** Abdominal pain.

ADVERSE REACTIONS/TOXIC EFFECTS

Neuroleptic malignant syndrome (NMS): hyperpyrexia, muscle rigidity, change in mental-status, irregular pulse, B/P, tachycardia, diaphoresis, cardiac dysrhythmias, elevated creatine phosphokinase, rhabdomyolysis, acute renal failure. Tardive dyskinesia: irreversible, involuntary, dyskinetic movements. Extension of action: drowsiness, sedation, tachycardia, hypotension, EPS.

NURSING IMPLICATIONS

BASELINE ASSESSMENT:

Renal and liver function tests should be done before therapy. Assess behavior, appearance, emotional status, response to environment, speech pattern, thought content.

INTERVENTION/EVALUATION:

Monitor for fine tongue movement (may be first sign of tardive dyskinesia, which may be irreversible: protrusion of tongue, puffing of cheeks, chewing/puckering of the mouth). Supervise suicidal risk pt closely during early therapy (as depression lessens, energy level improves, increasing suicide potential). Smallest prescription possible reduces risk of overdose. Assess for therapeutic response (greater interest in surroundings, improved self-care, increased ability to concentrate, relaxed facial expression). Monitor for potential NMS: fever, muscle rigidity, irregular B/P or pulse, altered mental status. Possible antiemetic effect may mask signs and symptoms of other conditions.

PATIENT/FAMILY TEACHING:

Change positions slowly to prevent hypotensive effect. Wear protective clothing, use sunscreens to protect from sunlight, ultraviolet light. Do not drive or perform tasks requiring alert response until assured that drug does not cause impairment. Consult physician before taking any other medications. Inform physician if become or plan to become pregnant; do not breast-feed.

secobarbital sodium

seek-oh-bar´bih-tall
(Seconal)

FIXED-COMBINATION(S):

W/amobarbital, a barbiturate (Tuinal)

CANADIAN AVAILABILITY:
Novosecobarb, Seconal

CLASSIFICATION

Sedative-hypnotic **(Schedule II)**

PHARMACOKINETICS

	ONSET	PEAK	DURATION
PO	15 min	—	1-4 hrs
IM	7-10 min	—	—
IV	1-3 min	—	15 min
Rectal	15-30 min	—	1-4 hrs

Variably absorbed after oral, parenteral administration. Rapidly, widely distributed. Protein binding: 46-70%. Metabolized in liver. Primarily excreted in urine. Half-life: 15-40 hrs.

ACTION

CNS depressant, producing all levels from mild sedation, hypnosis to deep coma.

USES

Short-term treatment of insomnia (up to 2 wks), preop sedation, routine sedation. Parenteral form used to control status epilepticus/acute seizure episodes, to facilitate intubation procedures, control of agitated behavior in psychosis, provide hypnosis for general, spinal, regional anesthesia. Used rectally to produce anesthesia in children.

STORAGE/HANDLING

Store oral form at room temperature. Refrigerate parenteral form, suppositories. Discard parenteral solution if precipitate forms or solution becomes cloudy.

PO/IM/IV/RECTAL ADMINISTRATION

PO:

1. Best absorbed if given on empty stomach, but may be given w/food.
2. Capsules may be emptied and mixed w/food.

PARENTERAL FORM:

1. Do not mix w/acidic solutions (produces precipitate).

IM:

1. May be diluted w/sterile water for injection, 0.9% NaCl, Ringer's injection. Do NOT use lactated Ringer's injection.
2. Do not inject more than 5 ml in any one IM injection site (produces tissue irritation).
3. Inject IM deep into gluteus maximus or lateral aspect of thigh.

IV:

1. Administer IV at rate not greater than 50 mg/15 seconds (1 ml of 5% concentration).
2. A too-rapid IV may produce marked respiratory depression, severe hypotension, apnea, laryngospasm, bronchospasm.
3. Monitor vital signs q3-5min during and q15min for 1-2 hrs after administration.
4. Inadvertent intra-arterial injection may result in arterial spasm w/severe pain, tissue necrosis. Extravasation in SubQ tissue may produce redness, tenderness, tissue necrosis. If either occurs, treat w/injection of 0.5% procaine solution into affected area, apply moist heat.

RECTAL:

1. Moisten suppository w/cold water before inserting well up into rectum.

INDICATIONS/DOSAGE ROUTES

NOTE: Reduce dosage in elderly, debilitated, impaired liver function.

Hypnotic:
PO/IM: Adults, elderly: 100-200 mg.
IM: Children: 3-5 mg/kg. **Maximum:** 100 mg.

Preop sedation:
PO: Adults, elderly: 100-300 mg given 1-2 hrs before surgery. **Children:** 50-100 mg.
IM: Children: 4-5 mg/kg.
RECTAL: Children over 3 yrs: 60-120 mg. **Children 6 mo-3 yrs:** 60 mg. **Children <6 mo:** 30-60 mg.

Status epilepticus:
IM/IV: Adults, elderly: 250-350 mg. If no response in 5 min, additional dose may be administered. Do not exceed total IV dosage of 500 mg.

Acute seizures:
IM/IV: Adults, elderly: 5.5 mg/kg. May repeat q3-4h as needed.

PRECAUTIONS

CONTRAINDICATIONS: History of porphyria, bronchopneumonia. **CAUTIONS:** Uncontrolled pain (may produce paradoxical reaction), impaired liver function. **PREGNANCY/LACTATION:** Readily crosses placenta; is distributed in breast milk. Produces respiratory depression in neonates during labor. May cause postpartum hemorrhage, hemorrhagic disease in newborn. Withdrawal symptoms may occur in neonates born to women who receive barbiturates during last trimester of pregnancy. **Pregnancy Category D.**

INTERACTIONS

DRUG INTERACTIONS: May decrease effects of glucocorticoids, digoxin, metronidazole, oral anticoagulants, quinidine, tricyclic antidepressants. Alcohol, CNS depressants may increase effect. May increase metabolism of carbamazepine. Valproic acid may decrease metabolism, increase concentration, toxicity. **ALTERED LAB VALUES:** May decrease bilirubin.

SIDE EFFECTS

FREQUENT: Drowsiness, sedation, residual "hangover" effect, lethargy, irritability, nausea, anorexia, muscle aches and pains, gastric distress. **OCCASIONAL:** Paradoxical CNS hyperactivity/nervousness in children, excitement/restlessness in elderly (generally noted during first 2 wks of therapy, particularly noted in presence of uncontrolled pain).

ADVERSE REACTIONS/TOXIC EFFECTS

Abrupt withdrawal after prolonged therapy may produce effects ranging from markedly increased dreaming, nightmares and/or insomnia, tremor, sweating, vomiting, to hallucinations, delirium, seizures, status epilepticus. Skin eruptions appear as hypersensitivity reaction. Blood dyscrasias, liver disease, hypocalcemia occur rarely. Overdosage produces cold, clammy skin, hypothermia, severe CNS depression, cyanosis, rapid pulse, Cheyne-Stokes respirations. Toxicity may result in severe renal impairment.

NURSING IMPLICATIONS

BASELINE ASSESSMENT:

Assess B/P, pulse, respirations immediately before administration. *Hypnotic:* Raise bed rails, provide environment conducive to sleep (back rub, quiet environment, low lighting). *Seizures:* Review history of seizure disorder (length, intensity, frequency, duration, level of consciousness). Observe frequently for recurrence of seizure activity. Initiate seizure precautions.

INTERVENTION/EVALUATION:

Assess sleep pattern of pt. Assess elderly/debilitated for paradoxical reaction, particularly during early therapy. Evaluate for therapeutic response. *Insomnia:* A decrease in number of nocturnal awakenings, increase in length of sleep duration time. *Seizures:* A decrease in number, frequency of seizures.

PATIENT/FAMILY TEACHING:

Drowsiness usually diminishes w/continued therapy. Do not abruptly withdraw medication following long-term therapy (may precipitate seizures). Avoid tasks that require alertness, motor skills until response to drug is established. Tolerance/dependence may occur w/prolonged use of high doses. Strict maintenance of drug therapy is essential for seizure control. Avoid alcohol.

selegiline hydrochloride

sell-eh´geh-leen
(Eldepryl)

CANADIAN AVAILABILITY:

Deprenyl, Eldepryl

CLASSIFICATION

Antiparkinson

PHARMACOKINETICS

Rapidly absorbed from GI tract. Crosses blood-brain barrier. Metabolized in liver to active metabolites. Primarily excreted in urine. Half-life: 16-69 hrs.

ACTION

Irreversibly inhibits monoamine oxidase type B activity. Increases dopaminergic action, assisting in reduction in tremor, akinesia (absence of sense of movement), posture and equilibrium disorders, rigidity of parkinsonism.

USES

Adjunctive to levodopa/carbidopa in treatment of Parkinson's disease.

PO ADMINISTRATION

May be given w/meals.

INDICATIONS/DOSAGE/ROUTES

NOTE: Therapy should begin w/lowest dosage, then be increased in gradual increments over 3-4 weeks.

Parkinsonism:
PO: Adults: 10 mg/day in divided doses (5 mg at breakfast and lunch). **Elderly:** Initially, 5 mg in morning. May increase up to 10 mg/day.

PRECAUTIONS

CONTRAINDICATIONS: None significant. **CAUTIONS:** Cardiac dysrhythmias. **PREGNANCY/LACTATION:** Unknown whether drug crosses placenta or is distributed in breast milk. **Pregnancy Category C.**

INTERACTIONS

DRUG INTERACTIONS: Fluoxetine may cause mania, serotonin syndrome (mental changes, restlessness, diaphoresis, diarrhea, fever). Meperidine may cause a potentially fatal reaction (e.g., excitation, sweating, rigidity, hypertension or hypotension, coma and death). Tyramine rich foods may produce hypertensive reactions. **ALTERED LAB VALUES:** None significant.

SIDE EFFECTS

FREQUENT: Nausea, dizziness, lightheadedness, faintness, abdominal discomfort. **OCCASIONAL:** Confusion, hallucinations, dry mouth, vivid dreams, dyskinesia (impairment of voluntary movement). **RARE:** Headache, generalized aches.

ADVERSE REACTIONS/TOXIC EFFECTS

Overdosage may vary from CNS depression (sedation, apnea, cardiovascular collapse, death) to severe paradoxical reaction (hallucinations, tremor, seizures). Impaired motor coordination (loss of balance, blepharospasm [eye blinking], facial grimace, feeling of heavy leg/stiff neck, involuntary movements), hallucinations, confusion, depression, nightmares, delusions, overstimulation, sleep disturbance, anger occurs in some pts.

NURSING IMPLICATIONS

INTERVENTION/EVALUATION:

Be alert to neurologic effects (headache, lethargy, mental confusion, agitation). Monitor for evidence of dyskinesia (difficulty w/movement). Assess for clinical reversal of symptoms (improvement of tremor of head/hands at rest, mask-like facial expression, shuffling gait, muscular rigidity.

PATIENT/FAMILY TEACHING:

Tolerance to feeling of lightheadedness develops during therapy. To reduce hypotensive effect, rise slowly from lying to sitting position and permit legs to dangle momentarily before standing. Avoid tasks that require alertness, motor skills until response to drug is established. Dry mouth, drowsiness, dizziness may be an expected response of drug. Avoid alcoholic beverages during therapy. Coffee/tea may help reduce drowsiness. Inform other physicians, dentist of Eldepryl therapy.

sertraline hydrochloride

sir´trah-leen
(Zoloft)

CLASSIFICATION

Antidepressant

PHARMACOKINETICS

Incompletely, slowly absorbed from GI tract (food increases absorption). Widely distributed. Protein binding: 87%. Undergoes extensive first-pass metabolism in liver to active compound. Excreted in urine, eliminated in feces. Half-life: 26 hrs.

ACTION

Blocks reuptake of neurotransmitter, serotonin at CNS neuronal presynaptic membranes, increasing availability at postsynaptic receptor sites.

USES

Treatment of major depressive disorders.

PO ADMINISTRATION

Give w/food or milk if GI distress occurs.

INDICATIONS/DOSAGE/ROUTES

Antidepressant:
PO: Adults: Initially, 50 mg/day w/morning or evening meal. May increase at intervals no sooner than 1 wk. **Elderly:** Initially, 25 mg/day. May increase by 25 mg q2-3days. **Maximum:** 200 mg/day.

PRECAUTIONS

CONTRAINDICATIONS: During or within 14 days of MAO inhibitor antidepressant therapy. **CAUTIONS:** Severe hepatic/renal impairment. **PREGNANCY/LACTATION:** Unknown whether drug crosses placenta or is distributed in breast milk. **Pregnancy Category B.**

INTERACTIONS

DRUG INTERACTIONS: May increase concentration, toxicity of highly protein bound medications (e.g., digoxin, warfarin). MAO inhibitors may cause serotonin syndrome (mental changes, restlessness, diaphoresis, shivering, diarrhea, fever), confusion, agitation, hyperpyretic convulsions. **ALTERED LAB VALUES:** May increase SGOT (AST), SGPT (ALT), total cholesterol, triglycerides. May decrease uric acid.

SIDE EFFECTS

FREQUENT: Nausea, headache, diarrhea, insomnia, dry mouth, sexual dysfunction (male), dizziness, tremor, fatigue. **OCCASIONAL:** Increased sweating, constipation, dyspepsia, agitation, flatulence, anorexia, nervousness, rhinitis, abnormal vision. **RARE:** Palpitations, paresthesia, rash, vomiting, frequent urination, twitching.

ADVERSE REACTIONS/TOXIC EFFECTS

None significant.

NURSING IMPLICATIONS

BASELINE ASSESSMENT:

For those on long-term therapy, liver/renal function tests, blood counts should be performed periodically.

INTERVENTION/EVALUATION:

Supervise suicidal-risk pt closely during early therapy (as depression lessens, energy level improves, increasing suicide potential. Assess appearance, behavior, speech pattern, level of interest, mood. Monitor pattern of daily bowel activity, stool consistency. Assist w/ambulation if dizziness occurs.

PATIENT/FAMILY TEACHING:

Dry mouth may be relieved by sugarless gum or sips of tepid water. Report headache, fatigue, tremor, sexual dysfunction. Avoid tasks that require alertness, motor skills until response to drug is established. Take w/food if nausea occurs. Inform physician if become pregnant. Avoid alcohol. Do not take over-the-counter medications w/o consulting physician.

---

temazepam

tem-az´eh-pam
(Restoril)

CANADIAN AVAILABILITY:

Restoril

CLASSIFICATION

Sedative-hypnotics

PHARMACOKINETICS

Well absorbed from GI tract. Widely distributed. Crosses blood-brain barrier. Protein binding: 96%. Metabolized in liver. Primarily excreted in urine. Half-life: 8-15 hrs.

ACTION

Enhances action of inhibitory neurotransmitter gamma-aminobutyric acid (GABA). Depressant effects occur at all levels of CNS.

USES

Short-term treatment of insomnia (up to 5 wks). Reduces sleep-induction time, number of nocturnal awakenings; increases length of sleep.

PO ADMINISTRATION

1. Give w/o regard to meals.
2. Capsules may be emptied and mixed w/food.

INDICATIONS/DOSAGE/ROUTES

Hypnotic:
PO: Adults >18 yrs: 15-30 mg at bedtime. **Elderly/debilitated:** 15 mg at bedtime.

PRECAUTIONS

CONTRAINDICATIONS: Acute narrow-angle glaucoma, acute alcohol intoxication. **CAUTIONS:** Impaired renal/hepatic function. **PREGNANCY/LACTATION:** Crosses placenta; may be distributed in breast milk. Chronic ingestion during pregnancy may produce withdrawal symptoms, CNS depression in neonates. **Pregnancy Category X.**

INTERACTIONS

DRUG INTERACTIONS: Alcohol, CNS depressants may increase CNS depressant effect. **ALTERED LAB VALUES:** None significant.

SIDE EFFECTS

FREQUENT: Drowsiness, sedation, rebound insomnia (may occur for 1-2 nights after drug is discontinued), dizziness, confusion, euphoria. **OCCASIONAL:** Weakness, anorexia, diarrhea. **RARE:** Paradoxical CNS excitement, restlessness (particularly noted in elderly/debilitated).

ADVERSE REACTION/TOXIC EFFECTS

Abrupt or too-rapid withdrawal may result in pronounced restlessness, irritability, insomnia, hand tremors, abdominal/muscle cramps, sweating, vomiting, seizures. Overdosage results in somnolence, confusion, diminished reflexes, coma.

NURSING IMPLICATIONS

BASELINE ASSESSMENT:

Assess B/P, pulse, respirations immediately before administration. Raise bed rails. Provide environment conducive to sleep (back rub, quiet environment, low lighting).

INTERVENTION/EVALUATION:

Assess sleep pattern of pt. Assess elderly/debilitated for paradoxical reaction, particularly during early therapy. Evaluate for therapeutic response: Decrease in number of nocturnal awakenings, increase in length of sleep.

PATIENT/FAMILY TEACHING:

Do not exceed prescribed dosage. Smoking reduces drug effectiveness. Do not abruptly withdraw medication following long-term use. Rebound insomnia may occur when drug is discontinued after short-term therapy. Avoid alcohol and other CNS depressants. Inform physician if you are or are planning to become pregnant.

thioridazine

thigh-or-rid´ah-zeen
(Mellaril-S)

thioridazine hydrochloride

(Mellaril)

CANADIAN AVAILABILITY:

Apo-Thioridazine, Mellaril, Novoridazine

CLASSIFICATION

Antipsychotic

PHARMACOKINETICS

Variably absorbed from GI tract. Widely distributed. Protein binding: >90%. Metabolized in liver to some active metabolites. Excreted in urine, eliminated in feces.

ACTION

Blocks postsynaptic dopaminergic receptors in brain. Possesses strong anticholinergic, sedative effects.

USES

Management of psychotic disorders, severe behavioral disturbances in children, including those w/excessive motor activity, conduct disorders. Used in short-term treatment of moderate to marked depression w/variable degrees of anxiety.

PO ADMINISTRATION

1. Dilute oral concentrate solution in water or fruit juice just before administration.
2. Do not crush, chew, or break tablets.

INDICATIONS/DOSAGE/ROUTES

Psychotic disorders:
PO: Adults: 50-100 mg 3 times/day in hospitalized pts. May gradually increase to 800 mg/day maximum. Dosage from 200-800 mg/day should be divided in 2-3 divided doses. Reduce dose gradually when therapeutic response is achieved.

Depression w/anxiety:
PO: Adults: 25 mg 3 times/day. **Total dose range/day:** 10 mg 2 times/day to 50 mg 3-4 times/day.

Usual elderly dosage (nonpsychotic):
PO: Elderly: Initially, 10-25 mg 1-2 times/day. May increase by 10-25 mg q4-7days. **Maximum:** 400 mg/day.

Moderate behavioral disturbances:
PO: Children 2-12 yrs: Initially, 10 mg 3 times/day in hospitalized children.

PRECAUTIONS

CONTRAINDICATIONS: Severe CNS depression, comatose states, severe cardiovascular disease, bone marrow depression, subcortical brain damage. **CAUTIONS:** Impaired respiratory/hepatic/renal/cardiac function, alcohol withdrawal, history of seizures, urinary retention, glaucoma, prostatic hypertrophy, hypocalcemia (increases susceptibility to dystonias). **PREGNANCY/LACTATION:** Crosses placenta; distributed in breast milk. **Pregnancy Category C.**

INTERACTIONS

DRUG INTERACTIONS: Alcohol, CNS depressants may increase CNS, respiratory depression, hypotensive effects. Tricyclic antidepressants, MAO inhibitors may increase sedative, anticholinergic effects. Antithyroid agents may increase risk of agranulocytosis. Extrapyramidal symptoms (EPS) may increase w/EPS producing medications. Hypotensives may increase hypotension. May decrease levodopa effects. Lithium may decrease absorption, produce adverse neurologic effects. **ALTERED LAB VALUES:** May cause EKG changes.

SIDE EFFECTS

Generally well-tolerated w/only mild and transient effects. **OCCASIONAL:** Drowsiness during early therapy, dry mouth, blurred vision, lethargy, constipation or diarrhea, nasal congestion, peripheral edema, urinary retention. **RARE:** Ocular changes, skin pigmentation (those on high doses for prolonged periods).

ADVERSE REACTIONS/TOXIC EFFECTS

Extrapyramidal symptoms appear dose-related (particularly high dosage) and are divided into 3 categories: Akathisia (inability to sit still, tapping of feet, urge to move around), parkinsonian symptoms (mask-like face, tremors, shuffling gait, hypersalivation), and acute dystonias: Torticollis (neck muscle spasm), opisthotonos (rigidity of back muscles), and oculogyric crisis (rolling back of eyes). Dystonic reaction may also produce profuse sweating, pallor. Tardive dyskinesia (protrusion of tongue, puffing of cheeks, chewing/puckering of the mouth) occurs rarely (may be irreversible). Abrupt withdrawal following long-term therapy may precipitate nausea, vomiting, gastritis, dizziness, tremors. Blood dyscrasias, particularly agranulocytosis, mild leukopenia (sore mouth/gums/throat) may occur. May lower seizure threshold.

NURSING IMPLICATIONS

BASELINE ASSESSMENT:

Avoid skin contact w/solution (contact dermatitis). Assess

behavior, appearance, emotional status, response to environment, speech pattern, thought content.

INTERVENTION EVALUATION:

Monitor B/P for hypotension. Assess for extrapyramidal symptoms. Monitor WBC, differential count for blood dyscrasias. Monitor for fine tongue movement (may be early sign of tardive dyskinesia). Supervise suicidal-risk pt closely during early therapy (as depression lessens, energy level improves, but suicide potential increases). Assess for therapeutic response (interest in surroundings, improvement in self-care, increased ability to concentrate, relaxed facial expression).

PATIENT/FAMILY TEACHING:

Full therapeutic effect may take up to 6 wks. Urine may darken. Do not abruptly withdraw from long-term drug therapy. Report visual disturbances. Sugarless gum or sips of tepid water may relieve dry mouth. Drowsiness generally subsides during continued therapy. Avoid tasks that require alertness, motor skills until response to drug is established.

thiothixene

thigh-oh-thick´seen
(Navane caps)

thiothixene hydrochloride

(Navane solution, injection)

CANADIAN AVAILABILITY:
Navane

CLASSIFICATION

Antipsychotic

PHARMACOKINETICS

	ONSET	PEAK	DURATION
IM	—	1-6 hrs	—

Well absorbed from GI tract, after IM administration. Widely distributed. Protein binding: 90-99%. Metabolized in liver. Primarily excreted in urine. Half-life: 34 hrs.

ACTION

Blocks postsynaptic dopamine receptors. Has alpha-adrenergic blocking effects; depresses release of hypothalamic, hypophyseal hormones.

USES

Symptomatic management of psychotic disorders.

STORAGE/HANDLING

Reconstituted solutions stable for 48 hrs at room temperature.

PO/IM ADMINISTRATION

PO:

1. Give w/o regard to meals.
2. Avoid skin contact w/oral solution (contact dermatitis).

IM:

1. Following parenteral form, pt must remain recumbent for 30-60 min in head-low position w/legs raised, to minimize hypotensive effect.
2. For IM injection, reconstitute 10 mg thiothixene hydrochloride w/2.2 ml sterile water for injection, yielding final solution of 5 mg/ml.
3. Inject slow, deep IM into upper outer quadrant of gluteus maximus or midlateral thigh.

INDICATIONS/DOSAGE/ROUTES

NOTE: Reduce dosage gradually to optimum response, then decrease to lowest effective level for maintenance. Replace parenteral therapy w/oral therapy as soon as possible.

Mild to moderate symptoms:
PO: Adults: 2 mg 3 times/day. May be increased gradually to 15 mg/day.

Severe symptoms:
PO: Adults: 5 mg 2 times/day. Increase gradually to 60 mg if needed. **Usual dose range:** 20-30 mg/day.
IM: Adults: 4 mg 2-4 times/day. May increase to maximum 30 mg/day. **Usual dose range:** 16-20 mg/day.

Usual elderly dosage (nonpsychotic):
PO: Elderly: Initially, 1-2 mg 1-2 times/day. May increase by 1-2 mg q4-7days. **Maximum:** 30 mg/day.

PRECAUTIONS

CONTRAINDICATIONS: Comatose states, circulatory collapse, CNS depression, blood dyscrasias. **EXTREME CAUTION:** History of seizures. **CAUTIONS:** Severe cardiovascular disorders, alcoholic withdrawal, pt exposure to extreme heat, glaucoma, prostatic hypertrophy. **PREGNANCY/LACTATION:** Crosses placenta; distributed in breast milk. **Pregnancy Category C.**

INTERACTIONS

DRUG INTERACTIONS: Alcohol, CNS depressants may increase CNS, respiratory depression, increase hypotension. Extrapyramidal symptom (EPS) producing medications may increase risk of EPS. May inhibit effects of levodopa. May increase cardiac effects w/quinidine. **ALTERED LAB VALUES:** May decrease uric acid.

SIDE EFFECTS

Hypotension, dizziness, and fainting occur frequently after first injection, occasionally after subsequent injections, and rarely w/oral dosage. **FREQUENT:** Transient drowsiness, dry mouth, constipation, blurred vision, nasal congestion. **OCCASIONAL:** Diarrhea, peripheral edema, urinary retention, nausea. **RARE:** Ocular changes, skin pigmentation (those of high doses for prolonged periods).

ADVERSE REACTIONS/TOXIC EFFECTS

Frequently noted extrapyramidal symptom is akathisia (motor restlessness, anxiety). Occurring less frequently is akinesia (rigidity, tremor, salivation, mask-like facial expression, reduced voluntary movements). Infrequently noted are dystonias: Torticollis (neck muscle spasm), opisthotonos (rigidity of back muscles), and oculogyric crisis (rolling back of eyes). Tardive dyskinesia (protrusion of tongue, puffing of cheeks, chewing/puckering of mouth) occurs rarely but may be irreversible. Risk is greater in female geriatric pts. Grand mal seizures may occur in epileptic pts (risk higher w/IM administration).

NURSING IMPLICATIONS

BASELINE ASSESSMENT:

Assess behavior, appearance, emotional status, response to environment, speech pattern, thought content.

INTERVENTION/EVALUATION:

Supervise suicidal-risk pt closely during early therapy (as depression lessens, energy level improves, increasing suicide potential. Monitor B/P for hypotension. Assess for peripheral edema behind medial malleolus (sacral area in bedridden pts). Assess stools; prevent constipation. Monitor for EPS, tardive dyskinesia (see Adverse Reactions) and potentially fatal, rare neuroleptic malignant syndrome: fever, irregular pulse or B/P, muscle rigidity, altered mental status. Assess for therapeutic response (interest in surroundings, improvement in self-care, increased ability to concentrate, relaxed facial expression).

PATIENT/FAMILY TEACHING:

Full therapeutic effect may take up to 6 wks. Report visual disturbances. Sugarless gum or sips of tepid water may relieve dry mouth. Drowsiness generally subsides during continued therapy. Avoid tasks that require alertness, motor skills until response to drug is established. Avoid alcohol and other CNS depressants.

tranylcypromine sulfate

tran-ill-cy´proe-meen
(Parnate)

CANADIAN AVAILABILITY:

Parnate

CLASSIFICATION

Antidepressant: MAO inhibitor

PHARMACOKINETICS

Well absorbed from GI tract. Metabolized in liver. Primarily excreted in urine. Half-life: 1.5-3 hrs.

ACTION

Inhibits MAO enzyme (assists in metabolism of sympathomimetic amines) at CNS storage sites. Levels of epinephrine, norepinephrine, serotonin, dopamine increased at neuron receptor sites, producing antidepressant effect.

USES

Symptomatic treatment of severe depression in hospitalized or closely supervised pts who have not responded to other antidepressant therapy, including electroconvulsive therapy.

PO ADMINISTRATION

Give w/food if GI distress occurs.

INDICATIONS/DOSAGE/ROUTES

PO: Adults, elderly: 20 mg daily (10 mg in morning, 10 mg in afternoon) for 2 wks. If no response, increase to 30 mg/day (20 mg in morning, 10 mg in afternoon) for 1 wk. Thereafter, reduce dosage gradually to maintenance level of 10-20 mg/day.

PRECAUTIONS

CONTRAINDICATIONS: Pts >60 yrs, debilitated/hypertensive pts, cerebrovascular / cardiovascular disease, foods containing tryptophan/tyramine, within 10 days of elective surgery, pheochromocytoma, congestive heart failure, history of liver disease, abnormal liver function tests, severe renal impairment, history of severe/recurrent headache. **CAUTIONS:** Impaired renal function, history of seizures, parkinsonian syndrome, diabetic pts, hyperthyroidism. **PREGNANCY/LACTATION:** Crosses placenta; unknown whether distributed in breast milk. **Pregnancy Category C.**

INTERACTIONS

DRUG INTERACTIONS: Alcohol, CNS depressants may increase CNS depressant effects. Tricyclic antidepressants, fluoxetine, trazodone may cause serotonin syndrome. May increase effect of oral hypoglycemics, insulin. B/P may increase w/buspirone. Caffeine containing medications may increase cardiac arrhythmias, hypertension. May precipitate hypertensive crises w/carbamazepine, cyclobenzaprine, maprotiline, other MAO inhibitors. Meperidine, other opioid analgesics may produce immediate excitation, sweating, rigidity, severe hypertension or hypotension, severe respiratory distress, coma, convulsions, vascular collapse, death. May increase CNS stimulant, vasopressor effects. Tyramine, foods w/pressor amines (e.g., aged cheese) may cause sudden, severe hypertension. **ALTERED LAB VALUES:** None significant.

SIDE EFFECTS

FREQUENT: Postural hypotension, restlessness, GI upset, insomnia, dizziness, lethargy, weakness, dry mouth, peripheral edema. **OCCASIONAL:** Flushing, increased perspiration, rash, urinary frequency, increased appetite, transient impotence. **RARE:** Visual disturbances.

ADVERSE REACTIONS/TOXIC EFFECTS

Hypertensive crisis may be noted by hypertension, occipital headache radiating frontally, neck stiffness/soreness, nausea, vomiting, sweating, fever/chilliness, clammy skin, dilated pupils, palpitations. Tachycardia/bradycardia, constricting chest pain may also be present. Antidote for hypertensive crisis: 5-10 mg phentolamine IV injection.

NURSING IMPLICATIONS

BASELINE ASSESSMENT:

Periodic liver function tests should be performed in those requiring high dosage and/or undergoing prolonged therapy.

MAO inhibitor therapy should be discontinued for 7-14 days before elective surgery.

INTERVENTION/EVALUATION:

Assess appearance, behavior, speech pattern, level of interest, mood. Monitor for occipital headache radiating frontally, and/or neck stiffness or soreness (may be first signal of impending hypertensive crisis). Monitor blood pressure diligently for hypertension. Assess skin temperature for fever. Discontinue medication immediately if palpitations or frequent headaches occur.

PATIENT/FAMILY TEACHING:

Antidepressant relief may be noted during first week of therapy; maximum benefit noted within 3 wks. Report headache, neck stiffness/soreness immediately. To avoid orthostatic hypotension, change from lying to sitting position slowly and dangle legs momentarily before standing. Avoid tasks that require alertness, motor skills until response to drug is established. Avoid foods that require bacteria/molds for their preparation/preservation or those that contain tyramine, e.g., cheese, sour cream, beer, wine, pickled herring, liver, figs, raisins, bananas, avocados, soy sauce, yeast extracts, yogurt, papaya, broad beans, meat tenderizers, or excessive amounts of caffeine (coffee, tea, chocolate), or over-the-counter preparations for hay fever, colds, weight reduction.

trazodone hydrochloride

tray´zeh-doan
(Desyrel)

CANADIAN AVAILABILITY:

Desyrel

CLASSIFICATION

Antidepressant

PHARMACOKINETICS

Well absorbed from GI tract. Protein binding: 89-95%. Metabolized in liver. Primarily excreted in urine. Half-life: 5-9 hrs.

ACTION

Selectively inhibits serotonin reuptake in brain. Alters serotonin receptor binding.

USES

Treatment of major depression often w/psychotherapy.

PO ADMINISTRATION

1. Give shortly after snack, meal (reduces risk of dizziness, lightheadedness).
2. Tablets may be crushed.

INDICATIONS/DOSAGE/ROUTES

Antidepressant:

PO: Adults: Initially, 150 mg daily in equally divided doses. Increase by 50 mg/day at 3-4 day intervals until therapeutic response is achieved. Do not exceed 400 mg/day for outpatients, 600 mg/day for hospitalized pts.

Usual elderly dosage:

PO: Elderly: Initially, 25-50 mg at bedtime. May increase by 25-50 mg q3-7days. **Range:** 75-150 mg/day.

PRECAUTIONS

CONTRAINDICATIONS: Recovery phase of MI, surgical pts, electroconvulsive therapy. **CAUTIONS:** Cardiovascular disease, MAO inhibitor therapy. **PREGNANCY/LACTATION:** Crosses placenta; minimally distributed in breast milk. **Pregnancy Category C.**

INTERACTIONS

DRUG INTERACTIONS: Alcohol, CNS depression producing medications may increase CNS depression. May increase effects of antihypertensives. May increase concentration of digoxin, phenytoin. **ALTERED LAB VALUES:** May decrease neutrophil, leukocyte counts.

SIDE EFFECTS

COMMON: Drowsiness, dry mouth, lightheadedness/dizziness, headache, blurred vision, nausea/vomiting. **OCCASIONAL:** Nervousness, fatigue, constipation, generalized aches and pains, mild hypotension.

ADVERSE REACTIONS/TOXIC EFFECTS

Priapism (painful, prolonged penile erection), decreased/increased libido, retrograde ejaculation, impotence have been noted rarely. Appears to be less cardiotoxic than other antidepressants, although arrhythmias may occur in pts w/preexisting cardiac disease.

NURSING IMPLICATIONS

BASELINE ASSESSMENT:

For those on long-term therapy, liver/renal function tests, blood counts should be performed periodically.

INTERVENTION/EVALUATION:

Supervise suicidal-risk pt closely during early therapy (as depression lessens, energy level improves, increasing suicide potential). Assess appearance, behavior, speech pattern, level of interest, mood. Monitor WBC and neutrophil count (drug should be stopped if levels fall below normal). Assist w/ambulation if dizziness or lightheadedness occurs.

PATIENT/FAMILY TEACHING:

Immediately discontinue medication and consult physician if priapism occurs. Change positions slowly to avoid hypotensive effect. Tolerance to sedative and anticholinergic effects usually develops during early therapy. Photosensitivity to sun may occur. Dry mouth may be relieved by sugarless gum, sips of tepid water. Report visual disturbances. Do not abruptly discontinue medication. Avoid tasks that require alertness, motor skills until response to drug is established. Avoid alcohol.

triazolam

try-a-zoe´lam
(Halcion)

CANADIAN AVAILABILITY:

Apo-Triazo, Halcion, Novotriolam

CLASSIFICATION

Sedative-hypnotic **(Schedule IV)**

PHARMACOKINETICS

Well absorbed from GI tract. Widely distributed (crosses blood-brain barrier). Protein binding: 89%. Metabolized in liver (undergoes first-pass liver extraction). Primarily excreted in urine. Half-life: 1.5-5.5 hrs.

ACTION

Enhances action of inhibitory neurotransmitter gamma-aminobutyric acid (GABA). Depressant effects occur at all levels of CNS.

USES

Short-term treatment of insomnia (up to 6 wks). Reduces sleep-induction time, number of nocturnal awakenings; increases length of sleep.

PO ADMINISTRATION

1. Give w/o regard to meals.
2. Tablets may be crushed.

INDICATIONS/DOSAGE/ROUTES

Hypnotic:
PO: Adults >18 yrs: 0.125-0.5 mg at bedtime. **Elderly:** 0.0625-0.125 mg at bedtime.

PRECAUTIONS

CONTRAINDICATIONS: Acute narrow-angle glaucoma, acute alcohol intoxication. **CAUTIONS:** Impaired renal/hepatic function. **PREGNANCY/LACTATION:** May cross placenta; may be distributed in breast milk. Chronic ingestion during pregnancy may produce withdrawal symptoms. CNS depression in neonates. **Pregnancy Category X.**

INTERACTIONS

DRUG INTERACTIONS: Alcohol, CNS depressants may increase CNS depressant effect. **ALTERED LAB VALUES:** None significant.

SIDE EFFECTS

FREQUENT: Drowsiness, sedation, headache, dizziness, nervousness, lightheadedness, incoordination, nausea. **OCCASIONAL:** Euphoria, tachycardia, abdominal cramps, visual disturbances. **RARE:** Paradoxical CNS excitement, restlessness, particularly noted in elderly, debilitated.

ADVERSE REACTIONS/TOXIC EFFECTS

Abrupt or too-rapid withdrawal may result in pronounced restlessness, irritability, insomnia, hand tremors, abdominal/muscle cramps, sweating, vomiting, seizures. Overdosage results in somnolence, confusion, diminished reflexes, coma.

NURSING IMPLICATIONS

BASELINE ASSESSMENT:

Assess B/P, pulse, respirations immediately before administration. Raise bedrails. Provide environment conducive to sleep (backrub, quiet environment, low lighting).

INTERVENTION/EVALUATION:

Assess sleep pattern of pt. Assess elderly/debilitated for paradoxical reaction, particularly during early therapy. Evaluate for therapeutic response to insomnia: A decrease in number of nocturnal awakenings, increase in length of sleep.

PATIENT/FAMILY TEACHING:

Smoking reduces drug effectiveness. Do not abruptly withdraw medication following long-term use. Rebound insomnia may occur when drug is discontinued after short-term therapy. Avoid alcohol.

trifluoperazine hydrochloride

try-floo-oh-pear´ah-zeen
(Stelazine)

CANADIAN AVAILABILITY:

Apo-Trifluoperazine, Stelazine

CLASSIFICATION

Antipsychotic

PHARMACOKINETICS

Variably absorbed after oral administration, well absorbed after IM administration. Widely distributed. Protein binding: >90%. Metabolized in liver to some active metabolites. Primarily excreted in urine.

ACTION

Blocks postsynaptic dopaminergic receptors in brain. Has strong extrapyramidal, antiemetic action; weak anticholinergic, sedative effects.

USES

Management of psychotic disorders, nonpsychotic anxiety.

STORAGE/HANDLING

Store oral solutions, parenteral form at room temperature. Slight yellow discoloration of solutions does not affect potency, but discard if markedly discolored or if precipitate forms.

PO/IM ADMINISTRATION

PO:

1. Add oral concentrate to 60 ml tomato or fruit juice,

milk, carbonated beverages, coffee, tea, water. May also add to semi-solid food.

IM:

1. **Parenteral administration:** Pt must remain recumbent for 30-60 min in head-low position w/legs raised, to minimize hypotensive effect.
2. Inject slow, deep IM into upper outer quadrant of gluteus maximus. If irritation occurs, further injections may be diluted w/0.9% NaCl or 2% procaine hydrochloride.

INDICATIONS/DOSAGE/ROUTES

NOTE: Decrease dosage gradually to optimum response, then decrease to lowest effective level for maintenance. Replace parenteral therapy w/oral therapy as soon as possible.

Psychotic disorders (hospitalized):
PO: Adults: 2-5 mg twice daily. Gradually increase to average daily dose of 15-20 mg (up to 40 mg may be required in severe cases). **Children 6-12 yrs:** 1 mg 1-2 times/day. Gradually increase to maximum daily dose of 15 mg.
IM: Adults: 1-2 mg q4-6h. Do not exceed 6 mg/24 hrs. **Children 6-12 yrs:** 1 mg 1-2 times/day.

Psychotic disorders (outpatient):
PO: Adults: 1-2 mg 2 times/day.

Nonpsychotic anxiety:
PO/IM: Adults: 1-2 mg 2 times/day.

Usual elderly dosage (nonpsychotic):
PO: Elderly: Initially, 1-5 mg 2 times/day. **Range:** 15-20 mg/day. **Maximum:** 40 mg/day.
IM: Elderly: Initially, 1 mg q4-6h as needed. **Maximum:** 6 mg/day.

PRECAUTIONS

CONTRAINDICATIONS: Severe CNS depression, comatose states, severe cardiovascular disease, bone marrow depression, subcortical brain damage. **CAUTIONS:** Impaired respiratory/hepatic/renal/cardiac function, alcohol withdrawal, history of seizures, urinary retention, glaucoma, prostatic hypertrophy, hypocalcemia (increases susceptibility to dystonias). **PREGNANCY/LACTATION:** Crosses placenta; distributed in breast milk. **Pregnancy Category C.**

INTERACTIONS

DRUG INTERACTIONS: Alcohol, CNS depressants may increase CNS, respiratory depression, hypotensive effects. Tricyclic antidepressants, MAO inhibitors may increase sedative, anticholinergic effects. Antithyroid agents may increase risk of agranulocytosis. Extrapyramidal symptoms (EPS) may increase w/EPS producing medications. Hypotensives may increase hypotension. May decrease levodopa effects. Lithium may decrease absorption, produce adverse neurologic effects. **ALTERED LAB VALUES:** May cause EKG changes.

SIDE EFFECTS

FREQUENT: Hypotension, dizziness, and fainting occur frequently after first injection, occasionally after subsequent injections, and rarely w/oral dosage. **OCCASIONAL:** Drowsiness during early therapy, dry mouth, blurred vision, lethargy, constipation or diarrhea, nasal congestion, peripheral edema, urinary retention. **RARE:** Ocular changes, skin pigmentation (those on high doses for prolonged periods).

ADVERSE REACTIONS/TOXIC EFFECTS

Extrapyramidal symptoms appear dose-related (particularly high dosage), and is divided into 3 categories: Akathisia (inability to sit still, tapping of feet, urge to move around), parkinsonian symptoms (mask-like face, tremors, shuffling gait, hypersalivation), and acute dystonias: Torticollis (neck muscle spasm), opisthotonos (rigidity of back muscles), and oculogyric crisis (rolling back of eyes). Dystonic reaction may also produce profuse sweating, pallor. Tardive dyskinesia (protrusion of tongue, puffing of cheeks, chewing/puckering of the mouth) occurs rarely (may be irreversible). Abrupt withdrawal following long-term therapy may precipitate nausea, vomiting, gastritis, dizziness, tremors. Blood dyscrasias, particularly agranulocytosis, mild leukopenia (sore mouth/gums/throat) may occur. May lower seizure threshold.

NURSING IMPLICATIONS

BASELINE ASSESSMENT:

Avoid skin contact w/solution (contact dermatitis). Assess behavior, appearance, emotional status, response to environment, speech pattern, thought content.

INTERVENTION/EVALUATION:

Monitor B/P for hypotension. Assess for extrapyramidal symptoms. Monitor WBC, differential count for blood dyscrasias. Monitor for fine tongue movement (may be early sign of tardive dyskinesia). Supervise suicidal-risk pt closely during early therapy (as depression lessons, energy level improves, increasing suicide potential). Assess for therapeutic response (interest in surroundings, improvement in self-care, increased ability to concentrate, relaxed facial expression).

PATIENT/FAMILY TEACHING:

Maximum therapeutic response occurs in 2-3 wks. Urine may darken. Do not abruptly withdraw from long-term drug therapy. Report visual disturbances. Sugarless gum or sips of tepid water may relieve dry mouth. Drowsiness generally subsides during continued therapy. Avoid tasks that require alertness, motor skills until response to drug is established. Avoid alcohol.

trihexyphenidyl hydrochloride

try-hex-eh-fen´ih-dill
(Artane)

CANADIAN AVAILABILITY:

Apo-Trihex, Artane, Novohexidyl

CLASSIFICATION

Anticholinergic, antiparkinsonism

PHARMACOKINETICS

	ONSET	PEAK	DURATION
PO	1 hr	2-3 hrs	6-12 hrs

Well absorbed from GI tract. Primarily excreted in urine. Half-life: 5.6-10.2 hrs.

ACTION

Blocks central cholinergic receptors (aids in balancing cholinergic and dopaminergic activity). Decreases salivation, relaxes smooth muscle.

USES

Adjunctive treatment for all forms of Parkinson's disease, including postencephalitic, arteriosclerotic, idiopathic types. Controls symptoms of drug-induced extrapyramidal symptoms.

PO ADMINISTRATION

1. May take w/o regard to food; give w/food if GI distress occurs.

2. Scored tablets may be crushed; do not crush or break sustained-release capsules.

INDICATIONS/DOSAGE/ROUTES

Parkinsonism:

NOTE: Do not use sustained-release capsules for initial therapy. Once stabilized, may switch, on mg-for-mg basis, giving a single daily dose after breakfast or 2 divided doses 12 hrs apart.

PO: Adults, elderly: Initially, 1 mg on first day. May increase by 2 mg/day at 3-5 day intervals up to 6-10 mg/day (12-15 mg/day in pts w/postencephalitic parkinsonism).

Drug-induced extrapyramidal symptoms:

PO: Adults, elderly: Initially, 1 mg/day. **Range:** 5-15 mg/day.

PRECAUTIONS

CONTRAINDICATIONS: Angle-closure glaucoma, GI obstruction, paralytic ileus, intestinal atony, severe ulcerative colitis, prostatic hypertrophy, myasthenia gravis, megacolon. **CAUTIONS:** Treated open-angle glaucoma, autonomic neuropathy, pulmonary disease, esophageal reflux, hiatal hernia, heart disease, hyperthyroidism, hypertension. **PREGNANCY/LACTATION:** Unknown whether drug crosses placenta; is distributed in breast milk. **Pregnancy Category C.**

INTERACTIONS

DRUG INTERACTIONS: Alcohol, CNS depressants may increase sedative effect. Amantadine, anticholinergics, MAO inhibitors may increase anticholinergic effects. Antacids, antidiarrheals may decrease absorption, effects. **ALTERED LAB VALUES:** None significant.

SIDE EFFECTS

NOTE: Elderly (>60 yrs) tend to develop mental confusion, disorientation, agitation, psychotic-like symptoms. **FREQUENT:** Drowsiness, dizziness, muscular weakness, dry mouth/nose/throat/lips, urinary retention, thickening of bronchial secretions. Sedation, dizziness, hypotension more likely noted in elderly. **OCCASIONAL:** Epigastric distress, flushing, visual disturbances, hearing disturbances, paresthesia, sweating, chills.

ADVERSE REACTIONS/TOXIC EFFECTS

Children may experience dominant paradoxical reaction (restlessness, insomnia, euphoria, nervousness, tremors). Overdosage in children may result in hallucinations, convulsions, death. Hypersensitivity reaction (eczema, pruritus, rash, cardiac disturbances, photosensitivity) may occur. Overdosage may vary from CNS depression (sedation, apnea, cardiovascular collapse, death) to severe paradoxical reaction (hallucinations, tremor, seizures).

NURSING IMPLICATIONS

BASELINE ASSESSMENT:

If pt is undergoing allergic reaction, obtain history of recently ingested foods, drugs, environmental exposure, recent emotional stress. Monitor rate, depth, rhythm, type of respiration; quality and rate of pulse. Assess lung sounds for rhonchi, wheezing, rales.

INTERVENTION/EVALUATION:

Be alert to neurologic effects: Headache, lethargy, mental confusion, agitation. Monitor children closely for paradoxical reaction. Assess for clinical reversal of symptoms (improvement of tremor of head/hands at rest, masklike facial expression, shuffling gait, muscular rigidity).

PATIENT/FAMILY TEACHING:

Avoid tasks that require alertness, motor skills until response to drug is established. Dry mouth, drowsiness, dizziness may be an expected response of drug. Avoid alcoholic beverages during therapy. Sugarless gum, sips of tepid water may relieve dry mouth. Coffee/tea may help reduce drowsiness.

valproic acid

val-pro´ick

(Depakene)

valproate sodium

(Depakene syrup)

divalproex sodium

(Depakote)

CANADIAN AVAILABILITY:

Divalproex sodium (Epival), valproic acid (Depakene)

CLASSIFICATION

Anticonvulsant

PHARMACOKINETICS

Well absorbed from GI tract. Protein binding: 90-95%. Metabolized in liver. Primarily excreted in urine. Half-life: 6-16 hrs (may be increased in decreased liver function, elderly, children <18 months).

ACTION

Directly increases concentration of inhibitory neurotransmitter gamma-aminobutyric acid (GABA). May also act on postsynaptic receptor sites.

USES

Prophylaxis of absence seizures (petit mal), myoclonic, tonic-clonic seizure control. Used principally as adjunct w/ other anticonvulsant agents.

PO ADMINISTRATION

1. Give w/food if GI distress occurs.
2. Do not crush, chew, or break enteric-coated tablets.
3. Do not mix solution w/carbonated drinks (may produce local mouth irritation, unpleasant taste).

INDICATIONS/DOSAGE/ROUTES

Anticonvulsant:
PO: Adults, elderly, children: Initially, 15 mg/kg daily (if dosage exceeds 250 mg daily, give in two or more equally divided doses). Increase at 1-wk intervals by 5-10 mg/kg daily until seizures are controlled or unacceptable effects occur. **Maximum daily dose:** 60 mg/kg.

PRECAUTIONS

CONTRAINDICATIONS: Hepatic disease. **CAUTIONS:** History of hepatic disease, bleeding abnormalities. **PREGNANCY/LACTATION:** Crosses placenta; is distributed in breast milk. **Pregnancy Category D.**

INTERACTIONS

DRUG INTERACTIONS: Alcohol, CNS depressants may increase CNS depressant effects. May increase risk of bleeding w/anticoagulants, heparin, thrombolytics, platelet aggregation inhibitors. May increase concentration of primidone. Carbamazepine may decrease concentration. Hepatotoxic medications may increase risk of hepatotoxicity. May alter phenytoin protein binding increasing toxicity. Phenytoin may decrease effect. **ALTERED LAB VALUES:** May increase SGOT (AST), SGPT (ALT), LDH, bilirubin.

SIDE EFFECTS

FREQUENT: Transient nausea, vomiting, indigestion (high incidence in children). **OCCASIONAL:** Abdominal cramps, diarrhea, or constipation. Sedation and drowsiness may be seen in those on adjunctive therapy.

ADVERSE REACTIONS/TOXIC EFFECTS

Hepatotoxicity may occur, particularly in the first 6 mo of therapy. May not be preceded by abnormal liver function tests, but may be noted as loss of seizure control, malaise, weakness, lethargy, anorexia, and vomiting. Blood dyscrasias may occur.

NURSING IMPLICATIONS

BASELINE ASSESSMENT:

Review history of seizure disorder (intensity, frequency, duration, level of consciousness). Initiate safety measures, quiet, dark environment. CBC, platelet count should be performed before and 2 wks after therapy begins, then 2 wks after maintenance dose is given.

INTERVENTION/EVALUATION:

Observe frequently for recurrence of seizure activity. Monitor liver function, CBC, platelet count. Assess skin for bruising, petechiae. Monitor for clinical improvement (decrease in intensity or frequency of seizures).

PATIENT/FAMILY TEACHING:

Do not abruptly withdraw medication following long-term use (may precipitate seizures). Strict maintenance of drug therapy is essential for seizure control. Drowsiness usually disappears during continued therapy. Avoid tasks that require alertness, motor skills until response to drug is established. Avoid alcohol.

venlafaxine

ven-lah-fah'zeen
(Effexor)

CLASSIFICATION

Antidepressant

PHARMACOKINETICS

Well absorbed from GI tract. Protein binding: 25-29%. Metabolized in liver to active metabolite. Primarily excreted in urine. Half-life: 3-7 hrs; metabolite: 9-13 hrs (increased in pts w/liver and/or renal disease).

ACTION

Potentiates CNS neurotransmitter activity. Inhibits reuptake of serotonin, norepinephrine (weakly inhibits dopamine reuptake).

USES

Treatment of depression w/psychotherapy.

PO ADMINISTRATION

1. May give w/o regard to food. Give w/food or milk if GI distress occurs.
2. Scored tablet may be crushed.

INDICATIONS/DOSAGE/ROUTES

NOTE: Decrease dose by 50% in pts w/moderate liver impairment; 25% in mild-moderate renal impairment (50% in pts on dialysis, withholding dose until completion of dialysis). When discontinuing the medication, taper slowly over 2 wks.

Depression:
PO: Adults, elderly: Initially, 75 mg/day in 2-3 divided doses w/food. May increase by 75 mg/day no sooner than 4 day intervals. **Maximum:** 375 mg/day in 3 divided doses.

PRECAUTIONS

CONTRAINDICATIONS: Hypersensitivity to venlafaxine. Children <18 yrs of age (safety unknown). Pts currently receiving MAO inhibitors (see Drug Interactions). **CAUTIONS:** Renal, hepatic impairment. History of mania, seizures, those w/metabolic or hemodynamic disease, hypertension, history of drug abuse. **PREGNANCY/LACTATION:** Unknown whether excreted in breast milk. **Pregnancy Category C.**

INTERACTIONS

DRUG INTERACTIONS: MAO inhibitors (MAOIs) may cause hyperthermia, rigidity, myoclonus, autonomic instability (including rapid fluctuations of vital signs), mental status changes, coma, extreme agitation. May cause neuroleptic malignant syndrome (wait 14 days after discontinuing MAOIs to start or wait 7 days after discontinuing venlafaxine before starting MAOIs). **ALTERED LAB VALUES:** May increase serum cholesterol, uric acid, alkaline phosphatase, SGOT (AST), SGPT (ALT), bilirubin, BUN. May decrease sodium, phosphate. May alter glucose, potassium.

SIDE EFFECTS

FREQUENT: Nausea, somnolence, headache, dry mouth. **OCCASIONAL:** Dizziness, insomnia, constipation, sweating, nervousness, asthenia (loss of strength, energy), ejaculatory disturbance, anorexia. **RARE:** Anxiety, blurred vision, diarrhea, vomiting, tremor, abnormal dreams, impotence.

ADVERSE REACTIONS/TOXIC EFFECTS

Sustained increase in diastolic B/P (10-15 mm Hg) occurs occasionally.

NURSING IMPLICATIONS

BASELINE ASSESSMENT:

Obtain initial weight and B/P.

INTERVENTION/EVALUATION:

Check B/P regularly for hypertension. Monitor weight and encourage small, frequent meals of favorite foods to prevent weight loss, esp. in underweight pts. Assess sleep pattern for insomnia. Check during waking hours for somnolence or dizziness and anxiety; provide assistance as necessary. Prescriptions should be for smallest amount possible to reduce risk of suicide. Supervise suicidal-risk pt closely during early therapy (as depression lessens, energy level improves, increasing suicide potential). Assess appearance, behavior, speech pattern, level of interest, mood for therapeutic response.

PATIENT/FAMILY TEACHING:

Take w/food. Do not increase, decrease, or suddenly stop medication. Venlafaxine may decrease appetite and cause weight loss. Do not drive or perform tasks that require alert response until certain drug does not cause impairment. Inform physician if breast-feeding, pregnant or planning to become pregnant. Avoid alcohol. Do not take any other medication including over-the-counter preparations w/o consulting physician. Report rash, hives, or other allergic responses promptly.

zolpidem tartrate

zewl′pih-dem
(Ambiem)

CLASSIFICATION

Sedative-hypnotic

PHARMACOKINETICS:

Rapidly absorbed from GI tract. Metabolized in liver; excreted in urine. Half-life: 1.4-4.5 hrs (increased in decreased liver function).

ACTION

Interacts with GABA receptor, inducing sleep w/fewer nightly awakenings, improvement of sleep quality.

USES

Short-term treatment of insomnia.

PO ADMINISTRATION

1. Do not break/crush capsule form.
2. For faster sleep onset, do not give w/or immediately after a meal.

INDICATIONS/DOSAGE/ROUTES

Hypnotic:
PO: Adults: 10 mg at bedtime. **Elderly, debilitated:** 5 mg at bedtime.

PRECAUTIONS

CONTRAINDICATIONS: None significant. **CAUTIONS:** Impaired hepatic function. **PREGNANCY/LACTATION:** Unknown whether drug crosses placenta or is distributed in breast milk. **Pregnancy Category B.**

INTERACTIONS

DRUG INTERACTIONS: Potentiated effects when used w/ other CNS depressants. **ALTERED LAB VALUES:** None significant.

SIDE EFFECTS

Generally well tolerated w/only mild and transient effects. **OCCASIONAL:** Residual hangover, headache, dizziness, drowsiness, lightheadedness.

ADVERSE REACTIONS/TOXIC EFFECTS

Overdosage may produce somnolence, confusion, slurred speech, severe incoordination, respiratory depression, coma. Abrupt withdrawal of drug after long-term use may produce weakness, facial flushing, sweating, vomiting, tremor. Tolerance/dependence may occur w/prolonged use of high doses.

NURSING IMPLICATIONS

BASELINE ASSESSMENT:

Assess B/P, pulse, respirations. Raise bed rails, lower bed, need call-light. Provide environment conducive to sleep (back rub, quiet environment, low lighting).

INTERVENTION/EVALUATION:

Assess sleep pattern of pt. Evaluate for therapeutic response to insomnia: a decrease in number of nocturnal awakenings, increase in length of sleep.

PATIENT/FAMILY TEACHING:

Do not abruptly withdraw med-ication following long-term use. Avoid alcohol, tasks that require alertness, motor skills until response to drug is established. Tolerance/dependence may occur w/prolonged use of high doses.

Index

Page numbers in *italics* refer to illustrations; numbers followed by t indicate tables.

► A

C

D

E

F

G

H

I

J

K

L

N

► O

P

Q

R

S

► T

U

V

► W

 X

 Y

 Z

ANA Standards of Psychiatric–Mental Health Nursing Practice

STANDARD I. ASSESSMENT
The psychiatric–mental health nurse collects client health data.

STANDARD II. DIAGNOSIS
The psychiatric–mental health nurse analyzes the assessment data in determining diagnoses.

STANDARD III. OUTCOME IDENTIFICATION
The psychiatric–mental health nurse identifies expected outcomes individualized to the client.

STANDARD IV. PLANNING
The psychiatric–mental health nurse develops a plan of care that prescribes interventions to attain expected outcomes.

STANDARD V. IMPLEMENTATION
The psychiatric–mental health nurse implements the interventions identified in the plan of care.

STANDARD V-A. COUNSELING
The psychiatric–mental health nurse uses counseling interventions to assist clients in improving or regaining their previous coping abilities, fostering mental health, and preventing mental illness and disability.

STANDARD V-B. MILIEU THERAPY
The psychiatric–mental health nurse provides, structures, and maintains a therapeutic environment in collaboration with the client and other health care providers.

STANDARD V-C. SELF-CARE ACTIVITIES
The psychiatric–mental health nurse structures interventions around the client's activities of daily living to foster self-care and mental and physical well-being.

STANDARD V-D. PSYCHOBIOLOGICAL INTERVENTIONS
The psychiatric–mental health nurse uses knowledge of psychobiological interventions and applies clinical skills to restore the client's health and prevent further disability.

STANDARD V-E. HEALTH TEACHING
The psychiatric–mental health nurse, through health teaching, assists clients in achieving satisfying, productive, and healthy patterns of living.

STANDARD V-F. CASE MANAGEMENT
The psychiatric–mental health nurse provides case management to coordinate comprehensive health services and ensure continuity of care.

STANDARD V-G. HEALTH PROMOTION AND HEALTH MAINTENANCE
The psychiatric–mental health nurse employs strategies and interventions to promote and maintain mental health and prevent mental illness.

STANDARD V-H. PSYCHOTHERAPY
The certified specialist in psychiatric–mental health nursing uses individual, group, and family psychotherapy, child psychotherapy, and other therapeutic treatments to assist clients in fostering mental health, preventing mental illness and disability, and improving or regaining previous health status and functional abilities.

STANDARD V-I. PRESCRIPTION OF PHARMACOLOGIC AGENTS
The certified specialist uses prescription of pharmacologic agents in accordance with the state nursing practice act, to treat symptoms of psychiatric illness and improve functional health status.

STANDARD V-J. CONSULTATION
The certified specialist provides consultation to health care providers and others to influence the plans of care for clients, and to enhance the abilities of others to provide psychiatric and mental health care and effect change in systems.

STANDARD VI. EVALUATION
The psychiatric–mental health nurse evaluates the client's progress in attaining expected outcomes.